CONTENTS

Community/
Public Health
Nursing

Promoting the Health of Populations

EDITION

7

MARY A. NIES, PhD, RN, FAAN, FAAHB
Director of Nursing Research and Professor College of Nursing
Joint Appointment MPH Program
Kasiska Division of Health Sciences
Idaho State University
Pocatello, Idaho

MELANIE McEWEN, PhD, RN, CNE, ANEF
Professor
University of Texas Health Science Center at Houston
Cizik School of Nursing
Houston, Texas

ELSEVIER

ELSEVIER

3251 Riverport Lane
St. Louis, Missouri 63043

Previous editions copyrighted 2015, 2011, 2007, 2001, 1997, and 1993.

Library of Congress Cataloging-in-Publication Control Number: 2018944741

Content Strategist: Jamie Blum
Senior Content Development Manager: Ellen Wurm-Cutter
Content Development Specialist: John Tomedi
Publishing Services Manager: Julie Eddy
Senior Project Manager: Rachel E. McMullen
Design Direction: Renee Duenow

Printed in Canada

Last digit is the print number: 9 8 7 6 5 4 3 2

Working together
to grow libraries in
developing countries

www.elsevier.com • www.bookaid.org

To Phil Yankovich, my husband, companion, and best friend, whose love, caring, and true support are always there for me. He provides me with the energy I need to pursue my dreams.

To Kara Nies Yankovich, my daughter, for whom I wish a happy and healthy life. Her energy, joy, and enthusiasm for life give so much to me.

To Earl (who passed away October 15, 2017, at the age of 92) and Lois Nies, my parents, for their never-ending encouragement and lifelong support. They helped me develop a foundation for creative thinking, new ideas, and spirited debate.

Mary A. Nies

To my husband, Scott McEwen, whose love, support, inspiration, and encouragement have been my foundation for more than 40 years. I can't wait to see what happens next!

Melanie McEwen

Mary A. Nies

Melanie McEwen

Mary A. Nies, PhD, RN, FAAN, FAAHB, is the Director of Nursing Research and Professor College of Nursing, Joint Appointment MPH Program, Kasiska Division of Health Sciences, Idaho State University. Dr. Nies received her diploma from the Bellin School of Nursing in Green Bay, Wisconsin; her BSN from the University of Wisconsin, Madison; her MSN from Loyola University, Chicago; and her PhD in Public Health Nursing, Health Services, and Health Promotion Research at the University of Illinois, Chicago. She completed a postdoctoral research fellowship in health promotion and community health at the University of Michigan, Ann Arbor. She is a fellow of the American Academy of Nursing and a fellow of the American Academy of Health Behavior. Dr. Nies co-edited *Community Health Nursing: Promoting the Health of Aggregates,* which received the 1993 Book of the Year award from the *American Journal of Nursing.* Her program of research focuses on the outcomes of health promotion interventions for minority and nonminority populations in the community. Her research is involved with physical activity and obesity prevention for vulnerable community populations.

Melanie McEwen, PhD, RN, CNE, ANEF, is a Professor at the University of Texas Health Science Center at Houston's Cizik School of Nursing. Dr. McEwen received her BSN from the University of Texas School of Nursing in Austin; her Master's in Community and Public Health Nursing from Louisiana State University Medical Center in New Orleans; and her PhD in Nursing from Texas Woman's University. Dr. McEwen has been a nursing educator for 30 years and is also the co-author of *Community–Based Nursing: An Introduction* (Elsevier, 2009) and co-author/editor of *Theoretical Basis for Nursing* (Wolters Kluwer, 2018).

ACKNOWLEDGMENTS

Community/Public Health Nursing: Promoting the Health of Populations could not have been written without sharing the experiences, thoughtful critique, and support of many people: individuals, families, groups, and communities. We give special thanks to everyone who made significant contributions to this book.

We are indebted to our contributing authors whose inspiration, untiring hours of work, and persistence have continued to build a new era of community health nursing practice with a focus on the population level. We thank the community health nursing faculty and students who welcomed the previous editions of the text and responded to our inquiries with comments and suggestions for the seventh edition. These people have challenged us to stretch, adapt, and continue to learn throughout our years of work. We also thank our colleagues in our respective work settings for their understanding and support during the writing and editing of this edition.

Finally, an enormous "thank you" to John Tomedi of Spring Hollow Press, Elsevier editors Ellen Wurm-Cutter and Jamie Blum, and project manager Rachel E. McMullen. Their energy, enthusiasm, encouragement, direction, and patience were essential to this project.

Mary A. Nies, PhD, RN, FAAN, FAAHB
Melanie McEwen, PhD, RN, CNE, ANEF

I would like to express appreciation for the chapter authors who have been with me since the very first edition of the textbook in 1993, namely:

- Patricia Burbank, *Chapter 7: Community Health Planning, Implementation, and Evaluation*
- Holly Cassells, *Chapter 5: Epidemiology; Chapter 6: Community Assessment*
- Susan Givens, *Chapter 16: Child and Adolescent Health*
- Jean Cozad Lyon, *Chapter 9: Case Management*

Mary A. Nies, PhD, RN, FAAN, FAAHB

CONTRIBUTORS

Cathy R. Arvidson, PhD, FNP-BC
Associate Professor
School of Nursing
Idaho State University
Pocatello, Idaho
Chapter 10: Policy, Politics, Legislation, and Community Health Nursing

Tonya Bragg-Underwood, DNP, FNP-BC, CNE
Associate Professor
School of Nursing
Western Kentucky University
Bowling Green, Kentucky
Chapter 20: Family Health

Carrie L. Buch, PhD, BSN, MS
Associate Professor
School of Nursing
Oakland University
Rochester, Michigan
Chapter 34: Home Health and Hospice

Patricia M. Burbank, DNSc, BS, MS
Associate Dean and Professor
College of Nursing
The University of Rhode Island
Kingston, Rhode Island
Chapter 7: Community Health Planning, Implementation, and Evaluation

Sarah G. Candler, MD, MPH
Assistant Professor
Baylor College of Medicine
Michael E. DeBakey Veterans Affairs Medical Center
Houston, Texas
Chapter 22: Veterans' Health

Holly B. Cassells, PhD, MPH, MN
Professor
School of Nursing and Health Professions
University of the Incarnate Word
San Antonio, Texas
Chapter 5: Epidemiology
Chapter 6: Community Assessment

Angelic Denise Chaison, PhD
Psychologist, Michael E. DeBakey Veterans Affairs Medical Center
Assistant Professor, Baylor College of Medicine
Houston, Texas
Chapter 22: Veterans' Health

Christina N. DesOrmeaux, BSN, MSN, PhD
Community Division Head
Community Nursing
The University of Texas at Houston Health Science Center
School of Nursing
Houston, Texas
Chapter 13: Cultural Diversity and Community Health Nursing
Chapter 30: School Health

Tina Doyle-Hines, LPC, NCC
U.S. Air Force, Retired
Former Veteran Counselor
UTH Cizik School of Nursing
Houston, Texas
Chapter 22: Veterans' Health

Stacy A. Drake, MSN, MPH, RN
Assistant Professor
Nursing Systems
The University of Texas Health Science Center at Houston
School of Nursing
Houston, Texas
Chapter 32: Forensic and Correctional Nursing

Allison P. Edwards, DrPH, MS, RN, CNE
Assistant Professor
Nursing Systems
The University of Texas Health Science Center at Houston
School of Nursing
Houston, Texas;
Board Member
Texas Board of Nursing
Austin, Texas
Chapter 21: Populations Affected by Disabilities

Rola El-Serag, MD
Medical Director Women Veteran's Program
Michael E. DeBakey Veterans Affairs Medical Center
Assistant Professor of Medicine
Baylor College of Medicine
Houston, Texas
Chapter 22: Veterans' Health

Melissa Domingeaux Ethington, BSN, MSN, PhD
Assistant Professor
Family Health
The University of Texas Health Science Center at Houston
School of Nursing
Houston, Texas
Chapter 16: Child and Adolescent Health

Ginette G. Ferszt, PhD, RN, PMHCNS-BC
Professor
College of Nursing
University of Rhode Island
Kingston, Rhode Island
Chapter 28: Violence

Lori A. Glenn, DNP, MS, CNM, RN
Clinical Associate Professor
McAuley School of Nursing
University of Detroit Mercy
Detroit, Michigan;
Nurse Midwife
Mid-Michigan Midwifery
Hurley Medical Center
Flint, Michigan
Chapter 17: Women's Health

Deanna E. Grimes, DrPH, RN, MSN, FAAN
Suzie Conway Endowed Professor in Nursing
Nursing Systems
The University of Texas Health Science Center at Houston
School of Nursing
Houston, Texas
Chapter 26: Communicable Diseases

Karyn Leavitt Grow, MS, BSN, RN
Director of Care Coordination Training
Clinical Development
Caravan Health
Berkeley, California;
Chief Nursing Officer
Manager, Case Management/Preadmission Screening
Sierra Surgery Hospital
Carson City, Nevada
Reno, Nevada
Chapter 9: Case Management

Jené M. Hurlbut, BSN, MSN, MS, PhD
Professor
Nursing
Roseman University of Health Sciences
Henderson, Nevada
Chapter 18: Men's Health

Joanna Lamkin, PhD
Postdoctoral Fellow
Veterans Affairs Health Services Research &
    Development, Houston Center of
    Excellence
Michael E. DeBakey Veterans Affairs
    Medical Center
Menninger Department of Psychiatry and
    Behavioral Sciences
Baylor College of Medicine
Veterans Affairs South Central Mental Illness
    Research, Education and Clinical Center
Houston, Texas
Chapter 22: Veterans' Health

Jean Cozad Lyon, PhD, MSN
Clinical Care Practitioner
ATOP2
HealthInsight
Reno, Nevada
Chapter 9: Case Management

Rex Marsau
U.S. Navy, Retired
Former Program Director
U.S. Vets
Houston, Texas
Chapter 22: Veterans' Health

Diane Cocozza Martins, MEd, MA, PhD
Professor
College of Nursing
University of Rhode Island
Kingston, Rhode Island
*Chapter 3: Thinking Upstream: Nursing
    Theories and Population-Focused Nursing
    Practice*
*Chapter 7: Community Health Planning,
    Implementation, and Evaluation*

Mary E. McBee, DNP, MSN, BSN, RN
Assistant Professor
Nursing Systems
The University of Texas Health Science
    Center at Houston
School of Nursing
Houston, Texas
Chapter 11: The Health Care System
Chapter 12: Economics of Health Care

Melanie McEwen, PhD, RN, CNE, ANEF
Professor
University of Texas Health Science Center at
    Houston
Cizik School of Nursing
Houston, Texas
Chapter 1: Health: A Community View
*Chapter 2: Historical Factors: Public Health
    Nursing in Context*
Chapter 11: The Health Care System
Chapter 12: Economics of Health Care

Cathy D. Meade, PhD, RN, FAAN
Senior Member
Population Science, Health Outcomes &
    Behavior
Moffitt Cancer Center;
Professor
Oncologic Sciences
University of South Florida
Tampa, Florida
Chapter 8: Community Health Education

Mary A. Nies, PhD, RN, FAAN, FAAHB
Director of Nursing Research and Professor
    College of Nursing
Joint Appointment MPH Program
Kasiska Division of Health Sciences
Idaho State University
Pocatello, Idaho
Chapter 1: Health: A Community View
Chapter 4: Health Promotion and Risk Reduction
Chapter 34: Home Health and Hospice

Julie Cowan Novak, DNSc, RN, CPNP
Executive Director
Neuro Developmental NICU Follow up Clinic
Sharp Mary Birch Hospital for Women and
    Newborns
San Diego, California;
Professor Emerita
Purdue University
West Lafayette, Indiana
Chapter 15: Health in the Global Community

Bridgette Crotwell Pullis, BSN, MS, PhD
Assistant Professor of Nursing, Director
The Veterans' Bachelor of Science in Nursing
    Program
Nursing Systems
The University of Texas Health Science
    Center at Houston
School of Nursing
Houston, Texas
Chapter 4: Health Promotion and Risk Reduction
Chapter 22: Veterans' Health

Robert Pullis
Houston, Texas
Chapter 22: Veterans' Health

Elda G. Ramirez, PhD, RN, FNP-BC
Professor of Clinical Nursing
Acute and Clinical Care
The University of Texas Health Science
    Center at Houston
School of Nursing
Houston, Texas
Chapter 29: Natural and Manmade Disasters

Bonnie Rogers, DrPH, COHN-S, LNCC
Director
NC Occupational Safety and Health and
    Education and Research Center
OHN Program
University of North Carolina
School of Public Health
Chapel Hill, North Carolina
Chapter 31: Occupational Health

Tamara Rose, BSN, MPH, PhD
Associate Dean
Nursing
Oregon Health and Science University
Klamath Falls, Oregon
Chapter 14: Environmental Health

**Mary Ellen Trail Ross, DrPH, MSN, RN,
GCNS-BC**
Associate Professor of Clinical Nursing
Department of Nursing Systems
The University of Texas Health Science
    Center at Houston
Houston, Texas
Chapter 19: Senior Health

Beverly Cook Siegrist, EdD, MS, BSN, CNE
Professor
School of Nursing
Western Kentucky University
Bowling Green, Kentucky
Chapter 20: Family Health
Chapter 33: Faith Community Nursing

Alison C. Sweeney, PsyD
Clinical Psychologist
Michael E. DeBakey Veterans Affairs
    Medical Center,
Assistant Professor
Menninger Department of Psychiatry and
    Behavioral Science
Baylor College of Medicine
Houston, Texas
Chapter 22: Veterans' Health

Lisa W. Thomas, DNP, MS, BSN
Assistant Professor, Clinical
Acute and Continuing Care
University of Texas Health Science Center;
Houston Research Nurse Consultant
Nursing Administration
TIRR Memorial Herman
Houston, Texas
Chapter 21: Populations Affected by Disabilities

Patricia L. Thomas, PhD, MS, BSN, ADN
Assistant Dean for Practice
Cook DeVos Health Science Center-Kirkhof
College of Nursing
Grand Valley State University
Grand Rapids, Michigan
Chapter 24: Rural and Migrant Health

Meredith Troutman-Jordan, PhD, MSN
Associate Professor
School of Nursing
University of North Carolina
Charlotte, North Carolina
Chapter 21: Populations Affected by Disabilities
Chapter 23: Homeless Populations
Chapter 25: Populations Affected by Mental Illness
Chapter 27: Substance Abuse

Lori Wightman, BSN, MSN, DNP
Chief Nursing Officer
System Administration
Regional Health
Rapid City, Michigan
Chapter 24: Rural and Migrant Health

ANCILLARY AUTHORS

Joanna E. Cain, BSN, BA, RN
President and Founder, Auctorial Pursuits,
    Inc.
Atlanta, Georgia
NCLEX Review Questions
Case Studies

Dulce Santacroce, DNP, RN, CCM
RN-BSN Coordinator
Touro University Nevada
Henderson, Nevada
PowerPoint Slides

Anna K. Wehling Weepie, DNP, RN, CNE, COI
Assistant Dean
Undergraduate Nursing and Professor
Allen College
Waterloo, Iowa
Test Bank

REVIEWERS

Lisa L. Capps, PhD, APN, FNP-BC
Assistant Professor
School of Nursing
Saint Xavier University
Chicago, Illinois

Michelle L. Gerrety, EdD, MSN, RN
Administrative Director, Academic Services
Director, St. Elizabeth School of Nursing
Division Coordinator, Nursing
Saint Joseph's College
Lafayette, Indiana

Jean Brewer Grantham, MSN, APRN, WHNP-BC
Instructor
Robert E. Smith School of Nursing
Delta State University
Cleveland, Mississippi

Meryle Gurmankin, PhD, RN, CSN, AHN-BC
Adjunct Faculty
School of Nursing and Health Sciences
LaSalle University
Philadelphia, Pennsylvania

Karen A. Ivantic, DNP, APRN-BC, APNP
Professor and Family Nurse Practitioner
Columbia College of Nursing
Milwaukee, Wisconsin

Susan K. Lee, PhD, MSN, RN
Nursing Consultant
Department of Education
Texas Board of Nursing
Austin, Texas

Sherry R. Lovan, PhD, MSN, RN
BSN Program Coordinator and Associate
    Professor
School of Nursing
Western Kentucky University
Bowling Green, Kentucky

Patricia S. Martin, MSN, RN
Assistant Professor
School of Nursing
University of Louisville
Louisville, Kentucky

Jill M. Nocella, PhD, APRN-BC
Associate Professor of Nursing
Department of Nursing
William Paterson University of New Jersey
Wayne, New Jersey

Dulce Anne Santacroce, DNP, RN, CCM
Assistant Professor
School of Nursing
Touro University Nevada
Henderson, Nevada

Marcia R. Scanlon, RN, DNP
Assistant Professor of Nursing
Department Chair of Nursing and Allied
    Health
Westfield State University
Westfield, Massachusetts

Terri Stone, MSN, MBA, RN
Assistant Professor of Nursing
Department of Nursing
Pennsylvania College of Technology
Williamsport, Pennsylvania

Deborah Lynn Sweeney, DNSc, RN
Associate Professor of Nursing
Division of Nursing
Baptist College of Health Sciences
Memphis, Tennessee

Dokagari Woods, PhD, RN
Assistant Professor and Undergraduate
    Program Director
Department of Nursing
Tarleton State University
Stephenville, Texas

More money is spent per capita for health care in the United States than in any other country ($9990 in 2015). The United States spent 17.8% of its gross domestic product on health care expenditures in 2015, reaching a record high of $3.2 trillion. It is one of the few industrialized countries in the world that lacks a program of national health services or national health insurance, so despite this spending, 8.8% of the nation lacks health insurance. In addition, many countries have far better indices of health, including traditional indicators such as infant mortality rates and longevity for both men and women, than does the United States.

Over the years, the most significant improvements in the health of the population have been achieved through advances in public health using organized community efforts, such as improvements in sanitation, immunizations, and food quality and quantity. Although access to health care services and individual behavioral changes are important, they are only components of the larger determinants of health, such as social and physical environments. The greatest determinants of health are still equated with factors in the community, such as education, employment, housing, and nutrition. The more money put into health care expenditures in the United States, the less money there is to improve these community factors.

UPSTREAM FOCUS

The traditional focus of many health care professionals, known as a *downstream focus,* has been to deliver health care services to ill people and to encourage needed behavioral change at the individual level. The focus of public/community health nursing has traditionally been on health promotion and illness prevention by working with individuals and families within the community. A shift is needed to an upstream focus, which includes working with aggregates and communities in activities such as organizing and setting health policy. This focus will help aggregates and communities work to create options for healthier environments with essential components of health, including adequate education, housing, employment, and nutrition, and will provide choices that allow people to make behavioral changes, live and work in safe environments, and access equitable and comprehensive health care.

Grounded in the tenets of public health nursing and the practice of public health nurses such as Lillian Wald, this seventh edition of *Community/Public Health Nursing: Promoting the Health of Populations* builds on the earlier works by highlighting an aggregate focus in addition to the traditional areas of family and community health, and thus promotes upstream thinking. The primary focus is on the promotion of the health of aggregates. This approach includes the family as a population and addresses the needs of other aggregates or population subgroups. It conceptualizes the individual as a member of the family and as a member of other aggregates, including organizations and institutions. Furthermore, individuals and families are viewed as a part of a population within an environment (i.e., within a community).

An aggregate is made up of a collective of individuals, be it a family or another group that, with others, makes up a community. This text emphasizes the aggregate as a unit of focus and how aggregates that make up communities promote their own health. The aggregate is presented within the social context of the community, and students are given the opportunity to define and analyze environmental, economic, political, and legal constraints to the health of these populations.

Community/public health nursing has been determined to be a synthesis of nursing and public health practice with goals to promote and preserve the health of populations. Diagnosis and treatment of human responses to actual or potential health problems comprise the nursing component. The ability to prevent disease, prolong life, and promote health through organized community effort is from the public health component. Community/public health nursing practice is responsible to the population as a whole. Nursing efforts to promote health and prevent disease are applied to the public, which includes all units in the community, be they individual or collective (e.g., person, family, other aggregate, community, or population).

PURPOSE OF THE TEXT

In this text, the reader is encouraged to become a student of the community, learn from families and other aggregates in the community how they define and promote their own health, and learn how to become an advocate of the community by working with it to initiate change. The student is exposed to the complexity and rich diversity of the community and is shown evidence of how the community organizes to meet change.

The use of language or terminology by clients and agencies varies in different parts of the United States, and it may vary from that used by government officials. The contributors to this text are a diverse group from various parts of the United States. Their terms vary from chapter to chapter and from those in use in local communities. For example, some authors refer to African Americans, some to blacks, some to European Americans, and some to whites. The student must be familiar with a range of terms and, most important, know what is used in his or her local community.

Outstanding features of this seventh edition include its provocative nature as it raises consciousness regarding the social inequalities that exist in the United States and how the market-driven health care system contributes to prevention of the realization of health as a right for all. With a focus on social justice, this text emphasizes society's responsibility for the protection of all human life to ensure that all people have their basic needs met, such as adequate health protection and income. Attention to the merits of population-focused care, or care that covers all people residing within geographic boundaries rather than only those populations enrolled in insurance plans, highlights the need for further reform of the systems of health reimbursement. Working toward providing health promotion and population-focused care to all requires a dramatic shift in thinking from individual-focused care for the practitioners of the future. The future paradigm for health care is demanding that the focus of nursing move toward population-based interventions if we are to forge toward the goals established in *Healthy People 2020*.

This text is designed to **stimulate critical thinking and challenge students to question and debate issues.** Complex problems demand complex answers; therefore the student is expected to *synthesize prior biophysical, psychosocial, cultural, and ethical arenas of knowledge.* However, experiential knowledge is also necessary, and the student is challenged to *enter new environments within the community* and gain new sensory, cognitive, and affective experiences. The authors of this text have integrated the concept of **upstream thinking,** introduced in the first edition, throughout this seventh edition as an important conceptual basis for nursing practice of aggregates and the community. The student is introduced to the individual and aggregate roles of community health nurses as they are engaged in a collective and interdisciplinary manner, working upstream, to facilitate the community's promotion of its own health. Students using this text will be better prepared to work with aggregates and communities in health promotion and with individuals and families in illness. Students using this text will also be better prepared to see the need to take responsibility for participation in organized community action targeting inequalities in arenas such as education, jobs, and housing and to participate in targeting individual health-behavioral change. These are important shifts in thinking for future practitioners who must be prepared to function in a population-focused health care system.

The text is also designed to increase the **cultural awareness** and **competency** of future community health nurses as they prepare to address the needs of culturally diverse populations. Students must be prepared to work with these growing populations as participation in the nursing workforce by ethnically and racially diverse people continues to lag. Various models are introduced to help students understand the growing link between social problems and health status, experienced disproportionately by diverse populations in the United States, and understand the methods of assessment and intervention used to meet the special needs of these populations.

The goals of the text are to provide the student with the ability to assess the complex factors in the community that affect individual, family, and other aggregate responses to health states and actual or potential health problems and to help students use this ability to plan, implement, and evaluate community/public health nursing interventions to increase contributions to the promotion of the health of populations.

MAJOR THEMES RELATED TO PROMOTING THE HEALTH OF POPULATIONS

This text is built on the following major themes:
- A social justice ethic of health care in contrast to a market justice ethic of health care in keeping with the philosophy of public health as "health for all"
- Integration of the concept of *upstream thinking* throughout the text and other appropriate theoretical frameworks related to chapter topics
- The use of population-focused and other community data to develop an assessment, or profile of health, and potential and actual health needs and capabilities of aggregates
- The application of all steps in the nursing process at the individual, family, and aggregate levels
- A focus on identification of needs of the aggregate from common interactions with individuals, families, and communities in traditional environments
- An orientation toward the application of all three levels of prevention at the individual, family, and aggregate levels
- The experience of the underserved aggregate, particularly the economically disenfranchised, including cultural and ethnic groups disproportionately at risk of developing health problems.

Themes are developed and related to promoting the health of populations in the following ways:
- The commitment of community/public health nursing is to an equity model; therefore community health nurses work toward the provision of the unmet health needs of populations.
- The development of a population-focused model is necessary to close the gap between unmet health care needs and health resources on a geographic basis to the entire population. The contributions of intervention at the aggregate level work toward the realization of such a model.
- Contemporary theories provide frameworks for holistic community health nursing practice that help students conceptualize the reciprocal influence of various components within the community on the health of aggregates and the population.
- The ability to gather population-focused and other community data in developing an assessment of health is a crucial initial step that precedes the identification of nursing diagnoses and plans to meet aggregate responses to potential and actual health problems.
- The nursing process includes, in each step, a focus on the aggregate, assessment of the aggregate, nursing diagnosis of the aggregate, planning for the aggregate, and intervention and evaluation at the aggregate level.
- The text discusses development of the ability to gather clues about the needs of aggregates from complex environments, such as during a home visit, with parents in a waiting room of a well-baby clinic, or with elders receiving hypertension screening, and to promote individual, collective, and political action that addresses the health of aggregates.
- Primary, secondary, and tertiary prevention strategies include a major focus at the population level.
- In addition to offering a chapter on cultural influences in the community, the text includes data on and the experience of underserved aggregates at high risk of developing health problems and who are most often in need of community health nursing services (i.e., low and marginal income, cultural, and ethnic groups) throughout.

ORGANIZATION

The text is divided into seven units. *Unit 1, Introduction to Community Health Nursing*, presents an overview of the concept of health, a perspective of health as evolving and as defined by the community, and the concept of community health nursing as the nursing of aggregates from both historical and contemporary mandates. Health is viewed as an individual and collective right, brought about through individual and collective/political action. The definitions of public health and community health nursing and their foci are presented. Current crises in public health and the health care system and consequences for the health of the public frame implications for community health nursing. The historical evolution of public health, the health care system, and community health nursing is presented, as well as the evolution of humans from wanderers and food gatherers to those who live in larger groups. The text also discusses the influence of the group on health, which contrasts with the evolution of a health care system built around the individual person, increasingly fractured into many parts. Community health nurses bring to their practice awareness of the social context; economic, political, and legal constraints from the larger community; and knowledge of the current health care system and its structural constraints and limitations on the care of populations. The theoretical foundations for the text, with a focus on the concept of upstream thinking, and the rationale for a population approach to community health nursing are presented. Recognizing the importance of health promotion and risk reduction when striving to improve the health of individuals, families, groups, and communities, this unit concludes with a chapter elaborating on those concepts. Strategies for assessment and analysis of risk factors and interventions to improve health are described.

Unit 2, The Art and Science of Community Health Nursing, describes application of the nursing process—assessment, planning, intervention, and evaluation—to aggregates in the community using selected theory bases. The unit addresses the need for a population focus that includes the public health sciences of biostatistics and epidemiology as key in community assessment and the application of the nursing process to aggregates to promote the health of populations. Application of the art and science of community health nursing to meeting the needs of aggregates is evident in chapters that focus on community health planning and evaluation, community health education, and case management.

Unit 3, Factors That Influence the Health of the Community, examines factors and issues that can both positively and negatively affect health. Beginning with an overview of health policy and legislation, the opening chapter in this unit focuses on how policy is developed and the effect of past and future legislative changes on how health care is delivered in the United States. This unit examines the health care delivery system and the importance of economics and health care financing on the health of individuals, families, and populations. Cultural diversity and associated issues are described in detail, showing the importance of consideration of culture when developing health interventions in the community. The influence of the environment on the health of populations is considered, and the reader is led to recognize the multitude of external factors that influence health. This unit concludes with an examination of various aspects of global health and describes features of the health care systems and patterns of health and illness in developing and developed countries.

Unit 4, Aggregates in the Community, presents the application of the nursing process to address potential health problems identified in large groups, including children and adolescents, women, men, families, and seniors. The focus is on the major indicators of health (e.g., longevity, mortality, and morbidity), types of common health problems, use of health services, pertinent legislation, health services and resources, selected applications of the community health nursing process to a case study, application of the levels of prevention, selected roles of the community health nurse, and relevant research.

Unit 5, Vulnerable Populations, focuses on those aggregates in the community considered vulnerable: persons with disabilities, veterans of the armed forces, the homeless, those living in rural areas including migrant workers, and persons with mental illness. Chapters address the application of the community health nursing process to the special service needs in each of these areas. Basic community health nursing strategies are applied to promoting the health of these vulnerable high-risk aggregates.

Unit 6, Population Health Problems, focuses on health problems that affect large aggregates and their service needs as applied in community health nursing. These problems include communicable disease, violence and associated issues, substance abuse, and a chapter describing nursing care during disasters.

Unit 7, Community Health Settings, focuses on selected sites or specialties for community health: school health, occupational health, faith community health, and home health and hospice. Finally, forensic nursing, one of the more recently added subspecialty areas of community health nursing, is presented in this unit, combined with correctional nursing content.

SPECIAL FEATURES

The following features are presented to enhance student learning:

- **Learning objectives.** Learning objectives set the framework for the content of each chapter.
- **Key terms.** A list of key terms for each chapter is provided at the beginning of the chapter. The terms are highlighted in blue within the chapter. The definitions of these terms are found in the glossary located on the book's Evolve website.
- **Chapter outline.** The major headings of each chapter are provided at the beginning of each chapter to help locate important content.
- **Theoretical frameworks.** The use of theoretical frameworks common to nursing and public health will aid the student in applying familiar and new theory bases to problems and challenges in the community.
- ***Healthy People 2020.*** Goals and objectives of *Healthy People 2020* are presented in a special box throughout the text. (The

updated *Healthy People 2020* information is new to this edition and based on the proposed objectives.)

- **Upstream thinking.** This theoretical construct is integrated into chapters throughout the text.
- **Case studies and application of the nursing process at individual, family, and aggregate levels.** The use of case studies and **clinical examples** throughout the text is designed to ground the theory, concepts, and application of the nursing process in practical and manageable examples for the student.
- **Research highlights.** The introduction of students to the growing bodies of community health nursing and public health research literature is enhanced by special boxes devoted to specific research studies.
- **Active learning exercises.** Selected learning activities are interspersed throughout the chapter to test students' knowledge of the content they've just read, helping provide clinical application and knowledge retention.
- **Photo novellas.** Numerous stories in photograph form depicting public health care in a variety of settings and with different population groups.
- **Ethical insights boxes.** These boxes present situations of ethical dilemmas or considerations pertinent to particular chapters.

NEW CONTENT IN THIS EDITION

- An increased focus on genomics—found in new **Genetics in Public Health boxes**—reflects growing scientific evidence supporting the health benefits of using genetic tests and family health history to guide public health interventions.

- A new chapter dedicated to the care of veterans has been added, reflecting the need for enhanced education and information related to the specific needs and issues for this special population.
- Most chapters contain new or updated **Research Highlights boxes** highlighting timely, relevant examples of the topics from recent nursing literature and **Ethical Insights boxes** that emphasize specific ethical issues.

TEACHING AND LEARNING PACKAGE

Evolve website: The website at http://evolve.elsevier.com/Nies/community is devoted exclusively to this text. It provides materials for both instructors and students.

- **For Instructors:** PowerPoint lecture slides, image collection, and more than 900 test bank questions with alternative item questions, as well as TEACH for Nurses, which contains detailed chapter Lesson Plans, including references to curriculum standards such as QSEN, BSN Essentials and Concepts, BSN Essentials for Public Health, and new and unique Case Studies.
- **For Students:** NCLEX-style multiple-choice review questions with correct answer rationales, and Case Studies with questions and answers.

1

Health: A Community View

Melanie McEwen and Mary A. Nies

OBJECTIVES

Upon completion of this chapter, the reader will be able to do the following:

1. Compare and contrast definitions of health from a public health nursing perspective.
2. Define and discuss the focus of public health.
3. Discuss determinates of health and indicators of health and illness from a population perspective.
4. List the three levels of prevention, and give examples of each.

5. Explain the difference between public/community health nursing practice and community-based nursing practice.
6. Describe the purpose of *Healthy People 2020* and give examples of the topic areas that encompass the national health objectives.
7. Discuss public/community health nursing practice in terms of public health's core functions and essential services.
8. Discuss public/community health nursing interventions as explained by the Intervention Wheel.

KEY TERMS

aggregates	health	primary prevention
community	health promotion	public health
community health	health-related quality-of-life (HRQOL)	public health nursing
community health nursing	population	secondary prevention
disease prevention	population-focused nursing	tertiary prevention

As a result of recent and anticipated changes related to health care reform, community/public health nurses are in a position to assist the U.S. health care system in the transition from a disease-oriented system to a health-oriented system. Costs of caring for the sick account for the majority of escalating health care dollars, which increased from 5.7% of the gross domestic product in 1965 to 17.8% in 2015 (National Center for Health Statistics [NCHS], 2017). Alarmingly, national annual health care expenditures reached $2.7 trillion in 2015, or an astonishing $8500 per person.

1

❤ HEALTHY PEOPLE 2020

Topic Areas

- Access to health services
- Adolescent health
- Arthritis, osteoporosis, and chronic back conditions
- Blood disorders and blood safety
- Cancer
- Chronic kidney disease
- Dementias, including Alzheimer
- Diabetes
- Disability and health
- Early and middle childhood
- Educational and community-based programs
- Environmental health
- Family planning
- Food safety
- Genomics
- Global health
- Health communication and health information technology
- Health care–associated infections
- Health-related quality of life and well-being
- Hearing and other sensory or communication disorders
- Heart disease and stroke
- HIV
- Immunization and infectious diseases
- Injury and violence prevention
- Lesbian, gay, bisexual, and transgender health
- Maternal, infant, and child health
- Medical product safety
- Mental health and mental disorders
- Nutrition and weight status
- Occupational safety and health
- Older adults
- Oral health
- Physical activity
- Preparedness
- Public health infrastructure
- Respiratory diseases
- Sexually transmitted diseases
- Social determinants of health
- Substance abuse
- Tobacco use
- Vision

From U.S. Department of Health and Human Services. *Healthy People 2020 topics & objectives—objectives A-Z.* Retrieved from <http://www.healthypeople.gov/2020/topicsobjectives2020/default.aspx>.

Health expenditures in the U.S. reflect a focus on the care of the sick. In 2015, $0.38 of each health care dollar supported hospital care, $0.23 supported physician/professional services, and $0.12 was spent on prescription drugs (more than double the proportion since 1980). The vast majority of these funds were spent providing care for the sick, and less than $0.03 of every health care dollar was directed toward preventive public health activities (NCHS, 2017). Despite high hospital and physician expenditures, U.S. health indicators such as life expectancy and infant mortality rate remain considerably below the health indicators of many other countries. This situation reflects a relatively severe disproportion of funding for preventive services

and social and economic opportunities. Furthermore, the health status of the population within the United States varies markedly across areas of the country and among groups. For example, the economically disadvantaged and many cultural and ethnic groups have poorer overall health status compared with middle-class Caucasians.

Nurses constitute the largest segment of health care workers; therefore they are instrumental in creating a health care delivery system that will meet the health-oriented needs of the people. According to a survey of registered nurses (RNs) conducted by the National Council of State Boards of Nursing (NCSBN, 2016), about 54.4% of approximately 2.5 million RNs employed full-time in the United States worked in hospitals during 2015 (down from about 66.5% in 1992). This survey also found that about 16%, or approximately 470,000, of all RNs worked in home, school, public/community health, or occupational health settings; 11% worked in ambulatory care settings; and 5.5% worked in nursing homes or other extended care facilities (NCSBN, 2016).

Between 1980 and 2015, the number of nurses employed in community, health, and ambulatory care settings more than doubled (NCSBN, 2016; USDHHS, HRSA, BHP, 2010). The decline in the percentage of nurses employed in hospitals and the subsequent increase in nurses employed in community settings suggests a shift in focus from illness and institutional-based care to health promotion and preventive care. This shift will likely continue into the future as alternative delivery systems, such as ambulatory and home care, employ more nurses (ANA, 2016; IOM, 2011; Rosenfeld & Russell, 2012).

Community/public health nursing is the synthesis of nursing practice and public health practice. The major goal of community/public health nursing is to preserve the health of the community and surrounding populations by focusing on health promotion and health maintenance of individuals, families, and groups within the community. Thus community/public health nursing is associated with health and the identification of populations at risk rather than with an episodic response to patient demand.

Public Health is often described as the art and science of preventing disease, prolonging life and promoting health through organized community efforts to benefit each citizen (Winslow, 1920). **The mission of public health is social justice, which entitles all people to basic necessities such as adequate income and health protection and accepts collective burdens to make it possible.** Public health, with its egalitarian tradition and vision, often conflicts with the predominant U.S. model of market justice that largely entitles people to what they have gained through individual efforts. Although market justice respects individual rights, collective action and obligations are minimal. An emphasis on technology and curative medical services within the market justice system has limited the evolution of a health system designed to protect and preserve the health of the population. Public health assumes that it is society's responsibility to meet the basic needs of the people. Thus there is a greater need for public funding of prevention efforts to enhance the health of our population.

Current U.S. health policies advocate changes in personal behaviors that might predispose individuals to chronic disease or accidents. These policies promote exercise, healthy eating, tobacco use cessation, and moderate consumption of alcohol. However, simply encouraging the individual to overcome the effects of unhealthy activities lessens focus on collective behaviors necessary to change the determinants of health stemming from such factors as poor air and water quality, workplace hazards, unsafe neighborhoods, and unequal access to health care. Because living arrangements, work/school environment, and other sociocultural constraints affect health and well-being, public policy must address societal and environmental changes, in addition to lifestyle changes, that will positively influence the health of the entire population.

With ongoing and very significant changes in the health care system and increased employment in community settings, there will be greater demands on community and public health nurses to broaden their population health perspective. The Code of Ethics of the American Nurses Association (ANA) (2015) promotes social reform by focusing on health policy and legislation to positively affect accessibility, quality, and cost of health care. Community and public health nurses therefore must align themselves with public health programs that promote and preserve the health of populations by influencing sociocultural issues such as human rights, homelessness, violence, disability, and stigma of illness. This principle allows nurses to be positioned to promote the health, welfare, and safety of all individuals.

This chapter examines health from a population-focused, community-based perspective. Therefore it requires understanding of how people identify, define, and describe related concepts. The following section explores six major ideas:
1. Definitions of "health" and "community"
2. Determinants of health and disease
3. Indicators of health and disease
4. Definition and focus of public and community health
5. Description of a preventive approach to health
6. Definition and focus of "public health nursing," "community health nursing," and "community-based nursing"

DEFINITIONS OF HEALTH AND COMMUNITY

Health

The definition of health is evolving. The early, classic definition of health by the World Health Organization (WHO) set a trend toward describing health in social terms rather than in medical terms. Indeed, the WHO (1958, p. 1) defined health as "a state of complete physical, mental, and social well-being and not merely the absence of disease or infirmity."

Social means "of or relating to living together in organized groups or similar close aggregates" (American Heritage College Dictionary, 1997, p. 1291) and refers to units of people in communities who interact with one another. "Social health" connotes community vitality and is a result of positive interaction among groups within the community, with an emphasis on health promotion and illness prevention. For example, community groups may sponsor food banks in churches and civic organizations to help alleviate problems of hunger and nutrition. Other community groups may form to address problems of violence and lack of opportunity, which can negatively affect social health.

In the mid-1980s, the WHO expanded the definition of health to emphasize recognition of the social implications of health. Thus health is:

the extent to which an individual or group is able, on the one hand, to realize aspirations and satisfy needs; and, on the other hand, to change or cope with the environment. Health is, therefore, seen as a resource for everyday life, not the objective of living; it is a positive concept emphasizing social and personal resources, and physical capacities.

(WHO, 1986, p. 73)

Saylor (2004) pointed out that the WHO definition considers several dimensions of health. These include physical (structure/function), social, role, mental (emotional and intellectual), and general perceptions of health status. It also conceptualizes health from a macro perspective, as a resource to be used rather than a goal in and of itself.

The nursing literature contains many varied definitions of health. For example, health has been defined as "a state of well-being in which the person is able to use purposeful, adaptive responses and processes physically, mentally, emotionally, spiritually, and socially" (Murray, Zentner, & Yakimo, 2009, p. 53); "The individual's total well-being. the regular patterns of people and their environments that result in maintaining wholeness and human integrity" (Roy, 2009, p. 3); "realization of human potential through goal-directed behavior, competent self-care, and satisfying relationships with others" (Pender, Murdaugh, & Parsons, 2011, p. 22); and a "state of physical, mental, spiritual and social functioning that realizes a person's potential and is experienced within a developmental context" (Greiner, 2014, p. 3).

The variety of characterizations of the word illustrates the difficulty in standardizing the conceptualization of health. Commonalities involve description of "goal-directed" or "purposeful" actions, processes, responses, functioning, or behaviors and the possession of "integrity," "wholeness," and/or "well-being." Problems can arise when the definition involves a unit of analysis. For example, some writers use the individual or "person" as the unit of analysis and exclude the community. Others may include additional concepts, such as adaptation and environment, in health definitions, and then present the environment as static and requiring human adaptation rather than as changing and enabling human modification.

For many years, community and public health nurses have favored Dunn's (1961) classic concept of wellness, in which family, community, society, and environment are interrelated and have an impact on health. From his viewpoint, illness, health, and peak wellness are on a continuum; health is fluid and changing. Consequently, within a social context or environment, the state of health depends on the goals, potentials, and performance of individuals, families, communities, and societies.

❓ ACTIVE LEARNING EXERCISE

Interview several community/public health nurses and several clients regarding their definitions of health. Share the results with your classmates. Do you agree with their definitions? Why or why not?

Community

The definitions of *community* are also numerous and variable. Baldwin and colleagues (1998) outlined the evolution of the definition of community by examining community health nursing textbooks. They determined that, before 1996, definitions of community focused on geographic boundaries combined with social attributes of people. Citing several sources from the later part of the decade, the authors observed that geographic location became a secondary characteristic in the discussion of what defines a community.

In recent nursing literature, community has been defined as "a collection of people who interact with one another and whose common interests or characteristics form the basis for a sense of unity or belonging" (Rector, 2017, p. 6); "a group of people who share something in common and interact with one another, who may exhibit a commitment with one another and may share a geographic boundary" (Lundy & Janes, 2016, p. 13); and "a locality-based entity, composed of systems of formal organizations reflecting society's institutions, informal groups and aggregates" (Shuster, 2012, p. 398).

Maurer and Smith (2013) further addressed the concept of community and identified three defining attributes: people; place; and social interaction or common characteristics, interests, or goals. Combining ideas and concepts, in this text, community is seen as a group or collection of individuals interacting in social units and sharing common interests, characteristics, values, and goals.

Maurer and Smith (2013) noted that there are two main types of communities: geopolitical communities and phenomenological communities. Geopolitical communities are those most traditionally recognized or imagined when the term *community* is considered. *Geopolitical communities* are defined or formed by natural and/or man-made boundaries and include cities, counties, states, and nations. Other commonly recognized geopolitical communities are school districts, census tracts, zip codes, and neighborhoods. *Phenomenological communities,* on the other hand, refer to relational, interactive groups. In phenomenological communities, the place or setting is more abstract, and people share a group perspective or identity based on culture, values, history, interests, and goals. Examples of phenomenological communities are schools, colleges, and universities; churches, synagogues, and mosques; and various groups and organizations, such as social networks.

A community of solution is a type of phenomenological community. A *community of solution* is a collection of people who form a group specifically to address a common need or concern. The Sierra Club, whose members lobby for the preservation of natural resource lands, and a group of disabled people who challenge the owners of an office building to obtain equal access to public buildings, education, jobs, and transportation are examples. These groups or social units work together to promote optimal "health" and to address identified actual and potential health threats and health needs.

Population and *aggregate* are related terms that are often used in public health and community health nursing. Population is typically used to denote a group of people with common personal or environmental characteristics. It can also refer to all of the people in a defined community (Williams, 2016). Aggregates are subgroups or subpopulations that have some common characteristics or concerns (Gibson & Thatcher, 2016). Depending on the situation, needs, and practice parameters, community health nursing interventions may be directed toward a community (e.g., residents of a small town), a population (e.g., all elders in a rural region), or an aggregate (e.g., pregnant teens within a school district).

DETERMINANTS OF HEALTH AND DISEASE

The health status of a community is associated with a number of factors, such as health care access, economic conditions, social and environmental issues, and cultural practices, and it is essential for the community health nurse to understand the determinants of health and recognize the interaction of the factors that lead to disease, death, and disability. It has been estimated that individual behaviors are responsible for about 50% of all premature deaths in the United States (Cassidy, Trujillo, & Orleans, 2015). Indeed, individual biology and behaviors influence health through their interaction with each other and with the individual's social and physical environments. Thus policies and interventions can improve health by targeting detrimental or harmful factors related to individuals and their environment. Fig. 1.1 shows the model of *Healthy People 2020,* which depicts the interaction of these determinants and shows how they influence health.

In a seminal work, McGinnis and Foege (1993) described what they termed "actual causes of death" in the United States, explaining how lifestyle choices contribute markedly to early deaths. Their work was updated a decade later (Mokdad et al., 2004). Leading the list of "actual causes of death" was tobacco, which was implicated in almost 20% of the annual deaths in the United States—approximately 435,000 individuals. Poor diet and physical inactivity were deemed to account for about 16.6% of deaths (about 400,000 per year), and alcohol consumption was implicated in about 85,000 deaths because of its association with accidents, suicides, homicides, and cirrhosis and chronic liver disease. Other leading causes of death were microbial agents (75,000), toxic agents (55,000), motor vehicle crashes (43,000), firearms (29,000), sexual behaviors (20,000), and illicit use of drugs (17,000).

Although all of these causes of mortality are related to individual lifestyle choices, they can also be strongly influenced by population-focused policy efforts and education. For example, the prevalence of smoking has fallen dramatically during the past two decades, largely because of legal efforts (e.g., laws prohibiting sale of tobacco to minors and much higher taxes), organizational policy (e.g., smoke-free workplaces), and education. Likewise, concerns about the widespread increase in incidence of overweight and obesity have led to population-based measures to address the issue (e.g., removal of soft drink and candy machines from schools, regulations prohibiting the use of certain types of fats in processed foods).

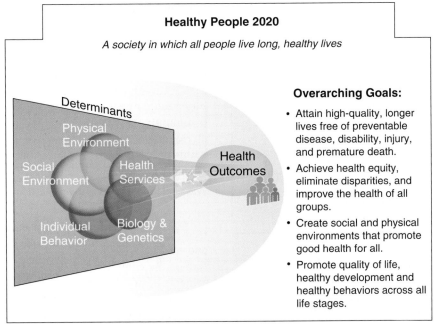

Healthy People 2020

A society in which all people live long, healthy lives

Determinants

Physical Environment

Social Environment

Health Services

Individual Behavior

Biology & Genetics

Health Outcomes

Overarching Goals:

- Attain high-quality, longer lives free of preventable disease, disability, injury, and premature death.
- Achieve health equity, eliminate disparities, and improve the health of all groups.
- Create social and physical environments that promote good health for all.
- Promote quality of life, healthy development and healthy behaviors across all life stages.

FIG. 1.1 Model: Healthy People 2020. (From U.S. Department of Health and Human Services Office of Disease Prevention and Health Promotion: *Federal interagency workgroup: the vision, mission, and goals of healthy people 2020, n.d.,* Retrieved from: https://www.healthypeople.gov/sites/default/files/HP2020Framework.pdf)

Public health experts have observed that health has improved over the past 100 years largely because people become ill less often (McKeown, 2003; Russo, 2015). Indeed, at the population level, better health can be attributed to higher standards of living, good nutrition, a healthier environment, and having fewer children. Furthermore, public health efforts, such as immunization and clean air and water, and medical care, including management of acute episodic illnesses (e.g., pneumonia, tuberculosis) and chronic disease (e.g., cancer, heart disease), have also contributed significantly to the increase in life expectancy.

Community and public health nurses should understand these concepts and appreciate that health and illness are influenced by a web of factors, some that can be changed (e.g., individual behaviors such as tobacco use, diet, physical activity) and some that cannot (e.g., genetics, age, gender). Other factors (e.g., physical and social environment) may require changes that will need to be accomplished from a policy perspective. Public health nurses must work with policy makers and community leaders to identify patterns of disease and death and to advocate for activities and policies that promote health at the individual, family, aggregate, and population levels.

INDICATORS OF HEALTH AND ILLNESS

A variety of health indicators are used by health providers, policy makers, and community health nurses to measure the health of the community. Local or state health departments, the Centers for Disease Control and Prevention (CDC), and the National Center for Health Statistics (NCHS) provide morbidity, mortality, and other health status–related data. State and local health departments are responsible for collecting morbidity and mortality data and forwarding the information to the appropriate federal-level agency, which is often the CDC. Some of the more commonly reported indicators are life expectancy, infant mortality, age-adjusted death rates, and cancer incidence rates.

Indicators of mortality in particular illustrate the health status of a community and/or population because changes in mortality reflect a number of social, economic, health service, and related trends (Shi & Singh, 2016). These data may be useful in analyzing health patterns over time, comparing communities from different geographic regions, or comparing different aggregates within a community.

When the national health objectives for *Healthy People 2020* were being developed, a total of 12 leading health indicators were identified that reflected the major public health concerns in the United States (see *Healthy People 2020* box). They are individual behaviors (e.g., tobacco use, nutrition, physical activity, and obesity), physical and social environmental factors (e.g., environmental quality, injury, and violence), and health systems issues (e.g., access to health services). Each of these indicators can affect the health of individuals and communities and can be correlated with leading causes of morbidity and mortality. For example, tobacco use is linked to heart disease, stroke, and cancer; substance abuse is linked to accidents, injuries, and violence; irresponsible sexual behaviors can lead to unwanted pregnancy as well as sexually transmitted diseases, including human immunodeficiency virus/acquired immunodeficiency syndrome (HIV/AIDS); and lack of access to health care can contribute to poor pregnancy outcomes, untreated illness, and disability.

HEALTHY PEOPLE 2020

Leading Health Indicator Topics

- Access to Health Services
- Clinical Preventive Services
- Environmental Quality
- Injury and Violence
- Maternal, Infant, and Child Health
- Mental Health
- Nutrition, Physical Activity, and Obesity
- Oral Health
- Reproductive and Sexual Health
- Social Determinants
- Substance Abuse
- Tobacco

From U.S. Department of Health and Human Services. *Healthy People 2020 leading health indicator topics*. Retrieved from https://www.healthypeople.gov/2020/Leading-Health-Indicators

Public health nurses should be aware of health patterns and health indicators within their practice. Each nurse should ask relevant questions, including the following: What are the leading causes of death and disease among various groups served? How do infant mortality rates and teenage pregnancy rates in my community compare with regional, state, and national rates? What are the most serious communicable disease threats in my neighborhood? What are the most serious environmental risks in my city?

The public health nurse may identify areas for further investigation and intervention through an understanding of health, disease, and mortality patterns. For example, if a school nurse learns that the teenage pregnancy rate in their community is higher than regional and state averages, the nurse should address the problem with school officials, parents, and students. Likewise, if an occupational health nurse discovers an apparent high rate of chronic lung disease in an industrial facility, the nurse should work with company management, employees, and state and federal officials to identify potential harmful sources. Finally, if a public health nurse works in a state-sponsored AIDS clinic and recognizes an increase in the number of women testing positive for HIV, the nurse should report all findings to the designated agencies. The nurse should then participate in investigative efforts to determine what is precipitating the increase and work to remedy the identified threats or risks.

DEFINITION AND FOCUS OF PUBLIC HEALTH AND COMMUNITY HEALTH

C. E. Winslow is known for the following classic definition of public health:

> Public health is the Science and Art of (1) preventing disease, (2) prolonging life, and (3) promoting health and efficiency through organized community effort for:
> (a) sanitation of the environment,
> (b) control of communicable infections,
> (c) education of the individual in personal hygiene,
> (d) organization of medical and nursing services for the early diagnosis and preventive treatment of disease, and

BOX 1.1   Core Public Health Functions

Assessment: Regular collection, analysis, and information sharing about health conditions, risks, and resources in a community.

Policy development: Use of information gathered during assessment to develop local and state health policies and to direct resources toward those policies.

Assurance: Focuses on the availability of necessary health services throughout the community. It includes maintaining the ability of both public health agencies and private providers to manage day-to-day operations and the capacity to respond to critical situations and emergencies.

From Institute of Medicine: *The future of public health,* Washington, DC, 1988, National Academy Press.

> (e) development of the social machinery to ensure everyone a standard of living adequate for the maintenance of health, so organizing these benefits as to enable every citizen to realize his birthright of health and longevity.
> **(Hanlon, 1960, p. 23)**

A key phrase in this definition of public health is "through organized community effort." The term *public health* connotes organized, legislated, and tax-supported efforts that serve all people through health departments or related governmental agencies.

The public health nursing tradition, begun in the late 1800s by Lillian Wald and her associates, clearly illustrates this phenomenon (Wald, 1971; see Chapter 2). After moving into the immigrant community in New York City to provide care for individuals and families, these early public health nurses saw that neither administering bedside clinical nursing nor teaching family members to deliver care in the home adequately addressed the true determinants of health and disease. They resolved that collective political activity should focus on advancing the health of aggregates and improving social and environmental conditions by addressing the social and environmental determinants of health, such as child labor, pollution, and poverty. Wald and her colleagues affected the health of the community by organizing the community, establishing school nursing, and taking impoverished mothers to testify in Washington, DC (Wald, 1971).

In a key action, the National Academy of Medicine (NAM), formerly called the Institute of Medicine (IOM) (1988) identified the following three primary functions of public health: *assessment, assurance,* and *policy development.* Box 1.1 lists each of the three primary functions and describes them briefly. All nurses working in community settings should develop knowledge and skills related to each of these primary functions.

The term **community health** extends the realm of public health to include organized health efforts at the community level through both government *and* private efforts. Participants include privately funded agencies such as the American Heart Association and the American Red Cross. A variety of private and public structures serves community health efforts.

Public health efforts focus on prevention and promotion of population health at the federal, state, and local levels. These efforts at the federal and state levels concentrate on providing support and advisory services to public health structures at the

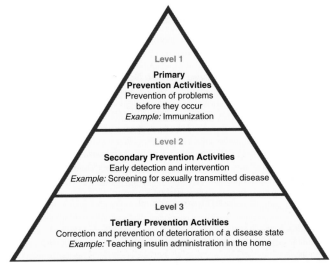

FIG. 1.2 The three levels of prevention.

local level. The local-level structures provide direct services to communities through two avenues:

- Community health services, which protect the public from hazards such as polluted water and air, tainted food, and unsafe housing
- Personal health care services, such as immunization and family planning services, well-infant care, and sexually transmitted disease (STD) treatment

Personal health services may be part of the public health effort and often target the populations most at risk and in need of services. Public health efforts are multidisciplinary because they require people with many different skills. Community health nurses work with a diverse team of public health professionals, including epidemiologists, local health officers, and health educators. Public health science methods that assess biostatistics, epidemiology, and population needs provide a method of measuring characteristics and health indicators and disease patterns within a community. In 1994 the American Public Health Association drafted a list of 10 essential public health services, which the U.S. Department of Health and Human Services later adopted. The updated list of essential services (CDC, 2014) appears in Box 1.2.

PREVENTIVE APPROACH TO HEALTH

Health Promotion and Levels of Prevention

Contrasting with "medical care," which focuses on disease management and "cure," public health efforts focus on health promotion and disease prevention. Health promotion activities enhance resources directed at improving well-being, whereas disease prevention activities protect people from disease and the effects of disease. Leavell and Clark (1958) identified three levels of prevention commonly described in nursing practice: primary prevention, secondary prevention, and tertiary prevention (Fig. 1.2 and Table 1.1).

Primary prevention relates to activities directed at preventing a problem before it occurs by altering susceptibility or reducing exposure for susceptible individuals. Primary prevention consists of two elements: general health promotion and specific protection. Health promotion efforts enhance resiliency and protective factors and target essentially well populations. Examples include promotion of good nutrition, provision of adequate shelter, and encouraging regular exercise. Specific protection efforts reduce or eliminate risk factors and include such measures as immunization, seat belt use, and water purification.

Secondary prevention refers to early detection and prompt intervention during the period of early disease pathogenesis. Secondary prevention is implemented after a problem has begun, but before signs and symptoms appear, and targets those populations that have risk factors. Mammography, blood pressure screening, scoliosis screening, and Papanicolaou tests are examples of secondary prevention.

Tertiary prevention targets populations that have experienced disease or injury and focuses on limitation of disability and rehabilitation. Aims of tertiary prevention are to keep health problems from getting worse, to reduce the effects of disease and injury, and to restore individuals to their optimal level of functioning. Examples include teaching how to perform insulin injections and disease management to a patient with diabetes, referral of a patient with spinal cord injury for occupational and physical therapy, and leading a support group for grieving parents.

Much of public health nursing practice is directed toward preventing the progression of disease at the earliest period or phase feasible using the appropriate level(s) of prevention. For example, when applying "levels of prevention" to a client with HIV/AIDS, a nurse might perform the following interventions:

- Educate students on the practice of sexual abstinence or "safer sex" by using barrier methods (primary prevention)
- Encourage testing and counseling for clients with known exposure or who are in high-risk groups; provide referrals for follow-up for clients who test positive for HIV (secondary prevention)
- Provide education on management of HIV infection, advocacy, case management, and other interventions for those who are HIV positive (tertiary prevention)

TABLE 1.1 Examples of Levels of Prevention and Clients Served in the Community

Definition of Client Served*	LEVEL OF PREVENTION		
	Primary (Health Promotion and Specific Prevention)	Secondary (Early Diagnosis and Treatment)	Tertiary (Limitation of Disability and Rehabilitation)
Individual	Dietary teaching during pregnancy Immunizations	HIV testing Screening for cervical cancer	Teaching new clients with diabetes how to administer insulin Exercise therapy after stroke Skin care for incontinent patients
Family (two or more individuals bound by kinship, law, or living arrangement and with common emotional ties and obligations [see Chapter 20])	Education or counseling regarding smoking, dental care, or nutrition Adequate housing	Dental examinations Tuberculin testing for family at risk	Mental health counseling or referral for family in crisis (e.g., grieving or experiencing a divorce) Dietary instructions and monitoring for family with overweight members
Group or aggregate (interacting people with a common purpose or purposes)	Birthing classes for pregnant teenage mothers AIDS and other STI education for high school students	Vision screening of a first-grade class Mammography van for screening of women in a low-income neighborhood Hearing tests at a senior center	Group counseling for grade-school children with asthma Swim therapy for physically disabled elders at a senior center Alcoholics Anonymous and other self-help groups Mental health services for military veterans
Community and populations (aggregate of people sharing space over time within a social system [see Chapter 6]; population groups or aggregates with power relations and common needs or purposes)	Fluoride water supplementation Environmental sanitation Removal of environmental hazards	Organized screening programs for communities (e.g., health fairs) Lead screening for children by school district	Shelter and relocation centers for fire or earthquake victims Emergency medical services Community mental health services for chronically mentally ill Home care services for chronically ill

AIDS, Acquired immunodeficiency syndrome; *HIV*, human immunodeficiency virus; *STI*, sexually transmitted infection.
*Note that terms are used differently in literature of various disciplines. There are not any clear-cut definitions; for example, families may be referred to as an aggregate, and a population and subpopulations may exist within a community.

Thinking Upstream

The concepts of prevention and population-focused care figure prominently in a conceptual orientation to nursing practice referred to as *thinking upstream*. This orientation is derived from an analogy of patients falling into a river upstream and being rescued downstream by health providers overwhelmed with the struggle of responding to disease and illness. The river as an analogy for the natural history of illness was first coined by McKinlay (1979), with a charge to health providers to refocus their efforts toward preventive and "upstream" activities. In a description of the daily challenges of providers to address health from a preventive versus curative focus, McKinlay differentiates the consequences of illness (*downstream* endeavors) from its precursors (*upstream* endeavors). The author then charges health providers to critically examine the relative weights of their activities toward illness response versus the prevention of illness.

A population-based perspective on health and health determinants is critical to understanding and formulating nursing actions to prevent disease. By examining the origins of disease, nurses identify social, political, environmental, and economic factors that often lead to poor health options for both individuals and populations. The call to refocus the efforts of nurses "upstream, where the real problems lie" (McKinlay, 1979) has been welcomed by community health nurses in a variety of practice settings. For these nurses, this theme provides affirmation of their daily efforts to prevent disease in populations at risk in schools, work sites, and clinics throughout their local communities and in the larger world.

ETHICAL INSIGHTS

Inequities: Distribution of Resources

In the United States, inequities in the distribution of resources pose a threat to the common good and a challenge for community and public health nurses. Factors that contribute to wide variations in health disparities include education, income, and occupation. Lack of health insurance is a key factor in this issue and a major rationale for health care reform efforts. Lack of insurance is damaging to population health, as low-income, uninsured individuals are much less likely than insured individuals to receive timely primary health care and preventive dental care.

Public health nurses are regularly confronted with the consequences of the fragmented health care delivery system. They diligently work to improve the circumstances for populations who have not had adequate access to resources largely because of who they are and where they live.

Ethical questions commonly encountered in community and public health nursing practice include the following: Should resources (e.g., free or low-cost immunizations) be offered to all, even those who have insurance that will pay for the care? Should public health nurses serve anyone who meets financial need guidelines, regardless of medical need? Should the health department provide flu shots to persons of all ages or just those most likely to be affected by the disease? Should nonresidents in the United States illegally or persons working on "green cards" receive the same level of health care services that are available to citizens? Who should have free or reduced-cost access to extremely expensive drugs such as those that treat hepatitis C, multiple sclerosis, or many forms of cancer, and who should bear the financial burden?

Access to health care is a goal for all. To this end, community and public health nurses must face the challenges and dilemmas related to these and other questions as they assist individuals, families, and communities dealing with the uneven distribution of health resources and the associated costs of health care.

Prevention versus Cure

Spending additional dollars for cure in the form of health care services does little to improve the health of a population, whereas spending money on prevention does a great deal to improve health. Getzen (2013) and others (Russo, 2015; Shi & Singh, 2016) note that there is an absence of convincing evidence that the amount of money expended for health care improves the health of a population. The real determinants of health, as mentioned, are prevention efforts that provide education, housing, food, a decent minimal income, and safe social and physical environments, as well as encouraging positive lifestyle choices. The United States spends more than one sixth of its wealth on health care or "cure" for individuals, likely diverting money away from the needed resources and services that would make a greater impact on health (NCHS, 2017 Shi & Singh, 2016).

U.S. policy makers must become committed to achieving improved health outcomes for the poor and vulnerable populations. With a limited health workforce and monetary resources, the United States cannot continue to spend vast amounts on health care services when the investment fails to improve health outcomes. In industrialized countries, life expectancy at birth is not related to the level of health care expenditures; in developing countries, longevity is closely related to the level of economic development and the education of the population (Russo, 2015; Shi & Singh, 2016).

The current health care system is currently in a flux following implementation of the Affordable Care Act (ACA) and subsequent efforts to "repeal and replace" it. These endeavors could actually be detrimental to the health of the population, as the focus on obtaining health insurance for more people may defer a large investment of the country's wealth from education and other developmental efforts that would positively affect the health of the population as a whole. Managed care organizations (MCOs) focus on prevention and have determined that the rate of health care cost increases have slowed among employees of large firms (Kongstvedt, 2013). Prevention programs may help reduce costs for those enrolled in MCOs, but it remains unclear who will provide services for those who are required to purchase insurance, those who are currently uninsured and may remain so, the poor, and other vulnerable populations. In addition, still to be determined is who will provide adequate schooling, housing, meals, wages, and a safe environment for the disadvantaged. Increasing health care spending may negatively affect efforts to address economic disparities by reducing investments in sufficient housing, employment, education, nutrition, and safe environments.

 ## Healthy People 2020

In 1979, the U.S. Department of Health and Human Services published a national prevention initiative titled *Healthy People: The Surgeon General's Report on Health Promotion and Disease Prevention*. The 1979 version established goals that would reduce mortality among infants, children, adolescents and young adults, and adults and increase independence among older adults. In 1990, the mortality of infants, children, and adults declined sufficiently to meet the goal. Adolescent mortality did not reach the 1990 target, and data systems were unable to adequately track the target for older adults (USDHHS, 2000).

Published in 1989, *Healthy People 2000* built on the first surgeon general's report. *Healthy People 2000* contained the following broad goals (USDHHS, 1989):

1. Increase the span of healthy life for Americans.
2. Reduce health disparities among Americans.
3. Achieve access to preventive services for all Americans.

The purpose of *Healthy People 2000* was to provide direction for individuals wanting to change personal behaviors and to improve health in communities through health promotion policies. The report assimilated the broad approaches of health promotion, health protection, and preventive services and contained more than 300 objectives organized into 22 priority areas. Although many of the objectives fell short, the initiative was extremely successful in raising providers' awareness of health behaviors and health promotional activities. States, local health departments, and private-sector health workers used the objectives to determine the relative health of their communities and to set goals for the future.

Healthy People 2010 emerged in January 2000. It expanded on the objectives from *Healthy People 2000* through a broadened prevention science base, an improved surveillance and data system, and a heightened awareness of and demand for preventive health services. This reflects changes in demographics, science, technology, and disease. *Healthy People 2010* listed two broad goals:

Goal 1: Increase quality and years of healthy life.
Goal 2: Eliminate health disparities.

The first goal moved beyond the idea of increasing life expectancy to incorporate the concept of **health-related quality of life (HRQOL)**. This concept of health includes aspects of physical and mental health and their determinants and measures functional status, participation, and well-being. HRQOL expands the definition of health—beyond simply opposing the negative concepts of disease and death—by integrating mental and physical health concepts (USDHHS, 2000).

The final review and analysis of the *Healthy People 2010* objectives showed decidedly mixed progress for the nation. Some 23% of the objectives were met or exceeded, and another 48% "moved toward target." Conversely, 24% of the objectives "moved away from target" (i.e., the indicators were worse than in the previous decade), and another 5% showed no change. Particularly concerning were the poor responses in two of the focus areas: Arthritis, Osteoporosis and Chronic Back conditions (Focus Area 2) and Nutrition and Overweight (Focus Area 19) "moved toward" or "achieved" less than 25% of their targets (USDHHS, 2012).

The fourth version of the nation's health objectives, *Healthy People 2020,* was published in 2010. *Healthy People 2020* is divided into 42 topic areas and contains numerous new objectives and updates for hundreds of objectives from the previous editions. The topic areas are listed in the "Healthy People 2020" box. The objectives and related information and materials can help guide health promotion activities and can be used to aid in community-wide initiatives (USDHHS, 2017). All health care practitioners, particularly those working in the community, should review the *Healthy People 2020* objectives and focus on the relevant areas in their practice. Practitioners should incorporate these objectives into programs, events, and publications whenever possible and should use them as a framework to promote healthy cities and communities. Selected relevant objectives are presented throughout this book to acquaint future community health nurses with the scope of the *Healthy People 2020* initiative and to enhance awareness of current health indicators and national goals (see www.healthypeople.gov for more information).

 ACTIVE LEARNING EXERCISE

Become familiar with *Healthy People 2020* (www.healthypeople.gov). Review objectives from several of the topic areas covered. How does your community compare with the groups, aggregates, and populations described? What objectives should be targeted for your community?

DEFINITION AND FOCUS OF PUBLIC HEALTH NURSING, COMMUNITY HEALTH NURSING, AND COMMUNITY-BASED NURSING

The terms *community health nursing* and *public health nursing* are often used synonymously or interchangeably. Like the practice of community/public health nursing, the terms are evolving. In past debates and discussions, definitions of "community health nursing" and "public health nursing" have indicated similar yet distinctive ideologies, visions, or philosophies of nursing. These concepts and a third related term—*community-based nursing*—are discussed in this section.

Public and Community Health Nursing

Public health nursing has frequently been described as the synthesis of public health and nursing practice. Freeman (1963) provided a classic definition of public health nursing:

> *Public health nursing may be defined as a field of professional practice in nursing and in public health in which technical nursing, interpersonal, analytical, and organizational skills are applied to problems of health as they affect the community. These skills are applied in concert with those of other persons engaged in health care, through comprehensive nursing care of families and other groups and through measures for evaluation or control of threats to health, for health education of the public, and for mobilization of the public for health action. (p. 34)*

Through the 1980s and 1990s, most nurses were taught that there was a distinction between "community health nursing" and "public health nursing." Indeed, "public health nursing" was seen as a subspecialty nursing practice generally delivered within "official" or governmental agencies. In contrast, "community health nursing" was considered to be a broader and more general specialty area that encompassed many additional subspecialties (e.g., school nursing, occupational health nursing, forensic nursing, home health). In 1980, the American Nurses Association (ANA) defined **community health nursing** as "the synthesis of nursing practice and public health practice applied to promoting and preserving the health of populations" (ANA, 1980, p. 2). This viewpoint noted that a community health nurse

directs care to individuals, families, or groups; this care, in turn, contributes to the health of the total population.

The ANA has revised the standards of practice for this specialty area (ANA, 2013). In the updated standards, the designation was again "public health nursing," and the ANA used the definition presented by the American Public Health Association (APHA) Committee on Public Health Nursing (1996). Thus, public health nursing is defined as "the practice of promoting and protecting the health of populations using knowledge from nursing, social, and public health sciences" (APHA, 1996, p. 5). The ANA (2013) elaborated by explaining that public health nursing practice "is population-focused, with the goals of promoting health and preventing disease and disability for all people through the creation of conditions in which people can be healthy" (p. 5).

Some nursing writers will continue to use *community health nursing* as a global or umbrella term and *public health nursing* as a component or subset. Others, as stated, use the terms interchangeably. This book uses the terms interchangeably.

 ACTIVE LEARNING EXERCISE

Ask several neighbors or consumers of health care about their views of the role of public health and community health nursing. Share your results with your classmates.

RESEARCH HIGHLIGHTS

Public Health Nursing Research Agenda

In 2010, a national conference was held to set a research agenda that would advance the science of public health nursing (PHN). The conference employed a multistage, multimethod, participatory developmental approach, involving many influential PHN leaders. Following numerous meetings and discussions, an agenda was proposed. The agenda was structured around four "High Priority Themes": (1) public health nursing interventions models, (2) quality of population-focused practice, (3) metrics of/for public health nursing, and (4) comparative effectiveness and public health nursing outcomes. The aim of the agenda is to help PHN scholars contribute to an understanding of how to improve health and reduce population health disparities by advancing the evidence base regarding the outcomes of practice and by influencing related health policy. The group encouraged the agenda's use to guide and inform programs of research, to influence funding priorities, and to be incorporated into doctoral PHN education through course and curriculum development. Ultimately, it is anticipated that PHN research will proactively contribute to the effectiveness of the public health system and create healthier communities.

Data from Issel, L. M., Bekemeier, B., & Kneipp, S. (2012). A public health nursing research agenda, *Public Health Nursing 29*, 330–342.

Community-Based Nursing

The term *community-based nursing* has been identified and defined in recent years to differentiate it from what has traditionally been seen as community and public health nursing practice. Community-based nursing practice refers to "application of the nursing process in caring for individuals, families and groups where they live, work or go to school or as they move through the health care system" (McEwen & Pullis, 2009, p. 6). Community-based nursing is setting specific, and the emphasis

BOX 1.3 The Scope and Standards of Practice for Public Health Nursing

The Scope and Standards of Practice for Public Health Nursing is the result of the collaborative effort between the American Nurses Association and the Quad Council of Public Health Nursing Organizations. The standards were originally developed in 1999 and were updated in 2013. The Scope and Standards of Practice, which are divided into Standards of Practice and Standards of Professional Performance, describe specific competencies relevant to the public health nurse and the public health nurse in advanced practice.

The Standards of Practice include six standards that are based on the critical thinking model of the nursing process, with competencies addressing each nursing process step. The implementation step is further broken down into specific public health areas, including coordination of services, health education and health promotion, consultation, and regulatory activities. The Standards of Professional Performance include the leadership competencies necessary in the professional practice of all registered nurses, but with additional standards specific to the public health nurse and advanced public health nurse roles. These standards include evidence-based practice and research, collaboration, resource utilization, and advocacy, with competencies specific to public health, such as building coalitions and achieving consensus in public health issues, assessing available health resources within a population, and advocating for equitable access to care and services.

Data from American Nurses Association: *Public health nursing: scope and standards of practice*, ed 2, Silver Spring, MD, 2013, Author. The standards can be purchased at: http://www.nursesbooks.org/Homepage/Hot-off-the-Press/Public-Health-Nursing-2nd.aspx

is on acute and chronic care and includes such practice areas as home health nursing and nursing in outpatient or ambulatory settings.

Zotti, Brown, and Stotts (1996) compared community-based nursing and community health nursing and explained that the goals of the two are different. Community health nursing emphasizes preservation and protection of health, and community-based nursing emphasizes managing acute or chronic conditions. In community health nursing, the primary client is the community; in community-based nursing, the primary clients are the individual and the family. Finally, services in community-based nursing are largely direct, but in community health nursing, services are both direct and indirect (Williams, 2016).

Community and Public Health Nursing Practice

Community and public health nurses practice disease prevention and health promotion. It is important to note that public health nursing practice is collaborative and is based in research and theory. It applies the nursing process to the care of individuals, families, aggregates, and the community. Box 1.3 provides an overview of the Standards for Public Health Nursing (ANA, 2013).

As discussed, the core functions of public health are assessment, policy development, and assurance. In 2003, the Quad Council of Public Health Nursing Organizations (Quad Council) closely examined the core functions and used them to develop a set of public health nursing competencies. These competencies were updated in 2011 and are summarized in Table 1.2 (Quad Council, 2011). Current and future community health nurses should study these competencies to understand

the practice parameters and skills required for public health nursing practice.

POPULATION-FOCUSED PRACTICE AND COMMUNITY/PUBLIC HEALTH NURSING INTERVENTIONS

Community/public health nurses must use a population-focused approach to move beyond providing direct care to individuals and families. Population-focused nursing concentrates on specific groups of people and focuses on health promotion and disease prevention, regardless of geographic location (Baldwin et al., 1998). The goal of population-focused nursing is "provision of evidence-based care to targeted groups of people with similar needs in order to improve outcomes" (Curley, 2016, p. 4). In short, population-focused practice (Minnesota Department of Health, 2003):

- Focuses on the entire population
- Is based on assessment of the population's health status
- Considers the broad determinants of health
- Emphasizes all levels of prevention
- Intervenes with communities, systems, individuals, and families

Whereas community and public health nurses may be responsible for a specific subpopulation in the community (e.g., a school nurse may be responsible for the school's pregnant teenagers), population-focused practice is concerned with many distinct and overlapping community subpopulations. The goal of population-focused nursing is to promote healthy communities.

Population-focused public health nurses would not have exclusive interest in one or two subpopulations, but instead would focus on the many subpopulations that make up the entire community. A population focus involves concern for those who do, and for those who do not, receive health services. A population focus also involves a scientific approach to community health nursing. Thus a thorough, systematic assessment of the community or population is necessary and basic to planning, intervention, and evaluation for the individual, family, aggregate, and population levels.

Public health nursing practice requires the following types of data for scientific approach and population focus: (1) the epidemiology, or body of knowledge, of a particular problem and its solution and (2) information about the community. Each type of knowledge and its source appear in Table 1.3. To determine the overall patterns of health in a population, data collection for assessment and management decisions within a community should be ongoing, not episodic.

Public Health Interventions

Public health nurses focus on the care of individuals, groups, aggregates, and populations in many settings, including homes, clinics, worksites, and schools. In addition to interviewing

TABLE 1.2   Summary of Tier 1 Public Health Nursing (PHN) Competencies (Generalist Public Health Nurses)

Domain	Community and Public Health Nursing Competencies
1. Analytic assessment skills	Identifies determinants of health and illness
	Uses epidemiological data and ecological perspective to identify health risks, needs, values, beliefs, resources, and relevant environmental factors
	Identifies variables that measure health and health conditions
	Uses valid and reliable methods and instruments for collecting data; develops data collection plan
	Identifies sources of public health data and information; collects, interprets, and documents data in understandable terms
	Uses valid and reliable data sources for comparisons
	Identifies gaps and redundancies in data sources
	Applies ethical, legal, and policy guidelines and principles in data collection, use, and dissemination
	Practices evidence-based public health nursing to promote the health of individuals, families, and groups
2. Policy development/program planning skills	Identifies policy issues relevant to health; describes the structure of the public health system and its impact on health
	Identifies the implications of policy options on public health programs
	Identifies outcomes of health policy relevant to PHN practice
	Collects information that will inform policy decisions; describes the legislative policy development process; identifies outcomes of current health policy
	Describes the structure of the public health system; identifies public health laws and regulations relevant to practice
	Participates as a team member to implement programs and policies
	Participates in teams to assure compliance with organizational policies
	Assists in design of evaluation plans
3. Communication skills	Assesses health literacy
	Communicates effectively in writing, orally, and electronically; communicates in a culturally responsive and relevant manner
	Solicits input when planning and delivering health care
	Uses a variety of methods to disseminate public health information
	Communicates effectively as a member of interprofessional team(s)
4. Cultural competency skills	Utilizes the social and ecological determinants of health to work effectively
	Uses concepts, knowledge, and evidence of the social determinants of health in the delivery of services
	Adapts PHN care on the basis of cultural needs and differences
	Explains factors contributing to cultural diversity
	Articulates benefits of a diverse public health workforce
	Demonstrates culturally appropriate public health nursing practice
5. Community dimensions of practice skills	Utilizes an ecological perspective in health assessment, planning, and interventions
	Identifies research issues at a community level; functions as a member of a participatory research team
	Identifies community partners for PHN practice
	Collaborates with community partners to promote health
	Partners effectively with key stakeholders and groups in care delivery
	Participates effectively in activities that facilitate community involvement
	Describes the role of government and the private and nonprofit sectors in the delivery of health services
	Utilizes community assets and resources to promote health and deliver care
	Seeks input into plans of care
	Supports public health policies, programs, and resources
6. Public health sciences skills	Incorporates public health and nursing science in the delivery of care
	Describes the historical foundation of public health and public health nursing
	Describes how programs contribute to meeting the core public health functions and the 10 essential services
	Uses basic descriptive epidemiological methods when conducting a health assessment
	Interprets research relevant to public health interventions
	Accesses public health and other sources of information using informatics and information technologies
	Identifies gaps in research evidence to guide public health nursing practice
	Complies with requirements of patient confidentiality and human subject protection
	Participates in research at the community level to build the scientific base of PHN

TABLE 1.2 Summary of Tier 1 Public Health Nursing (PHN) Competencies (Generalist Public Health Nurses)—cont'd

Domain	Community and Public Health Nursing Competencies
7. Financial planning and management skills	Describes the interrelationships among local, state, tribal, and federal public health and health care systems
	Describes the structure, function, and jurisdictional authority of organizational units within federal, state, tribal, and local public health agencies
	Adheres to the organization's policies and procedures
	Provides data for inclusion in a programmatic budget
	Describes the impact of budget constraints on the delivery of public health nursing care
	Provides input into budget priorities
	Provides data to evaluate care and services
	Adapts the delivery of PHN care on the basis of evaluation results
	Provides input into proposals for funding from external sources
	Applies basic human relations and conflict management skills in interaction with peers
	Utilizes public health informatics skills
	Provides input into contracts and other agreements for the provision of services
	Delivers PHN care within budgetary guidelines
8. Leadership and systems thinking skills	Incorporates ethical standards of practice as the basis of all interactions
	Applies systems theory to PHN practice
	Participates with stakeholders to identify vision, values, and principles of community action
	Identifies internal and external factors affecting PHN practice and services
	Uses individual, team, and organizational learning opportunities for personal and professional development
	Acts as a mentor, coach, or peer advisor for PHN staff; maintains personal commitment to lifelong learning and professional development
	Participates in quality initiatives
	Adapts the delivery of PHN care in consideration of changes in the health system and the larger social, political, and economic environment; maintains knowledge of current public health laws and policies

Modified from Quad Council of Public Health Nursing Organizations: *Public health nursing competencies*, Washington, DC, 2011, Author.

TABLE 1.3 Information Useful for Population Focus

Type of Information	Examples	Sources
Demographic data	Age, gender, race/ethnicity, socioeconomic status, education level	Vital statistic data (national, state, county, local); census
Groups at high risk	Health status and health indicators of various subpopulations in the community (e.g., children, elders, those with disabilities)	Health statistics (morbidity, mortality, natality); disease statistics (incidence and prevalence)
Services/providers available	Official (public) health departments; health care providers for low-income individuals and families; community service agencies and organizations (e.g., Red Cross, Meals on Wheels)	City directories; phone books; local or regional social workers; low-income providers' lists; local community health nurses (e.g., school nurses)

clients and assessing individual and family health, public health nurses must be able to assess a population's health needs and resources and identify its values. Public health nurses must also work with the community to identify and implement programs that meet health needs and to evaluate the effectiveness of programs after implementation. For example, school nurses were once responsible only for running first-aid stations and monitoring immunization compliance. Now they are actively involved in assessing the needs of their population and defining programs to meet those needs through activities such as health screening and group health education and promotion. The activities of school nurses may be as varied as designing health curricula with a school and community advisory group, leading support groups for elementary school children with chronic illness, advocating for emergency equipment (e.g., automatic external defibrillators) in gyms and athletic fields, and monitoring the health status of teenage mothers.

Similarly, occupational health nurses are no longer required to simply maintain an office or dispensary. They are involved in many different types of activities. These activities might include maintaining records of workers exposed to physical or chemical risks, monitoring compliance with Occupational Safety and Health Administration standards, teaching classes on health issues, acting as case managers for workers with chronic health conditions, and leading support group discussions for workers with health-related problems.

Private associations, such as the American Diabetes Association or the Red Cross, employ public health nurses for their organizational ability and health-related skills. Other public health nurses work with multidisciplinary groups of professionals, serve on boards of voluntary health associations such as the American Heart Association, work as case managers for insurance companies, and are members of health planning agencies and councils.

GENETICS IN PUBLIC HEALTH

Community-Based Research for the Prevention of Cardiovascular Disease

Cardiovascular disease (CVD) is the leading cause of death among Americans, and prevention of CVD should be a priority for all nurses. It has been established that CVD results from a complex interaction among modifiable factors including lifestyle choices and environmental influences, and non-modifiable factors such as age and race/ethnicity or genetics. A group of nurse researchers led by Fletcher (2011) presented a "call to action for nursing" to promote community-based research that focuses on the genetic factors that contribute to CVD. The team described the need to build capacity for participation in genetics research within communities through community engagement, particularly among vulnerable ethnic minority groups. The importance of identifying the genetic-environmental interactions that may led to clinical manifestation of CVD was stressed and a number of community-based interventions to prevent CVD were described.

Fletcher BJ, Himmelfarb CD, Lira MT, Meininger JC, Pradhan SR, Sikkema J: Global cardiovascular disease prevention: A call to action for nursing. *Journal of Cardiovascular Nursing*, 26, 45, 535-545.

The Public Health Intervention Wheel

The Public Health Intervention Model was initially proposed in the late 1990s by nurses from the Minnesota Department of Health to describe the breadth and scope of public health nursing practice (Keller et al., 1998). This model was later revised and termed the *Intervention Wheel* (Fig. 1.3) (Keller et al., 2004a; Keller et al., 2004b), and it has become increasingly recognized as a framework for community and public health nursing practice.

The Intervention Wheel contains three important elements: (1) it is population based; (2) it contains three levels of practice (community, systems, and individual/family); and (3) it identifies and defines 17 public health interventions. The levels of practice and interventions are directed at improving population health (Keller et al., 2004a). Within the Intervention Wheel, the 17 health interventions are grouped into five "wedges." These interventions are actions taken on behalf of communities, systems, individuals, and families to improve or protect health status. Table 1.4 provides definitions.

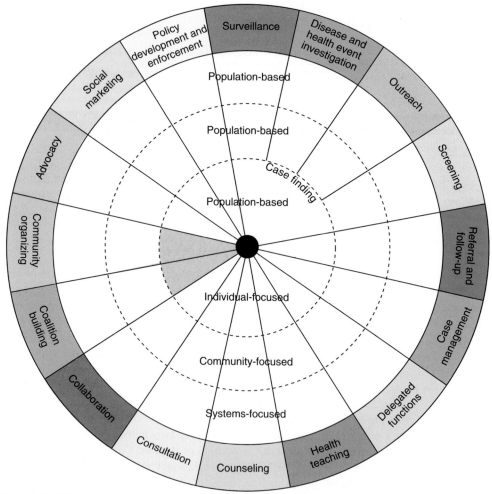

FIG. 1.3 Public Health Intervention Wheel. (Modified from Section of Public Health Nursing, Minnesota Department of Health: *Public health interventions*, 2001. Retrieved from: http://www.health.state.mn.us/divs/opi/cd/phn/docs/0301wheel_manual.pdf.)

The Intervention Wheel is further dissected into levels of practice, in which the interventions may be directed at an entire population within a community, a system that would affect the health of a population, and/or the individuals and families within the population. Thus each intervention can and should be applied at each level. For example, a systems-level intervention within "disease investigation" might be the community health nurse working with the state health department and federal vaccine program to coordinate a response to an outbreak of measles in a migrant population. An example of a population- or community-level intervention for "screening" would be public health nurses working with area high schools to give each student a profile of his or her health to promote nutritional and physical activity lifestyle changes to improve the student's health.

Finally, an individual-level implementation of the intervention "referral and follow-up" would occur when a nurse receives a referral to care for an individual with a diagnosed mental illness who would require regular monitoring of his or her medication compliance to prevent rehospitalization (Keller et al., 2004b).

PUBLIC HEALTH NURSING, MANAGED CARE, AND HEALTH REFORM

Shifts in reimbursement, the growth of managed care, and implementation and revision of the ACA have revitalized the notion of population-based care. Health insurance companies, governmental financing entities (e.g., Medicare, Medicaid), and MCOs use financial incentives and organizational structures in an attempt to increase efficiency and decrease health care costs. The foundation for managed care is management of health care for an enrolled group of individuals. This group of enrollees is the population covered by the plan who receive health services from managed care plan providers (Kongstvedt, 2013).

An understanding of enrolled populations and health care patterns is essential for managing health care services and resources effectively. Most MCOs have become sophisticated in identifying key subgroups within the population of enrollees at risk for health problems. Typically, managed care systems target subgroups according to characteristics associated with risk or use of expensive services, such as selected

TABLE 1.4 Public Health Interventions and Definitions

Public Health Intervention	Definition
Surveillance	Describes and monitors health events through ongoing and systematic collection, analysis, and interpretation of health data for the purpose of planning, implementing, and evaluating public health interventions
Disease and other health event investigation	Systematically gathers and analyzes data regarding threats to the health of populations, ascertains the source of the threat, identifies cases and others at risk, and determines control measures
Outreach	Locates populations of interest or populations at risk and provides information about the nature of the concern, what can be done about it, and how services can be obtained
Screening	Identifies individuals with unrecognized health risk factors or asymptomatic disease conditions
Case finding	Locates individuals and families with identified risk factors and connects them with resources
Referral and follow-up	Assists individuals, families, groups, organizations, and/or communities to identify and access necessary resources to prevent or resolve problems or concerns
Case management	Optimizes self-care capabilities of individuals and families and the capacity of systems and communities to coordinate and provide services
Delegated functions	Carries out direct care tasks under the authority of a health care practitioner as allowed by law
Health teaching	Communicates facts, ideas, and skills that change knowledge, attitudes, values, beliefs, behaviors, and practices of individuals, families, systems, and/or communities
Counseling	Establishes an interpersonal relationship with a community, a system, and a family or individual, with the intention of increasing or enhancing their capacity for self-care and coping
Consultation	Seeks information and generates optional solutions to perceived problems or issues through interactive problem solving with a community system and family or individual
Collaboration	Commits two or more persons or organizations to achieve a common goal by enhancing the capacity of one or more of the members to promote and protect health
Coalition building	Promotes and develops alliances among organizations or constituencies for a common purpose
Community organizing	Helps community groups to identify common problems or goals, mobilize resources, and develop and implement strategies for realizing the goals they collectively have set
Advocacy	Pleads someone's cause or acts on someone's behalf, with a focus on developing the community, system, and individual or family's capacity to plead their own cause or act on their own behalf
Social marketing	Utilizes commercial marketing principles and technologies for programs designed to influence the knowledge, attitudes, values, beliefs, behaviors, and practices of the population of interest
Policy development and enforcement	Places health issues on decision makers' agendas, acquires a plan of resolution, and determines needed resources, resulting in laws, rules, regulations, ordinances, and policies. Policy enforcement compels others to comply with laws, rules, regulations, ordinances, and policies

Modified from Keller LO, Strohschein S, Lia-Hoagberg B, Schaffer MA: *Population-based public health interventions: practice-based and evidence-supported. Part I*, St. Paul, MN, 2004a, Minnesota Department of Health, Center for Public Health Nursing.

clinical conditions, functional status, and past service use patterns.

In March 2010, President Obama signed the Patient Protection and Affordable Care Act (ACA) (PL 111-148) into law. The ACA served to expand insurance coverage for those uninsured and to help control health care costs. Expansion of coverage was accomplished by requiring individuals to purchase health insurance for themselves and their families, implementation of "exchanges" to increase options for individuals to purchase health insurance, and requiring more employers to offer health insurance to employees. Public programs (e.g., Medicaid and State Children's Health Insurance Program) were expanded to cover health care for those who could not afford to buy their own insurance. With the change of administration in 2017, it is anticipated that there will be significant revisions of the ACA with new federal and state-sponsored initiatives. Public health nurses must stay informed of these changes and work with groups and organizations to support legislation that will promote population health, reduce disparities, and better manage the costs of care.

The purpose of public health is to improve the health of the public by promoting healthy lifestyles, preventing disease and injury, and protecting the health of communities. In the past, shrinking public health resources have supported personal health services over community health promotion. In public health practice, the community is the population of interest. With the proposed changes to health care financing, the personal health care system will be under increasing pressure to provide the services that health departments previously provided. Traditionally served by public health, the most vulnerable populations will pose tremendous challenges for private health care providers. Public health agencies and providers will be responsible for partnering with private providers to care for these populations.

Providing population-based care requires a dramatic shift in thinking from individual-based care. Some of the practical demands of population-based care are the following:

1. It must be recognized that populations are not homogeneous; therefore it is necessary to address the needs of special subpopulations within populations.
2. High-risk and vulnerable subpopulations must be identified early in the care delivery cycle.
3. Nonusers of services often become high-cost users; therefore it is essential to develop outreach strategies.
4. Quality and cost of all health care services are linked together across the health care continuum. (Kaiser Family Foundation, 2013)

Nurses in community and public health have an opportunity to share their expertise regarding population-based approaches to health care for groups of individuals across health care settings. Today, health care practitioners require additional skills in assessment, policy development, and assurance to provide community public health practice and population-based service. Health care professionals should focus attention on promoting healthy lifestyles, providing preventive and primary care, expanding and ensuring access to cost-effective and technologically appropriate care, participating in coordinated and interdisciplinary care, and involving patients and families in the decision-making process. Public health nurses must work in partnership with colleagues in managed care settings to improve community health. Partnerships may address information management, cultural values, health care system improvement, and the physical environment roles in health and may require complex negotiations to share data. The partners may need to develop new community assessment strategies to augment epidemiological methods that often mask the context or meaning of the human experience of vulnerable populations.

SUMMARY

The health care system has been evolving from focusing on individuals in acute care settings to being more community based and population health directed. Nursing practice has changed in response, and today a growing proportion of nurses is working outside of hospitals. Public and community health nursing practice includes population-focused interventions that seek to improve the health and well-being of groups, aggregates, and communities.

This chapter has presented information on key concepts, including "health" and "community," and described the vital importance of addressing societal needs in order to improve population health. With widely recognized changes in population demographics, it is necessary that nurses be attuned to the determinants and indicators of health, health-promoting activities, and changes in the health care system. This includes efforts to promote access to more individuals and to understand the need to contain costs. With this knowledge and skills, public and community health nurses can influence health practices and policies that will positively affect the future health of individuals, families, groups, and communities.

EVOLVE WEBSITE

http://evolve.elsevier.com/Nies/community
- NCLEX Review Questions
- Case Studies

BIBLIOGRAPHY

American Heritage College Dictionary, ed 3 New York, 1997, Houghton Mifflin.

American Nurses Association: *A conceptual model of community health nursing,* Kansas City, MO, 1980, Pub No CH-10, ANA.

American Nurses Association: *ANA's Nurses by the Numbers*, 2016. Available from http://assets.1440n.net/16-238/10/.

American Nurses Association: *Public health nursing: scope and standards of practice*, Silver Spring, MD, 2013, American Nurses Publishing.

American Nurses Association: *Code of ethics for nurses, with interpretive statements*, Silver Spring, MD, 2015, American Nurses Publishing.

American Public Health Association: *Ad hoc committee on public health nursing: the definition and role of public health nursing practice in the delivery of health care*, Washington, DC, 1996, American Public Health Association.

Baldwin JH, Conger CO, Abegglen JC, et al.: Population-focused and community-based nursing: moving toward clarification of concepts, *Public Health Nurs* 15:12–18, 1998.

Cassidy EF, Trujillo MD, Orleans CT: Health and behavior. In Kovner AR, Knickman JR, editors: *Health care delivery in the United States*, ed 11, New York, 2015, Springer Publishing.

Centers for Disease Control and Prevention (CDC): *10 essential public health services*, 2014. Available from https://www.cdc.gov/nphpsp/essentialservices.html.

Curley ALC: Introduction to population-based nursing. In Curley ALC, Vitale PA, editors: *Population-based nursing: concepts and competencies for advanced practice*, ed 2, New York, 2016, Springer Publishing Co.

Dunn HL: *High level wellness*, Arlington, VA, 1961, RW Beatty.

Freeman RB: *Public health nursing practice*, ed 3, Philadelphia, 1963, WB Saunders.

Getzen T: *Health economics and financing*, ed 5, Hoboken, NJ, 2013, John Wiley & Sons.

Gibson ME, Thatcher EJ: Community as client: assessment and analysis. In Stanhope M, Lancaster J, editors: *Public health nursing: population-centered health care in the community*, ed 9, St. Louis, 2016, Elsevier.

Greiner PA: Health defined: objectives for promotion and prevention. In Edelman CL, Kudzma EC, Mandle CL, editors: *Health promotion throughout the life span*, ed 8, St. Louis, 2014, Elsevier.

Hanlon JJ: *Principles of public health administration*, ed 3, St. Louis, 1960, Mosby.

Institute of Medicine: *The future of nursing*, Washington, DC, 2011, National Academy Press.

Institute of Medicine: *The future of public health*, Washington, DC, 1988, National Academy Press.

Kaiser Family Foundation: *Health reform source*, 2013. Available from http://kff.org. Accessed March, 2017.

Kaiser Family Foundation: *Summary of the new health reform law*, Pub No. 8061, 2013. Available from http://kff.org/health-reform/factsheet/summary-of-the-affordable-care-act/. Accessed March, 2017.

Keller LO, Strohschein S, Lia-Hoagberg B, et al.: Population-based public health interventions: practice-based and evidence-supported. Part I, *Public Health Nurs* 21:453–468, 2004a.

Keller LO, Strohschein S, Schaffer MA, et al.: Population-based public health interventions: innovations in practice, teaching and management. Part II, *Public Health Nurs* 21:469–487, 2004b.

Keller LO, Strohschein S, Lia-Hoagberg B, et al.: Population-based public health interventions: a model for practice, *Public Health Nurs* 15:207–215, 1998.

Kongstvedt PR: *Essentials of managed health care*, ed 6, Burlington MA, 2013, Jones and Bartlett.

Leavell HR, Clark EG: *Preventive medicine for the doctor in his community*, New York, 1958, McGraw-Hill.

Lundy KS, Janes S: *Community health nursing: caring for the public's health*, ed 3, Boston, 2016, Jones & Bartlett.

Maurer FA, Smith CM: *Community/public health nursing practice: health for families and populations*, ed 5, St. Louis, 2013, Elsevier.

McEwen M, Pullis B: *Community-based nursing: an introduction*, ed 3, St. Louis, 2009, WB Saunders.

McGinnis MJ, Foege W: Actual causes of death in the United States, *JAMA* 270:2207–2212, 1993.

McKeown T: Determinants of health. In Lee PR, Estes CL, editors: *The nation's health*, ed 7, Boston, 2003, Jones & Bartlett.

McKinlay JB: A case for refocusing upstream: the political economy of illness. In Jaco EG, editor: *Patients, physicians, and illness*, ed 3, New York, 1979, The Free Press.

Minnesota Department of Health: *Definitions of population based practice*, 2003. Available from http://www.health.state.mn.us/divs/opi/cd/phn/docs/0303phn_popbasedpractice.pdf. Accessed March, 2017.

Mokdad AH, Marks JS, Stroup DF, et al.: Actual causes of death in the United States, *JAMA* 291:1238–1245, 2004.

Murray RB, Zentner JP, Yakimo R: *Health promotion strategies through the life span*, ed 8, Upper Saddle River, NJ, 2009, Prentice Hall.

National Center for Health Statistics: *Health, United States, 2016*, DHHS Publication No. 2017-1232, May, 2017. Available from https://www.cdc.gov/nchs/data/hus/hus16.pdf.

National Council for State Boards of Nursing (NCSBN): The 2015 national nursing workforce survey, *Jnl of Nsg Reg* 7(Suppl 1), 2016.

Pender NJ, Murdaugh CL, Parsons MA: *Health promotion in nursing practice*, ed 6, Upper Saddle River, NJ, 2011, Pearson Education.

Quad Council of Public Health Nursing Organizations: *Competencies for public health nurses*, 2011. Available from <http://www.achne.org/files/Quad%20Council/QuadCouncilCompetenciesforPublicHealth-Nurses.pdf>.

Rector C: *Community and public health nursing: promoting and protecting the public's health*, ed 9, Philadelphia, PA, 2017, Wolters Kluwer.

Rosenfeld P, Russell D: A review of factors influencing utilization of home and community-based long-term care: trends and implications to the nursing workforce, *Policy Polit Nurs Pract* 13:72–80, 2012.

Roy C: *The Roy adaption model*, ed 3, Upper Saddle River, NJ, 2009, Pearson.

Russo P: Population health. In Kovner AR, Knickman JR, editors: *Health care delivery in the United States*, ed 11, New York, 2015, Springer Publishing.

Saylor C: The circle of health: a health definition model, *J Holist Nurs* 22:98–115, 2004.

Shi L, Singh DA: *Delivering health care in America: a systems approach*, ed 6, Boston, 2016, Jones & Bartlett.

Shi L, Singh DA: *The nation's health*, ed 8, Boston, 2012, Jones & Bartlett.

Shuster GR: Community as client: assessment and analysis. In Stanhope M, Lancaster J, editors: *Public health nursing: population-centered health care in the community*, ed 8, St. Louis, 2012, Elsevier.

U.S. Department of Health and Human Services: *Health Resources and Services Administration: The registered nurse population: Initial findings 2008 national sample survey of registered nurses*. Available from: https://bhw.hrsa.gov/healthworkforce/rnsurvey/initialfindings2008.pdf.

U.S. Department of Health and Human Services: *Healthy People 2000 objectives*, Washington, DC, 1989, Author.

U.S. Department of Health and Human Services: *Healthy People 2010 objectives*, Washington, DC, 2000, Author.

U.S. Department of Health and Human Services: *Healthy People 2010: final review*, Washington, DC, 2012, Author. Available from <http://www.cdc.gov/nchs/data/hpdata2010/hp2010_final_review.pdf>.

U.S. Department of Health and Human Services: *Healthy People 2020 objectives*, 2017. Available from <http://www.healthypeople.gov/2020/about/default.aspx>.

Wald LD: *The house on Henry Street*, New York, 1971, Dover Publications.

Williams CA: Community and prevention-oriented, population-focused practice: the foundation of specialization in public health nursing. In Stanhope M, Lancaster J, editors: *Public health nursing: population-centered health care in the community*, ed 9, St. Louis, 2016, Elsevier.

Winslow CEA: The untilled field of public health, *Mod Med* 2:183, March, 1920.

World Health Organization: A discussion document on the concept and principles of health promotion, *Health Promot* 1:73–78, 1986.

World Health Organization: The first 10 years of the World Health Organization, *Chron WHO* 1:1–2, 1958.

Zotti ME, Brown P, Stotts RC: Community-based nursing versus community health nursing: what does it all mean? *Nurs Outlook* 44:211–217, 1996.

Historical Factors: Public Health Nursing in Context

*Melanie McEwen**

OBJECTIVES

Upon completion of this chapter, the reader will be able to do the following:

1. Describe the impact of aggregate living on population health.
2. Identify approaches to population health promotion from prerecorded historic to present times.
3. Understand historical events that have influenced population health.
4. Compare the application of public health principles to the nation's major health problems at the turn of the twentieth century (i.e., acute disease) with that at the beginning of the twenty-first century (i.e., chronic disease).
5. Describe two leaders in nursing who had a profound impact on addressing population health.
6. Discuss major contemporary issues facing community/public health nursing, and trace the historical roots to the present.

KEY TERMS

district nursing
Edward Jenner
Edwin Chadwick
Elizabethan Poor Law
endemic
epidemic
Flexner Report

Florence Nightingale
health visiting
House on Henry Street
John Snow
Joseph Lister
Lemuel Shattuck
Lillian Wald

Louis Pasteur
pandemic
Robert Koch
Sanitary Revolution
stages in disease history

An understanding of the historical factors that have influenced the evolution of population health may help explain current health challenges. This chapter examines the health of Western populations from early historic times to recent times and describes the evolution of modern health care. The role of public health nurses and concurrent challenges for improving the health of groups, aggregates, and communities are also discussed.

EVOLUTION OF HEALTH IN WESTERN POPULATIONS

Medical anthropologists use paleontological records and disease descriptions of primitive societies to speculate on the

interrelationship of early humans, probable diseases, and their environment. Historians have also documented the existence of public health activity (i.e., an organized community effort to prevent disease, prolong life, and promote health) since before recorded historical times. This section describes how aggregate living patterns and early public health efforts have affected the health of Western populations.

Aggregate Impact on Health

Polgar (1964) defined the following stages in disease history: hunting and gathering stage, settled villages stage, preindustrial cities stage, industrial cities stage, and present stage (Fig. 2.1). In these stages, growing populations, increased population density, and imbalanced human ecology resulted in changes in cultural adaptation. In each stage, humans created an ecological imbalance by altering their environment to

---

*The author would like to acknowledge the contribution of Tom H. Cook, who wrote this chapter for the previous edition.

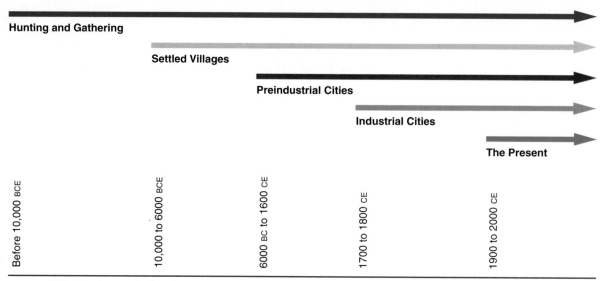

Hunting and Gathering

Settled Villages

Preindustrial Cities

Industrial Cities

The Present

Before 10,000 BCE

10,000 to 6000 BCE

6000 BC to 1600 CE

1700 to 1800 CE

1900 to 2000 CE

FIG. 2.1 Stages in the disease history of humankind. Stages overlap, and time periods are widely debated in the field of anthropology. Some form of each stage remains evident in the world today.

accommodate group living. This imbalance subsequently had a significant effect on aggregate health.

Although these stages are associated with the evolution of civilization, it is important to note that the information is limited by cultural bias. The stages depict the evolution of civilization from the perspective of the Western world. They consist of overlapping historical time periods, which anthropologists widely debate. However, the stages of human disease can provide a frame of reference to aid in determining the relationship among humans, disease, and environment from early historical times to the present. Furthermore, although the stages chronicle the general evolution in the Western world, it is important to realize that each stage still exists in civilization today. For example, Australian aborigines continue to hunt and gather food, and "settled villages" can readily be found in developing countries.

Public health nurses should be aware that populations from each stage consist of a variety of people with distinct cultural traditions and a broad range of health care practices and beliefs. For example, a nurse currently practicing in an American community may need to plan care for immigrants or refugees from a settled village or a preindustrial city. Public and community health nurses must recognize that the environment, the population's health risks, and the host culture's strengths and challenges affect the health status of each particular group.

Hunting and Gathering Stage

During the Paleolithic period, or Old Stone Age, nomadic and semi-nomadic people engaged in hunting and gathering, with generations of small aggregate groups wandering in search of food. Armelagos and Dewey (1978) reviewed how the size, density, and relationship to the environment of such people probably affected their health. These groups may have avoided many contagious diseases because the scattered groups were small, nomadic, and separated from other groups. Under these

conditions, diseases would not spread among the groups. Evidently the disposal of human feces and waste was not a great problem; the nomadic people most likely abandoned the caves they used for shelter once waste accumulated.

Settled Village Stage

Small settlements were characteristic of the Mesolithic period, or Middle Stone Age, and the Neolithic period, or New Stone Age. Wandering people became more sedentary and formed small encampments and villages. The concentration of people in these small areas caused new health problems. For example, people began to domesticate animals and live close to their herds, a practice that probably transmitted diseases such as salmonella, anthrax, Q fever, and tuberculosis (TB) (Polgar, 1964). These stationary people also domesticated plants, a change that may have reduced the range of consumable nutrients and may have led to deficiency diseases. They had to secure water and remove wastes, often leading to the cross-contamination of the water supply and the spread of waterborne diseases such as dysentery, cholera, typhoid, and hepatitis A.

Preindustrial Cities Stage

In preindustrial times, large urban centers formed to support the expanding population. Populations inhabited smaller areas; therefore exposure to preexisting problems expanded. For example, the urban population had to resource increased amounts of food and water and remove increased amounts of waste products. Some cultures developed elaborate water systems. However, waste removal via the water supply led to diseases such as cholera. Further, with the development of towns, rodent infestation increased and facilitated the spread of plague. People had more frequent close contact with one another; therefore the transmission of diseases spread by direct contact increased, and diseases such as mumps, measles, influenza, and smallpox became endemic (Polgar, 1964). Of significance,

TABLE 2.1 Disease Definitions

Types of Disease	Definition
Endemic	Diseases that are always present in a population (e.g., colds and pneumonia)
Epidemic	Diseases that are not always present in a population but flare up on occasion (e.g., diphtheria and measles)
Pandemic	The existence of disease in a large proportion of the population: a global epidemic (e.g., human immunodeficiency virus, acquired immunodeficiency syndrome, and annual outbreaks of influenza type A)

a population must reach a certain size to maintain a disease in endemic proportions (Table 2.1); for example, approximately 1 million people are needed to sustain measles at an endemic level (Cockburn, 1967).

Industrial Cities Stage

Industrialization caused urban areas to become denser and even more heavily populated. Increased industrial wastes, air and water pollution, and harsh working conditions took a toll on health. During the eighteenth and nineteenth centuries, there was an increase in respiratory diseases such as TB, pneumonia, and bronchitis and in epidemics of infectious diseases such as diphtheria, smallpox, typhoid fever, typhus, measles, malaria, and yellow fever (Armelagos and Dewey, 1978). Furthermore, exploration and imperialism spread epidemics of many diseases to susceptible populations throughout the world because settlers, traders, and soldiers moved from one location to another, introducing communicable diseases into native population groups.

Present Stage

Although infectious diseases no longer account for a majority of deaths in the Western world, they continue to cause many deaths in the non-Western world. They also remain prevalent among low-income populations and some ethnic minority groups in the West. Western diseases such as cancer, heart disease, obesity, hypertension, and diabetes are less common among populations from nonindustrial communities. These diseases typically appear when cultures adopt Western customs and transition into urban environments. Epidemiological studies suggest that common risk factors that contribute to chronic health conditions are changes in diet (e.g., increases in refined sugar and fats and lack of fiber), environmental alterations (e.g., use of motorized transportation and climate-controlled living and work sites), and occupational hazards. A rise in population and greater population density also increase mental and behavioral disorders.

In summary, disease patterns and environmental demands changed when wandering, hunting, and gathering aggregates grew into large populations and became sedentary. Humans had to adapt to more densely populated, largely urban existence with marked consequences for health. As a result, over time, the leading causes of death changed from infectious disease to chronic illness.

Evolution of Early Public Health Efforts

Traditionally, historians believed that organized public health efforts were eighteenth- and nineteenth-century activities associated with the Sanitary Revolution. However, modern historians have shown that organized community health efforts to prevent disease, prolong life, and promote health have existed since early human history.

Public health efforts developed slowly over time. The following sections briefly trace the evolution of organized public health and highlight the periods of prerecorded historical times (i.e., before 5000 BCE), classical times (i.e., 3000 to 200 BCE), the Middle Ages (i.e., 500 to 1500 CE), the Renaissance (i.e., fifteenth, sixteenth, and seventeenth centuries), the eighteenth century, the nineteenth century, and into the present day. It is important to note that, like the disease history of humankind, public health efforts exist in various stages of development throughout the world, and this brief history suggests a Western viewpoint.

Prerecorded Historic Times

From the early remains of human habitation, anthropologists recognize that early nomadic humans became domesticated and tended to live in increasingly larger groups. Aggregates ranging from extended families to larger communities inevitably shared episodes of life, health, sickness, and death. Whether based on superstition or sanitation, health practices evolved to ensure the survival of many aggregates. For example, primitive societies used elements of medicine (e.g., voodoo), isolation (e.g., banishment), and fumigation (i.e., use of smoke) to manage disease and thus protect the community for thousands of years (Hanlon and Pickett, 1990).

Classical Times

In the early years of the period 3000 to 1400 BCE, the Minoans devised ways to flush water and construct drainage systems. Circa 1000 BCE, the Egyptians constructed elaborate drainage systems, developed pharmaceutical preparations, and embalmed the dead. Pollution is an ancient problem. The biblical book of Exodus reported that "all the waters that were in the river stank," and in the book of Leviticus (believed to be written around 500 BCE), the Hebrews formulated the first written hygiene code. This hygiene code protected water and food by creating laws that governed personal and community hygiene such as contagion, disinfection, and sanitation.

Greece. Greek literature contains accounts of communicable diseases such as diphtheria, mumps, and malaria. The Hippocratic book *On Airs, Waters and Places,* a treatise on the balance between humans and their environment, may have been the only volume on this topic until the development of bacteriology in the late nineteenth century (Rosen, 2015). Diseases that were always present in a population, such as colds and pneumonia, were called endemic. When diseases such as diphtheria and measles presented fairly widespread outbreaks, the diseases were termed epidemic.

In practice, the Greeks emphasized the preservation of health, or good living, which the goddess Hygeia represented, and curative medicine, which the goddess Panacea personified.

Human life had to be in balance with environmental demands; therefore the Greeks weighed the importance of exercise, rest, and nutrition according to age, sex, constitution, and climate (Rosen, 2015).

Rome. Although the Romans readily adopted Greek culture, they far surpassed Greek engineering by constructing massive aqueducts, bathhouses, and sewer systems. For example, at the height of the Roman Empire, Rome provided its 1 million inhabitants with 40 gallons of water per person per day, which is comparable to modern consumption rates (Rosen, 2015). Inhabitants of the overcrowded Roman slums, however, did not share in public health amenities such as sewer systems and latrines, and their health suffered accordingly.

The Romans also observed and addressed occupational health threats. In particular, they noted the pallor of the miners, the danger of suffocation, and the smell of caustic fumes (Rosen, 2015) (Box 2.1). For protection, miners devised safeguards by using masks made of bags, sacks, membranes, and bladder skins.

In the early years of the Roman Republic, priests were believed to mediate diseases and often dispensed medicine. Public physicians worked in designated towns and earned money to care for the poor. In addition, they were able to charge wealthier patients a service fee. Much as in a modern health maintenance organization or group practice, several families paid a set fee for yearly services. Hospitals, surgeries, infirmaries, and nursing homes appeared throughout Rome. In the fourth century, a Christian woman named Fabiola established a hospital for the sick poor. Others repeated this model throughout medieval times (Donahue, 2011).

Middle Ages

The decline of Rome, which occurred circa 500 CE, led to the Middle Ages. Monasteries promoted collective activity to protect public health, and the population adopted protective measures such as building wells and fountains, cleaning streets, and disposing of refuse. The commonly occurring communicable diseases were measles, smallpox, diphtheria, leprosy, and bubonic plague. Physicians had little to offer in the management of diseases such as leprosy. The church took over by enforcing the hygienic codes from Leviticus and establishing isolation and leper houses, or leprosaria (Rosen, 2015).

A **pandemic** is the existence of disease in a large proportion of the population. One such pandemic, the bubonic plague, ravaged much of the world in the fourteenth century. This plague, or Black Death, claimed close to half the world's population at that time (Hanlon and Pickett, 1990). For centuries, medicine and science did not recognize that fleas, which were attracted to the large number of rodents inhabiting urban areas, were the transmitters of plague. Modern public health practices such as isolation, disinfection, and ship quarantines emerged in response to the bubonic plague (Box 2.2).

During the Middle Ages, clergymen often acted as physicians and treated kings and noblemen. Monks and nuns provided nursing care in small houses designated as structures similar to today's small hospitals. Medieval writings contained information on hygiene and addressed such topics as housing, diet, personal cleanliness, and sleep (Rosen, 2015). Box 2.3 presents an account of living conditions in the sixteenth century.

The Renaissance

Although the cause of infectious disease remained undiscovered, two events important to public health occurred during the Renaissance. In 1546, Girolamo Fracastoro presented a theory that infection was a cause and epidemic a consequence of the "seeds of disease." Then, in 1676, Anton van Leeuwenhoek described microscopic organisms, although he did not associate them with disease (Rosen, 2015).

The **Elizabethan Poor Law**, enacted in England in 1601, held the church parishes responsible for providing relief for the poor. This law governed health care for the poor for more than two centuries and became a prototype for later U.S. laws.

BOX 2.3 Life in an English Household in the Sixteenth Century

In the following account, Erasmus described how life in the sixteenth century must have affected health. Such accounts appeared in literature throughout the sixteenth century.

As to floors, they are usually made with clay, covered with rushes that grow in the fens and which are so seldom removed that the lower parts remain sometimes for twenty years and has in it a collection of spittle, vomit, urine of dogs and humans, beer, scraps of fish and other filthiness not to be named.

Quotation from Hanlon JJ, Pickett GE: *Public health administration and practice*, ed 9, St. Louis, MO, 1990, Mosby, p 25.

Eighteenth Century

Great Britain. The eighteenth century was marked by imperialism and industrialization. Unsanitary conditions remained a huge problem. During the Industrial Revolution, a gradual change in industrial productivity occurred. The industrial boom sacrificed many lives for profit. In particular, it forced poor children into labor. Under the Elizabethan Poor Law, parishes established workhouses to employ the poor. Orphaned and poor children were wards of the parish; therefore the parish forced these young children to labor in parish workhouses for long hours (George, 1925). At 12 to 14 years of age, a child became a master's apprentice. Those apprenticed to chimney sweeps reportedly suffered the worst fate because their masters forced them into chimneys at the risk of being burned and suffocated.

Vaccination was a major discovery of the times. In 1796, Edward Jenner observed that people who worked around cattle were less likely to contract smallpox. He concluded that immunity to smallpox resulted from an inoculation with the cowpox virus. Jenner's contribution was significant because approximately 95% of the population suffered from smallpox and approximately 10% of the population died of smallpox during the eighteenth century. Frequently, the faces of those who survived the disease were scarred with pockmarks.

The Sanitary Revolution's public health reforms were beginning to take place throughout Europe and England. In the eighteenth century, scholars used survey methods to study public health problems (Rosen, 2015). These surveys mapped "medical topographies," which were geographic factors related to regional health and disease. A health education movement provided books and pamphlets on health to the middle and upper classes, but it neglected "economic factors" and was not concerned with the working classes.

Nineteenth Century

Europe. During the nineteenth century, communicable diseases ravaged the population that lived in unsanitary conditions, and many lives were lost. For example, in the mid-1800s, typhus and typhoid fever claimed twice as many lives each year as the Battle of Waterloo (Hanlon and Pickett, 1990).

Edwin Chadwick called attention to the consequences of unsanitary conditions that resulted in health disparities that shortened life spans of the laboring class in particular. Chadwick contended that death rates were high in large industrial cities such as Liverpool, where more than half of all children born of working-class parents died by age 5. Laborers lived an average of 16 years. In contrast, tradesmen lived 22 years, and the upper classes lived 36 years (Richardson, 1887). In 1842, Chadwick published his famous *Report on an Inquiry Into the Sanitary Conditions of the Labouring Population of Great Britain*. The report furthered the establishment of the General Board of Health for England in 1848. Legislation for social reform followed, addressing prevailing concerns such as child welfare; factory management; education; and care for the elderly, sick, and mentally ill. Clean water, sewers, fireplugs, and sidewalks emerged as a result.

In 1849, a German pathologist named Rudolf Virchow argued for social action—bettering the lives of the people by improving economic, social, and environmental conditions—to attack the root social causes of disease. He proposed "a theory of epidemic disease as a manifestation of social and cultural maladjustment" (Rosen, 2015, p. 62). He further argued that the public was responsible for the health of the people; that social and economic conditions heavily affected health and disease; that efforts to promote health and fight disease must be social, economic, and medical; and that the study of social and economic determinants of health and disease would yield knowledge to guide appropriate action.

These principles were embodied in a public health law submitted to the Berlin Society of Physicians and Surgeons in 1849 (Rosen, 2015). According to this document, public health has as its objectives (1) the healthy mental and physical development of the citizen, (2) the prevention of all dangers to health, and (3) the control of disease.

A very critical event in the development of modern public health occurred in 1854, when an English physician, anesthetist, and epidemiologist named John Snow demonstrated that cholera was transmissible through contaminated water. In a large population afflicted with cholera, he shut down the community's water resource by removing the pump handle from a well on Broad Street and carefully documented changes as the number of cholera cases fell dramatically (Rosen, 2015).

United States. In the United States during the nineteenth century, waves of epidemics continued to spread. As in Europe, diseases such as yellow fever, smallpox, cholera, typhoid fever, and typhus particularly affected the poor. These illnesses spread because cities grew and the poor crowded into inadequate housing with unsanitary conditions.

Lemuel Shattuck, a Boston bookseller and publisher with an interest in public health, organized the American Statistical Society in 1839 and issued a *Census of Boston* in 1845. The census showed high overall mortality and very high infant and maternal mortality rates. Living conditions for the poor were inadequate, and communicable diseases were widely prevalent (Rosen, 2015). Shattuck's 1850 *Report of the Sanitary Commission of Massachusetts* outlined the findings and recommended modern public health reforms that included keeping vital statistics and providing environmental, food, drug, and communicable disease control information. Shattuck called for well-infant, well-child, and school-aged–child health care; mental health care; vaccination; and health education. Unfortunately, the report fell on deaf ears, and little was done to improve population health for many years. For example, a state board of health was not formed until 19 years after the report was issued.

ADVENT OF MODERN HEALTH CARE

Early public health efforts evolved slowly throughout the mid-nineteenth century. Administrative efforts, initial legislation, and debate regarding the determinants of health and approaches to health management began to appear on a social, economic, and medical level. The advent of "modern" health care occurred around this time, and nursing made a large contribution to the progress of health care. The following sections discuss the evolution of modern nursing, the evolution of modern medical care and public health practice, the evolution of the community caregiver, and the establishment of public health nursing.

Evolution of Modern Nursing

Florence Nightingale, the woman credited with establishing "modern nursing," began her work during the mid-nineteenth century. Historians remember Florence Nightingale for contributing to the health of British soldiers during the Crimean War and establishing nursing education. However, many historians failed to recognize her remarkable use of public health principles and distinguished scientific contributions to health care reform (Cohen, 1984; Grier and Grier, 1978).

Nightingale was from a wealthy English family, was well educated, and traveled extensively. She studied with Adolphe Quetelet, a Belgian statistician who taught her the discipline of social inquiry (Goodnow, 1933). Nightingale also had a passion for hygiene and health, and in 1851, at the age of 31 years, she trained in nursing at Kaiserswerth Hospital in Germany. She later studied the organization and discipline of the Sisters of Charity in Paris. Nightingale wrote extensively and published analyses of the nursing systems she studied in France, Austria, Italy, and Germany (Dock and Stewart, 1925).

In 1854, Nightingale responded to distressing accounts of a lack of care for wounded soldiers during the Crimean War. She and 40 other nurses traveled to Scutari, which was then a part of the Ottoman Empire. Nightingale was accompanied by lay nurses, Roman Catholic sisters, and Anglican sisters. Upon their arrival, the nurses learned that the British army's methods for treating the sick and wounded had created conditions that resulted in extraordinarily high death rates among soldiers. Indeed, one of Nightingale's greatest achievements was improving the management of these ill and wounded soldiers (Dossey, 2010).

During the Crimean War, cholera and "contagious fever" were rampant. Equal numbers of men died of disease and battlefield injury (Cohen, 1984). Nightingale found that allocated supplies were bound in bureaucratic red tape; for example, supplies were "sent to the wrong ports or were buried under munitions and could not be got" (Goodnow, 1933, p. 86).

Nightingale encountered problems reforming the army's methods for care of the sick because she had to work through eight military affairs departments related to her assignment. She sent reports of the appalling conditions of the hospitals to London. In response to her actions, governmental and private funds were donated to set up kitchens and a laundry and provided food, clothing, dressings, and laboratory equipment (Dock and Stewart, 1925).

Major reforms occurred during the first two months of her assignment. Aware that an interest in keeping social statistics was emerging, Nightingale realized that her most forceful argument would be statistical in nature. She reorganized the methods of keeping statistics and was the first to use shaded and colored coxcomb graphs of wedges, circles, and squares to illustrate the preventable deaths of soldiers. Nightingale compared the deaths of soldiers in hospitals during the Crimean War with the average annual mortality in Manchester and with the deaths of soldiers in military hospitals in and near London at the time (Fig. 2.2). Through her statistics she also showed that, by the end of the war, the death rate among ill soldiers during the Crimean War was no higher than that among well soldiers in Britain (Cohen, 1984). Indeed, Nightingale's careful statistics revealed that the death rate for treated soldiers decreased from 42% to 2%. Furthermore, she established community services and activities to improve the quality of life for recovering soldiers. These included rest and recreation facilities, study opportunities, a savings fund, and a post office. She also organized care for the families of the soldiers (Dock and Stewart, 1925).

After returning to London at the close of the war in 1856, Nightingale devoted her efforts to sanitary reform. At home, she surmised that if the sanitary neglect of the soldiers existed in the battle area, it probably existed at home in London. She prepared statistical tables to support her suspicions (Table 2.2).

In one study comparing the mortality of men aged 25 to 35 years in the army barracks of England with that of men the same age in civilian life, Nightingale found that the mortality of the soldiers was nearly twice that of the civilians. In one of her reports, she stated that "our soldiers enlist to death in the barracks" (Kopf, 1978, p. 95). Nightingale was very political and distributed her reports to members of Parliament and to the medical and commanding officers of the army (Kopf, 1978). Prominent leaders of the time challenged her reports. Undaunted, she rewrote them in greater depth and redistributed them.

In her efforts to compare the hospital systems in European countries, Nightingale discovered that each hospital kept incomparable data and that many hospitals used various names and classifications for diseases. She noted that these differences prevented the collection of similar statistics from larger geographic areas. These statistics would create a regional health–illness profile and allow for comparison with other regions. She printed common statistical forms that some hospitals in London adopted on an experimental basis. A study of the tabulated results revealed the promise of this strategy (Kopf, 1978) (Box 2.4).

Nightingale also stressed the need to use statistics at the administrative and political levels to direct health policy. Noting

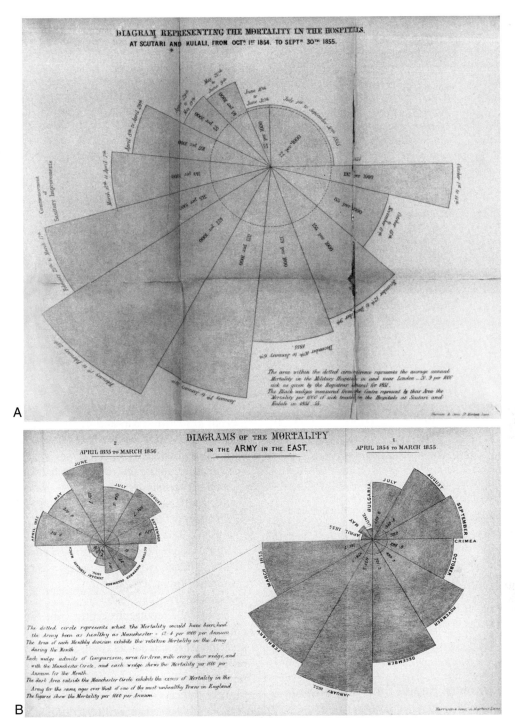

FIG. 2.2 (A) Coxcomb charts by Florence Nightingale. **(B)** Photographs of large, foldout charts from an original preserved at the University of Chicago Library. (**A** from Nightingale F: *Notes on matters affecting the health, efficiency and hospitalization of the British army,* London, 1858, Harrison and Sons; **B,** Public domain; courtesy University of Chicago Library.)

the ignorance of politicians and those who set policy regarding the interpretation and use of statistics, she emphasized the need to teach national leaders to use statistical facts. Nightingale continued the development and application of statistical procedures, and she won recognition for her efforts. The Royal Statistical Society made her a fellow in 1858, and the American Statistical Association made her an honorary member in 1874 (Kopf, 1978).

It is interesting to note that the paradigm for nursing practice and nursing education that evolved through Nightingale's work did not incorporate her emphasis on statistics and a sound research base. It is also curious that nursing education did not consult her writings and did not stress the importance of determining health's social and environmental determinants until much later.

TABLE 2.2 Nightingale's Crimean War Mortality Statistics: Nursing Research That Made a Difference*

Year	Deaths That Would Have Occurred in Healthy Districts Among Males of the Soldiers' Age†	Actual Deaths of Noncommissioned Officers and Men	Excess of Deaths Among Noncommissioned Officers and Men
1839	763	2914	2151
1840	829	3300	2471
1841	857	4167	3310
1842	888	5052	4164
1843	914	5270	4356
1844	920	3867	2947
1845	911	4587	3676
1846	930	5125	4195
1847	981	4232	3251
1848	987	3213	2226
1849	954	4052	3098
1850	919	3119	2200
1851	901	2729	1828
1852	915	3120	2205
1853	920	3392	2472
Total	13,589	58,139	44,550

*Number of deaths of noncommissioned officers and men also shows the number of deaths that would have occurred if the mortality were 7.7 per 1000—such as it was among Englishmen of the soldiers' age in healthy districts, in the years 1849 to 1853—which fairly represent the average mortality.
†The exact mortality in the healthy districts is 0.0077122, with use of the logarithm of 3.8871801.
From Grier B, Grier M: Contributions of the passionate statistician, *Res Nurs Health* 1:103–109, 1978. Copyright ©1978 by John Wiley & Sons, Inc. Reprinted by permission of John Wiley & Sons, Inc.

? ACTIVE LEARNING EXERCISE

Find two recent articles about Florence Nightingale. After reading the articles, list Nightingale's contributions to public health, public health nursing, and community health nursing.

Establishment of Modern Health Care and Public Health Practice

To place Nightingale's work in perspective, it is necessary to consider the development of health care in light of common education and practice during the late nineteenth and early twentieth centuries. Goodnow (1933) called this time a "dark age." Health sciences were underdeveloped, and bacteriology was unknown. Few medical schools existed at the time, thus apprenticeship was the path to medical education. The majority of physicians believed in the "spontaneous generation" theory of disease causation, which stated that disease organisms grew from nothing (Najman, 1990). Typical medical treatment included bloodletting, starving, using leeches, and prescribing large doses of metals such as mercury and antimony (Goodnow, 1933).

BOX 2.4 Nightingale's Use of Statistical Methods in Community Assessment

London's Southeastern Railway planned to remove St. Thomas' Hospital to enlarge the railway's right of way between London Bridge and Charing Cross. Nightingale applied her statistical method to the health needs of the community by conducting a community assessment. She plotted the cases served by the hospital, analyzed the proportion by distance, and calculated the probable impact on the community if the hospital were relocated to the proposed site. In her view, hospitals were a part of the wider community that served the needs of humanity. Kopf (1978) noted that this method of health planning and matching resources to the needs of the population was visionary and was not reapplied until the twentieth century.

Nightingale's uniform classification of hospital statistics focused on the importance of tabulating the classification of diseases in hospital patients and the need to identify the diseases that patients contracted in the hospital. These diseases, such as gangrene and septicemia, were later called *iatrogenic* diseases (Kopf, 1978). Considering the lack of surgical sanitation in hospitals at the time, it is not surprising that iatrogenic infection was rampant. For example, Goodnow (1933) illustrates the following unsanitary operating procedures:

Before an operation the surgeon turned up the sleeves of his coat to save the coat, and would often not trouble to wash his hands, knowing how soiled they soon would be! The area of the operation would sometimes be washed with soap and water, but not always, for the inevitability of corruption made it seem useless. The silk or thread used for stitches or ligatures was hung over a button of the surgeon's coat, and during the operation a convenient place for the knife to rest was between his lips. Instruments ... used for ... lancing abscesses were kept in the vest pocket and often only wiped with a piece of rag as the surgeon went from one patient to another. (pp. 471–472)

During the nineteenth century, the following important scientists were born: **Louis Pasteur** in 1822, **Joseph Lister** in 1827, and **Robert Koch** in 1843. Their research had a profound impact on health care, medicine, and nursing. Pasteur was a chemist, not a physician. While experimenting with wine production in 1854, he proposed the theory of the existence of "germs." Although his colleagues ridiculed him at first, Koch applied his theories and developed his methods for handling and studying bacteria. Subsequently, Pasteur's colleagues gave him acknowledgment for his work (Kalisch and Kalisch, 2004).

Lister, whose father perfected the microscope, observed the healing processes of fractures. He noted that when the bone was broken but the skin was not, recovery was uneventful. However, when both the bone and the skin were broken, fever, infection, and even death were frequent. He postulated the answer to his observation from Pasteur's work and suggested that something outside the body entered the wound through the broken skin, causing the infection (Goodnow, 1933). Lister's surgical successes eventually improved when he soaked the dressings and instruments in mixtures of carbolic acid (i.e., phenol) and oil.

In 1882, Koch discovered the causative agent for cholera and the tubercle bacillus. Pasteur discovered immunization in 1881 and the rabies vaccine in 1885. These discoveries were significant to the development of public health and medicine. However, physicians accepted these discoveries slowly (Rosen, 2015). For example, TB was a major cause of death in late nineteenth-century America and often afflicted its victims with chronic illness and disability. It was a highly stigmatized disease, and most physicians thought it was a hereditary, constitutional disease associated with poor environmental conditions. Hospitalization for TB was rare because the stigma caused families to hide their infected relatives. Without treatment, the communicability of the disease increased. The most common treatment was a change of climate (Rosen, 2015). Although Koch had announced the discovery of the tubercle bacillus in 1882, it was 10 years before the emergence of the first organized community campaign to stop the spread of the disease.

The case of puerperal (i.e., childbirth) fever illustrates another example of slow innovation stemming from scientific discoveries. Although Pasteur showed that *Streptococcus* caused puerperal fever, it was years before physicians accepted his discovery. However, medical practice eventually changed, and physicians no longer delivered infants after performing autopsies of puerperal fever cases without washing their hands (Goodnow, 1933).

Debates over the causes of disease occurred throughout the nineteenth century. Scientists discovered organisms during the latter part of the century, supporting the theory that specific contagious entities caused disease. This discovery challenged the earlier miasmic theory that environment and atmospheric conditions caused disease (Greifinger and Sidel, 1981). The new scientific discoveries had a major impact on the development of public health and medical practice. The emergence of the germ theory of disease focused diagnosis and treatment on the individual organism and the individual disease.

State and local governments felt increasingly responsible for controlling the spread of microorganisms. A community outcry for social reform forced state and local governments to take notice of the deplorable living conditions in the cities. In the New York City riots of 1863, the populace expressed their disgust for overcrowding; filthy streets; lack of provisions for the poor; and lack of adequate food, water, and housing. Local boards of health formed, taking responsibility for safeguarding food and water stores and managing the sewage and quarantine operation for victims of contagious diseases (Greifinger and Sidel, 1981).

The New York Metropolitan Board of Health formed in 1866, and state health departments formed shortly thereafter. States built large public hospitals that treated TB and mental disease with rest, diet, and quarantine. In 1889, the New York City Health Department recommended the surveillance of TB and TB health education, but physicians did not welcome either recommendation (Rosen, 2015). Despite their objections, in 1894 the New York City Health Department required institutions to report cases of TB and required physicians to do the same by 1897.

BOX 2.5   Scientific Theory/Single-Agent Theory

The emphasis on the use of scientific theory, or single-agent theory, in medical care developed into a focus on disease and symptoms rather than a focus on the prevention of disability and care for the "whole person." The old-fashioned family doctor viewed patients in relation to their families and communities and apparently helped people cope with problems in personal life, family, and society. American medicine adopted science with such vigor that these qualities faded away. Science allowed the physician to deal with tissues and organs, which were much easier to comprehend than the dynamics of human relationships or the complexities of disease prevention. Many physicians made efforts to integrate the various roles, but society was pushing toward academic science.

In 1883, The Johns Hopkins University Medical School in Baltimore, Maryland, formed under the German model that promoted medical education on the principles of scientific discovery. In the United States, the Carnegie Commission appointed Abraham Flexner to evaluate medical schools throughout the country on the basis of the German model. In 1910, the Flexner Report outlined the shortcomings of U.S. medical schools that did not use this model. Within a few years, the report caused philanthropic organizations such as the Rockefeller and Carnegie foundations to withdraw funding of poor-performing and scientifically "inadequate" medical schools, ensuring their closure. A "new breed" of physicians emerged who had been taught about "germ theory" and the "single agent theory" of disease causation (Greifinger and Sidel, 1981, p. 132) (Box 2.5).

Philanthropic foundations continued to influence health care efforts. For example, the Rockefeller Sanitary Commission for the Eradication of Hookworm formed in 1909. Hookworm was an occupational hazard among Southern workers. Implementation of preventive efforts to eradicate hookworm kept the workers healthy and thus proved to be a great industrial benefit. The model was so successful that the Rockefeller Foundation established the first school of public health, The Johns Hopkins School of Hygiene and Public Health, in 1916. The focus of this institution was the preservation and improvement of individual and community health and the prevention of disease through multidisciplinary activities.

Community Caregiver

The traditional role of the community caregiver or the traditional healer has nearly vanished in the West. However, medical and nurse anthropologists who have studied primitive and Western cultures are familiar with the community healer and caregiver role (McFarland and Wehbe-Alamah, 2015). The traditional healer (e.g., shaman, midwife, herbalist, or priest) is common in non-Western, ancient, and underdeveloped societies. Although traditional healers have always existed, professionals and many people throughout industrialized societies may overlook or minimize their role. The role of the healer is often integrated into other institutions of society, including religion, medicine, and morality. The notion that one person acts alone in healing may be foreign to many cultures; healers can be individuals, kin, or entire societies (Hughes, 1978).

Societies retain folk practices because they provide some repeated successes. Most cultures have a pharmacopeia and maintain therapeutic and preventive practices, and it is estimated that one-fourth to one-half of folk medicines are empirically effective. Indeed, many modern drugs are based on the medicines of primitive cultures (e.g., eucalyptus, coca, and opium) (Hughes, 1978).

Since ancient times, folk healers and cultural practices have both positively and negatively affected health. The late nineteenth- and early twentieth-century practice of midwifery illustrates modern medicine's arguably sometimes negative impact on traditional healing in many Western cultures (Smith, 1979). For example, traditional midwifery practices made women rise out of bed within 24 hours of delivery to help "clear" the lochia. Throughout the mid-1900s, in contrast, "modern medicine" recommended keeping women in bed after delivery, often for fairly extended periods (Smith, 1979).

🔍 RESEARCH HIGHLIGHTS

Historical Methodology for Nursing Research

Historiography is the methodology of historical research. It involves specialized techniques, principles, and theories that pertain to historical matters. *Historical research* involves interpreting history and contributing to understanding through data synthesis. It relies on existing sources or data and requires the researcher to gain access to sources such as libraries, librarians, and databases.

Historical research should be descriptive. It should answer the questions of who, what, when, where, how, and the interpretive why. Historians reconstruct an era using primary sources and interpret the story from that perspective. Historical research in nursing will enhance the understanding of current nursing practice and will help prepare for the future.

Adapted from Lusk B: Historical methodology for nursing research, *Image J Nurs Sch* 29:3555–3560, 1997.

Establishment of Public Health Nursing

Public health nursing as a holistic approach to health care developed in the late nineteenth and early twentieth centuries. Public and community health nursing in its current form evolved from home nursing practice, community organizations, and political interventions on behalf of families, groups, and populations as explained in this section.

England

Public health nursing developed from providing nursing care to the sick poor and furnishing information and through channels of community organization that enabled the poor to improve their own health status.

District Nursing. **District nursing** was first established in England. Between 1854 and 1856, the Epidemiological Society of London developed a plan that trained selected poor women to provide nursing care to the disadvantaged families within a community. The society theorized that nurses belonging to their patients' social class would be more effective caregivers and that more nurses would be available to improve the health of community residents (Rosen, 2015).

A similar plan was implemented by William Rathbone in Liverpool in 1859. After experiencing the excellent care a nurse gave his sick wife in his home, Rathbone strongly believed that nurses could offer the same care throughout the community. He developed a plan that divided the community into 18 districts and assigned a nurse and a social worker to each district. This team met the needs of their communities with respect to nursing, social work, and health education. The community widely accepted the plan. To further strengthen it, Rathbone consulted Nightingale about educating the district nurses. She assisted him by providing training for the district nurses, referring to them as "health nurses." The model was successful, and eventually voluntary agencies adopted the plan on the national level (Rosen, 2015).

Health Visiting. **Health visiting** to provide information to improve health is a parallel service based on the district nursing tradition. The Ladies Section of the Manchester and Salford Sanitary Association originated health visiting in Manchester in 1862. Prior to that time, it had been observed that providing health pamphlets alone had little effect on improving health; therefore this service enlisted home visitors to distribute health information to the poor.

In 1893, Nightingale pointed out that the district nurse should be a health teacher and a nurse for the sick in the home. She believed that teachers should educate "health missioners" for this purpose. The model charged the district nurse with providing care for the sick in the home and the health visitor with providing health information in the home. Eventually, government agencies sponsored health visitors, medical health officers supervised them, and the municipality paid them. Thus a collaborative model developed between government and voluntary agencies.

United States

In the United States, public health nursing developed from the British traditions of district nursing, health visiting, and home nursing. In 1877, the Women's Board of the New York City Mission sent a graduate nurse named Frances Root into homes to provide care for the sick. The innovation spread, and nursing associations, later called *visiting nurse associations,* were implemented in Buffalo in 1885 and in Boston and Philadelphia in 1886.

In 1893, nurses **Lillian Wald** and Mary Brewster established a district nursing service on the Lower East Side of New York City called the **House on Henry Street.** This was a crowded area teeming with unemployed and homeless immigrants who needed health care. The organization, later called the Visiting Nurse Association of New York City, played an important role in establishing public health nursing in the United States. Box 2.6 contains Wald's compelling account of her early exposure to the community where she identified public health nursing needs.

Wald (1971) described a range of services that evolved from the House on Henry Street. Nurses provided home visits, and patients paid carfare or a cursory fee. Physicians were consultants to Henry Street, and families could arrange a visit by calling the nurse directly, or a physician could call the nurse on the family's behalf. The nursing service adopted the philosophy of

BOX 2.6 Lillian Wald: The House On Henry Street

The following highlights from *The House on Henry Street*, published in 1915, bring Lillian Wald's experience to life:

A sick woman in a squalid rear tenement, so wretched and so pitiful that, in all the years since, I have not seen anything more appalling, determined me, within half an hour, to live on the East Side.

I had spent two years in a New York training-school for nurses . . . After graduation, I supplemented the theoretical instruction, which was casual and inconsequential in the hospital classes twenty-five years ago, by a period of study at a medical college. It was while at the college that a great opportunity came to me.

While there, the long hours "on duty" and the exhausting demands of the ward work scarcely admitted freedom for keeping informed as to what was happening in the world outside. The nurses had no time for general reading; visits to and from friends were brief; we were out of the current and saw little of life saved as it flowed into the hospital wards. It is not strange, therefore, that I should have been ignorant of the various movements which reflected the awakening of the social conscience at the time.

Remembering the families who came to visit patients in the wards, I outlined a course of instruction in home nursing adapted to their needs, and gave it in an old building in Henry Street, then used as a technical school and now part of the settlement. Henry Street then as now was the center of a dense industrial population.

From the schoolroom where I had been giving a lesson in bedmaking, a little girl led me one drizzling March morning. She had told me of her sick mother, and gathering from her incoherent account that a child had been born, I caught up the paraphernalia of the bedmaking lesson and carried it with me.

The child led me over broken roadways—there was no asphalt, although its use was well established in other parts of the city—over dirty mattresses and heaps of refuse—it was before Colonel Waring had shown the possibility of clean streets even in that quarter—between tall, reeking houses whose laden fire-escapes, useless for their appointed purpose, bulged with household goods of every description. The rain added to the dismal appearance of the streets and to the discomfort of the crowds which thronged them, intensifying the odors which assailed me from every side. Through Hester and Division Street[s] we went to the end of Ludlow; past odorous fishstands, for the streets were a market-place, unregulated, unsupervised, unclean; past evil-smelling, uncovered garbage-cans; and—perhaps worst of all, where so many little children played—past the trucks brought down from more fastidious quarters and stalled on these already overcrowded streets, lending themselves inevitably to many forms of indecency.

The child led me on through a tenement hallway, across a court where open and unscreened closets were promiscuously used by men and women, up into a rear tenement, by slimy steps whose accumulated dirt was augmented that day by the mud of the streets, and finally into the sickroom.

All the maladjustments of our social and economic relations seemed epitomized in this brief journey and what was found at the end of it. The family to which the child led me was neither criminal nor vicious. Although the husband was a cripple, one of those who stand on street corners exhibiting deformities to enlist compassion, and masking the begging of alms by a pretense at selling; although the family of seven shared their two rooms with boarders—who were literally boarders, since a piece of timber was placed over the floor for them to sleep on— and although the sick woman lay on a wretched, unclean bed, soiled with a hemorrhage two days old, they were not degraded human beings, judged by any measure of moral values.

In fact, it was very plain that they were sensitive to their condition, and when, at the end of my ministrations, they kissed my hands (those who have undergone similar experiences will, I am sure, understand), it would have been some solace if by any conviction of the moral unworthiness of the family I could have defended myself as a part of a society which permitted such conditions to exist. Indeed, my subsequent acquaintance with them revealed the fact that, miserable as their state was, they were not without ideals for the family life, and for society, of which they were so unloved and unlovely a part.

That morning's experience was a baptism of fire. Deserted were the laboratory and the academic work of the college. I never returned to them. On my way from the sickroom to my comfortable student quarters my mind was intent on my own responsibility. To my inexperience it seemed certain that conditions such as these were allowed because people did not know, and for me there was a challenge to know and to tell. When early morning found me still awake, my naive conviction remained that, if people knew things—and "things" meant everything implied in the condition of this family—such horrors would cease to exist, and I rejoiced that I had had a training in the care of the sick that in itself would give me an organic relationship to the neighborhood in which this awakening had come.

To the first sympathetic friend to whom I poured forth my story, I found myself presenting a plan which had been developing almost without conscious mental direction on my part.

Within a day or two a comrade from the training-school, Mary Brewster, agreed to share in the venture. We were to live in the neighborhood as nurses, identify ourselves with it socially, and, in brief, contribute to it our citizenship.

I should like to make it clear that from the beginning we were most profoundly moved by the wretched industrial conditions which were constantly forced upon us . . . I hope to tell of the constructive programmes that the people themselves have evolved out of their own hard lives, of the ameliorative measures, ripened out of sympathetic comprehension, and finally, of the social legislation that expresses the new compunction of the community.

From Wald L: *The house on Henry Street*, New York, 1971, Dover Publications (original work published 1915, Henry Holt), pp 1–9.

meeting the health needs of the population, which included the many evident social, economic, and environmental determinants of health. By necessity, this effort involved an aggregate approach that empowered people of the community.

Helen Hall, who later directed the House on Henry Street, wrote that the settlement's role was "one of helping people to help themselves" (Wald, 1971) through the development of centers of social action aimed at meeting the needs of the community and the individual. Community organization led to the formation of a great variety of programs, including youth clubs,

a juvenile program, sex education for local schoolteachers, and support programs for immigrants.

Additional programs such as school nursing were based on individual observations and interventions. Wald reported the following incident that preceded her successful trial of school nursing (1971):

I had been downtown only a short time when I met Louis. An open door in a rear tenement revealed a woman standing over a washtub, a fretting baby on her left arm, while with her right she rubbed at the butcher's aprons which she washed for a living.

"Louis," she explained, *"was bad."* He did not *"cure his head of lice and what would become of him, for they would not take him into the school because of it?"* Louis said he had been to the dispensary many times. He knew it was awful for a twelve-year-old boy not to know how to read the names of the streets on the lamp-posts, but *"every time I go to school Teacher tells me to go home."*

It needed only intelligent application of the dispensary ointments to cure the affected area, and in September, I had the joy of securing the boy's admittance to school for the first time in his life. The next day, at the noon recess, he fairly rushed up our five flights of stairs in the Jefferson Street tenement to spell the elementary words he had acquired that morning. (pp. 46–47)

Overcrowded schools, an uninformed and uninterested public, and an unaware Department of Health all contributed to social health neglect. Wald and the nursing staff at the settlement kept anecdotal notes on the sick children teachers excluded from school. One nurse found a boy in school whose skin was desquamating from scarlet fever and took him to the president of the Department of Health in an attempt to place physicians in schools. A later program had physicians screen children in school for 1 hour each day.

Twentieth Century. In 1902, Wald persuaded Dr. Ernest J. Lederle, Commissioner of Health in New York City, to try a school nursing experiment. Henry Street lent a public health nurse named Linda Rogers to the New York City Health Department to work in a school (Dock and Stewart, 1925). The experiment was successful, and schools adopted nursing on a widespread basis. School nurses performed physical assessments, treated minor infections, and taught health to pupils and parents.

In 1909, Wald mentioned the efficacy of home nursing to one of the officials of the Metropolitan Life Insurance Company. The company decided to provide home nursing to its industrial policyholders, and soon the United States and Canada used the program successfully (Wald, 1971).

The growing demand for public health nursing was hard to satisfy. In 1910, the Department of Nursing and Health formed at the Teachers College of Columbia University in New York City. A course in visiting nursing placed nurses at the Henry Street settlement for fieldwork. In 1912, the newly formed National Organization for Public Health Nursing elected Lillian Wald its first president. This organization was open to public health nurses and to those interested in public health nursing. In 1913, the Los Angeles Department of Health formed the first Bureau of Public Health Nursing (Rosen, 2015). That same year, the Public Health Service appointed its first public health nurse.

RESEARCH HIGHLIGHTS

Example of Historical Nursing Research

Thompson and Keeling (2012) presented an historical examination describing how public health nurses contributed to a significant decline in infant mortality in New England between 1884 and 1925. Analyzing archived data and documents from Providence, Rhode Island, they estimated that in the late nineteenth century, the mortality rate of children younger than 2 was between 15% and 20%. Furthermore, they reported that the health officials believed that of those infants and small children who died during those years, 40% to 50% died from digestive-related diseases (e.g., diarrhea).

The germ theory was not widely accepted until the early 1900s. Thus, in the late nineteenth century, nurses were trained to understand "elements of modern hygiene" (e.g., good nutrition, light, cleanliness). But following acceptance of the germ theory and epidemiological techniques for data analysis in the early 1900s, public health efforts shifted to consideration of factors, including biological, environmental, and economic, that contributed to the high infant mortality rate.

To address the problem of infant/child mortality, public health nurses focused on teaching low-income mothers how to care for and feed their children. The nurses worked in homes, "milk stations," and other creative settings to meet the identified needs. They set up and participated in "milk dispensaries," which provided pasteurized milk (rather than the widely available unrefrigerated milk—which was frequently days old). They also promoted breast-feeding and provided information on "infant hygiene" along with the milk. These and other efforts, including developing the role of a "children's special nurse," were effective, and the infant mortality rate dropped from 142/1000 to 102/1000 between 1907 and 1917.

From Thompson ME, Keeling AA: Nurses' role in the prevention of infant mortality in 1884–1925: health disparities then and now, *J Pediatr Nurs* 27:471–478, 2012.

At first, many public health nursing programs used nurses in specialized areas such as school nursing, TB nursing, maternal-child health nursing, and communicable disease nursing. In later years, more generalized programs have become acceptable. Efforts to contain health care costs include reducing the number of hospital days. With the advent of shortened hospital stays, private home health agencies provide home-based illness care across the United States.

The second half of the century saw a shift in emphasis to cost containment and the provision of health care services through managed care. Traditional models of public health nursing and visiting nursing from home health agencies became increasingly common over the next several decades, but waned toward the end of the century due to changes in health care financing.

� ACTIVE LEARNING EXERCISE

1. Research the history of the health department or visiting nurse association in a particular city or county.
2. Discuss with peers how Lillian Wald's approach to individual and community health care provides an understanding of how to facilitate the empowerment of aggregates in the community.

CONSEQUENCES FOR THE HEALTH OF POPULATIONS

An understanding of the consequences of the health care delivery system for population health is necessary to form conclusions about public health nursing from a historical perspective. Implications for the health of aggregates relate to new causes of mortality (i.e., *Hygeia*, or health promotion/care, vs. *Panacea*, or cure) and additional theories of disease causation.

Twenty-First Century

New Causes of Mortality

Since the middle of the twentieth century, the focus of disease in Western societies has changed from mostly infectious diseases to chronic diseases. Increased food production and better nutrition during the nineteenth and early twentieth centuries contributed to the decline in infectious disease–related deaths. Other factors were better sanitation through water purification, sewage disposal, improved food handling, and milk pasteurization. According to McKeown (2001) and Schneider (2017), the components of "modern" medicine, such as antibiotics and immunizations, had little effect on health until well into the twentieth century. Indeed, widespread vaccination programs began in the late 1950s, and antibiotics came into use after 1945.

The advent of chronic disease in Western populations puts selected groups at risk, and those groups need health education, screening, and programs to ensure occupational and environmental safety. Too often modern medicine still focuses on the single cause of disease (i.e., germ theory) and treating the acutely ill. As a result, many health providers treat the chronically ill with an acute care approach even though preventive care, health promotion, and restorative care are necessary and would likely be more effective in combating chronic disease. This expanded approach may develop under new systems of cost containment.

Hygeia versus Panacea

The Grecian Hygeia (i.e., healthful living) versus Panacea (i.e., cure) dichotomy still exists today. Although the change in the nature of health "problems" is certain, the roles of individual and collective activities in the prevention of illness and premature death are slow to evolve.

In 2010, about two thirds of the active physicians in the United States were specialists (U.S. Department of Health and Human Services, Agency for Healthcare Research and Quality [USDHHS/AHRQ], 2011). In recent years, medical education has increasingly focused on enhancing the education of primary care physicians (e.g., those specializing in internal medicine, obstetrics-gynecology, family medicine, and pediatrics) to meet the growing need for primary care. In addition to primary care, Hygeia (health promotion) requires a coordinated system that addresses health problems holistically with the use of multiple approaches and planning of outcomes for aggregates and populations. A redistribution of interest and resources to address the major determinants of health, such as food, housing, education, and a healthy social and physical environment, is critical (Shi and Singh, 2016).

Additional Theories of Disease Causation

As mentioned, the germ theory of disease causation is a unicausal model that evolved in the late nineteenth century. Najman (1990) reviewed the following theories of disease causation: the multicausal view, which considers the environment multidimensionally, and the general susceptibility view, which considers stress and lifestyle factors. Najman contended that each theory accounts for some disease under some conditions, but no single theory accounts for all disease. Other factors, such as literacy and nutrition, may reduce disease morbidity and mortality to a greater extent than medical interventions alone.

SOCIAL CHALLENGES AND PUBLIC HEALTH NURSING

Several social and political changes have occurred in the United States that have affected the development of public health nursing practice. During the twentieth century, the health of the client, nursing, health, and the environment were influenced by the development of health insurance and an emphasis on population-based focus.

The advent of and changes in health insurance dramatically altered health care delivery. The greatest health concerns at the beginning of the twentieth century were lost wages associated with sickness. The cost of health care was so low that there was little understanding of the need for health insurance. Between 1900 and 1920 there were minimal technological advances. Treatments available at the time, including surgery, were often performed in private homes.

During the 1920s and 1930s, the costs of health care rose. As the population moved from rural to urban settings, the delivery points for much of health care changed, moving from private homes to hospitals. Improved therapeutic options, more medications, the acceptance of medicine as a science, and the closure of underperforming medical schools during the 1920s increased the demand for health care and raised the associated cost (Rosenberg, 1987).

As hospitals began to expand and organize, they formed the American Hospital Association, whose leaders encouraged the development of health insurance plans. In 1929, the Committee of the Costs of Medical Care, a national group, produced a report that promoted voluntary insurance in the United States. That same year, Baylor Hospital in Dallas, Texas, joined with a local teachers' association to provide health care for those agreeing to pay a small monthly premium. In a short time, this relationship grew to include more employers and evolved into Blue Cross (Getzen, 2013; Sparer and Thompson, 2015). Improvements in medical technology and the growing practice of employers' offering health insurance in place of employee compensation during and after World War II further supported the expansion of private health insurance.

During the 1960s, politicians supported the development of federal and state health insurance for the poor and the elderly populations, subsequently enacting Medicare and Medicaid. As a result, since the 1970s most health care has been paid for with either public or private insurance plans. As a result of "third-party" reimbursement, costs grew steadily as much of the public paid little attention to charges because they were not directly responsible for payment. Consequently, the growth in available treatments because of improving technological advances, chronic disease associated with an aging

BOX 2.7 Ten Great Public Health Achievements—United States, 1900–2010

During the twentieth century, the health and life expectancy of persons living in the United States improved dramatically. It is important for nurses to realize that of the 30 years of life expectancy gained during the century, 25 years were attributable to public health efforts. During 1999, the Centers for Disease Control and Prevention published a series of articles outlining 10 of the great public health achievements of the twentieth century. In 2011, the agency published an update of highlights from the ensuing decade. Summarized here are the "Public Health Achievements" presented:

Vaccination/vaccine-preventable diseases—Widespread vaccination programs resulted in eradication of smallpox; elimination of polio in the Americas; and control of measles, rubella, tetanus, diphtheria, and a number of other infectious diseases in the United States. In the first decade of the twenty-first century, new vaccines (e.g., rotavirus, herpes zoster, hepatitis A, and human papilloma virus) were introduced and are having a significant, positive impact on population health.

Motor vehicle safety—Improvements in motor vehicle safety contributed to large reductions in traffic deaths. Improvements included efforts to make both vehicles and highways safer and to change personal behaviors (e.g., increase use of seat belts and child safety seats, reduce driving under the influence [DUI] offenses). Between 2000 and 2009, the death rate from motor vehicle accidents continued to decline, largely as a result of safer vehicles, safer roads, safer road use, and related policies (e.g., graduated driver's licenses).

Safer workplaces—Work-related health problems (e.g., coal worker's pneumoconiosis [black lung] and silicosis) were very significantly reduced during the twentieth century, as were severe injuries and deaths related to mining, manufacturing, construction, and transportation. Following legislation in 1980, safer workplaces resulted in further reduction of 40% in the rate of fatal occupational injuries by the end of the century.

Control of infectious diseases—Since the early 1900s, control of infectious diseases has resulted from clean water and better sanitation. Cholera and typhoid were major causes of illness and death in the early twentieth century and have been virtually eliminated today. Additionally, the discovery of antimicrobial therapy has been very successful in helping efforts to control infections such as tuberculosis, sexually transmitted infections, and influenza. Much of the efforts in the last decade of the twentieth century and the first of the twenty-first century focused on prevention and treatment of human immunodeficiency virus/acquired immunodeficiency syndrome (HIV/AIDS). Prevention/education efforts, along with enhanced screening for HIV, early diagnosis, and effective treatment, have resulted in reduction in transmission of the virus, along with enabling access to lifesaving treatment and care for those who are HIV positive and their partners.

Decline in deaths from coronary heart disease (CHD) and stroke—Since 1972, the death rate for CHD has decreased 51%. This improvement is largely the result of risk factor modification (e.g., smoking cessation, blood pressure control) coupled with early detection and better treatment. In the last decade, CHD deaths continued to decline, going from 195/100,000 to 126/100,000. Contributing to the ongoing reduction are better control of hypertension, reduction in elevated cholesterol and smoking, and improvement in treatment and available medications.

Safer and healthier foods—Since 1900, reduction in microbial contamination and increases in nutritional content have led to safer and healthier foods. Food fortification programs and enhanced availability of nutritional options have almost eliminated major nutritional deficiency diseases in the United States.

Healthier mothers and babies—Since 1900, infant mortality in the United States has decreased 90% and maternal mortality has decreased 99%. These improvements are the result of better hygiene and nutrition, availability of antibiotics, access to better health care, and advances in maternal and neonatal medicine. During the early twenty-first century, there has been a significant reduction in the number of infants born with neural tube defects, a change attributable to mandatory folic acid fortification of cereal grain products.

Family planning—Access to family planning and contraceptives has provided women with better social and economic opportunities and health benefits, including smaller families and longer intervals between children.

Fluoridation of drinking water—Fluoridation of drinking water began in 1945, and by 1999 about half of all Americans had fluoridated water. This achievement positively and inexpensively benefited both children and adults by preventing tooth decay. Indeed, fluoridation has been credited for reducing tooth decay by 40% to 70% in children and tooth loss by 40% to 60% in adults.

Tobacco control—Recognition in 1964 that tobacco use is a health hazard resulted in behavior and policy changes that eventually led to a dramatic decline in the prevalence of smoking among adults. The rate of smoking peaked in the 1960s, and by 2009 only about 20% of adults and youths were current smokers. Health policy efforts (e.g., prohibition of smoking in worksites, restaurants, and bars), dramatic increases in cigarette taxes, and prohibition of selling to youths have contributed to much of the recent decline.

Data from Centers for Disease Control and Prevention: Ten great public health achievements—United States, 1900-1999, *MMWR Morb Mortal Wkly Rep* 48(12):241–243, 1999; and Centers for Disease Control and Prevention: Ten great public health achievements—United States, 2001–2010, *MMWR Morb Mortal Wkly Rep* 60(19):619–623, 2001.

population, and negative lifestyle choices and other factors led to a dramatic number of individuals and families who were not able to afford health care because they could not afford health insurance.

The Patient Protection and Affordable Care Act (ACA) was passed in 2010 to help reduce some of the problems associated with access to health care. After implementation, the number of uninsured dropped dramatically, but costs continued to increase and access was still problematic for some.

Changes to the ACA are anticipated, but problems with costs and access will likely persist. Indeed, considerable attention on current public health initiatives, such as the *Healthy People 2020* campaign and further health care reform, focus on ensuring elimination of disparities in health care. Box 2.7 provides a summary of some of the dramatic effects of public health activities on the health of Americans during the last 100 years. The photo novella in this chapter illustrates community health nursing in the early and mid-twentieth century.

Group Immunization. Multiracial group of women and children in a housing project mobile clinic waiting for and receiving vaccinations. Scene contains a doctor and a nurse. (1972). (Courtesy of the Centers for Disease Control and Prevention Public Health Image Library [PHIL] Image #1661. Source: CDC/ Reuel Waldrop.)

A public health nurse performs health teaching. (Courtesy of the Library of Congress, Washington, DC.)

A visiting nurse outside a shack with a mother and two children. (Courtesy of the U.S. National Library of Medicine, History of Medicine Division. Order No. A017986.)

A public health nurse talks to a young woman and her mother about childbirth. (Courtesy of the U.S. National Library of Medicine, History of Medicine Division. Order No. A029980.)

A public health nurse immunizes farm and migrant workers in the 1940s. (Courtesy of the Library of Congress, Washington, DC.)

The Shanghai Mother's Club of the Child Welfare and Maternal Health Clinic. United Nations Relief and Rehabilitation Administration (UNRRA) Public Health Nurse Irene Muir instructs Nurse S. U. Zee on child bathing techniques. (Courtesy of the U.S. National Library of Medicine, History of Medicine Division. Order No. A016681.)

A public health nurse transports children to a clinic. (Courtesy of MedStar Visiting Nurse Association.)

⬛ RESEARCH HIGHLIGHTS
Example of Historical Nursing Research

Fairman's (1996) review of 150 fictional novels from 1850 to 1995 revealed how the image of nursing has changed over the past 140 years. The results showed that the image of nursing improved dramatically from the negative perception of the 1850s. Trained nurses became more common in the early 1900s, and novels began to depict strong, independent, female nurses. The positive image continued until the 1960s and 1970s, when novels presented the negative image of "bed hopping honeys." Popular literature showed the most negative image of nurses, and classics and children's literature showed a more positive image.

Adapted from Fairman PL: *Analysis of the image of nursing and nurses as portrayed in fictional literature from 1850 to 1995*, San Francisco, CA, 1996, University of San Francisco Dissertation Abstracts.

❓ ACTIVE LEARNING EXERCISE

Obtain copies of early articles from nursing journals (e.g., *American Journal of Nursing* dates from 1900). Discuss the health problems, medical care, and nursing practice these articles illustrated.

Collect copies of early nursing textbooks. Discuss the evolution of thoughts on pathology, illness management, and health promotion.

CHALLENGES FOR PUBLIC HEALTH NURSING

Public health nurses face the challenge of promoting the health of populations. They must accomplish this goal with a broadened understanding of the multiple causes of morbidity and mortality. The specialization of medicine and nursing has affected the delivery of nursing and health care. Well-prepared nurses must be aware of the increased technological advances that specialization has contributed to. These advances have resulted in an increase in the number of advanced practice nurses in the past several decades. It is anticipated that this growth will persist and likely expand (IOM, 2011).

The community need for a focus on prevention, health promotion, and home care may become more widespread with the changing patterns of health care cost reimbursement. Holistic care requires multiple dimensions and must have more attention in the future.

The need for education in public health nursing calls for a curriculum that prepares students to meet the needs of aggregates through population-based strategies that include an understanding of statistical data and epidemiology. Such a curriculum would move the focus from the individual to a broader population approach. Strategies would promote literacy, nutrition programs, prevention of overweight school-aged children, decent housing and income, education, and safe social and physical environments.

Health care services to individuals alone cannot solve today's health problems. All health care workers must learn to work with and on behalf of aggregates and help them build a constituency for the consumer issues they face.

A population focus for nursing addresses the health of all in the population through the careful gathering of information and statistics. A population focus will better enable community health nurses to contribute to the ethic of social justice by emphasizing society's responsibility for health (Beauchamp, 1986). Helping aggregates help themselves will empower people and create avenues for addressing their concerns.

⬛ RESEARCH HIGHLIGHTS
Example of Historical Nursing Research

An in-depth examination of all of the issues from 115 years of the *American Journal of Nursing* was undertaken to "explore the nurse's historical and contemporary role in promoting patient safety" (Kowalski and Anthony, 2017, p. 34). A detailed content analysis of almost 1100 articles outlined the evolution of nursing's emphasis and interventions related to safety.

The authors described how the "safety" focus moved from asepsis and the "newly understood germ theory" in the early decades of the twentieth century to preventing medication errors in the 1930s. During and after World War II, improving patient survival rates was emphasized, and in the 1950s, attention moved to progressive patient care and various levels of care (intensive, intermediate, long-term, or home care). During the 1960s and 1970s, focus turned to the increasing complexity of care related to technology and enhanced medication regimens and the associated safety problems. Hospital-acquired infections and medication and nursing procedure safety were emphasized in the 1980s and 1990s. Since 2000, safety attention has moved to systematic factors such as communication, patient–nurse ratios, provider skill mix, and shift work.

The authors identified three major themes related to patient safety throughout the 115 years: infection prevention, medication safety, and technology response. They described the concurrent processes and procedures that were implemented to improve patient safety, but concluded that much more work is needed.

Kowalski SL, Anthony M: Nursing's evolving role in patient safety, *Am J Nurs* 117(2):34–50, 2017.

⬛ SUMMARY

Western civilization evolved from the Paleolithic period to the present, and people began to live in increasingly closer proximity to one another; therefore they experienced a change in the nature of their health problems.

In the mid-nineteenth and early twentieth centuries, public health efforts and the precursors of modern and public health nursing began to improve societal health. Nursing pioneers such as Nightingale in England and Wald in the United States focused on the collection and analysis of statistical data, health care reforms, home health nursing, community empowerment, and nursing education. They established the groundwork for today's public health nurses.

Modern public health nurses must recognize and try to understand the philosophical controversies that influence society and ultimately their practice. These controversies include different opinions about what "intervention" means—specifically in regard to "cure" vs. "care."

Controversy also surrounds the significance of maintaining a focus on individuals, families, groups, or populations. Finally, public health nurses need to understand social determinants of health and to be part of the solution with regard to coming up with ways to address persistent health problems while addressing the critical problem of escalating health care costs.

EVOLVE WEBSITE

http://evolve.elsevier.com/Nies/community
- NCLEX Review Questions
- Case Studies

BIBLIOGRAPHY

Armelagos GK, Dewey JR: Evolutionary response to human infectious diseases. In Logan MH, Hunt EE, editors: *Health and the human condition*, North Scituate, MA, 1978, Duxbury Press.

Beauchamp DE: Public health as social justice. In Mappes T, Zembaty J, editors: *Biomedical ethics*, ed 2, New York, 1986, McGraw-Hill.

Centers for Disease Control and Prevention: Epidemiology of human plague in the United States, 1900-2012, *Emerg Infect Dis* 21(1): 16–22, 2015. Available from https://wwwnc.cdc.gov/eid/article/21/1/pdfs/14-0564.pdf.

Centers for Disease Control and Prevention: Investigation of and response to 2 plagues cases, Yosemite National Park, California, USA, 2015, *Emerg Infect Dis* 22(12):2045–2053, 2016. Available from https://wwwnc.cdc.gov/eid/article/22/12/pdfs/16-0560.pdf.

Cockburn TA: The evolution of human infectious diseases. In Cockburn T, editor: *Infectious diseases: their evolution and eradication*, Springfield, IL, 1967, Charles C Thomas.

Cohen IB: Florence Nightingale, *Sci Am* 250:128–137, 1984.

Dock LL, Stewart IM: *A short history of nursing: from the earliest times to the present day*, New York, 1925, Putnam.

Donahue MP: *Nursing: the finest art*, ed 3, St. Louis, MO, 2011, Mosby/Elsevier.

Dossey BM: *Florence Nightingale: mystic, visionary, healer*, Philadelphia, 2010, F.A. Davis Co.

Duffus RL: *Lillian Wald: neighbor and crusader*, New York, 1938, Macmillan.

Fairman PL: *Analysis of the image of nursing and nurses as portrayed in fictional literature from 1850 to 1995*, Dissertation Abstracts, University of San Francisco, 1996.

Garn SM: Culture and the direction of human evolution, *Hum Biol* 35:221–236, 1963.

George MD: *London life in the XVIIIth century*, New York, 1925, Knopf.

Getzen T: *Health economics and financing*, ed 5, Hoboken, NJ, 2013, John Wiley & Sons.

Goodnow M: *Outlines of nursing history*, Philadelphia, 1933, WB Saunders.

Greifinger RB, Sidel VW: American medicine: charity begins at home. In Lee P, Brown N, Red I, editors: *The nation's health*, San Francisco, 1981, Boyd and Fraser.

Grier B, Grier M: Contributions of the passionate statistician, *Res Nurs Health* 1:103–109, 1978.

Hanlon JJ, Pickett GE: *Public health administration and practice*, ed 9, St. Louis, 1990, Mosby.

Hughes CC: Medical care: ethnomedicine. In Logan MH, Hunt EE, editors: *Health and the human condition*, North Scituate, MA, 1978, Duxbury Press.

Institue of Medicine (IOM): *The future of nursing*, Wasthington, DC, 2011, National Academies Press.

Kalisch PA, Kalisch BJ: *American nursing: a history*, ed 4, Philadelphia, 2004, Lippincott,Williams & Wilkins.

Kopf EW: Florence Nightingale as statistician, *Res Nurs Health* 1:93–102, 1978.

Kowalski SL, Anthony M: Nursing's evolving role in patient safety, *Am J Nurs* 117(2):34–50, 2017.

McFarland MR, Wehbe-Alamah HB: *Leininger's Culture care diversity and universality: a worldwide nursing theory*, ed 3, Burlington, MA, 2015, Jones & Bartlett.

McKeown T: Determinants of health. In Lee P, Estes CL, editors: *The nation's health*, ed 6, Boston, MA, 2001, Jones & Bartlett.

Najman JM: Theories of disease causation and the concept of a general susceptibility: a review, *Soc Sci Med* 14A:231–237, 1990.

Nightingale F: *Notes on matters affecting the health, efficiency and hospitalization of the British army*, London, 1858, Harrison and Sons.

Polgar S: Evolution and the ills of mankind. In Tax S, editor: *Horizons of anthropology*, Chicago, 1964, Aldine.

Richardson BW: *The health of nations: a review of the works of Edwin Chadwickl*, vol 2, London, 1887, Longmans.

Rosen G: *A history of public health,* revised expanded edition, Baltimore, MD, 2015, Johns Hopkins University Press.

Rosenberg CE: *The care of strangers*, New York, 1987, Basic Books.

Schneider MJ: *Introduction to public health*, ed 5, Burlington, MA, 2017, Jones & Bartlett.

Shi L, Singh DA: *Delivering health care in America: a systems approach*, ed 6, Boston, MA, 2016, Jones & Bartlett.

Smith FB: *The people's health 1830-1910*, London, 1979, Croom Helm.

Sparer MS, Thompson FJ: Government and health insurance. In Knickman JR, Kovner AR, editors: *Health care delivery in the United States*, ed 11, New York, 2015, Springer Publishing Co.

U.S. Department of Health and Human Services, Agency for Healthcare Research and Quality: *The number of practicing primary care physicians in the United States*, 201. Available from <http://www.ahrq.gov/research/findings/factsheets/pcwork1.html>.

Wald L: *The house on Henry Street*, New York, 1971, Dover Publications (original work published 1915, Henry Holt).

3

Thinking Upstream: Nursing Theories and Population-Focused Nursing Practice

Diane Cocozza Martins

OBJECTIVES

Upon completion of this chapter, the reader will be able to do the following:

1. Differentiate between upstream interventions, which are designed to alter the precursors of poor health, and downstream interventions, which are characterized by efforts to modify individuals' perceptions of health.

2. Describe different theories and their application to community/public health nursing.
3. Critique a theory with regard to its relevance to population health issues.
4. Explain how theory-based practice achieves the goals of community/public health nursing by protecting and promoting the public's health.

KEY TERMS

conservative scope of practice
critical interactionism
critical theoretical perspective
health belief model (HBM)

macroscopic focus
microscopic focus
Milio's framework for prevention
self-care deficit theory

theory
upstream thinking

It may seem as if many community health problems are so complex, so multifaceted, and so deep that it is impossible for a nurse to make substantial improvements in health. Although nurses see persons in whom cancer, cardiovascular disease, or pulmonary disease has just been diagnosed, we know that their diseases began years or even decades ago. In many cases, genetic risks for diseases are interwoven with social, economic, and environmental risks in ways that are difficult to understand and more difficult to change. In the face of all these challenges, how can nurses hope to affect the health of the public in a significant way? How can the actions nurses take today reduce the current burden of illness and prevent illness in the next generation of citizens?

When nurses work on a complex community health problem, they need to think strategically. They need to know where to focus their time, energy, and programmatic resources. Most

likely they will be up against health problems that have existed for years, with other layers of foundational problems that may have existed for generations. If nurses use organizational resources in an unfocused manner, they will not solve the problem at hand and may create new problems along the way. If nurses do not build strong relationships with community partners (e.g., parent groups, ministers, local activists), it will be difficult to succeed. If nurses are unable to advocate for their constituencies in a scientifically responsible, logical, and persuasive manner, they may fail. In the face of these challenges and many more, how can nurses succeed in their goal to improve public health?

Fortunately, there are road maps for success. Some of those road maps can be found by reading a nursing history book or an archival work that tells the story of a nurse who succeeded in improving health by leveraging diplomacy skills or neighborhood power, such as Lillian Wald. Other road maps may be found in "success stories" that provide an overview of how a nurse approached a problem, mobilized resources, and moved strategically to promote change. This chapter addresses another road map for success: the ability to think conceptually, almost like a chess player, to formulate a plan to solve complex problems. Thinking conceptually is a subtle skill that requires you to understand the world at an abstract level, seeing the manifestations of power, oppression, justice, and access as they exist within our communities. Most of all, thinking conceptually means that you develop a "critical eye" for the community and understand how change happens at micro and macro levels.

This chapter begins with a brief overview of nursing theory, which is followed by a discussion of the scope of community health nursing in addressing population health concerns. Several theoretical approaches are compared to demonstrate how different conceptualizations can lead to different conclusions about the range of interventions available to the nurse.

THINKING UPSTREAM: EXAMINING THE ROOT CAUSES OF POOR HEALTH

I am standing by the shore of a swiftly flowing river and hear the cry of a drowning man. I jump into the cold waters. I fight against the strong current and force my way to the struggling man. I hold on hard and gradually pull him to shore. I lay him out on the bank and revive him with artificial respiration. Just when he begins to breathe, I hear another cry for help. I jump into the cold waters. I fight against the strong current and swim forcefully to the struggling woman. I grab hold and gradually pull her to shore. I lift her out onto the bank beside the man and work to revive her with artificial respiration. Just when she begins to breathe, I hear another cry for help. I jump into the cold waters. Fighting again against the strong current, I force my way to the struggling man. I am getting tired, so with great effort I eventually pull him to shore. I lay him out on the bank and try to revive him with artificial respiration. Just when he begins to breathe, I hear another cry for help. Near exhaustion, it occurs to me that I'm so busy jumping in, pulling them to shore, applying artificial respiration that I have no time to see who is upstream pushing them all in . . .(Adapted from a story told by Irving Zola as cited in McKinlay, J.B. (2012). A case for refocusing upstream: The political economy of illness. In P. Conrad & V. Leiter (Eds.), The sociology of health and illness: Critical perspectives (Ch 47, 9th ed.), New York: Worth.)

In his description of the frustrations in medical practice, McKinlay (1979) used the image of a swiftly flowing river to represent illness. In this analogy, doctors are so busy rescuing victims from the river that they fail to look upstream to see who is pushing patients into the perilous waters. Many things could cause a patient to fall (or be pushed) into the waters of illness. Refocusing upstream requires nurses to look beyond individual behavior or characteristics to what McKinlay terms the "manufacturers of illness." McKinlay discusses factors such

as tobacco products companies, companies that profit from selling products high in saturated fats, the alcoholic beverage industry, the beauty industry, exposure to environmental toxins, and occupationally induced illnesses. "Manufacturers of illness" are what push clients into the river. Cigarette companies are a good example of manufacturers of illness—their product causes a change for the worse in the health status of their consumers, and they take little to no responsibility for it. McKinlay used this analogy to illustrate the ultimate futility of "downstream endeavors," which are characterized by short-term, individual-based interventions, and challenged health care providers to focus more of their energies "upstream, where the real problems lie" (McKinlay, 1979, p. 9). Downstream health care takes place in our emergency departments, critical care units, and many other health care settings focused on illness care. Upstream thinking actions focus on modifying economic, political, and environmental factors that are the precursors of poor health throughout the world. Although the story cites medical practice, it is equally fitting to the dilemmas of nursing practice. Nursing has a rich history of providing preventive and population-based care, but the current U.S. health system emphasizes episodic and individual-based care. Chronic diseases are responsible for 70% of American deaths each year and accounts for 86% of U.S. health care costs (Centers for Disease Control and Prevention, 2017)

HISTORICAL PERSPECTIVES ON NURSING THEORY

Many scholars agree that Florence Nightingale was the first nurse to formulate a conceptual foundation for nursing practice. Nightingale believed that clean water, clean linens, access to adequate sanitation, and quiet would improve health outcomes (Ali Parani, 2016). However, in the years after her leadership, nursing practice became less theoretical and was based primarily on reacting to the immediacy of patient situations and the demands of medical staff. Thus hospital and medical personnel defined the boundaries of nursing practice. Once nursing leaders saw that others were defining their profession, they became proactive in advancing the theoretical and scientific foundations of nursing practice. Some of the early nursing theories were extremely narrow and depicted health care situations that involved only one nurse and one patient. Family members and other health professionals were noticeably absent from the context of care. Historically, this characterization may have been an appropriate response to the constraints of nursing practice and the need to emphasize the medically dependent activities of the nursing profession.

Although somewhat valuable, theories that address health from a microscopic, or individual, rather than a macroscopic, or global/social, perspective have limited applicability to community/public health nursing. Such perspectives are inadequate because they do not address social, political, and environmental factors that are central to an understanding of communities. More recent advances in nursing theory development address the dynamic nature of health-sustaining and/or health-damaging environments and address the nature of a collective (e.g., school, worksite) versus an individual client.

HOW THEORY PROVIDES DIRECTION TO NURSING

The goal of **theory** is to improve nursing practice. Chinn and Kramer (2015) stated that using theories or parts of theoretical frameworks to guide practice best achieves this goal. Students often find theory intellectually burdensome and cannot see the benefits to their practice of something so seemingly obscure. Theory-based practice guides data collection and interpretation in a clear and organized manner; therefore it is easier for the nurse to diagnose and address health problems. Through the process of integrating theory and practice, the student can focus on factors that are critical to understanding the situation. The student also has an opportunity to analyze the realities of nursing practice in relation to a specific theoretical perspective, in a process of ruling in and ruling out the fit of particular concepts (Schwartz-Barcott et al., 2002). Barnum (1998) stated, "A theory is like a map of a territory as opposed to an aerial photograph. The map does not give the full terrain (i.e., the full picture); instead it picks out those parts that are important for its given purpose" (p. 1). Using a theoretical perspective to plan nursing care guides the student in assessing a nursing situation and allows the student "to plan and not get lost in the details or side-tracked in the alleys" (J. M. Swanson, personal communication to P. Butterfield, May 1992).

As with other abstract concepts, different nursing writers have defined and interpreted theory in different ways. Several writers' definitions of theory are listed in Box 3.1. The lack of uniformity among these definitions reflects the evolution of thought and the individual differences in the understanding of relationships among theory, practice, and research. The definitions also reflect the difficult job of describing complex and diverse theories within the constraints of a single definition. Reading several definitions can foster an appreciation for the richness of theory and help the reader identify one or two particularly meaningful definitions. Within the profession, definitions of theory typically refer to a set of concepts and relational statements and the purpose of the theory. This chapter presents theoretical perspectives that are congruent with a broad interpretation of theory and correspond with the definitions proposed by Dickoff and James (1968), Torres (1986), and Chinn and Kramer (2015).

MICROSCOPIC VERSUS MACROSCOPIC APPROACHES TO THE CONCEPTUALIZATION OF COMMUNITY HEALTH PROBLEMS

Each nurse must find her or his own way of interpreting the complex forces that shape societies to understand population health. The nurse can best achieve this transformation by integrating population-based practice and theoretical perspectives to conceptualize health from a macroscopic rather than microscopic perspective. Table 3.1 differentiates between these two approaches to conceptualizing health problems.

The individual patient is the **microscopic focus**, whereas society or social economic factors influencing health status are the **macroscopic focus**. When the individual is the focus, the micro focus contains the health problem of interest (e.g., pediatric exposure to lead compounds). In this context, a microscopic approach to assessment would focus exclusively on individual children with lead poisoning. Nursing interventions would focus on the identification and treatment of the child and family. However, the nurse can broaden his or her view of this problem by addressing removal of lead sources in the home and by examining interpersonal and intercommunity factors that perpetuate lead poisoning on a national scale. A macroscopic approach to lead exposure may incorporate the following activities: examining trends in the prevalence of lead poisoning over time, estimating the percentage of older homes in a neighborhood that may contain lead pipes or lead-based paint surfaces, and locating industrial sources of lead emissions. These efforts usually involve the collaborative efforts of nurses from school, occupational, government, and community settings. Burbank and Martins (2010) discussed macro-level perspectives that provide nurses with the conceptual tools that empower clients to make health decisions on the basis of the interests of the community at large.

One common dilemma in community health practice is the tension between working on behalf of individuals and working on behalf of a population. For many nurses, this tension is exemplified by the need to reconcile and prioritize multiple daily tasks. Population-directed actions are often more global than the immediate demands of ill people; therefore they may sink to the bottom of the priority list. A community health nurse or nursing administrator may plan to spend the day on a community project directed at preventive efforts, such as screening programs, updating the surveillance program, or meeting with key community members about a specific preventive program. However, the nurse may actually end up spending the time responding to the emergency of the day. This type of reactive rather than proactive nursing practice prevents progress toward "big picture" initiatives and population-based programs. When faced with multiple demands, nurses must be vigilant in devoting a sustained effort toward population-focused projects. Daily pressures can easily distract the nurse from population-based nursing practice. Several nursing organizations focus on this population, and one

---

BOX 3.1 Definitions of Theory Proposed by Nursing Theorists

- "A systematic vision of reality; a set of interrelated concepts that is useful for prediction and control" (Woods and Catanzaro, 1988, p. 568).
- "A conceptual system or framework invented for some purpose; and as the purpose varies so too must the structure and complexity of the system" (Dickoff and James, 1968, p. 19).
- "A creative and rigorous structuring of ideas that projects a tentative, purposeful, and systematic view of phenomena" (Chinn & Kramer, 1999, p. 51).
- "A set of ideas, hunches, or hypotheses that provides some degree of prediction and/or explanation of the world" (Pryjmachuk, 1996, p. 679).
- "Theory organizes the relationships between the complex events that occur in a nursing situation so that we can assist human beings. Simply stated, theory provides a way of thinking about and looking at the world around us" (Torres, 1986, p. 19).

TABLE 3.1 Microscopic Versus Macroscopic Approaches to the Delineation of Community Health Nursing Problems

Microscopic Approach	Macroscopic Approach
Examines individual, and sometimes family, responses to health and illness	Examines interfamily and intercommunity themes in health and illness
	Delineates factors in the population that perpetuate the development of illness or foster the development of health
Often emphasizes behavioral responses to an individual's illness or lifestyle patterns	Emphasizes social, economic, and environmental precursors of illness
Nursing interventions are often aimed at modifying an individual's behavior by changing his or her perceptions or belief system	Nursing interventions may include modifying social or environmental variables (i.e., working to remove care barriers and improving sanitation or living conditions)
	May involve social or political action

organization, the Quad Council of Public Health Nursing, is composed of representatives from the following four public health/community health nursing organizations:

- Public Health Nursing Section of the American Public Health Association (PHN-APHA)
- Association of Community Health Nurse Educators (ACHNE)
- Association of Public Health Nurses (APHN)
- American Nurses Association Council on Nursing Practice and Economics (ANA)

The organizations emphasize system-level thinking in practice and the importance of improving health through the design and implementation of population-based interventions (Swider, Krothe, Reyes, and Cravetz, 2013).

A theoretical focus on the individual can preclude understanding of a larger perspective. Dreher (1982) used the term conservative scope of practice in describing frameworks that focus energy exclusively on intrapatient and nurse–patient factors. She stated that such frameworks often adopt psychological explanations of patient behavior. This mode of thinking attributes low compliance, missed appointments, and reluctant participation to problems in patient motivation or attitude. Nurses are responsible for altering patient attitudes toward health rather than altering the system itself, "even though such negative attitudes may well be a realistic appraisal of health care" (Dreher, 1982, p. 505). This perspective does not entertain the possibility of altering the system or empowering patients to make changes.

ASSESSING A THEORY'S SCOPE IN RELATION TO COMMUNITY HEALTH NURSING

Theoretical scope is especially important to community health nursing because there are many levels of practice within this specialty area. For example, a home health nurse who is caring for ill people after hospitalization has a very different scope of practice from that of a nurse epidemiologist or health planner. Unless a given theory is broad enough in scope to address health and the determinants of health from a population perspective, the theory will not be very useful to community health nurses. *Healthy People 2020* incorporated social determinants of health in the nation's health objectives (U.S. Department of Health and Human Services, 2017). Robert Wood Johnson Foundation addressed the need for a Culture of

Health that benefits everyone to ensure all people have equal opportunities to make healthy choices, whatever their circumstances (Robert Wood Johnson, 2017). Applying the terms *microscopic* and *macroscopic* to health situations may help nurses guide and stimulate theory development in community health nursing.

Although the concept of macroscopic is similar to the upstream analogy, the term *macroscopic* refers to a broad scope that incorporates many variables to aid in understanding a health problem. Upstream thinking would fall within this domain. Viewing a problem from this perspective emphasizes the variables that precede or play a role in the development of health problems. Macroscopic is the broad concept, and upstream is a more specific concept. These related concepts and their meanings can help nurses develop a critical eye in evaluating a theory's relevance to population health.

ACTIVE LEARNING EXERCISE

Review the ANA's definition of community health nursing practice and the APHA's definition of public health nursing practice. What do these definitions indicate about the theoretical basis of community health nursing? How does the theoretical basis of community health nursing practice differ from that of other nursing specialty areas?

REVIEW OF THEORETICAL APPROACHES

The differences among theoretical approaches demonstrate how a nurse may draw very diverse conclusions about the reasons for client behavior and the range of available interventions. The following section uses two theories to exemplify individual microscopic approaches to community health nursing problems; one originates within nursing and one is based in social psychology. Two other theories demonstrate the examination of nursing problems from a macroscopic perspective; one originates from nursing and another has roots in phenomenology.

The format for this review is as follows:
1. The individual is the focus of change (i.e., microscopic).
   a. Orem's self-care deficit theory of nursing
   b. The health belief model (HBM)

FIG. 3.1 Variables and relationships in the health belief model (HBM). (Redrawn from Rosenstock IM: Historical origins of the health belief model. In Becker MH, editor: *The health belief model and personal health behavior,* Thorofare, NJ, 1974, Charles B. Slack.)

2. Thinking upstream: Society is the focus of change (i.e., macroscopic).
   a. Milio's framework for prevention
   b. Critical social theory perspective

The Individual Is the Focus of Change
Orem's Self-Care Deficit Theory of Nursing

In 1958, Dorothea Orem, a staff and private duty nurse who later became a faculty member at Catholic University of America, began to formalize her insights about the purpose of nursing activities and why individuals required nursing care (Berbiglia and Banfield, 2014; Fawcett, 2001). Her theory is based on the assumption that self-care needs and activities are the primary focus of nursing practice. Orem outlined her self-care deficit theory of nursing and stated that this general theory is actually a composite of the following related constructs: the theory of self-care deficits, which provides criteria for identifying those who need nursing; the theory of self-care, which explains self-care and why it is necessary; and the theory of nursing systems, which specifies nursing's role in the delivery of care and how nursing helps people (Orem, 2001).

Application of Self-Care Deficit Theory. During a discussion about theory-based initiatives, a British occupational health nurse lamented over her nursing supervisor's intention to adopt Orem's self-care deficit theory. She was frustrated and argued that much of the model's assumptions seemed incongruous with the realities of her daily practice. Kennedy (1989) maintained that the self-care deficit theory assumes that people are able to exert purposeful control over their environments in the pursuit of health; however, people may have little control over the physical or social aspects of their work environment. On the basis of this thesis, she concluded that the self-care model is incompatible with the practice domain of occupational health nursing.

The Health Belief Model

The second theory that focuses on the individual as the locus of change is the health belief model (HBM). The model evolved from the premise that the world of the perceiver determines action. The model had its inception during the late 1950s, when America was breathing a collective sigh of relief after the development of the polio vaccine. When some people chose not to bring themselves or their children into clinics for immunization, social psychologists and other public health workers recognized the need to develop a more complete understanding of factors that influence preventive health behaviors. Their efforts resulted in the HBM.

Kurt Lewin's work lent itself to the model's core dimensions. He proposed that behavior is based on current dynamics confronting an individual rather than prior experience (Maiman and Becker, 1974). Fig. 3.1 outlines the variables and relationships in the HBM. The HBM is based on the assumption that the major determinant of preventive health behavior is disease avoidance. The concept of disease avoidance includes perceived susceptibility to disease "X," perceived seriousness of disease "X," modifying factors, cues to action, perceived benefits minus perceived barriers to preventive health action, perceived threat of disease "X," and the likelihood of taking a recommended health action. Disease "X" represents a particular disorder that a health action may prevent. It is important to note that actions that relate to breast cancer will be different from those relating to measles. For example, in breast cancer, a cue to action may involve a public service advertisement encouraging women to make an appointment for a mammogram. However, for measles, a cue to action may be news of a measles outbreak in a neighboring town.

Application of the Health Belief Model. Over the years, a number of writers have proposed broadening the scope of the HBM to address health promotion and illness behaviors (Kirscht, 1974; Pender, 1987) and to merge its concepts with other theories that describe health behavior (Cummings et al., 1980). The following section contains a brief personal account of the author's perceptions addressing the strengths and limitations of the model.

During my nursing education classes at the undergraduate level, I was exposed to a large number of nursing theories. The HBM was probably my least favorite. Most of the content was interesting, but I found it difficult applying the concepts to patients in the community and home settings. The model's focus on compliance was something that nurses with a critical theoretical perspective would have difficulty applying in their own clinical practice. My perception of the model changed a few years ago when my younger brother had pancreatic cancer diagnosed. This experience allowed me to see how the HBM could offer some insight into an individual's health behaviors. It helped me organize ideas about why people choose to accept or reject the instructions of well-intended nurses and doctors. Concepts such as perceived seriousness, perceived susceptibility, and cue to action afforded new insights into the dynamics of health decision making. I began to apply the model's concepts to guide my work with my family. My brother who became ill had smoked much of his life. Another brother also smoked. My family members believed that you are destined to follow a path of life and death, but this experience clearly modified their health beliefs. Until this point, my family members did not quit smoking because they did not perceive the susceptibility and seriousness of smoking; they belonged to a reference group that disdained most traditional medical practices and favored inaction over action. During the next several weeks, my siblings requested information on strategies that would help them quit smoking and hopefully decrease their chances for the development of cancer.

Over the years, I have become more skilled in assessing and identifying patient needs and issues and have gained a better appreciation for the strengths and limitations that any theoretical framework imposes on a situation.

Limitations of the HBM. The HBM places the burden of action exclusively on the client. It assumes that only those clients who have negative perceptions of the specified disease or recommended health action will fail to act. In practice, this model focuses the nurse's energies on interventions designed to modify the client's distorted perceptions.

The HBM offers an explanation of health behaviors that is similar to a mechanical system. Consulting the HBM, a nurse may induce compliance by using model variables as catalysts to stimulate action. For example, an intervention study based on HBM precepts sought to improve follow-up in clients with hypertension by increasing their perceived susceptibility to and seriousness of the dangers of hypertension (Jones et al., 1987). The study provided patients with education over the telephone or in the emergency department and resulted in a dramatic increase in compliance. However, the researchers noted that several patient groups, in particular, a group of patients without child care, failed to respond to the intervention. Studies such as these demonstrate the predictive abilities and the limitations of HBM concepts

(Lajunen and Rasanen, 2004; Lin et al., 2005; Mirotznik et al., 1998). The HBM was used for tobacco cessation health education by improving the knowledge, attitudes, and behaviors of tobacco users (Renuka and Pushpanjali, 2014).

The HBM may effectively promote behavioral change by altering patients' perspectives, but it does not acknowledge the health professional's responsibility to reduce or ameliorate health care barriers. The model reflects the type of theoretical perspective that dominated nursing education and behavioral health for many years. The narrow scope of the model is its strength and its limitation: nurses are not challenged to examine the root causes of health opportunities and behaviors in the communities we serve.

The Upstream View: Society Is the Focus of Change
Milio's Framework for Prevention

Nancy Milio conducted extensive research on tobacco policy (1985). Milio's approach to advancing people's health is seen in her seminal book, *Promoting Health through Public Policy*, and through her detailed studies of tobacco policy and Norwegian farm food policy (Draper, 1986). **Milio's framework for prevention** (1976) provides a complement to the HBM and a mechanism for directing attention upstream and examining opportunities for nursing intervention at the population level. Nancy Milio outlined six propositions that relate an individual's ability to improve healthful behavior to a society's ability to provide accessible and socially affirming options for healthy choices. Milio used these propositions to move the focus of attention upstream by challenging the notion that a main determinant for unhealthful behavior choice is lack of knowledge. She said that government and institutional policies set the range of health options, so community health nursing needs to examine a community's level of health and attempt to influence it through public policy. She noted that the range of available health choices is critical in shaping a society's overall health status. Milio believed that national-level policy making was the best way to favorably affect the health of most Americans rather than concentrating efforts on imparting information in an effort to change individual patterns of behavior.

Milio (1976) proposed that health deficits often result from an imbalance between a population's health needs and its health-sustaining resources. She stated that the diseases associated with excess (e.g., obesity and alcoholism) afflict affluent societies and that the diseases resulting from inadequate or unsafe food, shelter, and water afflict the poor. Within this context, the poor in affluent societies may experience the least desirable combination of factors. Milio (1976) cited the socioeconomic realities that deprive many Americans of a health-sustaining environment despite the fact that "cigarettes, sucrose, pollutants, and tensions are readily available to the poor" (p. 436). Propositions proposed by Milio are listed in Table 3.2.

Personal and societal resources affect the range of health-promoting or health-damaging choices available to individuals. Personal resources include the individual's awareness, knowledge, and beliefs and the beliefs of the individual's family and friends. Money, time, and the urgency of other priorities are also personal resources. Community and national locale strongly influence

TABLE 3.2   Application of Milio's Framework in Public Health Nursing

Milio's Proposition Summary	Population Health Examples
Population health results from deprivation and/or excess of critical health resources.	Individuals and families living in poverty have poorer health status compared with middle- and upper-class individuals and families.
Behaviors of populations result from selection from limited choices; these arise from actual and perceived options available, as well as beliefs and expectations resulting from socialization, education, and experience.	Positive and negative lifestyle choices (e.g., smoking, alcohol use, safe sex practices, regular exercise, diet/nutrition, seatbelt use) are strongly dependent on culture, socioeconomic status, and educational level.
Organizational decisions and policies (both governmental and nongovernmental) dictate many of the options available to individuals and populations and influence choices.	Health insurance coverage and availability are largely determined and financed by federal and state governments (e.g., Medicare and Medicaid) and employers (e.g., private insurance); the source and funding of insurance very strongly influence health provider choices and services.
Individual choices related to health-promoting or health-damaging behaviors are influenced by efforts to maximize valued resources.	Choices and behaviors of individuals are strongly influenced by desires, values, and beliefs. For example, the use of barrier protection during sex by adolescents is often dependent on peer pressure and the need for acceptance, love, and belonging.
Alteration in patterns of behavior resulting from decision making of a significant number of people in a population can result in social change.	Some behaviors, such as tobacco use, have become difficult to maintain in many settings or situations in response to organizational and public policy mandates. As a result, tobacco use in the United States has dropped dramatically.
Without concurrent availability of alternative health-promoting options for investment of personal resources, health education will be largely ineffective in changing behavior patterns.	Addressing persistent health problems (e.g., overweight/obesity) is hindered because most people are very aware of what causes the problem, but are reluctant to make lifestyle changes to prevent or reverse the condition. Often, "new" information (e.g., a new diet) or resources (e.g., a new medication) can assist in attracting attention and directing positive behavior changes.

Adapted from Milio N: A framework for prevention: changing health-damaging to health-generating life patterns, *American Journal of Public Health* 66:435–439, 1976.

societal resources. These resources include the availability and cost of health services, environmental protection, safe shelter, and the penalties or rewards for failure to select the given options.

Milio (1976) challenged health education's assumption that knowledge of health-generating behaviors implies an act in accordance with that knowledge. She proposed that "most human beings, professional or nonprofessional, provider or consumer, make the easiest choices available to them most of the time" (p. 435). Health-promoting choices must be more readily available and less costly than health-damaging options for individuals to gain health and for society to improve health status. Milio's framework can enable a nurse to reframe this view by understanding the historical play of social forces that have limited the choices available to the parties involved.

Comparison of the HBM and Milio's Conceptualizations of Health. Milio's health resources bear some resemblance to the concepts in the HBM. The purpose of the HBM is to provide the nurse with an understanding of the dynamics of personal health behaviors. The HBM specifies broader contextual variables, such as the constraints of the health care system, and their influence on the individual's decision-making processes. The HBM also assumes that each person has unlimited access to health resources and free will. In contrast, Milio based her framework on an assessment of community resources and their availability to individuals. By assessing such factors up front, the nurse is able to gain a more thorough understanding of the resources people actually have. Milio offered a different set of insights into the health behavior arena by proposing that many low-income individuals are acting within the constraints of their limited resources. bibthermore, she investigated beyond downstream focus and population health by examining the choices of significant numbers of people within a population.

Compared with the HBM, Milio's framework provides for the inclusion of economic, political, and environmental health determinants; therefore the nurse is given broader range in the diagnosis and interpretation of health problems. Whereas the HBM allows only two possible outcomes (i.e., "acts" or "fails to act" according to the recommended health action), Milio's framework encourages the nurse to understand health behaviors in the context of their societal milieu.

Implications of Milio's Framework for Current Health Delivery Systems. Through its broader scope, Milio's model provides direction for nursing interventions at many levels. Nurses may use this model to assess the personal and societal resources of individual patients and to analyze social and economic factors that may inhibit healthy choices in populations. Population-based interventions may include such diverse activities as working to improve the nutritional content of school lunches and encouraging political activity on behalf of health care reform (Hobbs et al., 2004; Milio, 1981).

Overall, current health care delivery systems perform best when responding to people with diagnostic-intensive and acute illnesses. Those people who experience chronic debilitation or have less intriguing diagnoses generally fare worse in the health care system despite efforts by community- and home-based care to "fill the gaps." Nurses in both hospital and community-based systems often feel constrained by profound financial and service restrictions imposed by third-party payers. These third parties often terminate nursing care after the resolution of the latest immediate health crisis and fail to cover care aimed toward long-term health improvements. Many health systems use nursing standards and reimbursement mechanisms that originate from a narrow, compartmentalized view of health.

TABLE 3.3	Comparison of Individual and Societal Levels of Change	
Individual Level	**Societal Level**	
The individual is the focus of change	Society/community is the focus of change	
Microscopic	Macroscopic	
Downstream activities emphasized	Upstream activities emphasized	
Theories:	Theories:	
1. Orem's self-care deficit theory of nursing	a. Milio's framework for prevention	
2. The health belief model (HBM)	b. Critical social theory perspective	

Personal behavior patterns are not simply "free" choices about "lifestyle" that are isolated from their personal and economic context. Lifestyles are patterns of choices made from available alternatives according to people's socioeconomic circumstances and how easily they are able to choose some over others (Milio, 1981). It is therefore imperative to practice nursing from a broader understanding of health, illness, and suffering. Public health nurses must often work at both the individual and societal levels. As Milio suggested, it is not only individual behaviors but the economic context as well. This can be seen in Table 3.3, which shows that the focus of change can be at the individual or society level.

Critical Theoretical Perspective

Similar to Milio's framework for prevention, critical theoretical perspective uses societal awareness to expose social inequalities that keep people from reaching their full potential. This perspective is devised from the belief that social meanings structure life through social domination. "A critical perspective can be used to understand the linkages between the health care system and the broader political, economic, and social systems of society" (Waitzkin, 1983, p. 5). According to Navarro (1976), in *Medicine Under Capitalism*, the health care system mirrors the class structure of the broader society. According to Conrad and Leiter (2012), a critical theoretical perspective is one that does not regard the present structure of health care as sacred. A critical theoretical perspective accepts no truth or fact merely because it has been accepted as such in the past. The social aspects of health and illness are too complex to use only one perspective. The critical theoretical perspective assumes that health and illness entail societal and personal values and that these values have to be made explicit if illness and health care problems are to be satisfactorily dealt with. This perspective is informed by the following values and assumptions:

- The problems and inequalities of health and health care are connected to the particular historically located social arrangements and the cultural values of society.
- Health care should be oriented toward the prevention of disease and illness.
- The priorities of any health care system should be based on the needs of the clients/population and not the health care providers.
- Ultimately, society itself must be changed for health and medical care to improve (Conrad and Leiter, 2012).

Stevens and Hall (1992) used critical theoretical perspective in nursing to address unsafe neighborhoods as well as economic, political, and social disadvantages of the communities we serve. They advocate for emancipator nursing actions for our communities. Proponents of this theoretical approach maintain that social exchanges that are not distorted by power imbalances will stimulate the evolution of a more just society (Allen et al., 1986). Critical theoretical perspective assumes that truth standards are socially determined and that no form of scientific inquiry is value free. Allen and colleagues (1986) stated, "One cannot separate theory and value, as the empiricist claims. Every theory is penetrated by value interests" (p. 34).

Application of Critical Theoretical Perspective. Critical theory has been applied to nursing in communities (Stevens and Hall, 1992). Application of a critical theoretical perspective can be seen when health care is used as a form of social control. The social control function in health care is used to get patients to adhere to norms of appropriate behavior. This is accomplished through the medicalization of a wide range of psychological and socioeconomic issues. *Medicalization* is identification or categorization of (a condition or behavior) as being a disorder requiring medical treatment or intervention. Examples include medicalization related to sexuality, family life, aging, learning disabilities, and dying (Conrad, 1975, 1992; Zola, 1972). Medicalization can incorporate many facets of health and illness care, from childbirth and allergies to hyperactivity and hospitals that have become dominated by the medical profession and its explanation of health and illness. When social problems are medicalized, there is often profit to be made. This can be seen when a patient readily receives a prescription for a medication before the root social cause of the illness is addressed by the health care provider. Using medical treatments for "undesirable behavior" has been implemented throughout history, including lobectomies for mental illness and synthetic stimulants for classroom behavior problems.

In this context, the nurse may examine how the concepts of power and empowerment influence access to quality child care (Kuokkanen and Leino-Kilpi, 2000). The nurse may contrast an organization's policies with interviews from workers who believe the organization is an impediment to achieving quality child care. Data analysis may also include an examination of the interests of workers and administration in promoting social change versus maintaining the status quo.

FIG. 3.2 McKinlay's model of continuum of health behaviors and corresponding interventions foci applied to tobacco use. (Data from McKinlay J: A case for refocusing upstream: the political economy of illness. In Gartley J, editor: *Patients, physicians and illness: a sourcebook in behavioral science and health,* New York, 1979, Free Press, pp 9–25.)

Wild (1993) used critical social theory to analyze the social, political, and economic conditions associated with the cost of prescription analgesics and the corresponding financial burden of clients who require these medications. Wild compared the trends in pharmaceutical pricing with the inflation rates of other commodities. The study stated that pharmaceutical sales techniques, which market directly to physicians, distance the needs of ill clients from the pharmaceutical industry. Wild's analysis specified nursing actions that a downstream analysis would not consider, such as challenging pricing policies on behalf of client groups.

Challenging Assumptions about Preventive Health Through Critical Theoretical Perspective. The HBM and Milio's prevention model focus on personal health behaviors from a disease avoidance or preventive health perspective; nurses may also analyze this phenomenon using critical social theory. Again, McKinlay's upstream analogy refers to health workers who were so busy fishing sick people out of the river that they did not look upstream to see how they were ending up in the water. Later in the same article, McKinlay (1979) used his upstream analogy to ask the rhetorical question, "How preventive is prevention?" (p. 22). He used this tactic to critically examine different intervention strategies aimed at enhancing preventive behavior. Fig. 3.2 illustrates McKinlay's model, which contrasts the different modes of prevention. He linked health professionals' curative and lifestyle modification interventions to a downstream conceptualization of health; the majority of alleged preventive actions fail to alter the process of illness at its origin. Political-economic interventions remain the most effective way to address population determinants of health and to ameliorate illness at its source.

McKinlay (1979) delineated the activities of the "manufacturers of illness—those individuals, interest groups, and organizations which, in addition to producing material goods and services, also produce, as an inevitable by-product, widespread morbidity and mortality" (pp. 9, 10). The manufacturers of illness embed desired behaviors in the dominant cultural norm and thus foster the habituation of high-risk behavior in the population. Unhealthy consumption patterns are integrated into everyday lives; for example, the American holiday dinner table offers concrete examples of "the binding of at-riskness to culture" (p. 12). The existing U.S. health care system, in a misguided attempt to help, devotes its efforts to changing the products of the illness manufacturers and neglects the processes that create the products. Manufacturers of illness include the tobacco industry, the alcohol industry, and multiple corporations that produce environmental carcinogens.

Waitzkin (1983) continued this theme by asserting that the health care system's emphasis on lifestyle diverts attention from important sources of illness in the capitalist industrial environment and "it also puts the burden of health squarely on the individual rather than seeking collective solutions to health problems" (p. 664). Salmon (1987) supported this position by noting that the basic tenets of Western medicine promote an understanding of individual health and illness factors and obscure the exploration of their social and economic roots. He stated that critical social theory "can aid in uncovering larger dimensions impacting health that are usually unseen or misrepresented by ideological biases. Thus the social reality of health conditions can be both understood and changed" (p. 75).

In the past decade, a critical theoretical perspective has been used with *symbolic interactionism,* a theory that focuses predominantly on the individual and the meaning of situations. **Critical interactionism** brings the two theories together to address some issues at both upstream and downstream levels to make health care system changes (Burbank and Martins, 2010; Martins and Burbank, 2011). Nurses can use both upstream and downstream approaches to address health issues through critical interactionism (Table 3.4).

Nurses in all practice settings face the challenge of understanding and responding to collective health within the context of a health system that allocates resources at the individual level. The Tavistock Group (1999) released a set of ethical principles that summarizes this juxtaposition by noting that "the care of individuals is at the center of health care delivery, but must be viewed and practiced within the overall context of continuing work to generate the greatest possible health gains for groups and populations" (pp. 2, 3). This perspective is an accurate reflection of Western-oriented thought, which generally gives individual health precedence over collective health. Although nurses can appreciate the concept of individual care at the center of health delivery, they should also consider transposing this principle. Doing so allows the nurse to consider a health care system that places the community in the center of health care and holds the goal of generating health gains for individuals. Fortunately, these worldviews of health delivery systems are not mutually exclusive, and nurses can understand the duality of health care needs in individuals and populations.

Issue	Downstream Focus	Upstream Focus	Critical Interactionism: An Upstream/Downstream Approach
Clients: Obesity rates	Individual behavior strategies to reduce weight Lifestyle changes Bariatric surgery nursing care	Health policy changes Vending machines in schools with healthier choices School lunch program modifications Target corporations that profit from obesity	Individual strategies with weight loss in conjunction with system changes Social marketing at both levels
Client or nurse: Workplace violence	Behavior change at individual level Workplace programs to reduce violence	Address organizational factors that promote workplace violence What organizational structures perpetuate workplace violence?	Change needed in knowledge and skills to address issue of workplace violence at both the downstream and upstream levels
Nurse: Workplace errors	Focus on individual: Root-cause analysis that has the individual as the focus Change the behavior of the individual nurse Reeducation of nurse with workplace error	System changes needed What system-level factors lead to workplace errors? What organizational structures perpetuate workplace errors?	A dual approach: Providers need changes in knowledge and skills to address root causes of workplace errors that move from individual to system level

TABLE 3.4 Critical Interactionism: Comparison of Upstream and Downstream Focuses

Data from Martins DC, Burbank P: Critical interactionism: an upstream-downstream approach to health care reform, *Advances in Nursing Science* 34(4):315–329, 2011.

 ACTIVE LEARNING EXERCISE

- Select a theory or conceptual model. Evaluate its potential for understanding health in individuals, families, a population of 400 children in an elementary school, a community of 50,000 residents, and 2000 workers within a corporate setting.
- Identify one health problem (e.g., substance abuse, domestic violence, or cardiovascular disease) that is prevalent in the community or city. Analyze the problem using two different theories or conceptual models. One should emphasize individual determinants of health, and another should emphasize population determinants of health. What are some differences in the way these different perspectives inform nursing practice?

ETHICAL INSIGHTS

Social Injustice in Community-Based Practice

Chafey (1996) refers to "putting justice to work in community-based practice" and notes that nursing has a rich historical legacy in social justice activities. Although social justice activities are alive and well in nursing practice, many leaders think that the continuing struggle for resources is taking its toll on the scope of social action within community health systems. In addition, the policies of the current federal administration often emphasize market justice values over social justice values. *Market justice* refers to the principle that people are entitled to valued ends (e.g., status, income) when they acquire them through fair rules of entitlement. In contrast, *social justice* refers to the principle that all citizens bear equitably in the benefits and burdens of society (Drevdahl et al., 2001). These are complex concepts that cannot be easily distilled into a clear set of rules or nursing policies. However, in the context of community health nursing, health (and consequently health care) is considered a right rather than a privilege. To the extent that certain citizens, by virtue of their income, race, health needs, or any other attribute, are unable to access health care, our society as a whole suffers. Nurses are well positioned to "stand on the shoulders" of yesterday's nursing leaders and act on behalf of justice in health care access for all citizens.

 HEALTHY PEOPLE 2020

Healthy People 2020 clearly moved to the population level with the addition of social determinants of health. This area was designed to identify ways to create social and physical environments that promote good health for all. All Americans deserve an equal opportunity to make the choices that lead to good health. But to ensure that all Americans have that opportunity, advances are needed not only in health care but also in fields such as education, child care, housing, business, law, media, community planning, transportation, and agriculture. Making these advances would involve working together to (1) explore how programs, practices, and policies in these areas affect the health of individuals, families, and communities; (2) establish common goals, complementary roles, and ongoing constructive relationships between the health sector and these areas; and (3) maximize opportunities for collaboration among federal-, state-, and local-level partners related to social determinants of health (U.S. Department of Health and Human Services, 2017).

The pictures in this chapter's photo novella present environmental health issues and efforts being taken by nurses to address them.

NURSES WORK IN ENVIRONMENTAL HEALTH IN A VARIETY OF WAYS

Open mine waste in the rural West can pose a continuing threat to local citizens. Nurses have been involved in advocacy efforts to ensure that citizens receive periodic screening for exposure to lead. Nurses can be active in policy efforts to prevent environmental disasters in the future.

A public health nurse inspects the site of an asphalt spill off a rural railway car. Hazardous materials spills often occur in remote areas away from health care services. Broad conceptual frameworks allow nurses to think upstream and incorporate environmental risks into the consideration of community health issues.

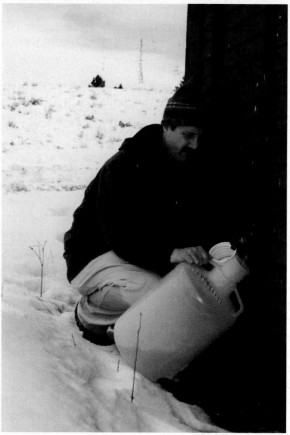

Citizens can be unaware of biological and chemical contaminants in their drinking water. Nurses are playing more active roles in water testing and in communicating the results of such tests to community members. When health is conceptualized broadly, nurses understand and view risk in new ways.

A public health nurse teaches a class on environmental health for local nurses. Environmental health is an important part of community health nursing's expanding practice.

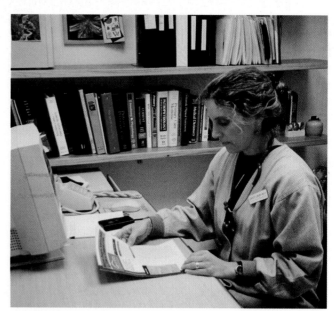

A nurse practitioner reviews educational materials addressing occupational and environmental health risks. By providing guidance for her clients, she is working to reduce risks and empower her clients to reduce their personal and community-based risks.

RESEARCH HIGHLIGHTS

Assessment of Hunger with the Homeless Populations

This study examined the relationship between nutritional status, food insecurity, and health risk among the population experiencing homelessness in Rhode Island (RI). A correlational study used a sample of 319 adults experiencing homelessness surveyed for access to emergency foods, shelters, and Supplemental Nutrition Assistance Program (SNAP). Participants completed a U.S. Department of Agriculture Food Security Module subset. Anthropometric measures included height, weight, and waist circumference. A 24-hour food diary was also collected. Findings indicated that participants had insufficient vegetables, fruit, dairy, and meat/beans but they had excessive amounts of fats. Almost 70% were overweight or obese. Ninety-four percent were food insecure, with 64% of this subset experiencing hunger. Only 55% were currently receiving SNAP benefits. Participants expressed concern about having no kitchen or ability to store or prepare food with their SNAP benefit.

The study results led to policy change in RI. The SNAP was expanded to include a *Restaurant Meals Program* so that the homeless, elderly, and disabled could use their SNAP benefits for prepared foods. This is now utilized across the state.

Adapted from Martins DC., et al.: Assessment of food intake, obesity and health risk among the homeless in Rhode Island, *Public Health Nursing* 32(5):453–461, 2015.

SUMMARY

Nursing and health service literature often focuses on health care access issues. This topic is interesting because tremendous disparities for access exist between insured and uninsured people in the United States. Access to care is associated with economic, social, and political factors, and, depending on individual and population needs, it can be a primary determinant of health status and survival. Structural variables, such as race-ethnicity, educational status, gender, and income, may be highly predictive of health status. These types of factors, which are also strongly grounded in the sociopolitical and economic milieu, identify risk factors for poor health and opportunities for community-based interventions.

Community health nurses have been instrumental in making many of the lifesaving advances in sanitation, communicable diseases, and environmental conditions that today's society takes for granted. Community health practice helps develop a broad context of nursing practice, because community environments are inherently less restrictive than hospital settings. Clarke and Cody (1994) compared the environmental characteristics in community-based settings with those in hospital-based settings. They proposed that the dynamic nature of community settings lends itself best to the education of professional nurses.

In a discussion addressing the future of community health nursing, Bellack (1998) differentiates between "nursing in the community" and "nursing with the community." This subtle reframing of the nursing role reinforces the notion that the health agenda originates from natural leaders, church members, local officials, parents, children, teens, and other community members. Forming and advancing a shared vision of health can be a formidable challenge for the nurse; as with any other complex issue, multiple viewpoints are the norm. Even "naming" health problems can be difficult, because different constituents are likely to see issues differently and pursue different lines of reasoning. However, allowing the genesis of change to occur from within the community is the essential challenge of nursing with the community. "Nursing with the community" efforts allow the nurse to create agendas that arise from community members rather than those imposed on community members. Listening, being patient, providing accurate and scientifically sound information, and respecting the experiences of community members are essential to the success of these efforts.

The nursing profession has advanced and with it so has the need to develop nursing theories that formalize the scientific base of community health nursing. The richness of community health nursing comes from the challenge of conceptualizing and implementing strategies that will enhance the health of many people. Likewise, nurses in this practice area must have access to theoretical perspectives that address the social, political, and environmental determinants of population health. The integration of population-based theory with practice gives nurses the means to favorably affect the health of the global community.

EVOLVE WEBSITE

http://evolve.elsevier.com/Nies/community
- NCLEX Review Questions
- Case Studies

BIBLIOGRAPHY

Ali Pirani SS: Application of Nightingale's theory in nursing practice, *Ann Nurs Pract* 3(1):1040, 2016.

Allen DG, Diekelmann N, Benner P: Three paradigms for nursing research: methodologic implications. In: Chinn P, editor: *Nursing research methodology: issues and implementation*, Rockville, MD, Aspen Publishers.

Barnum BS: *Nursing theory: analysis, application, evaluation*, ed 5, Philadelphia, 1998, Lippincott.

Bellack JP: Community-based nursing practice: necessary but not sufficient, *J Nurs Educe* 37(3):99–100, 1998.

Berbiglia V, Banfield B: Self-care deficit theory of nursing. In Alligood M, editor: *Nursing theorists and their work*, ed 8, St. Louis, 2014, Elsevier Mosby.

Berwick D, Davidoff F, Hiatt H, et al.: Refining and implementing the Tavistock principles for everybody in health care, *Br J Med* 323:616–620, 2000.

Burbank P, Martins DC: Symbolic interactionism and critical perspective: divergent or synergistic? *Nurs Philos* 11(1):25–41, 2010.

Centers for Disease Control and Prevention: *National Center for Chronic Disease Prevention and Health Promotion: chronic disease prevention, 2013, 2017*. Available from <http://www.cdc.gov/chronicdisease/overview/index.htm>.

Chafey K: Caring is not enough: ethical paradigms for community-based care, *N HC Perspect Community* 17(1):10–15, 1996.

Chinn PL, Kramer MK: *Knowledge development in nursing: theory and practice*, ed 9, St. Louis, 2015, Elsevier-Mosby.

Clarke PN, Cody WK: Nursing theory-based practice in the home and community: the crux of professional nursing education, *Adv Nurs Sci* 17(2):41–53, 1994.

Conrad P: The discovery of hyperkinesis: notes on the medicalization of deviant behavior, *Soc Probl* 23:12–21, 1975.

Conrad P: Medicalization and social control, *Annu Rev Sociol* 18:209–232, 1992.

Conrad P, Leiter V: *The sociology of heath and illness: critical perspectives*, ed 9, New York, Worth Publishing.

Cummings KM, Becker MH, Malie MC: Bringing the models together: an empirical approach to combining variables to explain health actions, *J Behav Med* 3:123–145, 1980.

Dickoff J, James P: A theory of theories: a position paper, *Nurs Res* 17:197–203, 1968.

Draper P: Nancy Milio's work and its importance for the development of health promotion, *Health Promot Int* 1(1):101–106, 1986.

Dreher M: The conflict of conservatism in public health nursing education, *Nurs Outlook* 30(9):504–509, 1982.

Drevdahl D, Kneipp S, Canales M, et al.: Reinvesting in social justice: a capital idea for public health nursing? *ANS Adv Nurs Sci* 24(2):19–31, 2001.

Fawcett J: The nurse theorists: 21st-century updates—Dorothea E. Orem, *Nurs Sci Q* 14(1):34–38, 2001.

Hobbs S, Ricketts T, Dodds J, et al.: Analysis of interest group influence on federal school meals regulations 1992 to 1996, *J Nutr Educ Behav* 36(2):90–98, 2004.

Jones PK, Jones SL, Katz J: Improving follow-up among hypertensive patients using a health belief model intervention, *Arch Intern Med* 147:1557–1560, 1987.

Kennedy A: How relevant are nursing models? *Occup Health* 41(12):352–354, 1989.

Kirscht JP: The health belief model and illness behavior. In Becker MH, editor: *The health belief model and personal health behavior*, Thorofare, NJ, 1974, Charles B. Slack.

Kuokkanen L, Leino-Kilpi H: Power and empowerment in nursing: three theoretical approaches, *J Adv Nurs* 31(1):235–241, 2000.

Lajunen T, Rasanen M: Can social psychological models be used to promote bicycle helmet use among teenagers? A comparison of the health belief model, theory of planned behavior and the locus of control, *J Safety Res* 35(1):115–123, 2004.

Lin P, Simoni J, Zemon V: The health belief mode, sexual behaviors, and HIV risk among Taiwanese immigrants, *AIDS Educ Prev* 17(5):469–483, 2005.

Maiman LA, Becker MH: The health belief model: origins and correlates in psychological theory. In Becker MH, editor: *The health belief model and personal health behavior*, Thorofare, NJ, 1974, Charles B. Slack.

Martins DC, Burbank P: Critical interactionism: an upstream-downstream approach to health care reform, *Adv Nurs Sci* 34(4):315–329, 2011.

Martins DC, Gorman K, Miller R, et al.: Assessment of food intake, obesity and health risk among the homeless in Rhode Island, *Public Health Nurs* 32(5):453–461, 2015.

McKinlay J: A case for refocusing upstream: the political economy of illness. In Gartley J, editor: *Patients, physicians and illness: a sourcebook in behavioral science and health*, New York, 1979, Free Press.

McKinlay JB: A case for refocusing upstream: the political economy of illness. In: Conrad P, Leiter V, editors: *the sociology of health and illness: critical perspectives*, ed 9, New York, Worth Publishing.

Milio N: A framework for prevention: changing health-damaging to health-generating life patterns, *Am J Public Health* 66:435–439, 1976.

Milio N: *Promoting health through public policy*, Philadelphia, 1981, FA Davis.

Milio N: Health policy and the emerging tobacco reality, *Soc Sci Med* 21(6):603–613, 1985.

Mirotznik J, Ginzler E, Zagon G: Using the health belief model to explain clinic appointment-keeping for the management of a chronic disease condition, *J Community Health* 23(3):195–210, 1998.

Navarro V: *Medicine under capitalism*, New York, 1976, Prodist.

Orem DE: *Nursing: concepts of practice*, ed 6, New York, 2001, Mosby.

Pender NJ: *Health promotion in nursing practice*, ed 2, Norwalk, CT, 1987, Appleton-Century-Crofts.

Pryjmachuk S: A nursing perspective on the interrelationship between theory, research, and practice, *J Adv Nurs* 23:679–684, 1996.

Renuka P, Pushpanjali K: Effectiveness of health belief model in motivating for tobacco cessation and improving knowledge, attitude, and behavior of tobacco users, *Cancer Oncology Res* 2(4):43–50, 2014.

Robert Wood Johnson Foundation: *Culture of health*. Available from http://www.cultureofhealth.org/ Accessed April 18, 2017.

Salmon JW: Dilemmas in studying social change versus individual change: considerations from political economy. In: Duffy M, Pender NJ, editors: *Conceptual issues in health promotion: a report of proceedings of a Wingspread Conference*, Indianapolis, IN, Sigma Theta Tau.

Schwartz-Barcott D, Patterson BJ, Lusardi P, et al.: From practice to theory: tightening the link via three fieldwork strategies, *J Adv Nurs* 39(3):281–289, 2002.

Stevens PE, Hall JM: Applying critical theories to nursing in communities, *Public Health Nurs* 9(1):2–9, 1992.

Swider SM, Krothe J, Reyes D, et al.: The Quad Council practice competencies for public health nursing, *Public Health Nurs* Nov/Dec 30(6):519–536, 2013.

Tavistock Group: A shared statement of ethical principles for those who shape and give health care: a working draft from the Tavistock Group, *Image J Nurs Sch* 31:2–3, 1999.

Torres G: *Theoretical foundations of nursing*, Norwalk, CT, 1986, Appleton-Century-Crofts.

U.S. Department of Health and Human Services: *Healthy People 2020: social determinants of health*, 2017. Available from <http://www.healthypeople.gov/2020/topicsobjectives2020/overview.aspx?topicid=39>.

Waitzkin H: A Marxist view of health and health care. In Mechanic D, editor: *Handbook of health, health care, and the health professions*, New York, 1983, Free Press.

Wild LR: Caveat emptor: a critical analysis of the costs of drugs used for pain management, *Adv Nurs Sci* 16:52–61, 1993.

Woods NF, Catanzaro M, editors: *Nursing research: theory and practice*, St. Louis, Mosby.

Zola I: Medicine as an institution of social control, *Sociol Rev* 20(4):487–504, 1972.

4

Health Promotion and Risk Reduction

Bridgette Crotwell Pullis and Mary A. Nies

OUTLINE

OBJECTIVES

Upon completion of this chapter, the reader will be able to do the following:

1. Discuss various theories of health promotion, including Pender's Health Promotion Model, the Health Belief Model, the Transtheoretical Theory, and the Theory of Reasoned Action.
2. Discuss definitions of health.
3. Demonstrate an understanding of the difference between health promotion and health protection.
4. Define risk.

5. Discuss the relationship of risk to health and health promotion activities.
6. Demonstrate an understanding of stratification of risk factors by age, race, and gender.
7. Discuss the influence of various factors on health.
8. List health behaviors for health promotion and disease prevention.
9. Relate the clinical implications of health promotion activities.

KEY TERMS

determinants of health	health protection	risk communication
health	portion distortion	risk reduction
health promotion	risk	

HEALTH PROMOTION AND COMMUNITY HEALTH NURSING

Since its inception, nursing has focused on helping individuals, groups, and communities maintain and protect their health. Florence Nightingale and other nursing pioneers recognized the importance of nutrition, rest, and hygiene in maximizing and protecting one's state of health. Though people are responsible for their health and medical care, they often seek advice from nurses in the community regarding health promotion and to help them make sense of the many, often competing recommendations that appear daily on TV, online, and in newspapers and magazines.

Green and Kreuter (1991) define **health promotion** as "any combination of health education and related organizational, economic, and environmental supports for behavior of individuals, groups, or communities conducive to health" (p. 2). Parse (1990) states that health promotion is that which is motivated by the desire to increase well-being and to reach the best possible health potential. This chapter's photo novella provides some examples of nurses engaging in health promotion.

HEALTH PROMOTION IN THE COMMUNITY

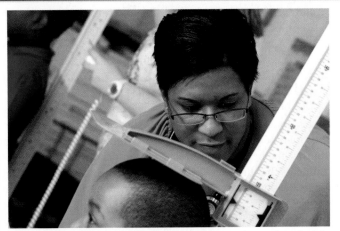

Elementary school screening: A nursing student takes height and weight measurements, which serve as a baseline to measure the growth rate of students.

A Veggie Fair in the community teaches children and their parents about the benefits of eating vegetables.

Elementary school screening: A nursing student securely holds the cuff as she takes this little boy's blood pressure.

Participants have fun educating children at the Veggie Fair, which will hopefully lead children and their parents to enjoy vegetables as a nutritious part of their daily diet.

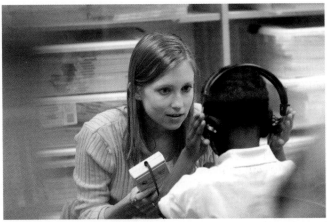

Elementary school screening: A nursing student watches and listens as she gives a hearing test.

Consider the clinical example about Jamie R. in Clinical Example 4.1. Jamie exemplifies this motivation to stay in her best health, at least at first glance. Let's look further into Jamie's health history.

Clinical Example 4.1

Jamie R. is a lifelong athlete. Married with three grown children, she rises at 4:20 each morning to go to the gym to swim for an hour before going to her job as an executive with a large company. A nonsmoker, Jamie rarely drinks alcohol and eats a diet consisting mostly of vegetables, grains, and fruit. Jamie's body mass index is in the normal range, and though her cholesterol and triglyceride levels are elevated, she does not require medication for this issue. After work, Jamie and her husband relax by walking their two dogs and reading. An early riser, Jamie is in bed by 9:30 almost every night. At 50 years of age, Jamie is youthful and energetic.

We all have friends like Jamie—people who seem to have an endless amount of energy and self-discipline. The rest of us, however, are typically less successful in achieving our health promotion goals.

When it comes to health practices, Jamie is a study in contradictions. Jamie's father had a myocardial infarction (MI) at the age of 48 years and died of an MI at the age of 50 years. Many of Jamie's paternal relatives have died of heart disease. Jamie's mother and one maternal aunt were each diagnosed with breast cancer in their early 50s. Though she has an annual physical examination by her family doctor and monitors her blood cholesterol and triglycerides, Jamie has never been screened for cardiac disease. Jamie receives the flu vaccine every year but has not had a tetanus-diphtheria vaccine booster in 14 years and has not had the shingles vaccine; though she sees her gynecologist yearly, she has had only one mammogram, 3 years ago.

In skipping annual mammograms and in not pursuing cardiac screening despite her high risk, Jamie is neglecting an important step in maintaining her health—health protection. **Health protection** consists of those behaviors in which one engages with the specific intent to prevent disease, to detect disease in the early stages, or to maximize health within the constraints of disease (Parse, 1990). Immunizations and cervical cancer screening are examples of health protection activities.

In discussing health promotion, it is helpful to define what is meant by **health**. One definition states that health is "being sound in body, mind, and spirit: freedom from physical disease or pain" (Merriam-Webster, 2009). As health promotion has become an important strategy to improve health, the way health is defined has shifted from a focus on the curative model to a focus on multidimensional aspects such as the social, cultural, and environmental facets of life and health (Benson, 1996). The well-known definition by the World Health Organization (WHO) states that health is "a state of complete physical, mental and social well-being, and not merely the absence of disease" (WHO, 2009). WHO also states that health is the extent to which an individual or group is able to realize aspirations, to satisfy needs, and to change or cope with the environment. In this aspect, health is viewed not only as an important goal but also as a resource for living (WHO, 1986).

❤ Healthy People 2020

Healthy People 2020 is the health promotion initiative for the nation. Developed through a consortium and managed by the U.S. Department of Health and Human Services (USDHHS), *Healthy People 2020* "challenges individuals, communities, and professionals, to take specific steps to ensure that good health, as well as long life, are enjoyed by all" (USDHHS, 2012).

The broad goals of *Healthy People 2020* are to attain high-quality, longer lives free of preventable disease, disability, injury, and premature death; achieve equity, eliminate disparities, and improve the health of all groups; create social and physical environments that promote good health for all; and promote quality of life, healthy development, and healthy behaviors across all life stages. Objectives toward achieving these goals are organized into 38 topic areas with corresponding priorities for action for each objective. Leading health indicators, or determinants of health, in each topic area help track progress toward meeting the goals of *Healthy People 2020*. A list of leading health indicators common to most of the topic areas is shown in Table 4.1. Fig. 4.1 illustrates the relationships among the determinants of health. The home page for *Healthy People 2020* can be accessed at http://www.healthypeople.gov/2020/. New topic areas such as sleep health, adolescent health, dementia, and genomics have been added.

❓ ACTIVE LEARNING EXERCISE

1. How has *Healthy People* changed? Get to know the *Healthy People 2020* proposed objectives at www.healthypeople.gov/hp2020/objectives/TopicAreas.aspx. Read over the new objectives and compare them with the *Healthy People 2010* objectives at www.healthypeople.gov/About/.
2. How did Americans do in meeting the *Healthy People 2010* objectives? Choose a focus area from *Healthy People 2010*, and access the periodic reviews for *Healthy People 2010*. What are the challenges to meeting the objectives? What are the strategies for meeting the objectives? Did the objective change for *Healthy People 2020*?

DETERMINANTS OF HEALTH

Biology is an individual's genetic makeup, family history, and any physical and mental health problems developed in the course of life. Aging, diet, physical activity, smoking, stress, alcohol or drug abuse, injury, violence, or a toxic or infectious agent may produce illness or disability, changing an individual's biology.

Behaviors are the individual's responses to internal stimuli and external conditions. Behaviors interact with biology in a common relationship, as one may influence the other. If a person chooses behaviors such as alcohol abuse or smoking, his or her biology may be changed as a result (e.g., liver cirrhosis, chronic obstructive pulmonary disease [COPD]). On the other hand, if an individual has a history of colon cancer in his or her family, the individual may choose to have regular screenings, thereby preventing advanced cancer and possibly death and changing his or her biology for the better. One's biology may affect behavior; if a person has hypertension or diabetes, he or

TABLE 4.1   Leading Health Indicators

Focus Area	Physical Activity	Overweight and Obesity	Tobacco USE	Substance Abuse	Responsible Sexual Behavior	Mental Health	Injury and Violence	Environmental Quality	Immunization	Access to Health Care
Access to quality health services	X	X	X	X	X	X	X		X	X
Arthritis, osteoporosis, and chronic back conditions	X	X					X			
Cancer	X	X	X	X	X			X	X	X
Chronic kidney disease	X	X	X							
Diabetes	X	X	X	X					X	X
Disability and secondary conditions	X	X	X	X		X			X	X
Educational and community-based programs	X	X	X	X	X	X	X	X	X	X
Environmental health								X		
Family planning				X	X			X		X
Food safety			X	X	X	X	X	X	X	X
Health communication	X	X	X	X	X	X	X	X		
Heart disease and stroke	X	X	X	X	X	X		X		
Human immunodeficiency virus			X	X	X	X		X		X
Immunization and infectious diseases										X
Injury and violence prevention			X	X	X	X	X			X
Maternal, infant, and child health	X	X	X	X	X	X	X		X	X
Medical product safety			X	X	X					
Mental health and mental disorders				X	X	X	X			X
Nutrition and overweight	X	X	X	X	X					X
Occupational safety and health							X	X		
Oral health	X	X	X	X	X		X	X		X
Physical activity and fitness	X	X	X	X	X	X		X	X	
Public health infrastructure	X	X	X	X	X	X	X	X	X	X
Respiratory diseases	X		X					X		
Sexually transmitted diseases			X	X	X	X				X
Substance abuse			X	X	X		X	X		X
Tobacco use		X	X	X						X
Vision and hearing										X

From Office of Disease Prevention and Health Promotion, U.S. Department of Health and Human Services: *Leading health indicators touch everyone, Healthy People 2010,* 2009. Retrieved from http://www.healthypeople.gov/2020/LHI/default.aspx.

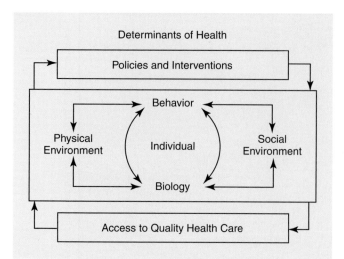

Determinants of Health

FIG. 4.1 The relationship among the determinants of health. (From U.S. Department of Health and Human Services: *Healthy People 2010: Understanding and improving health,* 2001. Retrieved from www.healthypeople.gov/Document/tableofcontents.htm#under.)

she may choose to begin an exercise regimen and to eat more healthfully.

Social environment includes interactions and relationships with family, friends, coworkers, and others in the community. Social institutions, such as law enforcement, faith communities, schools, and government agencies, are also part of the social environment, as well as housing, safety, public transportation, and availability of resources. The social environment has a great impact on the health of individuals, groups, and communities, yet it is complex in nature because of differing cultures and practices.

Physical environment is what is experienced with the senses—what is smelled, seen, touched, heard, and tasted. The physical environment can affect health negatively or positively. If there are toxic or infectious substances in the environment, this is certainly a negative influence on health. If the environment is clean with areas to recreate and play, this is a good influence on health.

Policies and interventions can have a profound effect on the health of individuals, groups, and communities. Positive effects such as policies against smoking in public places, seatbelt and child restraint laws, litter ordinances, and enhanced health care promote health. Policies are implemented at local, state, and national levels by many agencies, such as Transportation, Health and Human Services, Veterans' Affairs, Housing, and Justice departments.

Expansion of access to quality health care is essential to decrease health disparities and to improve the quality of life and the quantity of years of healthy life (USDHHS, 2013).

THEORIES IN HEALTH PROMOTION

Health promotion activities are broad in scope and in setting. Community health nurses and their clients engage in health promotion activities in workplace settings, schools, clinics,

and communities. The theories that are used most in health promotion are very diverse to accommodate the variety of settings, clients, and activities in community health. A working knowledge of theory is important in understanding why people act as they do and why they may or may not follow advice given to them by medical professionals and in helping clients progress from knowledge to behavior change. Some of the most frequently used health promotion theories and models are discussed here.

Pender's Health Promotion Model

Developed in the 1980s and revised in 1996, Pender's Health Promotion Model (HPM) explores the myriad biopsychosocial factors that influence individuals to pursue health promotion activities. The HPM depicts the complex multidimensional factors with which people interact as they work to achieve optimum health. This model contains seven variables related to health behaviors, as well as individual characteristics that may influence a behavioral outcome.

Pender's model does not include threat as a motivator, as threat may not be a motivating factor for clients in all age groups (Pender et al., Parsons, 2011). The HPM is depicted in Fig. 4.2.

Let's relate the HPM to Jamie R. in Clinical Example 4.1. The experience of having relatives who died of heart disease and cancer has probably increased her desire to engage in healthful behavior. Similarly, her busy schedule and lack of communication with her doctor may be reflected in her failure to obtain screenings or immunizations. Jamie has a habit of engaging in exercise and a high self-efficacy related to her success with exercise in the past. Jamie feels better after exercise, and she receives positive comments from significant others regarding her appearance, also increasing her motivation to exercise. Jamie works out in a lovely gym and is very committed to her workout routine. Jamie has found that working out first thing in the morning minimizes the competing demands that may keep her from exercising.

The Health Belief Model

Initially proposed in 1958, the Health Belief Model (HBM) provides the basis for much of the practice of health education and health promotion today. The HBM was developed by a group of social psychologists to attempt to explain why the public failed to participate in screening for tuberculosis (Hochbaum, 1958). Hochbaum and his associates had the same questions that perplex many health professionals today: *Why do people who may have a disease reject health screening? Why do individuals participate in screening if it may lead to the diagnosis of disease?* This research documented that information alone is rarely enough to motivate one to act. Individuals must know what to do and how to do it before they can take action. Also, the information must be related in some way to the individual's needs. One of the most widely used conceptual frameworks in health behavior, the HBM has been used to explain behavior change and maintenance of behavior change and to guide health promotion interventions (Champion and Skinner, 2008).

Individual Characteristics
and Experiences

Behavior-specific
Cognitions and Affect

Behavioral
Outcome

FIG. 4.2 The Health Promotion Model. (From Pender, N. [2009]. *The Health Promotion Model.* The University of Michigan School of Nursing. Retrieved from www.nursing.umich.edu/faculty/pender/chart.gif.)

The HBM has several constructs: perceived seriousness, perceived susceptibility, perceived benefits of treatment, perceived barriers to treatment, cues to action, and self-efficacy. These components can be found in Table 4.2. All of these constructs relate to the client's perception. How does the client perceive the seriousness of the condition? His or her susceptibility to the condition? The benefits of prevention or treatment? The barriers to prevention or treatment? The HBM is depicted in Fig. 4.3 (McEwen and Pullis, 2009).

Let's apply the HBM to Jamie. She may not perceive that she is susceptible to heart disease or breast cancer, or she may not perceive that there is a benefit of screening, or of treatment for heart disease or cancer—thus her failure to take up screening for these diseases.

The Transtheoretical Model

The Transtheoretical Model (TTM) combines several theories of intervention, giving its name. Table 4.3 lists the core constructs of the model, which also include the constructs of self-efficacy and the processes of change. The TTM is depicted in Fig. 4.4.

TABLE 4.2 Key Concepts and Definitions of the Health Belief Model

Concept	Definition
Perceived susceptibility	One's belief regarding the chance of getting a given condition
Perceived severity	One's belief regarding the seriousness of a given condition
Perceived benefits	One's belief in the ability of an advised action to reduce the health risk or seriousness of a given condition
Perceived barriers	One's belief regarding the tangible and psychological costs of an advised action
Cues to action	Strategies or conditions in one's environment that activate readiness to take action
Self-efficacy	One's confidence in one's ability to take action to reduce health risks

From Janz JK, Champion VL, Stretcher VJ: The health belief model. In Glanz K, Rimer BK, Lewis FM, editors: *Health behavior and health education: Theory, research, and practice,* San Francisco, CA, 2002, Jossey-Bass.

Individual Perceptions   Modifying Factors   Likelihood of Action

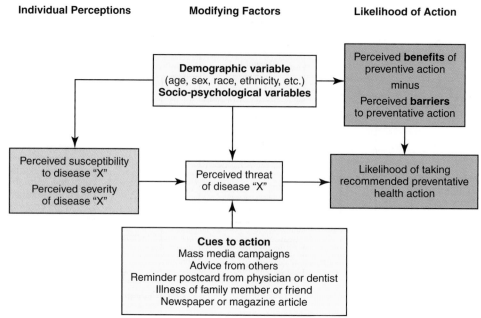

FIG. 4.3 The Health Belief Model. (From Becker, Maiman: Sociobehavioral determinants of compliance with health and medical care recommendations, *Medical Care* 13:10, 1975.)

TABLE 4.3	The Transtheoretical Model
Constructs	**Description**
Stages of Change	
Precontemplation	The individual has no intention to take action toward behavior change in the next 6 months. May be in this phase because of a lack of information about the consequences of the behavior or failure on previous attempts at change.
Contemplation	The individual has some intention to take action toward behavior change in the next 6 months. Weighing pros and cons to change.
Preparation	The individual intends to take action within the next month and has taken steps toward behavior change. Has a plan of action.
Action	The individual has changed overt behavior for less than 6 months. Has changed behavior sufficiently to reduce risk of disease.
Maintenance	The individual has changed overt behavior for more than 6 months. Strives to prevent relapse. This phase may last months to years.
Decisional Balance	
Pros	The benefits of behavior change
Cons	The costs of behavior change

Modified from Prochaska JO, Redding CA, & Evers KE: The transtheoretical model and stages of change. In Glanz K, Rimer B, Viswanath K, editors: *Health behavior and health education: Theory, research, and practice*, San Francisco, CA, 2008, Jossey-Bass, pp 97–121.

The TTM is based on the assumption that behavior change takes place over time, progressing through a sequence of stages. It also assumes that each of the stages is both stable and open to change. In other words, one may stop in one stage, progress to the next stage, or return to the previous stage.

The Transtheoretical Model and Change

Change is difficult, even for the most motivated of individuals. People resist change for many reasons. Change may:

- Be unpleasant (exercising)
- Require giving up pleasure (eating desserts or watching TV)
- Be painful (insulin injections)
- Be stressful (eating new foods)
- Jeopardize social relationships (gatherings with friends and family that involve food)
- Not seem important any more (older individuals or those with the ill effects of lifestyle choices, such as diabetes and hypertension)
- Require change in self-image (from couch potato to athlete) (Westberg and Jason, 1996).

Theory of Reasoned Action

Developed by Fishbein and Ajzen, the Theory of Reasoned Action (TRA) attempts to predict a person's intention to perform or not to perform a certain behavior (Montano and Kasprzyk, 2008). The TRA is based on the assumption that all behavior is determined by one's behavioral intentions. These intentions are determined by one's attitude regarding a behavior and the subjective norms associated with the behavior (Montano and Kasprzyk, 2008). One's attitude is determined by one's beliefs about the outcomes of performing the behavior, weighed by one's assessment of the outcomes. Consider Jamie R. for a moment. Jamie must believe strongly that exercise will have positive results, as she rises early and takes time from her busy schedule to work out daily. Conversely, Jamie may believe strongly that routine immunizations or health screenings will have negative results.

One's subjective norm is determined by one's normative beliefs, or whether or not important people in one's life approve or disapprove of the behavior under consideration, weighed

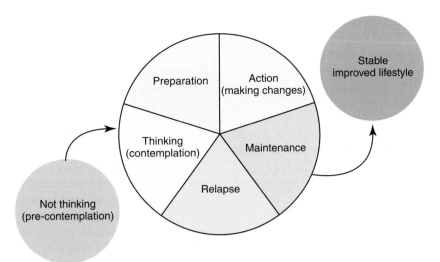

FIG. 4.4 The Transtheoretical Model. (From Prochaska J, DiClemente C: Transtheoretical therapy: Towards a more integrative model of change, *Psychotherapy: Theory, Research & Practice 19:* 276–288, 1982.)

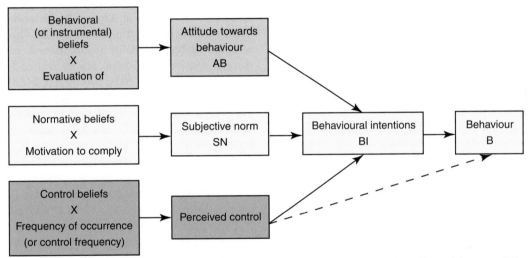

FIG. 4.5 The theory of reasoned action and the theory of planned behavior. (From Montano DE, Kaspryzyk D: Theory of reasoned action, theory of planned behavior, and the integrated behavioral model. In Glanz K, Rimer BK, Viswanath K, editors, *Health behavior and health education,* San Francisco, CA, 2008, Jossey-Bass, pp 67–96.)

by one's motivation to comply with those important persons (Montano and Kasprzyk, 2008). If Jamie believes that her husband or children think that she should get a mammogram, and if she is motivated to comply with their wishes, Jamie will have a positive subject norm regarding getting a mammogram.

Recently, the variable of perceived control has been added to the TRA to account for the amount of control an individual may have over whether or not he or she performs the behavior. With the addition of perceived control, the Theory of Planned Behavior was developed (Montano and Kasprzyk, 2008). Fig. 4.5 illustrates the TRA and the Theory of Planned Behavior.

RISK AND HEALTH

Oleckno defines **risk** as "the probability that a specific event will occur in a given time frame" (2002, p. 352). A risk factor is an exposure that is associated with a disease (Friis and Sellers,

2004). Jamie R. has an increased risk of heart disease and cancer. Jamie's risk factors include a family history of both of these diseases, work stress, her age, environmental exposures, and gender. There are known risk factors for some diseases, such as smoking and its association with lung cancer, as well as high blood pressure and heart disease. Some risk factors are assumed, such as cell phones and brain tumors. The three criteria for establishing a risk factor are as follows:

- The frequency of the disease varies by category, or amount of the factor. Lung cancer is more likely to develop in cigarette smokers than in nonsmokers and in those who smoke heavily than in those who smoke little.
- The risk factor must precede the onset of the disease. Cigarette smokers have lung cancer after they have been smoking for a while. If smokers had lung cancer before starting to smoke, this fact would cast doubt on smoking as a risk factor for lung cancer.

- The association of concern must not be due to any source of error. In any research study (especially one involving human behavior), there are many sources of error, such as study design, data collection methods, and data analysis. Other criteria that have been noted in the literature include strength of the association, consistency with repetition, specificity, and plausibility (Friis and Sellers, 2004).

In order to determine the health risks to individuals, groups, and populations, a risk assessment may be conducted. A *risk assessment* is a systematic way of distinguishing the risks posed by potentially harmful exposures. The four main steps of a risk assessment are hazard identification, risk description, exposure assessment, and risk estimation (Savitz, 1998).

THE RELATIONSHIP OF RISK TO HEALTH AND HEALTH PROMOTION ACTIVITIES

Health is directly related to the activities in which we participate, the food we eat, and the substances to which we are exposed daily. Where we live and work and our gender, age, and genetic makeup also affect health. In the assessment of risk regarding health and health promotion activities, there are two types of risks: modifiable risks and nonmodifiable risks. *Modifiable risk factors* are those aspects of a person's health risk over which he or she has control. Examples include smoking, leading a sedentary or active lifestyle, type and amount of food eaten, and the type of activities in which he or she engages (skydiving is riskier than bowling). *Nonmodifiable risk factors* are those aspects of one's health risk over which one has no or little control. Examples include genetic makeup, gender, age, and environmental exposures. A useful tool to help clients assess their family history for possible health risks is available at the U.S. Surgeon General's website at http://www.hhs.gov/familyhistory/. This assessment is easy to use and can create a dialogue between family members to discuss family health history. As the nurse assesses the various aspects of a client's health, it is important to evaluate behaviors that have a positive effect on the client's health, not only those behaviors that are detrimental to health. Healthful behaviors, such as maintaining an exercise regimen and following an eating plan, build self-efficacy and self-esteem. Positive health behaviors also provide a foundation on which a nurse can build to address unhealthful behaviors. If a client has been successful at smoking cessation, the confidence and self-efficacy learned from this change can be drawn upon to help him or her stick to a low-sodium, low-fat diet to address the hypertension.

Risk reduction is a proactive process in which individuals participate in behaviors that enable them to react to actual or potential threats to their health (Pender, 1996). Risk communication is the process through which the public receives information regarding possible or actual threats to health. Risk communication is affected by the way individuals and communities perceive, process, and act on their understanding of risk (Finnigan and Vinswanath, 2008). Individuals, groups, and communities receive information on health risks from many sources besides health care professionals today. The Internet is a newer source of risk communication for many community members, with 60% of Internet users accessing it for health information (Atkinson et al., 2009). Newspapers, periodicals, radio, TV, and billboards are long-standing sources of health information in public health. Though there are many sources of information on health risks available to the public, the quality varies widely in terms of the accuracy of the information presented (Hendrick et al., 2012; Kupferberg and Protus, 2011). The use of social media to communicate with audiences has also increased among public and private entities. Chat rooms, forums, Facebook, Twitter, and many specialized websites such as *Five Wishes*, which offers information on advance care planning, and nutrition websites such as *Eating Well* provide a wide range of information. Health care professionals are endeavoring to make risk communication as personalized and specific as possible for individuals, groups, and communities in an effort to improve uptake of screening and behavior change. Research has not shown personalized risk communication to be any more effective than traditional methods of risk communication (Edwards et al., Ahmed, 2013).

Approximately 50% of annual U.S. deaths occur as a result of modifiable or lifestyle factors (McGinnis and Foege, 1993; Mokdab et al., 2004). Fig. 4.6 depicts the leading causes of death and the numbers of deaths related to each. Those causes of death with the highest mortality (heart disease, cancer, stroke, and chronic respiratory disease) are all related to lifestyle factors (McGinnis and Foege, 2004; NRC and IOM, 2015). The relationship of lifestyle factors to mortality is so strong that medical care has been found to play a minor role in preventing premature deaths. (Schroeder, 2007) Table 4.4 details the relationship of the leading causes of death and common risk factors. A 2012 study found that people adopting healthful behaviors such as exercising, eating a healthful diet, not using tobacco, and maintaining a normal weight had a 66% lower risk of death than did those who did not adopt these behaviors (Loef and Walach, 2012).

Unfortunately many people experience a clustering of unhealthy lifestyle behaviors such as poor diet, physical inactivity, obesity, and smoking. The American Heart Association has developed a useful self-assessment of cardiovascular health. Life's Simple Seven (LS7) (http://www.heart.org/HEARTORG/Conditions/My-Life-Check---Lifes-Simple-7_UCM_471453_Article.jsp#.WOKWg2ckq70) is based on physical activity, diet, tobacco use, body weight, cholesterol, blood pressure, and blood sugar. This tool uses data entered by the user to derive a score and to offer feedback on areas needing improvement.

Tobacco and Health Risk

Smoking cessation is an important step in achieving optimum health. In the United States, smoking is the leading cause of preventable death, accounting for approximately one out of every five deaths, or 438,000 deaths, per year. Smoking is a causal factor in cancers of the esophagus, bladder, stomach, oral cavity, pharynx, larynx, cervix, and lung, with more than 90% of lung cancers in men and 80% of lung cancers among women attributable to smoking (Centers for Disease Control and Prevention [CDC], January 2, 2013). Smoking also has an economic impact, costing $97.2 billion annually in health care and lost productivity (American Lung Association, n.d.).

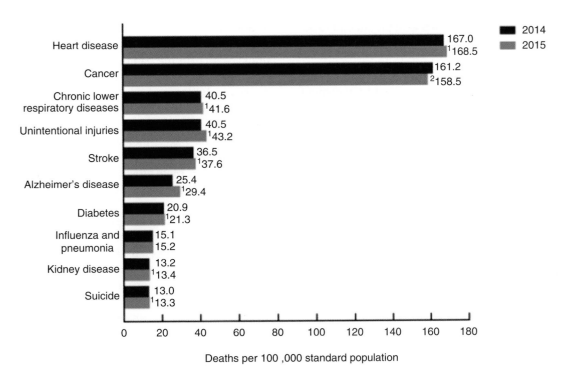

FIG. 4.6 Leading causes of death, United States, 2014–2015. (From Centers for Disease Control and Prevention, National Center for Chronic Disease: Age-adjusted death rates for the 10 leading causes of death in 2015: United States, 2014 and 2015. NCHS, National vital statistics system, Mortality. Retrieved from https://www.cdc.gov/nchs/products/databriefs/db267.htm.)

TABLE 4.4	Relationship Between Risk Factors and 10 Leading Causes of Death								
Cause of Death	Percentage of Total Deaths	Smoking	High-Fat, Low-Fiber Diet	Sedentary Lifestyle	High Blood Pressure	Elevated Cholesterol	Obesity	Diabetes	Alcohol Abuse
Heart disease	25	X	X	X	X	X	X	X	X
Cancer	23	X	X	X			X		X
Stroke	6	X	X		X	X	X		
Chronic obstructive pulmonary disease (COPD)	5	X							
Unintentional injury	5	X							X
Diabetes	3		X	X			X	X	
Alzheimer disease	3		X	X					
All other causes	29	X							

From Centers for Disease Control and Prevention. *Health United States 2010.* Retrieved from http://www.cdc.gov/heartdisease/statistical_reports.htm.

Most smokers are between the ages of 18 and 44 years, and more men than women smoke. In 2015, 16.7% of adult men and 13.6% of adult women were smokers. The prevalence of smoking is highest among American Indians/Alaskan Natives and Caucasians. Smoking is most common among adults who are less educated and adults who live below the poverty level. Kentucky, West Virginia, Oklahoma, and Mississippi have the highest rates of smokers, with Utah, California, and Idaho having the lowest rates (CDC, 2016). Persons with a disability smoke at a higher rate than do persons without a disability.

Gay, lesbian, and bisexual adults are more likely to smoke than straight Americans (CDC, 2016).

More than 70% of current smokers report that they would like to quit smoking (CDC, n.d.). Nicotine addiction is the most common form of chemical dependence in the United States. Smokers who are trying to quit experience withdrawal symptoms such as anxiety, increased appetite, irritability, and difficulty concentrating. These symptoms make quitting difficult, and most people relapse several times before being able to quit successfully. Nicotine replacement, pharmaceutical alternatives, hypnosis, and acupuncture may be helpful in the attempt to quit smoking. The American Cancer Society recommends the following steps to quit smoking:

- Make the decision to quit. Any change is scary, and smoking cessation is a big change, requiring a long-term commitment.
- Set a date to quit and choose a plan.
- Mark the date on your calendar.
- Tell your family and friends about the date, and ask for their support.
- Get rid of all tobacco products, ashtrays, and lighters in your environment.
- Stock up on oral substitutes such as sugarless gum, hard candy, fruit, and carrot sticks.
- Decide on a plan and prepare to implement it; register for the stop-smoking class, or see your doctor about nicotine replacement therapy or pharmaceutical alternatives.
- Practice saying "No thank you, I don't smoke."
- Think back to your previous attempts to quit and see what worked and what did not work.
- If you are taking bupropion or varenicline, take your medication each day of the week leading up to your quit day.
  Deal with withdrawal by:
- Avoiding temptation.
- Changing your habits. Walk when you are stressed or during breaks. Use hard candy, carrot sticks, or gum to satisfy the need to put something in your mouth. If you feel the urge to light up, tell yourself that you are going to wait 10 minutes before giving in. Usually, the urge will pass within that time.
- Staying off of tobacco is a lifelong process. Many former smokers state that they experienced strong desires to smoke after weeks, months, even years of smoking cessation. These unexpected cravings can be difficult to deal with.
- Remind yourself of the reasons why you quit.
- Wait out the craving. There is no such thing as just one cigarette or just one puff.
- Avoid alcohol.
- Begin an exercise program and work on eating a healthy diet to avoid gaining weight (American Cancer Society, 2016).

Information on quitting can be accessed at the CDC website at http://www.cdc.gov/tobacco/quit_smoking/how_to_quit/index.htm. The American Lung Association also has information on smoking cessation at http://www.lung.org/stop-smoking/. The American Cancer Society offers a quit-smoking guide at https://www.cancer.org/healthy/stay-away-from-tobacco/guide-quitting-smoking/deciding-to-quit-smoking-and-making-a-plan.html.

It is important to remember that smokers who are trying to quit smoking need support, and most families and loved ones want to help. The American Cancer Society has suggestions for supporting someone who is quitting smoking at https://www.cancer.org/healthy/stay-away-from-tobacco/helping-a-smoker-quit.html.

Teens are a population of concern regarding smoking. Though the rate of smoking has declined among Americans since the 1990s, more high school juniors and seniors smoke than do adults. Half of high school–aged smokers have tried to quit at least once. Those who start using tobacco in their teens have a harder time giving up smoking later in life. Most smokers pick up the habit at age 18, with very few initiating smoking after the age of 25 (American Cancer Society, 2012). A resource for teens who are trying to quit smoking is available at http://www.lung.org/associations/states/colorado/tobacco/not-on-tobacco/.

Only 4% to 7% of smokers are able to quit smoking on any attempt without pharmaceutical or other interventions to help them, so nurses must provide information and referrals to help clients access resources that help them to get off and to stay off tobacco.

Smokeless tobacco also poses a health threat. Commonly called *spit tobacco,* smokeless tobacco is a significant health threat and is not a safe substitute for smoking tobacco. Smokeless tobacco is known to be a cause of cancer and oral health problems. Smokeless tobacco causes nicotine addiction and dependence, and adolescents who use smokeless tobacco are more likely to take up smoking. Smoking bans may be increasing the use of smokeless tobacco as smokers use these products in settings where smoking is prohibited (CDC, 2014).

In the United States, 3% of adults use smokeless tobacco, with far more men (7%) than women (0.4%) using it. It is estimated that 6% of high school students use smokeless tobacco. Smokeless tobacco use is more common among young white males, with its heaviest use among those living in the southern or north central states and among blue collar workers, service workers, and laborers as well as the unemployed. American Indian/Alaska Natives are the heaviest users of smokeless tobacco, followed by whites. School nurses are in an important position to intervene early in the use of smokeless tobacco. Most smokeless tobacco use begins in middle school, and interventions to prevent or stop this habit are essential in the school setting (CDC, 2014).

The clinical implications of tobacco use are clear. First, community health nurses must ask about tobacco use at every clinic visit or home visit and look for teachable moments, when the client may be interested in discussing his or her tobacco habit (a respiratory illness or a scare with an oral lesion may prompt the client to reconsider the habit). Assess the client's tobacco use: "Do you use tobacco?" "What kind of tobacco (cigarettes, cigars, chewing tobacco, pipe) do you use?" "How much do you smoke (dip, chew)?" "Have you thought about quitting?" Explore with the client why he or she may or may not have considered giving up the tobacco habit and what options are available to help should he or she desire to quit. Refer the client to smoking cessation websites or other health care professionals for assistance in quitting. Chances are great that the client is very well acquainted with the health risks posed by tobacco but not with the options for helping him or her to quit. Encourage the client to attempt to give up tobacco, and encourage him or her in any attempts to decrease or stop the use of tobacco.

Alcohol Consumption and Health

Alcohol use is very common in our society. In 2010, half of Americans reported being current drinkers, with 5% reporting being heavy drinkers and 17% engaging in binge drinking.

Though only 6% of the U.S. population is addicted to alcohol, about 25% of the population drinks excessively. One in five adults reported drinking five or more drinks per day. Men are more likely (63%) than women (55%) to be current drinkers and to binge drink. Men are also more than twice as likely to suffer death or injury related to drinking. Nationally, women are nearly twice as likely as men to be lifetime abstainers, yet one in two women of childbearing age drinks alcohol (NIH, 2010).

Binge drinking is an unrecognized problem among women and girls. One in five high school–aged girls and one in eight adult women reported binge drinking. The intensity and frequency of binge drinking are similar among pregnant and non-pregnant women: about three times per month and six drinks per occasion (Marchetta et al., 2012). It takes less alcohol for females to become impaired than males because of body size and differences in the way alcohol is processed by females. About 7.6% of women use alcohol while pregnant, with about 1 in 20 women using alcohol heavily before discovering that they are pregnant. For both men and women, those aged 25 to 44 years had the highest prevalence of drinking. The drinking prevalence declines at age 44 years and declines steadily with age thereafter. Non-Hispanic white people have the highest drinking prevalence, with non-Hispanic white men being the heaviest drinkers (CDC, October 16, 2016).

Alcohol use, particularly heavy alcohol use, is responsible for many health problems such as liver disease and for unintentional injuries. *Excessive alcohol use* is drinking more than two drinks per day on average for men or more than one drink per day for women; *binge drinking* is drinking five or more drinks on a single occasion for men or four or more drinks in a single occasion for women. Binge drinking is the most common form of excess alcohol use in America. Most people who binge drink are not alcohol dependent. A *drink* is any drink containing 0.6 ounces or 1.2 tablespoons of pure alcohol. A drink is:

- 12 ounces of beer or wine cooler
- 8 ounces of malt liquor
- 5 ounces of wine
- 1.5 ounces of 80-proof distilled spirits or liquor (gin, rum, vodka, whiskey) (CDC, July 25, 2016)

The *Dietary Guidelines for Americans* states that alcohol should be consumed in moderation—no more than one drink per day for women and no more than two drinks per day for men (USDHHS, 2015). People who should not drink are those who:

- Are less than 21 years of age
- Are taking medications that can cause harmful reactions when mixed with alcohol
- Are pregnant or trying to become pregnant
- Are recovering from alcoholism or are unable to control the amount that they drink
- Have a medical condition that may be worsened by alcohol
- Are driving or planning to drive or to perform activities requiring coordination and concentration (USDHHS, 2015)

Responsible for 80,000 deaths annually, alcohol use is the third leading lifestyle-related cause of death for the nation. In 2006 there were more than 1.2 million emergency department visits for alcohol-related conditions. The short-term risks of alcohol consumption are usually due to binge drinking or excess drinking and include risky sexual behavior, violence, unintentional injuries from motor vehicle accidents, falls, firearms, and drowning. Miscarriage or stillbirth and alcohol poisoning are also possible immediate effects of excessive alcohol use. The long-term risks of alcohol use are neurological conditions such as dementia and stroke; cardiovascular problems such as MI, hypertension, and cardiomyopathy; psychiatric problems such as depression and anxiety; social problems such as unemployment and family dysfunction; cancer of the mouth, throat, liver, and breast; and liver disease, including cirrhosis and hepatitis. Pancreatitis and gastritis are other gastrointestinal consequences of long-term alcohol consumption (CDC, July 25, 2016).

The prevalence of underage drinking declined significantly when states established the minimum legal drinking age as 21 years, and those states with more stringent drinking laws have a lower prevalence of adult and underage binge drinking. Despite age limits for legal consumption of alcohol, alcohol is the number-one used and abused drug among U.S. youth. People aged 12 to 20 drink 11% of all alcohol consumed annually in the United States, 90% of it during binge drinking. Alcohol consumption contributes to more than 43,000 deaths among underage youth annually, and 20% of youth aged 12 to 20 reported drinking alcohol in 2011. Initiation to alcohol begins early: a national report found that 33% of eighth graders had tried alcohol and 13% had drunk alcohol in the previous month. Youth who start drinking prior to age 15 are six times more likely to experience alcohol dependence or abuse than those who begin drinking at or after 21 years of age. The prevalence of adult binge drinking behavior is strongly predictive of binge drinking behavior by college students living in the same state (CDC, October 20, 2016).

Clinical implications for health promotion related to alcohol consumption emphasize prevention of underage drinking and identifying and assisting groups and individuals at risk for alcohol abuse and dependence. A helpful resource for locating and contacting local agencies for alcohol treatment is the National Drug and Alcohol Treatment Referral Routing Service, available at 1-800-662-HELP. Alcohol Screening and Brief Intervention (SBI) consists of screening for those who are at risk for excessive alcohol consumption and providing brief counseling. In trauma centers and emergency departments where SBI has been implemented, medical costs and readmissions related to alcohol have been reduced (CDC, 2015).

Preventing underage drinking is a public health priority. Enforcement of the legal drinking age, as well as enforcement of bans on sales of alcohol to minors, is an important aspect of prevention. Increased excise tax on alcoholic beverages has also been found to decrease underage drinking. Education of both adults and youth regarding alcohol and the myriad of risks posed by underage alcohol consumption must accompany enforcement efforts. The "Too Smart to Start" program targets parents and caregivers of 9- to 13-year-olds. The goal of the program is to increase the percentage of youth and their caregivers who view underage drinking unfavorably (CDC, October 17, 2016).

Preventing excessive alcohol consumption must consider several prominent environmental factors:

- Alcohol is cheap.
- Alcohol is readily available.
- Americans are exposed to $4 billion of alcohol advertising per year.
- New alcohol products cater to youthful tastes and may promote underage drinking (U.S. Department of Justice, 2002).

Decreasing the morbidity and mortality related to overconsumption of alcohol requires a community-wide effort to address the problem on several fronts. Youth tend to model their drinking behavior after adults, and adults are often the source of alcohol for many youth, meaning that interventions must be aimed at the population across the lifespan. Interventions supported by research include:

- Increase taxes on alcohol—a 10% increase in price results in a 7% decrease in alcohol consumption.
- Decrease alcohol outlet density—higher outlet density is associated with greater alcohol consumption and negative impacts of alcohol.
- Hold alcohol retailers responsible for harm caused by inebriated or underage drinkers.

Diet and Health

Diet is one of the most modifiable of risk factors. A healthy diet contributes to the prevention of such chronic diseases as type 2 diabetes, hypertension, heart disease, and some cancers. With 17% of U.S. children 2 to 19 years and 36.5% of U.S. adults being obese (Ogden et al., 2016), diet is an important topic in health promotion. Americans are bombarded with nutrition information, and many are confused and have no idea how to apply the information regarding diet that they have received. As portion sizes get larger, Americans of all ages are spending more time engaged in inactive pursuits such as watching TV and using a computer. Commonly, the terms "portion" and "serving" are misused. A *portion* is the "amount of a single food item served in a single eating occasion." A meal or a snack is a single eating occasion, with the amount of green beans or roast beef on your plate being the portion. A *serving* is a "standardized unit of measuring foods" used in dietary guidelines. A cup or an ounce is an example of a serving size (CDC, 2006).

What does it mean to be overweight or obese? Both of these terms are used to indicate a condition of excess weight for height. Both terms also identify ranges of weight that have been found to be associated with an increased risk of certain diseases or conditions. The body mass index (BMI) is used to determine weight status in adults and children. The BMI takes both height and weight into account and has been found to correlate well with the amount of body fat present. An adult with a BMI of 25 to 29.9 is considered overweight, and an adult with a BMI of 30 or higher is considered obese. Though there are many contributing factors to overweight and obesity, controlling one's weight is a matter of balancing caloric intake with physical activity. Too many calories in and too few calories out eventually result in overweight. Fig. 4.7 illustrates this energy balance.

FIG. 4.7 Caloric balance equation. (From Centers for Disease Control and Prevention: *Overweight and obesity: An overview,* 2009. Retrieved from www.cdc.gov/nccdphp/dnpa/obesity/contributing_factors.htm.)

The rate of obesity in the United States was unchanged from 2003 to 2004 and 2011 to 2012; no state met the *Healthy People 2010* goal to reduce the obesity prevalence to 15%. California, Colorado, Massachusetts, Montana, Utah, Hawaii, and the District of Columbia had the lowest prevalence rates of between 20% and 25% (CDC, April 10, 2017). Persons aged 40 to 59 are most likely to be overweight in the United States (40.2%), and obesity rates vary among races and ethnicities. Non-Hispanic black persons have the highest rates of obesity (48.1%), followed by Hispanics (42.5%), and non-Hispanic whites (34.5%) (CDC, April 10, 2017. See Fig. 4.8 for specific details on trends in obesity.

Though most obese Americans could not be classified as low income, the prevalence of obesity among women rises as income decreases, with 42% of women whose income is at or below the poverty level being obese. The prevalence of obesity among women also rises as education level decreases. Among men, there is no correlation between obesity prevalence, education, or income level.

Obesity is also a concern for children. Since 1976 the prevalence of childhood obesity has increased, with 17% of children between the ages of 2 and 19 being obese. From 1999 to 2008 there was no trend in obesity prevalence for any age group among children. There are ethnic disparities in childhood obesity, with Mexican American adolescents having a significantly higher rate of obesity (21.9%) than non-Hispanic white adolescents (14.5%).

As rates of obesity have risen, so has the cost associated with the health comorbidities of obesity. It is well known that obesity is related to the most common causes of death—heart disease, stroke, some cancers, and type 2 diabetes. In 2008, medical costs associated with obesity were estimated to be approximately $147 billion, with obese persons each costing $1429 more in medical expenditures than individuals of normal weight. It is estimated that about 27% of the increase in health care spending between 1987 and 2001 was related to obesity, and about half of this cost was paid for by Medicare and Medicaid. An obese beneficiary

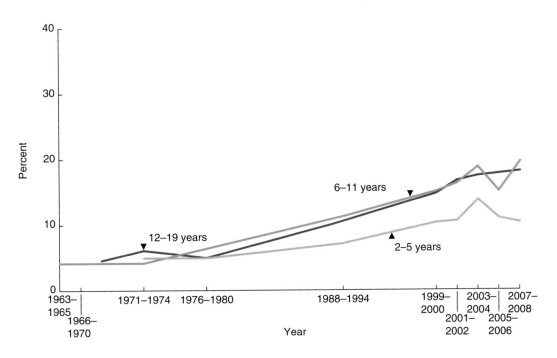

NOTE: Obesity is defined as body mass index (BMI) greater than or equal to sex- and age-specific 95th percentile from the 2000 CDC Growth Charts.

FIG. 4.8 Trends in obesity among children and adolescents: United States, 1963–2008. (From Ogden C, Carroll M: Prevalence of obesity among children and adolescents: United States, 1963–1965 through 2007–2008, 2010, NCHS Health E-Stat, 2010. Retrieved from – http://www.cdc.gov/nchs/data/hestat/obesity_child_07_08/obesity_child_07_08.htm. Data from CDC/NCHS, National Health Examination Surveys II [ages 6–11], III [ages 12–17] and National Health and Nutrition Examination Surveys [NHANES] I–III, and NHANES 1999–2000, 2001–2002, 2003–2004, 2005–2006, and 2007–2008.)

costs Medicare more than $600 more annually than a beneficiary of normal weight.

Fats are an essential nutrient for energy and serve many purposes in the body, but too much fat in the diet, especially trans-fats, saturated fats, and cholesterol, may increase the risk of heart disease (U.S. Department of Agriculture [USDA]/USDHHS, 2010). Trans-fatty acids are deleterious to health, leading to an increased risk for heart disease and stroke. The Food and Drug Administration revoked the "generally recognized as safe" status for trans-fatty acids on June 16, 2015, and gave food manufactures until June 2018 to remove trans-fats from their products. Most trans-fats are found in fried foods, margarine, pizza, and commercially prepared baked goods such as cookies. New York City instituted restrictions on trans-fatty acids in commercial eateries beginning July 1, 2007.

In 2013, the median intake of fruits and vegetables for adults in the United States was only 1.6 times per day. Only 70% of census tracts report having retail establishments that sell healthier food within the census tract or within 1 half-mile of the census tract boundary. Though the benefits of eating a diet rich in fruits and vegetables is well known, this trend is unchanged since 1996 (USDA/USDHHS, 2013). The CDC has information on incorporating fruits and vegetables into a daily diet at https://www.cdc.gov/healthyweight/healthy_eating/index.html.

Although the same eating plan is not appropriate for everyone, the USDA does make some key recommendations regarding a healthy diet based on a 2000 calorie per day intake, as follows:

- Select 2 cups of fruit and 2½ cups of vegetables per day. Select a variety of colors and types.
- Consume three or more 1-ounce-equivalent servings per day of whole-grain products.
- Consume 3 cups per day of fat-free or low-fat milk or milk products.
- Keep total fat intake to 20% to 35% of caloric intake.
- When choosing fats, emphasize lean meats, beans, poultry, and fat-free or low-fat milk products.
- Limit intake of trans-fatty acids or saturated fats.
- Choose fiber-rich fruits and vegetables often.
- Prepare beverages and foods with little added sugar.
- Consume less than 1 teaspoon of salt per day.
- Consume alcoholic beverages moderately—up to one drink per day for women and two drinks per day for men.

Special populations such as pregnant or lactating women, infants, children, older adults, athletic or very active adults, and adolescents have differing nutritional needs.

The USDA recommends that all Americans go to http://www.choosemyplate.gov/ to develop a personalized eating plan based on individual needs and preferences. *My Plate* (Fig. 4.9) was released in 2011, replacing the Food Guide Pyramid. This tool helps users easily translate the USDA guidelines into the kinds and amounts of food to eat each day. *My Plate* is

FIG. 4.9 *My Plate* logo. (From the United States Department of Agriculture. (n.d.). *My Plate* 2013, Retrieved from http://www.choosemyplate.gov/print-materials-ordering/graphic-resources.html.)

applicable to children as well as adults and is simple and fun enough that children can use it themselves. *My Plate* illustrates a healthful eating plan in a simple and familiar format—a place setting. The key messages of *My Plate* are that half of the plate should be fruits and vegetables; a quarter of the plate should be grains, and half of the grains consumed daily should be whole grain; one quarter of the plate should be protein; and a serving of a low-fat or nonfat dairy product should be included in each meal. Oils, a source of essential nutrients, are also included in *My Plate*, with the emphasis on oils low in trans-fats. The Choose My Plate homepage at http://www.choosemyplate.gov/ contains information on eating on a budget, weight management, and a food and activity tracker to help users balance food intake with activity. Many popular foods, such as pizza and spaghetti, are mixed dishes in that they do not fit into only one food group.

Studies confirm that eating away from home is associated with an increased likelihood of being overweight (Bauer et al., 2012 Rafferty). Busy families have more opportunities to eat away from home as the number of eateries has increased in recent years. The latest findings indicate that from 1999 to 2004, American families spent 45% of their food budget on foods eaten away from home (The Keystone Center, 2006). Though parental employment is a benefit to families, the stresses of balancing family and work demands affect nutrition and the kinds of foods consumed. Families with parents who work full time spend less time on food preparation, eat fewer family meals, eat more fast food, and spend less time encouraging healthful eating behaviors (Bauer et al., 2012). Men between ages 40 and 59 years consume the most food prepared away from home (Van der Horst et al., 2011). (This author can attest to the fact that when her 53-year-old husband is left to fend for himself at mealtime, he will most likely eat out.) Adolescents also consume a large amount of fast food, with 30% of adolescent males and 27% of adolescent females reporting eating fast food at least three times per week (Bauer et al., 2009). Among adults the percentage of calories consumed from fast food rises as weight status increases, with obese adults consuming the highest percentage of their calories from fast food (Fryar and Ervin,

2013). Economics can also determine the quality of a family's diet, with families with lower incomes having a poorer-quality diet than do families with higher incomes. Research has found that families with less money to spend on food eat diets lower in fruits and vegetables than do families who have more money to spend on food (Rehm et al., 2015).

Portions served in restaurants are larger than portions served at home, in some cases up to 40% larger. Convenience foods and prepackaged foods contain larger portion sizes than in the 1970s. When presented with a large portion size, individuals often unknowingly eat larger amounts than they would usually eat or than they intend to eat. This phenomenon, called **portion distortion**, occurs frequently when people are dining out (NHLBI, 2013). Portion control is an important aspect of weight management, and distortion of portion sizes makes this difficult task harder. There are several reasons why we tend to overeat when we eat away from home: foods presented in restaurants are high in energy density (high number of calories for a particular weight of food); restaurant foods are very palatable and there is a wide variety of this great-tasting food to choose from; and we want to get more food for our money, so we order the larger entrées (The Keystone Center, 2006).

For many people, eating at home all the time is impossible or impractical, and food is central to many social interactions. In order to consume fewer calories when eating out, one may:
- Patronize establishments that offer a variety of food choices and are willing to make substitutions or changes
- Order lower-fat steamed, broiled, baked, roasted, or poached items, or ask that an item be prepared in a lower-calorie way, such as grilled rather than fried
- Choose lower-calorie sauces or condiments, or do without them altogether
- Substitute colorful vegetables for other side dishes (such as French fries)
- Ask for half of the meal to be boxed to take home before the meal is brought to the table
- Share an entrée with someone
- Order a vegetarian meal
- Select a fruit for dessert

To decrease reliance on away-from-home foods, plan ahead and:
- Pack healthy snacks to avoid the use of vending machines
- Cook a healthful dinner at home, and make extra to pack for lunch the next day
- Purchase healthful foods when grocery shopping to pack for lunch, such as prepackaged salads, fresh fruits, vegetables, and low-calorie soups
- For travel or longer excursions, bring along nutritious foods that will not spoil, such as fresh fruits and vegetables, or pack a cooler with healthy foods

Various online communities and other support groups are available to help individuals manage their weight. Social media is harnessing the power of the Internet to help the public meet fitness goals. Sites such as Sparkpeople and Livestrong offer interactive and social networking opportunities. Group support is helpful for those who want them, whereas others prefer to have programs that they can implement on their own. The cost to join a weight management community ranges from free to moderate in price. Another popular option for weight control is the large selection of applications for mobile devices. With these applications it is possible to easily track foods eaten and calories expended throughout the day. Many are free and available for mobile devices.

Physical Activity and Health

There are many reasons why people engage in physical activity and exercise: for weight management, increased energy, or better appearance; to fit into those favorite jeans; to prevent development or worsening of a chronic health condition; to manage stress; to improve mood and self-esteem; or any combination of these reasons.

Several factors acting individually and in concert can affect the likelihood that one is physically active. Men are a little more likely to engage in leisure physical activity and are more likely to engage in strength training than are women. The percentage of adults who engage in leisure-time physical activity decreases with age, from its highest among adults aged 18 to 24 years. White adults and Asian adults are more likely to engage in leisure-time physical activity than are black and Hispanic adults. The percentage of adults participating in leisure-time physical activity increases with level of education; adults with advanced degrees are twice as likely to engage in some physical activity than are high school graduates. The percentage of adults who engage in regular leisure-time physical activity also increases with income level. Adults whose income is four times the federal poverty level are nearly twice as likely to engage in some form of regular leisure-time physical activity than are adults whose income is below the poverty level. Adults living in the southern region of the United States get the least amount of leisure-time physical activity (CDC, May 23, 2014).

As has been previously mentioned, one's surroundings also affect whether one will choose to exercise. The Walk Score has ranked cities across the United States for suitability for walking. So what makes a city walkable?

- A center: It may be a shopping center, park, or main street.
- Mixed use, mixed income: Businesses are located next to homes at all price points.
- Pedestrian-centric design: Businesses are close to the street to encourage foot traffic with parking in back.
- Density: The city is compact enough to allow businesses to flourish and for public transportation to run frequently.
- Parks and public spaces: There are plenty of public areas in which to gather.
- Nearby schools and workplaces: Schools and workplaces are close enough that most people can walk from home (Walk Score, 2013).

Research has found that one's environment is a significant factor in health promotion. Adults and adolescents living in neighborhoods with high walkability engage in significantly more walking and cycling than those living in neighborhoods with low walkability. As a result, the rates of obesity are lower in communities that are walkable than in communities that do not encourage physical activity (Brown et al., 2013; CDC, 2015; Slater et al., Chriqui, 2013).

How much exercise do I need? What counts as exercise? Nurses in the community hear these questions commonly as they educate the public on the need to increase physical activity. The answers to these questions depend on the age, physical condition, and gender of the client. The CDC website at https://www.cdc.gov/physicalactivity/basics/index.htm presents the amount of exercise recommended for adults and children. Videos on the website further explain and illustrate the use of these guidelines. People may feel overwhelmed by the idea that they must add one more demand to an already busy schedule, and some think, "I'm in such bad shape, I'll never be able to exercise." The most important idea is that one must take a first step to try exercise. Walking, biking, taking the stairs, swimming—there is something for everyone, and any exercise is better than none. Exercise may also be broken up into smaller blocks of time during the day if it is not possible or convenient to do it all at once. Physical activity can also be a family affair, with the entire family using the time to reconnect and have fun together. Walking has been found to be one of the most beneficial exercises. It does not require special skills or expensive equipment, and many people with disabilities are able to participate in a walking program using assistive devices. Walking is an easy form of physical activity to perform and to maintain. Walking is a safe activity with a lower likelihood of injury than more vigorous forms of exercise. And it is a good activity for those who are physically inactive, as it can be adapted to one's abilities, time, and circumstances.

⁉ ACTIVE LEARNING EXERCISE

1. How is your community doing in comparison with other communities? Prevalence and incidence rates for diseases or health conditions allow us to make comparisons between communities. Rates of activities such as smoking and physical activity allow us to make comparisons between communities regarding other areas of health promotion. Consider a community of which you are a member (e.g., your state, your county, your age group, or your school). Choose a health promotion topic that is of particular importance to your community of interest, such as sexual health, obesity, communicable disease, or physical activity. How does your community compare with a similar community in a different area of the state or the country? How does your community compare with a similar community in another part of the world?
2. View the Institute of Medicine series *Weight of the Nation* at http://theweightofthenation.hbo.com/. As you watch the series consider the following: What is the largest contributing factor to obesity among children? What interventions can you think of that would be effective in preventing or reducing obesity prevalence in your community? What are common barriers to preventing or reducing obesity among people across the lifespan? What negative effects will the United States as a whole face due to obesity?

Sleep

Sleep is an essential component of chronic disease prevention and health promotion, yet 74% of adults report having a sleeping problem one or more nights per week. One-quarter of the U.S. population reports that they occasionally do not get enough sleep, 39% report getting less than 7 hours of sleep

TABLE 4.5	How Much Sleep Do We Really Need?
Age	**Sleep Needs**
Newborns (1–2 mo)	10.5–18 hr
Infants (3–11 mo)	9–12 hr during night and 30-min to 2-hr naps, 1–4 hr a day
Toddlers (1–3 yr)	12–14 hr
Preschoolers (3–5 yr)	11–13 hr
School-aged children (5–12 yr)	10–11 hr
Teens (11–17 yr)	8.5–9.25 hr
Adults	7–9 hr
Older adults	7–9 hr

Used with permission of the National Sleep Foundation. For further information, please visit www.sleepfoundation.org/how-much-sleep-do-we-really-need.

per night, and 37% report being so sleepy during the day that it interferes with daily activities. Insufficient sleep is associated with diabetes, heart disease, obesity, and depression. Insufficient sleep contributes to 100,000 motor vehicle crashes each year and 15,000 deaths. Sleep requirements change as people age (Table 4.5), and depending on life circumstances, one may require more than the minimum hours listed. If a person is so tired or sleepy that it interferes with his or her daily activities, that person probably needs more sleep (National Sleep Foundation, n.d.).

As we age, sleep is often interrupted by pain, trips to the bathroom, medications, medical conditions, and sleep disorders. In order to get enough sleep, we must plan to set aside enough time for sleep. Preferably, this means that we can awaken naturally, without an alarm clock, ensuring adequate rest. The need for sleep is regulated by two processes. One is the number of hours we are awake. The longer we are awake, the stronger the desire is to sleep. The other process is the circadian biological clock in the brain, the suprachiasmatic nucleus, which responds to light. This clock makes us tend to be sleepy at night when it is dark and to be active during the day when it is light. The circadian rhythm is why we are sleepiest between 2:00 and 4:00 AM and 1:00 and 3:00 PM. The circadian rhythm also regulates the 24-hour cycle of the body. While we sleep, important hormones are released, memory is consolidated, blood pressure is decreased, and kidney function changes (National Sleep Foundation, n.d.).

One of the results of lack of sleep is drowsy driving. More than one-third of U.S. drivers admit to having fallen asleep while driving, and 4% have had an accident due to driving while drowsy. An estimated 1550 deaths result from driver fatigue annually. Sleep-related motor vehicle accidents are most common among young people, shift workers, men, and adults with children. Adults between 18 and 29 years of age are the most likely to drive when sleepy. The less people sleep, the greater their risk for being involved in a vehicular crash. People who sleep 6 to 7 hours per night are twice as likely to be involved in a crash as those sleeping 8 hours per night or more. People sleeping 4 to 5 hours have a four to five times higher risk of being involved in a sleep-related accident. Being awake for 18

hours produces the same degree of impairment as being legally intoxicated (National Sleep Foundation, 2013).

Practicing sleep hygiene will help achieve optimum sleep, as follows:

- Avoid caffeine and nicotine close to bedtime.
- Avoid alcohol, as it can cause sleep disruptions.
- Go to bed and get up at the same time every day.
- Exercise regularly, but finish all exercise and vigorous activity at least 3 hours before bedtime.
- Establish a regular, relaxing bedtime routine (a warm bath, reading a book).
- Create a dark, quiet, cool sleep environment.
- Have a comfortable mattress and bedding.
- Use the bed for sleep only; do not read, listen to music, or watch TV in bed.
- Avoid large meals before bedtime (National Sleep Foundation, n.d.).

Sleep assessment is an important nursing function. If a client reports snoring, apnea, restlessness, or insomnia, he or she may have a sleep disorder. Recommend keeping a sleep log that details how many hours are spent in sleep each night and any problems with sleep. If insufficient sleep is causing trouble concentrating or completing daily activities, recommend consulting a doctor, as a sleep disorder may be to blame. A sleep assessment tool and a list of sleep disorders and descriptions of each may be found at the National Sleep Foundation's website, at http://www.sleepfoundation.org/.

Because of the 24-hour-per-day nature of nursing, nurses are among many workers who must work night shifts. Negative physical effects of working nights include an increased risk for stroke and heart disease, increased development of metabolic syndrome, and irregular menstrual cycles. Sleep deprivation related to shift work can cause practice errors related to a lack of attention to detail, impaired psychomotor skills, and reduced coordination, among others.

Those who work night shifts often experience *shift work disorder*. Shift work disorder is caused by night shifts, rotating shifts, and sometimes morning shifts. It causes chronic sleep deprivation in which a person never catches up on needed sleep. This sleep deprivation affects one's health, safety, productivity, and quality of life. Many shift workers struggle with excess sleepiness during work or leisure hours that interferes with their ability to work, study, or engage in social activities.

The National Sleep Foundation has helpful ways to cope with shift work disorder at https://sleepfoundation.org/shift-work/content/living-coping-shift-work-disorder.

❓ ACTIVE LEARNING EXERCISE

How do people, groups, and populations meet health promotion goals? Interview someone who is successful at meeting his or her health promotion goals. For example: How did the person manage to keep his or her weight at a healthy level? How did the person stop smoking? How does he or she make time to exercise daily? Does the individual have a philosophy of health that helps him or her stay on track with health promotion goals? How does the individual incorporate health promotion into daily life? What advice does he or she have for others striving to achieve better health?

SUMMARY

Health promotion is an essential component to ongoing good health and well-being, yet many Americans have difficulty with one or more of the components of health promotion. Exercise, diet, sleep, and tobacco and alcohol use all affect our health. Nurses, particularly community health nurses, are in a position to assess and counsel clients on their health habits. Community health nurses also possess the unique combination of community familiarity and the knowledge and training to affect health at the policy level. As the environment is made safer and more walkable, or with a lower density of available alcohol or fast food, the community as a whole will benefit.

EVOLVE WEBSITE

http://evolve.elsevier.com/Nies/community

- NCLEX Review Questions
- Case Studies

BIBLIOGRAPHY

American Cancer Society: *Child and teen tobacco use*, November 8, 2012. Available from: <http://www.cancer.org/cancer/cancer-causes/tobaccocancer/childandteentobaccouse/child-and-teen-tobacco-use-child-and-teen-tobacco-use>. Accessed February 27, 2013.

American Cancer Society: *Guide to quitting smoking*, April 19, 2016. Available from: https://www.cancer.org/healthy/stay-away-from-tobacco/guide-quitting-smoking/deciding-to-quit-smoking-and-making-a-plan.html. Accessed April 7, 2017.

American Cancer Society: *Helping a smoker quit*, October 2016. Available from: https://www.cancer.org/healthy/stay-away-from-tobacco/helping-a-smoker-quit.html. Accessed April 7, 2017.

American Lung Association: *Quit smoking*, n.d. Available from: <http://www.lung.org/stop-smoking/>. Accessed January 9, 2014.

Atkinson LN, Saperstein LS, Pleis J: Using the internet for health-related activities: findings from a national probability sample, *J Med Internet Res* 11(1):e4, 2009.

Bauer KW, Hearst MO, Escoto K: Parental environments and work-family stress: associations with family food environments, *Soc Sci Med* 75:496–504, 2012.

Bauer KW, Larson NI, Nelson MC: Fast food intake among adolescents: secular and longitudinal trends from 1999-2004, *Prev Med* 48:284–287, 2009.

Benson H: *Timeless healing: the power and biology of belief*, New York, 1996, Scribner.

Brown BB, Smith KR, Hanson H: Neighborhood design for walking and biking: physical activity and body mass index, *Am J Prev Med* 44:23–238, 2013.

Burger KS, Kern M, Coleman KJ: Characteristics of self-selected portion sizes in young adults [electronic version], *J Am Diet Assoc* 107:611–1608, 2007.

Centers for Disease Control and Prevention: *Smoking cessation* (n.d.), January 2, 2013. Available from: <http://www.cdc.gov/tobacco/data_statistics/fact_sheets/cessation/quitting/index.htm>. Accessed August 22, 2013.

Centers for Disease Control and Prevention: *Do increased portion sizes affect how much we eat? Nutrition resources for health professionals*, May 2006. Available from <www.cdc.gov/nccdphp/dnpa/nutrition/pdf/portion_size_research.pdf>. Accessed April 20, 2009.

Centers for Disease Control and Prevention: *US obesity trends 1985-2007: overweight and obesity*, July 24, 2008. Available from: <www.cdc.gov/nccdphp/dnpa/obesity/trend/maps/index.htm>. Accessed April 19, 2009.

Centers for Disease Control and Prevention: *Quick stats: age 21 legal minimum drinking age. alcohol and public health*, September 3, 2008. Available from: <www.cdc.gov/alcohol/quickstats/mlda.htm>. Accessed May 04, 2009.

Centers for Disease Control and Prevention: *Incorporating eaten-away-from-home food into a healthy eating plan: nutrition resources for health professionals*, December 22, 2008. Available from: <www.cdc.gov/nccdphp/dnpa/nutrition/pdf/r2p_away_from_home_food.pdf>. Accessed April 13, 2009.

Centers for Disease Control and Prevention: *Excessive alcohol use and risks to women's health*, October 1, 2012. Available from: <http://www.cdc.gov/alcohol/fact-sheets/womens-health.htm>. Accessed February 28, 2012.

Centers for Disease Control and Prevention: *Ways to reduce cancer risk*, January 2, 2013. Available from: <http://www.cdc.gov/cancer/dcpc/prevention/other.htm>. Accessed February 25, 2013.

Centers for Disease Control and Prevention: *Smokeless tobacco use in the United States*, 2014. Available at https://www.cdc.gov/tobacco/data_statistics/fact_sheets/smokeless/use_us/index.htm. Accessed April 7, 2017.

Centers for Disease Control and Prevention: *Facts about physical activity*, May 23, 2014. Available from: https://www.cdc.gov/physicalactivity/data/facts.htm. Accessed April 17, 2017.

Centers for Disease Control and Prevention: *Alcohol screening*, April 21, 2015. Available from: https://www.cdc.gov/features/alcoholscreening/index.html. Accessed April 13, 2017.

Centers for Disease Control and Prevention: *Alcohol use and health*, July 25, 2016. Available from: https://www.cdc.gov/alcohol/fact-sheets/alcohol-use.htm. Accessed April 13, 2017.

Centers for Disease Control and Prevention: *Binge drinking*, October 16, 2016. Available from: https://www.cdc.gov/alcohol/fact-sheets/binge-drinking.htm. Accessed April 13, 2017.

Centers for Disease Control and Prevention: *Preventing excessive alcohol use*, October 17, 2016. Available at https://www.cdc.gov/alcohol/fact-sheets/prevention.htm. Accessed April 13, 2017.

Centers for Disease Control and Prevention: *Underage drinking*, October 20, 2016. Available from: https://www.cdc.gov/alcohol/fact-sheets/underage-drinking.htm. Accessed April 10, 2017.

Centers for Disease Control and Prevention: *Current Cigarette Smoking among adults in 2015*, December 1, 2016. Available from: https://www.cdc.gov/tobacco/data_statistics/fact_sheets/adult_data/cig_smoking/index.htm. Accessed April 3, 2017.

Centers for Disease Control and Prevention: *Prevalence of childhood obesity in the United States*, April 10, 2017. Available at https://www.cdc.gov/obesity/data/childhood.html. Accessed April 14, 2017.

Centers for Disease Control and Prevention, National Center for Chronic Disease Prevention and Health Promotion: *State indicator report on fruits and vegetables 2013*, November 6, 2008. Available at https://www.cdc.gov/nutrition/downloads/state-indicator-report-fruits-vegetables-2013.pdf. Accessed April 17, 2017. Available from: <apps.nccd.cdc.gov/5ADaySurveillance/displayV.asp>. Accessed April 13, 2009.

Centers for Disease Control and Prevention: *Trends in the prevalence of extreme obesity among US preschool-aged children living in low-income families, 1998-2010.* Available from: <http://www.cdc.gov/obesity/data/childhood.html/>. Accessed March 2013.

Centers for Disease Control and Prevention: *Prevalence of obesity among adults and youth: United States 2011-2014.* Available at https://www.cdc.gov/nchs/data/databriefs/db219.pdf. Accessed April 13, 2017.

Champion VL, Skinner CS: The health belief model. In Glanz K, Rimer BK, Viswanath K, editors: *Health behavior and health education: theory, research, and practice,* San Francisco, 2008, Jossey-Bass.

De Castro JM, King GA, Duarte-Gardea M: Overweight and obese humans overeat away from home, *Appetite* 59:204–211, 2012.

Edwards A, Naik G, Ahmed H: Personalised risk communication for informed decision making about screening tests (Review) [update], *The Cochrane Library* 2:CD001865, 2013.

Finklestein EA, Trogdon JG, Cohen JW: Annual medical spending attributable to obesity: payer- and service-specific estimates, *Health Aff* 289(5):w822–w831, 2009.

Finnigan JR, Vinswanath K: Communication theory and health behavior change. In Glanz KR, Rimer BK, Vinswanath K, editors: *Health behavior and health education,* ed 4, San Francisco, 2008, Jossey-Bass, pp 363–384.

Flegal K, Carroll O: Johnson Prevalence and trends among US adults, 1999-2000, *JAMA* 288:1723–1727, 2002.

Frank LS: Linking objectively measured physical activity with objectively measured urban form: findings from SMARTRAQ, *Am J Prev Med* 28:117–125, 2005.

Friis R, Sellers: *Epidemiology for public health practice,* London, 2004, Jones & Bartlett.

Fryar CD, Ervin RB: Caloric intake from fast food among adults: United States, 2007-2010. NCHS Data Brief No. 114, 2013. Available from: www.cdc.gov/nchs/data/databriefs/db114.htm. Accessed March 2013.

Fulkerson JA, Farbakhsh K, Lytle L: Away-from-home family dinner sources and associations with weight status, body composition and related biomarkers of chronic disease among adolescents and their parents, *J Am Diet Assoc* 111(112):1892–1897, 2011.

Green L, Kreuter M: *Health promotion and planning: an educational and environmental approach,* Mountain View, CA, 1991, Mayfield.

Hendrick PA, Ahmed OH, Bankier SS: Acute low back pain information online: an evaluation of quality, content, accuracy and readability of related websites, *Man Ther* 17:318–324, 2012.

Hochbaum G: *Public participation in medical screening programs: a socio-psychological study,* Washington, DC, 1958, U.S. Public Health Service.

Kupferberg N, Protus B: Accuracy and completeness of drug information in Wikipedia: an assessment, *J Med Libr Assoc* 99:310–313, 2011.

Loef M, Walach H: The combined effects of healthy lifestyle behaviors on all cause mortality: a systematic review and meta-analysis, *Prev Med* 55:163–170, 2012.

Marchetta CM, Denny CH, Floyd L: Alcohol use and binge drinking among women of childbearing age—United States, 2006-2010, *Morb Mortal Wkly Rep* 61:534–538, 2012.

McCrory MA, Fuss PJ, Hays NP, et al.: Overeating in America: association between restaurant food consumption and body fatness in healthy adult men and women, *Obes Res* 92:564–571, 1999.

McEwen M, Pullis B: *Community-based nursing: an introduction,* St. Louis, 2009, Saunders.

McGinnis JM, Foege WH: Actual causes of death in the United States, *JAMA* 270:2207–2212, 1993.

McGinnis JM, Foege WH: The immediate and the important, *JAMA* 291:1263–1264, 2004.

Medscape: *Help me make it through the night (shift).* Available from: http://www.medscape.com/viewarticle/757050. Accessed March 2013.

Merriam-Webster Online Dictionary: *Health,* March 2009. Available from: <www.merriam-webster.com/dictionary/health>. Accessed March 23, 2009.

Mokdab AH, Marks JS, Stroup DF, et al.: Actual causes of death in the United States 2000, *JAMA* 291:1238–1245, 2004.

Montano D, Kasprzyk D: Theory of reasoned action, theory of planned behavior, and the integrated behavioral model. In Glanz KR, editor: *Health behavior and health education: theory, research, and practice,* ed 4, San Francisco, 2008, Jossey-Bass, pp 67–96.

National Heart, Lung, and Blood Institute (NHLBI): *Portion Distortion,* February 2013. http://www.nhlbi.nih.gov/health/public/heart/obesity/wecan/portion/index.htm. Accessed January 2014.

National Institutes of Health: *Alcohol facts and statistics,* February 2017. Available at https://pubs.niaaa.nih.gov/publications/AlcoholFacts&Stats/AlcoholFacts&Stats.htm. Accessed April 10, 2017.

National Research Council (NRC) and Institute of Medicine (IOM): *Measuring the Risks and Causes of Premature Death: Summary of Workshops, H.G. Rhodes, rapporteur, Committee on Population, Division of Behavioral and Social Sciences and Education and Board on Health Care Services, Institute of Medicine,* Washington, DC, 2015, The National Academies Press.

National Sleep Foundation: *How much sleep do we really need?* n.d., 2013. Available from: <http://www.sleepfoundation.org/article/how-sleep-works/how-much-sleep-do-we-really-need>. Accessed January 28, 2010.

National Sleep Foundation: *Drowsy driving: facts and stats.* Available from: <http://drowsydriving.org/about/facts-and-stats/>. Accessed March 2013.

Office of Applied Studies: *The NSDUH report: alcohol dependence or abuse and age at first use.* Substance Abuse and Mental Health Services Administration: Rockville, MD.

Ogden C, Carroll C, Curtin LR, et al.: Prevalence of overweight and obesity in the United States, 1999-2004, *JAMA* 295:1545–1599, 2006.

Ogden C, Carroll MD, Flegal KM: *Prevalence of obesity in the United States: 2009-2010. NCHS Data Brief #82.* Available from: <http://www.cdc.gov/obesity/data/adult.html>. Accessed March 2013.

Ogden CL, Carroll MD, Lawman HG, et al.: Trends in obesity prevalence among children and adolescents in the United States, 1988-1994 through 2013-2014, *JAMA* 315(21):2292–2299, 2016. Centers for Disease Control and Prevention. Available https://www.ncbi.nlm.nih.gov/pubmed/?term=Ogden+CL%2C+Carroll+MD%2C+Lawman+HG%2C+Fryar+CD%2C+Kruszon-Moran+D%2C+Kit+BK%2C+et+al.+Trends+in+Obesity+Prevalence+Among+Children+and+Adolescents+in+the+United+States%2C+1988-1994+Through+2013-2014.+Jama+2016%3B315(21)%3A2292. Accessed April 13, 2017.

Ogden CL, Lamb MM, Carroll MD: Obesity and socioeconomic status in adults: United States, 2005-2008. NCHS data brief no. 50, 2010. Available from: <http://www.cdc.gov/nchs/data/databriefs/db50.pdf>. Accessed March 2013.

Oleckno W: *Essential epidemiology.* Prospects Heights, IL: Waveland Press.

Parse R: Health promotion and prevention: two distinct cosmologies, *Nurs Sci Q* 3:101, 1990.

Pender N: *Health promotion and disease prevention*, ed 3, Stamford, CT, 1996, Appleton & Lange.

Pender N, Murdaugh CL, Parsons MA: *Health promotion in nursing practice*, ed 6, Upper Saddle River, NJ, 2011, Pearson.

Rehm CD, Monsivais P, Drewnowski A: Relation between diet cost and Healthy Eating Index 2010 scores among adults in the United States 2007-2010, *Prev Med* 73:70–75, 2015.

Saelens B, Salis JF, Black JB, et al.: Neighborhood-based differences in physical activity: an environment scale evaluation, *Research and Practice* 93:43–54, 2003.

Savitz DR: Methods in chronic epidemiology. In Brownson RC, Remington PL, Davis JR, editors: *Chronic disease epidemiology and control*, Washington, DC, 1998, American Public Health Association, pp 27–54 .

Schroder H, Fito M, Cavas M: Association of fast food consumption with energy intake, diet quality, body mass index, and the risk of obesity in a representative Mediterranean population, *Br J Nutr* 98:1274–1280, 2007.

Schroeder SA: We can do better—Improving the health of the American people, *N Engl J Med* 357:1221–1228, 2007. https://doi.org/10.1056/NEJMsa073350.

Schwartz J, Byrd-Bredbrenner C: Portion distortion: typical portion sizes selected by young adults, *J Am Diet Assoc* 106:1412–1418, 2006.

Slater DJ, Nicholson L, Chriqui J: Walkable communities and adolescent weight, *Am J Prev Med* 44:164–168, 2013.

The Keystone Center: *The Keystone forum on away-from-home foods: opportunities for preventing weight gain and obesity*, Washington, DC, 2006, Author.

U.S. Department of Agriculture: *Choose my plate*.gov. Available from: <http://www.choosemyplate.gov/>. Accessed March, 2013.

U.S. Department of Agriculture, Center for Nutrition Policy and Promotion: *2010 Dietary guidelines for Americans*, ed 8, Author, 2015. Available from: https://health.gov/dietaryguidelines/2015/guidelines/. Accessed April 13, 2017.

U.S. Department of Agriculture and U.S. Department of Health and Human Services: Chapter 3. Foods and food components to reduce. In *Dietary guidelines for Americans*, Washington, DC, 2010, US Government Printing Office, pp 30–32.

U.S. Department of Health and Human Services: *About healthy people*, December 17, 2012. Available from: <http://www.healthypeople.gov/2020/about/default.aspx>. Accessed March, 2013.

U.S. Department of Health and Human Services: *Healthy People 2020: topics and objectives*, March 8, 2013. Available from: <http://www.healthypeople.gov/2020/topicsobjectives2020/default.aspx>. Accessed March 2013.

U.S. Department of Health and Human Services: *Step it Up! The surgeon general's call to action to promote walking and walkable communities*, 2015. Available at www.surgeongeneral.gov. Accessed April 17, 2017.

U.S. Department of Justice: *Drinking in America: myths, realities and prevention policies*. Available from: <http://www.udetc.org/documents/Drinking_in_America.pdf>. Accessed February 28, 2013.

Van der Horst K, Brunner TA, Siegrist M: Fast food and take-away food consumption are associated with different lifestyle characteristics, *J Hum Nutr Diet* 24:596–602, 2011.

Walk Score: *What makes a city walkable? Walkscore: find a walkable place to live*, 2013. Available from: <www.walkscore.com/rankings/what-makes-a-city-walkable.shtml>. Accessed January 9, 2014.

Westberg J, Jason H: Fostering healthy behavior: the process. In Woolf SH, Jonas S, Lawrence RS, editors: *Health promotion and disease prevention in clinical practice*, Baltimore, 1996, Williams & Wilkins.

World Health Organization: Health promotion: a discussion document on the concept and principles, *Public Health Rev* 14:245–254, 1986.

World Health Organization: *Mental health*, 2009. Available from: <www.who.int/topics/mental_health/en/>. Accessed March 23, 2009.

5

Epidemiology

Holly B. Cassells

OBJECTIVES

Upon completion of this chapter, the reader will be able to do the following:

1. Identify epidemiological models used to explain disease and health patterns in populations.
2. Use epidemiological methods to describe the state of health in a community or aggregate.
3. Calculate epidemiological rates in order to characterize population health.
4. Understand the use of epidemiological methods in primary, secondary, and tertiary prevention.
5. Evaluate epidemiological study designs for researching health problems.

KEY TERMS

age adjustment of rates
age-specific rates
analytic epidemiology
attack rates
cause-and-effect relationship
crude rates
descriptive epidemiology
ecosocial epidemiology
epidemiological triangle

epidemiology
incidence rates
infant mortality rate
morbidity rates
mortality rates
natural history of disease
person–place–time model
prevalence rate
proportionate mortality ratio

rates
risk
risk factors
screening
screening programs
standardization of rates
surveillance
web of causation

Epidemiology is the study of the distribution and determinants of health and disease in human populations (World Health Organization, 2017) and is the principal science of public health. It entails a body of knowledge derived from epidemiological research and specialized epidemiological methods and approaches to scientific research. Community health nurses use epidemiological concepts to improve the health of population groups by identifying risk factors and optimal approaches that reduce disease risk and promote health. Epidemiological methods are important for accurate community assessment and diagnosis and in planning and evaluating effective community interventions. This chapter discusses the uses of epidemiology and its specialized methodologies.

USE OF EPIDEMIOLOGY IN DISEASE CONTROL AND PREVENTION

Although epidemiological principles and ideas originated in ancient times, formal epidemiological techniques developed in the nineteenth century. Early applications focused on identifying factors associated with infectious diseases and the spread of disease in the community. Public health practitioners hoped to improve preventive strategies by identifying critical factors in disease development.

Specifically, investigators attempted to identify characteristics of people who had a disease such as cholera or plague and compared them with characteristics of those who remained healthy. These differences might include a broad range of personal factors, such as age, gender, socioeconomic status, and health status. Investigators also questioned whether there were differences in the location or living environment of ill people compared with healthy individuals and whether these factors influenced disease development. Finally, researchers examined whether common time factors existed (i.e., when people acquired disease). Use of this **person-place-time model** organized epidemiologists' investigations of the disease pattern in the community (Box 5.1). This study of the amount and distribution of disease constitutes **descriptive epidemiology.** Identified patterns frequently indicate possible causes of disease that public health professionals can examine with more advanced epidemiological methods.

In addition to investigating the person, place, and time factors related to disease, epidemiologists examine complex relationships among the many determinants of disease. This investigation of the causes of disease, or etiology, is called *analytic epidemiology.*

Even before the identification of bacterial agents, public health practitioners recognized that single factors were insufficient to cause disease. For example, while exploring the cholera epidemics in London in 1855, Dr. John Snow collected data about social and physical environmental conditions that might favor disease development. He specifically examined the contamination of local water systems. Snow also gathered information about people who became ill—their living patterns, water sources, socioeconomic characteristics, and health status. A comprehensive database helped him develop a theory about the possible cause of the epidemic. Snow suspected that a single biological agent was responsible for the cholera infection, although the organism, *Vibrio cholerae,* had yet to be discovered. He compared the death rates among individuals using one water well with those among people using a different water source. His findings suggested an association between cholera and water quality (Box 5.2).

The epidemiologist examines the interrelationships between host and environmental characteristics and uses an organized method of inquiry to derive an explanation of disease. This model of investigation is called the **epidemiological triangle** because the epidemiologist must analyze the following three elements: agent, host, and environment (Fig. 5.1). The development of disease depends on the extent of the host's exposure to an agent, the strength or virulence of the agent, and the host's genetic or immunological susceptibility. Disease also depends on the environmental conditions existing at the time of exposure, which include the biological, social, political, and physical environments (Table 5.1). The model implies that the rate of disease will change when the balance among these three factors is altered. By examining each of the three elements, a community health nurse can methodically assess a health problem, determine protective factors, and evaluate the factors that make the host vulnerable to disease.

Conditions linked to clearly identifiable agents, such as bacteria, chemicals, toxins, and other exposure factors, are readily explained by the epidemiological triangle. However, other models that stress the multiplicity of host and environmental interactions have developed, and understanding of disease has progressed. The "wheel model" is an example of such a model (Fig. 5.2). The wheel consists of a hub that represents the host and its human characteristics, such as genetic makeup, personality, and immunity. The surrounding wheel represents the environment and comprises biological, social, and physical dimensions. The relative size of each component in the wheel depends on the health problem. A relatively large genetic core represents health conditions associated with heredity. Origins of other health conditions may be more dependent on environmental factors (Mausner and Kramer, 1985). This model subscribes to multiple-causation rather than single-causation disease theory; therefore it is more useful for analyzing complex chronic conditions and identifying factors that are amenable to intervention.

After the discovery of the causative agents of many infectious diseases, public health interventions eventually resulted in a decline in widespread epidemic mortality, particularly in developed countries. The focus of public health then shifted to chronic diseases such as cancer, coronary heart disease, and diabetes during the past few decades. The development of these chronic diseases tends to be associated with multiple interrelated factors rather than single causative agents.

In studying chronic diseases, epidemiologists use methods that are similar to those used in infectious disease investigation, thereby developing theories about chronic disease control. Risk factor identification is of particular importance to chronic disease reduction. **Risk factors** are variables that increase the rate of disease in people who have them (e.g., a genetic predisposition) or in people exposed to them (e.g., an infectious agent or a diet high in saturated fat). Therefore their identification is critical to identifying specific prevention and intervention approaches that effectively and efficiently reduce chronic disease morbidity and mortality. For example, the identification of cardiovascular disease risk factors has suggested a number of lifestyle modifications that could reduce the morbidity risk before disease

---

BOX 5.1 Person–Place–Time Model

Person: "Who" factors, such as demographic characteristics, health, and disease status
Place: "Where" factors, such as geographic location, climate and environmental conditions, and political and social environment
Time: "When" factors, such as time of day, week, or month and secular trends over months and years

BOX 5.2 Example of the Epidemiological Approach

An early example of the epidemiological approach is John Snow's investigation of a cholera epidemic in the 1850s. He analyzed the distribution of person, place, and time factors by comparing the death rates among people living in different geographic sectors of London. His geographic map of cases, shown here, is an early example of the use of geographic information to formulate a hypothesis about the causes of an epidemic. Snow noted that people using a particular water pump had significantly higher mortality rates from cholera than people using other water sources in the city. Although the cholera organism was yet unidentified, the clustering of disease cases around one neighborhood pump suggested new prevention strategies to public health officials (i.e., that cholera might be reduced in a community by controlling contaminated drinking water sources). As an immediate response, in September 1854, Snow persuaded local leaders to remove the handle of the pump, which to this day can be seen on Broadwick Street in London (Snow, 1855.)

John Snow's map of London neighborhood showing location of cholera case cluster surrounding the Broad Street water pump. (Published by C. F. Cheffins, Lith, Southhampton Buildings, London, England, 1854. In Snow J, editor: *On the mode of communication of cholera*, ed 2, London, 1855, John Churchill. Retrieved from: http://www.ph.ucla.edu/epi/snow/snowmap1_1854_lge.html.)

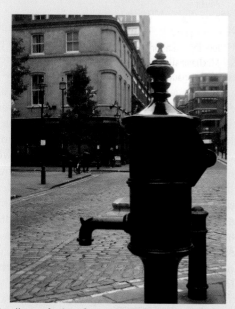

Replica of the famous Broad Street pump. Broadwick Street, London. (Photo courtesy of http://commons.wikimedia.org/wiki/File:John_Snow_memorial_and_pub.jpg, Creative Commons Attribution-Share Alike 2.0 Generic [CC BY-SA 2.0].)

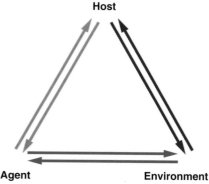

FIG. 5.1 Epidemiological triangle.

onset. Primary prevention strategies, such as dietary saturated fat reduction, smoking cessation, and hypertension control, were developed in response to previous epidemiological studies that identified these risk factors (Box 5.3). The **web of causation** model illustrates the complexity of relationships among causal variables for heart disease (Fig. 5.3).

A newer paradigm, **ecosocial epidemiology**, challenges the more individually focused risk factor approach to understanding disease origins. This ecosocial approach emphasizes the role of evolving macro-level socioenvironmental factors, including complex political and economic forces, along with microbiological processes, in understanding health and illness (Smith and Lincoln, 2011). Investigating the context of health will necessitate alternative research approaches, such as qualitative and ecological studies and studies of social institutions and processes.

TABLE 5.1 A Classification of Agent, Host, and Environmental Factors that Determine the Occurrence of Diseases in Human Populations

Factors	Examples
Agents of Disease—Etiological Factors	
A. Nutritive elements:	
Excesses	Cholesterol
Deficiencies	Vitamins, proteins
B. Chemical agents:	
Poisons	Carbon monoxide, carbon tetrachloride, drugs
Allergens	Ragweed, poison ivy, medications
C. Physical agents:	
Ionizing radiation	Sun exposure, medical imaging
Mechanical	Repetitive motion injury
D. Infectious agents:	
Metazoa	Hookworm, schistosomiasis, onchocerciasis
Protozoa	Amebae, malaria
Bacteria	Rheumatic fever, lobar pneumonia, typhoid, tuberculosis, syphilis
Fungi	Histoplasmosis, athlete's foot
Rickettsia	Rocky Mountain spotted fever, typhus, Lyme disease
Viruses	Measles, mumps, chickenpox, smallpox, poliomyelitis, rabies, yellow fever, human immunodeficiency virus
Host Factors (i.e., intrinsic factors)— Susceptibility or Response Influence Exposure to Agent	
A. Genetic	Cystic fibrosis, Huntington disease
B. Age	Alzheimer disease
C. Sex	Rheumatoid arthritis
D. Ethnic group	Tay-Sachs disease, sickle cell disease
E. Physiological state	Fatigue, pregnancy, puberty, stress, nutritional state
F. Prior immunological experience:	Hypersensitivity, protection
Active	Prior infection, immunization
Passive	Maternal antibodies, gamma globulin prophylaxis
G. Intercurrent or preexisting disease	Diabetes, liver dysfunction, hypertension
H. Human behavior	Personal hygiene, food handling, diet, interpersonal contact, occupation, recreation, use of health resources, tobacco use
Environmental Factors (i.e., extrinsic factors)—Influence Existence of the Agent, Exposure, or Susceptibility to Agent	
A. Physical environment	Geology, climate
B. Biological environment	
Human populations	Density
Flora	Sources of food, influence on vertebrates and arthropods, as a source of agents
Fauna	Food sources, vertebrate hosts, arthropod vectors
C. Socioeconomic environment	
Occupation	Exposure to chemical agents
Urbanization and economic development	Urban crowding, tension and pressures, cooperative efforts in health and education
Disruption	Wars, floods

Modified from Lilienfeld DE, Stoley PD: *Foundations of epidemiology*, New York, NY, 1994, Oxford University Press.

In turn, the examination of social and contextual origins will enlighten the interventions of public health practitioners.

For example, Buffardi et al. (2008) analyzed the ecosocial and psychosocial correlates of diagnosis of sexually transmitted infections (STIs) among young adults. Specifically, they examined STI diagnosis within "contextual conditions" such as low income, "housing insecurity," childhood physical or sexual abuse, intimate partner abuse, gang participation, personal history of having been arrested, and drug/alcohol use. It was determined that STIs were statistically associated with housing insecurity, exposure to crime, and having been arrested. The researchers concluded that ecosocial or contextual conditions strongly enhance STI risk by increasing sexual risk behaviors and likelihood of exposure to infection.

In another study, Phillips (2011) applied an ecosocial perspective when examining the effects of social/contextual factors

FIG. 5.2 Wheel model of human–environment interaction. (Redrawn from Mausner JS, Kramer S: *Mausner and Bahn epidemiology: an introductory text,* ed 2, Philadelphia, 1985, Saunders)

BOX 5.3 Coronary Heart Disease (Chd) Risk Factors Supported by Epidemiological Data From the Framingham Study

- Age
- Gender (male)
- Current cigarette smoking
- Hypertension
- High level of low-density lipoprotein (LDL) cholesterol
- Low level of high-density lipoprotein (HDL) cholesterol
- (Diabetes)[1]
- Family history of premature coronary heart disease[2]

[1]Diabetes is not included in the Framingham Global Risk Score but is now considered to be a coronary heart disease risk equivalent, meaning that persons with diabetes will be treated as intensively as those with coronary heart disease.
[2]Included in NCEP list of major risk factors but not in the Framingham Global Risk Score.
Data from the Executive summary of the third report of the National Cholesterol Education Program (NCEP) expert panel on detection, evaluation, and treatment of high blood cholesterol in adults (adult treatment panel III), *JAMA* 285:2486–2497, 2001. The 2013 recommendations from the American College of Cardiology/American Heart Association indicate these risk factors predict 10-year cardiovascular disease incidence (rather than CHD as in NCEP ATP III), *Circulation,* 2013. http://dx.doi.org/10.1161/01.cir.0000437741.48606.98, 2013.

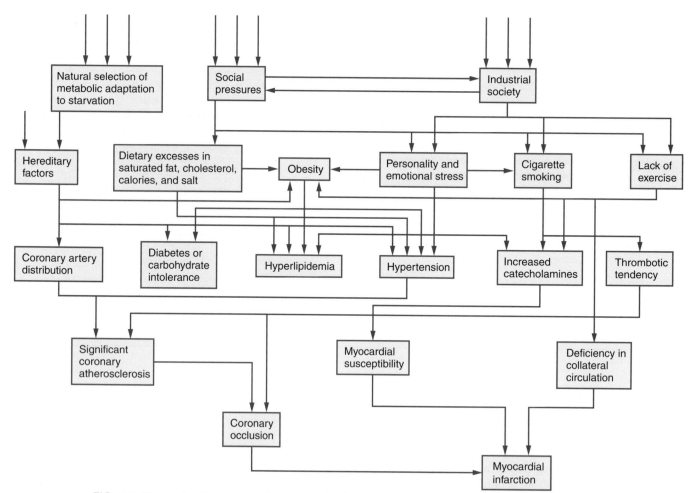

FIG. 5.3 The web of causation for myocardial infarction: A current view. (From Friedman GD: *Primer of epidemiology,* ed 5, New York, 2004, McGraw-Hill.)

on adherence to antiretroviral therapy (ART) among black men who tested positive for human immunodeficiency virus (HIV). He examined both individual factors (e.g., psychological state of mind, psychological distress, illicit drug use) and interpersonal/social contextual factors (e.g., partner status, housing status, patient–provider relationship, social capital [groups/networks]). He concluded that adherence to the medication regimen was strongly associated with homelessness and how well the individual tolerated the ART. Other factors included the individual's state of mind and illicit drug use. Practice implications included the observation that providers should assess social and behavioral factors and intervene accordingly. This would include identification of psychological distress or presence of substance abuse. He also suggested assessment of housing status and facilitation of effective patient–provider relationships to mitigate tolerability issues with ART.

CALCULATION OF RATES

The community health nurse must analyze data about the health of the community to determine disease patterns. The nurse may collect data by conducting surveys or compiling data from existing records (e.g., data from clinic facilities or vital statistics records). Assessment data often are in the form of counts or simple frequencies of events (e.g., the number of people with a specific health condition). Community health practitioners interpret these raw counts by transforming them into rates.

Rates are arithmetic expressions that help practitioners consider a count of an event relative to the size of the population from which it is extracted (e.g., the population at risk). Rates are population proportions or fractions in which the numerator is the number of events occurring in a specified period. The denominator consists of those in the population at the specified time period (e.g., per day, per week, or per year), frequently drawing on demographic data from the U.S. census. This proportion is multiplied by a constant (k) that is a multiple of 10, such as 1000, 10,000, or 100,000. The constant usually converts the resultant number to a whole number, which is larger and easier to interpret. Thus a rate can be the number of cases of a disease occurring for every 1000, 10,000, or 100,000 people in the population, as follows:

$$\text{Rate} = \frac{\text{Numerator}}{\text{Denominator}} = \frac{\text{Number of health events in a specified period}}{\text{Population in same area in same specified period}}$$

When raw counts or numbers are converted to rates, the community health nurse can make meaningful comparisons with rates from other cities, counties, districts, or states; from the nation; and from previous periods. These analyses help the nurse determine the magnitude of a public health problem in a given area and allow more meaningful and reliable tracking of trends in the community over time (Box 5.4).

Sometimes a ratio is used to express a relationship between two variables. A *ratio* is obtained by dividing one quantity

by another, and the numerator is not necessarily part of the denominator. For example, a ratio could contrast the number of male births to that of female births. *Proportions* can describe characteristics of a population. A proportion is often a percentage, and it represents the numerator as part of the denominator.

Morbidity: Incidence and Prevalence Rates

The two principal types of morbidity rates, or rates of illness, in public health are incidence rates and prevalence rates. Incidence rates describe the occurrence of new cases of a disease (e.g., tuberculosis, influenza) or condition (e.g., teen pregnancy) in a community over a given period relative to the size of the population at risk for that disease or condition during that same period. The denominator consists of only those at risk for the disease or condition; therefore known cases or those not susceptible (e.g., those immunized against a disease) are subtracted from the total population (Table 5.2):

$$\text{Incidence rate} = \frac{\begin{array}{c}\text{Number of new cases or events}\\\text{occurring in the population in a}\\\text{specified period}\end{array}}{\begin{array}{c}\text{Population at risk during same}\\\text{specified period}\end{array}} \times k$$

The incidence rate may be the most sensitive indicator of the changing health of a community because it captures the fluctuations of disease in a population. Although incidence rates are valuable for monitoring trends in chronic disease, they are particularly useful for detecting short-term changes in acute disease—such as those that occur with influenza or measles—in which the duration of the disease is typically short.

If a population is exposed to an infectious disease at a given time and place, the nurse may calculate the attack rate, a specialized form of the incidence rate. Attack rates document the number of new cases of a disease in those exposed to the disease. A common example of the application of the attack rate is food poisoning; the denominator is the number of people exposed to

TABLE 5.2	Examples of Rate Calculations	
Morbidity Rates	**Crude Rates**	**Specific Rates**
Incidence Rate $\dfrac{\text{Number of new cases in a given time period}}{\text{Population risk in the same time period}} \times 10{,}000$ $= \dfrac{75}{(4000 - 250 \text{ old cases})} = 0.02$ $0.02 \times 1000 = 20 \text{ per } 1000 \text{ per time period}$	**Crude Death Rate** $\dfrac{\text{Number of deaths in a year}}{\text{Total population size}} \times 100{,}000$ $= \dfrac{1720}{200{,}000} = 0.0086$ $0.0086 \times 100{,}000 = 860 \text{ per } 100{,}000 \text{ per year}$	**Infant Mortality Rate** $\dfrac{\text{Number of infant death} < 1 \text{ year of age}}{\text{Number of births in same year}} \times 1000$ $\dfrac{300}{45{,}000} = .00666 \times 1000 = 6.66 \text{ per } 1000 \text{ live births}$
Prevalence Rate $\dfrac{\text{Number of existing cases}}{\text{Total population}} \times 1000$ $\dfrac{250}{4000} = .0625$ $.0625 \times 1000 = 62.5 \text{ per } 1000$	**Crude Birth Rate** $\dfrac{\text{Number of births in a year}}{\text{Total population size}} \times 100{,}000$ $= \dfrac{2900}{200{,}000} = 0.0145$ $0.0145 \times 100{,}000 = 1450 \text{ per } 100{,}000 \text{ per year}$	**Fertility Rate** $\dfrac{\text{Number of live births}}{\text{Number of women aged 15–44 years}} \times 1000$ $\dfrac{35{,}000}{500{,}000} = .07 \text{ per women aged } 15 - 44 \text{ years}$ $.07 \times 1000 = 70 \text{ per } 1000 \text{ women aged } 15–44 \text{ years}$

a suspect food, and the numerator is the number of people who were exposed and became ill. The nurse can calculate and compare the attack rates of illness among those exposed to specific foods to identify the critical food sources or exposure variables.

A **prevalence rate** is the number of all cases of a specific disease or condition (e.g., deafness) in a population at a given point in time relative to the population at the same point in time:

$$\text{Prevalence rate} = \frac{\begin{array}{c}\text{Number of existing cases in}\\ \text{population at a specified point}\\ \text{in time}\end{array}}{\begin{array}{c}\text{Population at same specified}\\ \text{point in time}\end{array}} \times k$$

When prevalence rates describe the number of people with the disease at a specific point in time, they are sometimes called *point prevalences*. For this reason, cross-sectional studies frequently use them. *Period prevalences* represent the number of existing cases during a specified period or interval of time and include old cases and new cases that appear within the same period.

Prevalence rates are influenced by the number of people who experience a particular condition (i.e., incidence) and the duration of the condition. A nurse can derive the prevalence rate *(P)* by multiplying incidence *(I)* by duration *(D)*: (P = I × D). An increase in the incidence rate or the duration of a disease increases the prevalence rate of a disease. With the advent of life-prolonging therapies (e.g., insulin for treatment of type 1 diabetes and antiretroviral drugs for treatment of HIV), the prevalence of a disease may increase without a change in the incidence rate. Those who survive a chronic disease without cure remain in the "prevalence pot" (Fig. 5.4). For conditions such as cataracts, surgical removal of the cataracts permits many people to recover and thereby move out of the prevalence pot. Although the incidence has not necessarily changed, the reduced duration of the disease (because of surgery) lowers the prevalence rate of cataracts in the population.

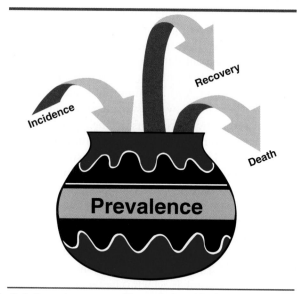

FIG. 5.4 Prevalence pot: The relationship between incidence and prevalence. (Redrawn from Morton RF, Hebel JR, McCarter RJ: *A study guide to epidemiology and biostatistics*, ed 3, Gaithersburg, MD, 1990, Aspen Publishers.)

Morbidity rates are not available for many conditions because surveillance of many chronic diseases is not widely conducted. Furthermore, morbidity rates may be subject to underreporting when they are available. Routinely collected birth and death rates, or **mortality rates**, are more widely available. Table 5.2 provides examples of calculating selected rates.

Other Rates

Numerous other rates are useful in characterizing the health of a population. For example, **crude rates** summarize the occurrence of births (i.e., crude birth rate), mortality (i.e., crude death rates), or diseases (i.e., crude disease rates) in the general population. The numerator is the number of events, and the denominator is the average population size or the population size at midyear (i.e., usually July 1) multiplied by a constant.

The denominators of crude rates represent the total population and not the population at risk for a given event; therefore these rates are subject to certain biases in interpretation. Crude death rates are sensitive to the number of people at the highest risk for dying. A relatively older population will probably produce a higher crude death rate than a population with a more evenly distributed age range. Conversely, a young population will have a somewhat lower crude death rate. Similar biases can occur for crude birth rates (e.g., higher birth rates in young populations).

This distortion occurs because the denominator reflects the entire population and not exclusively the population at risk for giving birth. Age is one of the most common confounding factors that can mask the true distribution of variables. However, many variables, such as race and socioeconomic status, can also bias the interpretation of biostatistical data. Therefore the nurse may use several approaches to remove the confounding effect of these variables on rates.

Age-specific rates characterize a particular age group in the population and usually consider deaths and births. Determining the rate for specific subgroups of a population and using a denominator that reflects only that subgroup remove age bias:

$$\text{Age specific rate} = \frac{\begin{array}{c}\text{Number of cases in a specific}\\\text{age category in population at}\\\text{a specified time}\end{array}}{\begin{array}{c}\text{Population in the same age}\\\text{category at the same}\\\text{specified time}\end{array}} \times k$$

To characterize a total population using age-specific rates, one must compute the rate for each category separately. The reason is that a single summary rate, such as a mean, cannot adequately characterize a total population. Specific rates for other variables can be determined in a similar fashion (e.g., race-specific or gender-specific rates) (Table 5.3).

Age adjustment or **standardization of rates** is another method of reducing bias when there is a difference between the age distributions of two populations. The nurse uses either the direct method or the indirect standardization method. The direct method selects a standard population, which is often the population distribution of the United States. This method essentially converts age-specific rates for age categories of the two populations to those of the standard population, and it calculates a summary age-adjusted rate for each of the two populations of interest. This conversion enables the nurse to compare the two rates as if both had the standard population's age structure (i.e., without the prior problem of age distortion).

The **proportionate mortality ratio** (PMR) method also describes mortality. It represents the percentage of deaths resulting from a specific cause relative to deaths from all causes. It is often helpful in identifying areas in which public health programs might make significant contributions to reducing deaths. In some situations, a high PMR may reflect a low overall mortality or reduced number of deaths resulting from other causes.

TABLE 5.3 Comparison of U.S. Mortality Rates—2014 (Preliminary)	
Death Rate	**Rate Per 100,000**
Crude death rate	823.7
Age-adjusted death rate	724.6
Age-specific death rates (years):	
<1 (infant)	588.0
1–4	24.0
5–14	12.7
15–24	65.5
25–34	108.4
35–44	175.2
45–54	404.8
55–64	870.3
65–74	1786.3
75–84	4564.2
≥85	13,407.9

Modified from National Center for Health Statistics: Deaths. Preliminary data for 2014, *National Vital Statistics Reports* 65(4):1–122, 2016. Retrieved from: http://www.cdc.gov/nchs/data/nvsr65/nvsr65_04.pdf.

Therefore the PMR requires consideration in the context of the mortality experience of the population.

$$\text{PMR} = \frac{\begin{array}{c}\text{Number of deaths resulting from a specific}\\\text{cause in a specific time period}\end{array}}{\begin{array}{c}\text{Total number of deaths in same}\\\text{time period}\end{array}} \times k$$

Table 5.4 summarizes the advantages and disadvantages of crude, specific, and adjusted rates. Numerous other rates assess particular segments of the population. One that is followed closely by public health professionals is the **infant mortality rate**, calculated by dividing the number of deaths in infants less than 1 year old by the number of live births for that period. This rate is considered a particularly sensitive indicator of the health of a community or nation and reflective of the care provided to women and children. Disparities in infant mortality rates can be seen within subgroups of the U.S. population, and the rate ranks 32 among 35 developed countries (Organisation for Economic Cooperation and Development [OECD], 2017). Although the United States achieved its *Healthy People 2020* goal of 6.0 per 1000, the 2014 rate, 5.8 per 1000, masks disparities within the population. Black infants experienced an infant mortality rate 2.24 times higher than white infants (11.0 vs. 4.9 per 1000 in 2014) (Centers for Disease Control and Prevention [CDC], 2016). Socioeconomic status and racial disparities, which are frequently associated with inadequate prenatal care, prematurity, adolescent pregnancy, and smoking, are key risk factors. Recent concern focuses on the steep rise in pregnancy-related maternal mortality from 10 per 100,000 in 1990 to 17.3 per 100,000 in 2013 (CDC, 2017). Again, racial differences were significant, with the presence of chronic conditions such as hypertension, diabetes, and heart disease likely playing a role. Table 5.5 provides a summary of the major public health rates. A standard epidemiology textbook contains more information.

TABLE 5.4   Advantages and Disadvantages of Crude, Specific, and Adjusted Rates

Rate	Advantages	Disadvantages
Crude	Actual summary rates	Populations vary in composition (e.g., age); therefore differences in crude rates are difficult to interpret
	Readily calculable for international comparisons (widely used despite limitations)	
Specific	Homogeneous subgroup	Cumbersome to compare many subgroups of two or more populations
	Detailed rates useful for epidemiological and public health purposes	
Adjusted	Summary statements	Fictional rates
	Differences in composition of group "removed," permitting unbiased comparison	Absolute magnitude dependent on chosen standard population
		Opposing trends in subgroups masked

Modified from Mausner JS, Kramer S: *Mausner and Bahn epidemiology: an introductory text*, ed 2, Philadelphia, 1985, W. B. Saunders.

TABLE 5.5   Major Public Health Rates

Rate Denominator	Rates	Usual	Factor Rate for United States, 2013
Total population	Crude birth rate = $\dfrac{\text{Number of live births during the year}}{\text{Average (midyear) population}}$	Per 1000 population	12.5
	Crude death rate = $\dfrac{\text{Number of deaths during the year}}{\text{Average (midyear) population}}$	Per 100,000 population	823.7
	Age-specific death rate = $\dfrac{\text{Number of deaths among people of a given age group during the year}}{\text{Average (midyear) population of the same age group}}$	Per 100,000 population	12.7 (5–14 yr) 404.8 (45–54 yr) 1786.3(65–75 yr)
	Cause-specific death rate = $\dfrac{\text{Number of deaths from a staed cause during the year}}{\text{Average (midyear) population of the same age group}}$	Per 100,000 population	167.0 (heart diseases) 185.6 (malignant neoplasms)
Women aged 15-44 yr	Fertility rate = $\dfrac{\text{Number of live births during the year}}{\text{Number of women 15 to 44 years of age in the same year}}$	Per 1000 women aged 15–44 yr	62.9
Live births	Infant mortality rate = $\dfrac{\text{Number of deaths during the year of children younger than 1 year of age}}{\text{Number of live births in the same year}}$	Per 1000 live births	5.82
	Neonatal mortality rate = $\dfrac{\text{Number of deaths during the year of children younger than 28 days}}{\text{Number of live births in the same year}}$	Per 1000 live births	3.9
	Maternal mortality rate (puerperal) = $\dfrac{\text{Number of deaths from pueperal causes during the year}}{\text{Number of live births in the same year}}$	Per 100,000 live births	17.3**
Live births and fetal deaths	Fetal death rate = $\dfrac{\text{Number of fetal deaths during the year}}{\text{Number of live births in the same year}}$	Per 1000 live births and fetal deaths	6.0*
	Perinatal mortality rate = $\dfrac{\text{Number of fetal deaths } (>28 \text{ wks plus infant } <7 \text{ days}) \text{ during the year}}{\text{Number of live births} >28 \text{ weeks in the same year}}$	Per 1000 live births and fetal deaths	6.2*

Modified from Mausner JS, Kramer S: *Mausner and Bahn epidemiology: an introductory text*, ed 2, Philadelphia, 1985, Saunders.
Rates from U.S. Department of Health and Human Services/National Center for Health Statistics: *Health, United States, 2015*. Retrieved from: http://www.cdc.gov/nchs/data/hus/hus15.pdf.
*2013 rate from National Center for Health Statistics: *Health, United States, 2015: with special features on racial and ethnic health disparities*. Retrieved from: http://www.cdc.gov/nchs/data/hus/hus15.pdf.
**Rate from Centers for Disease Control and Prevention: Deaths: final data for 2014, *National Vital Statistics Reports* 65(4):49, 2016. Retrieved from: http://www.cdc.gov/nchs/data/nvsr/nvsr65_04.pdf>

CONCEPT OF RISK

The concepts of risk and risk factor are familiar to community health nurses whose practices focus on disease prevention. Risk refers to the probability of an adverse event (i.e., the likelihood that healthy people exposed to a specific factor will acquire a specific disease). *Risk factor* refers to the specific exposure factor, such as cigarette smoke, hypertension, high cholesterol, excessive stress, high noise levels, or an environmental chemical. Frequently, the exposure factor is external to the individual. Risk factors may include fixed characteristics of people, such as age, sex, and genetic makeup. Although these intrinsic risk factors are not alterable, certain lifestyle changes may reduce their effect. For example, weight-bearing exercise and taking calcium and hormonal supplements may reduce the risk of osteoporosis for susceptible women.

Epidemiologists describe disease patterns in aggregates and quantify the effects of exposure to particular factors on the disease rates. To identify specific risk factors, epidemiologists compare rates of disease for those exposed with those not exposed. One method for comparing two rates is subtracting the rate of nonexposed individuals from the exposed. This measure of risk is called the *attributable risk*; it is the estimate of the disease burden in a population. For example, if the rate of non–insulin-dependent diabetes were 5000 per 100,000 people in the obese population (i.e., those weighing more than 120% of ideal body weight) and 1000 per 100,000 people in the nonobese population, the attributable risk of non–insulin-dependent diabetes resulting from obesity would be:

$$4000 \text{ per } 100,000 \text{ people} \left(\text{i.e., } \frac{5000}{100,000} - \frac{1000}{100,000} \right)$$

This means that 4000 cases per 100,000 people may be attributed to obesity. Thus a prevention program designed to reduce obesity could theoretically eliminate 4000 cases per 100,000 people in the population. Attributable risks are particularly important in describing the potential impact of a public health intervention in a community.

A second measure of the excess risk caused by a factor is the *relative risk ratio*. The relative risk is calculated by dividing the incidence rate of disease in the exposed population by the incidence rate of disease in the nonexposed population. In the previous example, a relative risk of 5 was obtained by dividing 5000/100,000 by 1000/100,000. This risk ratio suggests that an obese individual has a fivefold greater risk of diabetes than a nonobese individual. In general, a relative risk of 1 indicates no excessive risk from exposure to a factor; a relative risk of 1.5 indicates a 50% increase in risk; a relative risk of 2 indicates twice the risk; and a relative risk of less than 1 suggests that a factor may have a protective effect associated with a reduced disease rate.

The relative risk ratio forms the statistical basis for the risk factor concept. Relative risks are valuable indicators of the excess risk incurred by exposure to certain factors. They have been used extensively in identifying the major causal factors of many common diseases, and they direct public health practitioners' efforts to reduce health risks.

Community health nurses may apply the concept of relative risk to suspected exposure variables to isolate risk factors associated with community health problems. For example, a community health nurse might investigate an outbreak of probable foodborne illness. The nurse may compare the incidence rate among those exposed to potato salad in a school cafeteria with the incidence rate among those not exposed. The relative risk calculated from the ratio of these two incidence rates indicates the amount of excess risk for disease incurred by eating the potato salad. A community health nurse might also determine the relative risks for other suspected foods and compare them with the relative risk for potato salad. Attack rates are the calculated incidence rates for foods involved in foodborne illnesses. A food with a markedly higher relative risk than other foods might be the causal agent in a foodborne epidemic. The identification of the causal agent, or specific food, is critical to the implementation of an effective prevention program such as teaching proper food-handling techniques.

USE OF EPIDEMIOLOGY IN DISEASE PREVENTION

Primary Prevention

The central goals of epidemiology are describing the disease patterns, identifying the etiological factors in disease development, and taking the most effective preventive measures. These preventive measures are specific to the stage of disease progression, or the natural history of disease, from prepathogenesis through resolution of the disease process. When interventions occur before disease development, they are called *primary prevention*. Primary prevention relies on epidemiological information to indicate those behaviors that are protective, or those that will not contribute to an increase in disease, and those that are associated with increased risk.

Two types of activities constitute primary prevention. Those actions that are general in nature and designed to foster healthful lifestyles and a safe environment are called *health promotion*. Actions aimed at reducing the risk of specific diseases are called *specific protection*. Public health practitioners use epidemiological research to understand practices that are likely to reduce or increase disease rates. For example, numerous research studies have confirmed that regular exercise is an important health promotion activity that has positive effects on general physical and mental health. Immunizations exemplify specific protection measures that reduce the incidence of particular diseases.

Secondary and Tertiary Prevention

Secondary prevention occurs after pathogenesis. Those measures designed to detect disease at its earliest stage, namely screening and physical examinations that are aimed at early diagnosis, are *secondary prevention*. Interventions that provide for early treatment and cure of disease are also in this category. Again, epidemiological data and clinical trials determining effective treatments are crucial in disease identification. Mammography, guaiac testing of feces, and the treatment of infections and dental caries are all examples of secondary prevention.

Tertiary prevention focuses on limitation of disability and the rehabilitation of those with irreversible diseases such as diabetes and spinal cord injury. Epidemiological studies examine risk factors affecting function and suggest optimal strategies in the care of patients with chronic advanced disease.

Establishing Causality

As discussed earlier, a principal goal of epidemiology is to identify etiological factors of diseases to encourage the most effective prevention activities and develop treatment modalities. During the last few decades, researchers recognized that many diseases have not one but multiple causes. Epidemiologists who examine disease rates and conduct population-focused research often find multiple factors associated with health problems. For example, cardiovascular disease rates may vary by location, ethnicity, and smoking status. Even infectious diseases often require not only an organism but also certain behaviors or conditions to cause exposure. Determining the extent that these correlates represent associative or causal relationships is important for public health practitioners who seek to prevent, diagnose, and treat disease.

Definitively establishing causality—particularly in chronic disease—is a challenge. The following six criteria establish the existence of a **cause-and-effect relationship**:

1. **Strength of association:** Rates of morbidity or mortality must be higher in the exposed group than in the nonexposed group. Relative risk ratios, or odds ratios, and correlation coefficients indicate whether the relationship between the exposure variable and the outcome is causal. For example, epidemiological studies demonstrated a higher relative risk for heart disease among smokers than among nonsmokers.

2. **Dose–response relationship:** An increased exposure to the risk factor causes a concomitant increase in disease rate. Indeed, the risk of heart disease mortality is higher for heavy smokers than for light smokers.

3. **Temporally correct relationship:** Exposure to the causal factor must occur before the effect, or disease. For heart disease, smoking history must precede disease development.

4. **Biological plausibility:** The data must make biological sense and represent a coherent explanation for the relationship. Nicotine and other tobacco-derived chemicals are toxic to the vascular endothelium. In addition to raising low-density lipoprotein (LDL) and decreasing high-density lipoprotein (HDL) cholesterol levels, cigarette smoking causes arterial vasoconstriction and platelet reactivity, which contribute to platelet thrombus formation.

5. **Consistency with other studies:** Varying types of studies in other populations must observe similar associations. Numerous studies using different designs have repeatedly supported the relationship between smoking and heart disease.

6. **Specificity:** The exposure variable must be necessary and sufficient to cause disease; there is only one causal factor. Although specificity may be strong causal evidence in the case of infectious disease, this criterion is less important today. Diseases do not have single causes; they have multifactorial origins.

The exposure variable of smoking is one of several risk factors for heart disease. Few factors are linked to a single condition. Furthermore, smoking is not specific to heart disease alone. It is a causal factor for other diseases such as lung and oral cancers. Additionally, smoking is not "necessary and sufficient" to the development of heart disease, because there are nonsmokers who also have coronary heart disease. Therefore the causal criterion of specificity more frequently pertains to infectious diseases.

Although these criteria are useful in evaluating epidemiological evidence, it is important to note that causality is largely a matter of judgment. In reality, absolute causality is only rarely established. Rather, epidemiologists more commonly refer to suggested causal and associated factors. The effect of confounding variables makes it difficult to ascertain true relationships between the exposure and outcome variables. Confounding variables must be independently related to both the dependent variable and the independent variable. Therefore these third variables can distort the true relationship between the dependent and independent variables. For example, researchers frequently control for the confounding effect of exercise and age when they examine the relationship between diet and coronary heart disease. This is because persons with heart disease may exercise less and be older than those without heart disease; that is, there is both an independent relationship between exercise and heart disease and also between age and heart disease. Without controlling for these factors, it is not possible to know if the association between dietary fat and heart disease is real or if it can be attributed to differences in physical activity and age.

By measuring the confounding variable, the researcher can statistically account for its effect in the analysis (e.g., by using multiple logistical regression analysis or stratification). A biostatistics text contains a discussion of these methods. Alternatively, matching subjects in treatment and control groups with respect to the confounding variable minimizes the effects of the confounder. Again, standardization for variables such as age is another method for managing spurious associations, which makes true relationships more apparent. An understanding of such relationships facilitates the practitioner's interpretation and application of findings.

Screening

As explained previously, a central aim of epidemiology is to describe the course of disease according to person, place, and time. Observations of the disease process may suggest factors that aggravate or ameliorate its progress. This information also assists in determining effective treatment and rehabilitation options (i.e., secondary or tertiary prevention approaches).

The purpose of **screening** is to identify risk factors and diseases in their earliest stages. Screening is usually a secondary prevention activity because indications of disease appear *after* a pathological change has occurred. In all forms of secondary and tertiary prevention, the identification of illness prompts the nurse to consider which forms of upstream prevention could have interrupted disease development.

Community health nurses commonly conduct **screening programs**. Community health nurses may devote a large portion of their work activities to performing physical examinations; promoting client self-examination; or conducting screening programs in schools, clinics, or community settings. Although secondary prevention activities are important and provide vital information on community health status, they focus on detecting existing disease. In contrast, primary prevention and anticipatory guidance, which are hallmarks of community health nursing practice, attempt to prevent the development of disease.

Community health nurses should consider several guidelines for screening programs. First, nurses must plan and execute adequate and appropriate follow-up treatment for patients who test positive for the disease. It is critical that nurses identify how to contact patients with positive findings and where to refer them and then follow up with patients to determine whether they accessed care. Health fairs have been criticized for the lack of consistent follow-up of screening activities. Second, in the planning phase, the nurse should determine whether early disease diagnosis constitutes a real benefit to clients in terms of improved life expectancy or quality of life. Third, a critical prerequisite to screening is the existence of acceptable and medically sound treatment and follow-up. In the past, public health providers debated the ethical and practical arguments for implementing widespread HIV screening. Concern exists regarding the potential for stigmatic consequences for and discrimination against those who screen positively for a test; therefore people implementing screening programs should establish procedures for ensuring confidentiality. These procedures, in conjunction with the development of effective antiviral treatments, have encouraged earlier and more widespread identification of HIV-positive individuals.

A screening program's procedures must also be cost effective and acceptable to clients. Although colonoscopy is a routine and effective screening procedure for colon cancer, it is neither simple nor inexpensive. Although it is recommended periodically for all Americans with no known risk factors beginning at age 50 years, less than 60% of that group have undergone the procedure (CDC, 2013b). Annual screening using home fecal immunochemical tests (FIT) are not only cheaper but do not require bowel preparation, anesthesia, or transportation. Therefore non-DNA FITs are suggested by the U.S. Preventive Services Task Force as a more acceptable alternative to colonoscopy (Lin, et.al., 2016). In short, a nurse should consider whether or not to screen a population on the basis of the significant costs of screening programs and procedures, follow-up for clients who test positive, and subsequent medical care (Box 5.5).

When developing a screening program, the community health nurse also must evaluate issues related to the validity of the screening test. Detecting clients with disease is the purpose of screening, and *sensitivity* is the test's ability to do so correctly. Conversely, *specificity* is the extent to which a test can correctly

---

BOX 5.5   Guidelines For Screening Programs

- Screen for conditions in which early detection and treatment can improve disease outcome and quality of life.
- Screen populations that have risk factors or are more susceptible to the disease.
- Select a screening method that is simple, safe, inexpensive to administer, acceptable to clients, and has acceptable sensitivity and specificity.
- Plan for the timely referral and follow-up of clients with positive results.
- Identify referral sources that are appropriate, cost effective, and convenient for clients.
- Refer to evidenced-based screening recommendations published by the U.S. Preventive Services Taskforce (http://www.uspreventiveservicestaskforce.org/Page/Name/recommendations) and other organizations.

---

identify those who do not have disease. To obtain estimates of these two dimensions, the nurse must compare screening results with the best available diagnostic procedure. For a given test, the sensitivity and specificity tend to be inversely related to each other. When a test is highly sensitive, individuals without disease may be incorrectly labeled as testing positive. These false-positive results may cause stress and worry for clients and require further expense in the form of testing to confirm a diagnosis. With a highly sensitive test, specificity may be lower and the test may identify people as having the disease who are in fact disease free (i.e., more false-positive results). If the sensitivity is low (and the specificity high), more patients who have the disease will have negative test results. These patients will not be diagnosed and thus presumably will receive care later in the disease process.

Optimally, a screening test should be maximally sensitive and specific. To a large extent, this depends on the precision of the test and the stringency of the cutoff point established for determining a positive result. In the past, for example, the tuberculosis skin testing criterion was based exclusively on a skin reaction of 10 mm of induration. As a result, some persons with the disease were missed because their skin reactions were less than 10 mm (false-negative results), and some with 10 mm of reaction were identified as having the disease but further testing showed they did not have it (false-positive results). More recently, risk factors have been considered in addition to induration, creating a more sensitive and specific TB screening algorithm. Currently, high-risk individuals, such as those with HIV disease, are considered to have a positive skin test result with 5 mm of induration, which is more sensitive than the criteria of 15 mm set for those of low risk. Use of the more stringent 5-mm criterion among those with HIV will lead to fewer false-negative results, and use of the 15-mm cut point among low-risk individuals will lead to fewer false-positive results (CDC, 2016). Box 5.6 shows the formula for calculating sensitivity and specificity.

Sensitivity and specificity reflect the *yield* of a screening test, which is the amount of detected disease. One measure of yield is the *positive predictive value* of a test, which is the proportion of true-positive results relative to all positive test results. On the basis of Box 5.6, the formula is $\frac{a}{a+b}$. The positive predictive value depends on the prevalence of undetected disease in a population. Screening for a rare disease such as

BOX 5.6 Sensitivity and Specificity of a Screening Test

Screening Test Result	Those With Disease	Those Without Disease
Positive	True positives (a)	False positives (b)
Negative	False negatives (c)	True negatives (d)

$$\text{Sensitivity (in percent)} = \frac{\text{True positives}}{\text{All with disease}} - \frac{(a)}{(a+c)} \times 100$$

$$\text{Sensitivity (in percent)} = \frac{\text{True negative}}{\text{All without disease}} - \frac{(d)}{(b+d)} \times 100$$

phenylketonuria will yield a lower predictive value and more false-positive results. In phenylketonuria, a low predictive value is acceptable, because the false-negative result has very serious consequences. The predictive value is also affected by the nature of the screened population. Screening only the individuals at high risk for a disease will produce a higher predictive value and can be a more efficient way to identify those with health problems. For example, diabetes screening in an American Indian, Mexican American, or African American adult population should produce a higher predictive value than screening the general adult population.

Surveillance

In addition to screening, **surveillance** is a mechanism for the ongoing collection of community health information. Monitoring for changes in disease frequency is essential to effective and responsive public health programs. Identifying trends in disease incidence or identifying risk factor status by location and population subgroup over time allows the community health nurse to evaluate the effectiveness of existing programs and to implement interventions targeted to high-risk groups. Again, identifying new cases for calculating incidence rates is particularly useful in evaluating morbidity trends. However, this form of surveillance data is more difficult to collect, and public health practitioners can access the data only for selected diseases. Prevalence rates, mortality data, risk factor data, and hospital and health service data can help indicate a program's successes or deficiencies.

The Centers for Disease Control and Prevention (CDC) coordinates a system of data collection among federal, state, and local agencies. These groups compile numerous sets of data and base some of these data sets on the entire population (e.g., vital statistics data) and other collections on subsamples of the population (e.g., the National Health Interview Survey). The completeness of data reporting is variable because not all diseases are reportable. For example, practitioners are required to report only four sexually transmitted infections (i.e., HIV/AIDS, syphilis, gonorrhea, and chlamydia) to local and state health departments. Furthermore, not all practitioners report cases on a regular basis, and not all people with sexually transmitted infections actually seek care. Studies have indicated that practitioners also underreport childhood communicable diseases,

such as chickenpox and mumps. The CDC conducts studies that estimate the magnitude of this underreporting problem.

Practitioners have a continuing need for comprehensive and systematically collected surveillance data that describe the health status of national and local subgroups. They use this information to evaluate the impact of programs on specific groups in a community.

♥ HEALTHY PEOPLE 2020

Objectives for Data Collection and Reporting

PHI HP2020–7: Increase the proportion of population-based *Healthy People 2020* objectives for which national data are available for all major population groups.

PHI HP2020–8: Increase the proportion of *Healthy People 2020* objectives that are tracked regularly at the national level.

PHI HP2020–9: Increase the proportion of *Healthy People 2020* objectives for which national data are released within one year of the end of data collection.

PHI HP2020–10: Increase the percentage of vital events (births, deaths, fetal deaths) reported using the latest U.S. standard certificates of birth and death and the report of fetal death.

From U.S. Department of Health and *Human Services: Healthy People 2020: public health infrastructure,* n.d. Retrieved from: https://www.healthypeople.gov/2020/topics-objectives/topic/public-health-infrastructure/objectives.

For example, the effectiveness of *Healthy People 2020* depends on the availability of reliable baseline and continuing data to characterize health problems and evaluate goal achievement as listed in the *Healthy People 2020* box. *Healthy People 2020* addresses the ongoing need to extend the inclusiveness of such data collection systems (U.S. Department of Health and Human Services [USDHHS], n.d.). For example, simply documenting children's mortality rates resulting from injury is insufficient for the development of specific methods of injury prevention. Data on the number of injured children and the nature of injury (e.g., motor vehicle accidents, drowning, abuse) across the nation would increase the usefulness of surveillance information. The Health Indicators Warehouse has compiled indicator data for initiatives like Healthy People and the Center for Medicare Services so that health status and service quality can be monitored through April 2017 (National Center for Health Statistics, n.d.). Databases such as Health, United States, Healthy People, and Health Status Indicators available at the CDC webpage will be the primary source of evaluative information.

Nurses need to describe trends in health and illness according to a community's locale, demographics, and risk factor status to intervene effectively on behalf of the people. They must compare the data for their locale with those of a relevant neighboring area (e.g., a census tract, city, county, state, or nation) to gain perspective on the magnitude of a local problem (see Clinical Example 5.1). Ideally, the nurse should have access to surveillance data at several different levels over a given period. In some instances, community health nurses find it necessary to construct their own surveillance systems that are tailored to specific health conditions or available programs in their community. These smaller data collection systems help nurses evaluate programs when the data are readily accessible and are compatible with data from large city or statewide surveillance systems.

Clinical Example 5.1

In 1991, a cluster of neural tube defects (NTDs) occurred in babies born in Brownsville, Texas, within a span of 6 weeks. Investigation indicated a rate of 27.1 cases per 10,000 live births, in contrast to the U.S. rate of approximately 8 per 10,000 (Texas Department of Health, unpublished report, 1992). The Brownsville rate was more than three times the national rate and represented an increased risk in Hispanic women. This increased risk was partially attributable to cultural and environmental factors, including lower socioeconomic status and migrant farm work. The investigators implemented a surveillance program that obtained more accurate population-based data. Additionally, the program implemented folic acid supplementation in Texas counties along the Mexican border. NTD rates dropped to 13 per 10,000 after the supplementation effort.

Research suggests that 50% to 70% of NTDs may be preventable with folic acid supplementation. This finding supports the fortification of bread and cereal products; in January 1998, the U.S. Food and Drug Administration (FDA) mandated the addition of 140 µg of vitamin B per 100 g of most grain products. It is estimated that there has been a 24% reduction in the number of NTDs since grain fortification with folic acid began.

Dietary intake alone may be insufficient; also, the greatest risk to the fetus occurs within the first 3 to 8 weeks of pregnancy, a time when many women do not yet recognize their pregnancies. Therefore the CDC and U.S. Preventive Services Task Force recommend that all women of reproductive age consume 400 µg (0.4 mg) to 800 µg (0.8 mg) daily of synthetic folic acid in addition to dietary sources such as cereal or grain products, leafy green vegetables, and vitamin supplements.

From U.S. Preventive Services Task Force: Folic acid to prevent neural tube defects: preventive medication, 2009. Retrieved from: http://www.uspreventiveservicestaskforce.org/uspstf09/folicacid/folicacidrs.htm.

⬛ RESEARCH HIGHLIGHTS

Reducing Infant Mortality Rates Using the Perinatal Periods of Risk Model

The infant mortality rate is an accepted indicator for measuring a nation's health. The rate is representative of the health status and social well-being of any nation. Despite decreases in the past 50 years, infant mortality rates in the United States remain higher than in other industrialized countries. Using overall infant mortality rates to determine the effectiveness of interventions does not help communities focus on particular underlying factors contributing to the rates. Targeting interventions to the factors most responsible for the infant mortality rate should help reduce the rate more rapidly and effectively.

The Perinatal Periods of Risk (PPOR) model was developed to provide direction, focus, and suggestions for effective interventions. The model helps users identify and rank four factors as they contribute to the overall infant mortality rate: (1) mother's health before and between pregnancies, (2) maternal health care systems, (3) neonatal health care systems, and (4) infant health during the first year of life. The PPOR model is based on two major theoretical constructs: age of fetus-infant at death and birth weight. The PPOR model maps each death in a geographic region on the basis of birth weight and age at death, including fetal, neonatal, and postneonatal periods. The lowest birth weight infant deaths are combined into one cell named the maternal health cell. The three remaining groups are put into cells suggesting the primary preventive focus for that group: maternal health, newborn health, and infant health. Multiple interventions are important in reducing infant mortality, and the PPOR model guides prioritizing interventions based on the cell contributing the most to infant mortality rates (Peck et al., 2010).

The PPOR model has been used in several programs and research studies to improve mother and infant health. In one intervention study (Chao et al., 2010) the PPOR model was successfully used to improve birth outcomes in very-high-risk populations in the Antelope Valley area of Los Angeles County. On the basis of assessment findings per PPOR directives, efforts were made to infuse resources into the community and expand case management initiatives for high-risk mothers. Long-term findings indicated that the PPOR model was useful for identifying risk and social factors and that it helped mobilize community partnerships that resulted in widely improved birth outcomes.

Data from Chao SM, Donatoni G, Bemis C., et al.: Integrated approaches to improve birth outcomes: perinatal periods of risk, infant mortality review and the Los Angeles mommy and baby project, *Maternal and Child Health Journal* 14:827–837, 2010; Peck MG, Sappenfield WM, Skala J: Perinatal periods of risk: a community approach for using data to improve women and infants' health, *Maternal and Child Health Journal* 14:864–874, 2010.

As stated, epidemiologists describe the course of disease over time. These secular trends are changes that occur over years or decades, such as the fairly recent, significant decline in lung cancer deaths in men and the gradual increase in lung cancer deaths in women. Frequently, epidemiologists document the associated patterns of treatment and intervention. In many instances, studies conducted by clinical epidemiologists provide this information. Cancer registries are a form of surveillance that document the prevalence and incidence of cancer in a community and document its course, treatment, and associated survival rates. The Surveillance, Epidemiology and End Results (SEER) program of the National Cancer Institute compiles national cancer data from existing cancer registries covering approximately 28% of the U.S. population (National Cancer Institute, 2017).

Public health practitioners need to conduct community surveys of population segments to plan for the segments' health. For example, a survey of the disabled population that assesses prevalence may also evaluate the adequacy of current services and project future needs.

USE OF EPIDEMIOLOGY IN HEALTH SERVICES

Epidemiological approaches, such as the ones presented here, can be used to describe the distribution of disease and its determinants in populations. However, epidemiological principles are also useful in studying population health care delivery and in describing and evaluating the use of community health services. For example, analyzing the ratio of health care providers to population size helps determine the system's ability to provide care. The clients' reasons for seeking care, the clients' payment methods, and the clients' satisfaction with care are also informative. Regardless of whether community health nurses or other health services professionals collect these data, the information is essential for those who strive to improve clients' access to quality health care.

Health services epidemiology focuses on the population's health care patterns. In particular, public health practitioners are concerned with the accessibility and affordability of services and the barriers that may contribute to excess morbidity in at-risk groups. Traditionally, children are a vulnerable group, and they are a particular focus of health services research. Studies examining poverty rates and care access have underscored the need to expand insurance coverage to those who do not have private medical insurance and do not qualify for Medicaid programs or the State Children's Health Insurance Program.

Ultimately, nurses must apply epidemiological findings in practice. It is essential that they incorporate study results into prevention programs for communities and at-risk populations. Furthermore, the philosophy of public health and epidemiology dictates that nurses extend their application into major health policy decisions, because the aim of health policy planning is to achieve positive health goals and outcomes for improved population health.

A goal of policy development is to bring about desirable social changes. Epidemiological factors, history, politics, economics, culture, and technology influence policy development. The complex interaction of these factors may explain the challenges with application of epidemiological knowledge. Lung disease in the United States exemplifies the incomplete progress in implementing effective health policy. In the early 1950s, studies identified and conclusively linked cigarette smoking to lung cancer and heart disease (Doll and Hill, 1952). Beginning in the 1950s, public policies to address this health threat have included cigarette taxes, cigarette package warning labels, smoking restrictions in public areas, the institution of smoke-free workplaces, and restrictions on selling tobacco to minors. Despite the successes of the past 60 years, approximately 20% of Americans continue to smoke, with rates particularly high among young adults, suggesting a continued need for focused and effective public health policy. Community health nurses should exercise "social responsibility" in applying epidemiological findings, but doing so will require the active involvement of the consumer. Community health nurses collaborating with community members can combine epidemiological knowledge and aggregate-level strategies to effect change on the broadest scale.

EPIDEMIOLOGICAL METHODS

Two epidemiological methods—descriptive epidemiology and analytic epidemiology—are used by community health nurses. This section describes both and gives examples of how they are used in population health.

Descriptive Epidemiology

Descriptive epidemiology focuses on the amount and distribution of health and health problems within a population. Its purpose is to describe the characteristics of both people who are protected from disease and those who have a disease. Factors of particular interest are age, sex, ethnicity or race, socioeconomic status, occupation, and family status. Epidemiologists use morbidity and mortality rates to describe the extent of disease and to determine the risk factors that make certain groups more prone to acquiring disease.

In addition to "person" characteristics, the place of occurrence describes disease frequency. For example, certain parasitic diseases, such as malaria and schistosomiasis, occur in tropical areas. Other diseases may occur in certain geopolitical entities. For example, gastroenteritis outbreaks often occur in communities with lax water quality standards. Time is the third parameter that helps define disease patterns. Epidemiologists may track incidence rates over a period of days or weeks (e.g., epidemics of infectious disease) or over an extended period of years (e.g., secular trends in the cancer death rate).

These person, place, and time factors can form a framework for disease analysis and may suggest variables associated with high versus low disease rates. Descriptive epidemiology can then generate hypotheses about the cause of disease, and *analytic epidemiology* approaches can test these hypotheses (Box 5.7).

❓ ACTIVE LEARNING EXERCISE

Consult *Healthy People 2020* to find the national goals for selected causes of morbidity and mortality. Identify groups at an increased risk for these selected diseases. What are the approaches suggested by these documents for reducing the rates of disease? How can this information be useful in planning for your community?

🧬 GENETICS IN PUBLIC HEALTH

Community-Based Research for the Prevention of Anencephaly

A nurse-led investigation in Washington State exposed a cluster of infants born with anencephaly in a three county region between 2010 and 2015. Subsequent investigation revealed almost five times greater incidence of anencephaly in the counties in question when compared with rates the U.S. (9.5 per 10,000 in select Washington counties vs 2.1 per 10,000 nationwide). Preliminarily review showed that cases were much more commonly identified among Hispanic infants, suggesting that cultural and genetic factors were contributory. Among the risk factors identified were increased dietary consumption of non-fortified corn-based foods, rather than wheat-based products. Also noted were defects in folic acid metabolism among mothers of Hispanic ancestry.

Strategies to address and ultimately reduce the number of babies born with anencephaly were to enhance surveillance activities including both active and passive case finding, counseling to reduce risk factors including stressing the importance of folic acid intake, participating in research, and advocating policy change to protect patients from preventable birth defects,

Barron, S: Anencephaly: An ongoing investigation in Washington state. *AJN*, 116(3), 60-66.

BOX 5.7   **An Example of Descriptive Epidemiology**

The **p**erson–**p**lace–**t**ime model is illustrated by two measles outbreaks in Utah:

- *Person:* Initially, an unvaccinated 15-year-old student had contracted measles, likely from a trip to Europe. Subsequently, six more students contracted the illness.
- *Place:* Salt Lake County; three cases were "school transmission," and three cases were "household transmission."
- *Time:* The index case traveled to Europe during March 3–17, 2011. He attended school on March 21 and subsequently became ill. The other cases occurred between April 5 and April 17, 2011.

From Centers for Disease Control and Prevention: Two measles outbreaks after importation—Utah, March–June 2011, *Morbidity and Mortality Weekly Report* 62(12):222–225, 2013. Retrieved from: http://www.cdc.gov/mmwr/pdf/wk/mm6212.pdf.

Time Dimension

Present

Sample: Subjects sampled
from population-at-large at
one point in time

Advantages	Disadvantages
Quick to plan and conduct	Cannot calculate relative risk with prevalence data
Relatively inexpensive	
May provide preliminary indication of whether an association between a risk factor and disease exists	Temporal sequence of factor and outcome unknown
Provides prevalence data needed for planning health services	
Hypothesis generating	

FIG. 5.5 Cross-sectional, or prevalence, study.

Analytic Epidemiology

Analytic epidemiology investigates the causes of disease by determining why a disease rate is lower in one population group than in another. This method tests hypotheses generated from descriptive data and either accepts or rejects them on the basis of analytic research. The epidemiologist seeks to establish a cause-and-effect relationship between a preexisting condition or event and the disease (see previous section on causality). To determine this relationship, the epidemiologist may undertake two major types of research studies: observational and experimental.

Observational Studies

Epidemiologists frequently use observational studies for descriptive purposes, but they also use them to discover the etiology of disease. The investigator can begin to understand the factors that contribute to disease by observing disease rates in groups of people differentiated by experience or exposure. For example, differences in disease rates may occur in the obese compared with the nonobese, in smokers compared with nonsmokers, and in those with high stress levels compared with those with low stress levels. These characteristics (i.e., obesity, smoking, and stress) are called exposure variables.

Unlike experimental studies, observational studies do not allow the investigator to manipulate the specific exposure or experience or to control or limit the effects of other extraneous factors that may influence disease development. For example, life stress is related to depression. People with low socioeconomic status also have high depression rates. People with low socioeconomic status frequently experience greater life stresses; therefore the confounding factor of socioeconomic status makes it more difficult to demonstrate the effect of stress on depression. The three major study designs used in observational research are cross-sectional, retrospective, and prospective studies.

Cross-Sectional Studies. Cross-sectional studies, sometimes called prevalence or correlational studies, examine relationships between potential causal factors and disease at a specific time (Fig. 5.5). Surveys that simultaneously collect information about risk factors and disease exemplify this design. For example, the National Health and Nutrition Examination Survey (NHANES) has collected cross-sectional data regarding current dietary practices, physical status, and health in adults and children in the United States since the early 1960s (CDC, 2017). Data from the NHANES studies have been analyzed and compared over the years by a number of researchers and have provided important health information.

For example, NHANES studies have tracked contemporary behavior issues such as unsweetened beverage consumption in U.S. youth (Kit et al., 2013) and fast food in adults, showing recent declines in the total daily calories consumed from these sources. Although overall fast-food consumption has declined from approximately 13% of daily caloric intake to 11.3% in the period ending 2010, this decline was not shared by all groups, with non-Hispanic African Americans consuming more fast food than other groups, as did all persons who were overweight (Fryar and Ervin, 2013). NHANES has conducted interviews and physical examinations on youth, nutrient studies on children, and dietary surveys of older Americans, contributing important data that suggest risk factors that can be examined through more rigorous study designs.

Although a cross-sectional study can identify associations among disease and specific factors, it is impossible to make causal inferences because the study cannot establish the temporal sequence of events (i.e., the cause preceded the effect). For example, the NHANES was unable to determine whether high salt intake precedes hypertension—thus making it a causal factor—or whether they are unrelated. Therefore cross-sectional studies have limitations in discovering etiological factors of disease. These studies can help identify preliminary relationships that other analytic designs may explore further; therefore they are hypothesis-generating studies.

Time Dimension

Past

Sample: Subjects sampled
with regard to disease and
condition

Disease

No Disease

History of exposure
(i.e., risk factors)

Exposed   Not exposed
(a)   (c)

Exposed   Not exposed
(b)   (d)

Advantages

Can calculate odds ratio (OR),
which is an estimate of
relative risk:

$$OR = \frac{a}{a+c} \div \frac{b}{b+d} \overset{*}{=} \frac{ad}{bc}$$

(*If disease is rare.)

Requires fewer subjects than
prospective designs

Possible to study multiple risk
factors presumed to be related
to a disease

Less expensive and difficult to
conduct than a prospective study

Disadvantages

Incidence of disease cannot
be calculated

Selection of control group is
difficult

Relies on recall or records
for exposure information
that is subject to bias

Exposure ascertained after
disease occurs (i.e., temporal
relationship)

FIG. 5.6 Retrospective, or case-control, study.

Retrospective Studies. *Retrospective studies* compare individuals with a particular condition or disease and those who do not have the disease. These studies determine whether cases, or a diseased group, differ in their exposure to a specific factor or characteristic relative to controls, or a nondiseased group. To make unambiguous comparisons, investigators select the cases according to explicitly defined criteria regarding the type of case and the stage of disease. Investigators also select a control group from the general population that is characteristically similar to the cases (Fig. 5.6).

Frequently, people hospitalized for diseases that are not under study become controls if they do not share the exposure or risk factor under study. For example, a researcher may select patients with heart disease to be controls in a study of patients with lung cancer. However, this choice may introduce serious bias because the two groups often share the risk factor of smoking. The methods of data collection must be the same for both groups to prevent further introduction of bias into the study. Therefore it is desirable for interviewers to remain unaware of which subjects are cases and which are controls.

In retrospective studies, data collection extends back in time to determine previous exposure or risk factors. Investigators analyze study data by comparing the proportion of subjects with disease, or cases, who possess the exposure or risk factors with the corresponding proportion in the control group. A greater proportion of exposed cases than of exposed controls suggests a relationship between the disease and the risk factor.

Investigators often use retrospective study designs because these designs address the question of causality better than cross-sectional studies. Retrospective studies also require fewer resources and less data collection time than prospective studies. Many examples of *retrospective,* or *case-control,* studies exist in the literature. One classic example is Doll and Hill's (1952) investigation of risk factors for lung cancer. They compared exposure rates for cases in which lung cancer was diagnosed with those in the control group, in whom cancer was diagnosed outside the chest and oral cavity. The researchers recorded detailed smoking histories in all subjects. Compared with the controls, a significantly higher proportion of patients with lung cancer smoked. This study yielded the hypothesis that smoking may be etiologically related to lung cancer.

Prospective Studies. *Prospective studies* monitor a group of disease-free individuals to determine whether and when disease occurs (Fig. 5.7). These individuals, or the *cohort,* have a common experience within a defined period. For example, a birth cohort consists of all people born within a given period. The study assesses the cohort with respect to an exposure factor associated with the disease and thus classifies it at the beginning of the study. The study then monitors the cohort for disease development. The investigator compares

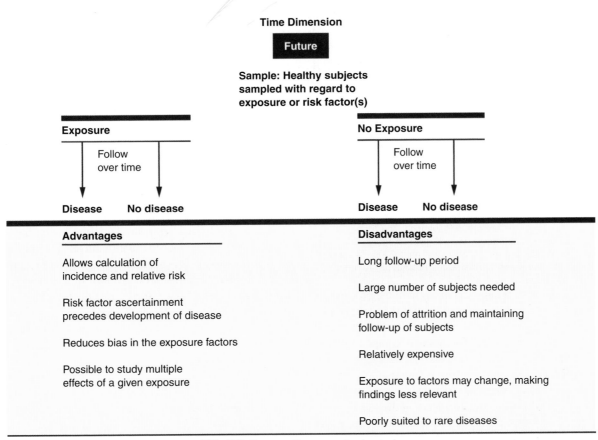

Time Dimension

Future

Sample: Healthy subjects sampled with regard to exposure or risk factor(s)

Exposure

Follow over time

Disease   **No disease**

No Exposure

Follow over time

Disease   **No disease**

Advantages	**Disadvantages**
Allows calculation of incidence and relative risk	Long follow-up period
	Large number of subjects needed
Risk factor ascertainment precedes development of disease	Problem of attrition and maintaining follow-up of subjects
Reduces bias in the exposure factors	Relatively expensive
Possible to study multiple effects of a given exposure	Exposure to factors may change, making findings less relevant
	Poorly suited to rare diseases

FIG. 5.7 Prospective, or cohort, study.

BOX 5.8 Comparison of Time Factors in Retrospective and Prospective Study Designs

Cohort Study

Girls with bacteriuria → Women with renal disease
Girls with sterile urine → Women without renal disease

Case-Control Study

Girls with bacteriuria ← Women with renal disease
Girls with sterile urine ← Women without renal disease

PAST--------------PRESENT (BEGINNING)--------------FUTURE

Comparison of time factors in prospective design (i.e., cohort) and retrospective design (i.e., case-control) approaches to studying the possible effect of childhood bacteriuria on renal disease in adult women.

---

the disease rates for those with a known exposure and the disease rates for those who remain unexposed. The study observes subjects prospectively; therefore it summarizes data collected over time by the incidence rates of new cases (Box 5.8). Again, comparing two incidence rates produces a measure of relative risk:

$$\text{Relative risk} = \frac{\text{Incidence rate among exposed}}{\text{Incidence rate among unexposed}}$$

The relative risk indicates the extent of excess risk incurred by exposure relative to nonexposure. A relative risk of 1 suggests no excess risk resulting from exposure, whereas a relative risk of 2 suggests twice the risk of having disease from exposure.

Prospective studies, or *longitudinal, cohort,* or *incidence* studies, are advantageous because they obtain more reliable information about the cause of disease than do other study methodologies. These studies establish a stronger temporal relationship between the presumed causal factors and the effect than do retrospective and cross-sectional studies. Calculations of incidence rates and relative risks provide a valuable indicator of the level of risk that exposure creates.

ETHICAL INSIGHTS

The Tuskegee Syphilis Study

In 1932 the U.S. Public Health Service (PHS) began a longitudinal-experimental study of 600 African American sharecroppers, 399 of whom had syphilis and 201 who did not. The study was conducted in one of the poorest counties of Alabama, and the subjects were unaware that they had syphilis; they were told they were being treated for "bad blood." Enticed by the promise of free medical care and meals, the subjects joined the study without knowledge of their disease, its treatment, or the study procedures. The experimental group was initially treated with ineffective doses of the treatments of the time—bismuth or mercury—and later with aspirin. Even when penicillin became available in the late 1940s, these subjects were actively denied treatment. For 40 years, these men were followed up by PHS investigators affiliated with the Tuskegee Institute and hospital, who claimed to be observing the differences in the progression of the disease in blacks in comparison with the control group. During the course of the study, many subjects died of syphilis or other causes, numerous wives became infected, and children were born with congenital syphilis.

In 1972, a former venereal disease interviewer, Peter Buxtun, "blew the whistle" on the study, and reports were published in newspapers. Only after the public became outraged about the unethical nature of the study did the

CDC and the PHS move to end it. In 1973, the National Association for the Advancement of Colored People won a $10 million class action suit on behalf of the subjects. In 1997, President Bill Clinton formally apologized to the few survivors and their families for the harm inflicted on these men and their families in the name of public health research.

The Tuskegee Study raises questions about how a study could proceed without informing and seeking consent of participants, how available treatment could be withheld, and how government researchers could pursue an unethical research plan without periodic review and questioning. Furthermore, the racial and discriminatory issues suggest disturbing questions for researchers and practicing nurses to contemplate, one being that the Tuskegee Study contributes to a legacy of distrust that minorities may harbor toward both the health care delivery system and research programs.

Data from Centers for Disease Control and Prevention: *The Tuskegee timeline*, 2013. Retrieved from: http://www.cdc.gov/tuskegee/timeline.htm; Infoplease: *The Tuskegee syphilis experiment*, 2005, Pearson Education. Retrieved from: www.infoplease.com/ipa/A0762136.html.

However, certain disadvantages are inherent in the prospective design. It is costly in terms of resources and staff to monitor a cohort over time, and lengthy studies result in subject attrition. Problems arising from the nature of chronic diseases may compound these logistical dilemmas. Frequently, chronic diseases have long latency periods between exposure and symptom manifestation. Furthermore, the onset of chronic conditions may be insidious, making it extremely difficult to document the incidence of disease. In addition, many diseases do not have a unifactorial cause (i.e., single variable) because many interacting factors influence disease. These problems do not negate the benefits of prospectively designed epidemiological studies; rather, they suggest a need to carefully plan and tailor a study specifically to the disease and the study's purpose.

The literature contains numerous prospective studies. In many cases, these studies have been instrumental in substantiating causal links between specific risk factors and disease. A classic example is a Doll and Hill cohort study of subjects who eventually developed lung cancer during the follow-up period (1956). Doll and Hill originally completed questionnaires on a cohort of physicians in Great Britain. Next, they classified the subjects according to several variables, emphasizing the number of cigarettes smoked. In 4½ years, they accessed death certificate data. These data revealed a higher mortality rate resulting from lung cancer and coronary thrombosis among smoking physicians compared with nonsmokers. The death rate for heavy smokers was 166 per 100,000 versus 7 per 100,000 for nonsmokers. Combining these two incidence rates in a measure of excess risk indicated that heavy smokers were 23.7 times more likely to develop lung cancer than nonsmokers:

$$\text{Relative risk} = \frac{\dfrac{166}{100,000} \div 7}{100,000} = 23.7$$

These findings in a prospective study provided strong epidemiological support for smoking as a risk factor for lung cancer.

Another well-known prospective study is the Framingham Heart Study, which has followed an essentially healthy cohort of Framingham, Massachusetts residents for more than 50 years. Findings from the study suggested that serum cholesterol level and other risk factors are associated with the future development of cardiovascular disease (Kramarow et al., 2013). The Framingham Study and subsequent "offspring studies" helped form the basis for later experimental studies aimed at reducing serum cholesterol through diet modification or drug therapy to ultimately lower the incidence rate of coronary heart disease.

The Nurses' Health Study was initiated in 1976 with 121,700 registered nurses, with the intent of examining the long-term consequences of oral contraceptives. The initial cohort still returns questionnaires every 2 years, and data have been collected on diet and nutrition, smoking, hormone use, and menopause as well as various chronic illnesses. In 1989 the Nurses' Health Study II was initiated to study lifestyle issues, contraception, and illness patterns in younger women, and in 2008 a third study was begun looking at similar issues in another cohort.

These studies continue to monitor nurses' changing health status and risk factors and to examine factors associated with the development of numerous health conditions in women, such as breast cancer and heart disease (Nurses' Health Study, 2017). For example, research using Nurses' Health Study data has determined that regular use of nonsteroidal antiinflammatory drugs (i.e., acetaminophen) does not reduce the incidence of skin cancer (Jeter et al., 2012) or breast cancer (Eliassen et al., 2009). Similarly, research from the nurses' health studies have shown that although consumption of sugar-sweetened beverages is associated with higher risk of type 2 diabetes, caffeine intake lowers the risk (Bhupathiraju et al., 2013). Last, the Nurses' Health Study suggested the deleterious effects of exposure to foods containing trans-fats. Groundbreaking research found a 50% increase in cardiovascular disease risk for women who consumed the highest trans-fat intakes (Willet et al., 1993). This initial finding set the stage for sweeping policy changes in FDA labeling of these fats on Nutrition Facts boxes on food packages, on restaurant menus in many cities, and an ultimate 2015 FDA determination that partially hydrogenated oils are not "Generally Recognized as Safe" (Curtis et al., 2016). These changes have led to a reduction in population levels of serum cholesterol.

Experimental Studies

Another type of analytic study is the experimental design, called the *randomized clinical trial* (Fig. 5.8). Epidemiological investigations apply experimental methods to test treatment and prevention strategies. The investigator randomly assigns subjects at risk for a particular disease to an experimental or a control group. The investigator observes both groups for the occurrence of disease over time, but only the experimental group receives intervention, although often the control group receives a placebo. The primary statistical analysis is based on "intention to treat," that is, all subjects remain assigned to the original treatment group, regardless of whether subjects may have decided on their own to discontinue or change their therapy. For example, if a subject in a drug trial who is assigned to the active medication experiences side effects possibly from this medication and therefore discontinues the medication, this subject still is considered to be within the active drug group for the purpose of statistical testing. The change in category from treatment to no treatment, or vice versa, is called a *crossover* and may decrease the likelihood of finding a significant effect for the active treatment.

Theoretically, it is possible to introduce a harmful exposure or risk factor as the experimental factor; however, ethical considerations usually prohibit the use of human subjects for these purposes. For example, it is unacceptable to require an experimental group to smoke cigarettes in an experiment; therefore the investigator uses case-control or cohort epidemiological designs. This limitation usually restricts experimental epidemiological studies to prophylactic and therapeutic clinical trials. Experimental studies testing vaccines and medications for safety and efficacy are examples.

The experimental design is also useful for investigating chronic disease prevention. Thus experimental studies may help evaluate community health nursing interventions. For example, they may help determine the effectiveness of a sex education program in preventing high rates of teenage pregnancy or the feasibility of an AIDS prevention program among intravenous drug users. Randomized trials were used to evaluate the Nurse-Family Partnership program, which established the long-term positive effects nurse home visits had on high-risk pregnant women and their children in comparison with those who did not receive home visits (Olds et al., 2014).

Time Dimension

Future

Sample: Participants randomized

Intervention

Follow over time

Disease   No disease

No intervention (i.e., placebo control or usual care)

Follow over time

Disease   No disease

Advantages	Disadvantages
With randomization, gives confidence that outcome is due to treatment or intervention and not to other unknown factors	Often impractical to conduct in human populations
Provides strongest evidence that a factor is causal when an effect is seen	Requires relatively long time to conduct and factors and/or disease may change unrelated to clinical trial

FIG. 5.8 Experimental study, or clinical trial.

CASE STUDY Application of the Nursing Process

Using an Epidemiological and Public Health Approach to Managing a Foodborne Outbreak

Nurses working in schools, daycare centers, camps, and other facilities where food is served must be cognizant of safe food-handling principles. Furthermore, they must be aware of the potential for transmitting disease if proper procedures are not followed. Outbreaks of foodborne illness must be assessed and managed, and often it is the community health nurse who initiates and participates in this process. The following is a scenario in which the nurse utilized the nursing process to analyze and intervene in such an epidemic.

Assessment

On Wednesday, October 4, the school nurse at Greenly Elementary School saw eight students who complained of abdominal cramping, diarrhea, and fever. Parents of the sick students were called, and the students were sent home. On Thursday, the nurse was alerted to a large number of absent students and teachers. Specifically, 62 students and 10 teachers were absent. Most reported diarrhea symptoms. Because the absentee rate of 10% exceeded the average daily rate of 4% for the 620-student school and because the nurse determined that the large number of diarrhea cases suggested an epidemic, the local public health department was notified.

Public health officials arrived at the school and began to assess students still at school and those who were recovering at home. Stool culture specimens were collected and sent to the state laboratory. Results indicated that the organism causing illness was in most cases *Shigella sonnei*, the most commonly found form of the bacteria. Persons with severe symptoms were referred to their physicians for possible antibiotic therapy. Food histories of meals eaten both at school and outside of school were taken.

Friday saw a continuing increase in absenteeism of students and staff reporting gastrointestinal illness. Public health specialists defined the criteria for identifying cases on the basis primarily of positive laboratory results, symptoms of diarrhea or vomiting, fever with nausea or abdominal pain, or all of these. Cafeteria staff were interviewed, and it was determined that one staff member had had diarrhea over the previous weekend but had returned to work on Monday. Public health staff continued to take dietary histories of affected and unaffected persons and constructed rates of illness for all foods served in the cafeteria beginning on Friday of the previous week. These data are displayed in the following table.

From the data, it can be seen that students who ate lunch at school on Tuesday and ate fajitas and salad had higher rates of illness than those who did not. Therefore it was concluded that the outbreak of *Shigella* could be attributed to a food source.

continued

CASE STUDY   Application of the Nursing Process—cont'd
Using an Epidemiological and Public Health Approach to Managing a Foodborne Outbreak

Diagnosis
Determining the likely cause of the outbreak was important in specifying a diagnosis and directing the planning of an intervention. The following diagnosis was formulated:

Increased risk for infectious diarrhea among elementary school children related to inadequate hygiene and food-handling practices as evidenced by a 19% increase in reported cases within a 4-day period.

Planning
The school nurse, in conjunction with public health specialists, determined that several groups should be targeted in order to eliminate the further spread of disease. They identified a need to assist families in understanding the nature of the disease, how to care for their children who were ill, and how to prevent the spread at home. Within the school, there was a need to review food-handling practices and the training that cafeteria workers received. Staff, including teachers, also required information about *Shigella* and how it should be prevented in the everyday lives of students. Needs of special ages and developmental levels of children were also important. A formal plan of what needed to be done, by whom, and when was drawn up. Research into the nature and prevention of *Shigella* was gathered from the CDC and the local health department, among other sources. Health department staff developed a plan to release information to the public about the prevention of gastrointestinal illnesses, as many of these diseases are easily spread and so many students were already ill.

Long-Term Goal
- An absence of cases of infectious diarrhea

Short-Term Goals
- Treatment and recovery of all identified cases of diarrhea
- Implementation of an effective program of hygienic practices among students and staff
- Implementation of a food-handling program for all cafeteria workers
- Adequate informing of the larger community in order to prevent spread of the epidemic

Intervention
The school nurse took a central leadership role, directing action within the school aimed at staff, students, and student families. Teaching of appropriate hand washing was stressed. Hand-washing facilities were inspected for soap, paper towels, and running water. Food preparation guidelines were reviewed with staff, and policies regarding remaining at home when ill were reiterated. The health department staff provided technical assistance and made recommendations. They informed community physicians about surveillance and reporting requirements and provided information regarding case identification and treatment regimens. Daycare centers and preschools were advised to watch for diarrhea outbreaks and to adhere to strict hand-washing and diaper-handling practices, as these facilities tend to be high-risk areas for the transmission of organisms such as *Shigella*. The media were contacted to elicit their help in disseminating correct and useful information to the community.

Evaluation
Immediate evaluation involved monitoring the decline in *Shigella* cases both within the school and in the larger community. The school nurse noted that rates of absenteeism returned to normal on the following Monday. She determined that all classes had received hygiene instruction within the following 2 weeks and that all teachers had received a flyer with specific information about *Shigella*, its care, and its prevention. She observed that bathrooms had filled soap dispensers, that friendly signs reminding students to wash hands were posted near sinks, and that students were given the opportunity to wash hands before lunch and snacks. The public health department likewise continued surveillance activities after encouraging physicians to collect and submit stool culture specimens for suspected cases and to report cases to the health department. Rates of diarrhea declined rapidly in the week after the school outbreak. The infection did not spread to other schools or community groups. This outcome can be attributed to successful epidemic management, yet surveillance remains critical if the public's health is to be protected.

Levels of Prevention
Primary
- Teach students and staff about hand washing and hygienic practices.
- Maintain a system that promotes safe food-handling practices.
- Exclude those with symptoms from school or food handling.

Secondary
- Collect stool culture specimens from all symptomatic individuals.
- Treat those with advanced diarrhea symptoms with antibiotics.
- Exclude those with positive culture results from food handling, and exclude those with symptoms from school.
- Advise families and individuals in the care of those with diarrhea.

Tertiary
- Treat and counsel those determined to be carriers of *Shigella*.

Information on *Shigella* infections is available at https://www.cdc.gov/shigella/index.html

Number Exposed by Meal and Food Item (*N* = 143)

EXPOSURE VARIABLE (FOOD EATEN)	NUMBER WHO ATE		NUMBER WHO DID NOT EAT		
	ILL (A)	NOT ILL (B)	ILL (C)	NOT ILL (D)	ODDS RATIO*
Ate on Monday	47	60	18	18	0.78
Ate on Tuesday:	63	57	3	20	7.37
Fajitas	57	52	8	26	4.56
Salad	44	21	24	54	4.7
Salsa	26	29	40	48	1.07
Tortillas	48	53	16	26	1.47
Beans	29	32	34	48	1.28
Milk	53	56	11	23	1.98
Ate on Wednesday	21	64	43	15	0.11

*Odds ratios were calculated with the formula: ad/bd.
Modified from Texas Department of Health: *Shigella* outbreak in an elementary school, *Dis Prev News* 55(6):1–3, 1995.

SUMMARY

Epidemiology offers the community health nurse methods to quantify the extent of health problems in the community and provides a body of knowledge about risk factors and their association with disease. At each step of the nursing process, epidemiological applications support the practice of the community health nurse. Compiling descriptive data from surveys or studies contributes to the nurse's understanding of the community's health level. In assessing community problems, epidemiological rates describe the magnitude of disease and provide support for community diagnoses. Epidemiological studies suggest interventions and their potential efficacy—information that is useful in planning prevention and intervention approaches. Evaluation studies using epidemiological methods, either reported in the literature or conducted by community health nurses, are essential for providing optimal research-based care.

LEARNING ACTIVITIES

ⓔ EVOLVE WEBSITE

http://evolve.elsevier.com/Nies/community

- NCLEX Review Questions
- Case Studies

BIBLIOGRAPHY

Bhupathiraju SN, Pan A, Malik VS: Caffeinated and caffeine-free beverages and risk of type 2 diabetes, *Am J Clin Nutr* 97:155–166, 2013.

Buffardi AL, Thomas KK, Holmes KK, et al.: Moving upstream: ecosocial and psychosocial correlates of sexually transmitted infections among young adults in the United States, *Am J Public Health* 98(5):1128–1136, 2008.

Centers for Disease Control and Prevention: *About the national health and nutrition examination survey*, 2013. Available from < www.cdc.gov/nchs/nhanes/about_nhanes.htm >.

Centers for Disease Control and Prevention: Vital signs: colorectal screening test use – United States 2012, *MMWR Morb Mortal Wkly Rep* 62:881–888, 2013. Available from < http://www.ncbi.nlm.nih.gov/pubmed/24196665 >.

Centers for Disease Control and Prevention: Deaths: preliminary report for 2014, *National Vital Statistics Report* 65(4):1–122, 2016. Available from < http://www.cdc.gov/nchs/data/nvsr/nvsr65/nvsr65_04.pdf >.

Centers for Disease Control and Prevention: *Tuberculosis skin testing*, 2016. Available from < http://www.cdc.gov/tb/publications/factsheets/testing/skintesting.htm >.

Centers for Disease Control and Prevention: *The Tuskegee timeline*, 2017. Available from < http://www.cdc.gov/tuskegee/timeline.htm >.

Curtis CJ, Clapp J, Goldstein G, et al.: How the nurses' health study helped Americans take the trans fat out, *Am J Public Health* 106:1537–1539, 2016.

Doll R, Hill AB: Study of the aetiology of carcinoma of the lung, *BMJ* 2:1271–1285, 1952.

Doll R, Hill AB: Lung cancer and other causes of death in relation to smoking, *BMJ* 2:1071–1081, 1956.

Eliassen AH, Chen WY, Spiegelman D, et al.: Use of aspirin, other nonsteroidal anti-inflammatory drugs and acetaminophen and risk of breast cancer among premenopausal women in the Nurses' Health Study II, *Arch Intern Med* 169:115–121, 2009.

Friedman GD: *Primer of epidemiology*, ed 4, McGraw-Hill: New York.

Fryar CD, Ervin RB: Caloric intake from fast food among adults: United States 2007-2010, *National Center for Health Statistics Data Brief* 114, 2013. Available from < http://www.cdc.gov/nchs/data/databriefs/db114.pdf >.

Jeter JM, Han J, Martinez ME: Non-steroidal anti- inflammatory drugs, acetaminophen and risk of skin cancer in the Nurses' Health Study, *Cancer Causes Control* 223:1451–1461, 2012.

Kit BK, Fakhouri TH, Park S, et al.: Trends in sugar-sweetened beverage consumption among youth and adults in the United States: 1999-2010, *Am J Clini Nutrition* 98(1):180–188, 2013.

Kramarow E, Lubitz J, Francis R: Trends in the coronary heart disease risk profile of middle-aged adults, *Annals of Epidemiology* 23:31–34, 2013.

Lin JS, Piper MA, Perdue LA, etal: Screening for colorectal cancer: updated evidence report and systematic review for the US Preventive Services Task Force, *JAMA* 315(23):2576–2594, 2016. https://doi.org/10.1001/jama.2016.3332.

Mausner JS, Kramer S: *Mausner and Bahn epidemiology: an introductory text*, ed 2, Saunders: Philadelphia.

Morton RF, Hebel JR, McCarter RJ: *A study guide to epidemiology and biostatistics*, ed 3, Aspen Publishers: Gaithersburg, MD.

National Cancer Institute: *Surveillance, epidemiology and end results program*, 2017. Available from < http://seer.cancer.gov/ >.

National Center for Health Statistics: *Health indicators warehouse*, 2017. Available from https://www.healthdata.gov/dataset/health-indicators-warehouse.

Nurses' Health Study: *History*, 2017. Available from < http://www.channing.harvard.edu/nhs/?page_id=70.www.nurseshealthstudy.org/about-nhs/history >.

Olds DL, Kitzman HJ, Knudtson MD, et al.: Effect of home visiting by nurses on maternal and child mortality: Results of a 2-decade follow-up of a randomized clinical trial, *JAMA Pediatrics* 168(9):800–806, 2014. https://doi.org/10.1001/jamapediatrics.2014.472. doi:10.1001/archpediatrics.2010.49.

Organisation for Economic Cooperation and Development (OECD): *Health status: infant mortality rates*, 2015. Available from 2017 https://data.oecd.org/healthstat/infant-mortality-rates.htm.

Phillips JC: Antiretroviral therapy adherence: testing a social context model among black men who use illicit drugs, *J Assoc Nurs AIDS Care* 22:100–127, 2011.

Smith MV, Lincoln AK: Integrating social epidemiology into public health research and practice for maternal depression, *Am Jnl of Public Health* 101:990–994, 2011.

Snow J: *On the mode of communication of cholera*, ed 2, London, 1855, Churchill. 18.

Texas Department of Health: Shigella outbreak in an elementary school, *Dis Prev News* 55(6):1–3, 1995.

U.S. Department of Health and Human Services: *Healthy People 2020*, n.d. Available from < http://www.healthypeople.gov/2020/topics objectives2020/default.aspx >. Accessed February 25, 2017 .

Willet WC, Stampfer MJ, Manson JE, et al.: Intake of trans fatty acids and risk of coronary heart disease among women, *Lancet* 341:581–585, 1993.

World Health Organization: *Health topics: epidemiology*. Available from http://www.who.int/topics/epidemiology/en/. Accessed February 25, 2017.

Community Assessment

Holly B. Cassells

OBJECTIVES

Upon completion of this chapter, the reader will be able to do the following:

1. Discuss the major dimensions of a community.
2. Identify sources of information about a community's health.
3. Describe the process of conducting a community assessment.
4. Formulate community and aggregate diagnoses.
5. Identify uses for epidemiological data at each step of the nursing process.

KEY TERMS

aggregate
census tracts
community diagnosis
community of solution

geographic community
metropolitan statistical areas
needs assessment
social system

vital statistics
windshield survey

The primary concern of community health nurses is to improve the health of the community. To address this concern, community health nurses use all the principles and skills of nursing and public health practice. This process involves using demographic and epidemiological methods to assess the community's health and diagnose its health needs.

Before beginning this process, the community health nurse must define the community. The nurse may wonder how he or she can provide services to such a large and nontraditional "client," but there are smaller and more circumscribed entities that constitute a community than towns and cities. A major aspect of public health practice is the application of approaches and solutions to health problems that ensure that the majority of people receive the maximum benefit. To this end, the nurse works to use time and resources efficiently.

Despite the desire to provide services to each individual in a community, the community health nurse recognizes the impracticality of this task. An alternative approach considers the community itself to be the unit of service and works collaboratively with the community using the steps of the nursing process. Therefore the community is not only the context or place where community health nursing occurs; it is the focus of community health nursing care. The nurse partners with

community members to identify community problems and develop solutions to ultimately improve the community's health.

Another central goal of public health practitioners is primary prevention, which protects the public's health and prevents disease development. Chapter 3 discusses how these "upstream efforts" are intended to reduce the pain, suffering, and huge expenditures that occur when significant segments of the population essentially "fall into the river" and require downstream resources to resolve their health problems. In a society greatly concerned about increasingly high health care costs, the need to prevent health problems becomes dire. In addition to reducing the occurrence of disease in individuals, community health nurses must examine the larger aggregate—its structures, environments, and shared health risks—to develop improved upstream prevention programs.

This chapter addresses the first steps in adopting a community- or population-oriented practice. A community health nurse must define a community and describe its characteristics before applying the nursing process. Then, the nurse can launch the assessment and diagnosis phase of the nursing process at the aggregate level and incorporate epidemiological approaches. Comprehensive assessment data are essential to directing effective primary prevention interventions within a community.

Gathering these data is one of the core public health functions identified in the Institute of Medicine's (2002) report on the future of public health. The community health nurse participates in assessing the community's health and its ability to deal with health needs. With sound data, the nurse makes a valuable contribution to health policy development and population-based interventions.

THE NATURE OF COMMUNITY

Many dimensions describe the nature of community. These include an aggregate of people, a location in space and time, and a social system (Box 6.1).

Aggregate of People

An **aggregate** is a community composed of people who have common characteristics. For example, members of a community may share residence in the same city, membership in the same religious organization, or similar demographic characteristics such as age and ethnic background. The aggregate of senior citizens, for example, comprises primarily retirees who frequently share ages, economic pressures, life experiences, interests, and concerns. This group lived through the many societal changes of the past 50 years; therefore they may possess similar perspectives on current issues and trends. Many elderly people share concern for the maintenance of good health, the pursuit of an active lifestyle, and the security of needed services to support a quality life. These shared interests translate into common goals and activities, which also are defining attributes of a common interest community. Communities also may consist of overlapping aggregates, in which case some community members belong to multiple aggregates.

Many human factors help delineate a community. Health-related traits, or risk factors, are one aspect of "people factors" to be considered. People who have impaired health or a shared predisposition to disease may join together in a group or community to learn from and support each other. Parents of disabled infants, people with acquired immunodeficiency syndrome (AIDS), or those at risk for a second myocardial infarction may consider themselves a community. Even when these individuals are not organized, the nurse may recognize that their unique needs constitute a form of community, or aggregate.

A **community of solution** may form when a common problem unites individuals. Although people may have little else in common with each other, their desire to redress problems brings them together. Such problems may include a shared hazard from environmental contamination, a shared health problem arising from a soaring rate of teenage suicide, or a shared political concern about an upcoming city council election. The

community of solution often disbands after problem resolution, but it may subsequently identify other common issues.

Each of these shared features may exist among people who are geographically dispersed or in close proximity to one another. However, in many situations, proximity facilitates the recognition of commonality and the development of cohesion among members. This active sharing of features fosters a sense of community among individuals.

Location in Space and Time

Regardless of shared features, geographic or physical location may define communities of people. Traditionally, a community is an entity delineated by geopolitical boundaries; this view best exemplifies the dimension of location. These boundaries demarcate the periphery of cities, counties, states, and nations. Voting precincts, school districts, water districts, and fire and police protection precincts set less visible boundary lines.

Census tracts subdivide larger communities. The U.S. Census Bureau uses them for data collection and population assessment. Census tracts facilitate the organization of resident information in specific community geographic locales. In densely populated urban areas, the size of tracts tends to be small; therefore data for one or more census tracts frequently describe neighborhood residents. Although residents may not be aware of their census tract's boundaries, census tract data help define and describe neighborhood communities.

⚡ RESEARCH HIGHLIGHTS

Using Community Participatory Research to Assess Substance Use in a Rural Community

Kulbok and colleagues (2012) employed a Community Participatory Model to guide the assessment of youth substance abuse in a rural Virginia county and the development of a prevention model. They integrated multiple assessment modalities that represent current public health nursing competencies. Specifically, this project engaged local community members and leaders with community health professionals in every step of the project, from planning the assessment to developing and evaluating the intervention. This process allowed public health nurses to integrate their knowledge of the local community with that gained from community partners and to develop a deeper understanding of substance use and its local ecological and cultural context.

Researchers used a geographic information system not only to map the location of youth substance use but also to pinpoint areas where preventive behaviors were more common. These maps helped specifically target the location for preventive interventions. Perspectives of the youth about key "teen places" were also geographically mapped. The project used the photographic charity Photovoice to capture participants' descriptions of local strengths as well as concerns and then employed the images to facilitate conversation about the nature of alcohol, tobacco, and substance use in the community. Qualitative data about youth beliefs about substance use were gathered from focus groups. These data were combined with descriptive information about the local population, the community environment, and local social systems and beliefs to develop a comprehensive picture of the local community. Involvement of a broad range of community members throughout the project planning enabled a more effective, culturally appropriate, and sustainable intervention to be developed for this rural community.

Data from Kulbok PA, Thatcher E, Park E, et al.: Evolving public health nursing roles: focus on community participatory health promotion and prevention, *Online J Issues Nurs* 17(2):1, 2012. Retrieved from http://nursingworld.org/MainMenuCategories/ANAMarketplace/ANAPeriodicals/OJIN/TableofContents/Vol-17-2012/No2-May-2012/Evolving-Public-Health-Nursing-Roles.html.

BOX 6.1 Major Features of a Community

- Aggregate of people
  The "who": personal characteristics and risks
- Location in space and time
  The "where" and "when": physical location frequently delineated by boundaries and influenced by the passage of time
- Social system
  The "why" and "how": interrelationships of aggregates fulfilling community functions

Current Smokers, Percent of Adults by tract, BRFSS 500 Cities Project 2014

FIG. 6.1 Current smokers, percent of adults by tract, BRFSS 500 Cities Project, 2014. Location, Rapid City, South Dakota. Community Commons. Retrieved from www.communitycommons.org.

A **geographic community** can encompass less formalized areas that lack official geopolitical boundaries. A geographic landmark may define neighborhoods (e.g., the East Lake section of town or the North Shore area). A particular building style or a common development era also may identify community neighborhoods. Similarly, a dormitory, a communal home, or a summer camp may be a community because each facility shares a close geographic proximity. Geographic location, including the urban or rural nature of a community, strongly influences the nature of the health problems a community health nurse might find there. Public health is increasingly recognizing that the interaction of humans with the natural environment and with constructed environments consisting of buildings and spaces, termed the *built environment*, is critical to healthy behavior and quality of life. The spatial location of health problems in a geographic area can be mapped with the use of geographic information system software, assisting the nurse to identify vulnerable populations and public health departments to develop programs specific to geographic communities. For example, public health practitioners can map the distribution of smoking, the prevalence of hypertension, or the presence of areas classified as "food deserts" to help specifically target areas for intervention (Fig. 6.1).

Location and the dimension of time define communities. The community's character and health problems evolve over time. Although some communities are very stable, most tend to change with the members' health status and demographics and the larger community's development or decline. For example, the presence of an emerging young workforce may attract new industry, which can alter a neighborhood's health and environment. A community's history illustrates its ability to change and how well it addresses health problems over time.

Social System

The third major feature of a community is the relationships that community members form with one another. Community members fulfill the essential functions of community by interacting in groups. These functions provide socialization, role fulfillment, goal achievement, and member support. Therefore a community is a complex **social system**, and its interacting members constitute various subsystems within the community.

These subsystems are interrelated and interdependent (i.e., the subsystems affect one another and affect various internal and external stimuli). These stimuli consist of a broad range of events, values, conditions, and needs.

A health care system is an example of a complex system that consists of smaller, interrelated subsystems. A health care system can also be a subsystem because it interacts with and depends on larger systems such as the city government. Changes in the larger system can cause repercussions in many subsystems. For example, when local economic pressures cause a health department to scale back its operations, many subsystems are affected. The health department may eliminate or cut back programs, limit service to other health care providers, reduce access to groups that normally use the system, and deny needed care to families who constitute subsystems in society. Almost every subsystem in the community must react and readjust to such a financial constraint.

Prevalent health problems also can have a severe impact on multiple systems. For example, the AIDS epidemic required significant funds for clients with this condition and for public education and prevention. It made unrelenting demands on many communities that were already strapped for funds to meet their citizens' basic health needs. In San Francisco, the allocation of funds for AIDS programs initially reduced funding for other programs, such as immunizations, family planning, and well-child care.

HEALTHY COMMUNITIES

Complex community systems receive many varied stimuli. The community's ability to respond effectively to changing dynamics and meet the needs of its members indicates productive functioning. Examining the community's functions and subsystems provides clues to existing and potential health problems. Examples of a community's functions include the provision of accessible and acceptable health services; educational opportunities; and safe, crime-free environments.

The model in Fig. 6.2 suggests assessment parameters that can help a nurse develop a more complete list of critical community functions. The community health nurse can then prioritize these functions from a particular community's perspective. Americans' views on health and healthy communities frequently reflect concern for quality-of-life issues over the absence of disease, and in particular safety and low levels of crime are of high priority. These findings are echoed in city-sponsored health surveys across the nation: ensuring safe and healthy environments that allow for healthy lifestyles, which include activity and nutritious food, is as important to residents as accessing quality health care.

Movements such as *Healthy Cities and Healthy Places* urge community members and leaders to bring about positive health changes in their local environments (CDC, 2014; World Health Organization, 2017). Involving many cities around the nation and world, these models stress the interconnectedness among people and the public and private sectors essential for local communities to address the causes of poor health. In particular, examining the role the "built environment" has on community health (e.g., its physical and environmental design) is an increasing priority (Robert Wood Johnson Foundation, 2017). Urban communities are encouraged to consider the health consequences of new policies and programs they introduce by

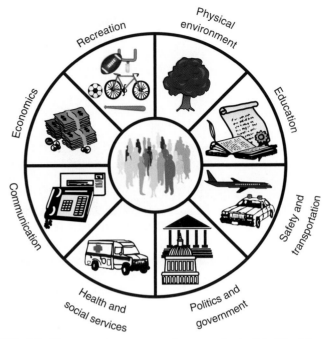

FIG. 6.2 Diagram of assessment parameters. (Modified from Anderson ET, McFarlane J: *Community as partner: theory and practice in nursing* ed 7, Philadelphia, PA, 2015, Wolters Kluwer.)

conducting health impact assessments (Pew Charitable Trusts, 2017). These assessments of projects, such as the potential impact of zoning decisions, transit systems, and sick leave policies, serve the important function of bringing a public health perspective to urban and civic initiatives.

Each community and aggregate presumably will have a unique perspective on critical health qualities. Indeed, a community or aggregate may have divergent definitions of health, differing even from that of the community health nurse. Nevertheless, nurses and health professionals work with communities in developing effective solutions that are acceptable to residents. Building a community's capacity to address future problems is often referred to as *developing community competence*. The nurse assesses the community's commitment to a healthy future, the ability to foster open communication and to elicit broad participation in problem identification and resolution, the active involvement of structures such as a health department that can assist a community with health issues, and the extent to which members have successfully worked together on past problems. This information provides the nurse with an indication of the community's strengths and potential for developing long-term solutions to identified problems.

ASSESSING THE COMMUNITY: SOURCES OF DATA

The community health nurse becomes familiar with the community and begins to understand its nature by traveling through the area. The nurse begins to establish certain hunches or hypotheses about the community's health, strengths, and potential health problems through this down-to-earth approach, called *shoe leather epidemiology*. The community health nurse must substantiate these initial assessments and impressions

WINDSHIELD SURVEY

Brookshire is a town of about 3500 in Southeast Texas.

Sugar mills and farms are the source of most jobs.

Accessible and affordable health care is a challenge. This van provides services to unskilled workers and area elders.

The economy of the town is predominantly agriculture and processing.

The car's thermometer shows 99°, evidence of a pervasive health threat in the summertime.

Much of the housing is substandard and suggests low-income families.

Many people live in small homes on multiple-acre lots.

Photos courtesy of University of Texas Health Science Center at Houston, School of Nursing, Community Health Division.

WINDSHIELD SURVEY—cont'd

The important determinants of a health community include a low crime rate, a good place to bring up children, good schools, a strong family life, good environmental quality, and a healthy economy. (iStock 540095516, 683792276, 504534788, 470237304, 638480042)

with more concrete or defined data before he or she can formulate a community diagnosis and plan.

Community health nurses often perform a community **windshield survey** by driving or walking through an area and making organized observations. See illustrations depicting an actual "windshield survey" in this chapter's photo novella. The nurse can gain an understanding of the environmental layout, including geographic features and the location of agencies, services, businesses, and industries, and can locate possible areas of environmental concern through "sight, sense, and sound." The windshield survey offers the nurse an opportunity to observe people and their role in the community. Box 6.2 provides examples of questions to guide a windshield survey assessment.

In addition to direct observational methods, certain public health tools become essential to an aggregate-focused

nursing practice. The analysis of demographic information and statistical data provides descriptive information about the population. Epidemiology involves the analysis of health data to discover the patterns of health and illness distribution in a population. Epidemiology also involves conducting research to explain the nature of health problems and identify the aggregates at increased risk. The rest of this section provides data sources and describes how the community health nurse can use demographic and epidemiological data to assess the aggregate.

? ACTIVE LEARNING EXERCISE

Walk through a neighborhood, and describe the sensory information (i.e., smells, sounds, and sights). How does each relate to the community's health?

BOX 6.2   Questions to Guide Community Observations During a Windshield Survey

1. Community vitality:
   - Are people visible in the community? What are they doing?
   - Who are the people living in the neighborhood? What is their age range? What is the predominant age (e.g., elderly, preschoolers, young mothers, or school-aged children)?
   - What ethnicity or race is most common?
   - What is the general appearance of those you observed? Do they appear healthy? Do you notice any people with obvious disabilities, such as those using walkers or wheelchairs, or those with mental or emotional disabilities? Where do they live?
   - Do you notice residents who are well nourished or malnourished, thin or obese, vigorous or frail, unkempt or scantily dressed, or well dressed and clean?
   - Do you notice tourists or visitors to the community?
   - Do you observe any people who appear to be under the influence of drugs or alcohol?
   - Do you see any pregnant women? Do you see women with strollers and young children?
2. Indicators of social and economic conditions:
   - What is the general condition of the homes you observe? Are these single-family homes or multifamily structures? Is there any evidence of dilapidated housing or of areas undergoing urban renewal? Is there public housing? What is its condition?
   - What forms of transportation do people seem to be using? Is there public transit? Are there adequate bus stops with benches and shade? Is transportation to health care resources available?
   - Are there any indicators of the kinds of work available to residents? Are there job opportunities nearby, such as factories, small businesses, or military installations? Are there unemployed people visible, such as homeless people?
   - Do you see men congregating in groups on the street? What do they look like, and what are they doing?
   - Is this a rural area? Are there farms or agricultural businesses?
   - Do you note any seasonal workers, such as migrant or day laborers?
   - Do you see any women hanging out along the streets? What are they doing?
   - Do you observe any children or adolescents out of school during the daytime?
   - Do you observe any interest in political campaigns or issues, such as campaign signs?
   - Do you see any evidence of health education on billboards, advertisements, signs, radio stations, or television stations? Do these methods seem appropriate for the people you observed?
   - What kinds of schools and day care centers are available?
3. Health resources:
   - Do you notice any hospitals? What kind are they? Where are they located?
   - Are there any clinics? Whom do they serve? Are there any family planning services?
   - Are there doctors' and dentists' offices? Are they specialists or generalists?
   - Do you notice any nursing homes, rehabilitation centers, mental health clinics, alcohol or drug treatment centers, homeless or abused shelters,

   wellness clinics, health department facilities, urgent care centers, mobile health vehicles, blood donation centers, or pharmacies?
   - Are these resources appropriate and sufficient to address the kinds of problems that exist in this community?
4. Environmental conditions related to health:
   - Do you see evidence of anything that might make you suspicious of ground, water, or air pollutants?
   - What is the sanitary condition of the housing? Is housing overcrowded, dirty, or in need of repair? Are windows screened?
   - What is the condition of the roads? Are potholes present? Are drainage systems in place? Are there low water crossings, and do they have warning signals? Are there adequate traffic lights, signs, sidewalks, and curbs? Are railroad crossings fitted with warnings and barriers? Are streets and parking lots well lit? Is this a heavily trafficked area, or are roads rural? Are there curves or features that make the roads hazardous?
   - Is there handicapped access to buildings, sidewalks, and streets?
   - Do you observe recreational facilities and playgrounds? Are they being used? Is there a YMCA/YWCA or community center? Are there any day-care facilities or preschools?
   - Are children playing in the streets, alleys, yards, or parks?
   - Do you see any restaurants?
   - Is food sold on the streets? Are people eating in public areas? Are there trash receptacles and places for people to sit? Are public restrooms available?
   - What evidence of any nuisances such as ants, flies, mosquitoes, or rodents do you observe? Are there stray animals wandering in the neighborhood?
5. Social functioning:
   - Do you observe any families in the neighborhoods? Can you observe their structure or functioning? Who is caring for the children? What kind of supervision do they have? Is more than one generation present?
   - Are there any identifiable subgroups related to one another either socially or geographically?
   - What evidence of a sense of neighborliness can you observe?
   - What evidence of community cohesiveness can you observe? Are there any group efforts in the neighborhood to improve the living conditions or the neighborhood? Is there a neighborhood watch? Do community groups post signs for neighborhood meetings?
   - How many and what type of churches, synagogues, and other places of worship are there?
   - Can you observe anything that would make you suspicious of social problems, such as gang activity, juvenile delinquency, drug or alcohol abuse, and adolescent pregnancy?
6. Attitude toward health and health care:
   - Do you observe any evidence of folk medicine practice, such as a botánica or herbal medicine shop? Are there any alternative medicine practitioners, such as healers or curanderos?
   - Do you observe that health resources are well utilized or underutilized?
   - Is there evidence of preventive or wellness care?
   - Do you observe any efforts to improve the neighborhood's health? Planned health fairs? Do you see advertisements for health-related events, clinics, or lectures?

Census Data

Every 10 years, the U.S. Census Bureau undertakes a massive survey of all American families. In addition to this decennial census, intermediate surveys collect specific types of information. These collections of statistical data describe the population characteristics of the nation within progressively smaller geopolitical entities (e.g., states, counties, and census tracts). The census also

describes large metropolitan areas that extend beyond formal city boundaries, called metropolitan statistical areas (MSAs). An MSA consists of a central city with more than 50,000 people and includes the associated suburban or adjacent counties, which yields a total metropolitan area with more than 100,000 people. Adjacent MSAs with their associated cities and counties constitute very large metropolitan regions called *combined statistical areas.* A census tract is one of the smallest reporting units. It usually consists of 3000 to 6000 people who share characteristics such as ethnicity, socioeconomic status, and housing class.

The census is extremely helpful to community health nurses familiarizing themselves with a new community. The census tabulates many demographic variables, including population size and the distribution of age, sex, race, and ethnicity. The American Community Survey, conducted annually, reports social data such as income, poverty, and occupational factors. Both data sets can be accessed through use of the Census Bureau's American Factfinder tools—available at http://factfinder2.census.gov/faces/nav/jsf/pages/index.xhtml—where the nurse can view several variables in combination (e.g., age and ethnicity). One can easily construct a community profile and compare trends with those in other communities. Note that variables that describe the community's health are not part of census data. However, census numbers are frequently used as denominators for morbidity and mortality rates (see Chapter 5).

The nurse analyzes and interprets data by comparing current and local census data with previous data and information from various locations to pinpoint key local differences and changes over time. The nurse can identify the attributes that make each community unique by comparing data for one census unit, such as a census tract or a city, with those of another community or the entire nation. These attributes provide clues to the community's potential vulnerabilities or health risks. For example, a community health nurse may review census reports and discover that a district has many elderly people. This knowledge directs the nurse toward further assessment of the social resources (i.e., housing, transportation, and community centers), health resources (i.e., hospitals, nursing homes, and geriatric clinics), and health problems common to aging people. By identifying the trends in the population over time, the community health nurse can modify public health programs to meet the changing needs of the community.

ETHICAL INSIGHTS

Attending to Nondominant Trends: "Hidden Pockets" of Need

Whereas most public health practitioners are attuned to the leading indicators or dominant trends in data, vital statistics or census data can suggest the existence of small "hidden pockets" of people with special needs. One nurse initially assessed her community as being in an upper-middle-class bracket. She was surprised to find 20 families living below the poverty level and 3 families living without running water. Although these 20 families made up far less than 1% of the community population, they nevertheless necessitated the attention of the community health nurse. Some may view a focus on such a minority segment as insignificant and in conflict with the "rule of utility," which posits "the greatest good for the greatest number." However, community health nursing practice combines principles of beneficence and social justice with utilitarianism, and thus small vulnerable segments of the community are considered legitimate clients of community health nursing. Indeed, social justice not only "gives moral privilege to the needs of the most vulnerable" but also suggests the amelioration of conditions that create social and economic disparities (Boutain, 2016). Furthermore, nurses recognize that this "hidden pocket" is a small piece of the total community and, as such, contributes to its overall health. By attending to these families' health needs, the nurse positively affects the health of the whole.

Vital Statistics

The official registration records of births, deaths, marriages, divorces, and adoptions form the basis of data in vital statistics. Every year, city, county, and state health departments aggregate and report these events for the preceding year. When compared with those from previous years, vital statistics provide indicators of population growth or reduction. In addition to supplying information about the number of births and deaths, registration certificates record the causes of death, which is useful in determining morbidity and mortality trends. Similarly, birth certificates document birth information (e.g., cesarean delivery, prenatal care, and teen mothers) and the occurrence of any congenital malformations. This information also is important in assessments of the community's health status.

Other Sources of Health Data

The U.S. Census Bureau conducts numerous surveys on subjects of government interest, such as crime, housing, and labor. Results of these surveys, the census reports, and vital statistics reports are usually available through public libraries and on the Internet. The National Center for Health Statistics (NCHS) compiles annual National Health Interview Survey data, which describe health trends in a national sample. The NCHS publishes reports on the prevalence of disability, illness, and other health-related variables. Specifically, the Behavioral Risk Factor Surveillance System is the world's largest telephone survey of U.S. citizens' health behaviors and risk factors. It tracks trends by nation, state, and year, with the goal of identifying emerging health problems. Data also are used to evaluate achievement of health objectives and develop prevention strategies. The Behavior Risk Factor Surveillance System's website allows one to compile graphs and maps to describe specific risk behaviors by state (http://www.cdc.gov/brfss/).

In addition to these important sources of information, community health nurses can access a broad range of local, regional, and state government reports that contribute to the comprehensive assessment of a population. Local agencies, chambers of commerce, and health and hospital districts collect invaluable information on their community's health. Local health planning agencies also compile and analyze statistical data during the planning process. The community health nurse can use all of these formal and informal resources in learning about a community or aggregate (Table 6.1). Box 6.3 lists additional information about sources of population health data.

Formal data collection does not exist for all community aspects; therefore many community health nurses must perform additional data collection, compilation, and analysis. For example, school nurses regularly use aggregate data from student records to learn about the demographic composition of their population. They conduct ongoing surveys of classroom attendance and causes of illness, which are essential to an effective school health program. Sometimes the nurse must screen the entire school population to discover the extent of a disease. Thus the school nurse is both a consumer of existent data and a researcher who collects new data for the assessment of the school community.

TABLE 6.1   Community Assessment Parameters

Parameter	Importance to chn	Source of information
Geography Topography Climate (e.g., extreme heat or cold)	Influences nature of health problems and access to health care	Almanac Chamber of commerce

Population
Size
Demographic character (e.g., aged or young)
Trends
Migration
Density
	Describes population served; suggests their health risks
	  and needs
	Suggests growth or decline
	Increases stress; may increase exposure to communicable
	  disease
		Census documents
		Chamber of commerce

Environment
Water (e.g., source, fluoridated)
Sewage and waste disposal
Air quality (e.g., ozone, pollutants)
Food quality and access
Housing (e.g., single-family or multifamily dwellings)
Animal control (e.g., exposure to rabies and other
  zoonotic diseases)
	Affects quality of life and nature of environmental health
	  problems
	Reflects community resources
	Suggests socioeconomic issues
		Local and state health departments
		Newspapers
		Local environmental action group
		Census documents

Industry Employment levels Manufacturing White collar vs. blue collar Income levels	Affects social class, access to health care, and resources Influences nature of health problems	Chamber of commerce Almanac Employment commission Census documents
Education Schools (e.g., physical plant, playground safety) Types of education Literacy rates Special education Health services Sex education School lunch programs (e.g., nutritious diets) After-school programs Daycare Access to higher education	Influences socioeconomic status, access to health care, and ability to read and understand health information	Census documents School districts and nurses
Recreation Parks and playgrounds Libraries Public and private recreation Special facilities	Reflects quality of life, resources available to community, and concern for the young and disadvantaged	Parks and recreation departments Newspapers

Religion
Churches and synagogues
Denominations
Community programs
Health-related programs and parish health programs
Community organizations
	Influences values in community by organizing common
	  interests and concerns
	Reflects involvement of members, community skills,
	  and resources for community needs
		Chamber of commerce
		Newspapers
		Community center newsletters

Communication Newspapers Neighborhood news Radio and television Telephone Internet Hotlines Medical media Public service announcements	Reflects concerns and needs of the community Contains networks and resources available for health-related use	Local libraries Newspapers Internet resources Local health department Medical and nursing societies
Transportation Intercity and intracity Handicapped Emergency transport	Affects access to services, food, and other resources Reflects resources available to community	Local bus and train services Local hospital emergency service

TABLE 6.1   Community Assessment Parameters—cont'd

Parameter	Importance to chn	Source of information
Public Services	Affects community security	Local police department
Fire protection	Reflects available resources	
Police protection		
Emergency medical services		
Rape treatment centers		
Utilities		
Political Organization	Reflects level of citizen activism, involvement, values, and concerns	Newspapers
Structure		Local political party organization
Method for filing positions	Mechanism for nurse activism and lobbying	Local board of elections
Responsibilities of positions		Local representatives
Sources of revenue		
Voter registration		
Community Development or Planning	Reflects community needs and concerns	Newspapers
Activities	Affects level of professionals' involvement in issues	Local and state planning board
Major issues		Local community organizations
Disaster Programs	Offers a level of preparedness, coordination, and available resources	Local American Red Cross office
American Red Cross		Local emergency coordinating council
Disaster plans	Influences resources and plans	Local fire department
Potential sources of disaster		
Health Statistics	Reflects health problems, trends, and state of community health	Local and state health department
Mortality		Health facilities and programs
Morbidity	Affects resources needed and CHN services provided	National vital statistics reports
Leading causes of death		National Center for Health Statistics reports
Births		Morbidity and Mortality Weekly Report
Social Problems	Affects health problems and amounts of required services	Local and state department of social services
Mental health issues	Influences CHN program priorities	
Alcoholism and drug abuse		Local mental health centers
Suicide		Local hotlines
Crime		Libraries
School dropout		
Unemployment		
Gangs		
Health Professionals	Influences available health resources and nature of CHN practice	Local and state health planning agencies
Number of physicians, dentists, and nurses per population		Health professional organizations
		Telephone directory
		Community service director
Health Professional Organizations	Provides support for CHN practice	Public health association
Community Services	Reflect available resources	Local United Way organization
(e.g., cost and eligibility, accessibility, and acceptability)		Local voluntary service directory
Institutional care (e.g., hospitals and nursing homes)		County hospital
Mental health care		Local health department
Ambulatory care		Telephone directory/Internet resources
Preventive health services		
Nursing services		
Welfare services		

CHN, Community health nursing.

NEEDS ASSESSMENT

The nurse must understand the community's perspective on health status, the services it uses or requires, and its concerns. Most official data do not capture this type of information. Data collected directly from an aggregate may be more insightful and accurate; therefore community health nurses sometimes conduct community needs assessments. There are several approaches to gathering subjective data; however, a nurse's careful planning of the process will contribute to its reliability and utility regardless of the method. Box 6.4 presents the required steps in conducting a needs assessment.

The strategy chosen for collecting needs assessment data depends on the size and nature of the aggregate, the purpose for collecting information, and the resources available to the nurse. In some cases, the nurse may survey a small sample of clients to measure their satisfaction with a program. In other situations, a large-scale community needs assessment may help the nurse

---

BOX 6.3 Retrieval of Data

Current data on U.S. population health are stored in many places. Finding the latest statistics at the local, state, or national level can be a challenging experience for a student, community health nurse, graduate student, or nurse researcher. However, statistics provide a necessary comparison in identifying the health status of an aggregate or population in a community. The following guidelines suggest places to begin a search.

Reference Librarian

The best place to start is in a school or community library or in a large university's health sciences library. Cultivate a relationship with the reference librarian and learn how to access the literature of interest (e.g., government documents) or how to perform computer-guided literature searches.

Government Documents

Local libraries have a listing of government depository libraries, which house government documents for the public. If the government document is not available at a local library, ask the reference librarian to contact a regional or state library for an interlibrary loan. The Library of Congress in Washington, D.C., has a *Directory of U.S. Government Depository Libraries*.

Health, United States

An annual publication of the National Center for Health Statistics (2017), *Health, United States* reports the latest health statistics for the country. It presents statistics in areas such as maternal–child health indicators (e.g., prenatal care, low birth weight, and infant mortality), life expectancy, mortality, morbidity (e.g., cancer incidence and survival, AIDS, and diabetes), environmental health indicators

(e.g., air pollution and noise exposure), and health system use (e.g., national health expenditures, health insurance coverage, physician contacts, and diagnostic and surgical procedures). Graphs and tables are easy to read and interpret with accompanying texts. Many statistics include a selected number of years to illustrate trends. Some statistics are compared with those from other countries and U.S. minority populations. (For more information, visit http://www.cdc.gov/nchs/hus/index.htm.)

Morbidity and Mortality Weekly Report (MMWR)

The CDC in Atlanta, Georgia, prepares this publication. State health departments compile weekly reports for the publication that outline the numbers of cases of notifiable diseases such as AIDS, gonorrhea, hepatitis, measles (rubeola), pertusis, rubella, syphilis, tuberculosis, and rabies and reports the deaths in 122 U.S. cities by age. It also reports accounts of interesting cases, environmental hazards, disease outbreaks, or other public health problems. Local and state health departments and many local and health sciences libraries house this weekly publication. A subscription is available at http://www.cdc.gov/mmwr/.

Centers for Disease Control and Prevention

The CDC compiles information on a range of topics, including health behavior, educational and community-based programs, unintentional injuries, occupational safety and health, environmental health, oral health, diabetes and chronic disabling conditions, communicable disease, immunizations, clinical preventive services, and surveillance and data systems. Data are reported in several publications and on the website: http://www.cdc.gov/.

BOX 6.4 Steps in the Needs Assessment Process

1. Identify aggregate for assessment.
2. Engage community in planning the assessment.
3. Identify required information.
4. Select method of data gathering.
5. Develop questionnaire or interview questions.
6. Develop procedures for data collection.
7. Train data collectors.
8. Arrange for a sample representative of the aggregate.
9. Conduct needs assessment.
10. Tabulate and analyze data.
11. Identify needs suggested by data.
12. Develop an action plan.

---

determine gaps in service. Although the process of needs assessment can indicate a program's strengths and weaknesses, it can also raise expectations for new services on the part of community members. Involving community members in the planning of the assessment builds trust and ownership in the process, and subsequently in the improvements that result. With the implementation of the U.S. Patient Protection and Affordable Care Act, nonprofit hospitals must conduct comprehensive community health needs assessments, often called *CHNAs*, which create an important opportunity to coordinate with public health agencies to more effectively make decisions and strategically plan to address local health needs (Community Commons, 2017; National Association of County and City Health Officials [NACCHO], 2017).

A first approach to gathering data is to interview *key informants* in the community. These may be knowledgeable residents, elected officials, or health care providers. It is essential that the community health nurse recognize that the views of these people may not reflect the views of all residents. A second approach is to hold a *community forum* to discuss selected questions. It is important for the nurse to carefully plan the meeting in advance to gain the most useful information. The community health nurse can also mail surveys to community members to elicit information from a more diverse group of people who may be unwilling or unable to attend a community forum. *Focus groups* are a third approach; these can be very effective in gathering community views, particularly for remote and vulnerable segments of a community and for those with underdeveloped opinionsNurses who conduct focus groups must carefully select participants, formulate questions, and analyze recorded sessions (University of Kansas, 2017). These sessions can produce greater interaction and expression of ideas than surveys and may provide more insight into an aggregate's opinions. In addition to encouraging community participation in the identification of assets and needs, focus groups may lay the groundwork for community involvement in planning the solutions to identified problems.

DIAGNOSING HEALTH PROBLEMS

The next step of the nursing process is synthesizing assessment data, in which the nurse plans to examine data and creates a list of all actual and potential problems. Then the nurse develops diagnostic statements about the community's health. These statements, or diagnoses, specify the nature and cause of an actual or potential community health problem and direct the community health nurses' plans to resolve the problem. Muecke

(1984) developed a format that assists in writing a **community diagnosis**. The diagnosis consists of four components: the identification of the health problem or risk, the affected aggregate or community, the etiological or causal statement, and the evidence or support for the diagnosis (Fig. 6.3). Each of these components has an important role to play in the nursing process. The problem represents a synthesis of all assessment data. The "among" phrase specifies the aggregate that will be the beneficiary of the nurse's action plan and whose health is at risk. The "related to" phrase describes the cause of the health problem and directs the focus of the intervention. All plans and interventions will be aimed at addressing this underlying cause. Last, the health indicators are the supporting data or evidence drawn from the completed assessment. These data can suggest the magnitude of the problem and have a bearing on prioritizing diagnoses. Other factors that assist the nurse in ranking the importance of diagnoses include the nature of the diagnosis, its potential impact on a broad range of community residents, and the community's perceptions of the health issue.

NURSING CARE GUIDELINES

Wellness Diagnosis

Sometimes nurses develop *wellness diagnoses*. These often focus on the individual, but can make a positive statement about the community's strengths. They are a variant on the North American Nursing Diagnosis Association's health promotion diagnoses. Wellness diagnoses address the potential of a segment of the population of the community to move toward a higher level of wellness and presume a certain level of readiness to change. For example, a wellness diagnosis might be written to describe a strength that should be reinforced and supported, as follows: *Increased potential for positive infant outcomes among teenage mothers related to effective parenting as evidenced by increased participation in mother–baby practice sessions and positive newborn-care behaviors.*

As in a community diagnosis, four components lead to a cohesive statement about health status.

Increased risk of _____
(disability, disease, etc.)

among _____ related to
(community or population)

_____ as demonstrated
(etiological statement)

in _____ .
(health indicators)

FIG. 6.3 Format for community health diagnosis. (Redrawn from Muecke MA: Community health diagnosis in nursing, *Public Health Nurs* 1:23–35, 1984. Used with permission of Blackwell Scientific Publications.)

BOX 6.5 Example of Outcomes Evaluation: A Community-Based Intervention to Promote Smoking Cessation

Matthews and colleagues (2013) reported the results of a community-based and culturally tailored smoking cessation program designed for lesbian, gay, bisexual, transgender (LGBT) people, a population with more than double the rate of smoking as heterosexuals and an increased risk for respiratory and cardiac disease. A series of smoking cessation classes designed for and marketed to the LGBT community were conducted for 198 individuals. Adapted from the American Lung Association's Freedom from Smoking curriculum, the intervention incorporated LGBT concerns related to the role of smoking in LGBT culture, stress due to homophobia as a smoking trigger, relationship between bar culture and smoking and alcohol, and the targeting of LGBT persons by the tobacco industry. Thirty separate small treatment groups were conducted in eight weekly sessions. Three of these included a peer-buddy program in the Call it Quits groups, and free nicotine replacement was available to all. Although only 42% completed treatment, 32.3% self-reported smoking cessation upon completion, with the 24% who used nicotine replacement having the highest cessation rates. These rates were consistent with general community programs; however, the authors cited the benefits of a tailored, culturally specific program and stressed the need to continue to address the formidable barriers to abstention faced by LGBT smokers in preventing relapses.

Data from Matthews AK, Chien-Ching L, Kuhns LM, et al.: Results from a community-based smoking cessation program for LGBT smokers, *J Environ Public Health, 2013,* Article ID 984508, https://doi:10.1155/2013/984508.

With a clear statement of the problem in the form of a diagnosis, the community health nurse is ready to begin the planning phase of the nursing process. Inherent in this phase is a plan for the intervention and its evaluation. Once again, epidemiological data can be useful as a basis for determining success. By comparing baseline data, national and local data, and other relevant indicators, the nurse can construct benchmarks to gauge achievement of program objectives. This step may entail the calculation of incidence rates if the goal is to reduce the development of disease, or primary prevention. Comparing data with national rates or with prevalence rates found in a local community may be other indicators of success. Reducing the presence of risk factors and documenting patterns of healthy behavior are other objective indices of successful programs.

It is evident that epidemiological data and methods are essential to each phase of the nursing process. The community health nurse compiles a range of assessment data that support the nursing diagnosis. Epidemiological studies support program planning by establishing the effectiveness of certain interventions

and their specificity for different aggregates. Finally, epidemiological data are important for the community health nurse's documentation of a program's long-term effectiveness. Box 6.5 provides an evaluation example.

ACTIVE LEARNING EXERCISE

1. Walk through a neighborhood, and compile a list of variables that are important to describe with demographic and epidemiological data. Write down hunches or preconceived notions about the nature of the community's population. Compare ideas with the collected statistical data.
2. Compile a range of relevant demographic and epidemiological data for the community by examining census reports, vital statistics reports, city records, and other library and agency sources.
3. Using the collected data, identify three community health problems and formulate three community health diagnoses.

CASE STUDY   Application of the Nursing Process

Assessment and Diagnosis

The following example demonstrates the process of collecting and analyzing data and deriving community diagnoses. It also exemplifies the multiple care levels within which community health nurses function: the individual client, the family, and the aggregate or community levels. In this scenario, the nurse identified an individual client health problem during a home visit, which provided the initial impetus for an aggregate health education program. Data collection expanded from the assessment of the individual to a broad range of literature and data about the nature of the problem in populations. The nurse then formulated a community-level diagnosis to direct the ensuing plan. This was subsequently implemented at the aggregate level and then evaluated.

School nurses frequently address a broad range of student health problems. In the West San Antonio School District, school nurses generally reserve several hours a week for home visits. In a recent case, a teacher expressed concern for a high school junior named "John" whose brother was dying of cancer. In a health class, John shared his personal fears about cancer, which caused his classmates to question their own cancer risks and how they might reduce them.

Assessment

The school nurse visited John's family and learned that the 25-year-old son had testicular cancer. Since his diagnosis 1 year earlier, he had undergone a range of therapies that were palliative but not curative; the cancer was advanced at the time of diagnosis. The nurse spent time with the family discussing care, answering questions, and exploring available support for the entire family.

At a school nurse staff meeting, the nurse inquired about her colleagues' experiences with other young clients with this type of cancer. Only one nurse remembered a young man with testicular cancer. The nurses were not familiar with its prevalence, incidence, risk factors, prevention strategies, or early detection approaches. The nurse recognized the high probability that high school students would have similar questions and could benefit from reliable information.

The school nurse embarked on a community assessment to answer these questions. The nurse first collected information about testicular cancer. Second, the nurse reviewed the nursing and medical literature for key articles discussing client care, diagnosis, and treatment. Epidemiological studies provided additional data regarding testicular cancer's distribution pattern in the population and associated risk factors.

The nurse learned that young men aged 20 to 35 years were at the greatest risk. Other major risk factors were not identified. It was learned that healthy young men do not seek testicular cancer screening and regular health care; they may be apprehensive about conditions affecting sexual function. These factors contribute to delays in detection and treatment. Although only an estimated 8850 new cases of testicular cancer will have been diagnosed in the United States in 2017, it is one of the most common tumors in young men. Furthermore, this cancer is amenable to treatment with early diagnosis (American Cancer Society, n.d.).

On the basis of these facts, the nurse reasoned that a prevention program would benefit high school students. However, to perform a comprehensive assessment, it was important that the nurse clarified what students did know, how comfortable they were discussing sexual health, and how much the subject interested them. Therefore the nurse approached the junior and senior high school students and administered a questionnaire to elicit this information. The nurse also queried the health teacher about the amount of pertinent cancer and sexual development information the students received in the classroom. The

nurse considered the latter an important prerequisite to dealing with the sensitive subject of sexual health. According to the health teacher, the students did receive instruction about physical development and psychosexual issues. Students expressed a strong desire for more classroom instruction on these subjects and more information on cancer prevention. However, they did not have sufficient knowledge of the beneficial health practices related to cancer prevention and early detection.

Key Assessment Data

- Health status of John's brother
- Knowledge, coping, and support resources of family
- Testicular cancer, its natural history, treatment and prevention, incidence, prevalence, mortality, and risk factors
- High school students' knowledge about cancer and its prevention
- Students' comfort level with discussing sexual health issues

Community Diagnosis

There is an increased risk of undetected testicular cancer among young men related to insufficient knowledge about the disease and the methods for preventing and detecting it at an early stage, as demonstrated by high rates of late initiation of treatment.

Planning

Clarifying the problem and its cause helped the nurse direct the planning phase of the nursing process and determine both long-term and short-term goals.

The long-term goal was:

- Students will identify testicular lesions at an early stage and seek care promptly.

The short-term goals were:

- Students will understand testicular cancer and self-detection techniques.
- Students will exhibit comfort with sexual health issues by asking questions.
- Male students will report regular testicular self-examination.

Planning encompassed several activities, including the discovery of recommended health care practices regarding testicular cancer. The nurse also sought to determine the most effective and appropriate educational approaches for male and female high school students. Identifying helpful community agencies was also an essential part of the process. The local chapter of the American Cancer Society provided valuable information, materials, and consulting services. A nearby nursing school's media center and faculty were also very supportive of the program.

After formalizing her objectives and plan, the nurse presented the project to the high school's teaching coordinator and principal. Their approval was necessary before the nurse could implement the project. After eliciting their enthusiastic support, the nurse proceeded with more detailed plans. She selected and developed classroom instruction methods and activities that would maximize high school students' involvement. The nurse also ordered a film and physical models for demonstrating and practicing testicular self-examination. She prepared group exercises designed to relax students and help them be comfortable with the sensitive subject matter. The nurse scheduled two 40-minute sessions dealing with testicular cancer for the junior-level health class. In a final step of the planning phase, she designed evaluation tools that assessed knowledge levels after each class session and measured the extent to which students integrated these health practices into their lifestyles at the end of their junior and senior years.

CASE STUDY Application of the Nursing Process—cont'd

Assessment and Diagnosis

The nurse was now ready to proceed with the implementation of a testicular cancer prevention and screening program. She initiated the assessment phase by identifying an individual client and family with a health need, and she extended the assessment to the high school aggregate. Her data collection at the aggregate level, for both the general and local high school populations, assisted in her community diagnosis. The diagnosis directed the development of a community-specific health intervention program and its subsequent implementation and evaluation.

Intervention

The nurse conducted the two sessions in a health education class. At the beginning of the class period, students participated in a group exercise, and the nurse asked them about their knowledge of testicular cancer. The nurse showed a film and led a discussion about cancer screening. In the second session, she demonstrated the self-examination procedure using testicular models and supervised the students while they practiced the procedure on the models. The nurse advised the male students about the frequency of self-examination. With the females, she discussed the need for young men to be aware of their increased risk, drawing a parallel to breast self-examination.

Evaluation

After completing the class sessions, the nurse administered the questionnaires she had developed for evaluation purposes. Analysis of the questionnaires indicated that knowledge levels were very high immediately after the classes. Students were pleased with the frank discussion, the opportunity to ask questions, and the clear responses to a sensitive subject. Teachers also offered positive feedback. Consequently, the nurse became a knowledgeable health resource in the high school.

Intermediate-term evaluation occurred at the end of the students' junior and senior years. The nurse arranged a 15-minute evaluation during other classes, which assessed the integration of positive health practices and testicular self-examinations into the students' lifestyles. At the end of the school year, the prevalence of regular self-assessment was significantly lower than knowledge levels. However, 30% of male students reported regularly practicing self-examinations at the end of 1 year, and 70% reported they had performed self-examination at least once during the past year.

The compilation of incidence data is ideal for long-term evaluation, and it documents the reduction of a community health problem. Testicular cancer is very rare; therefore incidence data are not reliable and may not be feasible to collect. However, for more prevalent conditions, objective statistics help reveal increases and decreases in disease rates, and these may be related to the strengths and deficiencies of health programs.

Levels of Prevention

The following are examples of the three levels of prevention as applied to this case study.

Primary
- Promotion of healthy lifestyles and attitudes toward sexuality
- Education about sexual health and the care of one's body

Secondary
- Self-examination to detect testicular cancer in its earliest stage
- Referral for medical care as soon as a lump or symptom is discovered
- Medical and surgical care to treat and cure testicular cancer

Tertiary
- Advanced care, including hospice services for those with incurable disease
- Support services and grief counseling to help families cope with loss of a loved one

SUMMARY

Communities form for a variety of reasons and can be homogeneous or heterogeneous in composition. To help them assess the nature of a given community, community health nurses study and interpret data from sources such as local government agencies, census reports, morbidity and mortality reports, and vital statistics. Nurses can gather valuable information about the causes and prevalence of health and disease in a community through epidemiological studies. On the basis of this information, the community health nurse can apply the nursing process, expanding assessment, diagnosis, planning, intervention, and evaluation from the individual client level to a targeted aggregate in the community.

ⓔ EVOLVE WEBSITE

http://evolve.elsevier.com/Nies/community
- NCLEX Review Questions
- Case Studies

BIBLIOGRAPHY

Boutain DM: Social justice in nursing: a review of the literature. In de Chesnay M, editor: *Caring for the vulnerable: Perspectives in nursing*, Boston, 2016, Jones and Bartlett.

Centers for Disease Control and Prevention: *About healthy places*, 2014. Available from <http://www.cdc.gov/healthyplaces/about. htm>.

Community Commons: *Community health needs assessment*, 2017. Available from <https://assessment.communitycommons. org/CHNA/About.aspx>.

Institute of Medicine: *The future of the public's health in the 21st century*, Washington, DC, 2002, National Academies Press.

Muecke MA: Community health diagnosis in nursing, *Public Health Nurs* 1:23–35, 1984.

National Association of County and City Health Officials: *Public Health Infrastructure and Systems, n.d.,* 2017. Available from <http://www.naccho.org/topics/infrastructure/mapp/chahealthreform.cfm>.

Pew Charitable Trusts: *Health impact project: about HIA, n.d.,* 2017. Available from <http://www.pewtrusts.org/en/projects >.

Robert Wood Johnson Foundation: *Built environment and health,* 2017. Available from <http://www.rwjf.org/en/our-focus-areas/topics/built-environment-and-health.html>.

University of Kansas: *the community toolbox: Assessing community needs and resources,* 2017. Available from <http://ctb.ku.edu/en/table-of-contents/assessment/assessing-community-needs-and-resources/conduct-focus-groups/main>.

World Health Organization: *Healthy cities,* 2017. Available from http://www.euro.who.int/en/health-topics/environment-and-health/urban-health/activities/healthy-cities.

Community Health Planning, Implementation, and Evaluation

Diane Cocozza Martins and Patricia M. Burbank

OBJECTIVES

Upon completion of this chapter, the reader will be able to do the following:

1. Describe the concept "community as client."
2. Apply the nursing process to the larger aggregate within a system's framework.
3. Describe the steps in the Health Planning Model.
4. Identify the appropriate prevention level and system level for nursing interventions in families, groups, aggregates, and communities.
5. Recognize major health planning legislation.
6. Analyze factors that have contributed to the failure of health planning legislation to control health care costs.
7. Describe the community health nurse's role in health planning, implementation, and evaluation.

KEY TERMS

certificate of need
community as client
health planning
Health Planning Model

Hill-Burton Act
key informant
National Health Planning and
  Resources Development Act

Partnership for Health Program
Regional Medical Programs

Health planning for and with the community is an essential component of community health nursing practice. The term health planning seems simple, but the underlying concept is quite complex. Like many of the other components of community health nursing, health planning tends to vary at the different aggregate levels. Health planning with an individual or a family may focus on direct care needs or self-care responsibilities. At the group level, the primary goal may be health education, and at the community level, health planning may involve population disease prevention or environmental hazard control.

Clinical Example 7.1 illustrates the interaction of community health nursing roles with health planning at a variety of aggregate levels.

Clinical Example 7.1

Maria Guitierrez is a registered nurse (RN) in a suburban middle school. During the course of the school year, she noted an increased incidence of sexually transmitted diseases (STDs) among the middle school students. After reviewing information in nursing journals, other professional journals, and Internet sources, Maria understood that there was a national increase in STDs among young adolescents. She found that significant numbers of adolescents are initiating sexual activity at age 13 and younger. The school nurse reviewed the Centers for Disease Control and Prevention (CDC) site on "Adolescent and School Health—Sexual Risk Behavior" (CDC, 2017). The CDC reported:

Many young people engage in sexual risk behaviors that can result in unintended health outcomes. For example, among U.S. high school students surveyed in 2015

- 41% had ever had sexual intercourse.
- 30% had had sexual intercourse during the previous 3 months, and, of these
- 43% did not use a condom the last time they had sex.
- 14% did not use any method to prevent pregnancy.
- 21% had drunk alcohol or used drugs before last sexual intercourse.
- Only 10% of sexually experienced students have ever been tested for human immunodeficiency virus (HIV).

Sexual risk behaviors place teens at risk for HIV infection, other sexually transmitted diseases (STDs), and unintended pregnancy:

- Young people (aged 13–24) accounted for an estimated 22% of all new HIV diagnoses in the United States in 2015.
- Among young people (aged 13–24) diagnosed with HIV in 2015, 81% were gay and bisexual males.
- Half of the nearly 20 million new STDs reported each year were among young people, between the ages of 15 to 24.
- Nearly 230,000 babies were born to teen girls aged 15–19 years in 2015 (CDC, 2017).

Maria reviewed the reasons for the increased STDs. Her assessment of the problem had several findings. LGBT sexual health issues were not being addressed. Sexually active teenagers do not use contraception regularly. Also, a variety of sexual misconceptions lead teens to believe they are invulnerable to STDs. Adolescents also find it difficult or embarrassing to obtain contraceptives that protect from not only pregnancy but also STDs. The suburb does not have a local family planning clinic, and area primary care providers are reluctant to counsel teenagers or prescribe contraceptives without parental permission. The nurse also discovered that several years earlier a group of parents had stopped an attempt by the local school board to establish sex education in the school system. The parents believed this responsibility belonged in the home.

Maria considered all of these factors in developing her plan of action. She met with teachers, officials, and parents. Teachers and school officials were willing to deal with this sensitive issue if parents could recognize its validity. In meetings, many parents revealed they were uncomfortable discussing sexuality with their adolescent children and welcomed assistance. However, they were concerned that teachers might introduce the mechanics of reproduction without giving proper attention to the moral decisions and obligations involved in relationships. The parents expressed their desire to participate in curriculum planning and to meet with the teachers instead of following a previous plan that required parents to sign a consent form for each student. In support of the parents, Maria asked a nearby urban family planning agency to consider opening a part-time clinic in the suburb.

Implementing such a comprehensive plan is time consuming and requires community involvement and resources. The nurse enlisted the aid of school officials and other community professionals. Time will reveal the plan's long-term effectiveness in reducing teen pregnancy.

This example shows how nurses can and should become involved in health planning. Teen pregnancy is a significant health problem and often results in lower education and lower socioeconomic status, which can lead to further health problems. The nurse's assessment and planned interventions involved individual teenagers, parents and families, the school system, and community resources.

This chapter provides an overview of health planning and evaluation from a nursing perspective. It also describes a model for student involvement in health planning projects and a review of significant health planning legislation.

OVERVIEW OF HEALTH PLANNING

One of the major criticisms of community health nursing practice involves the shift in focus from the community and larger aggregate to family caseload management or agency responsibilities. When focusing on the individual or family, nurses must remember that these clients are members of a larger population group or community and that environmental factors influence them. Nurses can identify these factors and plan health interventions by implementing an assessment of the entire aggregate or community. Fig. 7.1 illustrates this process.

The concept of "community as client" is not new. Lillian Wald's work at New York City's Henry Street settlement in the late 1800s exemplifies this concept. At the Henry Street settlement, Miss Wald, Mary Brewster, and other public health nurses worked with extremely poor immigrants.

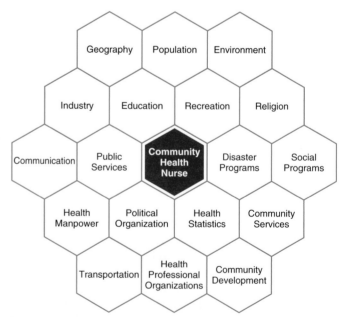

FIG. 7.1 The community as client. Chapter 6, Table 6.1, provides assessment parameters that help identify the client's assets and needs.

The increased focus on community-based nursing practice yields a greater emphasis on the aggregate as the client or care unit. However, the community health nurse should not neglect nursing care at the individual and family levels by focusing on health care only at the aggregate level. Rather, the nurse can use this community information to help him or her understand individual and family health problems and improve their health status. Table 7.1 illustrates the differences in community health nursing practice at the individual, family, and community levels. However, before nurses can participate in health care planning, they must be knowledgeable about the process and comfortable with the concept of community as client or care focus.

HEALTH PLANNING MODEL

A model based on Hogue's (1985) group intervention model was developed in response to this need for population focus. The Health Planning Model aims to improve aggregate health and applies the nursing process to the larger aggregate within a systems framework. Fig. 7.2 depicts this model. Incorporated into a health planning project, the model can help students view larger client aggregates and gain knowledge and experience in the health planning process. Nurses must carefully consider each step in the process, using this model. Box 7.1 outlines these steps. In addition, Box 7.2 provides the systems framework premises that nurses should incorporate.

Several considerations affect how nurses choose a specific aggregate for study. The community may have extensive or limited opportunities appropriate for nursing involvement. Additionally, each community offers different possibilities for health intervention. For example, an urban area might have a variety of industrial and business settings that need assistance, whereas a suburban community may offer a choice of family-oriented organizations, such as boys' and girls' "clubs" and parent–teacher associations, that would benefit from intervention.

A nurse should also consider personal interests and strengths in selecting an aggregate for intervention. For example, the nurse should consider whether he or she has an interest in teaching health promotion and preventive health or in planning for organizational change, whether his or her communication skills are better suited to large or small groups, and whether he or she has a preference for working with older adults or with children. Thoughtful consideration of these and other variables will facilitate assessment and planning.

TABLE 7.1 Levels of Community Health Nursing Practice

Client	Example	Characteristics	Health Assessment	Nursing Involvement
Individual	Lisa McDonald	An individual with various needs	Individual strengths, problems, and needs	Client–nurse interaction
Family	Moniz family	A family system with individual and group needs	Individual and family strengths, problems, and needs	Interactions with individuals and the family group
Group	Boy Scout troop Alzheimer support group	Common interests, problems, and needs Interdependency	Group dynamics Fulfillment of goals	Group member and leader
Population group	Patients with acquired immunodeficiency syndrome (AIDS) in a given state Pregnant adolescents in a school district	Large, unorganized group with common interests, problems, and needs	Assessment of common problems, needs, and vital statistics	Application of nursing process to identified needs
Organization	A workplace A school	Organized group in a common location with shared governance and goals	Relationship of goals, structure, communication, patterns of organization to its strengths, problems, and needs	Consultant and/or employee application of nursing process to identified needs
Community	Immigrant neighborhood Anytown, USA	An aggregate of people in a common location with organized social systems	Analysis of systems, strengths, characteristics, problems, and needs	Community leader, participant, and health care provider

FIG. 7.2 Health Planning Model.

BOX 7.1   Health Planning Project Objectives

I. Assessment
   A. Specify the aggregate level for study (e.g., group, population group, or organization). Identify and provide a general orientation to the aggregate (e.g., characteristics of the aggregate system, suprasystem, and subsystems). Include the reasons for selecting this aggregate and the method for gaining entry.
   A. Describe specific characteristics of the aggregate.
      1. *Sociodemographic characteristics:* Including age, sex, race or ethnic group, religion, educational background and level, occupation, income, and marital status.
      2. *Health status:* Work or school attendance, disease categories, mortality, health care use, and population growth and population pressure measurements (e.g., rates of birth and death, divorce, unemployment, and drug and alcohol abuse). Select indicators appropriate for the chosen aggregate.
      3. *Suprasystem influences:* Existing health services to improve aggregate health and the existing or potential positive and negative impact of other community-level social system variables on the aggregate. Identify the data collection methods.
   B. Provide relevant information from the literature review, especially in terms of the characteristics, problems, or needs within this type of aggregate. Compare the health status of the aggregate with that of similar aggregates, the community, the state, and the nation.
   C. Identify the specific aggregate's health problems and needs on the basis of comparative data collection analysis and interpretation and literature review. Include input from clients regarding their need perceptions. Give priorities to health problems and needs, and indicate how to determine these priorities.

II. Planning
   A. Select one health problem or need, and identify the ultimate goal of intervention. Identify specific, measurable objectives as mutually agreed on by the student and aggregate.
   B. Describe the alternative interventions that are necessary to accomplish the objectives. Consider interventions at each system level where appropriate (e.g., aggregate/target system, suprasystem, and subsystems). Select and validate the intervention(s) with the highest probability of success. Interventions may use existing resources, or they may require the development of new resources.

III. Intervention
   A. Implement at least one level of planned intervention when possible.
   B. If intervention was not implemented, provide reasons.

IV. Evaluation
   A. Evaluate the plan, objectives, and outcomes of the intervention(s). Include the aggregate's evaluation of the project. Evaluation should consider the process, product, appropriateness, and effectiveness.
   B. Make recommendations for further action based on the evaluation, and communicate them to the appropriate individuals or system levels. Discuss implications for community health nursing.

BOX 7.2   Systems Framework Premises

I. Each system is a goal-directed collection of interacting or interdependent parts, or subsystems.
II. The whole system is continually interacting with and adapting to the environment, or suprasystem.
III. There is a hierarchical structure (suprasystem, system, subsystems).
IV. Each system is characterized by the following:
   A. *Structure:* Arrangement and organization of parts, or subsystems.
      1. Organization and configuration (e.g., traditional vs. nontraditional; greater variability [no right or wrong and no proper vs. improper form]).
      2. Boundaries (open vs. closed; regulate input and output).
      3. Territory (spatial and behavioral).
      4. Role allocation.
   B. *Functions:* Goals and purpose of system and activities necessary to ensure survival, continuity, and growth of system.
      1. General.
         a. *Physical:* Food, clothing, shelter, protection from danger, and provision for health and illness care.
         b. *Affectional:* Meeting the emotional needs of affection and security.
         c. *Social:* Identity, affiliation, socialization, and controls.
      2. Specific: Each family, group, or aggregate has its own individual agenda regarding values, aspirations, and cultural obligations.
   C. Process and dynamics.
      1. *Adaptation:* Attempt to establish and maintain equilibrium; balance between stability, differentiation, and growth; self-regulation and adaptation (equilibrium and homeostasis).
         a. *Internal:* Families, groups, or aggregates.
         b. *External:* Interaction with suprasystem.
      2. Integration: Unity and ability to communicate.
      3. Decision making: Power distribution, consensus, accommodation, and authority.

Assessment

As discussed in Chapter 6 on assessment, it is essential to establish a professional relationship with the selected aggregate, which requires that a community health nurse first gain entry into the group. Good communication skills are essential to making a positive first impression. The nurse should make an appointment with the group leaders to set up the first meeting.

The nurse must initially clarify his or her position, organizational affiliation, knowledge, and skills. The nurse should also clarify mutual expectations and available times. Once entry into the aggregate is established, the nurse continues negotiation to maintain a mutually beneficial relationship.

Meeting with the aggregate on a regular basis will allow the nurse to make an in-depth assessment. Determining sociodemographic characteristics (e.g., distribution of age, sex, and race) may help the nurse ascertain health needs and develop appropriate intervention methods. For example, adolescents need information regarding nutrition, abuse of drugs and alcohol, and relationships with the opposite sex. They usually do not enjoy lectures in a classroom environment, but the nurse must possess skills to initiate small-group involvement and participation. An adult group's average educational level will affect the group's knowledge base and its comfort with formal versus informal learning settings. The nurse may find it more difficult to coordinate time and energy commitments if an organization is the focus group, because the aggregate members may be more diverse.

The nurse may gather information about sociodemographic characteristics from a variety of sources. These sources include observing the aggregate, consulting with other aggregate workers (e.g., the factory or school nurse, a Head Start teacher, or the resident manager of a high-rise senior citizen apartment building), reviewing available records or charts, interviewing members of the aggregate (i.e., verbally or via a short questionnaire), and interviewing a key informant. A **key informant** is a formal or informal leader in the community who provides data that are informed by his or her personal knowledge and experience with the community.

In assessing the aggregate's health status, the nurse must consider both the positive and negative factors. Unemployment or the presence of disease may suggest specific health problems, but low rates of absenteeism at work or school may suggest a need to focus more on preventive interventions. The specific aggregate determines the appropriate health status measures. Immunization levels are an important index for children, but nurses rarely collect this information for adults. However, the nurse should consider the need for influenza and/or pneumonia vaccines with older adults. Similarly, the nurse would expect a lower incidence of chronic disease among children, whereas older adults have higher rates of long-term morbidity and mortality.

Public health nursing (PHN) competencies include applying systems theory to PHN practice with communities and populations. This includes integrating systems thinking into public health practice and evaluating new approaches to public health practice that integrate organizational and systems theories (Quad Council of Public Health Nursing Organizations, 2017).

A systems analysis is needed when one is assessing the aggregate. The three levels of the system are the subsystem, the system, and the suprasystem. For example, a community health nurse working with incarcerated women in a prison needs to work at the three levels of the system to assist women planning to reunite with their children at release. The system is the group of women, the subsystem consists of the individual women, and the suprasytem would be the department of corrections and/or the state's department of social services.

The aggregate's suprasystem may facilitate or impede health status. Different organizations and communities provide various resources and services to their members. Some are obviously health related, such as the presence or absence of hospitals, clinics, private practitioners, emergency facilities, health centers, home health agencies, and health departments. Support services and facilities such as group meal sites or Meals on Wheels (MOW) for older adults and recreational facilities and programs for children, adolescents, and adults are also important. Transportation availability, reimbursement mechanisms or sliding-scale fees, and community-based volunteer groups may determine the use of services. An assessment of these factors requires researching public records (e.g., town halls, telephone directories, and community services directories) and interviewing health professionals, volunteers, and key informants in

the community. The nurse should augment existing resources or create a new service rather than duplicating what is already available to the aggregate.

A literature review is an important means of comparing the aggregate with the norm. For example, children in a Head Start setting, day care center, or elementary school may exhibit a high rate of upper respiratory tract infections during the winter. The nurse should review the pediatric literature and determine the normal incidence for this age range in group environments. Furthermore, the nurse should research potential problems in an especially healthy aggregate (e.g., developmental stresses for adolescents or work or family stresses for adults) or determine whether a factory's experience with work-related injury is within an average range. Comparing the foregoing assessment with research reports, statistics, and health information will help determine and prioritize the aggregate's health problems and needs.

The last phase of the initial assessment is identifying and prioritizing the specific aggregate's health problems and needs. This phase should relate directly to the assessment and the literature review and should include a comparative analysis of the two. Most important, this step should reflect the aggregate's perceptions of need. Depending on the aggregate, the nurse may consult the aggregate members directly or may interview others who work with the aggregate (e.g., a Head Start teacher). Interventions are seldom successful if the nurse omits or ignores the clients' input.

During the needs assessment, four types of needs should be assessed. The first is the expressed need or the need expressed by the behavior. This is seen as the demand for services and the market behavior of the targeted population. The second need is normative, which is the lack, deficit, or inadequacy as determined by expert health professionals. The third type of need is the perceived need expressed by the audience. Perceived needs include the population's wants and preferences. The final need is the relative need, which is the gap showing health disparities between the advantaged and disadvantaged populations (Issel, 2014).

Finally, the nurse must prioritize the identified problems and needs to create an effective plan. The nurse should consider the following factors when determining priorities:

- The aggregate's preferences
- Number of individuals in the aggregate affected by the health problem
- Severity of the health need or problem
- Availability of potential solutions to the problem
- Practical considerations such as individual skills, time limitations, and available resources

In addition, the nurse may further refine the priorities by applying a framework such as Maslow's (1968) hierarchy of needs (i.e., lower-level needs have priority over higher-level needs) or Leavell and Clark's (1965) levels of prevention (primary, secondary, and tertiary prevention). Primary prevention consists of health promotion and activities that protect the client from illness or dysfunction. Secondary prevention includes early diagnosis and treatment to reduce the duration and severity of disease or dysfunction. Tertiary prevention applies to irreversible disability or damage and aims to rehabilitate and restore an optimal level of functioning. Plans should include goals and activities that reflect the identified problem's prevention level.

Assessment and data collection are ongoing throughout the nurse's relationship with the aggregate. However, the nurse should proceed to the planning step once the initial assessment is complete. It is particularly important to link the assessment stage with other stages at this point in the process. Planning should stem directly and logically from the assessment, and implementation should be realistic.

An essential component of health planning is to have a strong level of community involvement. The nurse is responsible for advocating for client empowerment throughout the assessment, planning, implementation, and evaluation steps of this process. Community organization reinforces one of the field's underlying premises, as outlined by Nyswander (1956): "Start where the people are." Moreover, Labonte (1994) stated that the community is the engine of health promotion and a vehicle of empowerment. He describes five spheres of an empowerment model that focus on the following levels of social organization: interpersonal (personal empowerment), intragroup (small-group development), intergroup (community collaboration), interorganizational (coalition building), and political action. Paying attention to collective efforts and support of community involvement and empowerment, rather than focusing on individual efforts, will help ensure that the outcomes reflect the needs of the community and truly make a difference in people's lives.

Labonte's (1994) multilevel empowerment model allows us to consider both macro-level and micro-level forces that combine to create both health and disease. Therefore it seems that both micro and macro viewpoints on health education provide nurses with multiple opportunities for intervention across a broad continuum. In summary, health education activities that have an "upstream" focus examine the underlying causes of health inequalities through multilevel education and research. This allows nurses to be informed by a critical social perspective from education, anthropology, and public health and through community-based participatory research (Israel et al., 2005).

Successful health programs rely on empowering citizens to make decisions about individual and community health. Empowering citizens causes power to shift from health providers to community members in addressing health priorities. Collaboration and cooperation among community members, academicians, clinicians, health agencies, and businesses help ensure that scientific advances, community needs, sociopolitical needs, and environmental needs converge in a humanistic manner.

❓ ACTIVE LEARNING EXERCISE

You are working with U.S. veterans who have served in Iraq and Afghanistan. Refer to the U.S. Department of Veterans Affairs website (http://www.va.gov/health/) to review some health issues you should consider in your assessment.

Planning

As already stated, the nurse should determine which problems or needs require intervention in conjunction with the aggregate's perception of its health problems and needs and on the basis of the outcomes of prioritization. Then the nurse must identify the desired outcome or ultimate goal of the intervention. For example, the nurse should determine whether to increase the aggregate's knowledge level and whether an intervention will cause a change in health behavior. It is important to have specific and measurable goals and desired outcomes. Doing so will facilitate planning the nursing interventions and determining the evaluation process.

Planning interventions is a multistep process. First, the nurse must determine the intervention levels (e.g., subsystem, aggregate system, and/or suprasystem). A system is a set of interacting and interdependent parts (subsystems) organized as a whole with a specific purpose. Just as the human body can be viewed as a set of interacting subsystems (e.g., circulatory, neurological, integumentary), a family, a worksite, or a senior high-rise can also be viewed as a system. Each system then interacts with, and is further influenced by, its physical and social environment, or suprasystem (for example, the larger community).

Second, the nurse should plan interventions for each system level, which may center on the primary, secondary, or tertiary level of prevention. These levels apply to aggregates, communities, and individuals.

Third, the nurse should validate the practicality of the planned interventions according to available personal as well as aggregate and suprasystem resources. Although teaching is often a major component of community health nursing, the nurse should consider other potential forms of intervention (e.g., personal counseling, policy change, or community service development). Input from other disciplines or community agencies may also be helpful. Finally, the nurse should coordinate the planned interventions with the aggregate's input to maximize participation.

Goals and Objectives

Development of goals and objectives is essential. The goal is generally where the nurse wants to be, and the objectives are the steps needed to get there. *Measurable objectives* are the specific measures used to determine whether the nurse is successful in achieving the goal. The objectives are instructions about what the nurse wants the population to be able to do. In writing the objectives, the nurse should use verbs and include specific conditions (how well or how many) that describe to what degree the population will be able to demonstrate mastery of the task.

Because the objectives are specific and can be quantified, they may be used to measure outcomes. Objectives may also be referred to as *behavioral objectives* or *outcomes* because they describe observable behavior rather than knowledge. An example of the goals and measurable objectives for a city with a high rate of childhood obesity is shown in Box 7.3.

Intervention

The intervention stage may be the most enjoyable stage for the nurse and the clients. The nurse's careful preliminary assessment and planning should help ensure the aggregate's positive response

---

BOX 7.3 Program Goals and Objectives for Reduction of Childhood Obesity

GOAL
Reduce the rate of childhood obesity in the city of New Bedford.

OBJECTIVES
1. The percentage of children whose body weight exceeds the 98th percentile for age and height will be reduced to 5%.
2. All the children will be invited to join a 5, 2, 1 program:
   - Five fruits and vegetables per day
   - Two-hour limit on screen time (TV, video games, and computer) per day
   - One hour of physical activity per day
3. The food pyramid will be taught to all school nurses and health educators by the end of the school year.
4. The food pyramid will be presented and distributed to parents at all the summer health fairs.

---

to the intervention. Although implementation should follow the initial plan, the nurse should prepare for unexpected problems (e.g., bad weather, transportation problems, poor attendance, or competing events). If the nurse is unable to complete the intervention, the reasons for its failure should be analyzed. Interventions should be included from a range of strategies, including mass media (public service announcements, radio, television, billboards), general information dissemination (e.g., pamphlets, DVDs, CDs, posters), electronic information dissemination (e.g., websites, blogs, tweets, video stream), and public forums (e.g., town meetings, focus groups, discussion groups).

Evaluation

Evaluation is an important component for determining the success or failure of a project and understanding the factors that contributed to its success or failure. The evaluation should include the participant's verbal or written feedback and the nurse's detailed analysis. Evaluation includes reflecting on each previous stage to determine the plan's strengths and weaknesses (*process evaluation*). Process evaluation is also referred to as *formative evaluation*. It allows one to evaluate both positive and negative aspects of each experience honestly and comprehensively and whether the desired outcomes were achieved (*product evaluation*). Product evaluation is summative and can consist of end-of-intervention surveys and other tools that measure whether objectives have been met. *Summative evaluation* is another term for product evaluation and looks at outcomes. Evaluation should include adequacy, efficiency, appropriateness, and cost–benefit analysis. During both process and product evaluations, the nurse may ask the following questions:

- Was the assessment adequate?
- Were plans based on an incomplete assessment?
- Did the plan allow adequate client involvement?
- Were the interventions realistic or unrealistic in terms of available resources?
- Did the plan consider all levels of prevention?
- Were the stated goals and objectives accomplished?
- Were the participants satisfied with the interventions?
- Did the plan advance the knowledge levels of the aggregate and the nurse?

The intervention may have limited impact if the nurse fails to communicate follow-up recommendations to the aggregate upon completion of the project. Although follow-up activity is not necessary for all plans, most require additional interventions within the aggregate using community agencies and resources. A comprehensive health planning project involves a close working relationship with the aggregate and careful consideration of each step. Long-term evaluation may need to be done by those professionals working continuously with the aggregate to determine behavior changes and/or changes in health status.

◢ RESEARCH HIGHLIGHTS

What About the Children Playing Sports? Pesticide Use on Athletic Fields

Children come in contact with athletic fields on a daily basis. How these fields are maintained may have an impact on children's potential exposure to pesticides and associated health effects.

This is a cross-sectional, descriptive study that utilized a survey to assess playing field maintenance practices regarding the use of pesticides. Athletic fields ($N = 101$) in Maryland were stratified by population density and randomly selected.

A survey was administered to field managers ($n = 33$) to assess maintenance practices, including the use of pesticides. Analysis included descriptive statistics and generalized estimating equations.

Managers of 66 fields (65.3%) reported applying pesticides, mainly herbicides (57.4%). Managers of urban and suburban fields were less likely to apply pesticides than were managers of rural fields. Combined cultivation practice was also a significant predictor of increased pesticide use.

The use of pesticides on athletic fields presents many possible health hazards. Results indicate that there is a significant risk of exposure to pesticides for children engaged in sports activities. Given that children are also often concurrently exposed to pesticides as food residues and from home pest management, we need to examine opportunities to reduce their exposures. Both policy and practice questions are raised.

Data from Gilden R, Friedmann E, Sattler B., et al.: Potential health effects related to pesticide use on athletic fields, *Public Health Nursing* 29(3):198–207, 2012.

HEALTH PLANNING PROJECTS

Successful Projects

Student projects have used this health planning model with group, organization, population group, and community aggregates. Table 7.2 describes interventions with these aggregates at the subsystem, aggregate system, and suprasystem levels. Clinical Example 7.2 describes a successful project at a textile plant. Clinical Example 7.3 describes a crime watch program, and Clinical Example 7.4 involves clients in a rehabilitation group.

Clinical Example 7.2

Textile Industry

A nursing student studied a textile plant that had approximately 470 employees but did not have an occupational health nurse. The student nurse collected data and identified three major problems or needs by collaborating with management and union representatives. First, the student nurse observed

TABLE 7.2 Interventions by type of Aggregate and System Level

Project	Type of Aggregate	System Level for Intervention
Rehabilitation group	Group, organization	Subsystem and aggregate system
Textile industry	Population group	Aggregate system and suprasystem
Crime watch	Group, organization, and population group	Aggregate system and suprasystem
Bilingual students (case study)	Community	Aggregate system and suprasystem

TABLE 7.3 Unsuccessful Projects

Project	Problematic Step of Nursing Process
Group home for developmentally delayed	Assessment (i.e., mutual identification of health problems and needs)
Safe Rides program	Planning (i.e., mutual identification of goals and objectives)
Manufacturing plant	Evaluation (i.e., recommendations for follow-up) Implementation

that the most common, costly, and chronic work-related injury in plant workers was lower back injury. Second, some employees had concerns about possible undetected hypertension. Third, the first-aid facilities were disorganized and without an accurate inventory system. The student nurse planned and implemented interventions for all three areas.

On the suprasystem level, the student nurse formulated plans with the company's physicians and lobbied management to enact an employee training program on proper lifting techniques. The student nurse proposed creating specific and concise job descriptions and requirements to facilitate potential employees' medical assessments. In addition, the student nurse organized and clearly labeled the first-aid supplies and developed an inventory system. On the aggregate system level, the student nurse planned and conducted a hypertension screening program. Approximately 85% of the employees underwent screening, and 10 people had elevated blood pressure readings. These 10 people were referred for follow-up care, and hypertension was subsequently diagnosed in several of them.

In evaluating the project, management representatives recognized that a variety of nursing interventions could improve or maintain workers' health. Consequently, management hired the student nurse upon graduation to be the occupational health nurse.

Clinical Example 7.3
Crime Watch
Another nursing student was concerned with the rising incidence of crime in a community and organized a crime watch program. The student nurse met periodically with the police and local residents, or aggregate system. Interventions included posting crime watch signs in the neighborhood and establishing more frequent police patrols at the suprasystem level. Evaluation of the program revealed that the residents had greater awareness of and concern for neighborhood safety.

Clinical Example 7.4
Rehabilitation Group
After working at a senior citizens center for a few weeks, a student nurse began a careful assessment of the center's clients. The student nurse interviewed the center's clients and visited its homebound clients served by social workers and the MOW program. Several of the homebound clients

identified a need for socialization and rehabilitation. The center had recently purchased a van equipped to transport handicapped people in wheelchairs, which was a necessary factor in fulfilling this need.

After the student nurse assessed the clients' health and functional status and determined mutual goals, four of these homebound clients expressed a desire to attend a rehabilitation program at the center. The student nurse and the center's management initiated a weekly program based on the clients' needs, which included van transportation, a coffee hour, a noontime meal, an exercise class, and a craft class. Although some members were initially reluctant to participate and one man withdrew from the group, the group ultimately functioned very well. Evaluating this new program showed clearly that the student nurse made progress in meeting the goals of increased socialization and rehabilitation among elders at the center.

Unsuccessful Projects
Project failure is usually caused by problems with one or more steps of the nursing process. Usually the student does not discover problems until the evaluation phase. The following unsuccessful projects illustrate failures at different steps in the nursing process. Table 7.3 summarizes the identified problem areas for Clinical Examples 7.5 to 7.7.

Clinical Example 7.5
Group Home for Developmentally Delayed Adults
A nursing student worked with an aggregate of six women living in a group home for developmentally delayed citizens. The nursing student observed that the clients were all overweight, and she decided to establish a weight reduction program. She proceeded to meet with the women, chart their weight, and discuss their food choices on a weekly basis. After 8 weeks, her evaluation revealed that none of the women had lost weight and a few had actually gained weight. During the assessment phase the student failed to consider the women's perceptions of need. The women did not consider their weight a priority health problem, and their boyfriends provided positive reinforcement regarding their appearance.

Clinical Example 7.6
Safe Rides Program
One student nurse assessed a university student community through a questionnaire and identified a drinking and driving problem. Of those she surveyed, 77% admitted to driving under the influence of alcohol, and 16.5% stated they had been involved in an alcohol-related car accident. After

identifying the problem and determining student interest, the student nurse worked with the campus alcohol and drug resource center to plan and implement a program called Safe Rides. In this program, student volunteers would work a hotline and dispatch "on-call" drivers to pick up students who were unsafe to drive.

The student nurse resolved many potential complications before implementation (e.g., liability coverage for all participating individuals and expense funds for gasoline). The student nurse formulated a 12-hour training program that lasted 3 weeks to prepare student volunteers for the Safe Rides program. By the end of the semester, Safe Rides was ready to begin. However, the student nurse graduated at the semester's end, and her commitment had been the program's prime motivating force. Although others were committed and involved, the student nurse did not arrange for a replacement to coordinate and continue the program upon her departure. The Safe Rides program required ongoing coordination efforts, and no one fully implemented the program in the student nurse's absence.

Clinical Example 7.7
Manufacturing Plant

Even careful planning cannot always eliminate potential obstacles. For example, one student nurse chose to work in an occupational setting involving heavy industry. The occupational health nurse and the nurse's personnel supervisor both approved the student nurse's entry into the organization. After reviewing the literature, working with the nurse for several weeks, and assessing the organization and its employees, the student nurse concluded that back injury risk was a primary problem. She planned to reduce the risk factors involved in back injuries by distributing information about proper body mechanics in a teaching session.

The personnel manager resisted this plan. Although he recognized the need for education, he was initially unwilling to allow employees to attend the session on company time. The student nurse and manager reached a compromise by allowing attendance during extended coffee breaks. The personnel manager, however, canceled the program before the student nurse could implement the class; negotiations for a new union contract were forming, and there was high probability of a strike. This situation led management to deny any changes in the usual routine.

The student nurse proceeded appropriately and received clearance from the proper officials, but she could not anticipate or circumvent union problems. The student nurse could only share her information and concern with the nurse and the personnel manager and encourage them to implement her plan when contract negotiations were complete.

Discussion

Each of these projects attempted to address a particular level of prevention. Most of these examples focused on primary prevention and health promotion because they were conducted by students and limited by time available due to the length of the academic semester. Table 7.4 lists these projects and their prevention levels. However, the full-time community health nurse working with an aggregate (e.g., in the occupational health

TABLE 7.4   Level of Prevention for Each Project

Primary Prevention	Secondary Prevention	Tertiary Prevention
Textile industry	Textile industry	Rehabilitation group
Crime watch	Group home for developmentally delayed	
Manufacturing plant		
Safe Rides program		

setting) would target interventions for all three levels of prevention at a variety of system levels. It is useful to view nursing interventions with aggregates within a matrix structure to address all intervention opportunities. The matrix in Table 7.5 gives examples of how the occupational health nurse may intervene at all system levels and all prevention levels.

In practice, most interventions occur at the individual level and include all prevention levels. Interventions at the aggregate level are usually less common. For many community health nurses, time does not allow intervention at the suprasystem level. However, schools and schoolchildren are integral parts of the community system. Factors that affect the community's health also affect schoolchildren's health. For school nurses in these school districts, interventions at the suprasystem level may become a reality and improve the health of the community and the students. The suprasystem intervention can be used to reduce hunger and food insufficiency for all schoolchildren in a district. A school nurse working with students in the school office may note that the students are presenting with dizziness, headaches, or abdominal pain in the morning and may keep intervention at the individual level by treating the symptoms presented (e.g., with acetaminophen or food). However, the school nurse may investigate why the students are presenting with the symptoms especially on Monday mornings and may realize that lack of food in the homes is an issue. The nurse then would work to develop a breakfast program for the school district. This strategy is a good example of refocusing upstream by addressing the real source of problems.

These projects illustrate the variety of available opportunities for aggregate health planning. In addition, they exemplify the application of the nursing process within various aggregate types, at different systems levels, and at each prevention level. These examples demonstrate the vital importance of each step of the nursing process:

1. Aggregate assessments must be thorough. The textile industry project exemplifies this point. Assessments should elicit answers to key questions about the aggregate's health and demographic profile and should compare this information with information for similar aggregates presented in the literature.
2. The nurse must complete careful planning and set goals that the nurse and the aggregate accept. The rehabilitation group project illustrates the importance of mutual planning.
3. Interventions must include aggregate participation and must meet the mutual goals. The crime watch project exemplifies this point.
4. Evaluation must include process and product evaluation and aggregate input.

TABLE 7.5 Occupational Health: Levels of Prevention for System Levels

System Level	Primary Prevention	Secondary Prevention	Tertiary Prevention
Subsystem	Yearly physical examination for each employee	Regular blood pressure monitoring and diet counseling for each employee with elevated blood pressure	Referral for job retraining for employee with a back injury
Aggregate and group system	Incentive program to encourage departments to use safety devices	Weight reduction group for overweight employees	Support group for employees who are recovering from problems with alcohol or drug use
Suprasystem	Health fair open to the community and employees	Counseling and referral of community members with elevated blood pressure or cholesterol on the basis of health fair findings	Media advertising to encourage people with substance abuse problems to seek help and use community resources that provide assistance

GETTING INVOLVED IN HEALTH PLANNING

Nurses can support the health planning process to improve aggregate health care with awareness of, and involvement in, the political process. This involvement can consist of following health care legislation at the state and national levels, being an informed voter, contacting legislators on issues of concern, and participating in rallies and protests. (Photo Courtesy of Anthony Ricci, MD.)

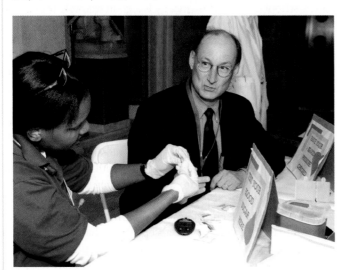

Student nurses also provide blood glucose screenings, with appropriate educational information regarding normal ranges, diet-controlled diabetes, and appropriate referral and treatment when necessary at the statehouse.

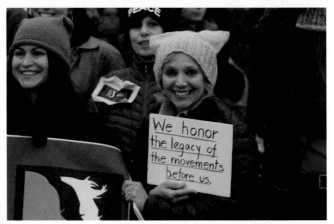

Nurses participate in Women's March on Washington. (Photo Courtesy Anthony Ricci MD.)

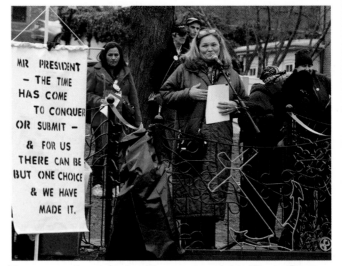

Nurses speak out for health care as a right. (Photo Courtesy Anthony Ricci, MD.)

HEALTH PLANNING MODELS IN PUBLIC HEALTH

According to Issel (2014), many planning programs to address public health problems began as environmental planning of water and sewer systems. Additional population-based planning became necessary with the advent of immunizations. Blum (1974) was the first to suggest how public health planning should be done. Perspectives on health planning range from systematic problem solving and an epidemiological approach to a social awareness approach.

Beginning in the mid-1980s the CDC began to develop and promote systematic methods for health planning in public health. These models were important for a structured approach to public health planning.

The PRECEDE-PROCEED model (Fig. 7.3) provides a structure for assessing health and quality-of-life needs. It also assists in designing, implementing, and evaluating health promotion and public health programs to meet those needs. PRECEDE (*P*redisposing, *R*einforcing, and *E*nabling *C*onstructs in *E*ducational *D*iagnosis and *E*valuation) assesses the diagnostic and planning process to assist in the development of focused public health programs. PROCEED (*P*olicy, *R*egulatory, and *O*rganizational *C*onstructs in *E*ducational and *E*nvironmental *D*evelopment) guides the implementation and evaluation of the programs (Green and Kreuter, 2005).

The PRECEDE-PROCEED framework is an approach to planning that examines factors contributing to behavior change. They are:

Predisposing factors: The knowledge, attitudes, behavior, beliefs, and values before intervention that affect willingness to change.

Enabling factors: The environment or community of an individual that facilitates or presents obstacles to change.

Reinforcing factors: The positive or negative effects of adopting new behavior (including social support).

PROCEED: Policy, Regulating or Resourcing, and Organizing for...

PRECEDE: Predisposing, Reinforcing and Enabling Constructs in Ecosystem Diagnosis and Evaluation

I. Planning

II.

III. Educational and Environmental Development... Evaluation

FIG. 7.3 Green's PRECEDE-PROCEED Model. Green's website provides assistance in guiding use and applications of this model at http://www.lgreen.net/index.html. (From Green LW, Kreuter MW: *Health program planning: An educational and ecological approach*, ed 4, 2004, McGraw-Hill.)

These factors require that individuals be considered in the context of their community and social structures, and not in isolation, in the planning of communication or health education strategies (Green and Kreuter, 2005).

PATCH

The Planning Approach to Community Health (PATCH) model was based on Green's PRECEDE (Green et al., 1980; Green and Kreuter, 2005). This model encouraged the idea that health promotion is a process that enables the population to have more control over its own health. An essential element of the PATCH model is community participation. Another element is the use of data to develop comprehensive health strategies. The PATCH model achieved this through mobilizing the community, collecting health data, selecting health priorities, developing a comprehensive intervention plan, and evaluating the process (Issel, 2014).

APEX-PH Program

The Assessment Protocol for Excellence in Public Health (APEX-PH) program began in 1987 as a cooperative project of the American Public Health Association, the Association of Schools of Public Health, the Association of State and Territorial Health Officials, the CDC, the National Association of County and City Health Officials (NACCHO), and the United States Conference of Local Health Officers. The APEX-PH is a voluntary process for organizational and community self-assessment, planned improvements, and continuing evaluation and reassessment. It is a true self-assessment and is intended to be more of a public endeavor involving the community as well as the public organizations (CDC, 2009).

MAPP Model

More recently, the CDC and NACCHO have released the MAPP (Mobilizing for Action Through Planning and Partnerships) model. The MAPP model is a health planning model that helps public health leaders facilitate community priorities about health issues and identify sources to address them. The first phase of MAPP is to mobilize the community; the second is to guide the community toward a shared vision for long-range planning; and the third is to conduct four assessments: identifying community strengths, local health systems, health status, and forces of change within the population (NACCHO, 2017).

> **? ACTIVE LEARNING EXERCISE**
>
> Select one of the following community diagnoses from your community: increased rates of violence, asthma, lead poisoning, SDIs, pediculosis, infected tattoos/piercings, childhood obesity, food insufficiency, or homelessness. Write a plan on how to address that diagnosis, including goals and objectives. What resources will be needed?

HEALTH PLANNING FEDERAL LEGISLATION

Health planning at the national, state, and local levels is another example of aggregate planning. Planning at any of these levels can be a broader extension of the suprasystem level and affects the individual, family, group, population, and organization levels. Again, upstream change can occur on these levels; for example, individual consumers and consumer groups have protested some managed-care practices at the suprasystem level because health policy can directly affect patient care.

Historically, nurses have influenced health planning only minimally at the community level, but health planning has a tremendous effect on nurses and nursing practice. It is necessary to understand planning on a suprasystem level; therefore the following section contains a review of past health planning efforts with projections for the future.

Hill-Burton Act

In 1946, Congress passed the Hospital Survey and Construction Act (Hill-Burton Act, PL 79-725) to address the need for better hospital access. This act provided federal aid to states for hospital facilities. A state had to submit a plan documenting available resources and need estimates to qualify for hospital construction and modernization funds under the Hill-Burton Act (Young and Kroth, 2018). In addition, each state had to designate a single agency for the development and implementation of the hospital construction plan. The Hill-Burton Act caused the expenditure of vast sums of money and resulted in an increase in the number of beds, especially in general hospitals. The act and its amendments focused only on construction.

Regional Medical Programs

The Hill-Burton Act provided construction-related planning, but it did not address coordination and care delivery directly. In response to recommendations from Dr. Michael DeBakey's national commission, the Heart Disease, Cancer, and Stroke Amendments of 1965 (PL 89-239) were enacted. This legislation was more comprehensive and established regional medical programs (RMPs).

The regional medical programs intended to make the latest technology for the diagnosis and treatment of heart disease, cancer, stroke, and related diseases available to community health care providers through the establishment of regional cooperative arrangements among medical schools, research institutions, and hospitals. The goals of these cooperative arrangements were to improve the health manpower and facilities available to the communities. The intent was to avoid interfering with methods of financing, hospital administration, patient care, or professional practice.

Although RMPs have been credited with the regionalization of certain services and the introduction of innovative approaches to organization and care delivery, some observers believed the reforms were not comprehensive enough. The RMPs did not partner with the existing federal and state programs; therefore there were gaps and duplication in service delivery, personnel training, and research (National Institute of Health, 2017).

Comprehensive Health Planning

Congress signed the Comprehensive Health Planning and Public Health Services Amendments of 1966 (PL 89-749) into law to broaden the previous legislation's categorical approach to health planning. Combined with the Partnership for Health Amendments of 1967 (PL 90-174), these amendments created the Partnership for Health Program (PHP). The PHP provided federal grants to states to establish and administer a local agency program to enact local comprehensive health care planning. The PHP's objectives were promoting and ensuring the highest level of health for every person and not interfering with the existing private practice patterns (Shonick, 1995).

To meet these objectives, the PHP formulated a two-level planning system. Under this system, each state had to designate a single health planning agency, or "A" agency. To play a statewide coordinating role, the "A" agency had to partner with an advisory council, which consisted largely of health care consumers. Meanwhile, the local "B" agencies formulated plans to meet designated local community needs, which could be any public or nonprofit private agency or organization. "A" agencies were to encourage the formation of local, comprehensive health planning "B" agencies, and federal grants were made available for that purpose (Shonick, 1995).

Although the comprehensive health plans were the first of these programs to mandate consumer involvement, they may have failed in their basic intent. The possible failure may have resulted from funding shortage, conflict avoidance in policy formulation and goal establishment, political absence, and provider opposition (e.g., American Medical Association, American Hospital Association, and major medical centers) (Shonick, 1995).

Certificate of Need

In response to increased capital investments and budgetary pressures, state governments developed the idea of obtaining prior governmental approval for certain projects through the use of a certificate of need (CON). New York State passed the first CON law in 1964, which required government approval of hospitals' and nursing homes' major capital investments. Eventually all states supported this CON requirement, and it ultimately became a component of health legislation (PL 93-641). In practice, state CON programs differ in structure and goals. These differences include program focus, decision-making levels, review standard scope, and appeals process exemption (Young and Kroth, 2018)

National Health Planning and Resources Development Act

Given the perceived failure of the comprehensive health planning programs, the federal government focused on a new approach to health planning. The government was greatly concerned with the cost of health care, which escalated dramatically after the end of World War II; the uneven distribution of services; the general lack of knowledge of personal health practices; and the emphasis on more costly modalities of care. The National Health Planning and Resources Development Act of 1974 (PL 93-641) (Endicott, 1975) combined the strengths of the Hill-Burton Act, RMPs, and the comprehensive health planning program to forge a new system of single-state and area-wide health planning agencies (Harlow, 2006).

The goals and purposes of the new law were to increase accessibility to as well as acceptability, continuity, and quality of health services; control over the rising costs of health care services; and prevention of unnecessary duplication of health resources. The new law addressed the needs of the underserved and provided quality health care. The provider and consumer were to be involved in planning and improving health services, and the law placed the system of private practice under scrutiny.

At the center of the program was a network of local health planning agencies, which developed health systems plans for their geographic service areas. The local agencies then submitted these plans to a state health planning and development agency, which integrated the plans into a preliminary state plan. The state agency presented this preliminary plan to a statewide health coordinating council for approval. The law required that the council consist of at least 16 governor-appointed members and that 50% of these members represent health system agencies and 50% represent consumers. One major function of this council was to prepare a state health plan that reflected the goals and purposes of the act. Once the council formulated a tentative plan, they presented it at public hearings throughout the state for discussion and possible revisions (Thorpe, 2002).

Despite careful deliberations by health planners with input from consumers, not all states accepted the health system plan at the grassroots level. A number of problems were encountered, and in time, the legislation failed to effect major change in the health care system. A significant problem was that the legislation had grandfathered in the entire health care system (i.e., health care delivery methods did not change). Although legislation mandated consumer involvement in the health system agency, it was often difficult to implement this aspect. Additionally, despite the mandated efforts by CON and required reviews, costs continued to rise and the health care system remained essentially unchanged (Thorpe, 2002).

Changing Focus of Health Planning

Health planning legislation is heavily influenced by the politics of the administration in power at any given time. The Reagan administration encouraged competition within the health care system. During the 1980s, the administration emphasized cost shifting and cost reduction with greater state power, less centralization of functions, and less national control. This approach represented the government's philosophical shift and combined it with a funding cutback from the Omnibus Budget Reconciliation Act in 1981. The result was a curtailment on federal health planning efforts at that time (Mueller, 1993). The cutbacks caused health system agencies to redefine their roles, and the federal government recommended eliminating these agencies.

A reduction in federal funding and the influence of medical lobbies caused the closure of some health system agencies. Those that remained open experienced a decrease in staff, a resulting drop in overall board functioning, and a reordering of priorities. In an effort to compensate for the decrease in federal funding, some health system agencies sought nonfederal funding or built coalitions to provide the necessary power base for change. Although the administration did not renew federal health planning legislation in the 1980s, it used other regulatory approaches to control costs. These included basing payments to Medicare on diagnosis-related groups, and, in the 1990s, the requirement by many individual states that their Medicaid recipients enroll in health maintenance organizations.

The Clinton administration's plan for health care reform included mechanisms to revitalize planning at the national level. The failure of Congress to pass the plan in 1994 gave planning efforts back to state and local agencies. As a result, most states have become very involved in various aspects of health planning. Indeed, there is considerable variation as many have statewide health plans, local health plans, and some other type of local health planning (American Health Planning Association [AHPA], 2009).

At the beginning of the twenty-first century, 36 states and the District of Columbia still required CON reviews for selected expenditures that include nursing homes, psychiatric facilities, and expensive equipment (AHPA, 2009). However, within these programs, requirements for approval are more liberal, expedited reviews are conducted, and certain projects are exempted from review, weakening the CON cost-containment mandate. Newer high-technology services (i.e., lithotripsy, gamma knives, and positron emission tomography) still need CON review in most states. Furthermore, it is anticipated that state CON programs will continue to assume a stronger role because states must increasingly monitor and report the quality of, cost of, and access to health care that managed care promised.

⚡ ACTIVE LEARNING EXERCISE

1. Attend a state or local health planning meeting. Observe the number of health care providers and consumers in attendance. Compare the meeting's issues with the goals of improving care quality and reducing health care costs.
2. Review the American Planning Association's Planning and Community Health Research Center Plan. Discuss which plans and policies improve the built environment in your community.

Affordable Care Act (ACA) of 2010

The ACA is a national health insurance program that requires all citizens to be covered by one or a combination of insurance programs (Rambur, 2015). This act put individuals, families, and small business owners in control of their health care. It reduced premium costs for millions of working families and small businesses by providing hundreds of billions of dollars in tax relief—the largest middle-class tax cut for health care in history. It also reduced what families will have to pay for health care by capping out-of-pocket expenses and requiring preventive care to be fully covered without any out-of-pocket expense. It kept insurance companies honest by setting clear rules that rein in the worst insurance industry abuses. And it prohibited insurance companies from denying insurance coverage because of a person's preexisting medical conditions while giving consumers new power to appeal insurance company decisions that deny doctor-ordered treatments covered by insurance (U.S. Department of Health and Human Services, 2017).

The U.S. government provides a website to understand the impact of this legislation for consumers, from pregnant women to older adults, at http://www.hhs.gov/healthcare/rights/index.html, as well as a timeline for the ACA at http://www.hhs.gov/healthcare/facts/timeline/index.html. The Kaiser Family Foundation (2017) offers a video that will be helpful for all patients.

The *Healthy People 2020* objectives support this notion. To help achieve improved health status for all, health planning needs a coordinated approach that combines public and private cooperation with an emphasis on supplies and services. Advances in planning models and the sophistication level of planners will affect future health planning efforts.

 ACTIVE LEARNING EXERCISE

Review the ACA and your state's plans for action if repealed.

CASE STUDY　Application of the Nursing Process

School Bilingual Program

José Mendez, a bilingual community health nursing student, worked with the school system in a community that had a large Portuguese subsystem. His primary responsibility was for students enrolled in the town's bilingual program. His contacts included the school nurse and the program teachers.

Assessment

José included the specific group of students, the members of the school system's organizational level, and the population group of the town's Portuguese-speaking residents in his assessment of the aggregate's health needs. José identified the subsystem's lack of primary disease prevention, specifically related to hygiene, dental care, nutrition, and lifestyle choices, by observing the children, interviewing teachers and community residents, and reviewing the literature. José's continued assessment and prioritization revealed that the problem was related to a lack of knowledge and not a lack of concern.

Diagnosis

Individual

- Inadequate preparation at home regarding basic hygiene, dental care, nutrition, and healthy lifestyles

Family

- Developing strengths toward self-care regarding basic hygiene, dental care, nutrition, and healthy lifestyles

Community

- Inadequate resources for communicating basics of hygiene, dental care, nutrition, and healthy lifestyles to the Portuguese community

Planning

The teachers and staff of the bilingual program helped contract and set goals, which reinforced the need for mutuality at this step in the process. A variety of alternative interventions were necessary to accomplish the following goals:

Individual

Long-Term Goal

- Students will regularly practice good hygiene, preventive dental care, good nutrition, exercise, and adequate sleep habits.

Short-Term Goal

- Students will learn the basics of good hygiene, preventive dental care, good nutrition, exercise, and adequate sleep habits.

Family

Long-Term Goal

- Families will regularly practice and teach their children good hygiene, preventive dental care, good nutrition, exercise, and adequate sleep habits.

Short-Term Goal

- Families will learn the basics of good hygiene, preventive dental care, good nutrition, exercise, and adequate sleep habits.

Community

Long-Term Goal

- Systematic programs will provide families and their children with education and information regarding the basics of good hygiene, preventive dental care, good nutrition, exercise, and adequate sleep habits.

Short-Term Goal

- Bilingual personnel will translate information into Portuguese, and program teachers will distribute it to families. This information will cover the basics of good hygiene, preventive dental care, good nutrition, exercise, and adequate sleep habits.

Intervention

- Sometimes nursing students' projects are more limited than the planning stage's ideal; in this case, interventions assessed only one grade level.

Individual

- The student nurse taught children many healthy lifestyle basics, including nutrition, hygiene, and dental care. Classes presented information in Portuguese and English.

Family

- All parents received a summary of the class content in both languages and in pictures.

Community

- The local teachers communicated the student nurse's activities to their state-level coordinators, and the coordinators incorporated the student nurse's materials into the bilingual program throughout the state.

Evaluation

Individual, Family, Community

This community health planning project had an impact on the individuals in the specific aggregate and had broader implications for the family system and the community suprasystem. The outcomes, or product, were hugely successful. Mutually identified goals and objectives influenced the development of the process and incorporated input from a variety of sources. The student nurse believed the resources and support for the bilingual program were adequate. Although the student nurse addressed only primary prevention, the continuing nature of the project will allow the teachers, the school nurse, and the families to assess problems related to the program's content. Future implementation may address secondary and tertiary prevention.

Questions

1. How would you evaluate this project?
2. How would you determine process and product evaluation?
3. What would you do differently?

NURSING IMPLICATIONS

Nurses must work collaboratively with health planners to improve aggregate health. Nurses can influence health planning at the local, state, or community level by fusing current technology with their knowledge of health care needs and skills gained through working with individuals, families, groups, and population groups. This is an example of "upstream interventions." Indeed, nurses may become directly involved in the planning process by participating in CON reviews or gaining membership on health planning councils. Even as students, nurses can begin to participate by engaging in aggregate-level projects, such as those outlined in this chapter, and by tracking health care legislation and contacting their legislators about important issues.

Increased nursing involvement is one method of strengthening local and national health planning. Nurses can use the Health Planning Model presented in this chapter to facilitate a systematic approach to improve aggregate health care. Nurses can assess aggregates from small groups through population groups; identify the group's health needs; and perform planning, intervention, and evaluations by applying this model. The health of individuals, families, and groups would improve if nurses reemphasized the larger aggregate.

■ SUMMARY

Community health nurses are responsible for incorporating health planning into their practice. Nurses' unique talents and skills, augmented by the comprehensive application of the nursing process, can facilitate population health improvement at various aggregate levels. Health planning policy and process constitute part of the knowledge base of the baccalaureate-prepared nurse. Systems theory provides one framework for nursing process application in the community. Interventions are possible at subsystem, system, and suprasystem levels using all three levels of prevention.

ⓔ EVOLVE WEBSITE

http://evolve.elsevier.com/Nies/community
- NCLEX Review Questions
- Case Studies

BIBLIOGRAPHY

American Health Planning Association: *National directory of health planning, policy, and regulatory agencies*, ed 20, Falls Church, VA, 2009, AHPA.

American Planning Association: Planning and community Health Research Center. Available at <http://www.planning.org/nationalcenters/health/>. Accessed June 07, 2017.

Blum HL: *Planning for health*, New York, 1974, Human Sciences Press.

Centers for Disease Control and Prevention: *Adolescent and school health: sexual risk behavior.* Available from: https://www.cdc.gov/healthyyouth/sexualbehaviors. Accessed June 2, 2017.

Congressional Budget Office: *American Health Care Act of 2017.* Available at https://www.cbo.gov/. Accessed June 6, 2017.

Endicott KL: National Health Planning and Resources Development Act of 1974: *PL 93–641, Public Health Rep* 90(3):i2, 1975. Available from: <http://www.ncbi.nlm.nih.gov/pmc/articles/PMC1435675/>. Accessed June 7, 2017.

Gilden R, Friedmann E, Sattler B, et al.: Potential health effects related to pesticide use on athletic fields, *Public Health Nurs* 29(3):198–207, 2012.

Green LW, Kreuter MW: *Health promotion planning: an educational and ecological approach*, ed 4, New York, 2005, McGraw-Hill.

Green LW, Kreuter MW, Deeds SG, et al.: *Health education planning: a diagnostic approach*, Palo Alto, CA, 1980, Mayfield Publishing.

Harlow JM: Government and other types of oversight. In Garber KM, editor: *The U.S. health care delivery system: fundamental facts, definitions, and statistics*, Chicago, 2006, American Hospital Association.

Heart Disease, Cancer, and Stroke Amendments of 1965: PL 89–239, 1965.

Hogue C: An epidemiologic approach to distributive nursing practice. In Hall JE, Weaver BR, editors: *Distributive nursing practice: a systems approach to community health*, ed 2, Philadelphia, 1985, Lippincott Williams & Wilkins.

Hospital Survey and Construction Act of 1946 (Hill-Burton Act): PL 79–725.

Israel BA, Eng E, Schulz AJ, editors: *Methods in community-based participatory research for health*, San Francisco, 2005, Jossey-Bass.

Issel LM: *Health program planning and evaluation*, ed 3, Burlington, MA, 2014, Jones and Bartlett.

Kaiser Family Foundation: *Health reform source*, 2017. Available from: http://www.kff.org/health-reform/video/health-reform-hits-main-street/. Accessed June 2, 2017.

Labonte R: Health promotion and empowerment: reflections on professional practice, *Health Educ Q* 21:253–268, 1994.

Leavell HR, Clark EG: *Preventive medicine for the doctor in his community*, New York, 1965, McGraw-Hill.

Maslow AH: *Toward a psychology of being*, New York, 1968, Van Nostrand Reinhold.

Mueller K: *Health care policy in the United States*, Lincoln, NE, 1993, University of Nebraska Press.

National Association of County and City Health Officials (NACCHO): MAPP, 2017. Available from: http://archived.naccho.org/topics/infrastructure/mapp/<. Accessed June 2, 2017.

National Institute of Health: *2017 Regional Medical Programs*, Washington DC, 2017, US National Library of Medicine. Available from: https://www.nlm.nih.gov/pubs/factsheets/rmp.html. Accessed June 02, 2017.

Nyswander DB: Education for health: some principles and their application, *Health Educ Mono* 14:65–70, 1956.

Partnership for Health Amendments of 1967: PL 90–174, 1967.

Quad Council of Public Health Nursing Organizations: American Public Health Association: PHN Section, ACHNE, APHN, ANA: *Quad council PHN competencies.* Available at: http://www.achne.org/files/Quad%20Council/QuadCouncilCompetenciesfor-PublicHealthNurses.pdf. Accessed June 02, 2017.

Rambur B: *Health care finance, economics and policy for nurses: a foundational guide*, New York, 2015, Springer Publishing Co.

Shonick W: *Government and health services: Government's role in the development of U.S. health services*, New York, 1930-1980, Oxford University Press.

Silverstein NG: Lillian Wald at Henry Street: 1893–1895, *ANS Adv Nurs Sci* 7:1–12, 1985.

Thorpe K: Cost containment. In Kovner A, Jonas S, editors: *Health care delivery in the United States*, ed 7, New York, 2002, Springer.

U.S. Department of Health and Human Services: About the affordable care act, 2017. Available from: https://www.hhs.gov/healthcare/about-the-aca/index.html. Accessed June 02, 2017.

U. S. Department of Veterans Affairs: Veterans Health Administration. Available at https://www.va.gov/health/. Accessed June 07, 2017.

U.S. Social Security Administration: Compilation of the Social Security laws: comprehensive health planning and public health services amendments of 1966: *PL 89–749*. Available from: http://uscode.house.gov/statutes/pl/89/749.pdf. Accessed June 07, 2017.

Young K, Kroth P: *Sultz & Young's Health care USA: Understanding its organization and delivery*, ed 9, Burlington, MA, 2018, Jones and Bartlett.

Community Health Education

Cathy D. Meade

OBJECTIVES

Upon completion of this chapter, the reader will be able to do the following:

1. Describe the goals of health education within the community setting.
2. Examine the nurse's role in community education within a sociopolitical and cultural context.
3. Select a learning theory, and describe its application to the individual, family, or aggregate.
4. Examine innovative and effective teaching and learning strategies that exemplify community-centered health education for the individual, family, or aggregate/group.
5. Compare and contrast Freire's approach to health education with an individualistic health education model.
6. Examine the importance of community engagement for affecting health disparities.
7. Outline a systematic process for developing culturally and literacy relevant health education materials, messages, media, and programs.
8. Relate and apply factors that enhance the suitability of health education materials, messages, media, and programs for an intended audience.
9. Prepare a meaningful teaching plan and evaluation criteria for the individual, family, and/or group.

KEY TERMS

autonomy
cognitive theory
community empowerment
community-based participatory
  methods
culturally effective care
health disparities

health education
health equity
health literacy
humanistic theories
learner verification
learning
materials, media, and messages

participatory action research (PAR)
Paulo Freire
problem-solving education
social justice
social learning theory

CONNECTING WITH EVERYDAY REALITIES

The nurse may be tempted to ask the following questions:

- Why does she keep smoking? She is pregnant.
- Why doesn't the 63-year-old man get his colonoscopy? His fecal occult blood test (I-FOBT) is abnormal.
- Why doesn't the teen take his diabetic medications (insulin) each day?
- Why aren't those parents thinking about the human papilloma virus (HPV) series for their kids?
- Why don't more women attend the clinic's cervical cancer screening? It's free!
- Why does the community have such an alarming rate of obesity?

Although these questions show the nurse's desire and good intentions to understand the link between health behavior and health education, they do not yield actionable answers or empower individuals, families, or groups. In fact, such questions negate critical root health issues and, rather, create a "blaming the victim" approach as recounted by Israel et al. (1994, 2013). Instead, the nurse should try to reframe the questions to get at reasons that help explain the behavior and that lend themselves to nursing actions. Consider these questions the nurse might ask instead:

- What life stressors get in the way of the expectant mom's quitting smoking for good? What stage of quitting might she be in? What social support could be offered to help her quit?
- What structural factors might be preventing this gentleman from getting a follow-up test (colonoscopy)? For example, is transportation a problem? Are the instructions clear? Might he view the colonoscopy procedure as scary? What beliefs might he have about the tests, for example, "that it has to do with my manhood"? Does he have money for the prep? What can I do better to verify that he understands the importance of the test?
- How does the teen with diabetes like to learn? What makes it difficult for him to remember to take his insulin? Are the needles a concern? Does he have worries about how his diabetes might affect his soccer game? What can I do to better connect my instructions to what is important to him in his everyday school and sports activities?
- What is hindering the parents from getting HPV immunizations for their kids? What have they heard about HPV? Could their religious beliefs play a role? Do they think their children will be sexually active sooner if they get the vaccination? Might the family be worried about side effects of the immunizations that they heard about from their relatives? How could I do a better job of explaining the importance of the importance of the HPV series in light of these concerns?
- What outreach methods might better attract the women to the free cervical cancer screening? Could a promotora help engage women and help them navigate the process? Are the materials and promotional flyers language specific?
- What social, physical, cultural, language, linguistic, or structural factors should be considered when developing nutrition messages? What role can I play to develop links with schools, grocery stores, churches, and community centers to better reach and teach families about nutritional interventions? How can community capacity be strengthened to advocate for greater access to healthier food in their grocery stores?

HEALTH EDUCATION IN THE COMMUNITY

Historically, teaching has been a significant nursing responsibility since Florence Nightingale's (1859) early work. Gardner (1936) emphasized that health teaching is one of the most fundamental nursing principles and that "a nurse, in even the most obscure position must be a teacher of no mean order." There is much support for the nurse's involvement in health education and health communications, including nurse practice acts, professional statements of the American Nurses Association (2013), The Joint Commission (2017), Quad Council of Public Health Nursing Organizations (2013), *Healthy People 2020* objectives (U.S. Department of Health and Human Services [USDHHS], n.d., available thfrom https://www.healthypeople.gov/2020/default.aspx).

Health education is an integral part of the nurse's role in the community for promoting health, preventing disease, and maintaining optimal wellness (Box 8.1). Moreover, the community is a vital link for the delivery of effective health care and offers the nurse multiple opportunities to provide appropriate health education within the context of a setting that is familiar to community members (Belone et al., 2016; Hébert et al., 2015; Meade et al., 2011; Meade et al., 2011).

The role of the nurse as health educator is especially important in light of the increasing diversity and demographically changing population in the United States, technological advancements in health care and communications, and attention on social determinants of health. Nurses are pivotal to improve the connection between scientific discovery and the delivery of interventions in the community and to advance **health equity** and **social justice** (Alcarz

---

BOX 8.1 Health Education Roles and Activities of the Nurse in the Community

- Advocate
- Administrator
- Caregiver
- Case manager
- Coach
- Collaborator
- Community care agent
- Consultant
- Counselor
- Culture broker
- Educator
- Facilitator of health-promoting behaviors
- Information agent and broker
- Innovator
- Liaison
- Mediator
- Navigator
- Negotiator
- Policy analyst, policy maker, or change agent
- Promoter of collaborative partnerships
- Promoter of self-care and self-efficacy
- Referral resource
- Researcher
- Sensitizer
- Social activist

American Nurses Association (2013), Clark (2015), Meade et al. (2014), Quad Council of Public Health Organizations (2011), Randall et al. (2017), Redman (2007), and Swider et al. (2013).

et al., 2016; Chu et al., 2008; Freeman, 2004; Marmot and Wilkinson 2000; Quinn et al., 2015; Thurman Pfitzinger-Lippe 2017). More than ever before, health education activities and services are taking place outside the walls of hospitals in such settings as missions, Young Men's/Women's Christian Associations, beauty and barber shops, grocery stores, truck stops, youth centers, homeless shelters, Veterans of Foreign Wars halls, churches, community-based clinics, health maintenance organizations, schools, worksites, shopping malls, senior centers, adult education/literacy centers, mobile health units, homes, libraries, etc. Further, health education activities are increasingly occurring via social media, e-health, and/or Internet-based communication channels (Glanz et al., 2015; Koskan et al., 2014). However, at the core of health education is the development of trusting relationships based on nurturing and healing interactions that heavily rely on **community-based participatory methods**. Such methods highlight community strengths and sustainable collaborations and partnerships (Balls-Berry et al., 2017; Braun et al., 2015; Gwede et al., 2010, 2015; Luque et al., 2012; Meade et al., 2011; Ross et al., 2016; Simmons et al., 2015; Wells et al., 2012).

Health education is any combination of learning experiences designed to predispose, enable, and reinforce voluntary behavior conducive to health in individuals, groups, or communities. Its goal is to understand health behavior and to translate knowledge into relevant interventions and strategies for health enhancement, disease prevention, and chronic illness management. Health education aims to enhance wellness and decrease disability; attempts to actualize the health potential of individuals, families, communities, and society; and includes a broad and varied set of strategies aimed at influencing individuals within their social environment for improved health and well-being (Green and Kreuter, 2005).

Kleinman (1978) described a social and cultural community health care system as one that bridges external factors (e.g., economic, political, and epidemiological) to internal factors (e.g., behavioral and communicative). This view of a sociocultural health care system firmly grounds health education activities within sociopolitical structures, especially within local environmental settings, and views the *community* as client (Holt et al., 2017; Kelly et al., 2017; Martinez et al., 2016; Meade et al., 2007, 2011; Ramaswamy et al., 2017). As such, because the community level is often the location of health prevention and health promotion programs, it is a significant and enriching venue for obtaining positive health outcomes. Nurses are uniquely qualified to influence the health and well-being of community members' health behaviors through original and inventive activities that incorporate culturally, linguistically, and educationally relevant health education and messaging due to their knowledge, competencies, and skills. They are able to take on leadership roles to expertly assess community assets and information gaps and put forward effective solutions to complex, multicausal community concerns to advance social justice (Kulbok et al., 2012; Thurman and Pfitzinger-Lippe, 2017).

It is paramount that community nurse educators address the myriad sociopolitical conditions that affect community health by placing value on the contributions of community members' strengths. Sustained cognitive and behavioral changes often rely heavily on engaging learners in becoming partners in their own health behavior and practice. For example, take a look at the community interventions directed toward empowerment and participatory approaches as remarked by the following writers:

Aranda et al. (2017), who reported that the use of participatory methods (15 focus groups among young people, ages 11–19) were helpful to generate discussions about sexual health. By making the topic more visible, they addressed the complex tensions in designing and delivering acceptable sexual health care services. As a result, the school nurse was instrumental in promoting a positive sexual health culture within the school setting; Kelly et al. (2017), who carried out in-depth interviews with incarcerated women to examine their experiences with Pap tests and how they followed up on abnormal results. A number of contextual factors elucidated in this work included Pap test abnormality as an all-inclusive phrase for women's health problems, the nature of these women's unstable lives, the structural challenges of money, and competing demands—all of which played a role in whether they followed up on abnormal Pap test results or with other health problems; Christy et al. (2016), who illustrated how the formation of sustainable community–academic partnerships led to the development of improved colorectal cancer screening rates that achieved national screening goals of 80% in community clinics through health education and provision of the Fecal Immunochemical Test; Kille et al. (2017), who conducted a content analysis of web-based advertisements among women, men, and transgender sex workers in Canada to help identify information that could inform the health and safety of Internet-based sex workers and their clients; and Irewall et al. (2016), who highlighted the value of a nurse-led, telephone-based intervention as being more efficient than usual care at improving blood pressure and low-density lipoprotein cholesterol levels at 12 months after hospital discharge, thus contributing to modifying patients' risk factors after stroke or transient ischemic attack.

In short, nurses have significant roles in providing contextually appropriate health education, which involves practical, useful, and scientifically sound methods that fit the lives and learning needs of diverse groups across the lifespan.

LEARNING THEORIES, PRINCIPLES, AND HEALTH EDUCATION MODELS

Learning Theories

Learning theories are helpful in understanding how individuals, families, and groups learn. The field of psychology provides the basis for most of these theories and illustrates how environmental stimuli elicit specific responses. Such theories can aid nurses to recognize the mechanisms that potentially modify knowledge, attitude, and behavior. Bigge and Shermis (2004) assert that **learning** is an enduring change that involves the modification of insights, behaviors, perceptions, or motivations. Although psychology textbooks describe learning theories in great detail, the following broad categories relate to the nursing application in a community setting: stimulus-response (S-R) conditioning (i.e., behavioristic), cognitive, humanistic, and social learning.

RESEARCH HIGHLIGHTS

An Examination of Intimate Partner Violence and Sexual Relationship Power Among Adolescents in South Africa

A nurse-led team (Teitelman et al., 2016) sought to explore the associations of intimate partner violence (IPV) and relationship power about sexual-risk behaviors and determine if these associations differed by gender among adolescents in South Africa. Their work required careful understanding of the landscape of gender-based sexual norms that often reflect social construction of masculinities and femininities. This perspective was important to understand possible gender inequities and associated sexual risks faced by adolescents. As background, the study built on prior work by Jemmott et al. (2010, 2015) that described a systematic approach to developing and testing an HIV/sexually transmitted infection health education intervention. This 12-hour educational intervention delivered to sixth graders was based on social cognitive theory, the theory of planned behavior, and extensive formative research and was delivered in the Xhosa language. A total of 1057 students took part in the intervention that was carried out in 18 schools in Cape Province, South Africa. Results showed that students retained risk-reduction knowledge, self-efficacy, and outcome expectancies and kept engaging in safer sexual behavior during follow-up at multiple time points.

The current study (Teitelman et al.) reported data from the 54-month follow-up among 786 adolescents who reported sexual debut (mean age = 16.9). The rationale for exploring this aspect of sexual health (IPV and sexual relationship power) is based on literature showing that low relationship power and victimization by IPV is linked to increased HIV risks among adult females and adolescent girls. The data were collected by paper/pencil questionnaires and assessed the adolescents' sexual risk behaviors (e.g., multiple partners in 3 months, condom use at last sex, IPV, and relationship power). IPV victimization was operationalized as "things that happened to you with a sexual partner while you were having an argument, e.g., physical, sexual and psychological threatening." Results showed that adolescent boys were less likely to report condom use at last sex ($p = .001$) and more likely to report multiple partners ($p < .001$). Also, as IPV increased, reported condom use decreased at last sex for girls, but for boys, it increased. Overall, boys reported lower total relationship power than girls, which may suggest a shift toward more progressive gender norms and gender parity in sexual decision-making power. Findings suggest that sexual risk-reduction interventions for adolescents in South Africa should be developed in light of the social context to reduce adolescent partner violence and sexual relationship power imbalances. It was suggested that interventions should integrate individual attitudes about IPV and interpersonal gender power dynamics, as well as draw on community-level intervention approaches to change harmful social gender norms that perpetuate inequalities. The authors related that HIV risk-reduction policies and programs need to be implemented to address IPV to promote gender equity and respectful and safe relationships among adolescents. It should be noted, though, that a limitation of the study was the use of self-report of behaviors and experiences. Yet, collectively, these studies point to the value of nurse-delivered health education and reinforce the need for future studies (both globally and here in the United States) that test the utility of theoretically driven health education interventions that discern key features that contribute to healthy behaviors.

Data from Teitelman AM, Jemmott AM, Bellamy SL., et al.: Partner violence, power and gender differences in South African adolescents' HIV/STI behaviors, *Health Psychology* 35(7):751–760, 2016. doi:10.1037/hea0000351; Jemmott JB, Jemmott LS, O'Leary A., et al.: School-based randomized controlled trial of an HIV/STD risk-reduction intervention for South African adolescents, *Archives of Pediatrics & Adolescent Medicine* 164(10):923–929, 2010. doi:10.1001/archpediatrics.2010.176; Jemmott JB, Jemmott LS, O'Leary A., et al.: HIV/ STI risk-reduction-intervention efficacy with South African adolescents over 54 months, *Health Psychology* 34(6):610–621, 2015. https://doi.org/10.1037/hea0000140

The nurse should remember that theories are not completely right or wrong. Different theories work well in different situations. Knowles (1989) relates that behaviorists program individuals through S-R mechanisms to behave in a certain fashion. **Humanistic theories** help individuals develop their potential in self-directing and holistic manners. Cognitive theorists recognize the brain's ability to think, feel, learn, and solve problems and train the brain to maximize these functions. Although social learning theory is largely a **cognitive theory**, it also includes elements of behaviorism (Bandura, 1977b). **Social learning theory's** premise is based on the idea that behavior explains and enhances learning through the concepts of efficacy, outcome expectation, and incentives. Clinical Example 8.1 applies various theories to a community intervention.

Clinical Example 8.1

Application of Characteristics of Adult Learners to the Development of a Community Support Group

This example illustrates the long-standing value of incorporating theoretical underpinnings in the development of community-engaged activities designed to meet specific learning needs. It provides a description of how nurses played an active role in bolstering the community capacity and health of their community. Although this account dates back to the 1980s, it serves as an important reminder of the value of applying learning theories to one's work and how such application leads to sustainability of efforts (a key goal of nursing actions!). It is common for nurses based in the community to be an educational resource for patients, families, and community members as they cope with health, wellness, and disease. Later in the chapter, another example is discussed, LUNA (Latinas Unidas por un Nuevo Amanecer, Inc.), a nonprofit organization whose mission is to provide support and offer culturally and linguistically relevant education to Hispanic breast cancer survivors and their families, and it is based on similar tenets.

As background, the author and another nursing colleague began a community education support group for individuals with amyotrophic lateral sclerosis (ALS), more commonly known as *Lou Gehrig's disease*, on the basis of an identified community need. ALS is an incurable degenerative neuromuscular disease that affects nerve and muscle function and the brain's ability to control muscle movement (see http://alsawi.org/ for more information about ALS). The support group was open to family members and friends. At that time, southeast Wisconsin did not have a support group. Community members provided feedback and identified the need for specific education topics and support for people with ALS. This initial dialogue provided the organizing framework for the inception of the first support group, and based on observations and interactions at the monthly meetings, an illustration of Knowles' assumptions follows:

Need to know: At the first support group meetings, the facilitators, both nurses, introduced possible topics by describing the reason for the discussion and the rationale for the selected subjects (e.g., common concerns of patients and family members and informal assessments based on conversations and the literature). To prepare for discussion, group members introduced themselves, and the nurses asked what they hoped to learn from the sessions. In some cases, members were unsure why they might want more information on given topics but indicated that they wanted to listen. Progression of the disease is variable; therefore the need to know was often facilitated by the nurses and other patients who already noted the importance of specific learning tasks (e.g., need for supportive care, assistive walking devices, financial planning, or information on assistive breathing devices).

Self-concept: A comfortable, informal, and trusting environment allowed patients to express feelings, emotions, and frustrations about the disease. Patients, family members, caregivers, and support persons were encouraged to express themselves. Over time, participants cultivated mutual respect and trust for one another as a result of many commonalities. Hugs were common as members began to understand that others had similar situations and concerns. Group members had an opportunity to share and speak about ways that they managed and coped with their disease (e.g., decisions about life support and feeding tubes). Even if their choices were not the same, participants recognized and acknowledged these decisions without imposing their own value judgments. Facilitators and group members soon became equal partners in the learning process. At the core of the meetings was the formation of therapeutic healing and respectful relationships.

Experiences: Some patients and family members had gone through other difficult life experiences and stressors (e.g., other illnesses or deaths in the family) and helped others cope with the management of ALS. Patients shared their strengths gained from such experiences with other support group members. Additionally, individuals and family members who were going through varying stages of the disease process shared their experiences (e.g., obtaining home care, selecting a computer, and managing swallowing and eating). They shared tips and time-saving strategies with one another and with newly diagnosed families and learned from those experiences.

Readiness to learn: Family members often take on many roles when someone becomes ill, especially with a chronic illness such as ALS. This redefinition of roles creates new learning opportunities; however, it can hinder learning if it is too overwhelming. For example, the well spouse may assume the roles of caregiver, parent, and financial supporter. It is helpful for nurses to identify resources to help the family cope with new roles (e.g., respite care).

Orientation to learning: Learning a variety of psychomotor skills is necessary to care for the patient with ALS (e.g., suctioning, positioning, using a feeding tube, and toileting). The time frame for learning such skills varies depending on the course of illness. Presenting information about such skills too early in the course of the disease may cause fear and anxiety. Families may be resistant to learning such tasks until the need is apparent. In some cases, the need may be evident at a crisis point (e.g., a fall, a choking incident, or severe respiratory distress). However, nurse facilitators of support groups can introduce these topics slowly by providing information via educational sessions, newsletters, e-mails, telephone calls, the Internet, printed brochures, blogs, FaceTime, discussion boards, and one-on-one discussions.

Motivation: Individuals and families often experience a shift in life goals when faced with ALS. Such shifts create new learning opportunities aimed at enhancing quality of life, promoting survivorship, and maintaining self-esteem. For example, a college professor with ALS kept his link to the university. He was highly motivated to continue his research work and supervise his graduate students. To continue his academic work, he learned to manage his breathing by using a ventilator, arranged transportation to the university, obtained nursing care, and created communication methods by using a computer to ensure that his students' work continued.

As a result of this initial local support group the ALS Association Wisconsin Chapter evolved and became an official ALS Association chapter in 1987. The chapter's mission is to "lead the fight to cure and treat ALS through global, cutting-edge research, and to empower people with ALS and their families to live fuller lives by providing them with compassionate care and support." Today, there are more than eight ALS Association Wisconsin Chapter–sponsored patient/caregiver support groups in Wisconsin as well as five additional support groups and meetings in Wisconsin. This is the result from just one meeting held by two nurses on a Saturday several decades ago in response to an unmet need in the community. Over the years, many community and family activities, health education programs, and fundraising events have brought significant awareness, scientific advancements, and patient services to individuals with ALS and their loved ones.

For more information on services, go to ALS national and state websites.

❓ ACTIVE LEARNING EXERCISE

In groups of three to four students, discuss how theoretical frameworks help explain health behavior. Identify the strengths and limitations of models that focus on individual health determinants versus models that encompass sociopolitical, environmental, and structural factors.

Knowles' Assumptions About Adult Learners

Knowles (1988, 1989) outlines several assumptions about adult learners. He contends that adults, like children, learn better in a facilitative, nonrestrictive, and nonstructured environment. Nurses who are familiar with these assumptions can develop teaching strategies that motivate and interest individuals, families, and groups and encourage active and full participation in the learning process. Nurses can help create a self-directing, self-empowering learning environment. The following characteristics affect learning: the client's need to know, concept of self, readiness to learn, orientation to learning, experience, and motivation. Table 8.1 expands on these characteristics.

TABLE 8.1   Characteristics of Adult Learners

Characteristics	Application to Health Education
Need to Know Adults must know why they need to learn.	The nurse explores the reasons that individuals, families, and groups want to learn. The nurse helps individuals recognize a need to learn.
Concept of Self Adults have a self-concept that developed from dependence to independence. It moves from others' direction to self-direction. Adults want to be capable of self-direction.	The nurse acknowledges that individuals, families, and groups are able to make choices and decisions. The nurse creates an environment in which patients can express themselves. The nurse recognizes that individuals, families, and groups can learn from their selected actions and can take self-direction and responsibility for such behaviors.
Experience Adults can draw on many life experiences. Such experiences are enriching and are powerful learning resources.	The nurse assesses individuals, families, and groups for life and worldview experiences related to health issues. The nurse helps facilitate connections between previous and present experiences. The nurse allows individuals, families, and groups to share experiences with others in a supportive manner. Experiential methods, problem solving, case methods, and problem-solving discussion can help uncover the learners' experiences. The nurse clarifies previous and present experiences; this is especially helpful with negative and/or positive past experiences.
Readiness to Learn Developmental tasks and social roles affect readiness to learn. The timing of learning experiences with developmental tasks is important.	The nurse assesses and identifies individual, family, and group roles (e.g., caregivers or single parents) and key developmental tasks. The nurse seeks to understand the impact of roles and tasks on learning. The nurse creates role-modeling experiences.
Orientation to Learning Learning is often present oriented and "now" based. Learning is directed to the immediate need and is problem centered.	The nurse assesses the learning needs of individuals, families, and groups on the basis of their learning priority. The nurse recognizes everyday stresses and hassles and addresses them within the learning context. The nurse provides health information, gives responses to their immediate needs, offers/provides health information, and offers problem-solving skills.
Motivation Internal drivers and factors are powerful motivators (e.g., self-esteem, life goals, quality of life, and responsibility).	The nurse determines individual, family, and group motivators. The nurse assesses for impediments that block motivation (e.g., poor self-esteem or lack of resources) and provides appropriate education, counseling, support, and referrals.

Modified from Knowles MS: *The making of an adult educator: an autobiographical journey,* San Francisco, 1989, Jossey-Bass; Knowles MS: *The modern practice of adult education: from pedagogy to andragogy,* Chicago, 1988, Cambridge Press.

TABLE 8.2   Health Belief Model*

Components	Example and Explanation
Perceived susceptibility*	Belief that disease state is present or likely to occur
Perceived severity*	Perception that disease state or condition is harmful and has serious consequences
Perceived benefits*	Belief that health action is of value and has efficacy
Perceived barriers*	Belief that health action is associated with hindrances (e.g., cost)
Self-efficacy	Belief that actions can be performed to achieve the desired outcome (one's confidence)
Modifying factors (demographic, psychosocial, structural)	Age, gender, education, experience, motivation
Cues to action	Influencing factors to get ready for action (e.g., educational materials, text messaging, billboards, newspapers, computer apps, blogs, reminder cues)

*For a more detailed description of the HBM and the original components, see Becker MH, editor: *The health belief model and personal health behavior,* Thorofare, NJ, 1974, Charles B. Slack.

Health Education Models

In addition to learning theories, the application of education theories and principles to situations involving individuals, families, and groups illustrates how ideas fit together, offers explanations for health behaviors or actions, and helps direct community nursing interventions. Such theoretical elements form the basis of understanding health behavior. Theoretical frameworks offer nurses an intervention blueprint that promotes learning and provides them with an organized approach to explaining concept relationships (Padilla and Bulcavage, 1991). It gives nurses the ability to assess an intervention's strength and impact. Importantly, theory and practice need to coexist, and the best theory is one often rooted from practice (Glanz et al., 2015).

Models of Individual Behavior

Two models that explain preventive behavior determinants are the Health Belief Model (HBM), which is presented in Table 8.2 (Becker et al., 1977; Hochbaum, 1958; Kegeles et al., 1965; Rosenstock, 1966), and the Health Promotion Model (HPM) (Pender et al., 2015). Both models are multifactorial;

are based on value expectancy; and address individual perceptions, modifying factors, and likelihood of action. The HBM is based on social psychology and has undergone much empirical testing to predict compliance on singular preventive measures. The initial purpose of the HBM was to explain why people did not participate in health education programs to prevent or detect disease, in particular, tuberculosis screening programs (Hochbaum, 1958). Subsequent studies addressed other preventive actions and factors related to adherence to medical regimens (Becker, 1974). Primarily, the HBM is a value expectancy theory that addresses factors that promote health-enhancing behavior. It is disease specific and focuses on avoidance orientation. The HBM considers perceived susceptibility, perceived severity, perceived benefits, perceived barriers, and other sociopsychological and structural variables (modifying factors). Self-efficacy, defined as the notion that an individual can act successfully on a given behavior to produce the desired outcome (Bandura, 1977a, 1977b), was later added to the HBM (Rosenstock et al., 1988; Strecher et al., 1986). In a meta-analysis (data combined from 18 studies with 2702 subjects), it was found that benefits and barriers were the strongest predictors of behaviors over time (Carpenter, 2010).

Champion and Skinner (2008) point out that one of the limitations of the HBM is the variability in measurement of the central HBM constructs, which include the inconsistent measurement of HBM concepts and the failure to establish the validity and reliability of the measures before testing. For example, applying similar construct measures across different behaviors, such as barriers for mammography and colonoscopy, may be quite different. The past decades have produced some good examples of HBM scale development (Champion et al., 2016, 2008; Rawl et al., 2012, 2015), yet caution in the application of the HBM to multicultural settings is warranted. It would be important to determine whether the overall assumptions of the HBM—assumptions related to the value of health and illness—are similar to those of the particular racial/ethnic group under study. Although the HBM identifies an array of variables important in explaining individual health, nurses should view these variables within a larger societal perspective. Checking for cultural distinctions is especially critical to the model's usefulness among diverse racial/ethnic groups (Brenner et al., 2015; Janz et al., 2002) and is even more important today in light of our demographically changing landscape.

Pender's HPM is a competence- or approach-oriented model first appearing in the nursing literature in 1982. The HPM brings together a number of constructs from expectancy value theory and social cognitive theory within a holistic nursing framework. Unlike the HBM, it does not rely on personal threat as a motivating factor. Rather, it aims to explain why individuals engage in health actions. The central focus of the model is based on individual characteristics and experience, behavior-specific cognitions and affect, and behavioral outcomes that can be assessed by the nurse and that serve as key points for nursing intervention (Pender et al., 2015). It is applicable across the lifespan and has been used to examine the multidimensional nature of persons interacting with their

TABLE 8.3 Health Promotion Model Components and Definitions*

Component	Definition-Example
Individual Characteristics and Experiences	
Prior behaviors	Amount and frequency of same/similar past behaviors
Personal factors (biological, psychological, and sociocultural)	Age, gender, sex, race/ethnicity, weight, body fat
	Personality, structure
	Socioeconomic status
Behavior – Specific Cognitions and Affect	
Activity-related affect	Subjective feeling of emotions before, during, or after the health behavior
Interpersonal influences	Interactions with family, peers, and nurses: perceptions about the behaviors
Situational factors	Perceptions of compatibility of life context or environmental determinants that make health-promoting options available and engaging
Perceived self-efficacy	Perceived ability to perform the necessary behaviors to achieve an outcome—judgment of personal capability
Perceived benefits of health-promoting behaviors	Perception of positive outcomes that can occur from health-promoting behavior (e.g., feel fit and toned)
Perceived barriers to health-promoting behaviors	Perception of things that obstruct health-promoting behaviors (e.g., money and transportation)
Commitment to plan of action	Intention to carry out a specific health behavior and identification of successful strategies to achieve it
Immediate competing demands and preferences	Alternative behaviors that influence a course of action just before intended occurrence of planned behavior (competing demands are alternative behaviors over which people have low control vs. competing preferences are alternative behaviors over which people have high control)
Behavioral Outcome	
Health-promoting behavior	Desired behavioral outcome, such as weight loss, improved decision making

*For a more comprehensive description and explanation of the HPM, see Pender NJ, Murdaugh CL, Parsons MA: *Health promotion in nursing practice*, ed 6, Englewood Cliffs, NJ, 2010, Prentice Hall; Pender NJ, Murdaugh C, Parsons MA., et al.: *Health promotion in nursing practice*, ed 7, 2015, Pearson.

physical and interpersonal environments. For example, it was used in studies to identify factors that enhance health-promoting behaviors of military spouses (Padden et al., 2013); to investigate the efficacy of how a "Girls on the Move" intervention could improve cardiovascular fitness among urban middle school girls (Robbins et al., 2013); and to examine ways to improve nutritional status and behaviors of overweight/obese women who presented at clinics in West Iran (Khodaveisi et al., 2017) Table 8.3 lists the main components of the HPM and supplies their definitions. The HBM and HPM can assist community health nurses in examining an individual's health choices and decisions for influencing health-related behaviors. The models offer nurses a cluster of variables that provide interesting insights into explaining health behavior. These variables are helpful cues. The nurse can consider them in planning programs, but should not try to fit an individual into all the categories. Simply put, models are aids that guide nurses in assessing patients and groups for the development, selection, and implementation of relevant educational interventions.

Try applying the model to your own life and health behaviors. Consider the following questions:

- Do you continually strive for improved health?
- Are you or your family susceptible to heart disease or obesity?
- Does a family history of cardiovascular disease motivate you or your family to exercise?
- What are your cholesterol and triglyceride numbers?
- Does looking fit and toned and having energy motivate you to exercise?
- Do work, school, or family responsibilities get in the way of your exercise plans?
- Has a family member, friend, or health provider recently reminded you of the benefits of exercise and encouraged you to start exercising?
- Do you believe you can initiate and incorporate an exercise program into your lifestyle, or do you need external reinforcement and cues?
- Does money, safety, or time pose any impediments to exercise?
- What would make exercise more appealing, such as a "running or walking club"?
- What do you see as the benefits to exercise, for example, looking and feeling better and having more energy?
- In modifying your health behaviors, how important is exercise compared with other behaviors (e.g., getting relief from work and school stresses, cutting down on snacks, spending quality time with your family and friends)?

Think about these questions and consider your answers. Talk about this behavior with your peers, and develop an exercise action plan that is personalized to your own priorities, needs, abilities, and interests.

Model of Health Education Empowerment

The HBM and HPM focus on individual strategies for achieving optimal health and well-being. The models are similar in that they are multifactorial; are based on the idea of value expectancy; and address individual perceptions, modifying factors, and likelihood of action. Although such approaches may be quite appropriate in changing individual behaviors, they do not necessarily address the complex relationships among social, structural, and physical factors in the environment, such as inadequate social support systems, racism, discrimination, and inaccessibility of health services (Devia et al., 2017; Israel et al., 2013; Minkler, 2012). Van Wyk (1999) suggests that nurses cannot assign power and control to the individual within the community, but, rather, that the "power" must be taken on by the individual and community with the nurse *guiding* this dynamic process. This process includes

examination of such factors as education, health literacy, gender, racism, social justice, and class and recognition of the structural and foundational changes that are needed to elicit change for socially and politically disenfranchised groups. Thus, knowledge is produced in a social context, and it is inextricably bound to relations of power. Therefore an appropriate and more relevant health education model may be one that embraces a broader definition of *health* and addresses social, political, and economic aspects of health. Such a theoretical perspective is highly congruent with current community health education practices because it supports learner participation, highlights community engagement, and emphasizes empowerment.

Freire: A Focus on Problem-Solving Education

Empowerment and literacy are two concepts that have a common history. The concept of empowerment can be traced back to **Paulo Freire**, a Brazilian educator in the 1950s who sought to promote literacy among the poorest of the poor and most oppressed members of the population. He based his work on a problem-solving approach to education, which contrasts with what he called the "banking education approach," which often places the learner in a passive role. **Problem-solving education** allows active participation and ongoing dialogue and encourages learners to be critical of and reflective about health issues. Freire suggested that when individuals assume the role of objects, they often become powerless and allow the environment to control them. However, when individuals become *subjects,* they influence environmental factors that affect their lives and community. Thus, community members, or subjects, are the best resources to elicit change (Freire, 2005).

Freire's methodology, often referred to as *critical consciousness,* involves not only education but also activism on the part of the educator. The basic tenet of Freire's work centers on empowerment; the contextualization of peoples' daily experiences; and collaborative, collegial dialogue in adult education. Freire's work speaks to a variety of action research applications, including those that relate to improving community health of marginalized populations. Freire's approach to health education increases health knowledge through a participatory group process and emphasizes establishing sustainable lateral relationships. This process explores the problem's nature and addresses the problem's deeper issues. The nurse serves as a central resource person and becomes an equal partner with other group members. Listening is a first essential step to understanding the issues. This exchange of ideas and concerns then creates a problem-posing dialogue to identify core problems or generative themes. As this process moves along, the group further delves into the root causes. Finally, the group co-creates relevant action plans that are suitably aligned with their lives (Freire, 2000).

Nurses can use health education as an empowering strategy to help people develop skills in problem solving, critical thinking, networking, negotiating, lobbying, advocacy, policy making, and information seeking to enhance health. Freire's approach may seem similar to health education's emphasis on helping people take responsibility for their health by providing them with information, skills, reinforcement, and support. However, Freire purports that knowledge imparted by the collective group is significantly more powerful than information provided by health educators. This learner-centered approach attempts to uncover the social and political aspects of problems and encourages group members to define and develop action strategies. Hence, there is keen recognition that health and behavior changes are multifaceted and usually do not have immediate solutions; therefore the term problem *posing*, rather than problem *solving*, better describes this empowerment process (Wallerstein et al., 2015). As Kark and Steuart (1962) once stated, "health education must achieve its ends through means that leave inviolate the rights of self-determination of the individuals and their community. The goal of **participatory action research** (PAR) is social change. PAR is also quite consistent with the role and responsibilities of nurses who are engaged in community health (Olshansky et al., 2005) and embraces the use of community-based participatory methods. What this means is that participation and action from stakeholders and knowledge about conditions and issues help facilitate strategies reached collectively (e.g., access to care, access to information). By way of definition, stakeholders are individuals, groups, or organizations that have common and direct interests and concern in a topic, situation, or health outcome. Some examples of the use of PAR include the following projects: Marsh et al., (2017) described the use of PAR to inform the creation of a community garden that functioned as a therapeutic place for end-of-life and bereavement support; Clements (2012) demonstrated how the use of PAR and photovoice was well suited as a framework within a community psychosocial recovery rehabilitation center in Winnipeg, Canada; and Zehbe et al. (2016) developed a PAR project in collaboration with 11 Ojibwa and Oji-Cree First Nations—Anishinaabe—communities in northwest Ontario, Canada, to promote cervical cancer screening through education that respectfully depicted female bodies, sexuality, and health behaviors through a First Nations lens.

ⓘ ACTIVE LEARNING EXERCISE

1. Identify a specific intended group in the community that you are interested in (e.g., medically underserved, homeless, seniors, pregnant women, new immigrants, deaf children, middle-school children).
   a. Describe the group's characteristics, learning needs, and strengths.
   b. Identify your methods for obtaining this information.
   c. Next, describe the application of Freire's empowerment education model to address health education priorities. How would you engage them in determining learning priorities?

Examples of Empowerment Education and Participatory Methods

To illustrate the use of empowerment principles, consider the following: Moya et al. (2017) related how photovoice was used as a participatory research method with participants experiencing homelessness in El Paso Texas, referred to as "The Voices and Images of the Residents of the Opportunity Center for the Homeless: A Visual Project on the Identity and Challenges Homeless Adults Face on the Border Region." Four themes that represented their experiences as well as their aspirations were depicted in their pictures: 1) broken systems, 2) invisibility, 3) opportunities and what works, and 4) growth and determination. The photographs were then shown at a gallery along with narratives. Along with the photographs, a "call to action" was formulated that asked the community, policy, and decision makers to commit to change in the current social, economic, and political conditions affecting individuals experiencing homelessness. As such, the use of photovoice offered an important and creative way to facilitate shared knowledge to achieve social change.

Luque et al. (2010) report the use of empowering processes based on Freire's popular education principles (Freire, 1968) and social cognitive theory, which focused on the constructs of environment, behavioral capability, observational learning, and self-efficacy (Bandura, 1977a, 1977b) for creating a barbershop training program about prostate cancer in an *urban* setting. By employing techniques borrowed from empowerment education (Wallerstein and Bernstein, 1988), barbers were engaged in group learning activities and problem-posing exercises designed around preferences and values related to prostate cancer health. Once the training and curriculum were completed among eight barbers, the team worked closely with the barbers to modify and create a supportive workplace environment for new health education tools (easy-to-read posters, brochures, DVD player, prostate cancer display model) to fuel discussions about prostate cancer health and decision making. Once the barbers were trained, structured surveys with barbershop clients ($N = 40$) were conducted. Results showed a significant increase in participants' self-reported knowledge of prostate cancer and an increased likelihood of discussing prostate cancer with a health care provider ($P < .001$). The barber-administered pilot intervention appeared to be an appropriate and viable communication strategy for promoting prostate knowledge to a priority population in a very convenient and familiar setting. Luque et al. (2015) further extended this work and evaluated the acceptability of barbershops for delivery of prostate cancer information among African Americans in a *rural* setting in Georgia and found high receptivity again for barbershops as a venue for health education Wells et al. (2012, 2015) reported on the use of community-based participatory research methods framed within a social construct theoretical framework to develop a low-literacy, navigator-delivered cervical cancer and HPV educational intervention. This program, based on empowerment principles, was designed to reach a rural Hispanic farmworker community in response to three gaps in care identified by a collaborating community clinical partner. The gaps were (1) delays in reporting results of Papanicolaou (Pap) tests to patients; (2) the need for navigated follow-up care for abnormal findings; and (3) the need for enhanced and consistent education about cervical cancer and HPV. The development of the lay navigation program was created on the basis of a long-standing community–academic collaboration between Catholic Mobile Medical Services and the Tampa Bay Community Cancer Network (TBCCN), a community network program funded by the National Cancer Institute (NCI). It was informed by formative research conducted with members of the farmworker community. Findings from the pilot were used to generate knowledge about evidence-based patient navigation programs in community-based settings, develop a set of low-literacy Spanish-language educational teaching cards, and guide the creation of a Spanish-language virtual patient educator—"an avatar" to be used with a lay navigator to educate women about cervical cancer and HPV. Overall, these projects that emphasize empowering principles illustrate the wide diversity of settings and methods that can be used to implement health education in the community. Think for a moment how empowerment approaches could be used in a health education outreach activity.

Community Empowerment

Community empowerment is a central tenet of community organization, whereby community members take on greater power to create change. It is based on community cultural strengths and assets. An empowerment continuum acknowledges the value and interdependence of individual and political action strategies aimed at the collective while maintaining the community organization as central (Minkler et al., 2012) As such, community organization reinforces one of the field's underlying premises as outlined by Nyswander (1956): "Start where the people are." Furthermore, Labonte (1994) states that the community is an engine of health promotion and a vehicle for empowerment. He describes five spheres of an empowerment model, which focus on the following levels of social organization: interpersonal (personal empowerment), intragroup (small-group development), intergroup (community), interorganizational (coalition building), and political action. A multilevel empowerment model allows us to consider both macro-level and micro-level forces that combine to create both health and disease. Therefore it seems that both micro and macro viewpoints on health education provide nurses with multiple opportunities for intervention across a broad continuum.

In summary, health education activities that respond to McKinlay's (1979) call to study "upstream," that is, to examine the underlying causes of health inequalities through multilevel education and research allow nurses to be informed by critical perspectives from education, anthropology, and public health. For more extensive readings on this topic, see *Methods in Community-Based Participatory Research for Health* (Israel et al., 2013), *Community Organizing and Community Building for Health and Welfare* (Minkler, 2012).

To effect change at the community level, nurses should become familiar with and knowledgeable about key concepts central to community organization (Table 8.4). This approach is an effective methodological tool that enables nurses to partner with the community; identify common goals; develop strategies; and mobilize resources to increase community empowerment, capacity, and community competence. Key concepts inherent in community health education programming are empowerment, principle of participation, issue selection, principle of relevance, social capital, and creation of critical consciousness (Minkler et al., 2012).

The development of LUNA in Tampa, Florida, as described in Clinical Example 8.2, illustrates how the basic tenets of community need and organization fueled the development of a locally initiated group. LUNA represents a grassroots initiative to meet the needs of the growing numbers of Hispanic cancer survivors and serves as a model for nurses, researchers, and community advocates working with underserved groups of cancer survivors (Siegel et al., 2015).

Clinical Example 8.2
Example of Community Empowerment-Collaboration-Participation: LUNA

More than a decade ago (2002), a Latina nurse (Melba Martinez, RN, BSN), who had been diagnosed with breast cancer in 1995, started the first grassroots support group for Latinas in west central Florida. The group began with five members and within the first year had 38 active members who attended monthly meetings. The group was initiated in response to an unmet need in the Tampa Bay area, that is, lack of education services for Latinas who had been diagnosed with breast cancer and who primarily spoke Spanish. Over the years, LUNA has created a network of more than 200 Latina survivors and has grown and become LUNA (Latinas Unidas por un Nuevo Amanecer, Inc.), a nonprofit organization whose mission is to provide emotional support and health education to cancer survivors and their families, friends, and caregivers from Latin communities of west central Florida .The organization primarily serves underserved, immigrant, low-income Latinas with limited English proficiency; assists with navigating the health care system; and functions as a community resource. LUNA draws on the tenets of community organization and empowerment fueled by problem-posing education. The three components of the LUNA model are (1) education (e.g., classes and presentations, Spanish cancer information, health care navigation, community outreach); (2) support (e.g., peer to peer, home, hospital and phone visits, communications); and (3) social reintegration (e.g., celebration of life events such as birthdays, cancer camps, walks, and other social events), similar to those of the startup of the ALS support group previously described.

Outcomes of LUNA

1. Campamento Alegria: The first-ever Spanish-language oncology camp for Latina cancer survivors. A biennial program designed to provide Latinas in whom cancer has been diagnosed a positive and unforgettable experience through a variety of activities that help sustain them through their cancer journey (Martinez et al., 2008). Campamento Alegria aims to serve 100 women who would otherwise not have the opportunity to participate in such activities. There are no fees for the patients/survivors for a 3-day/2-night stay at the retreat facility, meals and related activities, orientation, and reunion meeting.
2. Community education and outreach: Attendance at various community events and health fairs to increase breast cancer screening awareness and provide cancer information and resources in Spanish. These events are popular, and attendance increases each year.
3. Ongoing monthly educational support group meetings, now at two locations. Presentations and classes provided by Spanish-speaking health professionals on various survivorship issues and cancer-related topics.
4. Plans to develop a patient navigator program for Latina patients with newly diagnosed cancer.

The process for creating LUNA began with one nurse who, through dedication and dialogue with others in the same situation, began taking charge of the situation on the basis of input from other community members. From both her nursing and personal experiences, she knew how hard it was for Hispanic women in whom cancer was diagnosed to navigate the health care system, how difficult it is to take time for self-care, and how challenging it was for Hispanic women to talk about their fears. She recognized that Latinas with breast cancer should reach out to one another with understanding and compassion in their own language to move toward self-education and self-actualization. Since its inception, LUNA has partnered with various community-based organizations, hospitals, academic centers, churches, and other social support services to create a strong web of support. For example, LUNA has a strong partnership with researchers from the TBCCN, a community network program funded by the NCI's Center to Reduce Cancer Health Disparities, as well as with local hospitals. LUNA also has worked with researchers to understand the information needs of women undergoing chemotherapy and to transcreate a stress management program for Latinas undergoing chemotherapy (Martinez et al., 2016), which was evaluated in multisite clinical trial. LUNA represents a ground-up effort, which got its start because someone (a nurse) listened to the needs of Hispanic breast cancer survivors. It serves as an excellent model and reminder for nurses, researchers, and community advocates that the best ideas come from the "soul." For more information, view http://www.lunacancerfl.org/.

"Never doubt that a small group of thoughtful, committed citizens can change the world. Indeed, it is the only thing that ever has."

—Margaret Mead

Acknowledgments: Melba Martinez, RN, BSN, and Dinorah (Dina) Martinez-Tyson, MA, MPH, PhD

THE NURSE'S ROLE IN HEALTH EDUCATION

Although learning theories and health education models provide a useful framework for planning health interventions, the nurse's ability to facilitate the education process and become a partner with individuals and communities is inherently significant to the method's application (Clinical Example 8.3). At the core of health education is the therapeutic relationship between the nurse and individuals, families, and the community. Simply put, nurses hold the process together and are catalysts for change in delivering humanistic care. Nurses activate ideas, offer appropriate interventions, identify resources, and facilitate group empowerment. It is beyond the scope of this chapter to describe multiple communication techniques in detail, but the reader is reminded of the value of establishing inclusion and trust before delivering the health education content.

TABLE 8.4 **Community Engagement and Organization Practice**	
Key Concepts	**Application to Health Education (Nursing Actions)**
Empowerment Help individuals, families, and groups gain insight and mastery over life situations through problem solving and dialogue.	The nurse works with community members in identifying and defining issues and creates mechanisms for discussion and problem solving and identifying other factors that have an impact on everyday lives.
Principle of Relevancy Know what issues are important to community members (these may differ from the issues important to nurses).	The nurse holds "town hall meetings" and community group discussions to allow members to share concerns and important issues. The nurse encourages the community to define issues (*what is important to them*). The nurse facilitates communications with community members to help them make decisions about health programs and messages.
Principle of Participation Learn by doing.	The nurse encourages group support. The nurse recognizes that active rather than passive participation results in greater likelihood of attitude and behavior changes.
Issue Selection Identify problems that the community believes are specific, meaningful, and attainable.	The nurse uses problem-solving techniques to help group members identify relevant issues (e.g., group process activities, door-to-door surveys, charlas/talking circles).
Creation of Critical Consciousness Encourage relationships of equality and mutual respect among group members and educators to identify root problems and generate appropriate action plans.	The nurse uses problem-posing dialogue (Freire, 2005) to understand root issues and devises creative and innovative methods to transform situations.
Social Capital Foster relationships (networks) between community members (i.e., trust, engagement)	The nurse encourages community members to work together to improve social networks: they work together on a particular health gap in their community through partnership activities.

Modified from Wallerstein N, Minkler M, Carter-Edwards L., et al.: Improving health through community engagement organization and community building. In Glanz K, Rimer BK, Viswanath K, editors: *Health behavior: theory, research and practice*, ed 5, San Francisco, 2015, Jossey-Bass; Minkler M, editor: *Community organizing and community building for health and welfare*, ed 3, 2012, Rutgers University Press.

Clinical Example 8.3

Mr. Chen is new to the area and starts to visit the local neighborhood senior center weekly to play cards and have lunch with his brothers, who have lived in the area for a number of years. Adjacent to the senior center (men call it "the club") is a nurse-managed clinic, which was started more than 13 years ago by the college of nursing at the local university. The clinic offers education and free or low-cost screenings on a regular basis. Many community members take advantage of this convenient service for their primary care. Mr. Chen has limited resources, so this community resource provides him with valuable access to health care services and information. On his first visit to the clinic, his blood pressure is 174/92 mm Hg. He states that the public hospital that cared for him in another city treated him for high blood pressure for more than 7 years, that doctors prescribed several medications 6 months earlier, and that he received many written materials to read (they were all in English). Although he reads somewhat in English, he tells the nurse that it would have been nice to see materials in his familiar Chinese language

The nurse's assessment reveals that Mr. Chen takes his medication only when he does not "feel so good." He said his doctor advises him to take his medicines regularly, and he states that he takes them faithfully when he does not feel well. He tells the nurse that he remembers getting some educational booklets about his medications and "blood," but he found them too long and tiring to read. The nurse's educational assessment reveals that Mr. Chen has completed 8 years of schooling, does not read much, enjoys television over print, and likes to learn from pictures or from other people in groups. He states that he would really like to get his health information in easy English but would mostly prefer to get some easy materials in Chinese. His reading skills have not been verified by health providers. Yet it seems that he has taken the health instruction literally (e.g., he interprets "take regularly" to mean take consistently when "I don't feel right" vs. take the pills on a regular schedule).

To facilitate learning, the nurse establishes a teaching plan with Mr. Chen's input. This plan involves communicating health instructions in more relevant ways (e.g., using pictures, drawings, mnemonics, videotapes), providing word cards for him in Chinese with the help of the local translation services, and putting him in touch with county financial resources to assist in buying his medicines. The nurse also establishes a follow-up plan with a bilingual nurse to verify Mr. Chen's understanding of how to take his medications by asking him to repeat back in his own words when/how he takes them (teach-back methods). She also plans to develop a series of health education group classes for seniors at "the club" about health and wellness, with high blood pressure as one of the topics of discussion.

ENHANCING COMMUNICATION

The critical step of *inclusion* establishes the base for possible health action; it sets the relationship. What this means is that the nurse needs to be especially cognizant of those first introductory oral exchanges and interactions. Inclusion may simply entail greeting individuals, families, and groups in a warm fashion; offering comfort; and attending to their immediate concerns or worries. Education does not begin with the first instructional word. Rather, education begins with establishing an atmosphere conducive to learning, whereby a therapeutic trusting relationship forms the foundation for a healing relationship. If the nurse attends to *inclusion* first, individuals, families, and groups next begin to *trust* the nurse and thereby trust the *content* of the health education message. This trust is evident through active participation in and commitment to the education process.

It is important to note that the ongoing enhancement and refinement of nursing knowledge and skills to provide culturally effective care is critical to community health education. Nurses are fundamental in responding to diverse community members' everyday health concerns with meaningful, understandable, and actionable information. This involves taking time to get to know individuals, their families, and their everyday lived experiences.

Meleis (1999) describes culturally competent care as care that exhibits sensitivity to individuals based on their vast experiences and their responses, which are due to their backgrounds, sexual orientation, socioeconomic status, ethnicity, literacy, and cultural background. She depicts several properties that make up the "essence of health nurses" who deliver culturally competent care. First, they possess an explanatory system that values diversity. This is a system that is not drained by the constant attempt to interpret symbols, but rather is energized by the variations. Second, they show expert assessment skills to discern different and similar patterns of responses that help in planning appropriate educational interventions. Third, culturally competent nurses are aware of the diversity of communication patterns and how language and communication influence "trust within the relationship." Culturally effective professionals also recognize how marginalization may increase health risks for individuals and that using the expertise of insiders in the culture is a highly valued skill.

For more information on the provision of CLAS and health care standards, view the updated, enhanced 15 standards (USDHHS OMH, 2013) that represent a comprehensive series of guidelines to advance health equity, improve quality, and help eliminate health disparities (https://www.thinkculturalhealth.hhs.gov/). These standards were created in response to growing concerns about health inequities and the need for health care systems to reach increasingly diverse patient populations. The standards reinforce the ability of nurses and organizations to understand and respond well to the cultural and linguistic needs brought by patients and community members to the health care setting. Several standards have particular relevance to community nursing. For example, Standard 1 signifies the importance of providing effective, equitable, understandable, and respectful quality care and services, in light of diverse cultural health beliefs and practices, preferred languages, health literacy, and other communication needs. Standard 13 reinforces the need to partner with communities to design, implement, and evaluate policies, practices, and services to ensure appropriateness. To learn more about their application to nurses, visit the "blueprint" at https://www.thinkcultur alhealth.hhs.gov/clas/blueprint. "And remember: cultural competency and effectiveness is an ongoing journey that requires an openness to acknowledge what one does not know and the willingness to seek better ways to get the job done. It is a process, not simply a program or an end point. Consider health literacy as an ethical issue of concern in the community and how it contributes to health equity.

ETHICAL INSIGHTS

Ethical Issues Related to Health Education and Health Literacy

Health literacy—Do community members understand the printed, digital, and oral health messages communicated to them in terms of language, ease of reading, and linguistics? Are these communications helpful to their decision making? To address the national problem of health literacy, nurses should assess their roles as educators, information brokers, advocates, facilitators, collaborative problem solvers, and navigators. Nurses should consider the impact that the multitude of demands of the health care system has on client autonomy. To explain, health literacy universal precautions refers to strategies to reduce the complexity of health care, increase patient understanding of health information, and enhance support for patients of all health literacy. View the Agency for Healthcare Research and Quality website at https://www.ahrq.gov/professionals/quality-patient-safety/quality-resources/tools/literacy-toolkit/index.html.

Individual vs. collective/societal rights and responsibility for health—What communication factors should the nurse consider when balancing the health education needs of the individual against those of the collective (e.g., family and community)? What communication gaps can be bridged by the development and implementation of health information that is relevant culturally, linguistically, and in terms of literacy?

Social justice and equity—Do all community members enjoy equity in their access to health education and information? Does health information take into account the diversity of a demographically changing country? What types of materials are available for non–English-speaking clients? What strategies, programs, and interventions can be implemented to reduce the discovery-to-delivery disconnect? How can nurses reduce the demands of the health care system and implement navigation strategies?

Allocation of resources—In what way do policies promote and/or hinder promotion of health literacy? Do national/local government and corporate/institutional policies affect the availability, accessibility, and equitable distribution of information resources? In what way do current policies reward and support patient education? How can the nurse get involved in shaping and redirecting health policy and moving policy into practice? This includes policies at the institutional, community, local, and national levels.

Cultural effectiveness—What skills, knowledge, and experiences are necessary to the planning of health education within the context of people's history and everyday realities? The nurse should assess his or her abilities to approach health education tasks with confidence, compassion, competence, and cultural humility (Marks, 2009; USDHHS, 2013).

? ACTIVE LEARNING EXERCISE

Discuss the role of the nurse in health education. Outline specific activities and roles that the nurse can perform with regard to health education issues. Share with one another personal experience(s) relating to cultural effectiveness that might enhance/impede your education role.

FRAMEWORK FOR DEVELOPING HEALTH COMMUNICATIONS

Within the community, the nurse's intended audience may be an individual, family, group, or many segments of the community. Using a systematic approach to the development, design, and delivery of health education programs provides the nurse with an organized, user-friendly way to deliver health messages. Although nurses may select and use a variety of educational models, theoretical frameworks, and teaching and learning principles, the NCI suggests using the "Framework for Developing Health Communications" to create a variety of health education messages and programs (USDHHS, 2008).

This organizing framework has four stages (simplified from six) and is depicted by a circular loop that offers the opportunity for continuous assessment, feedback, and improvement. The framework has been used widely by the author to develop cancer education materials and media on such topics as smoking, prostate cancer, biobanking information, genetic counseling, breast and cervical cancer, stress management, and clinical trials (Brandon et al., 2012; Meade et al., 1994; Schapira et al., 1997; Scheer et al., in press; Sehovic et al., 2016; Simmons et al., 2011; Wells et al., 2015, 2012). This framework can be easily adapted to the design and development of all types of health education topics, such as diabetes, hypertension, HIV, and nutrition.

This framework is based on the principles of social marketing and health education and on mass communication theories, and it relies on intended audience assessment to guide the process. It is highly congruent with Freire's model of empowerment education, which encourages ongoing dialogue with potential consumers and users of health education services. Although this model focuses on communication strategies aimed at the programmatic level, the basic elements are applicable to individual, family, and group systems. The nurse should not expect to apply the model in a linear manner, but rather to move back and forth between the stages. These stages mirror the nursing process (assessment, planning, implementation, and evaluation) and provide a sequential and organized path for continuous assessment, feedback, and improvement so as to achieve a successful communication program. The ideas contained in this Framework for Developing Health Communications model are a practical schema for planning and implementing health education communications programs (see Clinical Example 8.4 and Fig. 8.1).

Stage I: Planning and Strategy Development

The planning stage provides the foundation for a communication program's planning process and is crucial in setting the stage for creating salient communications. Understanding the intended audience's learning needs and targeting the program or message to the audience are pivotal to activating effective health education. This step reinforces Freire's philosophical tenets of ascertaining the intended audience's needs and creating open dialogue. This stage also reduces expensive alterations once the program is under way.

Instructions: Think about a target group that you are currently working with and planning to deliver/create a health education program or message. Complete the exercise by asking yourself the following questions:

Questions to Ask	Action Plan
• **What is the overall intended message/goal?** (What are my reasons for planning this message? How do I know that it is needed or wanted by the audience?)	
• **Who is the intended audience?** (Write a brief statement describing the characteristics of the group.)	
• **What are the benefits of this message to the group?**	
• **What channels will I use to deliver the message?** (Provide a rationale.)	
• **Will I need to create materials?** (Are there available materials that are appropriate for the group?)	
• **How will I know if my message gets across to the audience?** (Did the audience respond? How many people were reached? Who responded?)	
• **Was there change?** (What are the reasons the message was or was not effective? What can be modified to strengthen the message?)	

FIG. 8.1 Planning your health education message.

Questions to Ask

- Who is the intended audience?
- What is known about the audience and from what sources?
- What are the communication and education objectives and goals?
- What evaluation strategies will the nurse use?
- What are the issues of most concern? (Note: These may not necessarily be health issues but may be important ones to link to the health issue when planning, e.g., safety, transportation.)
- What is the health issue of interest?

Collaborative Actions to Take

- Review available data from health statistics, census data, local sources, libraries, newspapers, and local or community stakeholders.
- Get community partners involved.
- Obtain new data (e.g., interviews, surveys, and focus groups using problem-posing dialogue format).
- Determine the intended group's needs and perceptions of health problems (i.e., identify audiences).
- Determine the community's assets and strengths:
  - Physical (e.g., gender, age, and health history)
  - Behavioral (e.g., lifestyle characteristics and health-related activities)
  - Demographic (e.g., income, years of schooling, language, and cultural characteristics)
  - Psychographics (e.g., beliefs, values, and attitudes)
  - Identify issues behind the issues and identify health knowledge gaps.
- Establish goals and objectives that are specific, attainable, prioritized, and time specific.
- Assess resources (e.g., money, staff, and materials).

Stage II: Developing and Pretesting Concepts, Messages, and Materials

The nurse's decisions in stage I can help guide him or her in selecting appropriate communication channels and producing effective and relevant materials. Consider how to reach the intended audience and use interesting and engaging supporting materials and media. *Channel* refers to how the nurse reaches communication sites (i.e., churches, clinics, missions, other nurses, or community-based organizations). *Format* refers to how the nurse communicates the health message (e.g., through individual or group discussion) (Table 8.5). Keep in mind that materials and media are the program's tools, not the program itself (Table 8.6). Education is a human activity and should not focus on audiovisuals exclusively. To ensure that messages are relevant and meaningful, the nurse can employ qualitative research methods (pretesting, learner verification) to obtain feedback about the understandability and acceptability of the materials. Learning now what works and does not work saves a lot of time and money later!

Questions to Ask

- What channels are best?
- What formats should be used?
- Are there existing resources?
- How can the nurse present the message?

TABLE 8.5   Teaching-Learning Formats

Teaching Format	Application to Health Education
Brainstorming session	Allows participants the freedom to generate ideas and discuss them in a group setting. Cultivates creativity. Fosters empowerment to allow members to identify the issue and find solutions.
Community-wide programs	Can reach large numbers of community members through a systematic plan. May include individual or group approaches with a defined intended audience.
Demonstration	Effective in learning perceptual motor skills. Aids in visual identification.
Group discussion/charlas	Members can learn from each other and receive support. Nurses can personalize teaching content to group needs. Ideal for groups combining patients and families. Nurses, health professionals, or lay members can lead the groups. Facilitator must be comfortable with group method and familiar with group characteristics.
Lecture	Varying group sizes can use formal oral presentations. Group members share expertise and experiences. Presenter must be comfortable and possess speaking ability. Requires organizational skills and ability to highlight key points in interesting and creative ways. A combination of lecture media may enhance learning. Audience participation is linked to the presenter's speaking style and ability. Audience feedback is limited.
Individual discussion	Allows individual assessment and identification of cultural barriers, physical impairments, learning needs, literacy, and anxiety. Promotes the tailoring of health education plans. Ideal to capture "teachable moments." Does not allow sharing and support from others. High cost in terms of staff time.
Role playing	Effective in influencing attitudes and opinions. Encourages problem-solving and critical thinking skills. Enhances learner participation. Some members may be hesitant to become involved.
Task force committee/community organizing meetings	Joins individuals with diverse backgrounds and expertise to achieve a goal. May represent many interests and perspectives.
Talking circles/charlas	May be held in convenient settings such as missions, homes, or service settings: engages people in small group discussions (Litvin et al., 2011).
Town hall meetings	Can offer shared experience in a familiar setting.

Data from Rankin SH., et al.: *Patient education in health and illness,* ed 5, Philadelphia, PA, 2005, Lippincott Williams and Wilkins, etc; Redman BK: *The practice of patient education: a case study approach,* ed 10, St. Louis, 2007, Elsevier; U.S. Department of Health and Human Services: *Making health communication programs work: a planner's guide, pink book,* Bethesda, MD, 2008, Office of Cancer Communications, National Cancer Institute. Available from: https://www.cancer.gov/publications/health-communication/pink-book.pdf.

- How will the intended audience react to the message?
- Will the audience understand, accept, and use the message?
- What changes can improve the message?

Collaborative Actions to Take

- Identify messages and materials.
- Decide whether to use existing materials or produce new ones.
- Select channels and formats.
- Develop relevant materials with the target audience.
- Pretest the message and materials and obtain audience feedback (e.g., through interviews, questionnaires, focus groups, and readability testing). Pretesting helps ensure comprehension, acceptability, and cultural relevance.

Stage III: Implementing the Program

At the third stage, the nurse introduces the health education message and program to the intended audience and reviews and revises necessary components. The nurse also analyzes the program and health message for effectiveness and tracks the mechanisms using process evaluation. This way of organizing the implementation process examines the procedures and tasks involved in the program or message, such as monitoring media, identifying the intended audience's interim reactions, and addressing internal functioning (e.g., work schedules and expenditures).

Questions to Ask

- How should the health education program/message be launched?
- How do we maintain interest and sustainability?
- How can we use process evaluation?
- What are the strengths of the health program?
- How can we keep on track within the timeline and budget?
- How can we find out whether we have reached the intended audience?
- How well did each step work (i.e., process evaluation)?
- Are we maintaining good relationships with our community partners?

Collaborative Actions to Take

- Work with community organizations, adult education centers, businesses, media, and other health agencies to enhance effectiveness.

TABLE 8.6   Materials and Media

Media	Considerations in Health Education Settings
Audio response system (ARS)	Allows high interactivity and participation among audience. Offers a data collection and assessment tool. Helps assess immediate understanding (Meade et al., 2015).
Audiotapes	Do not require reading. Portable and small. Individuals can use them at home in a comfortable setting and can replay and use them at their own pace. Economical. Helpful for individuals with visual difficulties or low literacy skills.
Bulletin boards	Inexpensive and easy to develop. Direct attention to a specific message; use few words.
Demonstrations	Helpful when conveying psychomotor skills; encourage patient involvement and tactile learning (e.g., penis model for condom placement or breast model to show breast self-examination, or use of a "mini" portable toilet to show how to collect a stool specimen using I-FOBT kit). Note: Our team has used this teaching tool at a variety of health fairs/classes and it is widely popular! No reading needed.
Exhibits and displays	Graphics offer appeal. Placement in high-traffic areas (e.g., waiting rooms and examination rooms) reaches wide audiences.
Flip charts, chalkboards, and whiteboards	Excellent format to enlarge teaching concepts or cue reader to salient points; graphics and diagrams may be added. Chalkboards are reusable; flip charts have replacement pads, so inexpensive.
Games, simulations, animations	Involve patients in a fun manner; involve the entire family. Highly effective with children. (Meppelink et al., 2015)
Graphics Drawings and visuals	Can convey important points in salient and visual fashion. Can aid understanding for low-literacy audiences. Visual messages should be pretested to ensure acceptability and understanding.
Journal clubs	Interactive process that facilitates understanding of varying concepts (e.g., health disparities, screening, literacy, science, technology). Brings into play perspectives from various stakeholders. (Vadaparampil et al., 2014)
Interactive media, e-health: conversational agents, tablets, kiosks	A variety of computer programs, talking touch screens, interactive kiosks, conversational agents, computer-assisted instructive media, mobile tablet technology based, etc. Algorithms and branching decisions can aid patients in motivation, decision making, problem solving, and fact acquisition (Badawy and Kuhns 2017; Fortmann et al., 2017; Miner et al., 2016; Sullivan et al., 2016; Wells et al., 2015; Zhang et al., 2017). Interactive patient education is increasingly commonplace via the Internet and a wide variety of technologies that bring information directly to people. Consider the use of varied eHealth technologies and assess patients' interests and preferences for receiving information, as well as their computer/technology use comfort level; e-coaching (Ritchie et al., 2016).
Models and real objects	Bring the teaching concept to the patient in a familiar way. Incorporate models and real objects into teaching.
Storytelling/playback theater/narratives	Reading is minimal. Encourages questions and elicits insights (Cueva et al., 2016; Moran et al., 2016; Scheer et al., in press; Smigelsky et al., 2016) Helpful in individual and group instruction and can also take shape as digital storytelling.
Overhead (acetate or digital, or other display media) data projector presentations/whiteboards/chalkboards	Useful in small- and large-group settings. Highlight key points and help patient focus ideas. Can use color and advance organizers, large type, and highlight key points; avoid busy and cluttered text.
Photographs, picture books, pictographs, and slide series (i.e., PowerPoint slides); photo-essay and photovoice Prezi presentations	Help promote understanding and empowerment by showing realistic images and real situations. Help patients make connections to their lives. May help elicit individual, relational, community, organizational, and societal levels of a socioecological model that inform health. Photographs may appear alone or in combination with other photographs, or slides or may be placed in an album (Cabassa et al., 2013; Choi, 2016; Flum et al., 2010; Holliday et al., 2016; Leung et al., 2017; Mabry et al., 2016;) PowerPoint slides are easily updated. Helpful for patients with limited literacy skills; offer visual presentation of concepts. Effective with an individual and with small groups (i.e., self-study or reflection). Easily updated.

TABLE 8.6 Materials and Media—cont'd

Media	Considerations in Health Education Settings
Printed materials (brochures, leaflets, or booklets)	Portable, widely available, and economical. Useful in reinforcing health concepts and interactions. Printed text continues to be a convenient and familiar way to send/receive information. Patients can set and adjust the pace and refer back to information later. Can be effective with individuals, families, groups, or community-wide dissemination. Materials written at simple levels can be effective and acceptable for both low-level and high-level readers (Brandon et al., 2016; Doak et al., 1998; Meade et al, 2015). Tailored materials are a promising strategy for health education that can be developed based on stages of behavioral change (Hawkins et al., 2008; Lee et al., 2017). Nurses should assess issues of readability, design, layout, cultural relevance, and appropriateness of content.
Programmed materials, self-help guides, workbooks	May involve printed materials combined with visuals to allow self-pacing. Helpful for learning facts. Nurse should assess individual or group to determine whether independent learning style is preferred. Can be easily personalized.
Teaching/flash cards	Portable, use few words, and offer visual interpretations. Can be easily personalized. The nurse can create them economically and update them easily. Effective with individual, small-group, or family instruction.
Television, radio and newspapers (mass media)	Reach large audiences within the community. Effective in conveying general health information in a user-friendly manner. Nurses can play an active role in disseminating health information via the local media. Effective in influencing attitudes and behaviors. Offer a familiar medium for viewers to learn about many health topics.
Telephones/smartphones/patient portals Text messaging	Automated phone systems: reminder phone calls, SMS, patient portals, telenursing (Coughlin et al., 2017; Young et al., 2014).
Videotapes, digital streaming, telenovella/YouTube	Combine audio and visual media to convey realistic images (Meade, 1996). Videotapes that incorporate a role-modeling concept can be used to convey a wide variety of health topics. Can offer closed-captioning for deaf audiences. Takes time to produce and update; may require access to audiovisual equipment and viewing sites. Computerized digital editing makes updating easier. Telenovella storytelling (Cueva et al., 2013).
Online resources (i.e., Internet, simple dial-up services, information, databases, bulletin board chat services, blogs, and World Wide Web)	Electronic information sources can link individuals, families, and groups to health. Can reach large audiences rapidly. Websites should be evaluated by nurses/providers for accuracy, credibility, and relevancy. New digital technologies and innovations can help consumers find health information, advice, and support, especially at-risk groups (Cueva et al., 2016).
Podcasts	Portable video technology that uses media broadcasts and can be accessed via the Internet and viewed on a personal computer or on a handheld device player (Bangia et al., 2017).
Social media	Online interactive discussions, blogs, social bookmarking, social news, Facebook, Twitter, social networking sites (Abramson et al., 2015; Bender et al., 2012; Chou et al., 2013; Koskan et al., 2014; Prestin et al., 2015; So et al., 2015).

Data from U.S. Department of Health and Human Services: *Making health communication programs work: a planner's guide, pink book*, Bethesda, MD, 2008, Office of Cancer Communications, National Cancer Institute. Available from: https://www.cancer.gov/publications/health-communication/pink-book.pdf

- Monitor and track progress.
- Establish process evaluation measures (e.g., follow up with users of the service, number of community members who used the service, and expenditures).

Stage IV: Assessing Effectiveness and Making Refinements

Outcome evaluation examines whether changes in knowledge, attitudes, and behavior did or did not occur as a result of the program. Together with the process evaluation, the data inform how well the program is functioning and direct future modifications. The nurse prepares for a new development cycle using information gained from audience feedback, communication channels, and the program's intended effect. This stage helps continually refine the health message and respond to the intended audience's needs. New information helps validate the program's strengths and allows for necessary modifications. Feedback is necessary to continually refine the message and direct new messages.

Questions to Ask

- What was learned?
- How can outcome evaluation be used to assess effectiveness?
- What worked well, and what did not work well?

- Has anything changed within the intended audience?
- How might we refine the methods, channels, or formats?
- Overall, what lessons were learned, and what modifications could strengthen the health education activity?

Collaborative Actions to Take

- Conduct outcome evaluations (e.g., randomized experiment, evaluation studies, definition of data needed for data collection).
- Reassess and revise goals and objectives.
- Modify unsuccessful strategies or activities.
- Generate continual support from businesses, health care agencies, and other community groups for ongoing collaboration and partnerships.

Clinical Example 8.4

The H. Lee Moffitt Cancer Center and Research Institute, or Moffitt, formed a partnership with Suncoast Community Health Centers, Inc., or Suncoast, in rural Hillsborough County, Florida. The partnership initially brought breast cancer education and screening services to Hispanic migrant and seasonal farmworkers and low-income rural women via Moffitt's Lifetime Cancer Screening Mobile Unit. Initiated by a cancer center physician who visited Suncoast, a federally funded, community-based center located about 30 miles south of Tampa, he was struck by the center's services and impressed with the clinic's dedication to reaching medically underserved populations. Suncoast consisted of multiple comprehensive federally qualified health care clinics in Plant City, Ruskin, Brandon, and Dover, Florida, and offered a wide range of primary health care services, yet it did not have mammography facilities. Moffitt was expanding its community outreach initiatives through mobile outreach services. Moffitt was a freestanding, private, nonprofit institution located at the University of South Florida campus in Tampa. An NCI-designated comprehensive cancer center in Florida, Moffitt is widely known for state-of-the-art treatment, novel research, ambulatory services, and advanced screening modalities. After a series of meetings between Suncoast and Moffitt's Lifetime Cancer Screening Center, the groups formed a partnership based on a mutual shared goal—to improve the breast health of high-risk and medically underserved women. Both parties determined that the goal was to develop and offer the community culturally appropriate education, accessible mammography service, and follow-up care.

Description of Health Issue and Intended Audience

Despite progress in the fight against cancer, many communities continue to bear a disproportionate share of the cancer burden. Cancer disparities very likely arise from the complex interplay of factors—that is, low socioeconomic status, low levels of education and literacy, social injustice, and poverty—that impede awareness about screening and follow-up care. Together, these factors affect access to care and cancer survival and yield an uneven distribution of cancer morbidity and mortality, which substantially affects marginalized populations (American Cancer Society, 2017; Braun et al., 2015; Chu et al., 2008; Meade et al., 2009) suggest that in the development of cancer outreach and screening programs, it is absolutely critical to layer on additional levels

of understanding of and sensitivity to the social, cultural, and political conditions of home countries, language and literacy needs, obstacles to basic health care access, cultural significance of gender and age roles, culturally mediated etiologic perceptions of disease, illness experiences, religiosity, and the sociopolitical nature of immigration situations. Such factors affect the design and meaning of health communication and health education. Our assessment revealed that many women did not appear for breast screenings because of a "fear of cancer" and uncertainty of how to navigate the health care system. Typically, many women did not seek preventive health care, but rather sought care for episodic acute illnesses. The lack of mammography screening and education for rural Hillsborough County's medically underserved women represented a health service gap. In particular, individuals may face a number of potential factors that get in the way of receiving acceptable mammography services. These factors may reflect limited access points to health care; low awareness of the importance of the screening; and language, literacy, and linguistic concerns. Educational and communication interventions and tools that address (1) unique value systems, (2) relevant and specific cultural and linguistic factors, and (3) access issues—as well as that capitalize on the strengths of the women—were warranted. Our experiences reminded us that women want and need information about breast health but that they also experience everyday struggles. As such, peer outreach/navigation can help deconstruct those concerns and better engage community members in their health.

What was required in Hillsborough County was the delivery of a culturally relevant health service in a geographically convenient area. Women aged 40 years and older were eligible for this service. The initial intended audience was primarily Hispanic migrant and seasonal farmworkers but also grew to include women from other diverse ethnic backgrounds (i.e., Haitian, rural white).

Goal: To prevent premature death and disability from breast cancer through early detection, screening, and culturally and linguistically relevant education.

Objectives: To increase education, mammograms, clinical breast examinations, and follow-up programs among medically underserved women in rural Hillsborough County.

Selecting Channels and Methods

Nurses selected a combination of channels to communicate health information about breast cancer, screenings, and early detection methods (e.g., community-based clinics, missions, social service agencies, health events, and fairs). Nurses conducted individual interactions at the mobile or stationary site at the screening center.

Nurses collected a variety of health materials and media about breast cancer from national, state, and local sources and determined that many of the printed materials were not culturally or educationally suited for the individuals the nurses were serving; for example, the materials were geared toward high reading levels, and few Spanish-language or Haitian Creole materials were available.

Developing Materials

Grants from Avon, National Alliance of Breast Cancer Organizations, Susan G. Komen for the Cure Florida Suncoast Affiliate, and NCI supported the development of English, Spanish, and Creole materials to educate women about breast health. Additionally, although translators were sporadically present, it became apparent that bilingual/bicultural staff was necessary. Ongoing dialogue with community members and clinics helped refine the screening process, the education component, and follow-up services to ensure effectiveness, efficiency, appropriateness, and timely follow-up.

Implementation

The mass media publicizes the services and disseminates human-interest stories, especially during October—Breast Cancer Awareness Month. The outreach workers posted flyers at a variety of sites (e.g., beauty shops, laundromats, missions, churches, grocery stores, churches, unemployment offices, and community centers). Twice per month, the mobile unit traveled to rural areas. There, staff greeted women and answered questions about the mammography procedure and follow-up.

Assessing Efficiency
Process Evaluation

A number of newspapers/flyers, television, and radio advertisements publicized the free or low-cost mammography service and highlighted the importance of breast health. Also, several human-interest stories emerged, which communicated the screening services to a wider audience. Since the onset of the program, increases in the number of staff involved in the program, the number of volunteers, and the number of funded projects that support the program enhanced its breadth and depth and sparked the development of new initiatives. Most notably, the TBCCN, an NCI-funded community network program center, a partnership of 28 community organizations, has increased the number of committed key stakeholders who have identified other areas of community need and outreach such as a need for cervical cancer navigation and increased colorectal cancer screening uptake (Davis et al., 2016; Gwede et al., 2013; Wells et al., 2015). As a result of an additional community partner needs assessment, (Gwede et al., 2010; Simmons et al., 2015) additional cancer education workshops, health events, and cancer services have been broadened and evaluated.

For example, funding for a Patient Research Navigation Program further augmented outreach efforts. Designed to eliminate barriers to cancer diagnosis and treatment, this project generated new knowledge for the advancement of an evidence-based, culturally and literacy appropriate, lay navigation program for community members who had a breast/colorectal cancer abnormality by evaluating timeliness to resolution of abnormality and enhancing timeliness to diagnosis and delivery of cancer care (Lee et al., 2017; Meade et al., 2015; Roetzheim et al., 2012; Wells et al., 2011).

Outcome Evaluation

During the mammography screening program's initial years, fewer than 200 women received mammography screening per year. The number of women screened approached more than 1000 per year in subsequent years. Currently, mammography services are provided at stationary screening sites at the cancer center (women use vouchers), and funding opportunities and institutional support sustain the program. The number of community partners has grown considerably, a reflection of enhanced community capacity and awareness. Regular health events are scheduled; refinement of screening services and follow-up are ongoing.

Feedback

Reports describing process and outcome evaluation and analysis provide a point of reference for continual improvements. Such reports apply knowledge and outline methods to enhance and improve the service's efficiency and effectiveness.

The mammography program has incorporated a network of outreach and educational components to reach rural migrant and seasonal farmworkers and other low-income women in south and east Hillsborough County. Although the program provided desired links to screening services and has formed successful community partnerships, it is important to develop and refine community empowerment strategies through outreach and education to sustain and widely disseminate the program. Building on this successful model of education and outreach (Meade 2014; Meade et al., 2009), the administrators of the program applied lessons learned for outreach to other high-risk populations, (e.g., Haitian and African American men and women) in the development of colorectal cancer screening initiatives (Gwede et al., 2013). A key lesson learned here is that community outreach, based on trust, respect, and mutual commitment, can fuel community-identified research priorities and lead to the testing and evaluating of evidence-based interventions for community benefit.

- Provide justification for continuing or ending the program.
- Summarize the health education program or message in an evaluation report.
- The reader is encouraged to think about how health education messages or programs can be planned using this model. The exercise in Fig. 8.1 can be helpful to organize your ideas.

HEALTH EDUCATION RESOURCES

A variety of health education materials, media, and resources are available from local, state, and national organizations and agencies. Such associations provide helpful information about services, educational materials, and links to support groups or self-help groups. Often, printed and electronic/digital materials are available for free or for a nominal cost. Nurses can help individuals, families, and groups find and access materials, services, or equipment loan programs and can become knowledgeable about community resources. Additionally, identifying gaps in services may help nurses create new resources. Some examples are:

- Local and regional hospitals, clinics, libraries, adult education centers, health education centers, media outlets, and businesses
- Local and state governmental sources (e.g., health departments and social service agencies); literacy associations (check the Internet for listings)
- Community-based organizations (i.e., advertised, nonadvertised, and those recommended by community leaders and stakeholders; National Association of Community Health Centers; parish nursing associations; faith-based organizations; social service agencies)
- Universities and colleges, community colleges, and academic nursing centers

- Professional organizations (e.g., American Public Health Association, National Association of Hispanic Nurses, National Black Nurses Association, National Student Nurses Association, Society for Behavioral Medicine)
- Commercial organizations (e.g., pharmaceutical companies, medical supply companies, and patient and health education companies); printed and electronic sources are often available
- Federal government sources (e.g., National Institutes of Health [NIH]; NCI; National Heart, Lung, and Blood Institute; OMH; CDC; National AIDS Clearinghouse; and Office on Smoking and Health) and related websites
- Voluntary agencies and their local affiliates (e.g., American Cancer Society, American Heart Association, Amyotrophic Lateral Sclerosis Association, American Diabetes Association, American Council for Drug Disorders, American Dairy Council, Alzheimer's Association, and American Lung Association)
- Internet searches
- Medline Plus Health Information (i.e., a service of the National Library of Medicine [NLM] for patient and consumer information) at medlineplus.gov

Can you think of another organization that you or a family member recently obtained information from relating to a health need? University or college libraries often provide information on beginning and advanced search strategies and are one of the most credible and accessible sources of information. The NLM, at www.nlm.nih.gov/hinfo.html, maintains extensive health-related bibliographies and offers links to the databases Medline Plus Health Information (http://www.nlm.nih.gov/medlineplus/), Household Products Database, Office of the Surgeon General, NIH Senior Health, and much more.

The nurse can locate many health resources through a variety of search engines on the Internet. As the World Wide Web continues to evolve as a major source of information exchange, an assessment of the quantity, quality, and broad nature of information must be undertaken See Google Medline Plus for an array of helpful aids: https://medlineplus.gov/evaluatinghealthinformation.html#cat_94. Key to the plethora of resources is gauging the appropriateness of the materials and media in consideration of literacy (see next section).

Health Literacy

In her 1944 text, *The Public Health Nurse in the Community,* Rue stated that the community's illiteracy level is an important factor in health program planning. This factor remains a significant issue in planning health education programs and materials. Low literacy is a problem of great magnitude in the United States and has serious implications across the continuum of health care. Consider Clinical Example 8.5.

Clinical Example 8.5

A 2-year-old is diagnosed with an inner ear infection and is prescribed an antibiotic. Her mother understands that her daughter should take the prescribed medication twice a day. After carefully studying the label on the bottle and deciding that it does not tell how to take the medicine, she fills the teaspoon and pours the antibiotic into her daughter's ear (Parker et al., 2003).

The nurse in a community setting who sees a sick child at the pediatric clinic might ask the following questions:

- Do the parents know the names of the medicines for their baby, how they work, and how and when to give them?
- In what way might teach-back methods (described later in this chapter) help the parents have a good understanding of how to administer the antibiotic?
- Will the parents know what to do if their baby gets a fever?
- Is the information in their preferred language?
- Do the parents know how to read a thermometer? Did I show them? Were they able to "show me back"?
- Do the mom and dad know who to call and under what conditions if their baby's condition worsens? Does the family have an understanding of what constitutes worsen? Will the parents know what action to take in case of a very high fever at 1:00 AM? Will they have the critical literacy skills to manage similar situations?

As background, the conceptual definitions of *health literacy* have evolved greatly over time. At one point, "literacy" was operationally defined as the ability to read and write at the fifth-grade level in any language and was measured on a continuum (National Literacy Act, 1991). Health literacy, on the other hand, is about empowerment, that is, having access to information, knowledge, and innovations. It is viewed as increasingly important for social, economic, and health development; is a key public health issue in the delivery of effective, safe health care; and calls for the development of national policies and programs and intervention tools by community practitioners.

 HEALTHY PEOPLE 2020

Health Literacy

Health literacy also is an essential component of *public health goals that aim to create social and physical environments for good health for all.* The recognition of this topic as a serious health issue subsequently resulted in the specific naming of topics, goals, and objectives in *Healthy People 2020,* entitled Health Communication and Health Information Technology (IT). The objectives in this topic area describe many ways in which health communication and health IT can have a positive impact on health, health care, and health equity. Examples especially pertinent to health education actions taken by nurses include delivering accurate, accessible, and actionable health information that is targeted or tailored to increasing health literacy skills, providing personalized self-management tools and resources, and following sound principles in the design of programs and interventions that result in healthier behaviors. See http://www.healthypeople.gov/2020/topicsobjectives2020/ for more information.

So what is health literacy? Health literacy is a constellation of skills needed to perform basic reading tasks required to function in the health care environment for accessing, understanding, and using information to make health decisions. For example, health literacy skills entail knowing when and where to go for health screenings; reading labels on prescription bottles; understanding public health messages about flu, Ebola, or Zika; text messaging while driving; completing health insurance forms; recognizing how to read food labels; and being aware of the expectations of research and clinical trials. *It might mean being able to understand, make sense, and apply the information contained in this book or chapter to the care of members of your community.*

Nutbeam (2009) proposed three levels for intervention that have individual and population benefits: (1) functional/basic literacy (focus on increasing basic reading/writing skills), (2) communicative/interactive literacy (focus on enhancing abilities to extract information and apply in new settings and with providers), and (3) critical literacy (focus on advancing skills to analyze information critically and use the information to control and manage life situations). Too often, he asserts, the provider's focus is on basic literacy rather than on critical literacy. The latter, he asserts, increases community members' empowerment abilities to successfully manage their everyday situations.

In 2004, the National Academy of Medicine (NAM), formerly called the Institute of Medicine (IOM) published a landmark report titled *Health Literacy: A Prescription to End Confusion* that relates that millions of U.S. adults are unable to read and act on the plethora of health instructions and messages (Nielsen-Bohlman et al., 2004). The definition of health literacy adopted by the NAM report is consistent with the *Healthy People 2020* program as follows: "the capacity to obtain, interpret and understand basic health information and services and the competence to use such information and services to enhance health." The NAM report lists a series of recommendations that offer the nurse a blueprint of action. Several recommendations emphasize the need for clear communication, stress the importance of involving consumers in the development of the health communications process, and relate the need to create culturally and linguistically appropriate health information. For more details on this report and other health literacy–related resources and roundtables, go to the NAM's website, www.nam.edu, and search for the term *health literacy*. The most recent health literacy roundtable centered on health communication with immigrants, refugees, and migrant workers. Pause for a moment now and consider the skills needed to read the words on this page, the skills needed to assimilate the information, and the skills needed to ultimately apply the information to your interactions with community members.

Nutbeam (2008) further emphasizes that health literacy from public health and health promotion perspectives should be conceptualized as an "asset." In this manner, strategies to promote literacy move beyond mere transmission of content to the promotion of skills that develop confidence in how to act on the information. This viewpoint regards health literacy as a critical component of empowerment by improving people's access to health information and their capacity to use it. Moreover, Peerson and Saunders (2009) hold that implicit in understanding the broad concepts of health literacy is that motivation and behavioral activation must be considered separate entities. Simply put, having knowledge does not necessarily equate to action. Therefore the quality of provider interactions and a greater awareness of and sensitivity to the possible impact of low literacy on individuals and communities is paramount (Nutbeam, 2008; Rowlands and Nutbeam, 2013).

Early research shows serious disparities between the reading levels of materials and patients' reading skills (Meade et al., 1994). Additionally, materials often failed to incorporate the intended audience's cultural beliefs, values, languages, and attitudes (Doak et al., 1998; Meade et al., 2007). Numerous studies show that low literacy affects utilization and access to health care services and costs (Levy and Janke, 2016; MacLeod et al., 2017; Morrison et al., 2014); decreases self-esteem and increases shame and stigma (Waite et al., 2008; Wolf et al., 2007); and adversely affects diabetes, cancer screenings, medication, HPV, blood pressure control, dialysis maintenance, cervical cancer, smoking, dental health, and use of patient portals (Bailey et al., 2014; Batista Ferrer et al., 2016; Coughlin et al., 2017; Davis et al., 2016; Green et al., 2013; Holtzman et al., 2014; McNaughton et al., 2014; Stewart, et al. 2017; Stewart et al., 2013; Tiraki and Yılmaz, 2017).

Additional studies reveal that health literacy affects participation in research and poses barriers to obtaining informed consent (Donovan-Kicken et al., 2012; Hughson et al., 2016) and affects the number of questions asked at medical visits (Aboumatar et al., 2013). Moreover a number of systematic reviews of health literacy studies offer additional evidence of the high prevalence of limited health literacy, increasingly complex medical systems, and need for high-level navigation skills for self-management of acute and chronic disease, promotion of health, and improvement of understanding of science and scientific research (Chesser et al., 2016; Chinn, 2011; Dewalt et al., 2004; Mancuso, 2009; Snow and Dibner 2016). Clearly, the past decades have seen many advances in translating research findings into public health practices to reduce health risks, yet such successes are not fully realized by all members of society representing various dimensions, including age, race and ethnicity, sexual identity and orientation, disability status, location/place, and/or socioeconomic status.

Guzys et al. (2015) suggests that too often the emphasis on health literacy is at the individual level. They contend that health literacy assessment and potential interventions need to shift and promote knowledge and skills for critical health literacy at a societal level. This paradigm shift offers a promising approach to improve community literacy whereby the inclusion of community members is a necessary requirement to coproduce an appropriate literacy framework reflective of societal influences. Similarly, McCormack et al. (2017) and Nutbeam et al. (2017) support the adoption of this broader social ecological perspective that embraces addressing individual educational interventions that are supported and enhanced by interventions at additional levels of societal influence.

As Hasnain-Wynia and Wolf (2010) point out, the intersection of health literacy and disparities in health care represents key contributors to high-quality, equitable health care. Although the exact relational mechanisms between literacy and health are unclear, it is known that individuals with very low literacy skills are at an increased risk for poor health, which contributes to health disparities. Paasche-Orlow and Wolf (2007) describe a conceptual causal model that aims to explain associations between limited health literacy and health outcomes that center on three distinct aspects of care: (1) access and utilization of health care, (2) patient–provider relationships, and (3) self-care. They point out that the relationship of literacy to health outcomes is not necessarily linear—as people exist within a sociocultural network—and suggest that health literacy be viewed as a "risk factor to be managed in clinical care." This being the case, nurses are ideally qualified and skilled to promote health in the community and address health literacy through the implementation of multiple strategies and techniques, as explained in the upcoming sections.

The Doaks (Leonard and Cecilia), who brought the literacy issue to the forefront in public health, describe the health community as a written culture. Unfortunately, many written instructions are "over the heads" of patients. There is a serious mismatch between the readability levels of health instructions and the reading skills of patients, but nurses can adapt the literacy levels of their instructions and reduce this mismatch. Techniques to reduce this mismatch are cogently outlined in the book *Teaching Patients with Low Literacy Skills* (Doak et al., 1996), which offers practical suggestions for preparing and evaluating materials. This book is not currently in print, but all chapters can be accessed through the Harvard health literacy website at https://www.hsph.harvard.edu/healthliteracy/resources/teaching-patients-with-low-literacy-skills/. This is a very helpful resource. The author has used the information contained in this book in the development of educational materials, community-based programs, and research interventions.

What steps can nurses employ to address health literacy in the community setting? Within Stage I of the Framework for Developing Health Communications model, the nurse can use assessment skills to determine the reading level of the intended audience. For example, the nurse could employ a number of informal and formal assessment measures to assess an individual's literacy skills. Informal measures include asking a series of simple questions to provide a better indication of his or her reading skills. For example: *Do you enjoy reading? What do you read? How often do you read? Where do you get your health information?* Although years of schooling completed can serve as a gauge of literacy, previous studies suggest that a three- to four-grade–level difference often exists between an individual's literacy level and years of education completed. The nurse could ask patients to read a paragraph from a health document aloud. Skilled readers enjoy reading, are fluent readers, understand content, interpret the meaning of words, and look up unfamiliar words. Limited readers read slowly, miss the intended meaning, take words literally, tire quickly from reading, and skip over uncommon words. Also, the nurse should ask the patients a few questions about the information they read. Readers should be able to answer questions about the material's content. Although these strategies are especially helpful to individuals with low literacy, people at all literacy levels prefer and better understand simply written, concise materials and are more motivated by materials that are relevant to their learning needs (Doak et al., 1998, 1996).

There has been ongoing attention to the development of literacy screening questions, but validation studies are needed before they become routine in clinical care (Chin et al., 2011;

Mancuso, 2009). Some formal instruments that have been used in health care settings to estimate academic skills include the Wide Range Achievement Test, Level IV (Wilkinson and Robertson, 2006) and the Rapid Estimate of Adult Literacy in Medicine (REALM), which assesses the ability to read common terms in English and is used as a brief literacy-screening tool (Davis et al., 1991, 1993, 2006). Please note that there is now a short form of the REALM (only seven terms—see https://www.ahrq.gov/professionals/quality-patient-safety/quality-resources/tools/literacy/index.html).

Although these instruments take only a few minutes to administer, few exist in Spanish or other languages. One short assessment tool, called the *Newest Vital Sign (NVS)*, created by Weiss et al. (2005), is available in English and Spanish as a six-question assessment tool based on an ice cream nutrition label and is a quick (3- to 5-minute) assessment. Another measure, the Test of Functional Health Literacy in Adults, long and short forms (TOFHLA and S-TOFHLA; Parker et al., 1995), also has been used in health settings with English- and Spanish-speaking/reading subjects (Kobayashi et al., 2015; Paasche-Orlow and Wolf, 2010; Soto Mas et al., 2015). For example, Robinson et al. (2011) administered the S-TOFHLA to 612 rural older adults with heart failure and found that inaccurate categorization of patients with low or marginal health literacy may occur when the test's time limits (7 minutes) are enforced. These findings reinforce that some health literacy instruments may not be useful with patients who have undetected and/or declining cognitive impairment. Further, although many new and translated health literacy measures have been reported, many health literacy measures have not been properly validated for racial/ethnic minorities, at-risk groups, and non–English language speaking groups (Haun et al., 2014; Nguyen et al., 2015).

Building on prior work (Chew et al., 2004; Wallace et al., 2006), Morris et al. (2006) developed the Single Item Literacy Screener: "How often do you need to have someone help when you read instructions, pamphlets, or other written material from your doctor or pharmacy (1 = never; 2 = rarely; 3 = sometimes; 4 = often; 5 = always)?" This particular item was found to be reasonably successful in detecting health literacy (in comparison with the TOFHLA), but only moderately sensitive. Yet it focuses on only one aspect of health literacy, which is reading materials. Recently, an "ability to read item," that is, How would you rate your ability to read? (1–5 scale from very poor to very good) performed the best, supporting use as a screening tool in safety-net systems caring for diverse populations among English/Spanish speakers (Bishop et al., 2016).

Other efforts in this field have centered on the development of tools that measure Internet-seeking abilities or e-health literacy (Norman and Skinner, 2006); assess general health skills across the dimensions of functional, communicative, and critical health, with such questions as "Do you need help to fill out official forms?" (Chinn and McCarthy, 2013); or gauge numeracy skills such as number sense, tables and graphs, probability, and statistics (Jacobs et al., 2016; Schapira et al., 2014). If you are interested in this topic, go to the *Health Literacy Toolshed,* an outstanding online database of health literacy measures compiled by the NLM in collaboration with Boston University, at https://www.nlm.nih.gov/news/health_literacy_tool_shed.html.

As one can see, there are many formal tools to measure reading level or word recognition, which in turn may be helpful to gauge an individual's health literacy. Yet the time needed to administer them in community-based settings greatly limits their use. Most importantly, these collective findings underscore that formal assessments should be secondary to the nurse's informal and ongoing assessments, which allow for verification of understanding about specific health content within a specific health context. Nurses need to be astute in their assessment of people's skills and to continually monitor the demands of the health care environment and make organizational adjustments as needed. Furthermore, Meade and Calvo (2001) continue to suggest asking patients and community members a series of simple questions on the topic of years of schooling and about their reading habits that will help gauge health literacy, followed by ongoing learner verification and teach-back methods. In this manner, health literacy can be viewed from both content and contextual outlooks.

The promising news here is that health literacy can be realized through health education (Nutbeam, 2009). Fundamental to implementing effective health education strategies is recognizing that health literacy needs to be viewed within its context, that is, the physical and social environment of health care settings (Rudd, 2013). As such, nurses play essential roles in their community outreach and engagement activities for conveying knowledge, deciphering motivations, adapting health education messages, making information accessible, promoting health decisions, and facilitating empowering processes to increase the useful uptake of information. As Sykes et al. (2013) point out, health literacy goes beyond merely the motivation and development of skills within the individual or community, but also entails a number of collaborative efforts at a structural level. It needs to become an organizational value integrated into all aspects of community planning and health operations and should be viewed as a relationship between individuals and their environment (Brach et al., 2012; Koh et al., 2013; Rudd, 2013; McCormack et al., 2016).

Helpful Tips for Effective Teaching

- Put patients at ease and establish rapport. Focus on inclusion and trust first.
- Assess reading skills using informal and formal methods.
- Determine what your patient/community member wants to know.
- Identify motivating factors for learning new information and behaviors.
- Stick with the essentials. Limit the number of concepts or key points. Focus on important critical and survival skills.

BOX 8.2 Patient Communication: Prostate Cancer and Treatment Options

Version A (harder to grasp – passive)

The doctor has recently communicated to the patient that he has localized prostate cancer, commonly labeled stage II. In addition to managing the anxieties associated with a life-threatening illness, patients with this disease must carefully consider the available treatment modalities and account for the potential effect each one may have on quality of life. Patients must seriously evaluate the benefits and adverse side effects of each treatment modality and determine the most efficacious intervention for their lifestyle.

Version B (easier to grasp – active)

You have just been told that you have early-stage prostate cancer. Choosing a treatment is hard, but it is important. Besides dealing with fears that often go along with having cancer, get to know about your treatment options:

- Learn about each treatment and how it may affect your life and your family.
- Get to know the benefits and side effects of each treatment.
- Ask questions. Write them down. Talk it over with your family.
- Choose the best treatment for you.

Modified from Doak CC, Doak LG, Root JH: *Teaching patients with low literacy skills,* ed 2, Philadelphia, PA, 1996, Lippincott Williams & Wilkins. (Chapter 10 on learner verification can now be accessed at the Harvard health literacy website: http://www.hsph.harvard.edu/healthliteracy/resources/teaching-patients-with-low-literacy-skills/).

- Set realistic goals and objectives. Take cues from your patients about what they want to learn and how to help them learn.
- Use clear and concise language. Avoid technical terms, if possible. For example, substitute *problem* for *complication.* Use *high blood pressure* instead of *hypertension,* or use *chance* instead of *possibility.* Do not needlessly simplify if the intended meaning is lost. Although the words *insulin* and *infection* are polysyllabic words, people with diabetes should get to be familiar with these terms (Box 8.2).
- Consider developing a glossary or vocabulary list for common words on the health topic. For example, in teaching a family about dental health, create a list of common words about the topic and words that might substitute well (e.g., flossing, toothbrush, cavity, decay, check-ups, x-rays).
- Space your teaching out over time, if possible. Incorporate health education activities into other activities. For example, ask women about their smoking habits at each prenatal visit. Relate teaching to their everyday concerns. Introduce HPV education into women's and men's health visits.
- Personalize health messages. Use the active voice. For example, instead of saying, "It is important that patients read labels if they want to cut down on fat and sodium intake," say, "Read the labels on foods to know what is in them. This will help you cut down on your fat and salt intake."
- Incorporate methods of illustration, demonstration, and real-life examples. Connect the health message to everyday events and real-life situations.
- Give and get. Review information often. Ask the patient questions before, during, and after teaching.
- Summarize often. Provide the patient with feedback. Obtain feedback from the patient.

TABLE 8.7   Components of Learner Verification (Checks the Suitability of the Message with Learners)

Components	Description
Attraction	Readers should be attracted to the message. For example, the cover should stimulate interest, and when possible, pictures should foster an identification that "tells me that this is important for my situation." Examples: • Is this material attractive/pleasing to you? • Overall, would you be likely to pick up and read this brochure?
Comprehension	Readers should be able to summarize the main points in their own words, not the vocabulary of the instruction. Examples: • What do you feel is the main point? • Are there any words that are not clear?
Acceptability	Readers need to perceive that the information is culturally acceptable for their lifestyle, situation, and background. Examples: • Is there anything that bothers you about this booklet? • In your opinion, who is this booklet for?
Persuasion	Readers need to feel that the instruction is significant for them. Example: • Do you think that the message in this booklet is important for you?
Self-efficacy	Is the message doable, and does the reader feel confident in carrying it out? Example: • Do you think you could do what is suggested in this booklet (e.g., cut down on cigarettes)?

- Be creative. Use your imagination to convey difficult concepts (e.g., use picture cards, drawings, objects, streaming videos, audiobooks, podcasts, flip charts, multimedia decision aids, photographs, embodied conversational agents, apps, photovoice, storytelling, use of metaphors).
- Use appropriate resources and materials to enhance teaching and convey ideas (e.g., picture cards, models, tablet devices, whiteboards).
- Praise patients, but do not patronize them. Let them know what they are doing right. Focus on their strengths and assets and what they bring to the teaching encounter.
- Be encouraging throughout the educational steps. We all like to be told what we are doing right.
- Allow time for patients and family members to think and ask questions.
- Remember that comprehension and understanding require time and practice. Ongoing feedback helps refocus the teaching encounter and can keep you on track.
- Employ "teach-back" methods. This means asking patients to state in their own words (i.e., teach back) key concepts, decisions, or instructions just discussed (Badaczewski et al., 2017; Byck and Sharif, 2017; Glascoe and Trimm 2014).
- Conduct learner verification (a process that checks suitability of information) to ensure understanding (Table 8.7).

- Evaluate the teaching plan, and keep adding new information to the interaction.
- Consider your environment and carry out a quick 10-item checklist to see if your institution is health literate as well (Kowalski et al., 2015)

Assess Materials: Become a Wise Consumer and User

Materials are collected, stored, and disseminated within community sites. In many instances, nurses distribute pamphlets, but patients either do not read them or review them only superficially.

People of this country have had so much pamphlet materials passed out to them free that some have lost respect for free literature. Health educators may have contributed to this delinquency by passing out health literature carelessly and indiscriminately. The nurse who expects the pamphlet to take the place of the health teacher is employing weak measures in the health education program.

(Rue, 1944, p. 215)

This statement continues to be true today. Moreover, many of today's pamphlets are even more complex and lengthier because of technological advances and health care innovations. Thus it is important that nurses evaluate health materials, including websites, before they disseminate them to or share them with individuals, families, or the general public. Health materials should strengthen previous teaching and should be used as an adjunct to health instruction.

Assess Relevancy of Health Materials

It is critical that nurses find and use materials, documents, and media that are appropriate for the intended target audience in community health education initiatives. Questions that the nurse should ask include the following:
- Do the materials match the intended audience?
- Are the materials appealing and culturally and linguistically relevant?
- Do they convey accurate and up-to-date information?
- Are the messages clear and understandable?
- Do the messages promote self-efficacy and motivation?

Fig. 8.2 provides an assessment guide for reviewing health materials that the author has used for gauging the appropriateness of materials. The nurse can use this guide in critiquing printed materials. Similarly, the nurse can make slight modifications in the tool and assess other types of health resources (e.g., booklets, videotapes, websites, and multimedia interactive modules). To use the tool, gather a few materials/media that are commonly used in the clinical setting where you are based. In a group or individually, begin to assess each category and critically assess the suitability for your intended audience. The tool allows the nurse to review health materials systematically for appropriateness for the intended target audience. The material assessment should focus on the following criteria: format/layout, type, verbal content, visual content, and aesthetic quality. This activity probably will take 10 to 15 minutes. It can also be used as a group activity with patients or community members. The feedback your users offer about the materials may surprise you!

Assessment of Health Education Materials

Name of material/media _____

Author _____

Intended target audience _____

Cost/availability/producer _____

> **Directions:** Assess your printed material using the following tool. Use the rating scale of 1-4 for each item in a major category. *1 = poor 2 = fair 3 = good 4 = very good N/A = not applicable.*
>
> For each category, give it an overall category rating of: *(+) effective* or *(–) not effective, (X) unsure*

Using the tool(s) that you brought to class, begin your review in groups of 2-3. Assess the material carefully to evaluate its suitability for your audience. Following your small group review, share your comments with others.

Category/criteria Comments   **Rating**

1 = Poor; 2 = Fair;
3 = Good; 4 = Very Good

Format/Layout
Organizational style _____
White/black space _____
Margins _____
Grouping of elements _____
Use of headers/advance organizers _____
Overall category rating of:
(+) effective _____ (–) not effective _____ (X) unsure _____

Type
Size _____
Style _____
Spacing _____
Overall category rating of:
(+) effective _____ (–) not effective _____ (X) unsure _____

Verbal Content
Clarity _____
Quantity _____
Relevancy to intended group _____
   (e.g., age, gender, race/ethnicity)
Use of active voice _____
Difficulty/readability level _____
Grade level _____
Accuracy _____
Currency _____
Overall category rating of:
(+) effective _____ (–) not effective _____ (X) unsure _____

Category/criteria   **Rating Comments**

1 = Poor; 2 = Fair;
3 = Good; 4 = Very Good

Visual Content
Tone/mood _____
Clarity _____
Cueing _____
Relevancy to intended group _____
   (e.g., age, gender, race/ethnicity)
Currency _____
Accuracy _____
Detail _____
Overall category rating of:
(+) effective _____ (–) not effective _____ (X) unsure _____

Aesthetic Quality/Appeal
Attractiveness _____
Color _____
Quality of production _____
Personalized instructions _____
Overall category rating of:
(+) effective _____ (–) not effective _____ (X) unsure _____

Comments:

Overall, based on your scoring of 1 to 4 and an evaluation of its effectiveness with the intended target audience, how suitable would you rate this educational tool? Circle one.

1 = poor: probably won't work with my intended audience. I would probably not ever use it.

2 = fair: has a low likelihood of success with my intended audience. I would use it rarely and only in combination with other sources.

3 = good: has a good likelihood of being suitable and relevant for about half of my intended audience. I would use it sometimes.

4 = very good: has a high likelihood of being suitable and relevant for most of my intended audience. I would most definitely use it!

FIG. 8.2 Assessment of health education materials.

CASE STUDY   Application of the Nursing Process
Selected Teaching Approaches and Learning Needs

The following case study and teaching plan provide an example of selected teaching approaches and learning needs for the individual, family, and community.

Emma Jackson, aged 33 years, receives ongoing health care at her neighborhood's community-based clinic, a federally funded community health center. She visits the nurse practitioner, and the nurse confirms that Mrs. Jackson is 2 months pregnant. She is married and has an 8-year-old son. Emma tells the nurse she smokes and wants to quit but she has been unable to quit since her last pregnancy. She tells the nurse, "I smoke when I get stressed. I have so many things on my mind." Her husband is also a smoker and has tried to quit at times as well. The nurse refers Mrs. Jackson to a community nursing student named Irene Green for counseling, education, and follow-up.

Assessment

Irene recognizes that smoking during pregnancy is detrimental for the unborn infant, unhealthy for Mrs. Jackson, and harmful for the 8-year-old child, who breathes the secondhand smoke (https://www.cdc.gov/reproductivehealth/maternalinfanthealth/tobaccousepregnancy/index.htm). Irene also knows that smokers often experience stages of readiness in their attempts to quit and that relapse is often part of the process (Prochaska and DiClemente, 1983). She notes that family and community support systems are important.

Irene assesses Mrs. Jackson on an individual level, as follows:

* Smoking history, smoking patterns, and previous attempts to quit
* Support systems (e.g., family, friends, and peers)
* Perceived barriers to quitting
* Perceived benefits to quitting
* Perceived priority in addressing this health issue vs. other everyday stresses
* Perceived effect of smoking behavior on family communication patterns
* Confidence and perceived efficacy in ability to quit

Assessment of other groups includes families, neighborhoods, churches, community organizations, and environmental messages that promote smoking cessation.

Diagnosis
Individual

* Health concerns related to smoking and personal stressors/triggers
* Desire for more information about ways to quit and stay smoke free

Family

* Effect and impact of smoking on family dynamics

Community

* Need for information about community programs and social support resources

Planning
Individual
Long-Term Goal

* Mrs. Jackson will quit smoking.

Short-Term Goals

* Mrs. Jackson will recognize that continued smoking is unhealthy for herself, her unborn infant, her young child, and her family.
* Mrs. Jackson will become aware of ways to enhance her confidence during smoking cessation.
* Mrs. Jackson will identify situations and stressors that influence her smoking patterns.
* Mrs. Jackson will learn two strategies to cope with stressful situations and will apply those strategies.

Family
Long-Term Goal

* Mr. and Mrs. Jackson will quit smoking and become a smoke-free family.

Short-Term Goals

* Mr. and Mrs. Jackson will acknowledge the benefits of a smoke-free environment.
* Mr. Jackson will recognize the need to quit smoking.
* The couple will recognize the need to support each other in smoking cessation.
* Mr. and Mrs. Jackson will identify and discuss specific supportive actions during the smoking cessation phases. The couple will enlist the support of another person or network.

Community
Long-Term Goals

* The community will support and endorse a smoke-free environment and publicize these efforts through billboards and other media.
* Community agencies and organizations will integrate smoking cessation and relapse programs and messages into their existing health-related activities.
* Cigarette advertising will cease.

Short-Term Goals

* A coalition of community members will develop and implement policies to support smoking cessation and relapse strategies.
* A consortium of health care agencies and community-based organizations will recognize the need to develop partnerships in creating smoking cessation strategies for the community and for high-risk groups.

Intervention
Individual

Planning interventions encourage self-expression, promote the use of adaptive coping mechanisms, offer positive reinforcement, disseminate appropriate smoking cessation strategies, and provide culturally and educationally relevant materials and media. The nurse applies the "five As" approach to smoking cessation counseling (Ask, Advise, Assess, Assist, and Arrange). Irene offers empowerment strategies to help Mrs. Jackson cope with her smoking cessation attempts and identifies daily hassles and stressors. Irene gives personalized smoking cessation messages and culturally and educationally appropriate materials and initiates a follow-up plan that is acceptable and doable on the basis of ongoing assessment and feedback (American College of Obstetrics and Gynecology, 2010; Brandon et al., 2012)

Family

Planning and interventions recognize the need for strong support systems within families. Irene provided education and counseling to promote family self-care and recognized that she must address and incorporate Mr. Jackson's support, or lack thereof, into the care plan. Irene makes links to community resources (e.g., health classes, support groups, and networking with other expectant mothers who have quit or are attempting to quit) to build Mrs. Jackson's support system.

Community

Planning and interventions implemented on an aggregate level identify key community leaders, agencies, legislators, and lay members who are committed to supporting smoking cessation/relapse initiatives at a sociopolitical level (e.g., creating smoking cessation/relapse initiatives at various community channels). Program initiatives assist community members in defining issues and solutions to the effects of smoking on individuals, families, and community groups.

CASE STUDY Application of the Nursing Process—cont'd

Selected Teaching Approaches and Learning Needs

Developing coalitions and partnerships among community-based organizations, health care groups, governmental agencies, and intended audience members through dialogue and increased awareness is essential.

Evaluation

Evaluation is systematic and continuous and focuses on the individual, family, and community.

Individual

An evaluation of Mrs. Jackson's smoking habits occurs within the health system and the community (clinics and Women, Infants, and Children Service). These groups address both process (decrease in number of cigarettes smoked) and outcome (quit or not quit) end points. Mrs. Jackson experiences an increase in her coping skills and support system, which is evident in her personalized care plan.

- Irene tailors smoking cessation messages to Mrs. Jackson to fit her everyday life and addresses negative affect, that is, negative emotional smoking triggers.
- Irene provides Mrs. Jackson with follow-up (e.g., telephone, letter, text messages, and follow-up visits).
- Irene also used a tablet (iPad) to promote knowledge of tobacco risk and cessation resources for pregnant women (Dotson et al., 2017).
- Irene provides educational resources for Mrs. Jackson (https://smokefree.gov/).

Readers are suggested to visit a virtual tour to enhance your counseling skills. See Smoking Cessation for Pregnancy and Beyond: A Virtual Clinic, a multimedia program that provides counseling guidance: https://www.smokingcessationand-pregnancy.org/.

Family

Care plans include supporting pattern development with family or significant other in smoking cessation initiatives.

- Irene assesses family health patterns and screens for other at-risk behaviors.
- Irene identifies and addresses family support and communication patterns in the care plan.

Community

Irene introduces smoking cessation and relapse programs and smoking prevention initiatives to at least two channels of dissemination (e.g., churches, schools, worksites, community-based clinics, restaurants).

- Smoking cessation/relapse messages are infused throughout the community by means of radio, television, and billboards.
- Community task forces and coalitions demonstrate a collaborative partnership among lay members, community leaders, organizers, and legislators to address smoking-related health issues.

Format/Layout

- Is the information organized clearly? Does it make sense?
- Do headers or advance organizers cue the reader? Headers help the reader visualize what is next.
- Is there a 50%/50% allocation of white and black space? This proportion gives the reader "breathing space."
- Is the information easy to read and uncluttered?

Type

- Is the type or font a readable size? Consider the age of your intended group and whether visual difficulties are likely.

Verbal Content

- Is the information current, accurate, and relevant to the intended group?
- Is the information culturally acceptable?
- Are difficult terms defined?
- Does the text reflect the racial and ethnic diversity and language of the intended audience?
- What is the reading level?

Visual Content

- Are the graphics accurate, current, and relevant and engaging to the intended group?
- Does cueing help the reader connect the printed words and pictures?
- Will the reader understand the intended meanings of the pictures?
- Is the information culturally acceptable?
- Are the pictures on the cover reflective of the material inside?
- Do the pictures reflect the target audience's racial and ethnic diversity?

Aesthetic Quality and Appeal

- Is the material appealing and engaging?
- Are there helpful special features (e.g., glossary, space for notes, and useful telephone numbers or websites)?

Assessment of Reading Level

Part of the written material's assessment is reading level. Many formulas are available to estimate the printed text's readability and grade level, including the SMOG readability formula.

Readability formulas are objective, quantitative tools that measure sentence and word variables. However, they do not consider factors such as motivation, experience, and need for information (Meade and Smith, 1991). Nor do they determine the effects of visuals or design factors that could influence readability and comprehension or address global text characteristics, including fluency, structure, and content of the text (Kauchak and Leroy, 2016). Formulas do estimate reading ease and provide helpful guidelines for assessing and rewriting health information. Two of the most commonly used formulas are the Flesch-Kincaid and the SMOG formulas. The Flesch-Kincaid Formula (Flesch, 1948) is a broad estimate of reading and is programmed into most computer software programs' grammar editing tools. To test a document's readability on your computer using the Flesch-Kincaid formula, search the term "readability statistic." You will be directed to a series of file and option tabs to reach grammar and spelling, and then readability statistics. The SMOG formula is shown in Resource 8D and is frequently used to calculate the readability estimate of health materials (McLaughlin, 1969).

Learner Verification

The best way to identify material suitability is to deliver the materials to the intended audience and obtain feedback about acceptability, understanding, and usefulness. Learner verification engages intended members in dialogue and helps uncover unsuitable aspects of the material (i.e., content, visuals, or format) (Doak et al., 1996). If the nurse discovers a need for new educational materials or media, he or she can incorporate Freirean principles to produce empowering products. The Freire approach supports learner participation in the development process, ensures that the learner is the active subject of the educational experience, and allows learners to define content and outcomes.

The process of learner verification helps identify the likelihood that the message is well suited to the audience. It involves verifying whether certain elements work well together to result in a good match of information for the learner. See Table 8.7 for a description of the specific elements and sample questions associated with each one.

The author and colleagues have used learner verification processes on many occasions, for example, to develop a series of education toolboxes on breast and cervical cancer and prostate cancer for Hispanic migrant and seasonal farmworkers and African American women and men. After holding a series of focus groups with members of the intended audience to elicit themes about health, illness, cancer, and prevention, we conducted learner verification measures. Through systematic questions and interviewing processes, we were able to collect information in the intended audience's own words to help shape and refocus the cancer issues (breast, cervical, and prostate) from their own perspective (African American men and women and Hispanic men and women farmworkers). Such verifying checks help assess the understanding of words and pictures; the acceptability of music, narrator, and pictures; the efficacy and persuasion of the message; and the overall attractiveness of the materials/media For example, we found that the word *prevention* was a term many men found difficult to grasp. What we found was that tuning up one's car was a familiar concept that could similarly be used to convey the importance of ongoing check-ups, as in maintaining prostate health. Similarly, the author and her colleagues used this approach to adapt smoking-relapse prevention materials for pregnant and postpartum women (Quinn et al., 2006), to develop stress management tools for Latinas undergoing chemotherapy (Meade, 2009), and to create biobanking education materials (Meade et al., 2015). Another useful example can be seen in the study by Hunter et al. (2012), who used learner verification techniques to clarify terminology, translation, preferred content, and illustrations for cervical cancer content for Mexican immigrant women. Their findings challenged the common simplification approaches often linked to teaching learners with low literacy and reinforced the need of learners to know more about their anatomy. Overall, the process of learner verification fits well within the framework of community-based participatory research methods, as outlined earlier in this chapter, and can be a very helpful qualitative tool for the nurse to use in gauging the suitability of his or her health education efforts.

⁉ ACTIVE LEARNING EXERCISE

1. Identify an issue of concern among community members (e.g., obesity, access to care, education of youth). Discuss sociopolitical issues that affect this issue and how it relates to health. Outline specific community-based participatory activities and roles that the community nurse can take on that can address this health issue. Identify at least two ways to promote community engagement on this topic. What educational resources might the nurse use?

2. Select a health education brochure or health website. Apply the assessment criteria presented to assess its appropriateness for an intended audience. Evaluate the relative strengths of the printed material or website and potential areas for improvement using learner verification questions. Describe how you and your group can make it more relevant for your audience. What can be improved? How could you involve your audience in its assessment?

SOCIAL MEDIA

Americans today are increasingly connected to the world of digital information. As such, nurses should consider the role of social media channels in connecting communities with reliable health information. Nurses should also think about how mobile health and e-health technologies might improve health outcomes of communities *Social media* refers to interactive Internet-based communication channels that allow users to create, share, comment on, and modify online content. It facilitates engagement and collaboration and has rapidly become a tool for health promotion and education (Alber et al., 2015). Social media platforms might include blogs, online discussion boards, microblogs such as Twitter, and video-sharing sites such as YouTube, Vimeo, and Flickr. In light of the growing number of people (both here in the United States and globally) who have mobile phones and use social media, such platforms may lend themselves to reaching diverse community constituents with important public health messages (O'Mara, 2012). It is estimated that most Americans (95%) own some type of a cell phone and most send and receive text messages (Pew Research Center, 2017). Ownership of smartphones is now 77%, up from about 35% since Pew Research Center's first survey of smartphone ownership in 2011. Given this widespread use of cell phones, social media text messaging offers a new and promising way to directly deliver health information to diverse groups in rural and urban areas.

Social media sites have the potential to facilitate interactive communications, increase the sharing of health information, and personalize and reinforce health messages, all of which in turn can empower community members to make informed health decisions (CDC, 2010). For example, Strasser et al. (2012) explored the use of social media (e.g., Facebook) to reduce IPV among gay men in Atlanta; Fortmann et al. (2017) explored the use of a series of text messages to improve glycemic control in Hispanics with type 2 diabetes; and Koskan et al. (2014) conducted a systematic review that reinforced the role of social media in cancer care (and most likely other areas of health). Further, in a study carried out in rural northern Kenya, Kazi et al. (2017) reported phone usage, ownership characteristics, and feasibility of text-based mHealth interventions (short messaging service [SMS]) among patients for enhancing maternal-child health (antenatal care immunizations). Notably, despite remoteness, most pregnant women and caregivers visiting for antenatal care and routine immunizations had some access to mobile phones, liked the idea of text messaging, and stated that they would use it if available. Hence, if designed appropriately, findings suggest that SMS may be an innovative way to engage women in their health and the health of their families.

Recently, Roland et al. (2017) examined the promulgation of online communities of practice that are emerging from interactions on social media using Twitter #Analytics. In particular, nurses in community health education settings are well poised to explore the utility of novel digital technology to connect individuals, families, and groups to communities of learning and to connect them with reliable and credible information, which has meaning for their everyday health concerns and needs.

SUMMARY

Teaching is a significant component of community health nursing, affecting virtually every nursing activity. The goal of health education is to facilitate a process that allows individuals, families, and groups to make well-informed decisions about health practices. An understanding of learning and the theoretical frameworks that explain behaviors and health actions is inherent in community health education. No single theory explains human behavior; the nurse must apply multiple theories and approaches.

Nurses must be knowledgeable about sociopolitical, cultural, environmental, and ecological forces affecting community health to ensure the success of health education strategies. Furthermore, relevant health education (classes, talking circles, support groups, individual/family instruction, health fairs, etc.) is based on the meeting of individual variables and social, structural, political, cultural, and economic factors within the larger community context. To create meaningful education interventions, nurses need to assess their audience(s) and their characteristics thoroughly and to employ systematic approaches when delivering health messages and programs. Implementing social

action strategies, such as advocating health-promoting lifestyles, creating an environment for problem-posing dialogue, and providing links to appropriate health resources, supports the philosophy of critical consciousness. Nurses can facilitate the principle of **social justice** by mastering health information delivery and committing themselves to creating empowerment strategies that equip individuals, families, and communities with knowledge and navigation skills for healthy lifestyles and environments.

Further, a variety of creative methods, materials, media, and mobile health technologies can support health education activities. Continual review and evaluation of such resources are essential to ensure cultural, linguistic, language, and literacy suitability. Embracing the notion that health education is an ongoing interactive process influenced by many internal and external factors is strategic to meeting the needs of individuals, families, and communities. As nurses, important contributions to the prevention of disease and the promotion of community health can be realized with an ongoing community health education mind-set and commitment to community empowerment and engagement strategies.

ⓔ EVOLVE WEBSITE

http://evolve.elsevier.com/Nies/community

- NCLEX Review Questions
- Case Studies

BIBLIOGRAPHY

Aboumatar HJ, Carson KA, Beach MC, et al.: The impact of health literacy on desire for participation in healthcare, medical visit communication, and patient reported outcomes among patients with hypertension, *J Gen Intern Med* 28:1469–1476, 2013.

Abramson K, Keefe B, Chou WY: Communicating about cancer through Facebook: a qualitative analysis of a breast cancer awareness page, *J Health Commun* 20(2):237–243, 2015. https://doi.org/10.1080/10810730.2014.927034. Epub 2014 Dec 13.

Alber JM, Bernhardt JM, Stellefson M, et al.: Designing and testing an inventory for measuring social media competency of certified health education specialists. Eysenbach G, ed, *J Med Internet Res* 17(9):e221, 2015. https://doi.org/10.2196/jmir.4943.

Alcaraz KI, Sly J, Ashing K, et al.: The ConNECT Framework: a model for advancing behavioral medicine science and practice to foster health equity, *J Behav Med*, Aug 10, 2016. [Epub ahead of print] PMID:27509892.

American Cancer Society: *Cancer facts and figures*, Atlanta, 2017, Author. https://www.cancer.org/research/cancer-facts-statistics/all-cancer-facts-figures/cancer-facts-figures-2017.html.

American College of Obstetricians and Gynecologists: *Smoking cessation during pregnancy*. Available from<http://www.acog.org/Resources_And_Publications/Committee_Opinions/Committee_on_Health_Care_for_Underserved_Women/Smoking_Cessation_During_Pregnanc>.

American College of Obstetricians and Gynecologists: *Smoking cessation during pregnancy*. Committee Opinion No. 471, *Obstet Gynecol* 116:1241–1244, 2010.

American Nurses Association (ANA): *Public health nursing: scope and standards of practice*, Washington, DC, 2013, American Nurse Publishing.

Aranda K, Coleman L, Sherriff NS, et al.: Listening for commissioning: A participatory study exploring young people's experiences, views and preferences of school-based sexual health and school nursing, *J Clin Nurs*, 2017 Jun 21. https://doi.org/10.1111/jocn.13936. [Epub ahead of print].

Badaczewski A, Bauman LJ, Blank AE, et al.: The progress and promise of health literacy research, *J Health Commun* 18(Suppl 1):5–8, 2013. https://doi.org/10.1080/10810730.2013.830042.

Badawy SM, Kuhns LM: Texting and Mobile Phone App Interventions for Improving Adherence to Preventive Behavior in Adolescents: A Systematic Review, *JMIR Mhealth Uhealth* 5(4):e50, Apr 19, 2017. https://doi.org/10.2196/mhealth.6837.

Bailey SC, Brega AG, Crutchfield TM, et al.: Update on health literacy and diabetes, *Diabetes Educ* 40(5):581–604, Sep-Oct 2014. https://doi.org/10.1177/0145721714540220. Epub 2014 Jun 19.

Balls-Berry JE, Billings H, Ernste L, et al.: Development of a self-directed, online-learning curriculum to increase community-engaged research in clinical and translational science, *J Clin Transl Sci* 1(2):135–139, Apr 2017. https://doi.org/10.1017/cts.2016.19.

Bandura A: Self-efficacy: toward a unifying theory of behavioral change, *Psychol Rev* 84:191–215, 1977.

Bandura A: *Social learning theory*, Englewood Cliffs, NJ, 1977b, Prentice Hall.

Bangia D, Shaffner DW, Palmer-Keenan DM: A point-of-purchase intervention using grocery store tour podcasts about omega-3s increases long-term purchases of omega-3-rich food items, *J Nutr Educ Behav* 49(6):475–480.e1, Jun 2017. https://doi.org/10.1016/j.jneb.2017.02.008. Epub 2017 Apr 1.

Batista Ferrer H, Trotter CL, Hickman M, et al.: Barriers and facilitators to uptake of the school-based HPV vaccination programme in an ethnically diverse group of young women, *J Public Health (Oxf)* 38(3):569–577, Sep 2016. Epub 2015 Jun 7.

Baur C: Calling the nation to act: implementing the national action plan to improve health literacy, *Nurs Outlook* 59:63–69, 2011.

Becker MH, editor: *The health belief model and personal health behavior*, Thorofare, NJ, 1974, Charles B. Slack.

Becker MH, Maiman LA, Kirscht JP, et al.: The health belief model and prediction of dietary compliance: a field experiment, *J Health Soc Behav* 18:348–366, 1977.

Belone L, Lucero JE, Duran B, et al.: Community-based participatory research conceptual model: community partner consultation and face validity, *Qual Health Res* 26(1):117–135, Jan 2016. https://doi.org/10.1177/1049732314557084. Epub 2014 Oct 31.

Bender JL, Wiljer D, To MJ, et al.: Testicular cancer survivors' supportive care needs and use of online support: a cross-sectional survey, *Support Care Cancer* 20(11):2737–2746, 2012. Epub 2012 March 3.

Bigge ML, Shermis SS: *Learning theories for teachers*, ed 6, Boston, 2004, Allyn & Bacon Classics.

Bishop WP, Craddock Lee SJ, Skinner CS, et al.: Validity of single-item screening for limited health literacy in english and spanish speakers, *Am J Public Health* 106(5):889–892, May 2016. https://doi.org/10.2105/AJPH.2016.303092. Epub 2016 Mar 17.

Brach C, Keller D, Hernandez LM, et al.: *Ten attributes of health literate health care organizations*, Washington, DC, 2012, Institute of Medicine of the National Academies.

Brandon TH, Simmons VN, Sutton SK, et al.: Extended self-help for smoking cessation: a randomized controlled trial, *Am J Prev Med* 51(1):54–62, 2016. https://doi.org/10.1016/j.amepre.2015.12.016.

Brandon TH, Simmons VN, Meade CD, et al.: Self-help booklets for preventing postpartum smoking relapse: a randomized trial, *Am J Public Health* 102:2109–2115, 2012.

Braun K, Stewart S, Baquet C, et al.: The national cancer institute's community networks program initiative to reduce cancer health disparities: outcomes and lessons learned, *Prog Community Health Partnersh* (9), *Special Issue* 2015, 21–32, 2015.

Brenner AT, Ko LK, Janz N, et al.: Race/ethnicity and primary language: health beliefs about colorectal cancer screening in a diverse, low-income population, *J Health Care Poor Underserved* 26(3):824–838, Aug 2015. https://doi.org/10.1353/hpu.2015.0075.

Byck H, Sharif I: Relationship between teach-back and patient-centered communication in primary care pediatric encounters, *Patient Educ Couns* 100(7):1345–1352, Jul 2017. https://doi.org/10.1016/j.pec.2017.02.022. Epub 2017 Feb 24.

Cabassa LJ, Nicasio A, Whitley R: Picturing recovery: a photovoice exploration of recovery dimensions among people with serious mental illness, *Psychiatric services (Washington, DC)* 64(9), 2013: https://doi.org/10.1176/appi.ps.201200503. doi:10.1176/appi.ps.201200503.

Carpenter CJ: A meta-analysis of the effectiveness of health belief model variables in predicting behavior, *Health Commun* 25(8):661–669, 2010 Dec. https://doi.org/10.1080/10410236.2010.521906.

Champion VL, Monahan PO, Springston JK, et al.: Measuring mammography and breast cancer beliefs in African American women, *J Health Psychol* 138:27–37, 2008.

Champion VL, Skinner CS: The health belief model. In: Glanz K, Rimer BK, Visnawath K, editors: *Health behavior and education: theory, research, and practice*, ed 4, San Francisco, Jossey-Bass, pp. 45–65.

Champion VL, Skinner CS: The health belief model. In Glanz K, Rimer BK, Viswanath K, editors: *Health behavior and health education: theories, research, and practice*, San Francisco, 2008, Jossey Bass.

Champion VL, Susan M, Rawl SM, et al.: Randomized trial of DVD, telephone, and usual care for increasing mammography adherence, *J Health Psychol* 21(6):916–926, Jun 2016.

Chesser AK, Keene Woods N, Smothers K, et al.: Health literacy and older adults: a systematic review, *Gerontology and geriatric medicine* 2, 2016, 2333721416630492. https://doi.org/10.1177/2333721416630492.

Chew LD, Bradley KA, Boyko EJ: Brief questions to identify patients with inadequate literacy, *Fam Med* 36:588–594, 2004.

Chin J, Lee EH, Son HJ, et al.: The process-knowledge model of health literacy: evidence from a componential analysis of two commonly used measures, *J Health Communication* 16(Suppl 3):222–241, 2011.

Chinn D, McCarthy C: All aspects of health literacy scale (AAHLS): developing a tool to measure functional, communicative and critical health literacy in primary healthcare settings, *Patient Educ Couns* 90:247–253, 2013.

Chinn D: Critical health literacy: a review and critical analyses, *Soc Sci Med* 73:60–67, 2011.

Choi J: Effect of pictograph-based discharge instructions on older adults' comprehension and recall: a pilot study, *Res Gerontol Nurs* 9(2):66–71, Mar-Apr 2016. https://doi.org/10.3928/19404921-20150513-05. Epub 2015 May 28.

Chou WY, Prestin A, Lyons C: Web 2.0 for health promotion: reviewing the current evidence, *Am J Public Health* 103(1), Jan 2013.

Christy S, Davis S, Williams K, et al.: A community-based trial of educational interventions with fecal immunochemical test for colorectal cancer screening uptake among Blacks in community settings, *Cancer* 122(21):3288–3296, Nov 2016. PMID: 27420119. PMCID: PMC5073009.

Chu KC, Chen Jr MS, Dignan MB, et al.: Parallels between the development of therapeutic drugs and cancer health disparity programs: implications for disparities reduction, *Cancer* 113:2790–2796, 2008.

Clark MJD: *Population and community health nursing*, ed 6, Englewood Cliffs, NJ, 2015, Prentice Hall.

Clements K: Participatory action research and photovoice in a psychiatric nursing/clubhouse collaboration exploring recovery narrative, *J Psychiatr Ment Health Nurs* 19:785–791, 2012.

Coughlin SS, Prochaska JJ, Williams LB, et al.: Patient web portals, disease management, and primary prevention, *Risk Manag Healthc Policy* 10:33–40, 2017. https://doi.org/10.2147/RMHP.S130431.

Cueva M, Kuhnley R, Lanier A, et al.: Promoting culturally respectful cancer education through digital storytelling, *Int J Circumpolar Health* 11(1):34–49, 2016. https://doi.org/10.18357/ijih111201616013.

Cueva M, Kuhnley R, Slatton J: Telenovela: an innovative colorectal cancer screening health messaging tool, *Int J Circumpolar Health* 72:21301, Aug 5, 2013.

Davis SN, Christy SM, Chavarria E, et al.: A randomized controlled trial of a multi-component targeted low-literacy educational intervention compared with a non-targeted intervention to boost colorectal cancer screening with fecal immunochemical testing in community clinics, *Cancer*, Dec 1, 2016. https://doi.org/10.1002/cncr.30481. [Epub ahead of print] PMID:27906448.

Davis TC, Crouch MA, Long SW, et al.: Rapid assessment of literacy levels of adult primary care patients, *Fam Med* 23(6):433–435, Aug 1991.

Davis TC, Long SW, Jackson RH, et al.: Rapid estimate of adult literacy in medicine: a shortened screening instrument, *Fam Med* 25:56–57, 1993.

Davis TC, Wolf MS, Arnold CL, et al.: Development and validation of the rapid estimate of adolescent literacy in medicine (REALM-Teen): a tool to screen adolescents for below-grade reading in health care settings, *Pediatrics* 118:1707–1714, 2006.

Devia C, Baker EA, Sanchez-Youngman S, et al.: Advancing system and policy changes for social and racial justice: comparing a Rural and Urban Community-Based Participatory Research Partnership in the U.S, *Int J Equity Health* 16(1):17, Feb 21, 2017. https://doi.org/10.1186/s12939-016-0509-3.

Dewalt DA, Berkman ND, Sheridan S, et al.: Literacy and health outcomes: a systematic review of the literature, *J Gen Intern Med* 19:1228–1239, 2004.

Doak CC, Doak LG, Root JH: *Teaching patients with low literacy skills*, ed 2, Philadelphia, 1996, Lippincott Williams & Wilkins. <http://www.hsph.harvard.edu/healthliteracy/files/2012/09/doakintro.pdf>.

Doak CC, Doak LG, Friedell GH: Improving comprehension for cancer patients with low literacy skills: strategies for clinicians, *CA Cancer J Clin* 48:151–162, 1998.

Doak LG, Doak CC, Meade CD: Strategies to develop effective cancer education materials, *Oncol Nurs Forum* 23:1305–1312, 1996.

Donovan-Kicken E, Mackert M, Guinn TD, et al.: Health literacy, self-efficacy, and patients' assessment of medical disclosure and consent documentation, *J Health Commun* 27:581–590, 2012.

Dotson JAW, Pineda R, Cylkowski H, Amiri S: Development and evaluation of an iPad application to promote knowledge of tobacco use and cessation by pregnant women, *Nurs Womens Health* 21(3):174–185, Jun–Jul 2017. https://doi.org/10.1016/j.nwh.2017.04.005.

Flesch RR: A new readability yardstick, *J Appl Psychol* 32:221–223, 1948.

Flum MR, Siqueira CE, DeCaro A, et al.: Photovoice in the workplace: a participatory method to give voice to workers to identify health and safety hazards and promote workplace change—a study of university custodians, *Am J Ind Med* 53(11):1150–1158, 2010. https://doi.org/10.1002/ajim.20873.

Fortmann AL, Gallo LC, Garcia MI, et al.: *Dulce digital: an mHealth SMS-based intervention improves glycemic control in hispanics with type 2 diabetes*, Jun 9, 2017. https://doi.org/10.2337/dc17-0230. pii: dc170230. [Epub ahead of print].

Freeman HP: Poverty, culture, and social injustice: determinants of cancer disparities, *CA Cancer J Clin* 54:72–77, 2004.

Freire P: *Pedagogy of the oppressed*, New York, 1970, Herder and Herder.

Freire P: *Education for critical consciousness*, New York, 2005, Continuum.

Gardner MS: *Public health nursing*, New York, 1936, Macmillan Co.

Geboers B, Brainard JS, Loke YK, et al.: The association of health literacy with adherence in older adults, and its role in interventions: a systematic meta-review, *BMC Public Health* 15:903, 2015. https://doi.org/10.1186/s12889-015-2251-y.

Glanz K, Rimer BK, Viswanath K, editors: *Health behavior: theory, research, and practice*, ed 5, (5). San Francisco, 2015, Jossey-Bass.

Glascoe FP, Trimm F: Brief approaches to developmental-behavioral promotion in primary care: updates on methods and technology, *Pediatrics* 133(5):884–897, May 2014. https://doi.org/10.1542/peds.2013-1859.

Green JA, Mor MK, Shields AM, et al.: Associations of health literacy with dialysis adherence and health resource utilization in patients receiving maintenance hemodialysis, *Am J Kidney Dis* 62(1):73–80, May 2013.

Green LW, Kreuter MW: *Health program planning: an educational and ecological approach*, ed 4, New York, 2005, McGraw-Hill.

Gwede CK, William CM, Thomas KB, et al.: Exploring disparities and variability in perceptions and self-reported colorectal cancer among three ethnic subgroups of US Blacks, *Oncol Nurs Forum* 37:581–591, 2010.

Gwede CK, Davis SN, Quinn GP: Meade CD and the tampa bay community cancer network (TBCCN) partners. (2013). Making It work: provider perspectives on improving communication strategies for colorectal cancer screening in federally qualified health centers, *J Cancer Educ* 28(4):777–783, Dec 2013.

Gwede CK, Koskan AM, Quinn GP, et al.: 2015 Patients' perceptions of colorectal cancer screening tests and preparatory education in Federally Qualified Health Centers, *J Cancer Educ* 30(2):294–300, Jun 2015. J Cancer Educ 2014 Sep 24. [Epub ahead of print] PMID: 25249181.

Gwede CK, Menard JM, Martinez-Tyson D: Community cancer network community partners. Strategies for assessing community challenges and strengths for cancer disparities participatory research and outreach, *Health Promot Pract* 11(6):876–887, Nov 2010.

Guzys D, Kenny A, Dickson-Swift V, et al.: A critical review of population health literacy assessment, *BMC Public Health* 15:215, Mar 4, 2015. https://doi.org/10.1186/s12889-015-1551-6.

Hasnain-Wynia R, Wolf MS: Promoting health care equity: is health literacy a missing link?, *Health Serv Res* 45(4):897–903, Aug 2010. https://doi.org/10.1111/j.1475-6773.2010.01134.x. PMCID: PMC2910560 NEW.

Haun JN, Valerio MA, McCormack LA, et al.: Health literacy measurement: an inventory and descriptive summary of 51 instruments, *J Health Commun* 19(Suppl 2):302–333, 2014. https://doi.org/10.1080/10810730.2014.936571.

Hawkins RP, Kreuter M, Resnicow K: Understanding tailoring in communicating about health, *Health Educ Res* 23(3):454–466, Jun 2008. Epub 2008 March 17.

Hébert JR, Braun KL, Meade CD, et al.: Community-based participatory research adds value to the national cancer institute's research portfolio, *Prog. Community Health Partnersh (9)*, Special Issue 1–4, 2015.

Hochbaum GM: *Public participation in medical screening programs: a sociopsychological study*, US Public Health Service Pub No 572, Washington, DC, 1958, 1589US Government Printing Office.

Holliday CE, Wynne M, Katz J, Ford C, Barbosa-Leiker C: A CBPR approach to finding community strengths and challenges to prevent youth suicide and substance abuse, *J Transcult Nurs*, Nov 25, 2016. pii: 1043659616679234. [Epub ahead of print].

Holt CL, Roth DL, Huang J, et al.: Longitudinal effects of religious involvement on religious coping and health behaviors in a national sample of African Americans, *Soc Sci Med* 187:11–19, Jun 15, 2017. https://doi.org/10.1016/j.socscimed.2017.06.014. [Epub ahead of print].

Holtzman JS, Atchison KA, Gironda MW, Radbod R, Gornbein J: The association between oral health literacy and failed appointments in adults attending a university-based general dental clinic, *Community Dent Oral Epidemiol* 42(3):263–270, Jun 2014. https://doi.org/10.1111/cdoe.12089. Epub 2013 Dec 24.

Hughson JA, Woodward-Kron R, Parker A, et al.: A review of approaches to improve participation of culturally and linguistically diverse populations in clinical trials, *Trials* 17(1):263, May 26, 2016. https://doi.org/10.1186/s13063-016-1384-3. ReviewPMID: 27229153.

Hunter J, Kelly PJ: Imagined anatomy and other lessons from learner verification interviews with Mexican immigrant women, *J Obstet Gynecol Neonatal Nurs* 41:E1–E12, 2012.

Israel BA, Checkoway B, Schulz A: Health education and community empowerment: conceptualizing and measuring perceptions of individual, organization, and community control, *Health Educ Q* 32:149–170, 1994.

Irewall AL, Ögren J, Bergström L, et al.: Nurse-led, telephone-based, secondary preventive follow-up after stroke or transient ischemic attack improves blood pressure and LDL cholesterol: results from the first 12 months of the randomized, controlled NAILED stroke risk factor trial, *PLoS One* 10(10):e0139997, Oct 16, 2015. https://doi.org/10.1371/journal.pone.0139997. eCollection 2015. PMID:26474055.

Israel BA, et al.: *Methods for community-based participatory research for health*, ed 2, San Francisco, 2013, Jossey-Bass.

Jacobsen PB, Phillips KM, Jim HS, et al.: Effects of self-directed stress management training and home-based exercise on quality of life in cancer patients receiving chemotherapy: a randomized controlled trial, *Psycho-Oncology* 22(6):1229–1235, 2012.

Jacobs EA, Walker CM, Miller T, et al.: Development and validation of the Spanish numeracy understanding in medicine instrument, *J Gen Intern Med* 31(11):1345–1352, Nov 2016. Epub 2016 Jun 16.

Janz NK, Champion VL, Strecher VJ: The health belief model. In Glanz K, Rimer BK, Lewis FM, editors: *Health behavior and education: theory, research and practice*, ed 2, San Francisco, 2002, Jossey-Bass, pp 45–66.

Jemmott JB, Jemmott LS, O'Leary A, et al.: School-based randomized controlled trial of an HIV/STD risk-reduction intervention for South African adolescents, *Arch Pediatr Adolesc Med* 164(10):923–929, 2010. https://doi.org/10.1001/archpediatrics.2010.176.

Jemmott JB, Jemmott LS, O'Leary A, et al.: HIV/STI risk-reduction-intervention efficacy with South African adolescents over 54 months, *Health psychology* 34(6):610–621, 2015. https://doi.org/10.1037/hea0000140.

Joint Commission on Accredditation of Healthcare Organization Resources, I: *Comprehensive accreditation manual for hospiitals: (CAMH) for hospitals: effective January 1, 2017*, 2017.

Jones PL, Baker JL, Gelaude D, et al.: Lessons learned from field-testing a brief behavioral intervention package for African American women at risk for HIV/STDs, *Health Promot Pract* 14:168–173, 2012.

Kark S, Steuart GW: *A practice of social medicine, a South African team's experiences in different African communities*, Edinburgh, E. & S. Livinstone, 1962.

Kauchak D, Leroy G: Moving beyond readability metrics for health-related text simplification, *IT Prof* 18(3):45–51, May-Jun 2016. https://doi.org/10.1109/MITP.2016.50. Published online 2016 May 25. PMC5044755 NIHMSID: NIHMS784261.

Kazi AM, Carmichael JL, Hapanna GW, et al.: Assessing mobile phone access and perceptions for texting-based mHealth interventions among expectant mothers and child caregivers in remote regions of Northern Kenya: a survey-based descriptive study, *JMIR Public Health Surveill* 3(1):e5, Jan 30, 2017. https://doi.org/10.2196/publichealth.5386.

Kegeles SS, Kirscht JP, Haefner DP: Survey of beliefs about cancer detection and Papanicolaou tests, *Public Health Rep* 80:815–823, 1965.

Kelly PJ, Hunter J, Daily EB, et al.: Challenges to pap smear follow-up among women in the criminal justice system, *J Community Health* 42(1):15–20, Feb 2017. https://doi.org/10.1007/s10900-016-0225-3.

Khodaveisi M, Omidi A, Farokhi S, et al.: The effect of pender's health promotion model in improving the nutritional behavior of overweight and obese women, *Int J Community Based Nurs Midwifery* 5(2):165–174, Apr 2017.

Killian L, Coletti M: The role of universal health literacy precautions in minimizing "Medspeak" and promoting shared decision making, *AMA J Ethics* 19(3):296–303, Mar 1, 2017. https://doi.org/10.1001/journalofethics.2017.19.3.pfor1-1703.

Kickbush IS: Health literacy: addressing the health and education divide, *Health Prom Intern* 16:289–297, 2001.

Kille J, Bungay V, Oliffe J, et al.: A content analysis of health and safety communications among internet-based sex work advertisements: important information for public health, *J Med Internet Res* 19(4):e111, Apr 13, 2017. https://doi.org/10.2196/jmir.6746.

Kleinman A: Concepts and a model for the comparison of medical systems as cultural systems, *Soc Sci Med* 12:85–93, 1978.

Knowles MS: *The modern practice of adult education: from pedagogy to andragogy*, Englewood Cliffs, NJ, 1988, Cambridge Adult Education.

Knowles MS: *The making of an adult educator : an autobiographical journey*, San Francisco, 1989, Jossey-Bass.

Kobayashi LC, Smith SG, O'Conor R, et al.: The role of cognitive function in the relationship between age and health literacy: a cross-sectional analysis of older adults in Chicago, USA, *BMJ Open* 5(4):e007222, 2015. https://doi.org/10.1136/bmjopen-2014-007222.

Koh HK, Brach C, Harris LM: A proposed 'health literate care model' would constitute a systems approach to improving patients' engagement in care, *Health Aff (Millwood)* 32:357–367, 2013.

Koskan A, Klasko L, Davis S, et al.: Usage and taxonomy of social media in cancer-related research: a systematic review, *Am J Public Health*, May 15, 2014. [Epub ahead of print]. PMID: 24832403; PMC4056246; NIHMS597977.

Krieger JL, Neil JM, Strekalova YA, et al.: Linguistic strategies for improving informed consent in clinical trials among low health literacy patients, *J Natl Cancer Inst* 109(3), Oct 28, 2016. pii: djw233. Print 2017 Mar.

Kowalski C, Lee SY, Schmidt A, et al.: The health literate health care organization 10 item questionnaire (HLHO-10): development and validation, *BMC Health Serv Res* 15:47, 2015. https://doi.org/10.1186/s12913-015-0707-5. Published online 2015 Feb 1. PMCID: PMC4332719.

Kulbok PA, Thatcher E, Park E: Evolving public health nursing roles: focus on community participation health promotion and prevention, *Online J of Issues in Nurs* 17:1–14, 2012.

Labonte R: Health promotion and empowerment: reflections on professional practice, *Health Educ Q* 21:253–268, 1994.

Lee JE, Lee DE, Kim K, et al.: Development of tailored nutrition information messages based on the transtheoretical model for smartphone application of an obesity prevention and management program for elementary-school students, *Nutr Res Pract* 11(3):247–256, 2017. https://doi.org/10.4162/nrp.2017.11.3.247.

Leung MM, Agaronov A, Entwistle T, et al.: Voices through cameras, *Health Promot Pract* 18(2):211–220, Mar 2017. https://doi.org/10.1177/1524839916678404. Epub 2016 Nov 21.

Levy H, Janke A: Health literacy and access to care, *J Health Commun* 21(Suppl):43–50, 2016. https://doi.org/10.1080/10810730.2015.1131776. PMCID: PMC4924568.

Lewin K: *The conceptual representation and the measurement of psychological forces*, Durham, NC, 1938, Duke University Press.

Litvin EB, Rojas A, Brandon TH, et al.: Cultural acceptability of a smoking relapse prevention intervention for pregnant women in puerto rico: providers' feedback, *Hispanic health care international* 9(3):117–126, 2011. https://doi.org/10.1891/1540-4153.9.3.117.

Luque JS, Rivers B, Kambon M, et al.: Barbers against prostate cancer: a feasibility study for training barbers to deliver prostate cancer education in an urban African American community, *J Cancer Educ*, Feb 10, 2010. [Epub ahead of print].

Luque JS, Roy S, Tarasenko YN, et al.: Feasibility study of engaging barbershops for prostate cancer education in rural african-american communities, *J Cancer Educ* 30(4):623–628, 2015. https://doi.org/10.1007/s13187-014-0739-2.

Luque JS, Castañeda H, Martinez-Tyson D, et al.: Formative research on HPV vaccine acceptability among Latina farmworkers, *Health Promot Pract* 13(5):617–625, 2012. 2011 [Epub ahead of print] PMID: 21881079 PMC3245360.

Mabry J, Farris PE, Forro VA, et al.: Environmental, behavioral, and cultural factors that influence healthy eating in rural women of childbearing age: findings from a photovoice study, *Glob Qual Nurs* 3, 2016. https://doi.org/10.1177/2333393615622176. 2333393615622176.

MacLeod S, Musich S, Gulyas S, et al.: The impact of inadequate health literacy on patient satisfaction, healthcare utilization, and expenditures among older adults, *Geriatr Nurs*, Jan 11, 2017. https://doi.org/10.1016/j.gerinurse.2016.12.003. pii: S0197-4572(16)30298-1. [Epub ahead of print].

Mancuso JM: Assessment and measurement of health literacy: an integrative review of the literature, *Nurs Health Sci* 11:77–89, 2009.

Marks R: Ethics and patient education: health literacy and cultural dilemmas, *Health Promot Pract* 10:328–332, 2009.

Marmot M, Wilkinson RG: *Social determinants of health*, Oxford, 2000, Oxford University Press.

Marsh P, Gartrell G, Egg G, et al.: End-of-Life care in a community garden: findings from a participatory action research project in regional Australia, *Health Place* 45:110–116, May 2017. https://doi.org/10.1016/j.healthplace.2017.03.006. Epub 2017 Mar 22.

Martinez Tyson DD, Jacobsen P, Meade CD: Understanding the stress management needs and preferences of Latinas undergoing chemotherapy, *J Cancer Educ* 31(4):633–639, Dec 2016. PMID: 25952939.

Maslow AH: *Motivation and personality*, ed 3, New York, 1987, Harper and Row.

Martinez D, Aguado Loi CX, et al.: Development of a cancer camp for adult Spanish-speaking survivors: lessons learned from Camp Alegria, *J Cancer Educ* 23(1):4–9, 2008.

McCormack L, Thomas V, Lewis MA, et al.: Improving low health literacy and patient engagement: A social ecological approach, *Patient Educ Couns* 100(1):8–13, Jan 2017. https://doi.org/10.1016/j.pec.2016.07.007. Epub 2016 Jul 4.

McLaughlin GH: SMOG grading—a new readability formula of reading, *Journal of Reading* 12(8):639–649, 1969.

McKinlay JB: Epidemiological and political determinants of social policies regarding the public health, *Soc Sci Med* 13A:541–558, 1979.

Meade CD: Producing videotapes for cancer education: methods and examples, *Oncol Nurs Forum* 23:837–846, 1996.

Meade CD, Calvo A: Developing community-academic partnerships to enhance breast health among rural and Hispanic migrant and seasonal farmworkers, *Oncol Nurs Forum* 28(10):1577–1584, 2001. PMID: 11759305.

Meade CD: Improving understanding of the informed consent process and document, *Semin Oncol Nurs* 15:124–137, 1999.

Meade CD, Rodriguez EM, Arevalo M, et al.: Introducing biospecimen science to communities: Tools from two cities, *Prog. Community Health Partnersh* 9 Special Issue 51–59, 2015.

Meade CD, Wells KJ, Arevalo M, et al.: Lay navigator model for impacting cancer health disparities, *J Cancer Educ Published online* 29(3):449–457, March 29, 2014. https://doi.org/10.1007/s13187-014-0640-z. PMID: 24683043; PMC4133280.

Meade CD, Smith CF: Readability formulas: cautions and criteria, *Patient Educ Couns* 17:153–158, 1991.

Meade CD, Menard J, Luque J: Creating community-academic partnerships for cancer disparities research and health promotion, *Health Promotion Practice* 12:456–462, 2011.

Meade CD, Calvo A, Rivera M: Focus groups in the design of prostate cancer screening information for Hispanic farmworkers and African American men, *Oncol Nursing Forum* 30:967–975, 2003.

Meade CD, Menard J, Martinez D, et al.: Impacting health disparities through community outreach: utilizing the CLEAN look (culture, literacy, education, assessment, networking), *Cancer Control* 14:70–77, 2007.

Meade CD, Menard J, Thervil C: Addressing cancer disparities through community engagement: improving breast health among Haitian women, *Oncol Nurs Forum* 36:716–722, 2009.

Meade CD, McKinney WP, Barnas G: Educating patients with limited literacy skills: the effectiveness of printed and videotaped materials about colon cancer, *Am J Public Health* 84:119–121, 1994.

Meleis AI: Culturally competent care, *J Transcult Nurs* 10:12, 1999.

Meppelink CS, van Weert JCM, Haven CJ, et al.: The Effectiveness of health animations in audiences with different health literacy levels: an experimental study, *J Med Internet Res* 17(1):e11, Jan 2015. https://doi.org/10.2196/jmir.3979. Published online 2015 Jan 13.

Miner AS, Milstein A, Schueller S, et al.: Smartphone-based conversational agents and responses to questions about mental health, interpersonal violence, and physical health, *JAMA Intern Med* 176(5):619–625, May 1, 2016. https://doi.org/10.1001/jamainternmed.2016.0400.

Minkler M, editor: *Community organizing and community building for health and welfare*, ed 3, Rutgers University Press, 2012.

McNaughton CD, Jacobson TA, Kripalani S: Low literacy is associated with uncontrolled blood pressure in primary care patients with hypertension and heart disease, *Patient Educ Couns* 96(2):165–170, 2014. http://doi.org/10.1016/j.pec.2014.05.007.

Moran MB, Frank LB, Chatterjee JS, et al.: A pilot test of the acceptability and efficacy of narrative and non-narrative health education materials in a low health literacy population, *J Commun Healthc* 9(1):40–48, 2016. Epub 2016 Feb 5.

Morris NS, MacLean CD, Chew LD: Single item literacy screener: evaluation of a brief instrument to identify limited reading ability, *BMC Fam Pract* 21, 2006.

Morrison AK, Schapira MM, Gorelick MH, et al.: Low caregiver health literacy is associated with higher pediatric emergency department use and nonurgent visits, *Acad Pediatr* 14(3):309–314, May-Jun 2014. https://doi.org/10.1016/j.acap.2014.01.004.

Moya EM, Chavez-Baray SM, Loweree J, et al.: Adults experiencing homelessness in the US–Mexico border region: a photovoice project, *Frontiers in Public Health* 5:113, 2017. https://doi.org/10.3389/fpubh.2017.00113.

The National Literacy Act of 1991: PL 102–173. [Go to http://eric.ed. gov/?id=ED341851, 1991. to download full-text document (28 pages)].

National Center for Education Statistics: *Technical report and data file user's manual for* 2003. National Assessment of Adult Literacy. NCES 2009476, August 11Available from http://nces.ed.gov/pubsearch/pubsinfo.asp?pubid=2009476 (2009).

Nielson-Bohlman L, Panzer A, Kindig D, editors: *Health literacy: a prescription to end confusion*, Washington, DC, 2014, National Academies Press.

Nightingale F: *Notes on nursing*, New York, 1859, Appleton-Century-Crofts.

Nguyen TH, Park H, Han HR, et al.: State of the science of health literacy measures: validity implications for minority populations, *Patient Educ Couns*, Jul 29, 2015 pii: S0738–3991(15)30021-5. https://doi.org/10.1016/j.pec.2015.07.013. [Epub ahead of print].

Norman C, Skinner HA: eHEALS: The eHealth Literacy Scale, *J Med Internet Res* 8(4):e27, 2006. https://doi.org/10.2196/jmir.8.4.e27.

Nutbeam D, McGill B, Premkumar P: Improving health literacy in community populations: a review of progress, *Health Promot Int*, Mar 28, 2017, https://doi.org/10.1093/heapro/dax015. [Epub ahead of print].

Nutbeam D: The evolving concept of health literacy, *Soc Sci Med* 67:2072–2078, 2008.

Nutbeam D: Defining and measuring health literacy: what can we learn from literacy studies? *Int J Public Health* 54(5):303–305, 2009.

Nyswander DB: Education for health: some principles and their application, *Health Educ Mono* 14:65–70, 1956.

Olshansky E, Sacco D, Braxter B, et al.: Participatory action research to understand and reduce health disparities, *Nurs Outlook* 53:121–126, 2005.

O'Mara B: Social media, digital video and health promotion in a culturally and linguistically diverse Australia, *Health Promot Int* 28(3):466–476, 2012.

Paasche-Orlow MK, Wolf MS: The causal pathways linking health literacy to health outcomes, *Am J Health Behav* 31(Suppl):S19–S26, 2007.

Paasche-Orlow MK, Wolf MS: Promoting health literacy research to reduce health disparities, *J Health Communication* 15(S2):34–41, 2010.

Padden DL, Connors RA, Posey SM, et al.: Factors influencing a health promoting lifestyle in spouses of active duty military, *Health Care Women Int* 34(8):674–693, 2013.

Padilla GV, Bulcavage LM: Theories used in patient/health education, *Semin Oncol Nurs* 7:87–96, 1991.

Parker EA, Israel BA, Williams M, et al.: Community action against asthma: examining the partnership process of a community-based participatory research project, *J Gen Intern Med* 18:558–567, 2003.

Parker RM, Baker DW, Williams MV, et al.: The test of functional health literacy in adults: a new instrument for measuring patients' literacy skills, *J Gen Intern Med* 10:537–541, 1995.

Pavlov IP: *Experimental psychology, and other essays*, New York, 1957, Philosophical Library.

Peerson A, Saunders M: Health literacy revisited: what do we mean and why does it matter? *Health Promot Int* 24:285–296, 2009.

Pender NJ, Murdaugh CL, Parsons MA: *Health promotion in nursing practice*, ed 6, Englewood Cliffs, NJ, 2010, Prentice Hall.

Pender NJ, Murdaugh C, Parsons MA, et al.: *Health promotion in nursing practice*, ed 7, Pearson, 2015.

Pew Research Center: Internet and Technology. Mobile Fact Sheets. Available http://www.pewinternet.org/fact-sheet/mobile/ Last updates January 2017.

Piaget J: *Adaptation and intelligence: organic selection and phenocopy*, Chicago, 1980, University of Chicago.

Prestin A, Vieux SN, Chou WY: Is online health activity alive and well or flatlining? findings from 10 years of the health information national trends survey, *J Health Commun* 20(7):790–798, 2015. https://doi.org/10.1080/10810730.2015.1018590. Epub 2015 Jun 4.

Prochaska JO, DiClemente CC: Stages and processes of self-change of smoking: toward an integrative model of change, *J Consult Clin Psychol* 51(3):390–395, 1983.

The Quad Council Practice Competencies for Public Health Nursing (PDF Download Available). fromhttps://www.researchgate.net/publication/260440165_The_Quad_Council_Practice_Competencies_for_Public_Health_Nursing [accessed Jul 3, 2017].

Quad Council of Public Health Organizations: *Core competencies for public health nurses*, Washington DC, 2011, Author.

Quinn G, Ellison BB, Meade C, et al.: Adapting smoking relapse-prevention materials for pregnant and postpartum women: formative research, *Matern Child Health J* 10:235–245, 2006.

Quinn GP, Sanchez JA, Sutton SK, et al.: Cancer and lesbian, gay, bisexual, transgender/transsexual, and queer/questioning populations (LGBTQ), *CA Cancer J Clin* 65(5):384–400, 2015. https://doi.org/10.3322/caac.21288.

Ramaswamy M, Lee J, Wickliffe J, et al.: Impact of a brief intervention on cervical health literacy: a waitlist control study with jailed women, *Prev Med Rep* 6:314–321, Apr 5, 2017. https://doi.org/10.1016/j.pmedr.2017.04.003. eCollection 2017 Jun.

Randall S, Crawford T, Currie J, et al.: Impact of community based nurse-led clinics on patient outcomes, patient satisfaction, patient access and cost effectiveness: A systematic review, *Int J Nurs Stud* 73:24–33, 2017, May 11. https://doi.org/10.1016/j.ijnurstu.2017.05.008. [Epub ahead of print].

Rankin SH, et al.: *Patient education in health and illness*, ed 5, Philadelphia, PA, 2005, Lippincott Williams and Wilkins. etc.

Rawl SM, Christy SM, Monahan PO, et al.: *Health Educ Res* 30(4):622–637, Aug 2015. https://doi.org/10.1093/her/cyv021. Epub 2015 May 28.

Rawl SM, Skinner CS, Perkins SM, et al.: Computer-delivered tailored intervention improves colon cancer screening knowledge and health beliefs of African Americans, *Health Educ Res* 5:868–885, 2012.

Rawl SM, Christy SM, Monahan PO, et al.: *Health Educ Res* 30(4):622–637, Aug 2015. https://doi.org/10.1093/her/cyv021. Epub 2015 May 28.

Rawl SM, Skinner CS, Perkins SM, et al.: Computer-delivered tailored intervention improves colon cancer screening knowledge and health beliefs of African Americans, *Health Educ Res* 5:868–885, 2012.

Redman BK: *The practice of patient education: a case study approach*, ed 10, St. Louis, 2007, Elsevier.

Ritchie CS, Houston TK, Richman JS, et al.: The E-Coach technology-assisted care transition system: a pragmatic randomized trial, *Transl Behav Med* 6(3):428–437, 2016. https://doi.org/10.1007/s13142-016-0422-8.

Robbins LB, Pfeiffer KA, Vermeesch A, et al.: "Girls on the move" intervention protocol for increasing physical activity among low-active underserved urban girls: a group randomized trial, *BMC Public Health* 13, 2013.

Robinson S, Moser D, Pelter MM: Assessing health literacy in heart failure patients, *J Card Fail* 17(11):887–892, 2011.

Roetzheim RG, Lee JH, Ferrante JM, et al.: Diagnostic resolution of cancer screening abnormalities at community health centers, *J Health Care Poor Underserved* 23:1280–1293, 2012. 2013.

Rogers CR: *A Carl Rogers reader*, Boston, 1989, Houghton Mifflin.

Roland D, Spurr J, Cabrera D: Preliminary evidence for the emergence of a health care online community of practice: using a netnographic framework for twitter hashtag analytics, *J Med Internet Res* 19(7):e252, Jul 14, 2017. https://doi.org/10.2196/jmir.7072.

Rosenstock I: Why people use health services, *Milbank Mem Fund Q* 44:94–127, 1966.

Rosenstock IM, Strecher VJ, Becker MH: Social learning theory and the health belief model, *Health Educ Q* 15(2):175–183, 1988.

Ross L, Johnson J, Smallwood SW, et al.: Using CBPR to extend prostate cancer education, counseling, and screening opportunities to urban-dwelling African-Americans, *Cancer Educ* 31(4):702–708, Dec 2016.

Rowlands G, Nutbeam D: Health literacy and the 'inverse information law', *Br J Gen Pract* 63(608):120–121, Mar 2013. https://doi.org/10.3399/bjgp13X664081. No abstract available. PMID:23561756.

Rudd RE: Needed action in health literacy, *J Health Psychol* 18(8):1004–1010, Aug 2013. Epub 2013 Jan 24.

Rue CB: *The public health nurse in the community*, Philadelphia, 1944, Saunders.

Schapira MM, Meade C, Nattinger AB: Enhanced decision-making: the use of a videotape decision-aid for patients with prostate cancer, *Patient Educ Couns* 30:119–127, 1997.

Schapira MM, Walker CM, Miller T, et al.: Development and validation of the numeracy understanding in Medicine Instrument short form, *J Health Commun* 19(Suppl 2):240–253, 2014. https://doi.org/10.1080/10810730.2014.933916. PMID:25315596.

Scheer CL, Nam K, Augusto B, et al.: *Assessment of a narrative intervention to promote genetic counseling for breast cancer survivors* (accepted).

Sehovic I, Gwede CK, Meade CD, et al.: A Web-based platform for educating researchers about bioethics and biobanking, *J Cancer Educ* 31(2):397–404, Jun 2016. PMID: 25773136. PMCID: PMC4573774.

Siegel RL, Fedewa SA, Miller KD, et al.: Cancer statistics for Hispanics/Latinos, 2015, *CA Cancer J Clin* 65(6):457–480, Nov-Dec 2015. https://doi.org/10.3322/caac.21314. Epub 2015 Sep 16.

Simmons VN, Quinn G, Litvin EB, et al.: Transcreation of validated smoking relapse-prevention booklets for use with Hispanic populations, *J Health Care Poor Underserved* 22:886–893, 2011.

Simmons VN, Fleming K, Koskan AM, et al.: Participatory evaluation of a community-academic partnership to inform capacity-building and sustainability, *Eval Program Plann* 52:19–26, 2015. https://doi.org/10.1016/jevalprogplan.2015.03.005. [Epub ahead of print]. PMID:25863014; PMC4509815.

Skinner BF: About Behaviorism. In *Vintage Books*, New York, 1976, Random House.

Smigelsky MA, Neimeyer RA, Murphy V, et al.: Performing the peace: using playback theatre in the strengthening of police-community relations, *Prog Community Health Partnersh* 10(4):533–539, 2016. https://doi.org/10.1353/cpr.2016.0061.

Smokefree.gov. U.S. Department of Health and Human Services Available from: https://smokefree.gov/

Snow CE, Dibner KA, editors: *Science literacy: concepts, contexts, and consequences. committee on science literacy and public perception of science; board on science education; division of behavioral and social sciences and education; national academies of sciences, engineering, and medicine*, Washington (DC), 2016 Oct, National Academies Press (US).

So J, Prestin A, Lee L, et al.: What do people like to "Share" about obesity? A content analysis of frequent retweets about obesity on twitter, *J Health Commun* 31(2):193–206, 2016. https://doi.org/10.1080/10410236.2014.940675. Epub 2015 Jun 18.

Soto Mas F, Ji M, Fuentes BO, et al.: The health literacy and ESL study: a community-based intervention for Spanish-speaking adults, *J Health Commun* 20(4):369–376, Apr 2015. https://doi.org/10.1080/10810730.2014.965368. Epub 2015 Jan 20.

Stewart DW, et al.: "Health literacy, smoking, and health indicators in African American adults.", *J Health Commun* 20(0 2):24–33, 2015. PMC. Web. 16 July 2017.

Stewart DW, Adams CE, Cano MA, et al.: Associations between health literacy and established predictors of smoking cessation, *Am J Public Health (2013)*, May 16, 2015. [Epub ahead of print].

Strasser SM, Smith M, Pendrick-Denney D: Feasibility study of social media to reduce intimate partner violence among gay men in metro Atlanta, *Georgia. West J Emerg Med* 13(3):298–304, 2012.

Strecher VJ, DeVellis BM, Becker MH: The role of self-efficacy in achieving health behavior change, *Health Educ Q* 13:73–92, 1986.

Sullivan PS, Driggers R, Stekler JD, et al.: Usability and acceptability of a mobile comprehensive HIV prevention app for men who have sex with men: a pilot study. Eysenbach G, ed, *JMIR mHealth and uHealth* 5(3):e26, 2017. https://doi.org/10.2196/mhealth.7199.

Sykes S, Wills J, Rowlands G, et al.: Understanding critical health literacy: a concept analysis, *BMC Public Health* 13:150, 2013.

Teitelman AM, Jemmott AM, Bellamy SL, et al.: Partner violence, power and gender differences in South African adolescents' HIV/STI behaviors, *Health Psychol* 35(7):751–760, 2016. https://doi.org/10.1037/hea0000351.

Thorndike EL: *Educational psychology*, New York, 1969, Arno Press.

Thurman W, Pfitzinger-Lippe M: Returning to the profession's roots: social justice in nursing education for the 21st Century, *ANS Adv Nurs Sci* 40(2):184–193, Apr/Jun 2017. https://doi.org/10.1097/ANS.0000000000000140.

Tiraki Z, Yılmaz M: Cervical cancer knowledge, self-efficacy, and health literacy levels of married women, *J Cancer Educ*, Jul 1, 2017. https://doi.org/10.1007/s13187-017-1242-3. [Epub ahead of print].

U.S. Department of Health and Human Services: *Making health communication programs work: a planner's guide, pink book*, Bethesda, MD, 2008, Office of Cancer Communications, National Cancer Institute. Available from https://www.cancer.gov/publications/health-communication/pink-book.pdf.

U.S. Department of Health and Human Services: *National action plan to improve health literacy*. Available from: https://health.gov/communication/hlactionplan/pdf/Health_Literacy_Action_Plan.pdf (direct link)

U.S. Department of Health and Human Services, Centers for Disease Control and Prevention, National Center for Chronic Disease Prevention and Health Promotion: *The health consequences of smoking: a report of the Surgeon General*. Office on Smoking and Health: Atlanta.U.S. Department of Health and Human Services, Public Health Services: Healthy People 2020, n.d. Available from https://www.healthypeople.gov/2020/default.aspx.

U.S. Department of Health and Human Services, Public Health Services, Office of Minority Health (OMH): *The national standards for culturally and linguistically appropriate services in health and health care (The National CLAS Standards)* https://minorityhealth.hhs.gov/omh/browse.aspx?lvl=2&lvlid=53

U.S. Department of Health and Human Services, Public Health Services, Office of Minority Health (OMH): *Enhanced national culturally and linguistically appropriate services (CLAS) standards*. Available from https://www.thinkculturalhealth.hhs.gov/clas/standards

view The Blueprint and National CLAS Standards https://www. thinkculturalhealth.hhs.gov/assets/pdfs/EnhancedCLASStandards Blueprint.pdf U.S. Department of Health and Human Services, Public Health Services, Tobacco use and Pregnancy. Available from https://www.cdc.gov/reproductivehealth/maternalinfanthealth/ tobaccousepregnancy/index.htm

Vadaparampil ST, Simmons VN, Lee JH, et al.: Journal clubs: an educational approach to advance understanding about CBPR and cancer health disparities, *J Cancer Educ* 29(1):122–128, Mar 2014. PMID 24078328.

Van Wyk NC: Health education as education of the oppressed, *Curationis* 22:29–34, 1999.

Waite KR, Paasche-Orlow M, Rintamaki LS, et al.: Literacy, social stigma, and HIV medication adherence, *J Gen Intern Med* 23:1367–1372, 2008. 9: 503–516, 2013.

Wallace LS, Rogers ES, Roskos SE, et al.: Brief report: screening items to identify patients with limited health literacy skills, *J Gen Intern Med* 21:874–877, 2006.

Wallerstein N, Bernstein E: Empowerment education: freire's ideas adapted to health education, *Health Educ Q* 15:379–394, 1988.

Wallerstein N, Minkler M, Carter-Edwards L, et al.: Improving health through community engagement, community organization and co.etmmunity building. In Glanz K, Rimer BK, Visnawath K, editors: *Health behavior: theory, research, & practice*, ed 5, San Francisco, 2015, Jossey-Bass, pp 277–300.

Weiss BD, Mays MZ, Martz W, et al.: Quick assessment of literacy in primary care: the newest vital sign, *Ann Fam Med* 3:514–522, 2005.

Wells KJ, Otero CV, Bredice M, et al.: Acceptability of a virtual patient educator for Hispanic women, *Hispanic Health Care International* 13(4):179–185, 2015. https://doi.org/10.1891/1540-4153.13.4.179.

Wells KJ, Meade CD, Calcano E: Innovative approaches to reducing cancer health disparities: the Moffitt Cancer Center patient Navigator research program, *J Cancer Edu* 26(4):649–657, Dec 2011.

Wells KJ, Quinn GP, Meade CD, et al.: Development of a cancer clinical trials multi-media intervention: clinical trials: are they right for you? *Patient Education and Counseling* 88(2):232–240, 2012.

Wertheimer M: *Productive thinking*, New York, 1959, Harper.

Wilkinson GS, Robertson GJ: *Wide range achievement test 4 professional manual*, Lutz, FL, 2006, Psychological Assessment Resources.

Wolf MS, Williams MV, Parker RM, et al.: Patients' shame and attitudes toward discussing the results of literacy screening, *J Health Commun* 12:721–732, 2007.

World Health Organization Commission on the Social Determinants of Health: *Achieving health equity: from root causes to fair outcomes*. World Health Organization: http://apps.who.int/iris/bitstream/10665/69670/1/interim_statement_eng.pdf

Zhang H, Jiang Y, Nguyen HD, et al.: The effect of a smartphone-based coronary heart disease prevention (SBCHDP) programme on awareness and knowledge of CHD, stress, and cardiac-related lifestyle behaviours among the working population in Singapore: a pilot randomised controlled trial, *Health and Quality of Life Outcomes* 15:49, 2017. https://doi.org/10.1186/s12955-017-0623-y.

Young H, Miyamoto S, Ward D, et al.: Sustained effects of a nurse coaching intervention via telehealth to improve health behavior change in diabetes, *Telemed J E Health* 20(9):828–834, 2014. https://doi.org/10.1089/tmj.2013.0326.

Zehbe I, Wood B, Wakewich P, et al.: on behalf of ACCSS group. Teaching tools to engage Anishinaabek First Nations women in cervical cancer screening: report of an educational workshop, *Health Edu J* 75(3):331–342, 2016. https://doi.org/10.1177/0017896915580446.

Case Management

Karyn Leavitt Grow and Jean Cozad Lyon

OBJECTIVES

Upon completion of this chapter, the reader will be able to do the following:

1. Define case management, care management, and care coordination and compare the differences.
2. Discuss the philosophy and guiding principles of case management.
3. Identify the origin and purpose of case management.
4. Identify the case management process.
5. Discuss the roles and characteristics of case management in a reformed health care environment.
6. Incorporate case management concepts into clinical practice settings.
7. Identify educational preparation and skills recommended for case managers.

KEY TERMS

care management
case management
chronic care management

transitional care management
continuum of care

patient-centered medical home
utilization review

OVERVIEW OF CASE MANAGEMENT

Case management is a term that describes a wide variety of patient care coordination programs in acute hospital and community settings. Case management is also referred to as *care management* and *care coordination*. These terms apply to community health settings that include patient-centered medical homes (PCMHs), occupational health, geriatric services, ambulatory care clinics, mental health settings, and outpatient primary care settings. Patient populations of all ages receive case management services.

159

Since the late 1980s and the 1990s, a variety of case management programs have emerged (Huber, 2002). From 1990 to 2005, case management evolved rapidly in response to changes in the health care environment and an increase in the number of managed care programs. Client service use reflects a greater emphasis on health care costs. Third-party payers evaluate the appropriate use of health care resources such as diagnostic tests, laboratory tests, length of hospital visits, and duration of home health care services. Health care providers, interested in close monitoring of resources, introduced various forms of case management programs.

More recently, health care evolved from a quantity-driven delivery system to a quality-driven system. In 2001, the National Academy of Medicine (NAM), formerly called the Institute of Medicine (IOM) published a report, *Crossing the Quality Chasm*. It recommended a redesign of the health care system to provide care that is safe, efficient, effective, timely, equitable, and patient centered. The report names care coordination as an essential function to reach these goals and improve health care quality (IOM, 2001). The Institute for Healthcare Improvement's Triple Aim Initiative is a framework of goals to optimize health system performance. The framework includes improving the patient experience, improving the health of populations, and reducing the per capita cost of health care.

Case management has emerged as an intervention strategy for quality improvement initiatives. A single definition of case management does not exist. The Case Management Society of America (CMSA) (2016) offers the following definition of case management:

Case management is a collaborative process of assessment, planning, facilitation, care coordination, evaluation and advocacy for options and services to meet an individual's and family's comprehensive health care needs through communication and available resources to promote patient safety, quality of care and cost effective outcomes. (p. 11)

The philosophy statement published by CMSA (2016) reads as follows:

Some hospitals, health maintenance organizations (HMOs), and other insurance companies inaccurately use the term case management to describe "utilization management," "managed care," or the method of monitoring and controlling service use within a system or care episode to control cost.

Case management programs, however, aim to provide a service delivery approach to ensure the following: cost-effective care, alternatives to institutionalization, access to care, coordinated services, and patient's improved functional capacity (Lyon, 1993) (Box 9.1). These goals apply to community health and acute care settings. Subsets of case management are care management, care coordination, and transitional care management (TCM).

Care Management

Care management consists of programs that apply systems, science, incentives, and information to improve medical practice and to allow clients and their support systems to participate in a

---

> **BOX 9.1   Possible Case Management Functions**
>
> - Identifying the target population
> - Determining screening and eligibility
> - Arranging services
> - Monitoring and follow-up
> - Assessing
> - Planning care
> - Reassessing
> - Assisting clients through a complex, fragmented health care system
> - Providing care coordination and continuity

---

collaborative process with a goal of improving medical, psychosocial, and behavioral health conditions more effectively. Care management is a concept that is evidence based, patient centered, and clinical care focused.

The overall goal of care management is to improve the coordination of services provided to clients who are enrolled in a care management program. Examples of groups of people who may be served by care management services are the elderly, children from low-income families who receive Medicaid services, and groups of people with chronic illnesses.

Care Coordination

Care coordination was identified in the NAM report *Crossing the Quality Chasm* as an essential function in improving health quality (IOM, 2001). It has also been recognized as an approach to integrate fragmented health care, improve the transitions of care between providers, and decrease the unnecessary utilization of resources and costs. Care coordination programs are those that target chronically ill persons at risk for adverse outcomes and expensive care and that meet their needs by filling the gaps in health care. They (1) identify the full range of medical, functional, social, and emotional problems that increase patients' risk of adverse health events; (2) address those needs through education in self-care, optimization of medical treatment, and integration of care fragmented by setting or provider; and (3) monitor patients for progress and early signs of problems. Such programs hold the promise of raising the quality of health care, improving health outcomes, and reducing the need for costly hospitalizations and medical care (Chen et al., 2000).

There are many definitions of care coordination. In its 2005 report *Closing the Quality Gap: A Critical Analysis of Quality Improvement Strategies, Volume 7: Care Coordination*, the Agency for Health Care Research and Quality (AHRQ) defines *care coordination* as:

The deliberate organization of patient care activities between two or more participants (including the patient) involved in a patient's care to facilitate the appropriate delivery of health care services. Organizing care involves the marshaling of personnel and other resources needed to carry out all required patient care activities, and is often managed by the exchange of information among participants responsible for different aspects of care. Care coordination is a process component and function of case management.

McDonald et al., 2005

And in the American Nurses Association (ANA) white paper titled *The Value of Nursing Care Coordination,* the term *care coordination* is defined as follows:

> *Care coordination is (a) a function that helps ensure that the patient's needs and preferences are met over time with respect to health services and information sharing across people, functions, and sites; and (b) the deliberate organization of patient care activities between two or more participants (including the patient) involved in a patient's care to facilitate the appropriate delivery of health care services. Additionally, the best coordination model is one in which a patient experiences primary care as delivered by an integrated, multidisciplinary team that explicitly includes at least one staff care coordinator.*

ANA, 2012

Transitional Care Management

Transitional care management (TCM) is the process of providing a postdischarge patient with a high or moderate risk of readmission a face-to-face visit with their practitioner within a defined period (7 to 14 days) and care coordination services to prevent readmissions and improve outcomes. The TCM care coordinator follows a patient posthospitalization to improve patient/caregiver understanding and self-management of new disease processes, discharge instructions, medication management, coordination of care and resources, and timely access and follow-up with the patient's primary care provider (DHHS and CMS, 2016).

The paper *Transitions of Care Measures* by the National Transition of Care Coalition (NTOCC, 2008) defines TCM as:

> *A set of actions designed to ensure coordination and continuity. They should be based on a comprehensive care plan and the availability of well-trained practitioners who have current information about the patient's treatment goals, preferences, and health or clinical status. They include logistical arrangements and education of patient and family, as well as coordination among the health professionals involved in the transition.*

In effect, transitions of care are a subpart of the broader concept of care coordination.

ORIGINS OF CASE MANAGEMENT

Case management has a long history with the mentally ill, elderly patients, and the community setting (Steinberg and Carter, 1983). Public health, mental health, and long-term care settings have implemented and studied case management services and have reported them in their literature for many years (Mahn and Spross, 1996; Weil and Karls, 1985).

Public Health

Community service coordination, which was a forerunner of case management, appeared in public health programs in the early 1900s. During this time, health care providers reported these community service and case management programs in the nursing literature. Programs focused on community education in sanitation, nutrition, and disease prevention became prevalent. Lillian Wald and Mary Brewster conducted many of these programs at the Henry Street Settlement House in New York City. The Metropolitan Life Insurance Company later expanded nursing services for individuals, families, and the community to include disease prevention and health promotion (Conger, 1999).

The concept of **continuum of care** originated after World War II to describe the long-term services required for discharged psychiatric patients (Grau, 1984). Service coordination evolved into case management, a term that first appeared in social welfare literature during the early 1970s.

Case Management in Behavioral Health

During the late 1960s and early 1970s, mental health care emphasized moving patients from mental health institutions back into the community (Crosby, 1987; Pittman, 1989). The Community Mental Health Center Act of 1963 placed federal approbation on deinstitutionalization, which emphasized the importance of community mental health services. Mental health providers began to move patients from large state institutions to the community.

Several problems resulted from the deinstitutionalization of mentally ill patients. In 1977, Congress acknowledged that many disabled people had been deinstitutionalized without basic needs, proper follow-up, or health care monitoring. Congress further recognized that a systematic approach to service delivery could have prevented many state hospital readmissions. Case management in community mental health helped avoid client service fragmentation (Pittman, 1989).

Care Management Tracking System (CMTS)

CMTS was developed to ensure that all patients are followed, that none are lost to follow-up, and that any patients who are not improving are identified and further interventions are initiated. These systems are often integrated into the electronic health record, or other organizations and clinics use a patient-tracking spreadsheet (University of Washington, 2017).

Case Management and the Elderly

Specific elderly services recognized that age-generic programs do not adequately assist older people. Many older people have special, population-specific health care needs. Thus case management services frequently target the elderly population, specifically homebound individuals or those with complex problems. However, not all older people who subscribe to multiple services require a case manager. Older adults may not need a case manager if they possess adequate functional status and can coordinate and access services for themselves, if they have family support, or if they have formal or informal caregivers who provide these functions for them.

Disease-Specific Case Management

Case management services are often provided for individuals who are identified as having medical conditions that are high-cost or high-volume acute and chronic illnesses. Examples are chronic obstructive pulmonary disease and chronic cardiac conditions such as congestive heart failure. The goal of disease-specific case management is to keep the individuals as healthy as possible and stable in their home environments. One particular goal is to decrease the frequency and length of hospital stays and consequently reduce health care costs.

PURPOSE OF CASE MANAGEMENT

Case management, care management, and care coordination are patient-centered and system-centered processes. Patient-centered case management improves self-management of chronic disease; helps the client or patient proceed through a complex, fragmented, and often confusing health care delivery system; and achieves specific client-centered goals. System-centered processes recognize that health care resources are finite. The upward spiral in health care costs leads third-party payers such as Medicare, managed care organizations, and commercial payers to demand cost-effective health care. Providers are reimbursed for care provided on the basis of value-based purchasing; this includes hospitals, skilled-nursing facilities, home health organizations, and practitioners. Client consumers insist on cost-effective, efficient, high-quality care. This demand forces health care providers to reevaluate the way they administer care, to emphasize quality improvement, and to focus on decreasing cost. Health care resources then become allocated to those populations with the greatest needs.

Case management is used to promote and integrate the coordination of clinical services, linking patients to community services and agencies. Case managers monitor resources used by clients, support collaborative practice and continuity of care, and enhance patient satisfaction (Yamamoto and Lucey, 2005).

Care Management

Care management has emerged as a primary means of managing the health of a defined population. The purpose of care management is to reduce health risks and cost of care for a defined population (AHRQ, 2015).

In the "Care Management Issue Brief: Implications for Medical Practice, Health Policy and Health Services Research," AHRQ highlights three key strategies to enhance care management for target populations:

(1) Identify population(s) with modifiable risks; (2) Align CM services to the needs of the population(s); and (3) Identify, prepare, and integrate appropriate personnel to deliver the needed services.

Care Coordination

Care coordination is an emerging process. It encompasses collaborating with the patient to develop a plan of care and patient-centered goals, working to develop improved chronic disease self-management skills, and providing coordination of services. AHRQ defines care coordination as

the deliberate organization of patient care activities between two or more participants (including the patient) involved in a patient's care to facilitate the appropriate delivery of health care

services. Organizing care involves the marshalling of personnel and other resources needed to carry out all required patient care activities, and is often managed by the exchange of information among participants responsible for different aspects of care.

McDonald, 2005

Utilization Review and Managed Care

Equity and cost effectiveness require management and allocation of available resources in a hospital, community, city, state, or particular health care client population. Utilization review (UR), as defined by CMSA, consists of the evaluation of medical appropriateness or medical necessity of care. This review ensures that patients receive the "right care at the right time" to improve clinical outcomes and lower costs (Stricker, n.d.).

Case management programs are often motivated by the need to evaluate, use, and allocate health care resources. Many case management programs evolved from UR departments. These departments showed that monitoring service use alone is insufficient for managing patient populations with diverse resource needs. Over time, the UR nurses assumed the additional case manager responsibilities.

ETHICAL INSIGHTS
Ethical Issues in Case Management

There are several ethical issues that a case manager should take into consideration when working with populations. Examples are as follows:

1. Right to privacy. Confidentiality of clients served must be maintained. Communicating patient information to others who are involved with the client's care must be done only with the client's knowledge and permission.
2. Health care resources are expensive and limited. The case manager must use appropriate, reliable, and accessible resources for individual clients or groups of clients with the same identified needs.
3. Respect for the client's rights to be informed about his or her care and services and to choose to receive services or not.
4. Clients have the right to know what resources are available to them and have the right to select providers of the resources.

TRENDS THAT INFLUENCE CASE MANAGEMENT

Numerous trends have influenced case management programs. During the 1970s, hospitals billed Medicare, Medicaid, and other third-party payers for client services and received reimbursement. Health care costs skyrocketed and rapidly became the basis for discussion and concern throughout the health care industry and the country. In 1983, PL 98-21 of the Social Security Amendments introduced the prospective payment system (PPS) in the acute care setting. Under the PPS, health care providers receive a fixed amount of money based on the relative cost of resources they use to treat Medicare patients within each diagnosis-related group. Other third-party payers followed this example and negotiated reimbursement schedules through preferred provider programs or managed care contracts (U.S. Department of Commerce, 1990).

Changes in Health Care Reimbursement

Title III of the Patient Protection and Affordable Care Act (Public Law 111-148), passed by Congress in March 2010, includes provisions that require improvement in the quality and efficiency of health care. The Centers for Medicare and Medicaid (CMS) have established value-based purchasing programs for hospitals, postacute providers, and practitioners. These programs link Medicare payments to quality performance, utilization of evidence-based practices, cost of care, and patient experience scores (CMS.gov 2017). Providers who participate and exceed in their relative scoring will be eligible for incentive payments; additionally, there are financial penalties for nonparticipating providers (Public Law 111-148, 2010).

To assist practitioners with success in the value-based reimbursement structure, CMS provides reimbursement for chronic care management programs and transitions of care programs.

Access to Health Care for More Americans

The Patient Protection and Affordable Care Act removes many barriers to health care for Americans. With insurance coverage available to people through employers or purchased through health care access networks, more Americans have insurance and have access to health care. These changes opened up opportunities for nurses working in case manager or care coordination roles. Case managers have developed and expanded their roles in working with diverse patient populations. These issues have influenced, and continue to influence, the expansion of case management services to control costs and distribute health care resources in a variety of settings.

EDUCATION AND PREPARATION FOR CASE MANAGERS

It is essential to determine what classification of health care provider is best qualified to provide case management services. Traditionally, case managers were social workers (SWs) who assumed the role of discharge planner. Client health care needs have become more complex, the need for ongoing patient assessment has emerged, and available resources have become more numerous and diverse; therefore nurses have become case managers. Several health care organizations exclusively employ SWs in case manager roles, others exclusively employ nurses in case management, and others use a combination of SWs and nurses, depending on the client population's needs. Combining the strength and knowledge of the nurse's clinical background with the SW's community service background can efficiently move a client through the complex health care system (Lyon et al., 1995).

Nurse Case Managers

Although both nurses and SWs have proved themselves to be excellent case managers, this chapter focuses on the nurse case manager in discussing educational requirements. A nurse case manager's optimum education level is debatable. The basic nursing education for case managers required by employers can vary. Some require a baccalaureate degree, and others do not. In some settings, a master's degree is required. Some programs are more interested in prior experience, continuing education, and case management certification than in the entry-level nursing degree. Education and experience requirements may vary, depending on the program's geographic location, specific client needs, and available staff.

Nurses with master's degrees and a focus in case management are readily available in urban settings. This gives facilities the opportunity to hire case managers who are academically prepared in theory and clinical experience. Rural areas that do not have master's-level academic programs are at a great disadvantage in recruiting and hiring qualified nurses. To fill the case manager role, rural facilities promote nurses to case management positions, provide them with continuing education programs, and offer them necessary job-related experience. Although this is not the ideal solution, it is often the only option for facilities that are smaller or in more remote parts of the United States.

Regardless of the educational requirements in the individual case management program, case managers need a minimum skill level to ensure success in the role. These skills include sound knowledge of reimbursement structures; knowledge of available resources within the institution, organization, or community; working knowledge of the identification and evaluation of quality outcomes; the ability to perform cost–benefit ratios; and an understanding of financial strategies. In addition to the required knowledge, the nurse case manager needs flexibility, creativity, excellent communication skills, and the ability to work autonomously.

Case Manager Certification Options

There are two options for case managers to become certified. The certifications are offered by the CMSA and by the American Nurses Credentialing Center (ANCC).

Commission for Case Manager Certification

The Commission for Case Manager Certification offers certification in case management. The certification granted is the Certified Case Manager (CCM) credential. Following are the requirements for applicants (Commission for Case Manager Certification, 2013):

- Licensed health care worker or a bachelor's degree in a health or human services field
- Twelve months experience supervised by a CCM, or 24 months as a full-time case manager, or 12 months as a supervisor of individuals who provide case management

American Nurses Credentialing Center

The ANCC offers certification in nursing case management. To be eligible to take the certification examination, applicants must:

- Hold a current, active registered nurse (RN) license within a state or territory of the United States or the professional, legally recognized equivalent in another country
- Have practiced the equivalent of 2 years full time as an RN

- Have a minimum of 2000 hours of clinical practice in case management nursing within the last 3 years
- Have completed 30 hours of continuing education in case management nursing within the last 3 years

Other Certifications. Several other certifications in specialty case management are available: disability management, health care quality, utilization management, managed care, and case management administrator certification. Case management professionals who are interested in obtaining certification should carefully research the options available for certification and should select the credentialing program that fits their work performed, education, and future career goals (CMSA, 2006).

CASE MANAGER SERVICES

Although case management programs differ in structure and design, case managers provide services regardless of the program's location. There is a consensus in the literature that there are six components to case management: client identification and engagement, assessment, care plan development, implementation and coordination of plan of care, monitoring and evaluation, and closure of professional services (CMSA, 2016). The focus of each of these functions varies depending on the case management model.

Examples of care coordination include assisting the client or family member with medical appointments, equipment acquisition, home meal delivery, home follow-up services (e.g., home health or public health nursing), appointment transportation, and medical insurance or Medicare form completion. The types of services differ depending on the location of the case management program, the population of clients, and the scope of case management services. Some case managers in managed care environments monitor whether the patient keeps medical appointments and follows the prescribed course of treatment.

Depending on the setting, community case management services continue for varying lengths of time. Some programs continue service coordination indefinitely for populations such as the high-risk elderly and the chronically ill. Other programs move clients' case management status from active to inactive when patients no longer require services. However, the status becomes active again if their conditions change. Case management services continue in the home health care setting until the client is discharged from the program. Care coordination in the primary health care delivery setting is increasingly being provided in PCMHs and primary care clinics. It is widely recognized that early intervention on the part of a case manager and appropriate referrals prevent costly complications and can result in better health outcomes (Thurkettle and Noji, 2003).

CASE MANAGER ROLES AND CHARACTERISTICS

The individual case manager's role will vary depending on the specific program's services. The role functions of case managers are defined by the CMSA as including assessment, planning, facilitation, coordination, monitoring, evaluation, and advocacy, achieved through collaboration with the client and others involved in the client's care (CMSA, 2016).

The ANCC (2009) describes the practice of a nurse case manager as follows:

Nurse case managers actively participate with their clients to identify and facilitate options and services, providing and coordinating comprehensive care to meet patient/client health needs, with the goal of decreasing fragmentation and duplication of care, and enhancing quality, cost-effective clinical outcomes. Nursing case management is a dynamic and systematic collaborative approach to provide and coordinate health care services to a defined population. Nurse case managers continually evaluate each individual's health plan and specific challenges and then seek to overcome obstacles that affect outcomes. A nurse case manager uses a framework that includes interaction, assessment, planning, implementation, and evaluation. Outcomes are evaluated to determine if additional actions such as reassessment or revision to a plan of care are required to meet clients' health needs. To facilitate patient outcomes, the nurse case manager may fulfill the roles of advocate, collaborator, facilitator, risk manager, educator, mentor, liaison, negotiator, consultant, coordinator, evaluator, and/or researcher.

Nurse case managers must be flexible. The health care environment experiences rapid change, and new regulations and reimbursement schedules frequently emerge. The health care provider must respond to these changes rapidly to remain competitive. It is an ideal job for the self-directed nurse who enjoys being involved in a larger health care team within the organization and in the larger community. CMSA (2016) defines the standards of case management practice (Box 9.2).

CASE IDENTIFICATION

Identification of case management clients occurs in many ways, and each program should determine the criteria for eligibility for case management services. These criteria depend on the services provided, the service's location, the population served, and whether the service is in an acute care or community setting. Some programs are diagnosis based and use many community health care resources; for example, clients with chronic obstructive pulmonary disease often require numerous hospitalizations. Programs may focus on a particular population (e.g., the elderly or chronically ill with a specific chronic condition) and establish criteria to identify which clients to target for services (e.g., the high-risk elderly who are chronically ill, recently discharged from a hospital setting, and would benefit from case management services).

All clients referred for case management must undergo screening to determine their appropriateness for inclusion in the program. Not all referred clients need the services of a nurse case manager. Often, a nurse can arrange community services or instruct the client and family in the most appropriate follow-up based on client need and program design. The screening

BOX 9.2 CMSA Standards of Case Management Practice

Client Selection Process for Case Management demonstrated by consistent use of high-risk screening criteria

Client Assessment using standard tools to assess health history; cognition; spiritual, cultural, and support systems; resources; and other components

Care Needs and Opportunities Identification that would benefit from case management intervention

Planning the identification of short-term, long-term, and ongoing needs and strategies to address those needs

Monitoring the ongoing assessment and documentation to measure the client's response to the plan of care

Outcomes demonstrating the efficacy, quality, and cost effectiveness of the case manager's intervention

Closure of Professional Case Management Services once established case-closure guidelines are met

Facilitation, Coordination, and Collaboration between the client and other stakeholders to achieve goals and maximize positive client outcomes

Qualifications for Case Managers, which are maintaining unrestricted licenses and certifications or involve a bachelor's or higher health degree from a nationally accredited school

Legal adherence to all local, state, and federal laws, as well as employer policies and practice

Confidentiality and Client Privacy, including consent for case management services

Ethical Behavior, including the five basic ethical principles—beneficence, nonmalfeasance, autonomy, justice, and fidelity

Advocacy for the client at the service delivery, benefits administration, and policy-making levels

Cultural Competency of the client's cultural and demographic diversity

Resource Management and Stewardship of the health care and financial resources for effective and efficient utilization

Professional Responsibilities and Scholarship to maintain current knowledge, competencies, and evidence-supported innovations

instrument must be comprehensive enough to determine which clients meet the program's criteria and user friendly enough to allow the screener to evaluate the clients rapidly to determine their appropriateness for the program. The screener should refer clients to more suitable services within the community if they are not appropriate candidates for a particular case management program.

THE REFERRAL PROCESS

The nurse may perform program referrals in a variety of ways. In the acute care hospital setting, referrals are usually based on patient diagnosis, extended length of stay, or rehospitalization. Internal mechanisms alert the case manager of the patient's admission (e.g., a computerized list). Patients are also screened at discharge for risk of readmission and referred to the TCM case manager as appropriate.

A variety of tools are used to identify people who would benefit from case management services. They include health-risk screening tools; evidence-based criteria; risk stratification through data management; and referrals from hospitals, health care providers, and families. Information is collected by the

case manager and analyzed to determine whether the individual being referred is a candidate for case management services (CMSA, 2005).

In community settings, referrals originate from a variety of sources, such as a client's family, a primary care provider, and a hospital case manager. These referrals may be written or verbal. Staff in community agencies can also make service referrals; for example, the American Heart Association or American Cancer Society may receive calls from clients and families requesting information and assistance.

APPLICATION OF CASE MANAGEMENT IN COMMUNITY HEALTH

Case management can be used in all community health settings, with interventions at the primary, secondary, and tertiary levels of prevention, according to the community program and population served. Nurses working as case managers in the community setting have diverse roles and responsibilities.

Primary Care
Chronic Care Management

The CMS have recently developed criteria and reimbursement for **chronic care management** (CCM) and TCM in the primary care setting. Patients are referred to the CCM program by a practitioner who has identified the patient as having two or more chronic conditions that put the patient at a high risk of functional decline or death within the next 12 months (CMS.gov, 2016). Care coordinators work with patients and their caregivers to improve self-management of the disease process via support and education and coordinate care to empower patients to access care appropriately and efficiently.

Transitional Care Management

TCM patients are referred by practitioners or hospital staff for follow-up face-to-face visits with the outpatient practitioner and care coordination services for 30 days post-discharge. Patients are educated about new medications, condition-specific processes, and discharge instructions. As mentioned, care is coordinated for the patient, including a follow-up face-to-face visit with a practitioner. The goal of this program is to improve patient outcomes, increase understanding of condition-specific issues, and decrease hospital readmissions (DHHS and CMS, 2016).

Patient-Centered Medical Home

The **patient-centered medical home** (PCMH) is a recent model of care developed to provide collaborative, quality-driven, safe primary care. The PCMH utilizes care coordination and case management processes to provide comprehensive, patient-centered, cost-effective, high-quality care (Henderson et al., 2012). In 2007, the report *Joint Principles of the Patient-Centered Medical Home,* sponsored by four medical professional organizations, described the seven principles or characteristics of the PCMH, which are listed in Box 9.3 (Patient-Centered Primary Care Collaborative, 2007).

BOX 9.3   Principles of a Patient-Centered Medical Home

The patient-centered medical home has the following seven characteristics:

- The patient's relationship with the primary care physician
- The physician-led, team-based care
- The patient as a "whole person" who requires comprehensive care at various stages of life
- Integration and coordination of care
- Quality and safety
- Improved access to care
- A payment system that accurately reflects the efforts and care provided by the team

PCMHs are a care delivery model that utilizes the care coordination process as a foundational principle. The five key functions of the PCMH are care that is comprehensive, patient centered, coordinated, accessible, and safe (AHRQ, 2017).

The American Academy of Family Physicians (AAFP, 2008) defines the PCMH as follows:

Transition away from a model of symptom and illness based episodic care to a system of comprehensive coordinated primary care for children, youth and adults. Patient centeredness refers to an ongoing, active partnership with a personal primary care physician who leads a team of professionals dedicated to providing proactive, preventive and chronic care management through all stages of life. These personal physicians are responsible for the patient's coordination of care across all health care systems facilitated by registries, information technology, health information exchanges, and other means to ensure patients receive care when and where they need it. With a commitment to continuous quality improvement, care teams utilize evidence-based medicine and clinical decision support tools that guide decision making as well as ensure that patients and their families have the education and support to actively participate in their own care. Payment appropriately recognizes and incorporates the value of the care teams, non-direct patient care, and quality improvement provided in a patient-centered medical home.

High-Risk Clinic Settings

There are many examples of health care settings that provide services to high-risk clients in which the nurse serves as case manager. A few examples are diabetic clinics, settings that provide health care services to high-risk perinatal clients, clients who have received transplants, dialysis settings, oncology clinics, and infusion centers. The case management services offered by the nurse are determined by the specific needs of the clients seen in these settings. The models of case management are also developed for the needs of the clients.

Public Health Clinic Settings

Depending on the services provided in the public health setting, the nurse has an opportunity to provide education, screening, and referrals as needed to the clients served. Examples of primary prevention include an antepartum clinic, where the nurse interacts with women and can teach about pregnancy, diet, and exercise during pregnancy.

Working with parents in pediatric settings, the nurse case manager can teach nutrition, growth, and development and provide anticipatory guidance (primary level of prevention). The nurse can also screen children for growth and development and make referrals as needed to the Women, Infants, and Children program and other specialty programs available in the area for the clients' needs (secondary prevention).

Nurses can also serve as case managers working with elderly clients, providing nutrition education (primary prevention), screening for hypertension (secondary prevention), and even assisting with medication management and care of chronic diseases (tertiary prevention). The opportunities for community health nurses to provide case management services are vast, depending on the location, the populations served, and the resources available in the community.

Occupational Health Settings

More employers are providing health screening and education to their employees to keep their work forces healthy. Community health nurses who work in occupational health settings are in a position to provide primary prevention in health education classes designed to meet the needs of the employees. These classes can be designed on the basis of the health status of workers and to prevent the types of injuries to which they are prone. The nurse in this setting can also provide primary prevention by offering influenza vaccines and other immunizations to keep the employees healthy.

Secondary prevention can be provided to employees through screening clinics for hypertension and other potential chronic illnesses or health problems to which the employees may be more susceptible because of the nature of work performed. Referrals can be made as needed for follow-up with these employees. The occupational health nurse would continue to follow these employees and case-manage any health issues that could affect the employees' ability to perform the duties of their jobs.

Case management for tertiary prevention can include keeping in touch with injured employees and monitoring their recovery, therapy, or other services that are provided to the employees in the process of returning to health and their jobs. The occupational health nurse who provides case management services to these employees offers them education, referrals as needed, and assistance in their recovery process.

Home Health and Hospice Settings

The community health nurse working in home health or hospice services is often assigned a case load of clients for whom he or she provides case management services. In both of these settings, the nurse case manager provides primary, secondary, and tertiary prevention to clients. These services are designed on the basis of the individual needs of clients and their families. Coordination of care, referrals, assessment, medication management, patient and family education, and the development of plans of care are just a few of the nursing functions that are provided through a case management model.

RESEARCH IN CASE MANAGEMENT

Case management research is increasing in the last decade, much of it as a result of the quality reforms in health care and the role of case management in these reforms. A literature search in *PubMed* and the *Cumulative Index to Nursing and Allied Health* found many categories of case management research. These include disease management, evidence-based practice, roles and functions, models, transitions of care, and roles in quality improvement initiatives. Specific research evaluating case management and quality improvement examined the roles of case management in transitions of care and readmissions, core measures, hospital-acquired conditions, and patient satisfaction. Other research evaluated the effect of case management on geriatric populations, disabled populations, and end-of-life situations. The documented studies describe the implemented programs and evaluate the program outcomes. An example is given in the Research Highlights box.

RESEARCH HIGHLIGHTS

Geriatric Care Management for Low-Income Seniors: A Randomized Controlled Trial

Counsell et al. (2007) conducted a randomized clinical control study of 951 adults 65 years or older with annual incomes less than 200% of the federal poverty level whose primary care physicians were randomly assigned to the intervention group (474 patients) or usual care (477 patients) in community-based health centers. The intervention consisted of 2 years of home-based care management by a nurse practitioner and SW, who collaborated with the primary care physician and a geriatrics interdisciplinary team and were guided by 12 care protocols for common geriatric conditions. Results of the study showed that integrated and home-based geriatric care management resulted in improved quality of care and reduced acute care utilization among a high-risk group, in comparison with community-based care. Improvements in health-related quality-of-life issues were mixed, and physical function outcomes did not differ between the groups.

Case management programs in all settings require further study. Terms used in case management programs should be defined for comparison in various clinical sites. Programs with similar organizational structures and services can then be compared among settings. Critical to the success of case management programs are the inclusion of costs and cost savings and the evaluation of quality outcomes. The researcher or case manager must report the program's description as well as the case manager's role and professional background. Well-defined patient and program outcomes are essential to the evaluation of case management programs. With the implementation of well-designed research with measurable outcomes, management in health care settings across the continuum of care can identify the most cost-effective programs for specific populations served.

CASE STUDY Application of the Nursing Process

Comprehensive Case Management Program

The following case study is an example of a comprehensive case management program. Case management programs and the served populations are diverse; this is only one example of case management implementation.

Bill Wilson is a 76-year-old white male. He recently relocated to the Reno area from Wisconsin to be closer to family. Bill was recently admitted to the hospital for treatment of chest pain, hypertension, and poor glucose control. The case manager contacts Judy, a nurse practitioner at the diabetic clinic, and asks her if she will accept Bill as a primary care client in the TCM program. Judy accepts Bill into the TCM program and makes an appointment tomorrow, the day after Bill's hospital discharge.

Past Medical History

Metabolic syndrome: obesity (310 pounds, 5'11" BMI 43.2)

Type 2 diabetes, poorly controlled, A1c 9.5 during hospitalization

Hypertension

Coronary artery disease with two stents placed 5 years ago after a myocardial infarction

Peripheral vascular disease, both lower legs; healing wound on right foot

Diabetic neuropathy, both feet

Decreased vision due to diabetic retinopathy

Assessment

Bill has a 10-year history of type 2 diabetes, poorly controlled, with an A1c of 9.5. He has been taking metformin 1000 mg oral twice a day. His blood glucose is often 200 to 250. He admits to forgetting his medication more than two times a week. He does not perform fingerstick glucose monitoring because of the cost of supplies and low vision problems.

Individual

Bill is a retired employee of Johnson and Johnson in Racine, Wisconsin. His monthly income with Social Security and other retirement is $1700 per month. Since Bill moved to Reno, he is residing in a one-bedroom apartment. His rent is $700 a month and includes utilities. He has a car and drives. He recently enrolled in a Medicare managed care program that includes medications.

Family

Bill was married for 45 years. He is now a widower. He is not currently in a relationship. He has two siblings, a brother and a sister. Both siblings live near their children in the Midwest. Bill moved to Reno to be close to his daughter, Sally, who is his only child. Sally resides in a single-family home with her husband, Harry, and their three teenage children. Sally is an electrical engineer, employed full time, and her husband is a university English professor.

Community

Because Bill is new to the community, he is not familiar with community services that are available. Judy will put him in contact with senior services that are available and will make referrals as appropriate.

Diagnosis

Judy saw Bill in the clinic. She took his history, performed a physical examination, and reviewed his discharge medications. With Bill, she developed a care plan with specific goals for Bill's health promotion and disease stabilization.

The diagnosis list included:

Type 2 diabetes, poorly controlled

Metabolic syndrome: obesity (increased body fat around the waist), hypertension, high blood glucose, elevated cholesterol level

continued

Comprehensive Case Management Program

Hypertension
Hyperlipidemia
Coronary artery disease
Peripheral vascular Disease
Diabetic neuropathy
Visual disturbance, retinopathy, and cataracts

Individual

Judy and Bill mutually agreed that he lacks knowledge on how to manage his diabetes. Bill often eats foods high in carbohydrates and fats. It is convenient for Bill to eat fast foods. Bill admits that he often forgets to take his medications. He also acknowledged that he does not understand his medications and which medication treats his chronic conditions. Bill has not seen an ophthalmologist in more than 5 years.

Bill has a limited income, but he thinks that he can live on his monthly income, especially now that he is on a Medicare managed care program that covers his medications.

Bill does not exercise and finds exercise boring.

Family

Bill's daughter, Sally, is concerned about him. She is busy with her job, but is available to assist him on the weekends. She is willing to assist him with meal preparation and invites him to her house for meals at least once a week.

Community

Bill is new to the community. He does not know what services are available for seniors in the area. Part of his care plan includes an introduction to community services and activities.

Planning
Individual

Bill is at risk for hospital readmission. He requires education to learn how to manage his chronic illnesses. Most importantly, Judy suggests that Bill begin the Diabetic Education course offered at the clinic. The program includes information on how to monitor and control his blood glucose. The program also includes healthy cooking classes to encourage the attendees to prepare healthy meals at home. Judy is also setting an appointment for Bill to meet with the program's pharmacist to learn about his medications.

Short-Term Goals

Bill and Judy agreed on short-term goals that include the following:
- Diabetic education classes that include healthy cooking. A meeting with the program's dietitian to identify specific goals for Bill's meal plan.
- A referral to a podiatrist who comes to the diabetic clinic three times a week to see patients, with the goal of the foot wound healing completely. Education on foot care, wearing socks, appropriate shoes, and foot inspection.
- A referral to an ophthalmologist for a complete eye examination.
- A referral to a local gym. Bill's Medicare managed care health program pays for the monthly membership.
- An appointment with an exercise physiologist at the gym to evaluate Bill's current physical condition and create an exercise plan for Bill. Because Bill finds exercise boring, the physiologist will work with Bill to develop an exercise program that will interest Bill to encourage continuation of the program.

Long-Term Goal

Bill's long-term goals include the following:
- Control of his type 2 diabetes, including an A1c less than 7.5
- Weight loss

- Continuation of the exercise program
- Continued follow-up with his primary care provider, Judy

Family
Short-Term Goal

Bill's daughter, Sally, wants to make sure that Bill has the diabetic testing supplies that he needs. She contacts the Medicare managed care program and requests that the testing supplies be provided. The company representative assures Sally that the supplies are covered. They will provide Bill with a glucometer and testing supplies. They will provide the products as soon as possible so Bill can learn how to do blood glucose monitoring while enrolled in the Diabetic Education program.

Long-Term Goal

The long-term goals that Bill's family want him to achieve include:
- Diabetes control
- Weight loss through diet and exercise
- Independent living in his own apartment
- Social interaction Community

Short-Term Goal

Judy will provide Bill with his referral information. Judy will also provide Bill with resources available in the community that he can explore.

Long-Term Goal

- Socialization in the community. Bill plans to start attending the church that his daughter and her family attend. He wants to explore the activities offered at the local senior center.
- Attendance at exercise, completion of the Diabetic Education program.

Intervention
Individual

Judy's primary focus for Bill is to stabilize and improve his chronic illnesses. Making referrals to podiatry, ophthalmology, diabetic education, and exercise physiologist.

Family

Bill has good support from his daughter and her family, who are involved in his life.

Community

Bill has a stable living environment. He is able to drive and explore the community resources that Judy has provided.

Evaluation
Individual

Judy and Bill work together as a team to evaluate his chronic disease management. As necessary, they make revisions in his care plan.

Family

Bill's family remains involved in his life. They are a strong source of social support for him.

Community

Judy will evaluate Bill's progress in becoming involved in community activities and services.

SUMMARY

Case management programs continue to emerge in all health care settings. These programs change as health care reform measures are initiated and the needs of the population change. A common need among all programs is to collect data on the efficacy of programs, measuring client and program outcomes to ensure that the services that are offered are meeting targeted goals. Staff who work as case managers should consider obtaining certification to develop common knowledge and skills among case management providers and better validate the services provided.

ⓔ EVOLVE WEBSITE

http://evolve.elsevier.com/Nies/community
- NCLEX Review Questions
- Case Studies

BIBLIOGRAPHY

Agency for Healthcare Research and Quality (AHRQ): 2017. Available from <https://www.pcmh.ahrq.gov/page/tools-implementing-pcmh>.

Agency for Healthcare Research and Quality (AHRQ): *Issue Brief: Implications for Medical Practice, Health Policy and Health Services Research*, 2015. Available from <www.ahrq.gov/sites/default/files/publications/files/caremgmt-brief.pdf>.

American Academy of Family Physicians (AAFP): 2008. Available from <www.AAFP.org>.

American Nurses Association: *The Value of Nursing Care Coordination, A Whitepaper of the American Nurses Association*, 2012. Available from <www.nursingworld.org>.

American Nurses Credentialing Center: *Case management nursing*, 2009. Available from <www.nursingworld.org>.

Case Management Society of America: *Philosophy of case management*, 2005. Available from <www.cmsa.org/ABOUTUS/Definitionof-CaseManagement/tabid/104/Default.aspx>.

Case Management Society of America: *Standards of practice for case management*, Little Rock, AR, 2016, Author.

Case Management Society of America: *State of the science paper: care coordination*, Greenberg, L, 2006.

Center for Health Care Strategies, Inc: *Fact Sheet: Care management definition and framework*, Hamilton, NJ, 2007, Author.

Chen A, Brown R, Archibald N, et al.: *Best practices in coordinated care*, March 2000. Available from <http://www.cms.hhs.gov/DemoProjectsEvalRpts/downloads/CC_Full_Report.pdf>.

CMS.gov: *Value-Based Programs*, 2017. https://www.cms.gov/Medicare/Quality-Initiatives-Patient-Assessment-Instruments/Value-Based-Programs/Value-Based-Programs.html.

CMS.gov: *Chronic Care Management Services*, 2016. https://www.cms.gov/Outreach-and-Education/Medicare-Learning-Network-MLN/MLNProducts/Downloads/ChronicCareManagement.pdf.

Commission for Case Manager: *Certification: Certified Case Manager (CCM) certification requirement*, 2009. Available from <www.ccmcertification.org>.

Conger MM: Nursing case management: a managed care organizational strategy. In Conger MM, editor: *Managed care: practice strategies for nursing*, Thousand Oaks, CA, 1999, Sage Publications.

Counsell SR, Callahan CM, Clark DO, et al.: Geriatric care management for low-income seniors, *JAMA* 298:2623–2633, 2007.

Crosby RL: Community care of the chronically mentally ill, *Journal of Psychosocial Nursing* 25(1):33–37, 1987.

Department of Health and Human Services (DHHS): *Center for Medicare and Medicaid Services. Transitional Care Management Services*. ICN 908628, December, 2016.

Ethridge PA, Nursing HMO: Carondelet St: Mary's experience, *Nurs Manage* 22(7):22–27, 1991.

Ethridge PA, Johnson S: The influence of reimbursement on nurse case management practice: Carondelet's experience. In Cohen EL, editor: *Nurse case management in the 21st century*, St. Louis, 1996, Mosby.

Ethridge PA, Lamb GS: Professional nursing case management improves quality, access, and costs, *Nurs Manage* 20(3):30–35, 1989.

Grau L: Case management and the nurse, *Geriatr Nurs* 5(8):372–375, 1984.

Greenberg E: *State of the science paper #3: care coordination. Case Management Society of America*, 2006.

Hartford Institute for Geriatric Nursing (HIGN): *Hartford Institute history*. n.d, April 14, 2013. Available from <www.hartfordign.org/About/History>.

Henderson S, Princell C, Martin CO: The patient centered medical home: this primary care model offers RNs new practice—and reimbursement—opportunities, *American Journal of Nursing* 112(12):54–59, 2012.

Huber DL: The diversity of case management models, *Lippincott's Case Manag* 7(6):212–220, 2002.

Institute for Healthcare Improvement: *IHI triple aim initiative*, 2013. Available from http://www.ihi.org/offerings/Initiatives/TripleAim/Pages/default.aspx.

Institute of Medicine: *Crossing the quality chasm*, 2001. Available from <http://nationalacademies.org/hmd/reports/2001/crossing-the-quality-chasm-a-new-health-system-for-the-21st-century.aspx>.

Mahn VA, Spross JA: Nursing case management as an advanced practice role. In Hamric AB, Spross JA, Hanson CM, editors: *Advanced nursing practice: an integrative approach*, Philadelphia, 1996, Saunders.

McDonald K, Sundaram V, Bravata D, et al.: *Closing the quality gap: A critical analysis of quality improvement strategies, Vol 7: Care coordination*, AHRQ Technical Reviews No. 9.7. Rockville, MD, 2005, Agency for Healthcare Research and Quality.

National Transition of Care Coalition: *Transition of Care Measures*, 2008. Available from http://www.ntocc.org/Portals/0/PDF/Resources/TransitionsOfCare_Measures.pdf.

Patient-Centered Primary Care Collaborative: *Joint principles of the patient-centered medical home*, 2007. Available from <http://www.aafp.org/dam/AAFP/documents/practice_management/pcmh/initiatives/PCMHJoint.pdf>.

Patient Protection and Affordable Care Act, Title III: *Improving the quality and efficiency of healthcare*, Public Law 111–148, 2010. Available from <www.gpo.gov>.

PCM Editorial Review Board: The PCM journal "think tank" on case management predictions for 2009, *Prof Case Manag* 13:299–301, 2008.

Pittman DC: Nursing case management: holistic care for the deinstitutionalized mentally ill, *J Psychosoc Nurs* 27(11):23–27, 1989.

Public Law 111-148, 2010. Available from <http://www.gpo.gov/fdsys/pkg/PLAW-111publ148/pdf/PLAW-111publ148.pdf>.

Shea SC: *Improving medication adherence: how to talk with patients about their medications*, Philadelphia, 2006, Lippincott Williams & Wilkins.

Shea SC: The "Medication Interest Model": An integrative clinical interviewing approach for improving medication adherence—part I: Clinical applications, *Prof Case Manag* 6(13):305–315, 2008.

Simmons WJ, White M: Case management and discharge planning: two different worlds. In Volland P, editor: *Discharge planning: an interdisciplinary approach to continuity of care*, Owings Mills, MD, 1988, National Health Publication.

Steinberg RM, Carter GW: *Case management and the elderly*, Lexington, MA, 1983, Lexington Books, DC Health.

Stricker P: *The role of utilization management in case management. n.d.* Available from <http://cmsa.org/individual/newsevents/healthtechnologyarticles/tabid/649/default.aspx>.

Thurkettle MA, Noji A: Shifting the healthcare paradigm: the case manager's opportunity and responsibility, *Lippincott's Case Manag* 8(4):160–165, 2003.

University of Washington, Psychiatry & Behavioral Sciences: *Care Management Tracking System (CMTS)*, 2017. https://aims.uw.edu/resources-library/care-management-tracking-system-cmts.

U.S. Department of Commerce/International Trade Administration: *Health and medical services: US industrial outlook*, Washington, DC, 1990, Author.

Weil M, Karls J: *Case management in human service practice*, San Francisco, 1985, Jossey-Bass.

Yamamoto L, Lucey C: Case management "within the walls": A glimpse into the future, *Crit Care Nurs Q* 28(2):162–178, 2005.

Policy, Politics, Legislation, and Community Health Nursing

*Cathy R. Arvidson**

OUTLINE

OBJECTIVES

Upon completion of this chapter, the reader will be able to do the following:
1. Discuss how the structure of government affects the policy development process.
2. Describe the legislative, judicial, and administrative (executive) processes involved in establishing federal, state, or local health policy.
3. Examine the power of nursing to influence and change health policy.
4. Discuss current health policy issues.
5. Identify the social and political processes that influence health policy development.
6. Discuss the nurse's role in political activities.
7. Discuss nursing's involvement in private health policy.

KEY TERMS

administrative agencies
Clara Barton
coalition
Florence Nightingale
government
health policy
institutional policies
Lavinia Dock
laws
Lillian Wald

lobby
lobbyist
Mary Breckenridge
nursing policy
organizational policies
organizations
policy
policy analysis
political action committee (PAC)
politics

public health law
public policy
Ruth Watson Lubic
social policy
Sojourner Truth
sovereign power
statutes
Susie Walking Bear Yellowtail
Sylvia Trent-Adams

*The author would like to acknowledge the contributions of Anita Finkelman, who wrote this chapter for the previous edition.

This chapter addresses the interrelationships of the processes through which health policies are determined and instituted. Politics and legislation are the routes through which public health policies are established. Policy, politics, and legislation are the forces that determine the direction of health programs at every level of government, as well as the private sector. These programs are crucial to the health and well-being of the nation, the state, the community, and the individual. Nurses influence the maintenance and improvement of the health of individuals, groups, and communities by contributing to policy and legislative advancement.

The health care delivery system, including nursing practice and research, is profoundly influenced by policies set by both government and private entities. Nurses who understand the system of health policy development and implementation can effectively interpret and influence policies that affect nursing practice; the health of individuals, families, groups, communities, and populations; and, when required, offer an international health perspective.

OVERVIEW: NURSES' HISTORICAL AND CURRENT ACTIVITY IN HEALTH CARE POLICY

The more a nurse knows about the political process, the more he or she tends to become involved. Individual nurses may become politically active on a local, state, or national level. Nurses may work collectively within a group such as the National Student Nurses Association, the American Nurses Association (ANA), and state boards of nursing to lobby for health causes. There are more than 4 million employed registered nurses (Kaiser Foundation, 2016). Together nurses can be patient advocates, change agents, and policy makers. Lawmakers respect nurses and thus are usually effective as consultants in both the legislative and executive branches at local, state, and federal levels. It is the hallmark of the U.S. system of government that citizens have the right to have an influential voice in the governance of the community. Nurses are able to communicate concerns about conditions and issues in health care, the health care needs of individuals and communities, and the profession of nursing. United, nurses can influence political leaders to make changes to the health care system that are beneficial to all. Nurses experienced in the political arena can mentor novices to it.

Many individual nurses in the past and present have been instrumental in working with legislation and politics. A few exemplary nurses who had an impact on public health are:

Florence Nightingale was the first nurse to exert political pressure on a government (Hall-Long, 1995). In the 1850s Nightingale was asked to establish the first nurse corps to tend the soldiers in the Crimea War. She transformed military health and knew the value of data in influencing policy. She was a leader who knew how to use the support of followers, colleagues, and policy makers. As discussed in Chapter 2, Nightingale collected and analyzed data about health services and outcomes, an activity that now is a critical element of public health.

Sojourner Truth beginning in the 1840s became an ardent and eloquent advocate for abolishing slavery and supporting women's rights. Her work helped transform the racist and sexist policies that limited the health and well-being of African Americans and women. She fought for human rights and lobbied for federal funds to train nurses and physicians (Masonet al., 2007).

Clara Barton was responsible for organizing relief efforts during the U.S. Civil War. In 1882, she successfully persuaded Congress to ratify the Treaty of Geneva, which allowed the Red Cross to perform humanitarian efforts in times of peace. This organization has had a lasting influence on national and international policies (Hall-Long, 1995; Kalisch and Kalisch, 2004).

Lavinia Dock was a prolific writer and political activist. She waged a campaign for legislation to allow nurses to control the nursing profession instead of physicians. In 1893, with the assistance of Isabel Hampton Robb and Mary Adelaide Nutting, she founded the politically active American Society of Superintendents of Training Schools for Nurses, which later became the National League for Nursing (Kalisch and Kalisch, 2004). She was also active in the suffrage movement, advocating that nurses support the woman's right to vote (Lewinson, 2007).

Lillian Wald's political activism and vision were shaped by feminist values. Working in the early 1900s, she recognized the connections between health and social conditions. She was a driving force behind the federal government's development of the Children's Bureau in 1912. Wald appeared frequently at the White House to participate in the development of national and international policy (Mason et al., 2007).

Mary Breckenridge worked to develop nursing in rural Kentucky in the 1920s, establishing the Frontier Nursing Service.

Susie Walking Bear Yellowtail was a Native American nurse who walked from reservation to reservation, working to improve health services for this population from the 1930s to 1960s. She also established the Native American Nurses Association.

Florence Wald was a nursing leader in establishing hospice care in the United States—modeled after similar services offered in the United Kingdom—in the 1970s.

Dr. Ruth Watson Lubic is a nurse-midwife who crusaded for freestanding birth centers in this country, being influential in the opening of New York City's first birthing center in 1975. After developing the birth center model through the Maternity Center Association in New York City, Dr. Lubic expanded the model to Washington, DC, where the infant mortality rate was twice the national average. In 1993, Lubic was awarded the MacArthur Fellowship Grant and, in 2001, the National Academy of Medicine's Lienhard Award (Lyttle, 2000; Rychnovsky 2011).

DEFINITIONS

Policy denotes a course of action to be followed by a government, business, or institution to obtain a desired effect. *Merriam-Webster's Dictionary* defines policy as "a definite course or method of action selected from among alternatives and in light of given conditions to guide and determine present and future decisions"

(Merriam-Webster, 2014). Policy encompasses the choices that a society, segment of society, or organization makes regarding its goals and priorities and the ways it allocates its resources to attain those goals. Policy choices reflect the values, beliefs, and attitudes of those designing the policy (Mason et al., 2016).

Public policy denotes precepts and standards formed by governmental bodies that are of fundamental concern to the state and the whole of the general public. The field of public policy involves the study of specific policy problems and governmental responses to them. Political scientists involved in the study of public policy attempt to devise solutions for problems of public concern. They study issues such as health care, pollution, and the economy. Public policy overlaps comparative politics in the study of comparative public policy with international relations in the study of foreign policy and national security policy, and with political theory in considering ethics in policy making. See the examples in Table 10.1.

Health policy is a statement of a decision regarding a goal in health care and a plan for achieving that goal. For example, to prevent an epidemic, a program for inoculating a population is developed and implemented, and priorities and values underlying health resource allocation are determined.

Nursing policy specifies nursing leadership that influences and shapes health policy and nursing practice. Nursing, and therefore nursing leadership, is shaped dramatically by the impact of politics and policy. Effective nursing leadership is a vehicle through which both nursing practice and health policy can be influenced and shaped.

Institutional policies are rules that govern worksites and identify the institution's goals, operation, and treatment of employees.

Organizational policies are rules that govern organizations and their positions on issues with which the organization is concerned (Mason et al., 2016).

A **political action committee (PAC)** is a fundraising group usually associated with an organization. Money is raised from the members with the purpose of financially supporting political causes. Organizations are allowed to support candidates, but only PACs are permitted to donate money to candidates or legislation (Mason et al., 2016).

Social policy is policy associated with individuals and communities. In very general terms, social policy can be defined as the branch of public policy that advances social welfare and enhances participation in society. Social safety nets, however, often contribute to social exclusion, especially in urban settings, instead of being universally accessible. In most Western societies, social protection usually depends on contributory social insurance schemes to which only regular job holders have access (either in their own right or as dependents). In the United States, this is particularly evident with respect to the way the health care system and Social Security retirement benefits work. Social justice argues that all individuals and groups receive fair treatment in society as well as impartially share in the benefits of that society (Almgren, 2012).

Administrative agencies are departments of the executive branch with the authority to implement or administer particular legislation.

Laws are rules of conduct or procedure; they result from a *combination* of legislation, judicial decisions, constitutional decisions, and administrative actions.

Public health law focuses on legal issues in public health practice and on the public health effects of legal practice. Public health law typically has three major areas of practice: police power, disease and injury prevention, and the law of populations. Statute, ordinance, or code prescribes sanitary standards and regulation for the purpose of promoting and preserving the community's health. Public health law consists of legislation, regulations, and court decisions enacted by government at the federal, state, and local levels to protect the public's health. This includes case law and treaties.

Statutes are any laws passed by a legislative body at the federal, state, or local level.

Organizations are associations that set and enforce standards in a particular area; a group of individuals who voluntarily enter into an agreement to accomplish a purpose.

A *professional association* (also called a *professional body, professional organization,* or *professional society*) is a nonprofit organization seeking to further a particular profession, the interests of individuals engaged in that profession, and the public interest. It is a volunteer group that seeks to join large numbers of individuals who have a significant wealth of knowledge and experience in a particular field such as the Association of Public Health. There are also pooled funds for lobbying purposes (Thomas, 1997). The roles of these professional organizations are viewed as maintaining the control and oversight of the professional occupation as well as safeguarding the public trust. There is an element of protecting the interests of the professional practitioners, as in a cartel or labor union. Inherent in these organizations is the promotion of general standards for the performance of its members and the expectation of continued professional development.

TABLE 10.1	Terminology Example
Topic	**Example**
Public policy	A local or regional effort to prevent the sale of tobacco or alcohol to minors. Public policy directs that the right to health of the majority must be preserved over individual freedoms and corporate interests.
Public health law	New York State Public Health Law §2164: "Every person in parental (statute) relation to a child in this state shall have administered to such child an adequate dose of an immunizing agent against poliomyelitis, mumps, measles, diphtheria, rubella, varicella, *Haemophilus influenza* type B, and hepatitis B. . ."
Common law	The Supreme Court decision in *Roe v. Wade,* making first-trimester abortion legal, is an example of how common law becomes enforceable.
Regulation	Reporting of communicable diseases to state and local health departments, which then report them to the Centers for Disease Control and Prevention.
Treaty	Multilateral treaty: Treaty to eliminate all forms of discrimination against women.

Many professional bodies are involved in the development and monitoring of professional educational programs and the updating of skills, and thus they perform professional certification to indicate that a person possesses qualifications in the subject area. Sometimes membership in a professional body is synonymous with certification, though not always. Membership in a professional body, as a legal requirement, can in some professions form the primary formal basis for gaining entry to and setting up practice within the profession. Professional bodies also act as learned societies for the academic disciplines underlying their professions.

A MAJOR PARADIGM SHIFT

Policy is based on values, and the first step in forming policy is identifying the issue. Therefore it would seem rational to define "health" as the starting point for any policy annexed to health care issues. Historically, health was defined in the context of infectious diseases. Current definitions encompass prevention and management of chronic conditions. The World Health Organization (WHO) considers health to be the state of complete physical, mental, and social well-being and not merely the absence of disease or infirmity. Despite this broad definition, it is only in the most recent decades that the WHO is refocusing on its initial definition as it attempts to deal with environmental issues such as nuclear contamination and industrial toxins in industrialized nations and the exploration of carcinogenic commercial products such as tobacco products. On a global level, the WHO is working to prevent, treat, and care for communicable diseases such as HIV/AIDS, tuberculosis, malaria, and, most recently, the Zika virus. In addition, WHO focuses on noncommunicable diseases such as heart disease, stroke, cancer, diabetes, and lung diseases, which are responsible for more than 70% of all deaths worldwide. WHO emphasizes promoting health through the life cycle, taking into account environmental risks and social determinants of health. Thus there is a realization that health is a basic human right and that health problems are linked to government actions and, hence, affect human rights.

Human rights violations occur when governments fail to provide their people with the infrastructure, services, and information necessary to promote health, reduce risk, and control disease. For example, for every year of education women have, their infant mortality is decreased by 10%; yet education of women is not a global reality.

On a national level, an example of changing emphasis is the Centers for Disease Control and Prevention (CDC). It is committed to achieving true improvements in people's lives by accelerating health impact and reducing health disparities. Box 10.1 describes this priority for the CDC. All people, and especially those at greater risk of health disparities, will achieve their optimal lifespan with the best possible quality of health in every stage of life. However, a shift in the paradigm of health concepts would necessitate a substantial reallocation of resources, because the vast majority of health spending is directed at medical care and biomedical research and, as such,

reflects a viewpoint of health care as a commodity. If one considers that in 2015 28.4 million people in the United States younger than 65 years had no health insurance and 4.5% of children were uninsured, it becomes clear that the health and human rights relationship is not yet reflected in our health policies (CDC, 2015). In addition, many people are underinsured. Their insurance coverage is not at the level it should be to cover full services or longer-term needs. The economics of health care are discussed further in Chapter 12.

The publication of *Healthy People 2000* by U.S. Surgeon General C. Everett Koop in 1990 led to a resurgence of interest by the federal government in the health and welfare of Americans. However, fiscal resources for public health interventions declined, and only marginal progress was made in meeting the goals. In early 2000, *Healthy People 2010* marked the beginning of the new millennium and an enhanced focus on population-based health promotion strategies (U.S. Department of Health and Human Services [USDHHS], 2000). Many *Healthy People 2020* objectives directly or indirectly involve health policy with enhanced focus on the social determinants of health and health policy (USDHHS, 2013) (see the Healthy People 2020 box).

Virtually all of the areas of *Healthy People 2020* have multiple policy-related objectives, and the Healthy People box lists only a few of them. Building on previous iterations, the updated 2020 version has four "over-arching goals" for 2020: attain high-quality, longer lives free of preventable disease, disability, injury, and premature death; achieve health equity, eliminate disparities, and improve the health of all age groups; create social and physical environments that promote good health for all; and promote quality of life, health development, and health behaviors across all life stages. The Healthy People 2020 box describes *Healthy People* content related to the public health infrastructure. Another forward-looking recommendation is making *Healthy People 2020* into a web-accessible database that is searchable and interactive and allows users to tailor the document to the public's needs. The intent is that enhanced focus on social determinants represents a "deliberate shift away from the perception that access to health care services will ever solve all of our health care problems" (USDHHS, 2013).

BOX 10.1 Strategic Plan Priorities for the Center of Disease Control Strategic Framework

Strategic Priority #1	Improve health security at home and around the world.
Strategic Priority #2	Better prevent the leading causes of illness, injury, disability, and death.
Strategic Priority #3	Strengthen public health and health care collaboration.

From Centers for Disease Control and Prevention: *CDC strategic framework*, 2016. Retrieved from https://www.cdc.gov/about/organization/strategic-framework/index.html

HEALTHY PEOPLE 2020

Content Related to Public Health Infrastructure

Goal

To ensure that federal, state, tribal, and local health agencies have the necessary infrastructure to effectively provide essential public health services.

Overview

Public health infrastructure is fundamental to the provision and execution of public health services at all levels. A strong infrastructure provides the capacity to prepare for and respond to both acute (emergency) and chronic (ongoing) threats to the nation's health. Infrastructure is the foundation for planning, delivering, and evaluating public health.

Why is Public Health Infrastructure Important?

Public health infrastructure includes three key components that enable a public health organization at the federal, tribal, state, or local level to deliver public health services. These components are:

- A capable and qualified workforce
- Up-to-date data and information systems
- Public health agencies capable of assessing and responding to public health needs

These components are necessary to fulfill the following 10 essential public health services:

1. Monitor health status to identify and solve community health problems.
2. Diagnose and investigate health problems and health hazards in the community.
3. Inform, educate, and empower people about health issues.
4. Mobilize community partnerships and action to identify and solve health problems.
5. Develop policies and plans that support individual and community health efforts.
6. Enforce laws and regulations that protect health and ensure safety.
7. Link people to needed personal health services and assure the provision of health care when otherwise unavailable.
8. Ensure competent public and personal health care workforces.
9. Evaluate effectiveness, accessibility, and quality of personal and population-based health services.
10. Research for new insights and innovative solutions to health problems.

Understanding Public Health Infrastructure

Public health infrastructure is key to all other topic areas in *Healthy People 2020*. It allows for and supports key goals of *Healthy People*, including the:

- Improvement of health
- Creation of environments that promote good health

- Promotion of healthy development and behaviors

Public health infrastructure, along with the 10 essential functions of public health, influences—and is influenced by—a number of factors, including the social and political environment. As such, public health infrastructure provides a useful framework for addressing the social determinants of health.

Emerging Issues in Public Health Infrastructure

Increasing attention to public health infrastructure has led to the identification of a number of emerging issues.

Tribal Public Health Infrastructure

Each tribe is an independent government that must adopt local strategies to meet its public health challenges; interventions must be tailored to the cultural beliefs and practices of each tribe. There are many ways tribal entities are served through the Indian Health Service, Tribal Epidemiology Centers, and national organizations; however, challenges remain.

Disparities in the Public Health Workforce

As minority populations in the United States increase, the country will need a more diverse public health workforce. Hispanics, American Indians and Alaska Natives, and African Americans are underrepresented in the public health workforce.

Accreditation of Public Health Agencies

In an effort to standardize services and improve performance, public health agencies are moving toward a voluntary national accreditation program. This program will highlight agencies' commitment to service and quality and provide a standard toward which all public health agencies can work.

Public Health Systems Research

Expanding the evidence base for community interventions and for the effective organization, administration, and financing of public health services is critical to the future development of public health infrastructure. The emerging field of public health systems and services research is playing an important role in the development of this evidence base; its role should be supported and expanded over the decade, with a strong focus on translating research into practice.

Public Health Law

Novel policies are being developed to address legal and political challenges resulting from new and re-emerging infectious diseases and increasing levels of chronic disease. New centers devoted to the study of public health law are adding to the body of knowledge in this critical area.

From U.S. Department of Health and Human Services: *Healthy People 2020,* 2013, Public Health Infrastructure. Retrieved from http://www.healthypeople.gov/2020/topicsobjectives2020/overview.aspx?topicid=35.

STRUCTURE OF THE GOVERNMENT OF THE UNITED STATES

Government is the structure of principles and rules determining how a state, country, or organization is regulated. Among its purposes are regulation of conditions beyond individual control and provision of individual protection through a population-wide focus. These tasks are accomplished through passage and enforcement of laws. Requirements of childhood immunizations for school attendance, disease vector control, and sewage treatment are examples of regulations to protect the health of the population.

Government can also be viewed as the sovereign power vested in a nation or state. **Sovereign power** is the independent and supreme authority of the nation or state. Historical documents describe the government's responsibility for health in the United States and the subsequent authority to enact laws (including health laws). These documents reflect the values of the country's founders. They give the government the authority to enact laws, but they also limit that power. The earliest of these statements was the Mayflower Compact, through which the Pilgrims committed themselves to making "just and equal laws" for the general good. The Declaration of Independence later established the doctrine of inalienable rights, life, liberty, and the pursuit of happiness.

TABLE 10.2	Government Branches

Branch of Government	Includes
Executive branch	The president, the vice president, and the administrative agencies
Legislative branch	The Senate and the House of Representatives (Congress)
Judicial branch	At the federal level: district courts, circuit courts, and the Supreme Court
	At the state level: state and county courts

BOX 10.2 An Example of the President's Response to a House Bill (A President May or May not Respond to a Bill)

State Children's Health Insurance Program (SCHIP)

H.R. 2 (and related bills H.R. 57, H.R. 72, and S. 275) became Public Law 111-3, The Children's Health Insurance Reauthorization Act of 2009. This was signed into law by President Barack Obama on February 4, 2009. It went into effect on April 1, 2009. This bill:

- Allows certain state plans under Titles XIX (Medicaid) or Title XXI (State Children's Health Insurance Program, referred to in this Act as CHIP) of the Social Security Act (SSA) that require state legislation to meet additional requirements imposed by this Act additional time to make required plan changes.
- Provides for coordination of CHIP funding for the 2009 fiscal year.
- Amends SSA Title XXI to reauthorize the CHIP program through FY2013 at increased levels.

See http://thomas.loc.gov/home/thomas.php for more information.

BOX 10.3 Administrative Agencies

One of the most dramatic changes in American government since the ratification of the Constitution is the growth of administrative agencies. Federal administrative agencies have broad power. They exercise all of the powers of government: executive, legislative, and judicial.

The U.S. Food and Drug Administration (FDA) is one such administrative agency. Its power is in regulating the pharmaceutical industry as well as the food industry.

However, it was not until the representatives of the individual states signed the Constitution of the United States that the federal government realized its sovereign power. At the same time that its power was realized, a limit to that power was placed on the federal government. The drafters of the Constitution sought to balance the need to empower the new federal government to "establish Justice, insure domestic Tranquility, provide for the common defense, promote the general Welfare, and secure the Blessings of Liberty" for its people but with limits on that power. That balance is achieved in several important ways.

The federal government is a government of limited powers, which means that for a federal action to be legitimate, it must be authorized. Only those actions that are within the scope of the Constitution, the supreme law of the land, are authorized. The Constitution separates governmental powers among the branches of government (Table 10.2).

Some examples of the separation of powers doctrine that are written into the U.S. Constitution are as follows:

- The legislature is prohibited from interfering with the courts' final judgments.
- The Supreme Court cannot decide a "political question"; the issue must be an actual case or controversy.
- Congress must present a bill to the president before it can become law (Box 10.2).
- The president needs consent of the Senate to appoint Supreme Court justices or to make treaties.
- The president and members of Congress are elected; the judiciary is appointed.

The Constitution not only set forth the responsibilities of the federal government but also provided for the individual citizen's rights and freedoms. These are contained in the first 10 amendments, which were added after the original Articles of the Constitution were ratified in 1787. These 10 amendments, added in 1791, are known as the *Bill of Rights*. The rights guaranteed in the Bill of Rights, such as those of free speech and freedom of religion, applied only to the laws and actions of the federal government. It would take another 72 years for these rights to be guaranteed within the states. "Liberty interests" and "privacy rights" have been found to exist by Supreme Court determinations and have become guiding principles in setting policy and enacting legislation. Note that these rights are applicable only to state or federal government's interaction with people. Violations of restrictions on rights such as free speech do not apply to nongovernmental entities, unless a specific law states otherwise.

The balance of powers is an important concept in the U.S. government. Federalism is the relationship and distribution of power between the national and the state governments. This balance flows directly from the text of the Constitution: "The powers not delegated to the United States by the Constitution, nor prohibited by it to the States, are reserved to the States respectively, or to the people." Box 10.3 highlights one of the changes in the federal government since the Constitution: the development of administrative agencies. This development has had a major impact on government functioning.

States retain powers not delegated to the federal government; therefore much of public health law is under state jurisdiction and, as a result, varies considerably from state to state. These powers to enact laws for the public welfare are referred to as the states' *police powers*. Additionally, states may delegate these powers to local governments. In the United States, legislative activities of the three levels of government (federal, state, and local) may vary greatly in their expectations, actions, and results. The state legislatures, for the most part, are directly involved in health care, yet the federal government influences health policy, directly and indirectly, through the financing of health care for many groups (e.g., Medicare, Medicaid), regulation activities (e.g., approval of drugs), and setting of standards (e.g., air quality).

Decisions affecting the public's health are made not only at every level of government but also in each branch of government. The separation and balance of powers, referred to as *checks and balances,* is as important to health as it is to the economic or military status of the country.

The legislative branch (i.e., Congress at the federal level; legislature, general assembly, or general court at the state level) enacts the statutory laws that are the basis for governance. The executive branch administers and enforces the laws, which are broad in scope, through regulatory agencies. These agencies, in turn, define more specific implementation of the statutes through rules and regulations (i.e., regulatory or administrative law). The judiciary body provides protection against oppressive governance and against professional malpractice, fraud, and abuse. Its function through the courts, both state and federal, is to determine the constitutionality of laws, interpret them, and decide on their legitimacy when they are challenged. Decisions of the U.S. Supreme Court are binding law for the nation. Decisions of an individual state's highest court are binding law within that state alone. The courts also have jurisdiction over specific infractions of laws and regulations.

OVERVIEW OF HEALTH POLICY

Public Health Policy

To review, public policy refers to decisions made by legislative, executive, or judicial branches of one of the three levels of government (local, state, or federal). These decisions are intended to direct or influence actions, behaviors, or decisions of others. Public health policies influence health care through the monitoring, production, provision, and financing of health care services. Everyone, from health care providers to consumers, is affected by health policies. Likewise, health policy influences corporations, employers, insurers, colleges of nursing, hospitals, clinics, producers and retailers of medical technology and equipment, and senior care facilities.

The authority for the protection of the public's health is largely vested with the states, and most state constitutions specifically delineate their responsibility. Municipal subdivisions of states, such as counties, cities, and towns, generally have the power of local control of the services, conferred by the state legislature. The responsibilities of local, state, and federal governments for health services may differ under varying circumstances, sometimes complicating attempts to determine the locus of political decision making. The supremacy of the state prevails in most instances; therefore the state is a critical arena for political action. An example is the state's authority to license health professionals and health care institutions.

Each state establishes policies or standards for goods or services that affect the health of its citizens. However, if the federal government or the local government imposes a higher standard than the state requires, the lower standard is negated by the higher standard. An example would be standardization of pasteurized milk. A state may hold to one standard, whereas interstate commerce, which is under federal jurisdiction, may dictate a higher standard that must be met by that state.

The federal government has a strong influence on the health services available in each state. Constitutionally, this authority is derived from the federal role in interstate commerce and through broad interpretation of the "general welfare" clause (e.g., Medicare and Medicaid). States vary considerably in resources allocated to provide health programs; therefore significant de facto authority derives from the promise of revenues or threats to remove funding (e.g., funds for interstate highway repair are

BOX 10.4 History of Several Examples of Government-Funded Health Care Legislation

- **1965:** The Social Security Act established both Medicare and Medicaid. Medicare was a responsibility of the Social Security Administration (SSA), whereas federal assistance to the state Medicaid programs was administered by the Social and Rehabilitation Service (SRS). SSA and SRS were agencies in the Department of Health, Education, and Welfare (HEW).
- **1977:** The Health Care Financing Administration (HCFA) was created under HEW to effectively coordinate Medicare and Medicaid.
- **1980:** HEW was divided into the Department of Education and the Department of Health and Human Services (HHS).
- **2001:** HCFA was renamed the Centers for Medicare and Medicaid Services (CMS). CMS is the federal agency that administers the Medicare and Medicaid programs.
- **2010:** The Patient Protection and Affordable Care Act was a very comprehensive attempt to improve access to care by providing health insurance to most of the nation's uninsured.
- **2012:** The Food and Drug Administration Safety and Innovation Act reauthorizes user fees for the FDA.
- **2016:** VA Health system rule change granting veterans direct access to care by nurse practitioners, certified nurse midwives, and clinical nurse specialists who work in the VA health system.

often tied to air quality requirements). Federal funds typically fund most health care programs fully or partially.

Compliance by states with federal program standards is voluntary, but the advantage of the revenue, which is withheld from the states that fail to comply, is seldom ignored. Programs such as a statistical reporting system of sexually transmitted infections and control are standardized across the country in response to the indirect but marked effect of federal funding.

Health Policy and the Private Sector

In addition to the public policy–making sector, health policies can be made through the private sector. For example, an insurance company or an employer can determine some of what illnesses and preventive care is covered by the insurance program, what drugs are included in the formulary, and how much to charge for an insurance policy. The private sector includes employers, professional organizations (e.g., American Hospital Association), nonprofit health care organizations (e.g., American Heart Association), and for-profit corporations that deliver, insure, or fund health care services outside government control. In particular, health insurance companies and managed care organizations are increasingly setting policies that affect a large number of individuals.

In the private sector, health policy evolves differently from in the public sector. One difference is that private health policy is largely influenced by theories of economics and business management, as compared with the social and political theories that predominate in the public sector. In the private sector economics is central, whereas in the public sector economics is but one of many factors. In the private sector decisions can be swift and are often proactive, whereas in the public sector decisions are slow, deliberate, and more reactive. Private-sector needs are determined by consumerism, market trends, and economics. Public-sector needs are determined by voting shifts, electoral realignment, and term limits. Box 10.4 provides the history of several critical examples of government-funded health care legislation.

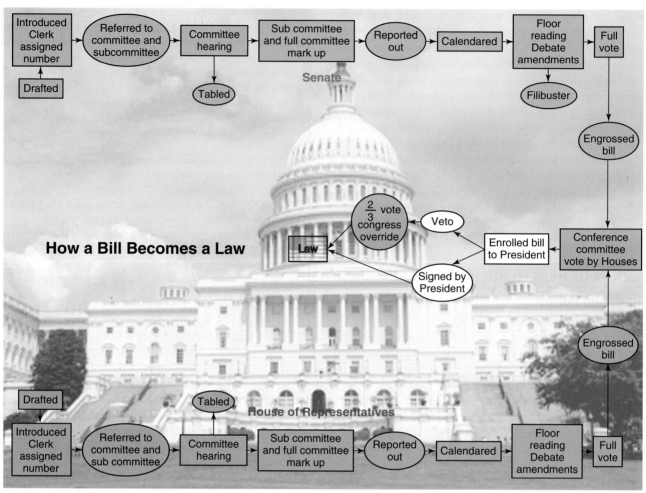

FIG. 10.1 How a bill becomes a law at the federal level. (Retrieved from http://publicdomain-clip-art.blogspot.com/2007_09_01_archive.html.)

The Legislative Process: How a Bill Becomes a Law

As stated in the previous section, there is a balance of powers within the government at both state and federal levels. The three branches of government, executive, judicial, and legislative, form a three-legged stool that is in equilibrium. Along with a separation of powers of the three branches of government, there is an additional mechanism that balances the power of the Congress: bicameralism (consisting of two houses). Bicameralism ensures that the power to enact laws is shared between the House of Representatives and the Senate. The procedure through which legislation must pass to eventually become law is similar for all legislative bodies in the country. Once a concept has been drafted into legislative language, it becomes a bill, is given a number, and moves through a series of steps. The bill's passage is sometimes smooth, but, more often than not, the bill is extensively altered through amendments or even "killed" (dropped from or stopped in the process).

In Congress and in the 49 states that have bicameral legislatures, a bill must succeed through the two legislative bodies, that is, the House of Representatives and the Senate (Fig. 10.1). Nebraska, which has a single-house legislature, is the exception. A bill that has moved successfully through the legislative process has one final hurdle, which is the chief executive's approval.

The approval may be a clear endorsement, in which case the governor or president signs it. If the executive neither signs nor vetoes it, the bill may become law by default. An explicit veto conclusively kills the bill, which then can be revived only by a substantial vote of the legislature to override the veto. This is another example of the checks and balances of the government process.

Issues that find their way into the legislative arena are commonly controversial, and proponents and opponents quickly align themselves. Defeating a bill is much easier than getting one passed; therefore the opposition always has the advantage.

Health legislation, which usually requires preventive action (e.g., toxic waste management) or creates a new service (e.g., nursing center organizations for Medicare recipients), is at a disadvantage from several standpoints. Few elected officials are knowledgeable about the health care field. Typically, they have staff who have more expertise in this area, and it is the staff who write legislation. Although health is readily recognized as a national resource, it is not easily quantified into the economic terms that make the issue easy to grasp. Health legislation is often costly to implement. As a result even legislation that has large bipartisan support may not pass due to the cost. Other disadvantages are the backgrounds, biases, and ambitions of each legislator. Despite these obstacles, good health laws can be passed when concerned nurses and other health care workers understand the legislative process and use it effectively. Nurses have been recognized as one of the most trusted professions. Nurses should educate their elected officials and function as expert tutors for them. In addition, this is yet another mode of intervention that nurses may perform on behalf of clients.

Major Legislative Actions and the Health Care System

An examination of the major legislative actions that federal and state governments have taken and recognition of their influence on health and health care delivery are critical to understanding the evolution of the health care system in the United States. Throughout the twentieth century, the U.S. Congress enacted bills that had a major influence on the private and public health care subsystems. Legislation pertaining to health increased in scope in each decade of the twentieth century, with the goal of improving the health of populations and coping with changing health care needs. During the last two decades, concerns about an increase in health care costs and the growth of managed care stimulated even more legislation. The Patient Protection and Affordable Care Act (ACA) was signed into law in March 2010 with a plan to increase health care coverage to previously uninsured Americans. The ACA had many supporters and opponents, resulting in much debate even after its implementation. Indeed, health care reform/health insurance reform was a major issue during both the 2012 and 2016 presidential elections. The Supreme Court also reviewed a major case related to the health care reform legislation, tying all levels of government to this landmark legislation—administrative, legislative, and judicial. The Court decision did not lead to major changes in the health care reform law. At the time of publication, the debate continues on introducing new legislation to repeal and replace the ACA. Issues of affordability, preexisting conditions, requirements for citizens to buy health insurance, and tax credits are being discussed.

Federal Legislation

This section describes some of the landmark federal laws that have influenced health services and health care professionals. They are listed in Table 10.3.

Pure Food and Drugs Act of 1906: This act established a program to supervise and control the manufacture, labeling, and sale of food. Subsequent legislation included meat and dairy products, pharmaceuticals, cosmetics, toys, and household products. Since 1927, the U.S. Food and Drug Administration (FDA) has administered elements of this act.

Children's Bureau Act of 1912: The Children's Bureau was founded to protect children from the unhealthy child labor practices of the time and to enact programs that had a positive effect on children's health. In 1921, the Sheppard-Towner Act extended children's health care programs by providing funds for the health and welfare of infants.

Social Security Act of 1935 and its amendments (1965, 1972): The Social Security Act and its subsequent amendments have had a far-reaching effect on health care for many groups. The Social Security Administration (SSA) provides wel-

TABLE 10.3 Critical Federal Legislation Related to Health Care

Year(s)	Legislation or Other Government Action
1906	Pure Food and Drugs Act
1912	Children's Bureau Act
1921	Sheppard-Towner Act
1935	Social Security Act
1944	Public Health Act
1945	McCarren-Ferguson Act
1946	Hill-Burton Act
1953	Establishment of the Department of Health, Education and Welfare as a cabinet-status agency; in 1980 establishment of U.S. Department of Education as separate from Department of Health and Human Services
1956	Health Amendments Act
1964	Nurse Training Act
1965	Social Security Act amendments: Title XVIII Medicare, Title XIX Medicaid
1970	Occupational Safety and Health Act
1972	Social Security Act amendments: Professional Standards Review Organization; further benefits under Medicare and Medicaid, including dialysis
1973	Health Maintenance Act
1974	National Health Planning Resources Act
1981, 1987, 1989, 1990	Omnibus Budget Reconciliation Acts
1982	Tax Equity and Fiscal Responsibility Act
1985	Consolidated Omnibus Budget Reconciliation Act
1988	Family Support Act
1990	Health Objectives Planning Act
1996	Health Insurance Portability and Accountability Act
1996	Welfare Act
2003	Nurse Reinvestment Act
2004	Medicare Reinvestment Act
2008	Mental Health Parity and Addictions Equity
2010	Patient Protection and Affordable Care Act

fare for high-risk mothers and children. Benefits were later expanded to include health care provisions for older adults and the handicapped. This major governmental action was the enactment of legislation for Medicare and Medicaid.

Medicare, Title XVIII Social Security Amendment (1965): This federal program, administered by the Centers for Medicare and Medicaid Services (CMS; formerly Health Care Financing Administration [HCFA]), pays specified health care services for all people 65 years of age and older who are eligible to receive Social Security benefits. People with permanent disabilities and those with end-stage renal disease are also covered. The objective of Medicare is to protect older adults and the disabled against large medical outlays. The program is funded through a payroll tax of most working citizens. Individuals or providers may submit payment requests for health care services and are paid according to Medicare regulations. See Chapter 12 for more information on Medicare.

Medicaid, Title XIX Social Security Amendment (1965): This combined federal and state program provides access to care for the poor and medically needy of all ages. Each state is

TABLE 10.4   2013 Federal Poverty Guidelines* for the 48 Contiguous States and the District of Columbia

Family Size	Gross Yearly Income ($)	Gross Monthly Income ($)	Approximate Hourly Income ($)
1	12,060	1005	5.81
2	16,240	1353	7.81
3	20,420	1702	9.82
4	24,600	2050	11.83
5	28,780	2398	13.84
6	32,960	2747	15.85
7	37,140	3095	17.86
8	41,320	3344	19.30
Over 8 add per child	+4,180	+348	+$

*Federal poverty guidelines: Typically, in January or February of each year the federal government releases an official income level for poverty called the Federal Poverty Income Guidelines, often informally referred to as the "federal poverty level." The benefit levels of many low-income assistance programs are based on these poverty guidelines.
From *Federal Register* 82(19):8831–8832, 2017.

allocated federal dollars on a matching basis (i.e., 50% of costs are paid with federal dollars). Each state has the responsibility and right to determine the services to be provided and the dollar amount allocated to the program. Basic services (e.g., ambulatory and inpatient hospital care, physical therapy, laboratory, radiography, skilled nursing, and home health care) are required to be eligible for matching federal dollars. States may choose from a wide range of optional services, including drugs, eyeglasses, intermediate care, inpatient psychiatric care, and dental care. Limits are placed on the amount and duration of service. Unlike Medicare, Medicaid provides long-term care services (e.g., nursing home and home health) and personal care services (e.g., chores and homemaking). In addition, Medicaid has eligibility criteria based on level of income. Table 10.4 provides the U.S. Department of Health and Human Services (HHS) poverty guidelines for 2013. The Medicaid population has complex needs, and managed care organizations may not always be able to provide optimum services to these beneficiaries. See Chapter 12 for more information on Medicaid.

Public Health Act of 1944: The Public Health Act consolidated all existing public health legislation into one law. Since then, many new pieces of legislation have become amendments. Some of its provisions, either in the original law or in amendments, provided for or established the following:

- Health services for migratory workers
- Family planning services
- Health research facilities
- National Institutes of Health
- Nurse training acts
- Traineeships for graduate students in public health
- Home health services for people with Alzheimer disease
- Prevention and primary care services
- Rural health clinics
- Communicable disease control

McCarren-Ferguson Act of 1945: The McCarren-Ferguson Act has had a major influence on the insurance industry through giving states the exclusive right to regulate health insurance plans (Knight, 1998). No federal government agency is solely responsible for monitoring insurance, as this supervision is in the hands of state governments. Some federal agencies are involved in insurance reimbursement; however, the structure of the benefit program for federal employees and military personnel, Medicare, and Medicaid allows Congress to pass laws that can override state health insurance laws if the laws do not meet certain criteria.

Hill-Burton Act of 1946: The Hill-Burton Act authorized federal assistance in the construction of hospitals and health centers with stipulations about services for the uninsured. As a result, hospitals with obligations to care for the uninsured were built in towns and cities across the United States. Through these measures, hospital care became more accessible, but by the late 1990s, the high cost of health care, combined with decreasing lengths of stay and increasing use of primary care, forced the closure of many of the hospitals built with Hill-Burton funds.

Health Amendments Act of 1956: The Health Amendments Act, Title II, authorizes funds to aid registered nurses (RNs) in full-time study of administration, supervision, or teaching. In 1963, the Surgeon General's Consultant Group on Nursing noted that there were still too few nursing schools, nursing personnel were not put to good use, and there was limited nursing research. As a result, in 1964, the Nurse Training Act provided funds for loans and scholarships for full-time study for nurses and funds for construction of nursing schools. Since this time, additional legislation has funded nursing education; even the Patient Protection and Affordable Care Act of 2010 provides some funding opportunities.

Occupational Safety and Health Act of 1970: The Occupational Safety and Health Act focuses on the health needs and risks in the workplace and environment. It continues to provide critical programs important to the workplace and the community. See Chapter 30 for more information on both the Occupational Safety and Health Act and the Occupational Safety and Health Administration.

Health Maintenance Organization (HMO) Act of 1973: The HMO Act provided grants for HMO development. The act required that employers offer federally qualified HMOs as a health care coverage option to employees and established that states were responsible for the oversight of HMOs. Although initially it was not successful in stimulating HMO growth, this legislation has had a long-term effect on the growth of managed care.

National Health Planning and Resources Act of 1974: The National Health Planning and Resources Act assigned the responsibility for health planning to the states and local health systems agencies. In addition, it required health care facilities to obtain prior approval from the state for expansion in the form of a certificate of need.

Omnibus Budget Reconciliation Acts (1981, 1987, 1989, and 1990): The Omnibus Budget Reconciliation Acts were each enacted in response to the huge federal deficit. They have influenced funding for nursing homes, home health agencies, and hospitals and have set up guidelines and regulations about several issues, including a move from process to outcome evaluation, use of restraints, and prescription drugs for Medicaid recipients.

Tax Equity and Fiscal Responsibility Act of 1982: The Tax Equity and Fiscal Responsibility Act was a major amendment to the Social Security Act of 1935, establishing the prospective payment system for Medicare, the diagnosis-related group (DRG) system. This law changed health care radically by introducing a new reimbursement method. See Chapter 12 for more information on DRGs.

Consolidated Omnibus Budget Reconciliation Act of 1985: The Consolidated Omnibus Budget Reconciliation Act (COBRA) is a federal law that affects health care delivery and reimbursement. It requires all hospitals with emergency services that participate in Medicare to treat any client in their emergency services, whether or not that client is covered by Medicare or has the ability to pay. This legislation includes requirements for Medicaid services for prenatal and postnatal care to low-income women in two-parent families in which the primary spouse is unemployed. Another important requirement of COBRA focuses on the problem of the loss of health insurance when a person loses his or her job. With the growing number of unemployed, COBRA is even more important. Employers who terminate an employee must continue benefits for the employee and dependents for a specified period if the employee had health benefits before the termination. COBRA is an example of how a federal law can affect state health care practices. The federal government must determine who receives federal Medicare funds; therefore COBRA provides the opportunity for the federal government to legislate health care delivery at the state level.

Family Support Act of 1988: The Family Support Act expanded coverage for poor women and children and required states to extend Medicaid coverage for 12 months to families who have increased earnings but are no longer receiving cash assistance. This act also required states to expand Aid to Families with Dependent Children (AFDC) coverage to two-parent families in which the principal wage earner is unemployed.

Health Objectives Planning Act of 1990: The Health Objectives Planning Act was initiated in response to the 1979 report *Healthy People: The Surgeon General's Report on Health Promotion and Disease Prevention.* After that report, the federal government began to take a directive approach in identifying and monitoring national health care goals. *Healthy People 2000, Healthy People 2010,* and *Healthy People 2020* are also results of this act.

Health Insurance Portability and Accountability Act of 1996: The Health Insurance Portability and Accountability Act (HIPAA) addressed several issues. The law offered protections for patient privacy and confidentiality. Critical insurance issues were the portability of coverage and limits on the restrictions health plans place on coverage for preexisting conditions. This law established that insurers cannot set limits on coverage of longer than 12 months. This is a complex law, but it has been important for consumers with preexisting conditions. It should be noted that 2010 health care reform legislation has eliminated HIPAA applicability to preexisting conditions, and this change went into effect in 2014.

Welfare Reform Act of 1996: The Welfare Reform Act placed restrictions on eligibility for AFDC, Medicaid, and other federally funded welfare programs. The Welfare Reform law decreased the number of people on welfare and forced many individuals to take low-paying jobs, many of which do not offer health insurance. Between 1994 and March 1999, welfare rolls dropped 47% (DeParle, 1999). Many individuals, particularly underserved women and children, subsequently lost Medicaid coverage. In 2012 this became the Temporary Assistance for Needy Families.

The State Child Health Improvement Act (SCHIP) of 1997: This has been a critical law, providing insurance for children and families who cannot afford health insurance. This law has been very important to children's health. The law was extended several times and then it was not renewed by the Bush administration. The program was renewed by the Obama administration in the Children's Health Insurance Reauthorization Act of 2009. See Box 10.2 (referred to as CHIP or SCHIP if "state" is included).

Medicare Modernization Act of 2003: The Medicare Modernization Act was the most significant law in 40 years for senior health care. After being implemented in January 2006, the law provided seniors and people living with disabilities some prescription drug benefit coverage, more choices, and better benefits.

Nurse Reinvestment Act of 2003: The Nurse Reinvestment Act is significant because it is a response to the critical nursing shortage that has been present across the country. Funding is provided to increase enrollments and the number of practicing nurses.

Mental Health Parity and Addictions Equity Act of 2008: A similar act was passed in the 1990s, but it was not an effective law. Improving the earlier law, this act mandates that if a group health plan includes medical/surgical benefits and mental health benefits and/or substance use disorder benefits, the financial requirements (e.g., deductibles and copayments) and treatment limitations (e.g., number of visits or days of coverage) that apply to mental health benefits must be no more restrictive than the predominant financial requirements or treatment limitations that apply to substantially all medical/surgical benefits.

Patient Protection and Affordable Care Act of 2010: The Patient Protection and Affordable Care Act of 2010, also called the *Health Care Reform Act,* is an extremely complex and comprehensive piece of legislation. One of the primary intents of the act is to reduce the number of uninsured Americans, and a number of provisions directly address this intent. For example, it requires all U.S. citizens and legal residents to have qualifying health coverage, whether provided through employers, individually purchased, or provided by federal plans (i.e., Medicare, Medicaid, CHIP). It also dramatically changes eligibility requirements for Medicaid, allowing coverage of childless adults with incomes up to 133% of the federal poverty line, and expands CHIP. Furthermore, it subsidizes premiums for lower- and middle-income families and requires coverage of dependent adult children up to age 26 for those with group policies (Kaiser Family Foundation, 2016).

The Health Care Reform Act included significant insurance changes. For example, it (1) establishes high-risk pools to provide health coverage to individuals with preexisting conditions; (2) prohibits insurers from placing lifetime limits on the dollar value of coverage; (3) prohibits insurers from disallowing coverage for some individuals because of preexisting health conditions and dropping policyholders when they get sick; and (4) requires health plans to provide some types of preventive care and screenings without consumer cost-sharing (i.e., copayments or coinsurance). The legislation creates programs to foster nonprofit, member-run health insurance companies that can offer health insurance; to establish state-based health insurance exchanges through which individuals and small businesses can buy coverage; and to permit states to form compacts that will allow insurers to sell policies in any participating state.

Funds for government-financed elements (i.e., Medicare, Medicaid, CHIP) are to be provided through a combination of new fees and taxes and a variety of cost-saving measures. For example, there will be taxes on indoor tanning and new Medicare taxes for people in high-income brackets. The act requires fees for pharmaceutical companies and medical devices as well as penalties for individuals who do not obtain health insurance. To cut costs, there are significant cuts to the Medicare Advantage program and modifications and reductions in Medicare spending. It also enhances efforts to reduce administrative costs, streamline care, and reduce fraud and abuse.

Until passage of the Patient Protection and Affordable Care Act of 2010, the focus of federal legislation was on either prevention of illness through influencing the environment, such as the Occupational Safety and Health Act of 1970, or provision of funding to support programs that influence health care, as demonstrated in the Social Security Act of 1935. Beginning with the Sheppard-Towner Act of 1921 and continuing to the present, federal grants have increased the involvement of state and local governments in health care. The involvement of the federal government through fiscal allocations to state and local governments provided money for programs not previously available to states and local areas. Similar services became available in all states. Funds supporting these services were accompanied by regulations that applied to all recipients. Many state and local government programs were developed on the basis of availability of federal funds. The involvement of the federal government through funding has served to standardize public health policy in the United States (Pickett and Hanlon, 1990).

The health reform legislation of 2010 was strongly influenced by the rising numbers of uninsured and underinsured U.S. citizens. Since the implementation of the ACA the rate of uninsured citizens has fallen from 16.6% in 2013 to 10% in 2016 (Kaiser, 2016). These changes do not mean that the country now has universal health care coverage. The United States continues to be the only major developed country to not have universal health care coverage. The ACA has not reduced the cost of health care as promised. Medicaid expansion has been rejected by 19 states despite the federal support. The ACA is being debated with the Trump administration, promising to repeal and replace it.

Role of State Legislatures

State governments are also directly involved in health care policy, legislation, and regulation. State governments focus particularly on financing and delivery of services and oversight of insurance. The latter has become important as managed care has grown. The 1988 report titled *Future of Public Health* from the National Academy of Medicine (NAM), formerly called the Institute of Medicine (IOM)—noted that it is the state's responsibility to see that functions and services necessary to address the mission of public health are in place throughout the state. The NAM framed the public health enterprise in terms of three functions: assessment, policy development, and assurance. Further the NAM reported in *The Future of the Public's Health in the 21st Century* (IOM, 1988) six areas of action and change:

1. Adopting a population health approach that considers the multiple determinants of health
2. Strengthening the governmental public health infrastructure, which forms the backbone of the public health system
3. Building a new generation of intersectoral partnerships that also draw on the perspectives and resources of diverse communities and actively engage them in health action
4. Developing systems of accountability to assure the quality and availability of public health services
5. Making evidence the foundation of decision making and the measure of success
6. Enhancing and facilitating communication within the public health system (e.g., among all levels of the governmental public health infrastructure and between public health professionals and community members) (IOM, 1988)

The Centers for Disease Control and Prevention (CDC) describes the 10 essential public health services that all communities should have:

- Monitor health status to identify and solve community health problems.
- Diagnose and investigate health problems and health hazards in the community.
- Inform, educate, and empower people about health issues.
- Mobilize community partnerships and action to identify and solve health problems.
- Develop policies and plans that support individual and community health efforts.
- Enforce laws and regulations that protect health and ensure safety.
- Link people to needed personal health services and assure the provision of health care when otherwise unavailable.
- Assure competent public and personal health care workforces.
- Evaluate effectiveness, accessibility, and quality of personal and population-based health services.
- Research for new insights and innovative solutions to health problems.

ACTIVE LEARNING EXERCISE

Review your state's legislative agenda. Identify bills that relate to health care, and from those bills, identify any bills that might affect community or public health. Discuss the bills in small groups—their impact in general and how nursing might be involved.

PUBLIC POLICY: BLUEPRINT FOR GOVERNANCE

Policy is directed by values. It articulates the guiding principles of collective endeavors, establishes direction, and sets goals. It influences and, in turn, is influenced by politics. Policy directives may become realized or obstructed at any stage in the political process.

Policy Formulation: The Ideal

In ideal circumstances, authorized authoritative bodies (e.g., state health departments, USDHHS, CMS) rationally determine actions to create, amend, implement, or rescind health care policy. These groups decide what is right or best and then develop the political strategies to effect the desired outcomes. Whether a particular policy is advocated or adopted depends on the degree that a group or society as a whole may benefit without harm or detriment to subgroups. Of all the seemingly endless limitless factors that may influence policy formation, group need and group demand should be the strongest determinants. The premises supporting the goals of health policy should be equitable distribution of services and the guarantee that the appropriate care is given to the right people, at the right time, and at a reasonable cost.

Policy Formulation: The Reality

In the real world, policy for health care exemplifies both conflict and social change theories. Health policy is the product of continuous interactive processes in which interested professionals, citizens, institutions, industries, and other interested groups compete with one another for health care dollars and policy initiatives. They also compete with one another for the attention of various branches of government. The most obvious and prominent among these is the legislative branch, although policy is also made through regulatory mechanisms and court decisions. Health policy may also be derived from the recommendations of fact-finding commissions established by the legislative or executive branch or nongovernmental organizations such as the NAM and may also be influenced by judicial decisions.

Health policy is rarely created through discrete, momentous determinations in relation to single problems or issues. It often evolves slowly because changes in the social beliefs and values that underlie established policy develop within the context of actual service delivery. Once a direct health care service is offered, especially an official tax-funded service, discontinuing is often difficult. Existing programs create tradition by establishing vested interest and a sense of entitlement on the part of the public. An example is the annual updating of the childhood and adolescent vaccination schedule recommended by the CDC. This is also an example of cooperation between professional organizations and government agencies to promote the well-being of individuals and communities (Box 10.5).

Steps in Policy Formulation and Analysis

The tangible formulation of public policy begins with the most critical step, which is defining the issue or describing the problem and placing it on the legislative agenda. This process includes cost–benefit analysis. Health policy analysis determines those who benefit and those who experience a loss as the result of a policy. These considerations are critical in order to develop health policies that are as fair as possible to all who are affected. Then legislation is finalized, typically developed by legislative staff. The bill then winds its way through the process in the legislative body at either the state or federal level. This includes a cost analysis of the bill at the federal level by the Congressional Budget Office. If the bill is passed and is signed by either a governor or the president, it becomes law. The next step is the commitment of resources, most often through the passage of legislation, and the development of regulations, which is done by a governmental agency assigned to ensure implementation of a bill that becomes law. A regulatory schedule for the implementation of the law is formulated. Then, an evaluation process is designed that satisfies regulatory and legislative remedies, should they be needed. Analysis of health policy is an objective process that identifies the sources and consequences of policy decisions in the context of the factors that influence them.

A 30-day window of opportunity is typical for public input into the development of regulations. Written comments about a political issue are made part of the public record. To facilitate correspondence, websites have been set up to promote contacting agencies, governmental organizations, and political figures. Nurses need to be aware of some of the important websites. furthermore, many legislators may have their own web pages so that the nurse can easily access their offices.

The Internet can provide almost unlimited access to information. However, access to information does not ensure its quality or credibility. The user is responsible for evaluating the information and separating quality information from misinformation. Nurses need to be information and communication technology literate. *Technology literacy* is the ability of an individual, working independently and with others, to responsibly,

---

BOX 10.5 **Recommended Childhood and Adolescent Immunization Schedule: United States**

The Advisory Committee on Immunization Practices (ACIP) annually reviews the recommended childhood and adolescent immunization schedule to ensure that the schedule is current with changes in vaccine formulations and reflects revised recommendations for the use of licensed vaccines, including those newly licensed. It is the only federal government body that provides written recommendations for the routine administration of vaccines for children and adults in the civilian population. Recommendations and format of the childhood and adolescent immunization schedule for February 2017 were approved by ACIP, and the American Academy of Family Physicians.

From Centers for Disease Control and Prevention: Recommended immunization schedules for persons 0–18 years—United States, 2017, *Morbidity and Mortality Weekly Report*, 2017, 66(5):134–135. Retrieved from http://www.cdc.gov/vaccines/schedules/hcp/index.html

appropriately, and effectively use technology tools to access, manage, integrate, evaluate, create, and communicate information. Technology fluency builds on technology literacy and is demonstrated when nurses apply technology to real-world experiences, adapt to changing technologies, modify current and create new technologies, and personalize technology to meet personal needs, interests, and learning style.

> **? ACTIVE LEARNING EXERCISE**
>
> Participate in a group organized around a public health issue (e.g., disposable diapers, toxic waste, or fluoride).

THE EFFECTIVE USE OF NURSES: A POLICY ISSUE

The Health Resources and Services Administration (HRSA) provides general resources and information to the public and for use in the development of policy by the government. The nursing workforce development programs administered by the HRSA through Public Health Service Act Title VIII funding provide federal support for nurse workforce development. Title VIII provides the largest source of federal funding for nursing education at the undergraduate and graduate levels and favors institutions that educate nurses for practice in rural and medically underserved communities. These programs provide loans, scholarships, traineeships, and programmatic support for nursing students and for nurses who are continuing their education in graduate programs.

An issue that is vital to effective health care delivery relates to nurse staffing. The current nursing shortage has been a topic of concern of nurses for many years and is now a health care crisis. This crisis has taken a strange course as a result of the economic crisis in the United States. Many nurses who were due to retire did not; some nurses who were working part time returned to full-time work; and some nurses who had not been employed in nursing returned to the field. These changes reduced the shortage and have also had a negative impact on new graduates obtaining positions. In addition, in some areas of the country, hospital administrators decided that as there are more new graduates, they could focus on hiring graduates with bachelor's degrees instead of associate-degree graduates—who have therefore had more difficulty obtaining jobs. Compounding the problem is the fact that nursing colleges and universities across the nation are struggling to expand enrollment to meet the rising demand for nursing care. A shortage of nursing faculty and changing demographics contribute to the concern that all 50 states will experience a shortage of nurses in the next few years. In February 2017 Congress introduced the Title VIII Nursing Workforce Reauthorization Act of 2017, which will reauthorize and improve nursing workforce programs, supporting practice in rural and medically underserved communities, as well as providing support for advanced nursing education, diversity, National Nurse Service Corps, nurse faculty loan forgiveness, and geriatric education (ANA, 2017).

NURSES' ROLES IN POLITICAL ACTIVITIES

The Power of One and Many

RNs are the largest health care professional group. One in 44 women voters is an RN. Why are nurses not more politically active? Taylor (2016) examined nurses' motivation for public policy involvement. Reasons nurses become involved in health policy included becoming engaged in an issue, family history of political activity, connection with other nurses, having an influential mentor, and being part of a professional organization. More effort needs to be given to educate nurses about the importance of being informed on health policy issues and to encourage them to be politically active. Exposure to positive role models is particularly important. Nurses must obtain the tools to overcome factors that impede involvement. Nurses most often identify positive role models as the major influence that assisted them to become politically active in the profession. Professional organizations offer a connectiveness that can support the nurse in engaging in political activities. Therefore mentorship from the student level up to the expert level is important. Box 10.6 describes responses to a survey used by Winter and Lockhart (1997) about what methods were useful in developing awareness in the profession, policy, and politics.

Nurses as Change Agents

The public, as well as the government, recognizes the nursing profession as indispensable, necessary, and a valuable national resource. In their advocacy role, nurses are seen as professionals whose knowledge, skills, and caring concern are used to promote both the individual's and the community's well-being. Nurses have a unique status in caring for patients; they are interpreters of the health care system to the public, and government-funded programs influence their professional activities. The private business sector is also involved. Therefore public health nurses must know how to participate in the political process. To do this effectively, they need a sound knowledge of the community, state, and national government organization and function and a clear understanding of how these bodies collectively interact to influence policy. Nurses must know how to influence the creation of health care legislation and how to contribute to the election and appointment of key officials.

Although there are more nurses than physicians, hospital administrators, insurance administrators, or other health care professionals, nursing traditionally has not been seen as having major political influence because of a lack of public policy consensus within the nursing community. Unity within professional organizations, coalitions, and lobbying efforts is changing this perception. Policy is fundamental to governance; therefore nurses need to know about the formation of public policy and the acts of government and its agencies. Tables 10.5 and 10.6 give sources of information on these issues.

Nurses must become invested and competent in health policy. This includes communicating with elected officials at the local, state, and federal levels. This may be done through writing letters, emails, or doing personal visits. Contacting legislators gives the nurse the opportunity to "tell their story" in how the issue affects nursing practice. In addition, belonging to a professional organization, serving on advisory boards, speaking publicly, and contributing to a PAC all engage the nurse in effecting policy change. By engaging others affected by an issue, nurses can bring voice to their concerns (Kostas-Polston et al., 2015).

Nurses and Coalitions

When two or more groups join to maximize resources, increasing their influence and improving their chances of success in achieving a common goal, they have formed a coalition. Coalitions of health care providers often work on issues such as family violence and fluoridation of water supplies. An outstanding example of such cooperative action is the establishment of rehabilitation programs for health professionals whose practice has been impaired by substance abuse or mental health problems.

Nursing and consumer groups often form coalitions to advance their shared interests in health promotion. The ANA joined 16 other organizations (e.g., American College of Nurse Practitioners, American Red Cross, Department of Veterans Affairs, and Sigma Theta Tau) in the 1990s to form a coalition called Nurses for a Healthier Tomorrow. This organization has grown to a membership of 43 organizations. Responding to concerns about a potentially dangerous shortage of nurses, this coalition hopes to raise funds for a national advertising campaign designed to recruit new nurses and encourage existing ones to remain in the profession. The campaign focuses on the message that nurses are essential to the health care team and that they save health care dollars. The campaign shows that an increased demand exists for nurses, both in specialty areas and outside the hospital (NHT, 2014).

Nurses as Lobbyists

A lobbyist is a person who, voluntarily or for a fee, represents himself or herself, another individual, an organization, or an entity before the legislature. A lobbyist typically represents special-interest groups. The term derives from the fact that lobbyists usually stay in the areas (lobbies) next to the Senate and House chambers, seeking to speak with legislators and their aides as they walk to and from the chambers, or as lobbyists await legislative action that might affect their interests.

To lobby is to try to influence legislators; it is an art of persuasion. Influencing lawmakers to pass effective health legislation requires the participation of individual nurses and nursing organizations. There are currently more than 100 national nursing organizations. Many also have state chapters. Professional organizations make advocacy easier for members through the use of the Internet. Policy action centers are now part of many organizations' websites. Email alerts can be sent instantly to members residing in targeted districts to contact their legislators on a particular bill or issue. By entering one's postal zip code and pushing a button, one can sign a template letter and send it to one's legislator.

The goal of the first contact with an official is to establish that the nurse is a concerned constituent as well as a credible source of information on health issues. The image of nurses caring for people is a definite advantage at this point. Nurses are considered the most ethical of all health care providers and are considered to be trustworthy (Robert Wood Johnson Foundation, 2012). In communities in which nurses have already established strong political credentials, their colleagues will be more readily accepted. An individual who establishes a reputation as a reliable and accurate resource as a lobbyist has substantial influence.

Legislators rely heavily on lobbyists to educate them on issues, and they usually want to hear from all sides before taking a position on an issue. The official must trust the lobbyists to give accurate, though predictably biased, information. Information needs to be timely and up to date.

Each official represents a constituency with varied needs and interests, and each vote must be weighted within this context. The positions taken by legislators will not always be to an individual or organization's liking. Evaluation of their performance should be based on their overall voting pattern, not just on individual votes. Many organizations regularly tally and publish the records of each federal legislator on all issues related to nursing and health. This information can be helpful in evaluating elected officials. Collective action by nursing and health care organizations is critical to meeting their goals. Professional associations monitor legislative activity related to relevant health issues and link the process to their membership. This continual surveillance

TABLE 10.5 Sources for Legislative Information

Government Level	Information Available	Location
Federal	Background of members of Congress Congressional committee assignments Congressional terms of service Congressional news House/Senate vote tabulations Bills in process or legislated (bill number needed) Health and nursing issues in Congress	Congressional Directory Government documents section of selected public or university libraries *Congressional Quarterly Weekly Report* U.S. representative or senator (may have local office) *The American Nurse* ANA 600 Maryland Ave SW Suite 100 Washington, DC 20024 (202) 554-4444
	American Nurses Association Political Action Committee (ANA-PAC) Public health issues in U.S. Congress	*The American Nurse* ANA (see above) *The Nation's Health* American Public Health Association (APHA) 1015 15th St NW Washington, DC 20005 (202) 789-5600
State	Bills in process or legislated (bill number needed) Health and nursing issues in state legislature State political action committees for nursing	State representative or senator (may have local office) State nurses association (SNA) (for location, see April directory issue of the *American Journal of Nursing*) National League for Nursing

TABLE 10.6 Sources For Electoral Information

Government Level	Information Available	Location
State	State government operations Political subdivisions Legislative information telephone number State election laws and procedures Campaign finance reports	Secretary of State (state capitol) Office of Lieutenant Governor (state capitol)
County or municipal	Similar to state as appropriate to local government Political jurisdictions for each household address	County clerk (county courthouse) City clerk (city hall)
General	Government information Political jurisdictions for each household address Names of current office holders in local jurisdictions	County clerk (county courthouse) City clerk (city hall)

of the legislative environment is critical because even seemingly minor amendments can have profound effects on health issues. Thorough legislative surveillance requires the participation of people who are knowledgeable about nursing, health care, and the political intricacies of the legislative process. Some of the nursing organizations that have full-time lobbyists who work in Congress are the ANA, the American Academy of Nursing, and the National League for Nursing. State associations also work with state legislators. State legislative contacts become the eyes, ears, and voices of their professional organizations.

These associations can then provide testimony and comment on relevant state and federal issues. However, regardless of the effectiveness of association lobbyists in promoting the interests of nurses and society, they always need grassroots cooperation to truly influence decisions. In the final analysis, a sufficiently high number of communications from individual constituents, via email messages, telephone calls, and letters, has the greatest influence. Lobbying is an ongoing activity for health policy issues influencing nursing and health care delivery. Box 10.7 provides an overview of the lobbying process.

❓ ACTIVE LEARNING EXERCISE

1. With a group of two or three, meet with an elected official for a 15-minute appointment to ask about the official's concerns and priorities. Remember to refer to the "ABCs of Lobbying" prior to meeting with the official.
2. Visit the American Nurses Association website and explore its political action section at http://nursingworld.org/MainMenuCategories/Policy-Advocacy. What type of information is available?
3. Visit the American Public Health Association website for information about policy outcome evaluation at https://www.apha.org/policies-and-advocacy. Review the various evaluation programs to gain an understanding of policy outcome evaluation.

Nurses and Political Action Committees

PACs have been important sources of collective political influence since the 1970s. These nonpartisan entities promote the election of candidates believed to be sympathetic to their interests. PACs are established by professional associations, businesses, and labor organizations and are highly regulated by

BOX 10.7 ABCs of Lobbying on a State Level

Before the Meeting
- Appointments will have been made with your legislator(s) for the lobby cay. Tell the staff that you are a constituent and what issue(s) you would like to discuss with your representative. If your legislator is unavailable, you may have a scheduled appointment with a member of the legislative staff.
- If possible, put together a delegation of nurses to attend the meeting. A number of individuals from the legislator's district who are concerned about the same issue will make a big impression. Take along students from their districts because legislators are impressed with their participation.

Preparing for the Meeting
- Establish your agenda and goals. For example, focus on educating the legislators on the profession of nurse midwifery, the legislation that this group would like them to sponsor, the concerns about the malpractice insurance crisis, and the benefit to women's and children's health. Nurse practitioners (NPs) would focus on the cost–benefit of NPs as primary care providers in all settings, including health care homes.
- Research your legislator's stance before the meeting. It is important that you know your official's position so that you can present your stance more effectively and can have an intelligent discussion.
- Meet with the delegation (e.g., midwives, NPs) that will participate in the lobbying. It is important that you review what each person will say during the meeting. Select someone as the group leader, and make a list of points to be made and questions to be asked by each person.
- Prepare materials. Review the packet of information you will leave with your legislator. It is important to include your name and phone number in the packet so that your legislator will have a contact person for more information. Leaving a business card would be appropriate.

During the Meeting
- Be on time for your meeting.
- Be concise and diplomatic. Keep your presentation short and to the point.
- Be a good listener. Look for indications of your legislator's views, and watch for opportunities to provide useful information in order to strengthen or counter particular views.
- Stress why the issues concern you and others in your district.
- Don't be intimidated. Your legislator is in office to serve you. It is important to have a general knowledge of the issues, but you don't have to know every little detail. If he or she asks a question that you do not know the answer to, simply say that you do not know but are willing to find out. Find out the best way to get the information to him or her (fax, email, or a follow-up phone call).

After the Meeting
- Write a follow-up letter. After your visit, write a letter thanking your legislator for his or her time.
- Stay in contact with your legislator. Remember: Your goal is to strengthen advanced practice nurse relationships with your legislators.

Modified from New York State Association of Licensed Midwives (NYSALM). *The Voice of Midwives* letter.

federal and state laws that stipulate how they may contribute financially to campaigns. The advantage of a PAC is that small donations from many members add up to a significant donation to a campaign fund in the name of the organization. This gains the attention of the candidate and earns goodwill for the group.

Valid concern exists about the correlation of major PAC contributions and legislators' votes on special-interest legislation.

However, as long as PACs are a reality of political life, nurses need to recognize their power and support those that are committed to electing candidates sympathetic to health care issues.

Most national associations of health care providers, including nursing organizations, have PACs. Among the more powerful are those representing hospitals, nursing homes, health insurers, home health agencies, and pharmaceutical companies. A PAC that makes major political contributions is the American Medical Political Action Committee, sponsored by the American Medical Association. State medical associations also have strong PACs. This means that organized medicine has a powerful influence on national and state elections and on health care legislation at both levels.

Nurses and Campaigning

Helping someone win an election is a sure way of gaining influence. All candidates are grateful for campaign assistance and usually remember to thank those who have helped. Although campaign contributions are commonly thought of as financial, they can also take the form of participation in campaign activities. Nurses are frequently unable to contribute much money, but they can provide these invaluable services. For the novice, veteran campaigners are eager to help develop the necessary skills. Initially, a volunteer can address or stuff envelopes for mailings. The volunteer can also invite friends and neighbors for a social gathering to meet the candidate, thereby providing an opportunity to discuss issues of concern with constituents. Telephone banks help a candidate identify supporters, opponents, and the critical undecided voters. This last group can make a difference on Election Day and is courted by all candidates. The telephone interviews are highly structured and easily handled by inexperienced campaign workers. Direct contact with potential voters may occur later in the form of house-to-house block walks or poll work on Election Day. The confidence that this process requires comes with experience and a strong commitment to the candidate and the cause. Hosting a social function to allow nurse colleagues to meet the candidate is a welcome contribution to the campaign. Nurses are substantial in number, and their voting record is humanistic; therefore they are valued as a political force. Government employees may be restricted by policies that limit or disallow political activism. Nurses employed at any level of government should be aware of such prohibitions.

Nurses and Voting Strength

With over 4 million members, nurses make up the largest profession in health care (Kaiser, 2016). Therefore if every RN voted, their influence on health policy would be tremendous. If the nursing profession is to meet the challenges of the twenty-first century and work as a profession to positively influence the health of populations, political action is necessary, and an understanding of the factors that motivate or impede political action is needed (Winter and Lockhart, 1997).

Nurses in Public Office

President Donald Trump named Sylvia Trent-Adams, PhD, RN, on April 20, 2017, as acting surgeon general. Sylvia Trent-Adams is the first nurse to hold the position.

The Office of the Surgeon General is within the Office of the Assistant Secretary for Health and is responsible for the Commissioned Corps. In addition, the surgeon general is an advisor on public health and scientific issues. The surgeon general also is a spokesperson for certain focused public health issues.

Other women who have been active in the federal government are Carolyn Davis, who in 2001 served as the administrator of the Health Care Financing Administration (renamed the CMS); Shirley Chater, commissioner of the SSA; and Patricia Montoya, commissioner for Children, Youth, and Families. Virginia Trotter Betts, who served as the president of the ANA, was also the senior advisor on nursing and policy to the secretary of HHS in Washington, DC.

Likewise, Dr. Beverly Malone resigned as president of the ANA in 1999 to assume the position of deputy assistant secretary of the HHS. In this capacity, she advised the assistant secretary for the HHS, Dr. David Satcher, in program and political matters, policy and program development, and setting of legislative priorities. Lastly, Janet Heinrich is associate administrator of the HRSA's Bureau of Health Professionals, and Michele Richardson is the senior advisor for national workforce diversity in the Bureau of Health Professions (NLN, 2010).

In the 114th Congress, the number of nurses serving was three. This is a major achievement for nursing. It provides a direct voice for nursing concerns and nursing expertise–related health care in general. The Congressional Nursing Caucus provides a nonpartisan forum for the discussion of issues that affect the nursing profession. It also allows members of Congress, nurses, and nonnurse members who care about these issues to come together to address them.

In the future, more nurses need to run for public office at all three levels of government. Whether serving as political appointees or career bureaucrats, nurses have much to offer. New nurses should accept the challenge of helping advance the nursing practice and the nation's health.

⍰ ACTIVE LEARNING EXERCISE

1. Serve as a volunteer in a campaign for a candidate who is supportive or potentially supportive of public health or nursing issues, or volunteer for a political party.
2. Invite an elected official who is sympathetic to nurses to speak to the local chapter of the National Student Nurses Association to discuss the political process and health policy.
3. Invite an elected official to spend a day engaging in appropriate activities with a public health nurse or nursing student. Take black-and-white photos for press use.

HEALTH CARE REFORM AND RESTRUCTURING OF THE HEALTH CARE INDUSTRY

Health care reform was a major topic of discussion during the 2016 presidential election. With the election of President Trump and significant Republican majorities in both the Senate and the House, it appears that health care reform will continue to be a headline. After the failed attempt at comprehensive reform during the early years of the Clinton presidency, politicians recognized some of the major concerns and issues and addressed them proactively. For example, strong opposition from many health care provider groups (e.g., physicians) and health care industry groups (e.g., insurers, pharmaceutical companies, hospitals) led to failure of the Clinton plan. In 2009, congressional leaders early on sought ways to attract leaders of these groups and persuade them to support reform measures, although passage of health care reform was not easy and there continues to be variable support for the initiatives in the legislation.

A great deal of debate on what should be included in reform was evident throughout 2009. Major items of contention included whether to require all Americans to purchase coverage (i.e., a health insurance mandate), whether there would be a "government option" whereby people could elect to be covered by an extension of Medicare (or another similar program sponsored and funded by the government), whether government funds would pay for abortions, and how all of the changes and mandates would eventually be financed. After much public and private debate, in March 2010, the House of Representatives rather reluctantly passed the bill that the Senate had approved in late 2009, and President Obama signed it into law on March 23, 2010.

Although the 2010 Patient Protection and Affordable Care Act remains extremely controversial, health care reform is a nursing issue, and few nurses will argue with the statement that reform is needed in the health system in the United States. In virtually every practice arena, nurses see the inequalities and inadequacies that diminish the nation's level of wellness. Recognition of these problems is important to discussions of reform, and changing policies and targeting popular beliefs that create barriers to reform are essential in correcting the inequalities and inadequacies.

These are some of the areas targeted by the Health Care Reform Act. For example, insurers will no longer be able to drop coverage for those who are seriously ill because the act prohibits health insurance plans from placing lifetime limits on coverage and prohibits insurers from rescinding coverage for those who are diagnosed with chronic or life-threatening conditions. Additionally, mechanisms to reduce administrative costs are encouraged (Kaiser Family Foundation, 2016).

Popular sentiments about governmental control over health care have mirrored attitudes concerning the government's role in general; this was very evident during the debates over reform. The politically viable range of cost-control measures available to public programs has been limited to cutbacks in payments to providers rather than limits on the demand for clinical services or limits on individual choice

At the same time the United States is implementing health care reform, the country is also coping with the health problems of today's military veterans. When these soldiers are discharged, they continue to require care, often for complex physical and mental issues. According to the Kaiser Family Foundation (2016):

Given the growing need for providing health care and related benefits to the nation's service members, policymakers will continue to focus on strengthening both the Department of Defense [DoD] Military Health System and the Department

of Veterans Affairs (VA) health care system, which operate in parallel and in conjunction with each other. There is also greater emphasis in policy circles on ensuring a "seamless transition" process for service members moving from active duty into the VA health care system. Areas of focused attention include coordination between health and other benefits offered by the DoD and the VA, improving care for injured service members, and easing the transition from combat service to other military or civilian life.

Nurses encounter veterans in all types of community and public health settings. Knowledge about these problems and health policies changes is important to providing effective care in the community.

On December 4, 2016, the Department of Veterans Affairs published a final ruling giving veterans direct access to care by nurse practitioners, certified nurse midwives, and clinical nurse specialists. Through this ruling these advanced practice RNs are able to have full practice authority when practicing at VA health care centers across the country.

RESEARCH HIGHLIGHTS

National Sample of Registered Nurses

The Division of Nursing, a component of the HRSA, helps direct policy through the National Sample Survey of Registered Nurses. Conducted nine times since 1977, this survey was done most recently in March 2008, and preliminary findings were released in 2010. The national survey looks at trends in demographics, employment, education, and compensation among RNs. Here are some of the findings:

- Number of licensed RNs in the United States grew by almost 5.3% between 2004 and 2008, to a new high of slightly more than 3 million.
- Average age of RNs climbed to 47 years, the highest average age since the first comparable report was published in 1980.
- Average annual earning for RNs was $66,973.
- Real earnings (comparable dollars over time) have grown almost 16% since 2004.
- The share of RNs whose initial nursing education was a bachelor's degree in nursing rose from 31% to 33.7% between 2004 and 2008.
- Employment in nursing rose to almost 85% of RNs with active licenses, the highest since 1980.
- The number of RNs with master's or doctorate degrees rose to more than 400,000, an increase of 32% from 2000.

Data from Health Resources and Services Administration: *The registered nurse population: Initial findings from the 2008 national sample survey of registered nurses,* Washington, DC, 2010, Author.

NURSES AND LEADERSHIP IN HEALTH POLICY DEVELOPMENT

As the role of nurses in changing health care policy increases in importance, more nurses are needed who are equipped for this challenge. A strong cadre of nursing leaders who have the vision for change is essential to promoting nursing's policy agenda. National fellowships and internships are available for nurses who are interested in taking leadership roles

The Robert Wood Johnson Health Policy Fellowship is a 1-year career development program for midcareer health professionals. The goal of this program is to help its fellows gain an understanding of the health policy process and contribute to the formulation of new policies and programs. Robert Wood Johnson Health Policy fellows are selected from academic faculties from diverse disciplines, including medicine, dentistry, nursing, public health, health services administration, economics, and social services. After an extensive orientation on the legislative and executive branches of government, the fellows work with a member of Congress or on a congressional health committee.

The President's Commission on White House Fellowships offers 20 fellowships each year to professionals, including nurses, early in their careers; the average age of participants is 33 years. The White House fellows participate in an education program that involves working with government officials, scholars, journalists, and private-sector leaders to explore U.S. policy in action. Nurses who have been White House fellows may work at the CMS and the Office of Science and Technology Policy, among others (White House, n.d.). These fellowship programs are competitive, but strong leaders are desperately needed.

Nursing should also incorporate private health policy into its policy agenda. Nurses can influence private health care organizations from internal and external positions. From an internal perspective, nurses hold important management positions in health care organizations. This placement allows them to have direct involvement in policy setting. Nurses also support and use nursing research that demonstrates positive clinical and economic outcomes. All of these activities serve to validate the importance of nursing within the health system (Pulcini et al., 2000).

External strategies that nurses can use to influence private health policy include participation in discussions regarding quality care and cost of care (Pulcini et al., 2000). Nurses should monitor the quality ratings of health care organizations and suggest changes that would improve care. Nurses also are developing entrepreneurial practices to provide lower-cost services for underserved groups. Nurses need to do more to request that nursing services be reimbursable under all types of health care coverage plans and programs. Interprofessional care is a key topic today, and nurses need to work with other health care providers to build teams that can influence private policy.

ACTIVE LEARNING EXERCISE

Look at a current public health issue that affects your community, including an understanding of the causes, effect on the public, and possible solutions. Influence its resolution through any of the following activities:

1. Write a succinct letter to the editor of a local newspaper.
2. Write a position paper and submit it to the "opinion page" of a local newspaper.
3. Write to elected or appointed officials whose jurisdiction may be influential on the issue.
4. Meet with an elected or appointed official to discuss the issue in groups of two or three. Write a one-page summary of your "talking points" to leave with the official.
5. Call in to a radio talk show about the issue.
6. Volunteer to speak on the issue to appropriate consumer or professional groups.

SUMMARY

Historically, nurses have been able to make significant differences in the quality of life experienced by the members of the communities in which they serve. By understanding how government works, how bills become laws, and how legislators make decisions, nurses can influence policy decisions through individual efforts such as electronic letter writing, social networking, participation in political campaigns, and selection of candidates who support policies conducive to improving the health and welfare of all citizens. When organized in lobbying groups, coalitions, and PACs, or when holding office, nurses can be a powerful force that brings about change in the delivery and quality of the health care of aggregates.

ⓔ EVOLVE WEBSITE

http://evolve.elsevier.com/Nies/community
- NCLEX Review Questions
- Case Studies

BIBLIOGRAPHY

Almgren G: *Health care, politics, policy and services*, New York, 2012, Springer.

American Nurses Association: ANA advises on health care reform, *Capital Update* 11(8):1, 1993.

American Nurses Association (ANA), 2017. http://nursingworld.org/MainMenuCategories/Policy-Advocacy. www.nursingworld.org/Function/ menucategory/aboutANA.aspx.

Centers for Disease Control and Prevention: *Ten essential services for public health*, 2015. Retrieved from: https://www.cdc.gov/stltpublichealth/hop/pdfs/Ten_Essential_Public_Health_Services_2011-09_508.pdf.

DeParle J: States struggle to use windfall born of shifts in welfare law, *New York Times*, August 29, 1999.

Hall-Long BA: Nursing's past, present, and future political experiences, *Nurs Health Care Perspect* 16(1):24–28, 1995.

Health Resources and Services Administration: *The registered nurse population: initial findings from the national 2008 sample survey of registered nurses*. Washington, DC, HRSA.

Henry J, Kaiser Family Foundation: *Military and veterans' health care*, http://www.kaiseredu.org/Issue-Modules/Military-and-Veterans-Health-Care/Background-Brief.aspx.

Institute of Medicine: *Future of public health*, Washington, DC, 1988, The National Academies Press.

Kaiser Family Foundation, 2016. From: <http://kff.org/>.

Kalisch PA, Kalisch BJ: *American nursing: a history*, ed 4, Philadelphia, 2004, Lippincott Williams & Wilkins.

Knight W: *Managed care: what it is and how it works*, Gaithersburg, MD, 1998, Aspen Publishers, Inc.

Kostas-Polston E, Thanavaro J, Arvidson CR, Taub LFM: Advanced practice nursing: shaping health through policy, *J Am Assoc Nurse Pract* 27(1):11–20, 2015.

Lewinson SB: A historical perspective on policy, politics and nursing. In Mason DJ, Leavitt JK, Chaffee MW, editors: *Policy and politics in nursing and health care*, ed 7, Philadelphia, 2007, Saunders.

Litman T: *Health, politics and policy*, ed 5, Albany, NY, Delmar.

Lyttle B: Humanizing childbirth, *Am J Nurs* 100(10):52–53, 2000.

Mason DJ, Leavitt JK, Chaffee MW: Policy and politics: a framework for action. In *Policy and politics in nursing and health care*, ed 7, St. Louis, 2007, Saunders.

Merriam-Webster: *Merriam-Webster Dictionary*, 2014. Retrieved from: http://www.merriam-webster.com/dictionary/policy.

National League for Nursing, 2010. http://www.nln.org/newsletter/aug092010.htm.

Nurses for a Healthier Tomorrow: *Mission/purpose*, 2014. http://www.nursesource.org/mission.html.

Pickett G, Hanlon JJ: *Public health administration and practice*, ed 9, St. Louis, 1990, Mosby.

Pulcini J, Mason DJ, Cohen SS, et al.: Health policy and the private sector: new vistas for nursing, *Nurs Health Care Perspect* 21(1):22–28, 2000.

Robert Wood Johnson: *Enduring trust: nurses again top Gallup's poll on honesty and ethics*, 2012. Retrieved from: http://www.rwjf.org/en/blogs/human-capital-blog/2012/12/enduring_trust_nurs.html.

Rychnovsky J: Dr. Ruth Lubic, a timeliness and tireless visionary for childbearing families, *J Obstet Gynecol Neonatal Nurs* 40(5): 509–511, 2011.

Taylor M: Impact of advocacy initiatives on nurses' motivation to sustain momentum in public policy advocacy, *J Prof Nurs* 32(3): 235–245, 2016.

Thomas J: Introduction, *Library Trends* 46(2), 1997.

U.S. Department of Health and Human Services: *Healthy People 2010*. Conference ed. Washington, DC, USDHHS.

U.S. Department of Health and Human Services: *Centers for Medicare and Medicaid Services: FY 2017 budget in brief*, 2017. Available from: <https://www.hhs.gov/about/budget/fy2017/budget-in-brief/index.html.

U.S. Department of Health and Human Services: Office of Disease Prevention and Health Promotion. *Healthy People 2020*, 2013, Accessed January 22, 2014 at http://www.healthypeople.gov/2020/about/history.aspx.

U.S. Department of Health and Human Services, Health Resources and Services Administration: Accessed May 1, 2017.

U.S. Department of Health and Human Services: Secretary's Advisory Committee on National Health Promotion and Disease Prevention for 2020: Healthy People 2020, phase I report. Available from: https://www.healthypeople.gov/sites/default/files/PhaseI_0.pdf

White House: White House Fellows. Retrieved from: https://www.whitehouse.gov/participate/fellows

Winter MK, Lockhart JS: From motivation to action: understanding nurses' political involvement, *Nurs Health Care Perspect* 18(5): 244–250, 1997.

11

The Health Care System

Melanie McEwen and Marie E. McBee

OUTLINE

OBJECTIVES

Upon completion of this chapter, the reader will be able to do the following:
1. Describe the organization of the public health care subsystem at the federal, state, and local levels.
2. Compare and contrast the scopes of the private health care subsystem and the public health care subsystem.

3. Describe the roles of the members of the interprofessional health care team.
4. Discuss the relationship of critical health care issues to the health care organization and health care providers.
5. Discuss future concerns for the health care delivery system.

KEY TERMS

accreditation
Agency for Healthcare Research and
  Quality (AHRQ)
client rights
community health center
complementary and alternative
  therapies
electronic health record/electronic
  medical record
health disparities

Health Plan Effectiveness Stat
  Information Set (HEDIS)
managed care
managed care organizations
Medicaid
Medicare
National Committee for Quality
  Assurance (NCQA)
outcomes measures

Patient Protection and Affordable
  Care Act (ACA)
patient rights
patient-centered medical homes
public health
quality care
telehealth
The Joint Commission
voluntary agencies

OVERVIEW: THE HEALTH CARE SYSTEM

The health care system of the United States is dynamic, multifaceted, and not comparable with any other health care system in the world. It is regularly praised for its technological breakthroughs, frequently criticized for its high costs, continues to experience major problems with its quality, and often is difficult to access for those most in need. This chapter describes the major components of the health care system, critical health care organization and provider issues, and the role of government in public health and health care reform and presents a futuristic perspective.

COMPONENTS OF THE HEALTH CARE SYSTEM

The current health care system consists of private and public health care subsystems (Fig. 11.1). The private health care subsystem includes personal care services from various sources, both nonprofit and profit, and numerous voluntary agencies. The major focus of the public health subsystem is prevention of disease and illness. These subsystems are not always mutually exclusive, and their functions sometimes overlap.

With the rapid growth of technology and increased demands on the private and public health care subsystems, health care

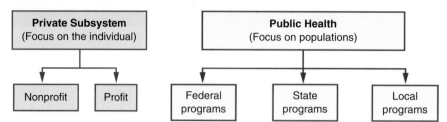

FIG. 11.1 U.S. health care system.

costs have become prohibitive. Cost-effectiveness and cost containment have become critical driving forces as health care delivery system changes are made; however, cost-effectiveness often conflicts with the provision of quality care. Additionally, considerable attention to "health care reform" and subsequent passage of the **Patient Protection and Affordable Care Act (ACA)** in 2010 have demonstrated the critical importance of access to health care for all Americans, but the enormous challenges that accompany that desire remain. There continues to be a need to apply the vast resources and tools available and to focus science and information technology in a way that will improve effectiveness and efficiency and produce high-quality health care (IOM, 2012a).

Public health nursing requires an understanding of the mission, organization, and role of both the private and the public health care subsystems and the contexts within which they function to effectively collaborate with health care providers and organizations to reach health goals. An organizational framework in which private and voluntary organizations and the government work collaboratively to prevent disease and promote health is essential. Public health nurses are in a unique position to provide leadership and facilitate change in the health care system that will help improve health and safety for all.

Private Health Care Subsystem

Most personal health care services are provided in the private sector. Services in the private subsystem include health promotion, prevention and early detection of disease, diagnosis and treatment of disease with a focus on cure, rehabilitative-restorative care, and custodial care. These services are provided in clinics, physicians' offices, hospitals, hospital ambulatory centers, skilled care facilities, and homes. Increasingly, these private-sector services are available through **managed care organizations** (MCOs).

Private health care services in the United States began with a simple model. Physicians provided care in their offices and made home visits. Patients were admitted to hospitals for general care if they experienced serious complications during the course of their illness. Currently, a variety of highly skilled health care professionals provide comprehensive, preventive, restorative, rehabilitative, and palliative care. Interprofessional teams have become more important. A broad array of services is available, ranging from general to highly specialized, with multiple delivery configurations.

Personal care provided by physicians and other health care professionals is delivered under the following five basic models:
1. The solo practice of a physician in an office continues to be present in many communities.

2. The single-specialty group model consists of physicians in the same specialty who pool expenses, income, and offices.
3. Multispecialty group practice provides for interaction among specialty areas.
4. The integrated health maintenance model has prepaid multispecialty physicians.
5. The **community health center**, developed through federal funds in the 1960s, addresses broader inputs into health such as education and housing.

Managed care has become a dominant paradigm in health care, affecting many aspects of health care delivery. Managed care involves capitated payments for care rather than fee-for-service. Health care providers, including physicians, hospitals, community clinics, and home care providers, are integrated in a system such as a health maintenance organization. See Chapter 12 for a more detailed discussion of managed care and reimbursement.

Though change in the configuration of the health care system is common, some of the newer changes relate more to the community than in the past. For example, more physician practices are joining together to form multispecialty groups, and hospitals are buying practices to expand their market into the community. The solo practice is fading. In addition, there are more advanced nurse practitioners (ANPs) and physician's assistants (PAs) who are assuming primary practice roles in a variety of settings, including community clinics, retail health clinics, and home health, and many who are opening their own practices. **Patient-centered medical homes** are practices that offer a team approach to assist in coordination of care for positive outcomes, providing comprehensive primary care. This model, which is connected to health care reform, is relatively new, and thus its long-term success is unknown. As health care reform legislation continues to be debated and modified, additional changes will likely occur.

Voluntary Agencies

Voluntary or nonofficial agencies refer to the nongovernmental, nonprofit entities that support health care provision and sometimes direct health services. **Voluntary agencies** are a part of the private health care system that developed in the United States at about the same time that the government was assuming responsibility for public health. During the 1700s and early 1800s, voluntary efforts to improve health were virtually nonexistent, because early settlers from Western Europe were not accustomed to participating in organized charity. Immigration expanded to include slaves from Africa and people from Eastern Europe, and their well-being received little attention.

Toward the end of the nineteenth century, new immigrants brought a heritage of social protest and reform. Wealthy businesspeople, such as the Rockefellers, Carnegies, and Mellons, responded to the needs of the poor and set up foundations that provided funds for charitable endeavors, including health. District nurses, such as Lillian Wald, established nursing practices in the large cities for the poor and destitute. These services were not exclusively focused on illness, but also on work conditions, health, communicable diseases, living conditions, and language skills. Voluntary initiatives from philanthropically focused families remain an important resource even into the twenty-first century. An example is the Gates Foundation, which is very active in health care concerns, particularly from a global perspective.

Voluntary agencies can be classified into those dealing with the following categories of health (Hanlon and Pickett, 1990):

a. Specific diseases, such as the American Diabetes Association, American Cancer Society, and National Multiple Sclerosis Society
b. Organ or body structures, such as the National Kidney Foundation and the American Heart Association
c. Health and welfare of special groups, such as the National Council on Aging and the March of Dimes
d. Particular phases of health, such as the Planned Parenthood Federation of America

Philanthropic groups also support research and programs. Many professional organizations, such as the American Medical Association, the American Nurses Association, the American Hospital Association, and the American Public Health Association, as well as many other professional organizations, have a significant role in advocacy and in providing professional expertise.

Voluntary organizations are major sources of help in the prevention of disease, promotion of health, treatment of illness, advocacy, consumer education, and research. For example, private and voluntary organizations currently support clients with human immunodeficiency virus (HIV). In many cities, the Chicken Soup Brigade provides meals for clients with HIV who are unable to cook for themselves, and HIV support groups exist in most larger communities. Services for the homeless such as meals, temporary housing and housing during the winter, medical care, and job support are common in most large cities. Overlap of services often occurs among the numerous private, voluntary, and public agencies. The private and public agencies provide a wide array of services, but sometimes duplication causes them to not be cost effective.

Voluntary agencies and organizations play a very important role in health care delivery. Indeed, it is anticipated that the emerging health care system will become an amalgam of different public and private forces that will work together to provide integrated, resource-conscious, population-based services. Further, the system needs to become more innovative and diverse in how it responds to health problems and more concerned with disease prevention and promotion of health in order to address the very significant disparities in health care (AHRQ, 2015).

ACTIVE LEARNING

Identify a voluntary agency or organization and review its website. What services does it offer? How does the agency collaborate with other groups and organizations? How is the agency/organization funded? How does it interface with the local public health agency? What information is available to consumers and professionals? With classmates, set up a site visit.

Public Health Subsystem

Although not explicitly addressing health or health care, the U.S. Constitution mandates that the federal government "promote the general welfare of its citizens." The public health subsystem therefore is required by law to address the health of populations by promoting their "general welfare." Legal provisions at the local, state, and federal levels of government direct the establishment, implementation, and evaluation of these activities. At the federal level, Congress enacts laws and writes rules and regulations. The various departments of the executive branch implement and administer them. Interpretations of, and amendments to, the Constitution, as well as Supreme Court decisions over time, have changed and enlarged the role of the federal government in health activities.

Federal policies and practices have had a significant influence on local and state governments in meeting health and social problems, and many laws have been enacted to respond to changing health needs and concerns. Coordination of federal services under several agencies culminated in the establishment of the Department of Health, Education, and Welfare under President Eisenhower in 1953. In 1979, this department was separated into the Department of Education and the Department of Health and Human Services (HHS). Currently, HHS is the second largest department of the federal government; only the Department of Defense is larger.

Public health refers to the efforts organized by society to protect, promote, and restore the people's health. Public health programs, services, and institutions emphasize the prevention of disease and address the health needs of the population as a whole. Public health activities typically respond to changing technology and social values, but the goals remain the same (i.e., to reduce the amount of disease, premature death, and disease-produced discomfort and disability).

The public health subsystem is concerned with the health of the population and a healthy environment. The scope of public health is broad and encompasses activities that promote good health. The public health subsystem is organized into multiple levels (i.e., federal, state, and local) to establish laws, rules, and regulations to protect the public and to more effectively provide services to those who are unable to obtain health care without assistance. Fig. 11.2 provides an overview of this system, specifically for the state of Ohio, although the basic organization will be similar across states.

Federal-Level Subsystem

Most health-related activities at the federal level are implemented and administered by the HHS, which consists of

FIG. 11.2 The public health system in Ohio. (From Health Policy Institute of Ohio: *Ohio public health basics*, 2012, p. 4. Retrieved from http://www.healthpolicyohio.org/wp-content/uploads/2014/01/publichealthbasics_final012520131.pdf)

11 major agencies (Box 11.1). This department is divided into 10 regions and is directed by the secretary of Health and Human Services. The secretary is assisted by numerous undersecretaries and assistant secretaries (USDHHS, 2017). The surgeon general is the principal deputy to the assistant secretary of HHS. In spring 2017, Rear Admiral Sylvia Trent-Adams became one of the first nurses to serve as "acting" surgeon general in a role she held for several months; she is currently a deputy surgeon general..

In addition to HHS, many federal agencies perform activities related to health. For example, the Department of Education is involved with health education and school health. The Department of Agriculture administers the inspection of meat and milk and provides funds for the Women, Infants, and Children program (supplemental nutrition), the food stamp program, and the school-based nutrition program. Other federal agencies of interest to public health nurses are the U.S. Environmental Protection Agency, the Occupational Safety and Health Administration, the Veterans Administration, and the Federal Emergency Management Agency.

The scope of health services of the federal-level subsystem targets the following major health areas: the general population,

special populations, and international health. For the general population, federal activities include protection against hazards, maintenance of vital and health statistics, advancement of scientific knowledge through research, and provision of disaster relief. In recent years, public health efforts have been directed toward changing behaviors by fostering healthy eating habits, encouraging exercise, and preventing or reducing tobacco, drug, and alcohol use. Other programs have provided nutritional food and food stamps to individuals and families to ensure adequate food intake.

Services for special populations include protection of workers against hazardous occupations and work conditions and health care for military veterans, Native Americans, Alaska natives, federal prisoners, and members of the armed services. In addition, the federal government provides special services for children, older adults, the mentally ill, and the vocationally handicapped.

In the international arena, the federal government works with other countries and international health organizations such as the World Health Organization and the Red Cross.

BOX 11.1 Structure of the U.S. Department of Health and Human Services

The USDHHS is composed of many agencies that provide different services related to U.S. health care. Among them are the following:

- The **Administration for Community Living** combines the Administration on Aging—the agency responsible for coordinating home- and community-based services for older persons and their caregivers—and the Office on Disability and the Administration on Developmental Disabilities in a single agency, with enhanced policy and program support for cross-cutting initiatives to serve these populations.
- The **Centers for Medicare and Medicaid Services** administers Medicare and Medicaid programs.
- The **Administration for Children and Families** provides family assistance (welfare), child support, Head Start, and other programs to strengthen the family unit.
- The **Centers for Disease Control and Prevention (CDC)** conducts and supports programs directed at preventing and controlling infectious diseases; they assist states during epidemics. In addition, they provide services related to health promotion and education and professional development and training. The CDC includes the **Agency for Toxic Substances and Disease Registry**, which serves the public by using the best science, taking responsive public health actions, and providing trusted health information to prevent harmful exposures and diseases related to toxic substances.
- The **Food and Drug Administration** provides surveillance over the safety and efficacy of foods, pharmaceuticals, and other consumer goods.
- The **Healthcare Resources and Services Administration** is concerned with the development of health services programs and facilities. The Division of Nursing is in this unit. A major focus of this agency is funding grants for nursing education and training.
- The **Indian Health Service** provides health services for Native Americans and Alaska Natives.
- The **National Institutes of Health (NIH)** performs and supports research programs. The focus of these efforts is to develop and extend the scientific knowledge base related to their respective areas. The National Institute for Nursing Research, which is part of NIH, focuses on nursing research.
- The **Substance Abuse and Mental Health Services Administration** awards grants and funds research related to problems with substance abuse and mental health.
- The **Agency for Healthcare Quality and Research** works to improve quality, safety, efficiency, and effectiveness of health care services for all Americans.

These entities combine efforts to monitor health and diseases and to promote various health programs throughout the world.

The current HHS maintains a strategic plan (USDHHS, 2015). The goals for 2015–2018 are:

- Strengthen health care
- Advance scientific knowledge and innovation
- Advance health, safety, and well-being of the American people
- Ensure the efficiency, transparency, accountability, and effectiveness of HHS programs

The HHS has been deeply involved in implementation of the ACA. This has included oversight of the state exchanges, awarding funding to meet the law's requirements; measuring program performance to ensure program integrity; and informing the public of requirements, mandates, and results. Changes brought by subsequent changes to the ACA will also likely require supervision of the HHS.

State-Level Subsystem

States are responsible for the health of their citizens and are the central authorities in the public health care system. The organization and activities of public health services vary widely among the states. A health commissioner or secretary of health is typically appointed by the governor and directs most state health agencies. The health officer is usually a physician with a degree and experience in public health. In some states, the health officer directs the state's health department. Many states have boards of health, which determine policies and priorities for allocation of funds. Staffing of the state agency varies among states; however, in comparison with other state programs, state health programs usually have a large staff.

The state health department does not exist in a vacuum. The United States requires an integrated system so that both federal and state levels work to the benefit of all citizens. Thus the state health departments are highly dependent on the federal level for resources and guidance. For example, funds contributed by the federal government to Medicaid, which is jointly funded by the federal government and states, have been changed over time and vary with respect to beneficiaries and services covered by each state. This has had a major impact on services that states can provide to their most vulnerable citizens.

One of the major provisions of the ACA resulting in large numbers of Americans receiving health care coverage was through the expansion of Medicaid; however, each state was allowed to determine whether they would accept this expansion. Ultimately, 31 states and the District of Columbia elected to extend Medicaid coverage through the ACA and 19 chose not to (Familiesusa.org, 2017). Without major legislative changes involving the ACA, it is anticipated that more states will elect to expand Medicaid to other beneficiaries with federal assistance.

Cooperation between the state and federal levels of the health care system has also been brought to the forefront with efforts to plan for bioterrorism and disasters. According to the scope of health services, the state-level subsystem is responsible for its own public health laws; therefore state policy varies widely. Factors that affect the level of state services include state-legislated or mandated services; political factors related to division of power between state and local health departments (LHDs); and competition among officials, providers, and the business community.

As discussed in previous chapters, the three core functions of public health are assessment, policy development, and assurance (IOM, 1988). Assessment activities include the collection of data pertaining to vital statistics, health facilities, and human resources; epidemiological activities, such as communicable disease control, health screening, and laboratory analyses; and participation in research projects. In the area of policy development, states formulate goals, develop health plans, and set standards for local health agencies. Assurance activities involve inspection in a variety of areas, licensing of health professionals and organizations, health education, environmental safety, and resource development.

Local Health Department Subsystems

LHDs are generally responsible for the direct delivery of public health services and protection of the health of citizens, although not all communities/counties have LHDs. State and local (i.e., city and county) governments delegate the authority to conduct these activities. The organization of LHDs varies widely depending on community size, economics, partnerships with the private health care system, health care facilities, business support, health care needs, transportation, and the number of citizens requiring public health care. Some LHDs function as district offices of the state health department; others are responsible to local government and the state; and still others—particularly those in large cities—are autonomous. An LHD may be a separate agency or a division within an agency, such as the HHS.

A health officer or administrator appointed by local government directs the LHD. At least half of the states require that the health officer of an LHD have a medical degree. An interdisciplinary team carries out the activities of the department. Public health nurses and health inspectors represent the two largest groups of professional staff members. Other professional staff members include dentists, social workers, epidemiologists, nutritionists, and health educators.

According to the designated scope of services, the LHD subsystem is responsible for monitoring the health status and meeting the health needs of their constituents. This includes identifying unmet needs and taking actions to meet these needs. Most services to groups and individuals are provided at the local level. These services fall into the following four major categories:

Community health services include control of communicable disease such as surveillance and immunizations, maternal-child health programs, nutrition services, and education. Health promotion education is directed toward changing behavior; individuals are encouraged to eat healthy foods; exercise more; and decrease their use of tobacco, drugs, and alcohol. Other programs provide nutritious food and food stamps to individuals and families. A major activity of LHDs is to perform preventive screening for potential problems throughout the lifespan of their community members.

Environmental health services include food hygiene such as inspection of food-producing and food-processing plants and restaurants; protection from hazardous substances; control of waste, air, noise, and water pollution; and occupational health. The objective of these activities is to provide a safe environment.

Personal health services provide care to individuals and families in clinics, schools, and correctional institutions. In many areas, home health care services are provided through the LHD.

Mental health services are provided through LHDs in many communities. These services are supported by funds offered by local and regional mental health and mental retardation facilities and programs. See Chapter 24 for more information on community-based mental health care.

LHDs establish local health codes, fund public hospitals such as city and/or county hospitals, and provide services to populations and individuals at risk who often lack health insurance. Programs and services for state health departments and LHDs vary among jurisdictions. The services provided reflect the values of the residents and officials, available resources, and perceived needs of their respective populations within their state and local area. Although the goals of the public health subsystem do not change, the programs and services evolve to meet the changing needs of the public.

Several provisions of the ACA addressed improvement of quality and access to care. For example, the law promoted establishment of local consortiums of health care providers to coordinate health care services for low-income uninsured and underinsured populations. It also substantially increased funds for community health centers and financed development of school-based health centers and nurse-managed health clinics.

Summary of Public Health's Three Levels

In the preceding description of the three government levels that provide public health services (i.e., local, state, and federal), distinctive and overlapping roles have been discussed. The federal government has been assuming a larger role in the protection of the population through regulation and funding. It finances specific programs such as Medicare and categorical programs for mothers and infants and provides direct care to special populations, for example, military veterans. States establish health codes, regulate the insurance industry, and license health care facilities and personnel. States also provide funds for services offered through Medicaid. Direct care activities funded by state health departments may include care in mental hospitals, state medical schools, and associated hospitals. LHDs are the primary agencies that provide direct services to communities, families, and individuals.

> **? ACTIVE LEARNING**
>
> 1. Describe the organization of the state and local health departments.
> 2. Visit the local health department and learn what services are provided. How do these services relate to *Healthy People 2020* objectives?
> 3. Identify regional and state health services and providers.

Health Care Providers

Providers of health care are individuals, groups, and organizations that deliver or support health care services. This section describes the different types of health care providers, including provider organizations, health care professionals, and nontraditional providers.

Provider Organizations

The following are examples of health care provider organizations:

- Hospital
- Clinic
- Physician practice
- Ambulatory care center
- Home health agency
- Long-term care facility
- Skilled nursing facility
- Rehabilitation center
- Hospice service
- Public health department
- School health clinic

- Birthing center
- Ambulatory surgical center
- Occupational health clinic
- Crisis clinic
- Community health center
- Retail health clinics located in retail stores, supermarkets, and pharmacies
- Any other type of organization that provides health care within the community

Health care provider organizations are undergoing tremendous changes. This is particularly true of hospitals, many of which are merging, consolidating, and closing. These changes have an impact on the entire community health system. With the increasing shift to ambulatory and primary care (see Box 11.2), hospital stays have shortened, and the patients who are admitted to the hospital are more acutely ill and require more intensive care. Consequently, reduced hospital stays result in more home care admissions or more discharges to long-term care facilities or skilled nursing units for short-term recovery and rehabilitation.

ETHICAL INSIGHTS

Universal Health Care

Universal health care coverage has been a topic of interest in the United States at least since the 1960s. The United States is the only developed country that does not have some form of universal health insurance. Although the ACA significantly reduced the number of uninsured individuals, there were 28 million people without health care coverage by the end of 2016 (Kaiser Family Foundation, 2016). Thus universal health coverage remains elusive. Clients without health coverage have a direct impact on communities, and health care providers should consider the following questions: Is health care a right of all citizens? Who is responsible for determining the right to health care access? What additional reforms will be necessary to resolve these questions? These are difficult questions, particularly in light of the growing problem of health care disparities in the United States.

BOX 11.2   Primary Care and Primary Prevention

"*Primary health care* is essential health care based on practical, scientifically sound, and socially acceptable methods and technology made universally accessible to individuals and families in the community through their full participation and at a cost that the community and country can afford to maintain at every stage of their development in the spirit of self-reliance and self-determination.... It is the first level of contact of individuals, the family, and the community with the national health system bringing health care as close as possible to where people live and work." (World Health Organization, 1978)

A physician, nurse practitioner, or physician's assistant may provide primary health care. Generally, the primary care provider's practice is in family medicine, internal medicine, or pediatrics. The primary care provider is responsible for health maintenance and for treatment of common illnesses and may refer clients to specialists as needed.

Primary prevention is a type of intervention that promotes health and prevents disease. Primary prevention includes immunizations and contraception, as well as promotion of good nutrition, exercise, and healthy lifestyle choices (e.g., avoidance of tobacco, limitation of alcohol).

How do these definitions compare? The WHO definition and the definition of primary care that is usually used in the United States are similar. Primary prevention is an intervention that is used in primary care services.

Health Care Professionals

The health care team has been growing and evolving significantly over the last decade, with members of the team taking on new responsibilities. There is greater emphasis today in all types of health care settings on using interprofessional teams to better coordinate care and to promote effective outcomes. The community particularly needs an interprofessional approach, because clients often have complex needs. Interprofessional teams have been recommended by the National Academy of Medicine (NAM), formerly called the Institute of Medicine (IOM) (2015a) and others. Indeed, working on interprofessional teams has been identified as a core competency for health care professions. Further, in recent years, there has been a push to move to more interprofessional education (IOM, 2015a; Interprofessional Professional Education Collaborative [IPEC], 2011; World Health Organization [WHO], 2010).

The following is a brief review of the major types of professional and nonprofessional members of the health care team:

- *Registered Nurse (RN):* This appears to be a simple designation, but different educational routes (i.e., diploma, associate degree, baccalaureate degree) exist to obtain a license to practice as an RN. In addition, many nurses now obtain master's degrees and doctorates. These advanced degrees provide nurses with the opportunity to do more independent practice, teach, and conduct research. Nurses represent the largest group of professionals providing health services, and they practice in all types of health settings. State legislatures determine licensure requirements and enact nurse practice acts. State boards of nursing are the administrative arm for implementation of these laws and regulations.
- *Advanced Nurse Practitioner (ANP):* This is a nurse who has obtained education beyond a baccalaureate degree and has studied content related to primary care or acute care. ANPs specialize in such areas as adult health, pediatrics, neonatology, gerontology, and psychiatric nursing. An ANP may work in a clinic, the community, a private practice, the home, a hospital, or a long-term care facility (i.e., any setting in which health care is provided). With health care reform raising the demand for primary care, it is expected that ANPs will provide more and more primary care.
- *Clinical Nurse Leader (CNL):* Clinical nurse leader is a new position that requires a master's degree. The CNL is a provider and manager of care at the point of care for individuals and cohorts and does not have a clinical specialty in the master's program. The types of positions that CNLs are taking are variable, though many are in acute care settings.
- *Clinical Nurse Specialist (CNS):* The clinical nurse specialist, who has a master's degree in a specialty area, provides acute care and guides other nursing staff in providing care. There are many fewer CNSs in clinical practice today, as the ANP role has become more common.
- *Nurse-Midwife (NM):* A nurse-midwife is a nurse who has completed an additional educational program focused on midwifery. NMs work in all types of settings in which women's health and obstetrical services are provided, and they may be very active in community health services.

- *Certified Registered Nurse Anesthetist (CRNA):* A CRNA has a master's or doctoral degree that educates them to provide anesthesia, often under a doctor's supervision. They typically work in hospitals, outpatient surgery centers, and physicians' offices.
- *Licensed Practical Nurse (LPN) or Licensed Vocational Nurse (LVN):* LPNs and LVNs perform some specific nursing functions and play a critical role in providing direct client care. They have high school degrees and additional training (usually 1 year) and work in all types of settings, typically under the direct supervision of an RN or a physician. They may work in hospitals, long-term care facilities, clinics, and homes.
- *Physician (MD or DO):* A physician has a medical degree; most physicians specialize in a specific area of practice (e.g., internal medicine, surgery, pediatrics, gynecology).
- *Physician Assistant (PA):* The PA is a "physician extender" who provides medical services under the supervision of a licensed physician. The role was developed in the 1960s in response to a shortage of primary care physicians in certain areas. PAs often work in primary care, but many specialize.
- *Registered Dietitian (RD):* This health care professional assesses the client's nutritional status and needs. RDs work in hospitals, long-term care facilities, clinics, community health centers, and homes.
- *Social Worker (SW):* SWs assist clients and their families with problems related to reimbursement, access to care, housing, care in the home, transportation, and social problems. They are discharge planners, particularly in acute care facilities or hospitals, often as case managers; however, they work in all types of settings. SWs may also have education to specialize in counseling. SWs are employed in many community agencies to help clients with a variety of needs, such as housing, ensuring that food is accessible, transportation, vocational assistance, medical equipment, and counseling.
- *Occupational Therapist (OT):* OTs assist clients with impaired functions or disabilities to reach the clients' maximum level of physical and psychosocial independence. They work in all types of settings, including with clients in their homes through home health agencies.
- *Speech-Language Pathologist:* Speech-language pathologists assist clients who need rehabilitative services related to speech, hearing, and language/communication disorders, as well as swallowing disorders. They work in all types of settings, including with clients in their homes through home health agencies.
- *Physical Therapist (PT):* PTs help clients who are experiencing musculoskeletal problems. These providers focus on maximizing physical functioning and work in all types of settings (e.g., hospitals, long-term care/rehabilitation, home health).
- *Pharmacist:* Pharmacists prepare and dispense medications. Pharmacists have become much more involved in educating clients about medications and in monitoring and evaluating the effects of medications. They work in all types of settings, including hospitals and community pharmacies.
- *Respiratory Therapist (RT):* RTs provide care to clients with respiratory illnesses. They use oxygen therapy, intermittent positive-pressure respirators, artificial mechanical ventilators, and inhalation therapy. Most RTs work in hospitals and long-term care, but they are becoming more common in home health care.
- *Chiropractor:* Chiropractors are concerned with improving the function of the clients' nervous system by means of various treatment modalities (e.g., spinal manipulation, diet, exercise, and massage). Chiropractors are mostly community based.
- *Paramedical Technologists:* Paramedical technologists work in various medical technology areas (e.g., radiology, nuclear medicine, and other laboratories).
- *Unlicensed Assistive Personnel (UAP):* Members of the health care team known as unlicensed assistive personnel have caused some controversy in last few years; however, the UAP is a critical member of the team. UAPs provide direct client care, supervised by RNs. The amount of education and training of UAPs is highly variable. UAPs work not only in acute care and long-term care but also for home health agencies.

Nontraditional Health Care Providers

Nontraditional health care providers deliver alternative or complementary therapies. During the last two decades, consumers have become more interested in this type of care and have demanded that it be available.

Although many large medical centers are now developing programs and centers that offer complementary therapies, reimbursement for these services is lagging. The National Institutes of Health (NIH) supports research focused on a wide array of alternative therapies and their effects on health and disease, and in 1998 established the National Center for Complementary and Alternative Medicine to meet the need. The name was recently changed to "National Center for Complementary and Integrative Health" to reflect recognition of the importance of incorporation of nontraditional therapies in health care. **Complementary and alternative therapies** provided by a variety of health care providers are extremely wide ranging. They include mediation, massage therapy, herbal therapy, healing touch, energetic healing, yoga, acupuncture, and acupressure. Ethnic healers, such as *curanderos,* and folk healers are also found in some communities. Training and licensure requirements for alternative therapists vary, but will probably become more standard as their care becomes more accepted. Many nurses have incorporated alternative therapies into their practices and seek educational opportunities on a wide range of associated topics.

CRITICAL ISSUES IN HEALTH CARE DELIVERY

Quality Care

Quality care has been a concern of consumers and providers for decades. Quality care is a difficult concept to define and more difficult to measure. In 1996, President Clinton established the Advisory Commission on Consumer Protection and Quality to address a number of issues that had been identified. This commission produced a report that supported improvement in consumer power and rights, a focus on vulnerable populations, promotion of accountability, reduction in errors, and an increase in health care safety. Further, they promoted evidence-based practice and enhanced investment in information systems (President's Advisory Commission on Consumer Protection and Quality in the Health Care Industry, 1999).

This report stimulated a series of more in-depth explorations of the health care delivery system. Key among them was the NAM's "Quality Chasm" series. In their series, the NAM defined *quality* as "the degree to which health services for individuals and populations increase the likelihood of desired health outcomes and are consistent with current professional knowledge" (IOM, 2001a, p. 232). This series has had a major impact on the U.S. health care delivery system and highlights of a number of the key reports are presented in Table 11.1.

The **Agency for Healthcare Research and Quality (AHRQ)** is the main federal organization that works to improve the safety and quality of the health care system. Following the 1999 NAM report "To Err Is Human," AHRQ led the response to improving the safety of health care. This was largely through funding research to make care safer and to improve quality by publishing materials to educate health care systems and professionals to put research into practice and through generation of measures and data to be used by providers and policymakers (AHRQ, 2017).

Among their numerous programs and initiatives, AHRQ support efforts for clinicians and providers include clinical guidelines and recommendations, the Team STEPPS program (Strategies and Tools to Enhance Performance and Patient Safety), and evidence-based education and training. With respect to quality and safety reports, AHRQ administers the "Consumer Assessment of Healthcare Providers and Systems" (CAHPS). CAHPS is a survey and reporting entity that collects data and provides reports and detailed information on consumers' experiences with specific aspects of their health plans and providers. This type of survey provides data that help purchasers of plans compare and contrast plans and allows informed consumers to select providers (AHRQ, 2017). Finally AHRQ publishes research and reports specifically related to health care disparities, quality, and evidence-based practice. These reports can be used by policymakers and others to make critical decisions about funding and promotion of research endeavors.

Accreditation

Accreditation is one means to assess the quality of services and care of the organization. Specific minimum standards must be met by an organization to obtain accreditation. Indeed, accreditation serves the purpose of instilling public confidence in a program, institution, or organization (NAM, 2016). Purchasers of care, including insurers and MCOs, are concerned about the accreditation status of health care organizations when they negotiate reimbursement contracts. Other entities, such nursing schools and medical schools, which use health care organizations for clinical sites, are also concerned with accreditation status.

Many groups provide accreditation for health care providers and health care organizations. For example, **The Joint Commission** was founded in 1951 to promote health care

quality through setting and maintaining standards for hospitals. Their work has evolved over the ensuing decades, and The Joint Commission currently accredits and/or certifies more than 21,000 organizations in the United States, including hospitals, home care agencies, long-term care facilities, ambulatory care centers, and laboratories (The Joint Commission, 2017).

The **National Committee for Quality Assurance (NCQA)** began in 1990 and oversees accreditation programs for individual physicians, health plans, and medical groups, including MCOs (NCQA, 2017). During the accreditation process, the NCQA collects data for a widely used set of performance measures, the **Health Plan Effectiveness Data and Information Set (HEDIS)**. HEDIS collects data on about 90% of health care plans to measure performance and consumer satisfaction; thus it allows consumers—including insurers—to compare performance of health plans and providers to regional and national benchmarks. Of note, Medicare uses HEDIS for their Medicare Advantage plans (CMS, 2017).

Currently, quality care monitoring focuses on improvement. Quality data are no longer hidden and will continue to be available when new methods are developed to assess improvement on the basis of outcomes. With the improvement approach, **outcomes measures** have moved to the forefront. Accrediting organizations require outcomes data, which they use to assess overall performance. Practitioners use outcomes to identify the treatment goals with the client. "Report cards" are used to compare and contrast health care organizations and health care plans. These report cards are available to the consumer, providers, and insurers. Medicare in particular has been increasing the number of its quality initiatives. Among the Medicare quality initiatives are:

- CMS Core Measures
- Quality Payment Program
- Merit-based Incentive Payment System (MIPS)
- Marketplace Quality Incentives
- ESRD Quality Incentive Program
- Skilled Nursing Facility (SNF) Quality Reporting Program

Managed Care

Managed care refers to any method of health care delivery designed to reduce unnecessary use of services, improve cost containment or cost-effectiveness, and ensure high-quality care. Managed care is currently one of the predominant forces in health care delivery. It affects health care organizations, health care providers, and reimbursement and has a direct influence on what care is provided and by whom, where, when, and whether it is to be provided. Chapter 12 provides additional information on managed care and reimbursement.

Information Technology

The development and utilization of information technology (IT) over the last decade has been phenomenal. Clinical staff members use computers and related technologies in all health care settings. For example, encouragement of widespread implementation of the **electronic health record (EHR)/ electronic medical record (EMR)** was promoted by the Health Information Technology for Economic and Clinical

TABLE 11.1	National Academy of Medicine—Landmark Reports on Quality in Health Care
Report Title (year)	**Major Findings and Recommendations**
To Err Is Human: Building a Safer Health System (1999)	Medication errors contribute to 44,000–98,000 deaths each year in the United States (more than motor vehicle accidents or breast cancer).
	Reported that errors largely result from system failures.
	Health care systems must focus on error prevention and promote changes to improve processes that will promote patient safety.
Crossing the Quality Chasm (2001a)	Among the findings was that the health care system is fragmented, poorly organized, does not use resources well, and quality varies considerably.
	The health care system needs improvement because of new technologies, rapid availably of information, and new treatments.
	Concerns were raised related to the rise in the number of people with multiple chronic conditions.
	Recommendations included the promotion of evidence-based care, more attention to patients' need for information, and improved access to clinical expertise.
	Report strongly supported enhanced use of information technology.
Leadership by Example (2003a)	Focused on government-funded programs: Medicare, Medicaid, CHIP, Dept. of Defense's TRICARE, VA program, and Indian Health Services.
	Report noted that federal leadership is needed to coordinate efforts and promote quality, and there is a notable lack of consistence in performance measurements.
	Recommended a more systematic approach to promote quality and to use technology in government-funded programs.
Who Will Keep the Public Healthy? (2003b)	Focused on the effects of globalization, travel, and technological advances and demographic changes on public health.
	Pointed out the need to address public health problems and educate public health professionals to meet current and future needs.
	Recommendations emphasized informatics, genomics, cultural competence, community-based participatory research, global health, and ethics.
Health Professions Education (2003c)	Education of health professionals is viewed as a bridge to quality care.
	Identified core competencies for all health professions: provide patient-centered care, work in interprofessional teams, employ evidence-based practice, apply quality improvement strategies, and utilize informatics.
Priority Areas for National Action: Transforming Health Care Quality (2003d)	The IOM identified 20 "priority areas" to be developed and/or addressed through an evidence-based approach to improve quality. Among the processes and issues were care coordination, health literacy, frailty of old age, medication management, and treatment for tobacco dependence.
	Among the health conditions/diagnoses identified as priority areas were nosocomial infections, obesity, asthma, diabetes, hypertension, stroke, major depression, and pregnancy/childbirth.
Future Directions for the National Healthcare Quality and Disparities Reports (2010)	Updated priority areas focusing on disparities.
	Areas to include were patient and family engagement, population health, safety, care coordination, palliative care, overuse of care, and improvement of access to care.
Future of Nursing: Leading Change, Advancing Health (2011)	This report addresses barriers that prevent nurses from being effectively used in the rapidly changing health care system.
	Among the main recommendations were that nurses should practice to the full extent of their education and training and that nurses should be encouraged to achieve higher levels of education and training.
Improving Diagnosis in Health Care (2015)	Diagnostic errors affect an estimated 5% of Americans each year; 6%–17% of adverse events in hospitals are the result of diagnostic errors. Reducing diagnostic errors is one of the new efforts to improve quality and safety in health care.
	Recommendations included the following: 1) promote more effective teamwork among health care professionals, patients, and family members; 2) ensure that health information technology supports patients and providers during the diagnostic process; 3) establish work systems and culture to support diagnostic processes and improvements; and 4) develop a system that facilitates learning from diagnostic errors and near misses.

Health, which was a component of the American Recovery and Reinvestment Act of 2009. The EHR/EMR allows for systematization of the collection of patient health information within a digital format that can be shared across health care settings and among providers through network-connected information systems. The ACA strongly supported expansion of the EHR, as has the CMS. Although EHR support and usage have climbed exponentially as a result of these efforts, there have been several issues with the widespread implementation. These issues include high associated costs, software deficiencies, difficulties with interfaces between and among systems, privacy concerns, and liability issues. Despite these concerns and issues, the EHR will continue to evolve and should eventually promote better-quality, safer, and more effective and efficient health care delivery.

Telehealth is another avenue in which IT is expanding within health care. Use of telehealth means that clients can receive care via technology, such as computer, video, or interactive television. The IOM (2012b) identified "telehealth" as a key component in ensuring access to health care services in isolated geographic areas. Further, they suggested that telehealth technologies will enhance the ability to better meet the health care needs of those in rural parts of the country, as well as for those in other underserved aggregates.

The Internet has opened doors for consumers and providers, and health information access has expanded rapidly. Although information availability to millions of people has been enhanced, resulting in an explosion of knowledge regarding health and health issues, the quality of this information is sometimes questionable. Providers must address the source and content of information on the Internet.

Social media, likewise, has become a more common source of information and is being widely used to share information about health. This can include health promotion and prevention activities and strategies. Individuals share a great variety of information now through social media, and this venue could be used in more organized efforts to get information out to the public. Finally, smartphones are a rapidly growing resource for engaging the community. Examples include employment of applications (apps) that track weight, exercise, and other health issues (e.g., heart function, blood glucose levels, hypertension).

Consumerism and Patient Rights

The growth of managed care and concerns over cost and value have increased the strength of consumerism. Over the past decade, the Baby Boomer generation has been subsidizing the health care system and paying more in premiums than it has taken out in claims. However, growing concern exists that, as this generation ages, it will demand more care than previous generations. Consumers are now critical of the health care system and demand changes as they encounter problems. Health care organizations, individual providers, and insurers recognize the importance of the consumer voice. *Client-* or *customer-centered health care* is a term that has become commonly used in health care, and more effort has been made to provide the consumer with information.

Patient or client rights are an important health care issue that individual states and the federal government have addressed through legislation. Patient rights have evolved over time and include access to medical records and the right to keep them private (through Health Insurance Portability and Accountability Act). In the United States a number of attempts have been made to enshrine a patients' bill of rights in law, including a bill rejected by Congress in 2001. The ACA included efforts to promote patients' rights, but it was not fully implemented.

Many states have promoted laws or regulations protecting patients. Further, health care facilities often have a "patients' bill of rights." Typically, a patients' bill of rights is a list of guarantees or promises for those receiving care at that facility or by providers. Generally included are guarantees of confidentiality, promises of access to information, fair treatment, informed consent, and autonomy over decisions, among other rights. Other patients' rights issues that are vitally important that continue to be discussed and debated are information disclosure, physician and provider choice, direct access to specialists, reimbursement for emergency care, and reimbursement denial.

Coordination and Access to Health Care

Health care providers often function in isolation from one another and provide fragmented services. Although multiple services are available for the wellness–illness continuum, coordination is lacking. Services range from office-clinic, home care, adult day care, acute care institutions, and specialized institutions to skilled nursing facilities. The services provided by one agency or one provider do not help the individual transit, or move, across boundaries and receive services offered by others. "Handoffs," when patients are transferred from one provider (e.g., individual provider, unit, agency) to another, are a time of increased risk for errors, reducing the quality of care. In addition, the services tend to be geographically separated, and each agency has different criteria for access. Further, the focus of services has not kept pace with the changing needs of individuals and populations. Millions of Americans lack access to health care services, and inadequate financial resources are a deterrent to available health services. Interprofessional teams can address many of these concerns and improve care in the community.

The current health care system continues to be pluralistic and competitive, and it provides fragmented and uncoordinated care. Private care agencies and institutions are in competition with one another for clients, health professionals, and resources. Even with recent reforms, two hospitals in the same geographic area may be competing for the same clients, whereas other communities may not have a hospital at all, may have only minimal services, or may lack essential services such as obstetrics. Hospital home care programs are in direct competition with private or public home care agencies. Hospitals diversify services to become economically viable; therefore they compete with ambulatory care providers for the ambulatory market. Public health services can be viewed as indirectly competing for resources. This fragmentation and duplication must be overcome to provide coordinated, collaborative, and accessible service to all citizens.

Disparity in Health Care Delivery

Health disparities refer to observable or quantifiable differences in the presence of disease, health outcomes, or access to health care among different groups or populations. In the United States, health disparities have long been recognized as particularly problematic among ethnic minorities, including blacks, Native Americans, and Hispanics. Research indicates that often these groups have a higher prevalence of chronic conditions and higher rates of mortality and poorer health outcomes when compared with the white population. Further, it is recognized that in addition to racial or ethnic group, health disparities adversely affect those based on such factors as socioeconomic status; age; mental health; cognitive, sensory, or physical disability; sexual orientation or gender identity; or geographic location.

For example, the Kaiser Family Foundation (2016) noted that blacks and American Indian and Alaska Native adults have a higher prevalence of asthma, diabetes, and cardiovascular disease than whites. Variations in HIV diagnoses and death rates from AIDS are very pronounced, with blacks experiencing over 8 and 10 times higher rates of HIV and AIDS diagnoses than whites. Further, infant mortality rates are significantly higher for blacks and American Indians and Alaska Natives compared to whites; African Americans and Latinos are also approximately twice as likely to develop diabetes. Finally, black males have the shortest life expectancy compared with other groups.

Disparities in health care provision have been observed, particularly related to cancer, cardiovascular disease, HIV/AIDS, diabetes, and mental illness. To address this problem, more cross-cultural education for health care professionals, including nurses, is needed to improve awareness of cultural and social factors and their impact on health care.

? ACTIVE LEARNING

1. Review the current National Health Care Quality Report and the National Disparities Report. They can be accessed at http://www.ahrq.gov/research/findings/nhqrdr/index.html. What frameworks or matrices are used to structure the report? What is the status of health care quality and disparities? What can you learn that would affect planning for health care services in a community?

2. Discuss how critical health care issues (e.g., managed care, quality care, fraud and abuse, diversity, and disparity) affect health care organizations in the community.

3. Cite examples of health care consumerism in the local community. What are their histories?

4. Give a personal reaction to health care fraud and abuse. How should the principles found in the Code for Nurses apply in practice?

5. Visit the following site on health care reform: https://www.hhs.gov/healthcare/about-the-aca/index.html. Review the elements of the law and current status. Discuss implications for nursing in the community. Also review http://www.helpingyoucare.com/21950/hhs-provides-tool-to-find-out-how-the-presidents-health-care-law-benefits-you-your-state. HHS provides this site for comparisons.

FUTURE OF PUBLIC HEALTH AND THE HEALTH CARE SYSTEM

Many changes are occurring in the health care system. With implementation of the ACA, the health care system is required to set limits on the care provided; identify criteria for the use of technology; and determine which conditions will be treated, which interventions are effective, and who should receive the care. The health care reform debate, however, is far from over, and additional changes are likely in the near future. Questions that continue to be important are:

- What health care services should be provided?
- Who should have access to health care services?
- Who should pay for health care services?
- How can costs of health care be reduced?
- How should health care be delivered?
- What is the role of the government?

The importance of health promotion, disease prevention, and a population-based approach to health care is becoming increasingly recognized. There is recognition of the need for widespread use of the EHR, which, to be effective, must incorporate care provided in the community. The roles of health care organizations, practitioners, and the government must address the public health component of the system. There is also the problem of the need to address new and emerging threats such as the problems from the opioid crisis, increasing gang violence, and health conditions such as the Zika virus. Finally, local, state, and national political leaders must continue to manage the health of the population and the need to reduce levels of health care expenditures.

Futurists rarely identify the public health subsystem as a component of the health care system, but this situation is changing. Indeed, the history of the public health subsystem's involvement with the poor and disenfranchised is a major influence on inattention to their problems. Furthermore, focus on environmental influences on the population, such as air quality, is critical for the future health of any nation.

Nursing has also been involved in change. The *Future of Nursing* (IOM, 2011) focused on how the nursing profession might fit into the change process. The key messages in this report were as follows:

1. Nurses should practice to the full extent of their education and training.
2. Nurses should achieve higher levels of education and training through an improved education system that promotes seamless academic progression.
3. Nurses should be full partners with physicians and other health professionals in redesigning health care in the United States.
4. Effective workforce planning and policy making require better data collection and an improved information infrastructure.

This report offered eight recommendations, many of which are already having a major impact. One of the most significant to date is the drive to increase the number of nurses with bachelor's of science nursing (BSN) degrees by developing more RN-BSN opportunities. Public health has been one area of health care that often has required a BSN for its entry positions, though with the nursing shortage this situation has been moderated some. Increasing the number of nurses with BSN degrees would help fill empty positions that require a BSN degree. The role of the ANP, as commented on earlier, is also expanding. The IOM report supported significant change, emphasizing these aspects of quality, access, and value:

- The need for patient-centered care
- The need for stronger primary care services
- The need to deliver more care in the community
- The need for seamless, coordinated care
- The need for reconceptualized roles for health professionals
- The need for interprofessional collaboration

Predicting future trends in human values is more difficult than predicting scientific discoveries or the patterns of disease. The past two decades have brought a significant shift in thinking about the future of the health care system. Consumer rights and further efforts to control or limit health care costs while improving access will be critical issues to be resolved in the future. How these decisions, and implementation of health care reform law, will affect public health is unclear.

SUMMARY

The health care system is complex and changes quickly. Federal, state, and local legislation and policies affect the system, and understanding the legislation and its effect on the health care delivery system is critical for any nurse. In addition, the implementation and pending changes to the ACA have demonstrated how important it is for health care providers to understand the reimbursement system and to learn how to advocate for their clients.

The many different types of health care organizations and health care providers also affect the health care system. Interprofessional care will be necessary for providers to achieve success in the system and to ensure that the client receives cost-effective, high-quality care. There are many concerns about health care, including cost, access, the number of uninsured, quality, and health care fraud and abuse. Resolving these problems will not be an easy task, but it must be done. Understanding the system helps as health care providers learn to function in the rapidly changing system.

EVOLVE WEBSITE

http://evolve.elsevier.com/Nies/community
- NCLEX Review Questions
- Case Studies

BIBLIOGRAPHY

Agency for Healthcare Research and Quality: *National Healthcare Disparities Report*, 2015. Available from: https://www.ahrq.gov/research/findings/nhqrdr/nhqdr15/index.html.

Agency for Healthcare Research and Quality: *Consumer assessment of health plans*, 2017. Available from: https://www.ahrq.gov/cahps/index.html.

Centers for Medicare and Medicaid Services (CMS): *Medicare Advantage HEDIS Public Use Files*, 2017. https://www.cms.gov/Research-Statistics-Data-and-Systems/Statistics-Trends-and-Reports/MCRAdvPartDEnrolData/MA-HEDIS-Public-Use-Files.html.

FamiliesUSA: *A 50-state look at Medicaid expansion*, 2017. Accessed from http://familiesusa.org/product/50-state-look-medicaid-expansion.

Hanlon G, Pickett J: *Public health administration and practice*, ed 9, St. Louis, 1979, Mosby.

Institute of Medicine: *The future of public health*, Washington, DC, 1988, National Academies Press.

Institute of Medicine: *To err is human: building a safer health system*, Washington, DC, 1999, National Academies Press.

Institute of Medicine: *Crossing the quality chasm*, Washington, DC, 2001a, National Academies Press.

Institute of Medicine: *Envisioning the national health care quality report*. Washington, DC, 2001, National Academies Press.

Institute of Medicine: *Leadership by example*, Washington, DC, 2003a, National Academies Press.

Institute of Medicine: *Who will keep the public healthy?*, Washington, DC, 2003b, National Academies Press.

Institute of Medicine: *Health professions education*, Washington, DC, 2003c, National Academies Press.

Institute of Medicine: *Priority areas for national action: transforming health care quality*, Washington, DC, 2003d, National Academies Press.

Institute of Medicine: *Future directions for the national healthcare quality and disparities reports*, Washington, DC, 2010, National Academies Press.

Institute of Medicine: *The future of nursing: leading change, advancing health*, Washington, DC, 2011, National Academies Press.

Institute of Medicine: *Best care at lower costs: the path to continuously learning health care in America*, Washington, DC, 2012a, National Academies Press.

Institute of Medicine: *The role of telehealth in an evolving health care environment: workshop summary*, Washington, DC, 2012b, National Academies Press.

Institute of Medicine: *Measuring the impact of interprofessional education on collaborative practice and patient outcomes*, Washington, DC, 2015a, National Academies Press. https://www.nap.edu/download/21726.

Institute of Medicine: *Improving diagnosis in health care*, Washington, DC, 2015b, National Academics Press.

Interprofessional Professional Education Collaborative (IPEC): *Core competencies for interprofessional collaborative practice: report of an expert panel*, 2011. Available from: < www.aacn.nche.edu/education-resources/IPECReport.pdf >.

Kaiser Family Foundation: *Key Facts about the Uninsured population*, 2016. Available from: http://www.kff.org/uninsured/fact-sheet/key-facts-about-the-uninsured-population/.

Kaiser Family Foundation: *Disparities in health and health care: five key questions and answers*, 2016. http://www.kff.org/disparities-policy/issue-brief/disparities-in-health-and-health-care-five-key-questions-and-answers/.

Kaiser Family Foundation: *Health reform*, 2017. Available from: http://www.kff.org/healthreform/ upload/ 8061.pdf 2010b. http://www.kff.org/health-reform.

National Academy of Sciences, Engineering, and Medicine, Health and Medicine Division. *Exploring the role of accreditation in enhancing quality and innovation in health professions education*, Washington, DC, 2016, National Academies Press. https://www.nap.edu/read/23636/chapter/1.

National Committee for Quality Assurance: *National Committee for Quality Assurance: Accreditation*, 2017. http://www.ncqa.org/hedis-quality-measurement.

National Quality Forum: National priorities partnership. Available from: http://www.qualityforum.org/Setting_Priorities/NPP/National_Priorities_Partnership.aspx.

President's Advisory Commission on Consumer Protection and Quality in the Health Care Industry: *Quality first: better health care for all Americans*, Washington, DC, 1999, U.S. Government Printing Office.

The Joint Commission: *About the Joint Commission*, 2017. https://www.jointcommission.org/facts_about_the_joint_commission/.

U.S. Department of Health and Human Services: *Strategic plan*, 2015. https://www.hhs.gov/about/strategic-plan/index.html.

U.S. Department of Health and Human Services: *HHS agencies and offices*, 2017. https://www.hhs.gov/about/agencies/hhs-agencies-and-offices/index.html.

U.S. Department of Health and Human Services: *Healthy people* 2020. Washington, DC, 2010, US Government Printing Office.

World Health Organization: *Framework for action on interprofessional education and collaborative practice*, 2010. Available from: http://apps.who.int/iris/bitstream/10665/70185/1/WHO_HRH_HPN_10.3_eng.pdf?ua=1.

World Health Organization: *Declaration of Alma Ata*. Available from: http://www.who.int/publications/almaata_declaration_en.pdf.

12

Economics of Health Care

Melanie McEwen and Marie E. McBee

OUTLINE

OBJECTIVES

Upon completion of this chapter, the reader will be able to do the following:
1. Discuss factors that influence the cost of health care.
2. Identify terms used in the financing of health care.
3. Discuss public financing of health care.
4. Discuss private financing of health care.
5. Discuss health insurance plans.
6. Describe trends in health care financing.
7. Describe the effects of economics on health care access.
8. Identify the future of health care economics.

KEY TERMS

access
actuarial classifications
adverse selection
ambulatory care
capitated reimbursement
carrier
carve-out service
coinsurance
copayment
cost containment

cost shifting
current procedural terminology (CPT) codes
deductible
diagnosis-related group (DRG)
effectiveness
flexible spending account (FSA)
gatekeepers
health care providers
health insurance plans

health maintenance organization (HMO)
health savings account (HSA)
high-deductible health plans (HDHP)
indemnity plan
managed care groups
managed care plans
mandates
Medicaid

Medicare	Patient Protection and Affordable	premiums
Medigap insurance	Health Care Act (ACA)	primary care provider
outcomes	point-of-service (POS)	prospective payment system (PPS)
out-of-pocket expenses	preferred provider organization (PPO)	

Economics represents the science of allocation of resources. Resources are commonly known as *goods or services,* for example, health care services. Economics affects all aspects of health care. Nurses have traditionally avoided the arena of health care economics, preferring to focus on the actual, direct care of the client. So strong is the feeling of social justice that some nurses express a reluctance to be informed of the individual client's health care financing source for fear that this knowledge will influence their care. Public health nurses who deal with the medically underserved have had more experience in this area. However, even these nurses may have only rudimentary knowledge.

Health care costs continue to rise and consume a greater percentage of our nation's resources. Indeed, health care is currently about 18% of the gross domestic product (GDP) of the United States and is anticipated to rise to 20% in only a few years (CMS, 2017). As a result, nursing can no longer ignore the intricacies of health care financing. The health of individuals, families, and aggregates is significantly influenced by economics. Economically disadvantaged individuals who have difficulty obtaining the basics, such as food and shelter, are less likely to have access to health care. Passage of the Patient Protection and Affordable Care Act (PL 111-148) in 2010 dramatically influenced health care access, resulting in many more individuals having insurance coverage. Indeed, most citizens have health insurance, whether provided by their employers, through private purchase, or, for those from low-income groups, through state and federal government sources (e.g., Medicare, Medicaid, Children's Health Insurance Plan [CHIP]). This change, however, is not to universal health care coverage—many still remain uninsured.

This chapter focuses on the economics of health care. It specifically discusses factors that influence health care costs, terminology of health care financing, and trends in health care economics and their impact on population health. This chapter also addresses the future of health care financing. Box 12.1 presents terms and definitions that are important to the discussion of these topics.

FACTORS INFLUENCING HEALTH CARE COSTS

Historical Perspective

Until the 1930s, the predominant method of individual health care financing in the United States was self-payment. Health care providers charged a fee for the services they rendered, and the patient paid these out-of-pocket expenses. The price of the service was under the control of the provider and generally represented the cost of providing that service. A certain amount of "charity" services was expected. The assumption was that those who could pay would pay and those who could not pay should receive care and pay what they could. The concept of public financing of health care for a specific aggregate was restricted and varied from geographic area to area until the term *public health* came into common use.

The following types of hospitals existed until the mid-twentieth century:

Public hospitals, which received public funds and served the health care needs of the entire population, regardless of ability to pay

Private hospitals, which cared mainly for those whose ability to pay was greater than that of the general population

For-profit hospitals, which were limited in number, received funds from investors, and cared for those who could definitely pay

Over time there has been growth in private and for-profit hospitals, resulting in large national hospital corporations that then expanded into offering more nonacute services.

This system worked well as long as those who could pay outnumbered those who could not. During the Great Depression, with more than 25% of the population out of work, the number of those capable of paying for health care was greatly reduced. Because public financing of health care was limited, hospitals, physicians, and other providers of health care went bankrupt.

In 1929, schoolteachers in Dallas, Texas, negotiated a prepaid health provision contract with Baylor Hospital. The teachers paid a sum of money each month, which guaranteed them access to health care through the hospital. The concept of insurance for health care proved extremely successful for Baylor Hospital. By 1939, this insurance plan had grown to include other groups and hospitals and became Blue Cross-Blue Shield (Momanyi, 2014).

Health insurance, or the idea of paying a small fee for guaranteed health care, appealed to the public. Societal concerns were mainly focused on sick care and acquisitions of curative therapies whenever needed. A public view that health insurance would provide freedom from fear that illness would impoverish them developed and prevails today. Health care providers envisioned guaranteed payment for their services (Higgins, 1997). During World War II, faced with a limited workforce and governmental restrictions on wages, employers began to see health insurance as a means of supplying workers' benefits without granting a wage increase.

To extend this same "insurance" to the general population, the Social Security Act of 1935 was amended in 1965 to create Medicare and Medicaid. Medicare provided indemnity insurance to those over the age of 65 years, and Medicaid, a state-administered health plan, provided a source for financing health care for some of the poor and the disabled.

BOX 12.1 Terminology Used in Health Care Financing

The financing of health care has given rise to new terminology. Nurses, as providers of care and consumers of services, need to be knowledgeable about these terms to improve their understanding of health care financing.

Terms pertaining to consumers:

Access—Ability to obtain health care services in a timely manner, at a reasonable cost, by a qualified practitioner, and at an accessible location.

Carve-out service—A service (e.g., mental health care) provided within a standard benefit package but delivered exclusively by a designated provider or group.

Charges—The posted prices of provider services.

Coinsurance—Cost sharing required by a health plan whereby the individual is responsible for a set percentage of the charge for each service.

Copayment—Cost sharing required by the health plan whereby the individual must pay a fixed dollar amount for each service.

Deductible—Cost sharing whereby the individual pays a specified amount before the health plan pays for covered services.

Fee schedule—List of predetermined payment rates for medical services.

Flexible spending account (FSA) or health savings account (HSA)—A mechanism by which an employee may pay for uncovered health care expenses through payroll deductions using pretax dollars.

Gatekeeper—Person in a managed care organization who decides whether a patient will be referred for specialty care. Doctors, nurses, nurse practitioners, and physician assistants function as gatekeepers.

Health care provider—An individual or institution that provides medical services (e.g., physicians, hospitals, or laboratories).

Health maintenance organization (HMO)—A managed care plan that acts as an insurer and sometimes a provider for a fixed prepaid premium. HMOs usually employ physicians.

Health plan—An insurance plan that pays a predetermined amount for covered health services.

High-deductible health plans (HDHP)—Insurance plan that uses cost sharing (i.e., high deductibles) to encourage employees to select plans with lower premiums. The intent is to encourage health care consumers to become more proactive in health care decisions from a financial perspective.

Indemnity plan—A health plan that pays covered services on a fee-for-service basis.

Managed care plan—A health plan that uses financial incentives to encourage enrollees to use selected providers who have contracted with the plan.

Medicaid—Joint federal- and state-funded programs that provide health care services for low-income people.

Medicare—A health insurance program for people who are older than 65 years of age, are disabled, or have end-stage renal disease.

Medicare Advantage—Part of Medicare by which recipients may choose to enroll in a coordinated care plan, private fee-for-service, or medical savings account plan created by the Balanced Budget Act of 1997.

Medigap insurance—Privately purchased individual or group health insurance plan designed to supplement Medicare coverage.

Out-of-pocket expenses—Payment made by the individual for medical services.

Point-of-service (POS) plan—A managed care plan that combines prepaid and fee-for-service plans. Enrollees may choose to use the services of an uncontracted provider by paying an increased copayment.

Portability—The guarantee that an individual changing jobs continues to receive health care coverage with the new employer without a waiting period or having to meet additional deductible requirements.

Preferred provider organization (PPO)—A health plan that contracts with providers to furnish services to the enrollees of the plan. Usually no insurance copayment is required.

Premium—Amount paid periodically to purchase health insurance benefits.

Primary care provider—A generalist physician, typically a family physician, internist, gynecologist, or pediatrician, who provides comprehensive medical services.

Terms pertaining to providers:

Ambulatory care—Medical services provided on an outpatient basis in a hospital or clinic setting.

Capitation—Payment mechanism that pays health care providers a fixed amount per enrollee to cover a defined set of services over a specified period, regardless of actual services provided.

Care management—Process used to improve quality of care by analyzing variations in and outcomes for current practice in the care of specific health conditions.

Cost containment—Reduction of inefficiencies in the consumption, allocation, or production of health care services.

Customary charge—Physician payment based on a median charge for a given service within a 12-month period.

Diagnosis-related group (DRG)—A system of payment classification for inpatient hospital services based on the principal diagnosis, procedure, age and gender of the patient, and complications.

Effectiveness—Net health benefit provided by a medical service or technology for a typical patient in community practice.

Full capitation—A stipulated dollar amount established to cover the cost of all health care services delivered for a person.

Maximum allowable costs—Specified cost level established by the health plan.

Outcome—The consequences of a medical intervention in a patient.

Physician's current procedural terminology (CPT) codes—A list of codes for medical services and procedures performed by physicians and other health care providers that has become the health care industry's standard for reporting physician procedures and services.

Practice guidelines—An explicit statement of what is known and believed about the benefits, risks, and costs of particular courses of medical action intended to assist decisions made by practitioners, patients, and others about appropriate health care for specific and clinical conditions.

Utilization review—A formal prospective, concurrent, or retrospective assessment of the medical necessity, efficiency, and appropriateness of health care services.

Terms pertaining to third-party payers:

Actuarial classification—Classification of enrollees that is determined by use of the mathematics of insurance, including probabilities, to ensure adequacy of the premium to provide future payment.

Administrative costs—Costs that the insurer incurs for utilization review, marketing, medical underwriting, agents' commissions, premium collection, claims processing, insurer profit, quality assurance activities, medical libraries, and risk management.

Adverse selection—Procedure in which a larger proportion of people with poorer health status enroll in specific plans or options. Plans that enroll a subpopulation with lower-than-average costs are favorably selected.

Capital cost—Depreciation, interest, leases and rentals, taxes, and insurance on tangible assets.

Carrier—An organization that contracts with the CMS to administer claims processing and make Medicare payments to health care providers.

Cost contract—Arrangement between a managed health care plan and the CMS for reimbursement of the costs of services provided.

Cost shifting—The cost of uncompensated care is passed on to the insured, resulting in higher costs for those with insurance coverage.

Mandate—A state or federal statute or regulation that requires coverage for certain health services.

Risk assessment—Statistical method used to estimate claims costs of enrollees.

As a result of these health care resources, a significant majority of the population was protected by indemnity health care insurance from various sources. The early indemnity plans lacked an incentive for limitation of use and had few or no provisions for health promotion. The emphasis was placed on illness care, providers received a fee only when a service was rendered, and all costs of services were reimbursed. Insulated from rising health care costs, health care consumers demanded complex and technologically advanced services whenever illness struck. These demands for costly services represented the major driving force in rising health care costs.

By the 1980s, the first efforts to curtail health care costs were made by the federal government. With institution of the **prospective payment system (PPS)**, hospital reimbursement for Medicare patients was based on a classification system that identified costs according to diagnosis and client characteristics—**diagnosis-related groups (DRGs)**. The PPS prompted an evolution toward managed care, dramatically altering health care financing through the end of the twentieth century and into the first decade of the twenty-first century. Despite containment efforts, however, costs of health care and, consequently, health insurance, have continued to rise.

The spiraling health care costs, starting from the mid-1960s and persisting into the twenty-first century, were fueled by the presence of very rapid technological advances, society's sense of entitlement to these therapies, a guaranteed payer, and the prevailing medical orientation toward curative measures. Prior to implementation of Medicare and Medicaid, national health expenditures represented less than 5% of the GDP. Fifty years later, however, costs have risen exponentially, as described previously.

Use of Health Care

According to economic principles, the existence of a desirable product, the demand for the product, and the availability of financial funding influence the use of the product. Health care is the product, and the demand for this product increases when the need expands and funding is available. In an attempt to reduce unnecessary utilization, insurance plans began to limit coverage for certain services and people; thus the move toward "managed care." Restrictions on use of health care, such as the establishment of a "gatekeeper," limited patient provider choice, requirement of preauthorization for some services, limited coverage for preexisting illnesses, and exclusion of those participants whose use was deemed exorbitant, have been instituted. However, these restrictions had only limited success in curbing health care costs. Consumers were activated by these changes made by managed care, protesting them, and in many instances alterations were made.

Despite recognition of the problem of increasing health care costs and multiple attempts to address it, spending for health care in the United States is more than double that of many other developed countries (i.e., those in the Organization for Economic Cooperation and Development [OCED]). Indeed, average per capita spending in 2015 was $3625 (8.9% of GDP) for OCED countries, compared with $8713 (17.6% of GDP) in the United States (OCED, 2016). In contrast, Canada, which was tenth highest per capita spending in the OCED, spent $4351 per person on health care. Because the approach in the U.S. health care system is reimbursement with multiple insurers, both private and public, expenses for health care vary according to types of care and sources of funding.

Lack of Preventive Care

Until recently, little to no incentive has existed to prevent illness or promote health. Curative measures have traditionally been the focus of health care. Soaring health care costs and an improved knowledge of health have heightened the public's awareness of their obligation to assume responsibility for their health by amending many unhealthy behaviors. As a result, more people are demanding preventive health care from the provider and their health care contractors. Public financing of health care has increased funding for such preventive care as screening tests, periodic examinations, and immunizations. Use of these preventive health services has increased, but significant disparities persist in relation to ethnic background and economic status (National Center for Health Statistics [NCHS], 2017). There continues to be a gap between the amount of funding available for preventive treatment modalities and funding for curative treatments.

Lifestyle and Health Behaviors

A healthy lifestyle does not ensure good health but has been shown to contribute to longevity and productivity (Harvard Medical School, 2009). The five leading causes of death and illness can be positively affected by changes in lifestyle. Studies have now found that a low-fat diet, exercise, maintaining of an optimal body weight, smoking cessation, and stress reduction can modify or even prevent many chronic illnesses. Smoking cessation reduces the incidence of lung cancer. Seat belt use decreases the severity of injuries incurred during moving vehicle accidents. Indeed, effective treatment of illness must often be coupled with a change in lifestyle. In the near future, access to expensive and unique medical treatment will probably be influenced less by the patient's ability to pay and more by the person's commitment to compulsory lifestyle changes. For example, legislation has levied "sin taxes" on products whose use has been associated with chronic illnesses. Examples include addition of taxes on cigarettes and other tobacco products, large soft drinks, alcoholic beverages, and certain cooking oils. Income from these taxes is intended to be used to care for, prevent, and conduct research on chronic illnesses.

Significant changes in lifestyle have taken place in the past 30 years. The current "smoke-free" environment appears shocking when contrasted to the nonchalant attitude toward smoking that was pervasive in the 1940s, 1950s, and 1960s. The advent of the Health Belief Model and Pender's Health Prevention Model has given rise to numerous studies into methods of achieving lifestyle changes. The total effects of these changes are just now being seen with dramatic reductions in lung cancer and chronic lung diseases. Meanwhile, the health care system must continue to contend with the results of years of unhealthy lifestyles; most striking is the concerning rise in overweight and obesity and the abuse of opioid medications.

Health care funding is changing to provide more funding for preventive services. Some insurance plans provide monetary incentives, such as reduction in insurance premiums, for those who participate in behavioral changes toward a healthier lifestyle. Medicare will pay for many screening procedures performed for specific persons at specified times (Centers for Medicare and Medicaid Services [CMS], 2017b). Funding for behavioral changes, however, is often limited, inadequate, or unavailable. Similarly, weight loss programs, support groups for smoking cessation, and participation in relaxation programs are not usually considered reimbursable treatment regimens, but more expensive pharmaceutical interventions are reimbursable.

Societal Beliefs

With the advent of such wonders as penicillin and insulin, society began to believe that the eradication of disease was just a few years away. More and more resources were dedicated to this elusive search. Armed with the belief that disease would soon be eliminated, society had limited interest in preventive care. The general belief was that making more money available for health care would lead to better health care and the greater likelihood that illness would be cured. Society has viewed insurance as an economic shield protecting against all disease and illness. The belief in cure rather than prevention, combined with this financial safety net, encouraged society to become a passive participant in health care. The feeling "I don't have to worry, I have insurance" became the pervasive societal thought (Sloan, 2004).

Health care professionals also were slow to embrace preventive care. Most efforts were directed toward curing illness. With what seemed to be an unending source of financing for curative care, illness prevention seemed counterproductive.

As health care costs accelerated at an alarming rate and technological advances did not keep up with the increase in illnesses, the health of society had to become a collaborative effort between society itself and the health care industry. Although the United States spends more money on health care than any other industrialized country, it ranks significantly behind many other countries in health status indicators (NCHS, 2017; OECD, 2017). People still expect the health care system to cure them when they are ill, but there is now an increase in preventive care interest, including interest in health education, health promotion, and behavioral changes. Research into barriers and facilitators to lifestyle changes has increased, but it is not funded at the same level as curative measures (OECD, 2017). As discussed in Chapter 11, the United States continues to spend more money on health care and yet has lower-quality health care than many other countries (Fineberg, 2012).

Technological Advances

Modern society has come to expect miraculous technological advances. In response to this expectation, and supplied with funding from various sources, technological advances have become too numerous to mention. The United States leads the world in laboratory and clinical research. People come from all over the world for education and to train in leading American centers for excellence. The United States exceeds other industrialized countries in the availability and use of these technological advances. Such advances can save the lives of people who would otherwise die.

These advances, although remarkable, are expensive. It has been widely suggested that in the United States, 20% of the population consumes 80% of the health care resources; the reality is probably closer to one-third of the population consuming two-thirds of the resources (CMS, 2012). As the health care dollar shrinks, these advances raise ethical questions involving health care access and rationing. Restriction on technology can significantly reduce the cost of health care, but the delays, inconvenience, and limitations to care with rationing would be strongly resisted by most Americans. An example of a growing technology area is telehealth:

> Telehealth has already started to play an even more important role, especially as we move away from the traditional fee for service system and toward new models of care, including accountable care organizations (ACOs), patient-centered medical homes (PCMHs), and other strategies that focus on outcomes. At the same time, the costs of telehealth technologies are dropping and [they are] becoming even easier to use. These technologies are becoming more widely prevalent in the marketplace, more accessible, and consequently, can be adopted more easily than perhaps 5 or 10 years ago. The pace of technological innovation is accelerating, but the cost of innovation is falling.
>
> **(Institute of Medicine [IOM], 2012, p. 7)**

Telehealth has implications for public health as it expands care and access to specialists into the community. A key to success will be the cost factor.

Aging of Society

Health care expenditures rise with age, dramatically so at older ages. According to the latest population projections, individuals older than 65 years constituted about 14.1% of the total population in 2015; this proportion is expected to almost double by the year 2050 (U.S. Census Bureau, 2015). As people live longer, the percentage of those older than 85 years is also increasing. Therefore the number of those consuming the greatest amount of health care resources will rise more rapidly than the number of those who provide the monetary support for these resources. For example, the cost of care for Alzheimer disease and related dementias is considerable, and the rate of such dementias is expected to rise as Baby Boomers age, with the expectation that cost for this care—which in 2010 was between $159 and $215 billion, depending on what factors were included—is expected to double by 2040 if no effective treatment or cure is found for the diseases (NIH-supported study, 2013).

Pharmaceuticals

A relatively new phenomenon that has influenced health care economics is the utilization of drugs, both over-the-counter and prescription drugs. New drugs are improving health outcomes and quality of life. These new drugs and new uses for older drugs are curing some illnesses, preventing or delaying other chronic diseases, and hastening recovery from yet other illnesses. As a result, during the last several decades, costs of prescription drugs have risen dramatically and have become a significant part of health expenditures. Seniors in particular are affected because many have chronic illnesses that require daily medications.

In 2003, to help alleviate the costs of prescriptions for seniors, Medicare added a pharmaceutical benefit for enrollees. With implementation of the Medicare Prescription Drug and Modernization Act (Medicare Part D), all Medicare recipients are eligible to purchase insurance coverage to offset the costs of prescription drugs. As with other health care services, once a funding source has been established, utilization and costs increase. One result is that as of 2016, about 10% of health care expenditures in the United States is for pharmaceuticals, and these expenditures continue to rise (NCSL, 2017).

Shift to For-Profit Health Care

The final contributor to the increase in health care costs is a national shift from nonprofit health care to for-profit health care. This has given rise to the term *health care industry*. More and more large, for-profit organizations are taking over smaller community organizations. As the emphasis is on profit, mechanisms of achieving higher reimbursement have been developed, which have had an effect on health care costs.

Health Care Fraud and Abuse

Health care fraud has been an ongoing problem. The billions of dollars spent on health care and the struggles for control between providers, consumers, and health care organizations have increased the risk of fraud and abuse. The Federal Bureau of Investigation (FBI) estimates that health care fraud costs the United States tens of billions of dollars annually (FBI, 2017). The FBI is the primary agency that handles this fraud. Though all areas of health care and all payers experience fraud, Medicare and Medicaid have the highest levels (National Health Care Anti-Fraud Association [NHCAA], 2016). A number of actions have been taken to address this problem. Among them are the False Claims Act Amendments of 1986, which allow private citizens to collect a percentage of recovered funds if they report fraudulent Medicare claims and monies are recovered as a result. The Health Insurance Portability and Accountability Act (HIPAA) contains a set of provisions that address fraud, including a Fraud and Abuse Control Program, the Medicare Integrity Program, and the Health Care Fraud and Abuse Data Collection Program. Each of these programs is designed to address concerns over health care fraud. In addition, HIPAA legislation dramatically raised funding for fraud enforcement activities (HHS/OIG, 2017).

Major health care fraud and abuse incidents have influenced the most vulnerable of the population (i.e., the mentally ill and older adults). For example, overbilling and unnecessary visits in home health care were reported across the United States, resulting in widespread reforms to Medicare reimbursement for home health services (Infante and McAnaney, 2004). Other significant abuses in recent years relate to ambulance/emergency

---

BOX 12.2 Medicare Fraud

What is Medicare fraud?
- Billing Medicare for services not received
- Billing Medicare for services other than those received
- Use of another's Medicare card to obtain services
  Be suspicious if providers tell you:
- Medicare wants you to have this service
- They know how to get Medicare to pay for service
- The more services provided, the cheaper they are
  Be suspicious if providers:
- Change copayment of Medicare-approved services
- Advertise "free" consultations to those with Medicare
- Claim they represent Medicare
- Use pressure to persuade you of the need for high-priced services
- Use telemarketing as a marketing tool
  Whenever you receive a Medicare payment notice, review it for errors. Make sure Medicare was not billed for services not received.

Modified from Centers for Medicare and Medicaid Services: *Help fight Medicare fraud.* Retrieved from https://www.medicare.gov/Pubs/pdf/10111-Protecting-Yourself-and-Medicare.pdf

---

transportation, overbilling/kickbacks, opioid prescription abuse, addiction treatment programs, money laundering, and compounding pharmacies (FBI, 2017).

The ACA included additional provisions to reduce fraud and abuse in public programs. It encouraged screening of providers and enhanced oversight for initial claims for durable medical equipment suppliers. The law required Medicare and Medicaid program providers and suppliers to establish compliance programs and developed a database to share fraud and abuse information among federal and state programs. Finally, it increased penalties for submitting false claims and increases funding for antifraud activities (Kaiser Family Foundation, 2013). Box 12.2 describes consumer tips related to health care fraud and abuse.

PUBLIC FINANCING OF HEALTH CARE

As the popularity and benefits of employer-provided insurance plans were recognized during the depression and post-WWII years, it became evident that the health care of some segments of society was being neglected. During the 1960s, a pervasive thrust for social justice in the public and political arenas presented the ideal opportunity for governmental participation in health care financing. In 1965, the federal government under President Lyndon Johnson enacted the first movement toward universal health care coverage. Titles XVIII and XIX, amendments to the Social Security Act, created Medicare and Medicaid, respectively.

Medicare

Medicare is a federal entitlement program that is totally funded by a combination of payroll taxes, general federal taxes and beneficiary premiums. This program is intended to help cover the costs of health care for people 65 years of age and older and people who are disabled, have end-stage renal disease, or have been diagnosed with amyotrophic lateral sclerosis (ALS). Medicare is divided into four parts. Medicare Part A is basically hospital insurance. Services covered by Medicare Part A include inpatient care in hospitals and skilled nursing facilities (not unskilled or long-term care). It also covers hospice care and some home health care. Most U.S. residents are eligible for premium-free Medicare Part A benefits when they reach age 65, on the basis of their own or their spouse's employment. Although Medicare Part A is an entitlement program, the enrollee must pay a **deductible** for health services. The Part A deductible is the beneficiary's only cost for up to 60 days of Medicare-covered inpatient hospital care in a benefit period. Beneficiaries have to pay an additional copayment per day for days 61 through 90, and this copayment increases per day for hospital stays beyond the ninetieth day in a benefit period. The Centers for Medicare & Medicaid Services (CMS) website (http://www.cms.gov) provides current information on costs for beneficiaries.

Those individuals who are eligible for Medicare Part A may *purchase* Medicare Part B for a monthly fee. Medicare Part B is medical insurance that helps pay for out-of-pocket costs related to physician services, hospital outpatient care, durable medical equipment, and other services, including some home health care. The monthly premium paid by beneficiaries enrolled in Medicare Part B has changed over time. Premiums are now prorated, based on income, and in 2017 ranged from the standard of $134/month to a high of $428/per month for individuals earning above $214,000 or couples earning above $428,000 per year. In addition to the monthly premium, Part B requires subscribers to pay deductibles and coinsurance (CMS, 2017b). The CMS website provides current information on these costs.

Medicare Part C, also known as the *Medicare Advantage plans,* is optional "gap" coverage provided by private insurance companies that are approved by, and under contract with, Medicare and may include health maintenance organizations (HMOs) and preferred provider organizations (PPOs). Covered services vary by plan and may include vision, hearing, and dental care, as well as other services and supplies not covered by Medicare Parts A, B, and D. Costs vary by plan, and to be eligible, the

individual must have Medicare Parts A and B and must live in the service area of the plan (CMS, 2017b). Enrollment in Medicare Advantage plans has grown steadily, and more than 25% of Medicare beneficiaries are enrolled in these programs.

Medicare Part D was initiated in 2006 to help defray the costs of prescription drugs. Like Parts B and C, Medicare Part D is optional, and if eligible Medicare recipients choose this option, they must enroll in an approved prescription drug plan. Most participants in Medicare Part D pay a monthly premium, a yearly deductible, and copayments, with out-of-pocket costs based on the plan selected and drugs used. In addition to these costs, the enrollee is responsible for cost of prescription drugs once the total costs reach a certain amount in a year, which vary. This is termed the *coverage gap* or *donut hole.* When the enrollee's out-of-pocket total for drugs reaches a particular level, Medicare will pay 95% of the costs of any further prescription drugs. The CMS website provides current information on the amounts to be paid. Fig. 12.1 shows current and projected Medicare costs for each of the four major parts.

Medicaid

Title XIX of the Social Security Act established the Medicaid Program. Medicaid is a public welfare assistance program that was initially designed to finance health care coverage for the indigent. Eligibility for this program, a joint venture with state and federal funding, is determined by each state. Initially Medicaid was intended to focus benefits to children, pregnant women, the disabled, and impoverished elders. This changed dramatically, however, with implementation of the ACA, as funds were made available to provide health care for all adults below the poverty line—within states that elected to participate.

The federal government sets baseline eligibility requirements for Medicaid. State governments that wish to provide care to more citizens through this program can alter the eligibility requirements. For example, the federal government

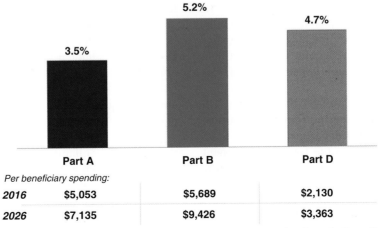

Average Annual Growth in Medicare Beneficiary Costs for Part A, Part B, and Part D Between 2016 and 2026

	Part A	Part B	Part D
	3.5%	5.2%	4.7%
Per beneficiary spending:			
2016	$5,053	$5,689	$2,130
2026	$7,135	$9,426	$3,363

FIG. 12.1 Average annual growth in Medicare beneficiary costs for Part A, Part, B, and Part D between 2016 and 2026. (Adapted from Kaiser Family Foundation: *The facts on Medicare spending and financing,* 2017. Retrieved from http://www.kff.org/medicare/issue-brief/the-facts-on-medicare-spending-and-financing/.)

may set 100% of poverty as an eligibility requirement, but an individual state may set the requirement as 110% of poverty. This means that a family living in that state can have an income slightly above the federal standard and still qualify for Medicaid.

The federal government **mandates** covered services, but state governments may provide more services. Mandated services covered by Medicaid for eligible recipients include inpatient and outpatient hospital care, physician's services, vaccines for children, family planning services, rural health clinic services, home health care, laboratory and radiography services, and Early and Periodic Screening, Diagnosis, and Treatment services for children younger than 21 years. Care provided by pediatric and family nurse practitioners is covered. Optional services that states may elect to provide include optometrist services and glasses, intermediate care facilities for the mentally disabled, rehabilitation, physical therapy, and hospice (CMS, 2017c).

Aside from Medicaid, many children younger than 18 years are eligible for CHIP. Established in 1997, CHIP is a program that provides insurance for children of low-socioeconomic families who do not qualify for Medicaid. Like Medicaid, the program is administered by the states, which share the cost with the national government. The ACA required expansion of Medicaid and CHIP to cover many of those who were previously uninsured.

The final decision as to whether Medicaid would be expanded in a state was determined by each state. The law covered payment of services for newly eligible Medicaid beneficiaries until 2016; the federal government will pay 90% of the cost for several more years. Initially, 32 states and the District of Columbia opted for Medicaid expansion and 19 did not (Families U.S.A., 2017). It is anticipated that more of the "opt-out" states will reconsider in the future, however, and elect to expand Medicaid coverage to more citizens.

Governmental Grants

Unlike individual health care services, governmental grants are directed toward funding large populations and different aggregates. Historically, the bulk of health promotion and disease-preventive measures has been limited to this arena of public health care. All three levels of government provide the major contribution of funding for these programs. On the national level the U.S. Department of Health and Human Services (HHS) administers this funding.

A variety of funding grants are available through the HHS (USDHHS, 2017). These "health-specific" grants are administered through the public health department at each state or community level. A large part of the federal government funding provided to the states is through "block grants." These "blocks" of funds are provided to the states to affect the health of the public as a whole. There are specific restrictions on how these monies can be spent, including limitations on the population that receives the services and what types of programs are to be funded. The states use these monies to provide for the care of the public within these restrictions. Depending on the health needs of the state, these monies may be spent to

provide direct aggregate care, but most often they are used for health promotion activities that are directed at a larger percentage of the population. Each level of government may make funds available for a specific health need of the members of the community.

To ensure that the needs of the community are being addressed, health care providers and programs may be required to compete for these funds. Proposals, grant applications, or requests must be submitted, reviewed, and prioritized. Funds are allocated on the basis of need and program merit. This type of funding is directed toward the population in general and not to specific individuals. When the funding is no longer provided, the programs cease, leading to lack of continuity of care. Historically, the funding priorities are closely related to the achievement of the *Healthy People 2020* objectives. Limitations on the amounts provided are related to available governmental resources.

> **? ACTIVE LEARNING**
>
> Interview an official from your local health department about finances. Identify strengths and weaknesses. Consider solutions for one of the weaknesses.

PHILANTHROPIC FINANCING OF HEALTH CARE

A limited amount of the nation's health care bill is paid by philanthropic sources, whose priorities are usually capricious and oriented toward research or treatment/interventions related to a specific disease or population aggregate. Eligibility for services through these associations is generally limited to the specific disease or population of interest, as with the American Heart Association, March of Dimes, or Susan Komen Foundation. Few direct services are rendered, and these services are approved on individual case considerations. Ancillary health care needs such as transportation, parental housing, or wigs may be addressed. Informational and research activities constitute the majority of services provided by these types of organizations. The organizations fund many educational programs that increase awareness of specific diseases, screening procedures, and preventive measures.

An example of a philanthropic national organization designed to provide care for a specific population group is the Shriners Hospitals for Children (http://www.shrinershospitalsforchildren.org). The services and costs related to this care, including transportation, are often provided to the eligible individual free of charge. The only requirement for care is meeting criteria set by the supporting organization.

Some of the private, nonprofit entities or associations that provide philanthropic services include professional associations such as the American Medical Association, the American Dental Association, and the American Nurses Association. Key groups that support research related to health care, health care delivery, and policy making are the Robert Wood Johnson Foundation (http://www.RWJF.org), the Kaiser Family Foundation (http://www.KFF.org), and the Pew Charitable Trusts (http://www.Pewtrusts.org). Examples of disease-specific, philanthropic organizations that provide important, patient-focused education, information, and other resources include the American Cancer Society (http://www.Cancer.org), the Alzheimer's Association (http://www.Alz.org), and the American Diabetes Association (http://www.Diabetes.org).

PRIVATE HEALTH CARE INSURANCE

Historical Perspective

During the 1930s, in an effort to provide care and avoid bankruptcy, health care providers began to establish health insurance plans. One of the most recognizable of these early plans is Blue Cross and Blue Shield. Blue Cross/Blue Shield was instituted by an agreement between Baylor University Hospital in Dallas and the Dallas area public school teachers. Those enrolled in the plan, called *enrollees*, paid a monthly fee for a guarantee of health care. Baylor providers delivered services to the enrollees and collected payment from the health insurance plan. The insurance plan paid fees plus its administrative costs from money collected from the enrollees (Young and Kroth, 2018).

Throughout the Depression and World War II, when prices and wages were frozen, industries began to offer health care insurance as a "fringe benefit" to employees. In 1953, as a further employer incentive to offer health care coverage to employees, money spent on health insurance was declared tax-exempt. Over the years, workers' union groups began to negotiate for these benefits. With more available financial resources and the patient largely insulated from the costs, health care expenditures increased. Further, reimbursement based on operational expenses represented a strong incentive for health care expansion (Higgins, 1997). Private, employer-based insurance became the prevailing model in the United States. This persisted even through implementation of Medicare and Medicaid in the mid-1960s. For the most part, until passage and implementation of the ACA, reasons for lack of health care insurance were costs, change in employment, or changes in eligibility such as change in marital status or death of spouse or parent. Even though the United States has an employer-based insurance system, only about half of Americans obtain insurance from their place of employment in 2015 (down from more than 60% in 2012) (Kaiser Family Foundation, 2017a). Despite provisions from the ACA, smaller businesses typically find it more costly to provide coverage, and many businesses do not provide coverage for part-time employees. Indeed, despite attempts at controlling them, annual insurance premiums (combined worker and employer contributions) in 2016 averaged more than $18,000 for a family ($6400 for an individual) (Kaiser Family Foundation, 2017b).

Types of Health Care Plans

The early Blue Cross and Blue Shield plan was an example of an indemnity plan. This plan paid all of the costs of covered services provided to the enrollee. The enrollee enjoyed free choice of provider and services. Indemnity plans preserved the enrollee's right of choice and allowed the person to manage his or her own health care. These plans became very costly because there were no incentives for cost containment. Although indemnity plans are still available, the monthly cost of enrollment has increased to exorbitant amounts, making them cost prohibitive. In an effort to support these plans while preserving freedom of choice, mechanisms of cost sharing were introduced. These cost-sharing methods include copayment, deductible amounts, and coinsurance. All of these methods represented efforts to have the enrollee share in the cost of health care.

As health care costs escalated, variations in health care insurance plans were developed. Industries and corporations, the major providers of insurance coverage, began to look for a more economical means of providing health care to their employees. Kaiser Permanente decided to assemble their own health care programs. They built hospitals, hired physicians, and provided health care services to their employees. In an effort to market this concept, Dr. Paul Elwood coined the phrase health maintenance organization (HMO) (Higgins, 1997). HMOs were designed to provide more comprehensive care, but this type of program lacks enrollee freedom of choice. In HMO plans, preventive care is covered and encouraged, but specialty care is somewhat restricted, and HMOs are encouraged to reduce costs by providing only the most necessary services. This loss of choice led to a decrease in the popularity of HMOs. In the United States, the number of HMO plans peaked in the mid-1990s, when about 31% of the population was enrolled in them, and they continue to represent a small portion of the plans. In early years, HMOs were considerably less expensive than other insurance plans, but the difference is now relatively small. In 2010, about 19% of enrollees selected HMO plans, but their popularity has continued to decline, as in 2016 only 15% selected HMOs (Kaiser Family Foundation, 2017b).

In an effort to compete with the HMO, physicians and hospitals organized the independent practice model (IPM). The IPM was a separate entity that provided services to enrollees of one insurance company. This model evolved into the preferred provider organization (PPO). These types of insurance plans negotiated with health care providers for services at a reduced rate in exchange for a guaranteed increase in consumers. A negotiated reimbursement rate allows the cost of the plan to be somewhat controlled. Plan enrollees are offered cost incentives for choosing health care from within the plan's network of health care providers. Because they receive a specific amount of reimbursement, regardless of the rendered services, providers have an incentive to be conscious of the costs of the services provided (Young and Kroth, 2018). PPOs are more flexible than HMOs, but to receive full benefits, the covered individual must use network providers. PPOs are somewhat more expensive than HMO plans (about $90 month on average), but they are the most common type of insurance plan in the United States. Although down from 60% of all plans in 2009, in 2016, almost half (48%) of private insurance plans were PPOs.

Point-of-service (POS) plans combine elements of the HMO and the PPO. In POS plans, the covered individual designates an in-network physician as the primary health care provider (PCP). If the individual goes outside the network for care, he or she will be responsible for most of the costs unless referred by the PCP. POS plans were common during the early years of the twenty-first century (about 12% in 2008), but interest dropped off over time. In 2016, about 9% of all insurance plans were POS plans (Kaiser Family Foundation, 2017b).

High-deductible health plans (HDHP) began in the early 2000s as a method to involve the consumer in health care decisions. The intent was to encourage employees to select plans with lower premiums but more pronounced up-front cost sharing (i.e., higher deductibles). One incentive is to have the health care consumer become more involved in health care decisions from an economic standpoint and to "shop around" for lower-cost care. Many HDHPs included **health savings accounts (HSAs),** which are tax-free contributions that employees may make to a fund to cover their health care expenses (Young and Kroth, 2018). By 2016, HDHPs have become the second most prevalent insurance plan and represent about 29% of all plans in the United States (Kaiser Family Foundation, 2017b).

GENETICS IN PUBLIC HEALTH

Health Insurance and Genetic Discrimination

The National Library of Medicine (2018) explains that "genetic discrimination occurs when people are treated differently by their employer or insurance company because they have a gene mutation that causes or increases the risk of an inherited disorder." Discrimination with respect to hiring or the ability to get health and life insurance is a common concern of people who seek or are offered genetic testing. These fears may keep them from getting genomics-based tests or participating in research to develop new tests or therapies.

There are federal laws specifically designed to protect people against genetic discrimination. The most comprehensive of these is the Genetic Information Nondiscrimination Act (GINA). GINA has been in effect since 2009 and prohibits genetic discrimination by making it illegal for health insurance providers to use or require genetic information to make decisions about a person's insurance eligibility or coverage. GINA also prevents genetic discrimination in employment, because employers are forbidden to use a person's genetic information in hiring or promotion decisions.

It is important to realize that GINA does not extend to those in the U.S. military or those receiving health benefits through the Veterans Health Administration or Indian Health Service. In addition, it does not protect against genetic discrimination for life, disability, or long-term care insurance.

Portions of other laws are also applicable to the prevention of genetic discrimination. Among them are the Health Insurance Portability and Accountability Act, the ACA, and the Americans with Disabilities Act.

Adapted from National Human Genome Research Institute: *Genetic discrimination,* 2017. Retrieved from https://www.genome.gov/10002077/; U.S. National Library of Medicine: *What is genetic discrimination?* 2018. Retrieved from https://ghr.nlm.nih.gov/primer/testing/discrimination

Private Insurance

Costs of private health insurance are staggering, often prohibitively high, even when sharing the costs with employers. There are, of course, millions of Americans who are self-employed or who do not work for a company that provides health insurance for all employees. This is the group that has been the focus of the ACA's "health exchanges." The health exchanges are the government-regulated marketplace for health insurance plans. Some of the health exchanges were developed and monitored by the individual state after implementation of the ACA, but

most states opted to use the federally designed exchange (Shi and Singh, 2015). In the individual marketplace, through the exchanges, individuals can chose between four tiers of standardized plans: bronze, silver, gold, or platinum. Costs of the plans vary based on cost-sharing levels selected and other actuarial factors. Because of the costs, many plans are subsidized through tax credits or other mechanisms (Young and Kroth, 2018).

Reimbursement Mechanisms of Insurance Plans
Retrospective Reimbursement

When insurance plans were initially offered, the customary method of reimbursement was a fee for the service rendered, or retrospective reimbursement. Calculation of the fee was based on the cost of providing the service. Included in this "umbrella" of costs were such things as salaries, supplies, equipment, building depreciation, utilities, and taxes. Cost-based reimbursement encouraged inflated prices and fraud. Physicians were encouraged to overtreat patients, and participants were encouraged to overuse the health care system (Shi and Singh, 2015).

Prospective Reimbursement

Prospective reimbursement, or the prospective payment system (i.e., the PPS), a concept derived from the HMO method of payment, was implemented as a financial alternative to cost-based reimbursement. In the PPS, care, no matter what the provider's cost, is reimbursed to hospitals according to a predetermined amount. The federal government introduced this method of reimbursement for Medicare in 1983, and an immediate savings was noted. The prospective reimbursement rates are based on diagnoses and patient characteristics and are designated by the term diagnosis related group (i.e., DRGs). These factors are represented by codes, following the *International Classification of Diseases, Tenth Edition,* or ICD-10 (CDC, 2017).

For determination of the prospective amount, Medicare depends on the DRG to calculate the reimbursement. The amount to be paid to the provider is determined according to the client's primary and secondary diagnoses, age, gender, and complications. This amount is deemed adequate compensation for treatment of the client's health issues. If the provider, at first limited to hospitals but later other types of providers, can provide the treatment for less than this amount, a profit is made. If the required services cost more than this amount, then the provider incurs a loss (Young and Kroth, 2018).

Implementation of the PPS led to a reduction in Medicare costs but did not result in overall health care cost savings as intended. Hospitals developed **cost shifting** as a means of supplementing the loss of Medicare funding. Private insurance's reimbursement continued to be cost-based. Therefore hospitals could include the loss from caring for Medicare patients in their cost. Private insurance companies were paying for the cost of providing care to their enrollees and to Medicare patients.

Only a few years after implementation of the PPS by Medicare, private health care plans followed the government's lead. In an effort to ensure appropriate reimbursement, more sophisticated methods of calculating the relative cost of health care were developed. **Actuarial classifications** ensured that adequate **premiums** were charged for the projected health care needs of those enrolled, and other means of cost control began

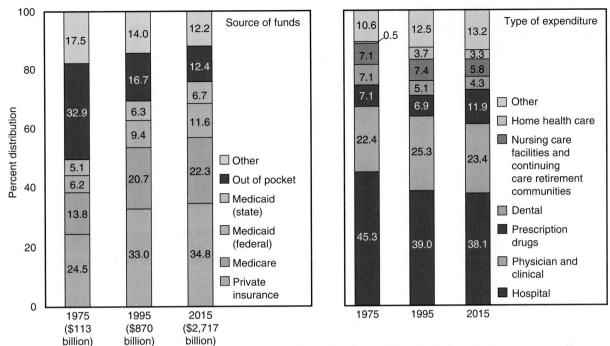

NOTE: Personal health care expenditures are outlays for goods and services relating directly to patient care.

FIG. 12.2 Personal health care expenditures: Source of funds/type of expenditure. (Modified from Department of Health and Human Services, Centers for Medicare and Medicaid Services, Office of Actuary, National Health Statistics Group: *Health, United States, 2016—individual charts and tables: spreadsheet, PDF, and PowerPoint files,* 2017. Retrieved from https://www.cdc.gov/nchs/hus/contents2016.htm#fig23.)

to emerge. Managed care groups negotiated with health care providers to render care for a specified amount of reimbursement based on community ratings modified by group-specific demographics. Prospective reimbursement creates incentives to control costs but also leads to instances of undertreatment and underuse of the system.

Similarly, physician services are given current procedural terminology (CPT) codes. Coding of the patient's illness determines reimbursement. Specialists in coding, as well as computer programs, are employed by both third-party payers and service providers. Third-party payers' code specialists scrutinize the claims for the appropriate data to support the code. Service provider code specialists are paid to ensure that the code is as accurate as possible to obtain the higher reimbursement. The appropriateness of services is based on the diagnosis code. For example, spirometry is appropriate (reimbursable) when the patient's diagnosis code indicates a variety of pulmonary and nonpulmonary conditions. Specialists in coding can quickly identify these codes, thus increasing payment for services. Physician visits, or CPT codes, are reimbursed on the basis of the documentation of the degree of "medical decision making" and time spent with the patient. Computerized medical record programs increase the ability to ensure that the visit can be reimbursed at the highest rate possible. This development has changed health care practices to the utilization of services that are low in costs and higher in reimbursement. High-cost services are limited or are not offered.

Fig. 12.2 illustrates how the nation's health care dollar is spent and the sources of funding for key years.

Covered Services

Until implementation of the ACA, insurance plans designated the types of services for which a plan would be financially responsible. When first developed, health insurance was meant to be a means of protecting an individual or family from economic catastrophe should a serious illness occur. Once an employee's fringe benefits included health insurance coverage, expanded benefit packages were developed. The scope of covered services began to widen to include such things as physician's office visits, medication, and dental costs. Unions began to negotiate for such expansion of covered medical services in lieu of additional wages.

When health care costs increased, so did the price of enrollment into the insurance plans. Industries began to refuse to pay these higher premium rates. Workers became disgruntled when their employers passed the cost of increased rates to them. To curtail the escalating premium price, insurance companies began to limit the covered services and dictate the conditions under which these services would be covered. Sites of care delivery changed. More treatments were required to be delivered outside the hospital or in ambulatory care clinics or ambulatory surgical centers. The patient was held financially responsible for "uncovered" services. Providers were pressured to comply with these requirements. Providers began to modify the delivery of health care to accommodate for these changes. After implementation of the PPS and various managed care options, the rate of hospitalization declined dramatically and the number of outpatient services increased.

All of these changes resulted in conflicts among providers, patients, employers, and the insurance plans, particularly when services deemed necessary by the consumer and provider were denied insurance coverage. Employers looked to the insurance

TABLE 12.1   Consumer Advantages and Disadvantages of Insurance Reimbursement Plans

Type	Advantages	Disadvantages
Indemnity Fee for service	No gatekeeper Unlimited choice of providers Full access to all services	High premiums Potential for overuse No incentive for cost containment
Managed care	"Credentialed" providers promote quality assurance	
Health maintenance organization (HMO)	Comprehensive care/primary care provider to oversee all care Lower premium	Restricted to plan provider except for emergencies Potential for lower-quality care to maximize costs
	No or reduced deductibles or copayment	Gatekeeper referral needed to see specialist
Preferred provider organization (PPO)	Greater selection of providers than with HMO Expedited provider reimbursement Lower premiums	Most expensive premiums Additional cost for out-of-plan provider Potential for lower-quality care to maximized costs
Point of service (POS)	More flexibility than HMO Comprehensive services with plan	Deductible required 20%–50% copayment for out-of-network services Primary care provider referral may be needed for specialized care
High-deductible health plan (HDHP)	Lower deductibles Encourages consumer involvement Often have health savings account to help defray costs	Higher out of pocket when services are utilized Must monitor medical expenses to determine when deductible is met

companies to provide health care services at a reasonable price. Insurance companies searched for ways to control costs, and providers searched for ways to deliver needed care within the confines of the health care policy. Table 12.1 describes some of the advantages and disadvantages of insurance reimbursement plans.

COST CONTAINMENT

Limiting health care costs is an imperative. All recent presidents have recognized that spiraling health care costs have eroded an already suffering economy. The public's increasing demand for care has increased costs, and the costs need to be controlled. This concept is known as **cost containment**. Numerous attempts to control costs have been made over the years, but none has been more than marginally successful.

Historical Perspective of Cost Containment

In addition to implementation of the PPS, health insurers and governmental sources attempted in the mid-1980s to curtail unnecessary proliferation of medical technology by requiring a certificate of need for additions to current health care buildings or services. To further reduce use, hospital records were reviewed for the appropriateness of care provided. Admission and treatment of hospitalized patients were reviewed by peer standard review organizations. Physicians and other medical personnel reviewed the hospital records and counseled the attending physician about unnecessary or excessively lengthy stays in the hospital as well as unwarranted services.

ETHICAL INSIGHTS

Cost Containment: How Will You Make Decisions?

You are the gatekeeper meeting with others in your community health organization to determine what services to provide to clients. You have $400,000 to divide among the needs. Who of the following clients will receive the required treatment? Who will not?

- A child with broken leg needs physical therapy (estimated cost: $10,000).
- A 55-year-old man requires knee replacement surgery and physical therapy (estimated cost: $40,000).
- A 76-year-old woman requires hip replacement (estimated cost: $40,000).
- A 32-year-old woman with leukemia requires a bone marrow transplant (estimated cost: $350,000).
- The community clinic needs new equipment for laboratory tests (estimated cost: $60,000).
- There is need for a new nurse who can act as a case manager for patients with complex diseases (estimated cost: $75,000 per year).
  Questions to consider:
- How does the American Nurses Association Code of Ethics apply to this case?
- What factors should be considered in the decision?
- How much does the cost of treatment affect the decision?
- How much does the age of the patient affect the decision?
- Is social justice a factor in the decision?

The cost reduction, as a result of prospective payment and other efforts, gave rise to managed care. Unable to shift costs to other entities, and with a predetermined reimbursement rate, providers searched for the most cost-effective mechanism of care provision. Greater ability to predict the cost of care enabled health care plans to negotiate the best value for their premiums.

Current Trends in Cost Containment

The managed care form of health care financing changed economic incentives and forced health care providers to rethink health management decisions. Treatment recommendations may be tied more to "Can you afford this?" rather than "This is best for you." Costs of the service rendered, rather than enhancement of revenue through service provision, must be considered. These economic or cost-containment incentives can be divided into the following broad categories: **capitated reimbursement**, access limitation, and rationing.

Capitated Reimbursement

The growing visibility of managed care models and their associated success in cost containment through the use of prospective reimbursement to influence provider practice gave rise to various arrangements that link health care financing to service delivery such as managed care. Managed care organizations create partnerships with health care providers using financial incentives to prevent overuse. Statistical norms, practice parameters, and population data determine the capitated, or maximum, payment for services. This is the maximum reimbursement amount that the health care provider will receive for the provision of care. The actual cost of provision of care does not affect the reimbursement. Health care providers must provide appropriate medical care while being cognizant of health care costs. As a reward for conservative practices, health care providers may receive a specified amount of money or a percentage of the agreed reimbursement if services are delivered below the limit set by the third-party payer. Providers whose services are inadequate or exceed this limit may be excluded from the network.

RESEARCH HIGHLIGHTS

Hospital Readmissions from Home Health Care Before and After Change to Prospective Payment System

In an effort to control the Medicare home health expenditure, home health reimbursement was changed from a fee-for-service system to a prospective payment system (PPS). This changed the reimbursement from a per-visit fee to episodes of care. Each episode of care begins on the first billable day and proceeds for a period of 60 days. Reimbursement is based on the diagnosis and type and level of care predicted to be required.

Through the use of a comprehensive evaluative tool, the Outcome and Assessment Information Set, a client is placed in a home health resource group (HHRG). Payment for services is based on the HHRG. Another important factor is that payment is received in two parts: 60% at the start of care and 40% after the episode of care is completed. Adjustments in final payment are made according to changes in the client's condition and may result in more or less than anticipated.

Anderson and colleagues (2005) studied unplanned hospital readmissions, which are an aspect of adverse change in patient condition or outcome. This study was designed to compare characteristics of clients rehospitalized during home health care before and after the institution of PPS.

The researchers determined that it was difficult to conclude whether PPS has any negative effect on home health care patient outcomes. Post-PPS clients were judged to be sicker at the time of rehospitalization and were almost twice as likely to be readmitted for another diagnosis. The investigators concluded that, since the institution of PPS, the hospital length of stay has decreased, with the result that clients are sicker at time of discharge.

The study shows that the first 2 weeks after hospital discharge are the most critical. Payments for home health services are suspended at the time of readmission, pending a client's return to home health care after rehospitalization. If the client does not return to home health care and the agency has completed five visits, 60% of the payment will awarded. If the agency has not completed the five visits, only 11% of the amount will be awarded. This arrangement might serve as an incentive for agencies to increase the number of visits after the initial hospital discharge but not after the second discharge.

Data from Anderson MA, Clarke MM, Helms LB, et al.: Hospital readmission from home health care before and after prospective payment. *J Nurs Scholarsh* 37(1):73–79, 2005.

Cost Containment Through Access Limitation

All third-party payers, or insurance plans, control access to health care through designation of covered services. Managed care organizations designate the type of covered services and specify the conditions under which the service is covered. Some services may only be accessed upon approval or referral from physicians who are used as gatekeepers. The enrollee must choose a primary care provider and consult this provider for a referral before seeking specialty services. Without this referral, the enrollee is financially responsible for the service. Even with the referral, choices may be limited to the providers who have contracted with the managed care plan.

Managed care plans may require that less costly health care modalities or medications be used. Exceptions to these modalities require justification. More technologically advanced and expensive treatments may be accessed under the most stringent conditions. Preauthorization requirements determine the medical necessity of the service. The process is so complex that the client may not be aware that the service is not covered until the reimbursement for the service is denied.

Cost Containment Through Rationing

Rationing is best described as determining the most appropriate use of health care or directing the health care where it can do the most good. Clinical Example 12.1 dramatizes the problem.

Clinical Example 12.1

A middle-aged woman was diagnosed with ovarian cancer. She was covered by Medicaid, lived alone in subsidized housing, and had a distant relative in another state. After surgery some years ago, she used home health services through the city home health agency. After conventional and high-dose chemotherapy failed, her physician recommended autologous bone marrow transplantation, which was considered experimental at the time. The procedure was approved and performed. Medical costs exceeded $200,000, but the patient died 2 months later.

Was the treatment in the Clinical Example a wise use of medical resources? Health care is not an exact science; too many variables exist. What appears to be the best course of action for one is not the best course of action for another. Making accurate treatment decisions is difficult, and the ramifications of a mistake are great. Complex socioeconomic factors also must be considered. Health care providers and third-party payers, including the federal government, are currently investigating the outcomes of health care practices to determine what methods, if any, can be instituted to improve the accuracy of these choices. Research into the area of treatment outcomes has led to major changes in treatments, many of which are quite costly. This situation presents a dilemma when decisions must be made as to their use.

TRENDS IN HEALTH FINANCING

The public's demand for affordable health care has created a new environment for health care financing. The ACA dramatically changed a number of things, particularly with respect to eligibility for Medicaid and regarding what is included in health insurance plans. Indeed, one of the significant elements of the ACA was the inclusion of the essential health benefits that must be covered in plans offered in the exchanges. Among the essential benefits are ambulatory care, emergency services, hospitalization, pregnancy/maternity and newborn care, mental health and substance use disorder services, and preventive care (healthcare.gov, 2017). It has been argued that requiring everyone to purchase all of these benefits has resulted in increasing the costs for all, even if the purchaser does not want or need the benefit.

Competition among health care providers and third-party payers has led to new and innovative health care. Outpatient services, patient education packages, electronic health records, and telehealth are just a few of these innovations. Increased competition has required insurance plans to be sensitive to the needs of the employee organizations and their enrollees. Individualized plans of covered services can be created. Enrollees can choose the plan that provides them with the services they desire at a selected cost. Health care providers advertise to ensure that the consumer selects an insurance plan that includes their services. Some providers, such as hospitals, campaign for inclusion in a plan.

Despite implementation of the ACA, along with the other measures described here, health care costs have continued to increase. Major changes are still needed, and indeed inevitable, as the status quo is not sustainable. Although more Americans have health insurance now than before implementation of the ACA, the costs of both insurance and of health care per se have continued to rise (Shi and Sing, 2015; Young and Kroth, 2018). Coupled with concerns over evolving demographics (i.e., aging of the Baby Boomers and resultant expansion of Medicare costs), it is apparent that more policy changes and interventions need to take place. Some of the more commonly described are mentioned here.

Cost Sharing

Aware of the amount that the employer is willing to contribute for basic coverage, a third-party payer or insurance plan may propose several options, giving the employee freedom to choose services desired. Employees willing to pay may be able to increase the covered services not provided by the basic plan. This arrangement is known as *cost sharing*. Cost sharing may also require the consumer to pay a greater portion of the bill for covered services in return for lower premiums. Enrollees may opt to pay a higher premium for the freedom to choose providers, or elimination of the gatekeeper. This can result in increased consumer control of health care.

Health Care Alliances

The creation of powerful regional or statewide insurance purchasing pools, or health alliances, is seen as one of the means of reform for the health care industry. The alliance would define basic benefits that all insurers would have to offer to everyone at the same price, regardless of health status. These alliances would not regulate insurance prices. Health alliances would collect premiums and help consumers choose among competing insurers and plans. The consumer's choice would be based on published, simple, standard information about benefits and outcomes of the different available plans. Plans would have to compete by offering better outcomes or lower cost. Insurers would have to contract with providers who find ways of delivering cost-efficient care. Medicare is currently participating

in health care alliances. Enrollees are given a choice between traditional Medicare, Parts A and B, and Medicare Advantage.

Self-Insurance

Many organizations, such as large companies and governmental entities (e.g., school districts or municipalities), have used health care information collected by insurance plans to self-insure their employees. This development has enabled industries and other types of organizations to reduce the administrative cost of insurance. Unlike the large industrial HMOs, self-insured status organizations administer their own health care plan and purchase health care services from an established insurance plan. In these cases the organizations or businesses are relying on a healthy employee population that will require less health care. The organization or business that uses self-insurance takes a risk and needs to ensure that it can cover any major costs. Health care reform will require that there be sufficient funds to cover these costs.

Health Savings Accounts and Flexible Spending Accounts

Another source of funding for uncovered services are the HSA (mentioned earlier) and the flexible spending account (FSA). Both are set up during insurance determination by the employee. With both the HSA and the FSA, the employee determines how much he or she will have to spend for uncovered services and arranges to have this amount deducted from his or her paycheck; these monies are "pretax." When these services are incurred, the employee pays for them with this account. There are some differences between the two types of accounts. First, the HSA is associated with high-deductible health plans (HDHP) and the funds are "owned" by the employee. In contrast, the FSA is set up by the employer through any health insurance plan and is "owned" by the employer. For the FSA, the employee continues to pay into the account until the estimated amount is reached. If the employee overestimates the cost, the remaining amount is forfeited. For HSAs, both the employer and employee contribute to the fund, and the balance does not expire (i.e., unused amounts will remain in the account to be used in subsequent years). Finally, there are limits to the amount of pretaxed funds that can be put into each account. In 2017, FSAs were limited to $2,600; contributions to HSAs were limited to $6,750 for a family with a HDHP.

Reimbursement for Health Promotion and Disease Prevention Initiatives

Unfortunately, until recent years, reimbursement for health promotion and disease prevention has been limited. Whereas, most health insurance plans, both private and public, pay for screening procedures, funding or reimbursement for treatment modalities such as support groups for smoking cessation, home safety evaluation, and relaxation techniques has been sporadic. Obesity is one of this nation's most common health problems, yet the costs of weight loss programs are rarely reimbursed.

Research into barriers and facilitators to changes in lifestyle continues to be funded well below curative treatment research. Lifestyle change interventions are slow to be developed and even more difficult to implement and evaluate. Mandated services required by the ACA include such preventive services as counseling for management of obesity, prevention of sexually transmitted diseases, and tobacco cessation. Until these types of interventions are directly financed, they most likely will not become widely implemented. With the rise in obesity there have been state proposals, and some have been initiated, to incentivize healthy eating habits, such as taxing the sale of sodas and putting calorie counts on restaurant menus. This type of approach relies heavily on policy and subsequent legislation and causes some people to protest because they consider it invasion of their personal decisions. Many businesses, such as restaurants and large fast-food chains, have added calorie and nutritional information to their menus.

> ### ❓ ACTIVE LEARNING
>
> 1. Evaluate a family's health care coverage. Investigate the type of coverage and the ability of this coverage type to meet the needs of the family. Would another type of insurance coverage meet more of the family's needs? What prohibits their ability to obtain this coverage?
> 2. Interview public health nurses employed in a public health department about their perception of funding for health promotion/disease prevention.

HEALTH CARE FINANCING REFORM

It was estimated that in 2011, before implementation of the ACA, about 18% of nonelderly Americans were uninsured (Kaiser Family Foundation, 2016). Underinsurance, likewise, has been a problem, as the underinsured cannot fully cover their health needs. Certain racial/ethnic groups have higher rates for both uninsurance and underinsurance. The ranking of such groups from highest to lowest rate of noninsurance is Hispanic, black/non-Hispanic, Asian, multiracial, and white/non-Hispanic (Kaiser Family Foundation, 2016). After implementation of many provisions of the ACA, by 2016 more than 17 million additional people had obtained health care coverage, dropping the percentage of uninsured Americans to about 10% (Kaiser Family Foundation, 2016).

Lack of insurance is the major factor associated with lack of access to medical care. Uninsured adults are more than three times as likely as insured adults to go without needed medical care (NCHS, 2017). In order to appreciate the potential impact of health care reform, one can look at the issue of lack of insurance among young adults:

> *The uninsured rate among young adults, ages 19 to 25, has improved slightly in the last year. The share of young adults that were uninsured decreased from 30.0% in 2010 to 27.9% in 2011, due in part to the ACA provision allowing them to remain on a parent's private health plan until age 26. The change in coverage for this age group accounted for about 40% of the overall decline in the number of uninsured. However, young adults continue to have a high uninsured rate.*
>
> ***(Kaiser Family Foundation, 2012, p. 9)***

The National Academy of Medicine (NAM), formerly called the Institute of Medicine (IOM) (2012) notes that health literacy and communication will be key factors in success as consumers try to figure out the key elements of the ACA and to use the exchanges to obtain insurance if their employers are not providing this information directly. The success of this process will affect access to health care.

Access to Health Care

Access to health care is a complex situation that is defined by the circumstances of the individual. The primary concern is inadequate access to health care, which leads to unnecessary illness. Most Americans want to believe that the best possible health care will be available for them and their family members at any time, regardless of their age, sex, race, or ability to pay. Anything that obstructs this pursuit can be considered a barrier to health care.

Financial support for health care, through either private insurance coverage or participation in government programs, is the mechanism that is largely responsible for access. Lack of a source for health care financing due to lack of insurance coverage, preexisting conditions, unapproved care, and physicians who do not participate in the health plan available to the patient represent the most common factors attributed to difficulty in obtaining care. Other impediments to health care access are physical barriers, including structural inaccessibility, lack of appropriate equipment, hours of operation, convenient transportation, inadequate services when needed, and inability to communicate.

Inequality in the distribution of health care services represents another type of physical barrier. Even those with insurance coverage may be unable to locate participating health care providers. Opportunities to seek health care, especially preventive health care, during work hours is often discouraged by employers, although this situation is gradually changing as some employers recognize that preventive care can reduce overall costs. Rural areas and inner cities have been recognized as medically underserved for many years. Government incentives for increasing available medical services in these areas have not solved the problem.

Sociological barriers to health care access exist among poor and ethnic Americans. Poor outpatient diagnosis and treatment, increased use of emergency departments for primary care, and reluctance to hospitalize are possible explanations. Language and fear of reprisals have become important sociological barriers. Many of the poor and uninsured are illegal aliens, and seeking medical attention, even during illnesses, may have severe repercussions. Disparities are discussed later in the text.

Historical Perspective

National health insurance is not a new concept. European countries began a social model of health insurance in the early 1900s. In 1916, President Theodore Roosevelt advocated enactment of a form of national medical coverage. President Franklin Roosevelt wanted national health insurance to be part of the Social Security Act of 1935, but that provision did not pass (Higgins, 1997). During the administration of President Lyndon Johnson, however, a modified form of national health insurance, Medicare and Medicaid, was instituted.

Before the 1930s, most Americans were uninsured. Most health care providers considered it their duty to donate time and services to charity. Hospitals and clinics maintained charity wards. Society believed that those who could, and those who could not, should help themselves. The enactment of governmental entitlement programs, coupled with the availability of health care insurance as a benefit of one's occupation, helped change this belief. Quickly, the pervasive societal view was that those who could not help themselves should get government assistance or go to work (Higgins, 1997).

As discussed previously, in the 1960s Medicare and Medicaid brought about national health insurance coverage for older adults, the disabled, and those living below the poverty level—particularly children. Expansion of Medicaid with CHIP in the 1990s expanded care coverage for children of the "working poor," or those whose employers did not provide insurance.

Efforts to address access to health care reemerged in the 1990s, when Bill Clinton attempted to reform the health care system, ensure coverage, and reduce health care costs. The initiative was headed by Hillary Clinton, but after about a year of debate and numerous proposals, the Clinton plan failed to reach a consensus. This was attributed to widespread opposition from various health care provider groups and organizations as well as lack of public support. Continuing rising costs combined with eroding access through the early 2000s contributed to the election of Barak Obama and a new mandate to enact health care reform. After considerable debate, Congress passed the Patient Protection and Affordable Care Act (PL111-148), also known as the *Affordable Care Act*, which was signed into law March 23, 2010. Although the ACA did not ensure "universal coverage," it was originally estimated that when fully implemented, an additional 32 million people would have access to health insurance coverage (Kaiser Family Foundation, 2013).

The ACA was an extremely complex piece of legislation, and the final version of the bill exceeded 2000 pages. Among the law's provisions are mandating that all citizens obtain health insurance, expanding Medicaid eligibility, subsidizing insurance premiums for low-income purchasers, prohibiting denial of coverage for preexisting conditions, and establishing health insurance exchanges. Costs for expansion of coverage and subsidies would be offset by a combination of taxes and fees, reduction in payments for Medicare and Medicaid services and prescription drugs, and enhanced efforts to reduce Medicare fraud and abuse. Box 12.3 outlines some of the major provisions covered in the ACA.

The ACA remains highly controversial, and additional legislative and legal challenges are anticipated. All health care providers and consumers should remain alert to both short- and long-term changes. Additional information about the ACA can be found in Chapters 10 and 11.

BOX 12.3 Key Provisions of the Patient Protection and Affordable Care Act (P.L. 111-148)

Individual Mandate—Requires U.S. citizens and legal residents to have qualifying health coverage.

Employer Requirements—Requires employers with more than 50 employees to offer coverage or vouchers for full-time employees; requires employers with more than 200 employees to enroll employees into health insurance plans offered by the employer.

Expansion of Medicaid—Expands Medicaid to all individuals under age 65 with incomes up to 133% of the federal poverty line.

Expansion of CHIP—Requires states to maintain current income eligibility levels for children enrolled in the Children's Health Insurance Plan (CHIP) until 2019.

Premium and Cost-Sharing Subsidies to Individuals—Creates insurance exchanges to provide premium credits and subsidies to individuals and families with incomes between 133% and 400% of the federal poverty level.

Changes to Private Insurance—Establishes a temporary national high-risk pool to provide health coverage to individuals with preexisting medical conditions; establishes a process for reviewing increases in health plan premiums and requires justification of increases; provides dependent coverage for children up to age 26 years for all individual and group policies; prohibits health plans from placing lifetime limits on the dollar amount of coverage and from rescinding coverage; establishes a website to help residents identify health coverage options; permits states to form health care choice compacts and allow insurers to sell policies in any state participating in the compacts.

Cost Containment Provisions—Requires rules to simplify health insurance administration by adopting a single set of rules for payment, verification, and claims status; restructures payments to Medicare Advantage plans; reduces waste, fraud, and abuse in public programs by allowing providers to have screening-enhanced oversight periods for new providers and suppliers; increases penalties for submitting false claims.

Prevention and Wellness—Improves prevention by covering preventive services and eliminating cost sharing for preventive services in Medicare and Medicaid; requires qualified health plans to provide preventive services, recommended immunizations, preventive care for infants, children, and adolescents, and additional preventive care and screening for women; provides grants for small employers who establish wellness programs; requires chain restaurants and foods sold from vending machines to disclose the nutritional content of each item.

Modified from The Henry J. Kaiser Family Foundation: *Summary of coverage provisions in the Patient Protection and Affordable Care Act*, 2013. Retrieved from http://www.kff.org/health-costs/issue-brief/summary-of-coverage-provisions-in-the-patient/

❓ ACTIVE LEARNING

1. Learn more about changes in health care reimbursement due to health care reform by visiting https://www.cms.gov/cciio/index.html. This CMS website is the Center for Consumer Information and Insurance Oversight. What type of information is provided? What is the value of this information to consumers?
2. Investigate the ACA from the points of view of the consumer, health care provider, and third-party payer and community health. How has it affected the concerns of each of these constituents? What more needs to be done?
3. Examine the status of health care reform implementation in your state. How has the community been informed about changes? Has this been effective? How is it affecting community health in your state?

Societal Perceptions

Health care for all is a concept that most Americans support. Most people state that health care should be one of those necessities available to all without consideration of what it costs; however, when discussion turns to actually doing this, most people become concerned about the implications. Efforts to provide universal coverage through increased governmental involvement in health care have failed because of a number of factors, including rejection of much higher taxes, objection to paying for care for noncitizens, concerns over access and availability, and fears of rationing.

The ongoing dilemma is how to provide health care to all Americans in a way that is acceptable and affordable. Other countries provide their citizens with universal health care, but there are aspects of this care that are unpopular with U.S. society. The most concerning or pressing problem relates to funding sources, because significant tax increases would be necessary to provide coverage for all. Furthermore, the United States already spends much more of our resources on health care than any other country; adding more costs is enormously concerning.

Furthermore, waiting several months for nonemergency treatment, lack of choice of treatment, and inaccessibility or unavailability of diagnostic and treatment modalities are not acceptable to most Americans. Indeed, most Americans want assurance that all of the health care services that they and their families need, now and in the future, will be available no matter what the condition, age of the patient, job status, or ability to pay. The debate and measures to address the problem of health care financing are ongoing. All nurses—and citizens—need to become familiar with the issues.

ROLES OF THE PUBLIC HEALTH NURSE IN THE ECONOMICS OF HEALTH CARE

Researcher

Nurses need to be engaged in research about the provision of efficient, cost-effective health care. Nurses are in a pivotal role to investigate culturally sensitive treatment modalities, health education, disease prevention, and factors to change behaviors. Health promotion and disease prevention are more cost effective than curative treatment modalities. Public health nurse researchers need to investigate, develop, and evaluate the effectiveness of health promotion and disease prevention. Research on health promotion intervention outcomes, program cost/benefit analysis, and health informatics are just a few of these areas.

Educator

Health education is the foundation of public health nursing practice. Public health nurses agree that knowledge empowers clients to actively participate in their health care. Funding for this education is provided primarily through public, governmental entities (e.g., schools). Educational plans for individuals are rare. In the area of health care economics, the nurse needs to demonstrate the value of this education. Outcome measures for health education need to be established.

Provider of Care

Any service delivered by the nurse needs to be appropriate, necessary, and cost effective. Nurses in all areas of practice need to be cost-conscious. Judicious application of the nursing process is imperative. An accurate assessment is the foundation for an appropriate nursing diagnosis. Goals for care, jointly established between members of the community and the community health nurse, will guide the choice of interventions. Evaluation, using previously developed outcome measures, will lead to appropriate modifications of the plan.

Nurses can serve as program service providers, health education providers, and health program participants. Nurses need to participate in the grant proposal process, design, and evaluation for these programs. They need to be familiar with and participate in the statistical information gathering process that serves as the basis for determining community health need.

Advocate

Nurses must become more involved in the economics of health care. Too often, nurses are cognizant of the effects of changes in health care economics but feel powerless to act. Increasing knowledge of health care funding and policy making will empower nurses to advocate for the type of funding that provides appropriate care to obtain the greatest good. The large number of nurses gives our occupation potential political clout. Nurses need to utilize this political power to influence health care funding. Nurses need to advocate for increase in health promotion/disease prevention funding from both public and private sectors. Nurses need to plan programs, seek funding, and evaluate program effectiveness through outcome measures. Nurses need to constantly seek sources of funding for health programs through any available sources.

BEST CARE AT LOWER COST

In 2012, the NAM published a report entitled *Best Care at Lower Cost: The Path to Continuously Learning Health Care in America*. Building on its earlier work in relation to quality care (discussed in Chapter 11), the NAM was asked to examine a critical concern.

Health care in America presents a fundamental paradox. The past 50 years have seen an explosion in biomedical knowledge, dramatic innovation in therapies and surgical procedures, and management of conditions that previously were fatal, with ever more exciting clinical capabilities on the horizon. Yet, American health care is falling short on basic dimensions of quality, outcomes, costs, and equity.

(IOM, 2013, p. 1)

Among the factors that are pushing this examination is the fact that there is an estimated $750 billion waste of resources in the health care system, meaning that the United States loses this amount of money that could be spent on improved health care outcomes. We need best care at lower cost, not higher cost. Compared with other countries, the United States is paying more for less poorer outcomes. The system has to manage the complexity that continues to grow and at the same time slow down ever-escalating costs. Citizens want quality care that is evidence based, but the system is not managing this well.

> **? ACTIVE LEARNING**
>
> In small groups review the Institute of Medicine report *U.S. Health in International Perspective: Shorter Lives, Poorer Health* (2013). Divide up the content. Discuss this report from perspectives of the health care delivery system, quality care, diversity, and cost of care. The report is fully accessible and can be downloaded from https://www.ncbi.nlm.nih.gov/books/NBK115854/pdf/Bookshelf_NBK115854.pdf https://www.ncbi.nlm.nih.gov/pubmed/24006554 https://www.nap.edu/catalog/13497/us-health-in-international-perspective-shorter-lives-poorer-health.

■ SUMMARY

Health care economics is influencing health care practice at all levels. Nurses in the community must become aware of the economics of health care to practice in this new era. Patient outcomes are quickly being seen as a measurement for health care financing. As the health care system evolves toward health promotion and disease prevention, nursing will play a pivotal role. Public health nurses, whose domain of practice has encompassed these areas, will be in the forefront of this change. This chapter has presented the basics of health care economics and its importance in providing effective, quality care in all settings, including the community. An understanding of these elements is essential to the practice of nursing. This is an extremely complex subject with innovations and changes coming every day. To be effective, the nurse must be attentive to these developments.

ⓔ EVOLVE WEBSITE

http://evolve.elsevier.com/Nies/community

- NCLEX Review Questions
- Case Studies

BIBLIOGRAPHY

Centers for Disease Control and Prevention (CDC): *International classification of diseases, tenth revision, clinical modification (ICD-10-CM)*, 2017. Available from: https://www.cdc.gov/nchs/icd/icd10cm.htm.

Centers for Medicare and Medicaid Services (CMS): *National health expenditure data*, 2017a. https://www.cms.gov/research-statistics-data-and-systems/statistics-trends-and-reports/nationalhealthexpenddata/nhe-fact-sheet.html.

Centers for Medicare and Medicaid Services (CMS): *Medicare and you*, 2017b. Available from: https://www.medicare.gov/medicare-and-you/medicare-and-you.html.

Centers for Medicare and Medicaid Services (CMS): *Medicaid Benefits*, 2017c. Available from: https://www.medicaid.gov/medicaid/benefits/index.html.

Centers for Medicare and Medicaid Services (CMS): *Chronic conditions among Medicare beneficiaries*, 2012. Available from: https://www.cms.gov/Research-Statistics-Data-and-Systems/Statistics-Trends-and-Reports/Chronic-Conditions/Downloads/2012Chartbook.pdf.

Centers for Medicare and Medicaid Services: *Medicare fraud: detection and prevention tips*, n.d, 2012. Available from: <www.medicare.gov/FraudAbuse/Tips.asp.>.

Families U.S.A.: *A 50-State Look at Medicaid Expansion*, 2017. Available from: http://familiesusa.org/product/50-state-look-medicaid-expansion.

Federal Bureau of Investigation: *Health care fraud*, 2017. Available from: http://www.fbi.gov/about-us/investigate/white_collar/health-care-fraud. https://www.fbi.gov/investigate/white-collar-crime/health-care-fraud.

Fineberg H: A successful and sustainable health care system—how to get there from here, *N Engl J Med* 366:1020–1027, 2012.

Harvard Medical School: The numbers game: Risk factors, lifestyle and longevity, *Harv Men's Health Watch* 13:8, 2009.

Healthcare.gov: *What marketplace health insurance plans cover*, 2017. Accessed from: https://www.healthcare.gov/coverage/what-marketplace-plans-cover/.

Higgins W: How did we get this way? *Health Care Econ* 11:35, 1997.

Infante M, McAnaney K: Home health agencies can avoid fraud charges with compliance plans, *Hosp Home Health* 21(5):49–51, 2004.

Institute of Medicine: *The role of telehealth in an evolving health care environment: a workshop summary*, Washington, DC, 2012, National Academies Press.

Institute of Medicine: *Facilitating state health exchange communication through the use of health literate practices: workshop summary*, Washington, DC, 2013, National Academies Press.

Institute of Medicine: *Best care at lower cost: the path to continuously learning health care in America*, Washington, DC, 2012, National Academies Press. Available http://nationalacademies.org/hmd/reports/2012/best-care-at-lower-cost-the-path-to-continuously-learning-health-care-in-america.aspx.

Kaiser Family Foundation: *Health insurance coverage of the total population*, 2017a. Available http://www.kff.org/other/state-indicator/total-population/.

Kaiser Family Foundation: *Employer medical benefits, 2016: Annual survey*, 2017b. Available from: http://www.kff.org/report-section/ehbs-2016-section-one-cost-of-health-insurance/.

Kaiser Family Foundation: *The uninsured: a primer*, 2016. Available from: http://files.kff.org/attachment/Report-The-Uninsured-A%20Primer-Key-Facts-about-Health-Insurance-and-the-Unisured-in-America-in-the-Era-of-Health-Reform.

Kaiser Family Foundation: *Summary of the Affordable Care Act*, 2013. Available from: http://www.kff.org/health-reform/fact-sheet/summary-of-the-affordable-care-act/.

Kaiser Family Foundation: *The uninsured: a primer*, 2012. Available from: https://kaiserfamilyfoundation.files.wordpress.com/2013/01/7451-08.pdf.

Momanyi B: *Blue cross and blue shield of Texas handbook of Texas online*, Published by the Texas State Historical Association, http://www.tshaonline.org/handbook/online/articles/djbcz accessed January 11, 2014.

National Health Care Anti-Fraud Association: *Health care fraud: a serious and costly reality for all Americans*, 2016. Available from: https://www.nhcaa.org/resources/health-care-anti-fraud-resources/the-challenge-of-health-care-fraud.aspx.

National Center for Health Statistics: *Health. United States*, 2017. Available from: https://www.cdc.gov/nchs/data/nhis/earlyrelease/insur201611.pdf.

NIH-supported study finds U.S. dementia care costs as high as $215 billion in 2010: *NIH News*, April 3, 2013. Available from: <http://www.nih.gov/news/health/apr2013/nia-03.htm>.

National Conferences of State Legislatures (NCSL): *Pharmaceuticals: costs and pricing*, 2017. http://www.ncsl.org/research/health/pharmaceuticals/costs-and-pricing.aspx.

Organization for Economic Co-operation and Development (OECD): *Health data 2015*, 2016. Available from: http://www.oecd.org/health/health-systems/Focus-Health-Spending-2015.pdf.

Shi L, Singh DA: *Delivering health care in America: a systems approach*, ed 6, Burlington, MA, 2015, Jones & Bartlett Learning.

Sloan T: Consumer-driven to nowhere: study throws cold water on recent efforts to beat health care cost inflation, *Mod Healthcare* 34(49):21, 2004.

U.S. Census Bureau: *Current population survey*, 2015. Available from: https://www.census.gov/newsroom/facts-for-features/2015/cb15-ff09.html.

U.S. Department of Health and Human Services (USDHHS): *Grants and funding*, 2017. Available from: https://www.hhs.gov/grants/grants/index.html.

U.S. Department of Health and Human Services/Office of Inspector General (HHS/OIG): *Health Care Fraud and Abuse Control Program Report*, 2017. https://www.oig.hhs.gov/reports-and-publications/hcfac/.

Young KM, Kroth PJ: *Shultz & Young's Health Care USA: Understanding its organization and delivery*, ed 9, Burlington, MA, 2018, Jones & Bartlett Leaning.

13

Cultural Diversity and Community Health Nursing

*Christina N. DesOrmeaux**

OBJECTIVES

Upon completion of this chapter, the reader will be able to do the following:

1. Critically analyze racial and cultural diversity in the United States.
2. Analyze the influence of sociocultural, political, economic, ethical, and religious factors that influence the health of culturally diverse individuals, groups, and communities.
3. Identify the cultural aspects of nursing care for culturally diverse individuals, groups, and communities.
4. Apply the principles of transcultural nursing to community health nursing practice.

*The author would like to acknowledge the contribution of Carrie L. Buch, who wrote this chapter for the previous edition.

KEY TERMS

biomedical

cultural competence

cultural imposition

cultural negotiation

cultural stereotyping

culture

culture-bound syndrome

culture shock

culture specific

culture universal

culturological assessment

dominant value orientation

ethnocentrism

Leininger's theory of culture care
   diversity and universality

magicoreligious

naturalistic

norms

poverty

religion

socioeconomic status

spirituality

subculture

transcultural nursing

value

yin-yang theory

CULTURAL DIVERSITY

Cultural diversity is a multifaceted and complex concept that refers to the differences among people, especially those related to values, attitudes, beliefs, norms, behaviors, customs, and ways of living. It is essential that all nurses understand how cultural groups view life processes, how cultural groups define health and illness, how healers cure and care for members of their respective cultural groups, and how the cultural background of the nurse influences the way in which care is delivered. Nurses in community health settings also need to understand the diversity or differences that occur in families, groups, neighborhoods, communities, and public and community health care organizations.

TRANSCULTURAL PERSPECTIVES ON COMMUNITY HEALTH NURSING

Nurses' knowledge of culture and cultural concepts improves the health of the community by enhancing their ability to provide culturally competent care. Cultural competence is respecting and understanding the values and beliefs of a certain cultural group so that one can function effectively in caring for members of that cultural group. Culturally competent community health nursing requires that nurses understand the lifestyle, value system, and health and illness behaviors of diverse individuals, families, groups, and communities. Nurses should also understand the culture of institutions that influence the health and well-being of communities. Nurses who have knowledge of, and an ability to work with, diverse cultures are able to devise effective interventions to reduce risks in a manner that is culturally congruent with community, group, and individual values.

The "Standards of Practice for Culturally Competent Nursing Care" established by the Expert Panel on Global Nursing and Health (2010) provides important guidelines to help nurses provide culturally competent care. The 12 standards are:

1. Social justice
2. Critical reflection
3. Knowledge of cultures
4. Culturally competent practice
5. Cultural competence in health care systems and organizations
6. Patient advocacy and empowerment
7. Multicultural workforce
8. Education and training in culturally competent care
9. Cross-cultural communication
10. Cross-cultural leadership
11. Policy development
12. Evidence-based practice and research

In the United States, metaphors such as *melting pot* describe the cultural diversity that characterizes the population. Although there is a tendency to identify the federally defined racial and ethnic minority groups when referring to the cultural aspects of community health nursing, all individuals, families, groups, communities, and institutions, including nurses and the nursing profession, have cultural characteristics that influence community health. When planning and implementing health care, community health nurses need to balance cultural diversity with the universal human experience and common needs of all people.

POPULATION TRENDS

The population of the United States is becoming increasingly diverse. In recent years, the populations within the federally defined minority groups have grown faster than the population as a whole. In 1970, minority groups accounted for 16% of the population. By 2017, this share had increased to 38.7% (U.S. Census Bureau, 2017). Assuming that current trends continue, the U.S. Census Bureau (2015) projects that by 2060 minorities will account for more than 56% of the total population.

Furthermore, the numbers of certain minority groups, such as Hispanics, are growing considerably faster than those of whites and other groups. In 2017, estimates of population by race and ethnicity were: white 61.3%; Hispanic or Latino, 17.8%; black/African American, 13.3%; Asian, 5.7%; American Indians and Alaska Natives, 1.3%; other, 0.6% (U.S. Census Bureau, 2017). If current demographic trends continue, the United States will have the following population composition by the year 2060: white, 43.6%; Hispanic or Latino, 28.6%; black/African American, 14.3%; Asian, 9.3%; American Indians and Alaska Natives, 1.3% and other or combination, 2.9% (U.S. Census Bureau, 2015).

Although the nursing profession has representatives from diverse groups, minorities are generally underrepresented. Currently about 83% of registered nurses in the United States are white/non-Hispanic. Estimates for each minority group are as follows: African American, 6.0%; Hispanic, 3.0%; Asian and Pacific Islander, 5.0%; and Native American and Alaska Native, 1.0% (American Association of Colleges of Nursing, 2016).

Additionally, each minority group is distributed differently around the country. African American nurses are more likely to be found in the South, Hispanics in the West or South (i.e., especially states bordering Mexico), and Asian and Pacific Islanders in the West or Northeast. Native American and Alaska Native nurses are predominantly in states with Native American reservations.

The United States has grown and achieved its success largely through immigration. Since 2010, more than 6 million legal immigrants have come to United States (U.S. Department of Homeland Security, 2016). In 2014, the U.S. population included almost 42.3 million foreign-born individuals, or 13.3% of the total population (U.S. Census Bureau, 2015). Among those foreign born, 52% were born in Mexico/Latin America, 26% in Asia, 14% in Europe, and the remaining 8% in other regions of the world (Pew Research Center, 2015b). The number of immigrants and refugees in the United States is projected to continue to increase.

In addition, people from other countries continue to seek treatment in U.S. hospitals, particularly for cardiovascular, neurological, and cancer care. Furthermore, U.S. nurses have the opportunity to travel abroad to work in a variety of health care settings in the international marketplace. In the course of a nursing career, it is possible to encounter foreign visitors, international university faculty members, international high school and university students, family members of foreign diplomats, immigrants, and refugees. Moreover, members of some cultural groups desire culturally relevant health care that incorporates their specific beliefs and practices. A growing expectation exists among members of certain cultural groups that health care providers will respect their "cultural health rights." However, this expectation frequently conflicts with the unicultural, Western biomedical worldview taught in most U.S. educational programs. Therefore a serious conceptual problem exists within nursing in that nurses are expected to know, understand, and meet the health needs of these culturally diverse individuals, groups, and communities without adequate preparation.

♥ HEALTHY PEOPLE 2020

Selected Objectives Related to Cultural Health

- Increase the proportion of all degrees awarded to members of underrepresented racial and ethnic groups among the health professions, allied and associated health profession fields, the nursing field, and the public health field
- Reduce the proportion of adults who are obese
- Reduce the overall cancer death rate
- Reduce the rate of new cases of end-stage renal disease (ESRD)
- Reduce the rate of lower-extremity amputations in persons with diabetes
- Reduce coronary heart disease and stroke deaths
- Reduce pregnancy rates among adolescent females
- Reduce low-birth-weight (LBW) and very-low-birth-weight (VLBW) infants
- Reduce human immunodeficiency virus incidence among adults and adolescents
- Reduce hospitalizations for sickle cell disease among children age 9 years and under
- Achieve and maintain effective vaccination coverage levels for universally recommended vaccines among young children
- Reduce past-month use of illicit substances
- Reduce firearm-related deaths
- Improve health, fitness, and quality of life through daily physical activity

From U.S. Department of Health and Human Services: *Healthy People 2020: Topics and objectives,* (n.d.) Retrieved from http://www.healthy-people.gov/2020/topicsobjectives2020/default.aspx

CULTURAL PERSPECTIVES AND *HEALTHY PEOPLE 2020*

Healthy People 2020 identifies priority areas and objectives. By developing a set of national health targets, which includes eliminating racial and ethnic disparities in health, U.S. health officials, together with state and local officials and members of the private sector, set goals to improve the quality and increase the years of healthy life for all Americans (U.S. Department of Health and Human Services [USDHHS], 2018).

The *Healthy People 2020* objectives embrace and focus on ways to close the gaps in health outcomes. Particularly targeted are racial and ethnic disparities in areas such as diabetes, acquired immunodeficiency syndrome (AIDS), heart disease, infant mortality rates, cancer screening and management, and immunizations. The objectives bring focus on disparities among racial and ethnic minorities, women, youth, older adults, people of low income and education, and people with disabilities (USDHHS, 2018). The *Healthy People 2020* box lists selected objectives from *Healthy People 2020* specific to cultural health issues.

The aims of *Healthy People 2020* are the promotion of healthy behaviors, promotion of healthy and safe communities, improvement of systems for personal and public health, and prevention and reduction of diseases and disorders. The initiative is a tool for monitoring and tracking health status, health risks, and use of health services.

Addressing Racial and Ethnic Disparities in Health Care

As in many nations, people in the United States who come from various racial, ethnic, cultural, and socioeconomic backgrounds often experience marked disparities in health care. The occurrence of many diseases, injuries, and other public health problems is disproportionately higher in some groups; access to health care may be more restricted, and the overall quality of health care is deemed inferior, for people from certain racial, ethnic, and cultural populations. Although the overall health of the U.S. population has improved during the past several decades, research reveals that all people have not shared equally in those improvements. For example, 25.6% of Hispanic adults and 20.5% of African American adults report that they are in fair or poor health, compared with 15.7% of non-Hispanic whites (Kaiser Family Foundation, 2016).

Primary care provides the foundation for the health care system, and research indicates that having a usual source of care increases the chance that people will receive adequate preventive care and other important health services. Data from the Agency for Healthcare Research and Quality (2017) reveal the following facts:

White Americans are more likely to have health insurance (9% uninsured) than either African Americans (14.6% uninsured) or Hispanics (25.9% uninsured).

Thirty percent of Hispanics and 20% of African Americans lack a usual source of health care (compared with fewer than 16% of whites).

Hispanic children are nearly three times as likely as non-Hispanic white children to have no usual source of health care.

African Americans (16%) and Hispanic Americans (13%) are more likely to rely on hospitals or clinics for health care than are whites (8%).

During the past two decades, health disparities have become the focus of numerous federal, state, and local government studies, and one of the major goals of *Healthy People 2020* is to achieve health equity, eliminate disparities, and improve the health of all groups (USDHHS, 2018). Therefore it is essential to look at how to overcome these and other identified factors that contribute to poorer health among members of some minority groups. A survey by the Commonwealth Fund (2007) found that disparities in health care can be reduced or even eliminated when adults have health care insurance and a medical home, which is defined as "a health care setting that provides patients with timely, well-organized care and enhanced access to providers." According to the survey, when adults have insurance and a medical home, "their access to needed care, receipt of routine preventive screenings, and management of chronic conditions improve substantially."

GENETICS IN PUBLIC HEALTH

Genetic Risk Assessment for Cancer: Racial and Ethnic Disparities

Racial and ethnic disparities in deaths attributable to cancer vary considerably for some types of cancer. This is particularly true for breast cancer for African American females, prostate cancer for African American males, and colon cancer for both African American men and women. Despite the widespread recognition of the importance of genetic risk assessment and testing, evidence-based practice guidelines are not followed uniformly in many instances.

Although use of genetic testing and risk assessment among specific populations has increased overall, there are differences based on racial and socioeconomic situations. Underhill and colleagues (2016) pointed out that although African American and Hispanic women have higher rates of hereditary-associated cancers (e.g. breast cancer), they are less likely than White women to be tested for genetic markers. This results in disparities in cancer prevention and early detection. The authors point out that nurses should recognize risk factors for hereditary cancers and refer for genetic testing per established clinical guidelines when appropriate.

Underhill ML, Jones T, Habin K: Disparities in cancer genetic risk assessment and testing, *Oncology Nursing Forum* 43(4):519–523, 2016.

ACTIVE LEARNING

Examine the vital statistics of a community, and compare differences in morbidity and mortality rates for whites and racial and ethnic subgroups. What data are available according to racial and ethnic heritage? What data are missing?

TRANSCULTURAL NURSING

In 1959, Madeleine Leininger, a nurse-anthropologist, used the term **transcultural nursing** to define the philosophical and theoretical similarities between nursing and anthropology. In 1968, Leininger proposed her theory-generated model, and, in 1970, she wrote the first book on transcultural nursing, *Nursing and Anthropology: Two Worlds to Blend* (Leininger, 1970). According to Leininger (1978), transcultural nursing is "a formal area of study and practice focused on a comparative analysis of different cultures and subcultures in the world with respect to cultural care, health and illness beliefs, values, and practices with the goal of using this knowledge to provide culture-specific and culture-universal nursing care to people" (p. 493). **Culture specific** refers to the "particularistic values, beliefs, and patterning of behavior that tend to be special, 'local,' or unique to a designated culture and which do not tend to be shared with members of other cultures" (Leininger, 1991, p. 491), whereas **culture universal** refers to the commonalities of values, norms of behavior, and life patterns that are similarly held among cultures about human behavior and lifestyles and form the bases for formulating theories for developing cross-cultural laws of human behavior" (Leininger, 1991, p. 491).

Although many nurse-scholars have developed theories of nursing, **Leininger's theory of culture care diversity and universality** is the only one that gives precedence to understanding the cultural dimensions of human care and caring. Leininger's theory is concerned with describing, explaining, and projecting nursing similarities and differences focused primarily on human care and caring in human cultures. Leininger used worldview, social structure, language, ethnohistory, environmental context, and the generic or folk and professional systems to provide a comprehensive and holistic view of influences in cultural care and well-being. The following three models of nursing decisions and actions may be useful in providing culturally congruent and competent care (Andrews and Boyle, 2016; Leininger, 1978, 1991, 1995; Leininger and McFarland, 2002):

1. Culture care preservation and maintenance
2. Culture care accommodation and negotiation
3. Culture care repatterning and restructuring

Among the strengths of Leininger's theory is its flexibility for use with individuals, families, groups, communities, and institutions in diverse health systems. Leininger's Sunrise Model depicts the theory of cultural care diversity and universality and provides a visual representation of the key components of the theory and the interrelationships among its components (Fig. 13.1).

The term *cross-cultural nursing* is sometimes used synonymously with *transcultural nursing*. The terms *intercultural nursing* and *multicultural nursing* are also used. Since Leininger's early work, many nurses have contributed significantly to the advancement of nursing care of culturally diverse clients, groups, and communities, and some of their contributions are mentioned in this chapter.

One of the major challenges that community health nurses face in working with clients from culturally diverse backgrounds is overcoming individual **ethnocentrism**, which is a person's tendencies to view his or her own way of life as the most desirable, acceptable, or best and to act in a superior manner toward individuals from another culture. Nurses also must beware of **cultural imposition**, which is a person's tendency to impose his or her own beliefs, values, and patterns of behavior on individuals from another culture. When clients' cultural values and expressions of care differ from those of the nurse, the nurse must exercise caution to ensure that mutual goals have been established.

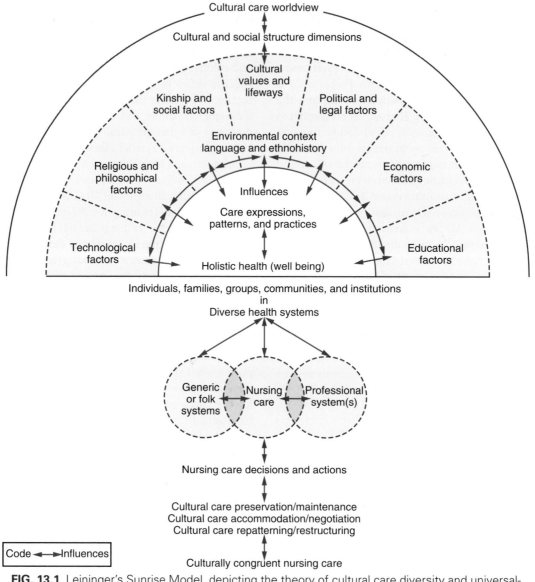

FIG. 13.1 Leininger's Sunrise Model, depicting the theory of cultural care diversity and universality. (From Leininger MM: *Culture, care, diversity, and universality: A theory of nursing*, New York, 1991, National League for Nursing Press.)

OVERVIEW OF CULTURE

In 1871, the English anthropologist Sir Edward Tylor was the first to define the term *culture*. According to Tylor (1871), culture is the complex whole, including knowledge, beliefs, art, morals, law, customs, and any other capabilities and habits acquired by virtue of the fact that one is a member of a particular society. Culture represents a person's way of perceiving, evaluating, and behaving within his or her world, and it provides the blueprint for determining his or her values, beliefs, and practices. Culture has four basic characteristics:

1. It is learned from birth through the processes of language acquisition and socialization.
2. It is shared by members of the same cultural group.
3. It is adapted to specific conditions related to environmental and technical factors and to the availability of natural resources.
4. It is dynamic.

Culture is an all-pervasive and universal phenomenon. However, the culture that develops in any given society is always specific and distinctive, encompassing the knowledge, beliefs, customs, and skills acquired by members of that society. Within cultures, groups of individuals share beliefs, values, and attitudes that are different from those of other groups within the same culture. Ethnicity, religion, education, occupation, age, sex, and individual preferences and variations bring differences. When such groups function within a large culture, they are termed *subcultural groups*.

The term **subculture** is used for fairly large aggregates of people who share characteristics that are not common to all members of the culture and that enable them to be a distinguishable subgroup. Ethnicity, religion, occupation, health-related characteristics, age, sex, and geographic location are frequently used to identify subcultural groups. Examples of

U.S. subcultures based on ethnicity (e.g., subcultures with common traits such as physical characteristics, language, or ancestry) include African Americans, Hispanics, Native Americans, and Chinese Americans. Subcultures based on religion include members of the more than 1200 recognized religions, such as Catholics, Jews, Mormons, Muslims, and Buddhists. Those based on occupation include health care professionals (e.g., nurses and physicians), career military personnel, and farmers. Those based on health-related characteristics include the blind, hearing impaired, and mentally challenged. Subcultures based on age include adolescents and older adults, and those based on sex or sexual preference include women, men, lesbians, and gay men. Those based on geographic location include Appalachians, Southerners, and New Yorkers. Lastly, military veterans are another very common subculture that shares distinct needs and values (see Chapter 22).

Culture and the Formation of Values

According to Leininger (1995), value refers to a desirable or undesirable state of affairs. Values are a universal feature of all cultures, although the types and expressions of values differ widely. Norms are the rules by which human behavior is governed and result from the cultural values held by the group. All societies have rules or norms that specify appropriate and inappropriate behavior. Individuals are rewarded or punished as they conform to or deviate from the established norms, respectively. Values and norms, along with the acceptable and unacceptable behaviors associated with them, are learned in childhood.

Every society has a dominant value orientation, a basic value orientation that is shared by the majority of its members as a result of early common experiences. In the United States, the dominant value orientation is reflected in the dominant cultural group, which is made up of white, middle-class Protestants, typically those who came to the United States at least two generations ago from Northern Europe. Members of the dominant cultural group are sometimes referred to as *white Anglo-Saxon Protestants,* a term that reflects their ancestry and religious beliefs. In the United States, the dominant cultural group places emphasis on educational achievement, science, technology, individual expression, democracy, experimentation, and informality.

Although an assumption is sometimes made that the term *white* refers to a homogeneous group of Americans, a rich diversity of ethnic variation exists among the many groups that constitute the dominant majority. Countries of origin include those of Eastern and Western Europe (e.g., Ireland, Poland, Italy, France, Sweden, and Russia). The origins of people in Canada, Australia, New Zealand, and South Africa can ultimately be traced to Western Europe. Appalachians, Amish, Cajuns, and other subgroups are also examples of whites who have cultural roots that are recognizably different from those of the dominant cultural group.

Values and norms vary, sometimes significantly, among various cultural groups. According to Kluckhohn and Strodtbeck (1961), several basic human problems exist for which all people must find a solution. They identified the following five questions related to values and norms:

1. What is the character of innate human nature (human nature orientation)?
2. What is the relationship of the human to nature (person–nature orientation)?
3. What is the temporal focus (i.e., time sense) of human life (time orientation)?
4. What is the mode of human activity (activity orientation)?
5. What is the mode of human relationships (social orientation)?

Human Nature Orientation

Innate human nature may be good, evil, or a combination of good and evil. Some believe that life is a struggle to overcome a basically evil nature; they consider human nature to be unalterable or able to be perfected only through great discipline and effort. For others, human nature is perceived as fundamentally good, unalterable, and difficult or impossible to corrupt.

According to Kohls (1984), the dominant U.S. cultural group chooses to believe the best about a person until that person proves otherwise. Concern in the United States for prison reform, social rehabilitation, and the plight of less fortunate people around the world is a reflective perception of the belief in the fundamental goodness of human nature. Recent scientific advances, such as advances in stem cell research and genome studies, have necessitated consideration of ethical quandaries regarding human nature. Questions emerge as to whether science can or should pursue activities that could alter the basic human orientation.

Person–Nature Orientation

The following three perspectives examine the ways in which the person–nature relationship is perceived:

- Destiny, in which people are subjugated to nature in a fatalistic, inevitable manner
- Harmony, in which people and nature exist together as a single entity
- Mastery, in which people are intended to overcome natural forces and to put them to use for the benefit of humankind

Most Americans consider humans and nature clearly separated; this is an incomprehensible perspective for many individuals of Asian heritage. The idea that a person can control his or her own destiny is alien to many individuals of culturally diverse backgrounds. Many cultures believe that people are driven and controlled by fate and can do very little, if anything, to influence it. The dominant U.S. cultural group, by contrast, has a mastery perspective.

For example, the reader should consider three individuals in whom hypertension has been diagnosed, each of whom embraces one of the values orientations described. The person whose values orientation is destiny may say, "Why should I bother watching my diet, taking medication, and getting regular blood pressure checks? High blood pressure is part of my genetic destiny and there is nothing I can do to change the outcome. There is no need to waste money on prescription drugs and health checkups." The person whose values orientation embraces harmony may say, "If I follow the diet described and use medication to lower my blood pressure, I can restore the balance and harmony that were upset by this illness. The emotional stress I've been feeling indicates an inner lack of harmony that needs to be balanced." The person whose values orientation leads to belief in active mastery may say, "I will overcome this hypertension no matter what. By eating the right foods, working toward stress reduction, and conquering the disease with medication, I will take charge of the situation and influence the course of my disease."

Time Orientation

People can perceive time in the following three ways:

- *The focus may be on the past, with traditions and ancestors playing an important role in the client's life.* For example, many Asians, Native Americans, East Indians, and Africans hold particular beliefs about ancestors and tend to value long-standing traditions. In times of crisis, such as illness, individuals with a values orientation emphasizing the past may consult with ancestors or ask for their guidance or protection during the illness.
- *The focus may be on the present, with little attention paid to the past or the future.* Individuals with this focus are concerned with the current situation, and they perceive the future as vague or unpredictable. Nurses may have difficulty encouraging such individuals to prepare for the future (e.g., to participate in primary prevention measures).
- *The focus may be on the future, with progress and change highly valued.* Individuals with a future focus may express discontent with the past and present. In terms of health care, they may inquire about the "latest treatment" and the most advanced equipment available for a particular problem.

The dominant U.S. cultural group is characterized by a belief in progress and a future orientation. This combination implies a strong task or goal focus. The group has an optimistic faith in what the future will bring. Change is often equated with improvement, and a rapid rate of change is usually normal.

Activity Orientation

There are different values orientations concerning activity. Philosophers have suggested the following three perspectives:

Being, in which a spontaneous expression of impulses and desires is largely nondevelopmental in nature

Growing, in which the person is self-contained and has inner control, including the ability to self-actualize

Doing, in which the person actively strives to achieve and accomplish something that is regarded highly

The person with a doing orientation often directs the doing toward achievement of an externally applied standard, such as a code of behavior from a religious or ethical perspective. The Ten Commandments, Pillars of Islam, Hippocratic Oath, and Nightingale Pledge are examples of externally applied standards.

The dominant cultural value is action oriented, with an emphasis on productivity and being busy. As a result of this action orientation, Americans have become proficient at problem solving and decision making. Even during leisure time and vacations, many Americans value activity.

Social Orientation

Variations in cultural values orientation are also related to the relationships that exist with others. Relationships may be categorized in the following three ways:

Lineal relationships: These exist by virtue of heredity and kinship ties. These relationships follow an ordered succession and have continuity through time.

Collateral relationships: The focus is primarily on group goals, and family orientation is important. For example, many Asian clients describe family honor and the importance of working together toward an achievement of the group versus a personal goal.

Individual relationships: These refer to personal autonomy and independence. Individual goals dominate, and group goals become secondary.

The social orientation among the dominant U.S. cultural group is toward the importance of the individual and the equality of all people. Friendly, informal, outgoing, and extroverted members of the dominant cultural group tend to scorn rank and authority. For example, nursing students may call faculty members by their first names, clients may call nurses by their first names, and employees may fraternize with their employers.

When making health-related decisions, clients from culturally diverse backgrounds rely on relationships with others in various ways. If the cultural values orientation is lineal, the client may seek assistance from other members of the family and allow a relative (e.g., parent, grandparent, or elder brother) to make decisions about important health-related matters. If collateral relationships are valued, decisions about the client may be interrelated with the influence of illness on the entire family or group. For example, among the Amish, the entire community is affected by the illness of a member because the community pays for health care from a common fund. Members join together to meet the needs of the client and family for the duration of the illness, and the roles of many in the community are likely to be affected by the illness of a single member.

In another example, there are approximately 11.4 million undocumented residents living in the United States as of January 2012 (Baker and Rytina, 2013). These individuals often create their own social groups which may fear that attempting to access the health care system may lead to deportation, and they often have "underground" or private access to home remedies and pharmaceuticals for their health care. As a result, they often enter the formal health care system via emergency departments when their health status has declined considerably (KFF, 2017).

A values orientation that emphasizes the individual is predominant among the dominant cultural majority in the United States. Decision making about health and illness is often an individual matter, with the client being responsible, although members of the nuclear family may participate to varying degrees.

Culture and the Family

The family remains the basic social unit in the United States. Although various ways exist to categorize families, the following are commonly recognized types of constellations in which people live together in society:

- Nuclear (i.e., husband, wife, and child or children)
- Nuclear dyad (i.e., husband and wife alone, either childless or with no children living at home)
- Single parent (i.e., either mother or father and at least one child)
- Blended (i.e., husband, wife, and children from previous relationships)
- Extended (i.e., nuclear plus other blood relatives)
- Communal (i.e., group of men and women with or without children)
- Cohabitation (i.e., unmarried man and woman sharing a household with or without children)
- Lesbian, gay, bisexual, transgender (i.e., same-gender couples, individuals that identify with another gender, with or without children)

In addition to structural differences in families cross-culturally, accompanying functional diversity may exist. For example, among extended families, kin residence sharing has long been recognized as a viable alternative to managing scarce resources, meeting child care needs, and caring for a handicapped or older family member.

The family constellations associated with teen parenting are unique and provide a special socialization context for infants. For example, Hispanic teen mothers receive more child care help from grandmothers and peers than do white teen mothers. Among African Americans and Puerto Ricans, the presence of the maternal grandmother ameliorates the negative consequences of adolescent childbirth on the infant. In addition, grandmothers are more responsive and less punitive in their interactions with the infant than their daughters (Andrews and Boyle, 2016). Three-generational households can have an influence on the infant's development: by influencing the mother's knowledge about development and providing other more responsive social interactions with the infant.

Families from diverse backgrounds are often characterized as being more conservative in terms of sex roles and parenting values and practices than white families. For example, traditional Japanese American and Mexican American families are family centered, enforce strict gender and age roles, and emphasize children's compliance with authority figures (Giger, 2017). Children of culturally diverse backgrounds are involved in family interactions that differ from those of children from the dominant U.S. cultural group. The values of children of immigrants typically evolve, depending on how far removed they are from the country of origin. These children may detach from their cultural traditions, becoming more individually focused or autonomous—often to the dismay of the elders in the family. Often the language of the ancestors is forgotten or, in certain subcultures, forbidden to be spoken, so that the children may assimilate to the dominant culture.

Relationships that may seem apparent sometimes warrant further exploration by nurses interacting with clients from culturally diverse backgrounds. For example, the dominant cultural group defines siblings as two people with the same mother, the same father, the same mother and father, or the same adoptive parents. In some Asian cultures, a sibling relationship is defined as involving infants who are breastfed by the same woman. In other cultures, certain kinship patterns, such as maternal first cousins, are sibling relationships. In some African cultures, anyone from the same village or town may be called "brother" or "sister" (Andrews and Boyle, 2016; Giger, 2017).

When providing care for infants and children, the nurse must identify the primary provider of care because this individual may or may not be the biological parent. For example, among some Hispanic groups, female members of the nuclear or extended family (e.g., sisters or aunts) are sometimes the primary providers of care. In some African American families, the grandmother may be the decision maker and primary caregiver of the children (Andrews and Boyle, 2016).

CULTURE AND SOCIOECONOMIC FACTORS

No single indicator can adequately capture all facets of economic status for entire populations, but measures such as median or average annual income, employment rate, poverty rate, and net worth are most often used. The economic status of most individuals, especially children, is better reflected by the pooled resources of family or household members than by their individual earnings or incomes. Socioeconomic status (SES) is a composite of the economic status of a family or unrelated individuals based on income, wealth, occupation, educational attainment, and power. It is a means of measuring inequalities based on economic differences and the manner in which families live as a result of their economic well-being. Most families with racially or ethnically diverse backgrounds have a lower SES than the population at large, with a few exceptions (e.g., Cuban Americans and subgroups of Asian Americans).

Poverty is another factor that dramatically influences health and well-being. National poverty data are calculated through the use of the official U.S. Census Bureau definition of poverty, which has remained standard since its initial introduction in the mid-1960s. Under this definition, poverty is determined by comparing pretax cash income with the poverty threshold, which adjusts for family size and composition. Table 13.1 provides an overview of the poverty thresholds according to size of family and number of related children under age 18 years residing in the home. The poverty guidelines are issued each year by the USDHHS. The guidelines are a simplification of the poverty threshold for administrative purposes, such as determining financial eligibility for federal programs (e.g., Head Start, National School Lunch, Medicaid, Aid to Families with Dependent Children) (U.S. Census Bureau, 2016).

According to the U.S. Census Bureau per Colby and Ortman (2015), the poverty rate in 2015 was 13.5%, down 1.2% from 2014. The distribution of the poor varies considerably on the basis of certain factors such as age, race or ethnicity, and marital status. For example, 24.1% of the African American population, 11.4% of the Asian population, and 21.4% of the Hispanic population live in poverty. In addition, children under 6 years of age

TABLE 13.1 **Poverty Thresholds ($) For 2016 by Size of Family and Number of Related Children Under 18 Years**

Size of Family Unit	None	RELATED CHILDREN UNDER 18 YEARS							
		One	Two	Three	Four	Five	Six	Seven	Eight or More
One person under 65 years	12,486								
One person 65 years and over	11,511								
Two people: Householder under 65 years	16,072	16,543							
Two people: Householder 65 years and over	14,507	16,480							
Three people	18,774	19,318	19,337						
Four people	24,755	25,160	24,339	24,424					
Five people	29,854	30,288	29,360	28,643	28,205				
Six people	34,337	34,473	33,763	33,082	32,070	31,470			
Seven people	39,509	39,756	38,905	38,313	37,208	35,920	34,507		
Eight people	44,188	44,578	43,776	43,072	42,075	40,809	39,491	39,156	
Nine people or more	53,155	53,413	52,702	52,106	51,127	49,779	48,561	48,259	46,400

Note: The poverty thresholds are updated each year with the use of the change in the average annual Consumer Price Index for All Urban Consumers (CPI-U).

From U.S. Census Bureau: *Poverty thresholds by size of family and number of children, 2016,* 2016. Retrieved from https://www.census.gov/data/tables/time-series/demo/income-poverty/historical-poverty-thresholds.html

are particularly vulnerable to poverty, with 21% of all U.S. children in this age group being poor (Colby and Ortman, 2015).

Distribution of Resources

Status, power, and wealth in the United States are not distributed equally throughout society. Rather, a small percentage of the population enjoys most of the nation's resources, primarily through ownership of multibillion-dollar corporations, large pieces of real estate in prime locations, and similar assets. The U.S. population has traditionally been divided into the following three social classes: upper, middle, and lower. SES may be calculated by considering a variety of factors, but it is customarily determined by examining factors such as total family income, occupation, and educational level.

A disproportionate number of individuals from the racially and ethnically diverse subgroups are members of the lower socioeconomic class, whereas a larger percentage of members of the dominant cultural group belong to the upper and middle socioeconomic classes. The United States has socioeconomic stratification; therefore the idealization of America as the land of opportunity often applies more to members of the upper and middle classes than to those of the lower class. The outcome of social stratification is social inequality. For example, school systems, grocery stores, and recreational facilities vary significantly between the inner city, which has a high percentage of minority residents, and the suburbs, where the residents are overwhelmingly of European ancestry.

For many years, health care settings and health care access have been the subject of study and concern regarding distribution of resources, with members of racial and ethnic minority groups compellingly pointing out the inequalities. Because financing of health care in the United States largely relies on a combination of federally funded insurance (i.e., Medicare) and employer-provided health insurance, those from the highest SES groups and elders tend to receive the best health care. In contrast, those from low-SES groups (i.e., those without health insurance or with Medicaid) tend to receive less health care. Thus, in the United States, SES largely determines access to health care as well as the quality of care received.

Education

One of the components considered in determining SES is educational level. Educational attainment is perhaps the single most important factor. In recent years, there has been an improvement in the level of education among those who have historically been less educated (e.g., elders, women, minorities). For example, women now have a higher rate of high school completion than do men. Also, in 2013, dropout rates for both African Americans and Hispanics have reached all-time lows (Fry, 2014).

❓ ACTIVE LEARNING

1. Visit an inner-city grocery store and compare its quality, prices, customer services, and variety of products with those of a suburban grocery store.
2. Watch prime-time television and note the racial and ethnic diversity that is present during the commercials. During the program, note the roles played by racially and ethnically diverse characters. Are they heroes or heroines or the "bad guys"? What are their occupations, SES, religions, and lifestyles?
3. Skim a popular magazine for references to racially and ethnically diverse subgroups. What is being written? Is the nature of the article favorable or unfavorable?

CULTURE AND NUTRITION

Long after assimilation into U.S. culture has occurred, many members of various ethnic groups continue to follow culturally based dietary practices and eat ethnic foods. Often, neighborhood food markets and ethnic restaurants are established soon after the arrival of a new group of immigrants to the United States. The ethnic restaurant is commonly a place for members of a cultural group to meet and mingle, and customers from the dominant cultural group may be of secondary interest. Food is an integral part of cultural identity that extends beyond dietary preferences.

Nutrition Assessment of Culturally Diverse Groups

Factors that must be considered in a nutrition assessment include the cultural definition of food, frequency and number of meals eaten away from home, form and content of ceremonial meals, amount and types of food eaten, and regularity of food consumption. Twenty-four-hour dietary recalls or 3-day food records traditionally used for assessment may be inadequate when dealing with clients from culturally diverse backgrounds. Standard dietary handbooks may fail to provide culture-specific diet information, because nutritional content and exchange tables are usually based on Western diets. Another source of error may originate from the cultural patterns of eating. For example, among low-income urban African American families, elaborate weekend meals are frequent, whereas weekday dietary patterns are markedly more moderate (Giger, 2017).

Although community health nurses may assume that *food* is a culture-universal term, they may need to clarify its meaning with the client. For example, certain Latin American groups do not consider greens, an important source of vitamins, to be food and fail to list intake of these vegetables on daily records. Among Vietnamese refugees, dietary intake of calcium may appear inadequate because low consumption rates of dairy products are common among members of this group. However, they commonly consume pork bones and shells, providing adequate quantities of calcium to meet daily requirements (Giger, 2017).

Food is only one part of eating. In some cultures, social contacts during meals are restricted to members of the immediate or extended family. For example, in some Middle Eastern cultures, men and women eat meals separately, or women are permitted to eat with their husbands but not with other males. Among some Hispanic groups, the male breadwinner is served first, then the women and children eat. Etiquette during meals, use of hands, type of eating utensils (e.g., chopsticks or special flatware), and protocols governing the order in which food is consumed during a meal all vary cross-culturally.

Dietary Practices of Selected Cultural Groups

Cultural stereotyping is the tendency to view individuals of common cultural backgrounds similarly and according to a preconceived notion of how they behave. However, not all Chinese like rice, not all Italians like spaghetti, and not all Mexicans like tortillas. Nevertheless, aggregate dietary preferences among people from certain cultural groups can be considered (e.g., characteristic ethnic dishes and methods of food preparation, including use of cooking oils); the reader is referred to nutrition texts on the topic for detailed information about culture-specific diets and the nutritional value of ethnic foods.

Religion and Diet

Cultural food preferences are often interrelated with religious dietary beliefs and practices. As indicated in Table 13.2, many religions have proscriptive dietary practices, and some use food

TABLE 13.2 Dietary Practices of Selected Religious Groups

Religion	Dietary Practice
Hinduism	All meats are prohibited.
Islam	Pork and intoxicating beverages are prohibited.
Judaism	Pork, predatory fowl, shellfish, other water creatures (fish with scales are permissible), and blood by ingestion (e.g., blood sausage and raw meat) are prohibited. Blood by transfusion is acceptable. Foods should be kosher (meaning "properly preserved"). All animals must be ritually slaughtered by a shochet (i.e., quickly with the least pain possible) to be kosher. Mixing dairy and meat dishes at the same meal is prohibited.
Mormonism (Church of Jesus Christ of Latter-day Saints)	Alcohol, tobacco, and beverages containing caffeine (e.g., coffee, tea, colas, and select carbonated soft drinks) are prohibited.
Seventh-Day Adventism	Pork, certain seafood (including shellfish), and fermented beverages are prohibited. A vegetarian diet is encouraged.

as symbols in celebrations and rituals. Knowing the client's religious practice as it relates to food makes it possible to suggest improvements or modifications that will not conflict with religious dietary laws.

Fasting and other religious observations may limit a person's food or liquid intake during specified times. For example, many Catholics fast or abstain from meat on Ash Wednesday, and each Friday during the season of Lent, Muslims refrain from eating during the daytime hours for the month of Ramadan but are permitted to eat after sunset, and Mormons refrain from ingesting all solid foods and liquids on the first Sunday of each month.

⁇ ACTIVE LEARNING

Dine at an ethnic restaurant. While dining, notice the type of cultural heritage in restaurant decor and information about the culture available from the menu, placemats, or elsewhere in the restaurant. Ask the owner or manager about the history of the restaurant.

CULTURE AND RELIGION

According to the *2014 U.S. Religious Landscape Study*, 70.6% of U.S. citizens identify with Christian faiths, 5.9% non-Christian faiths, and 22.8% unaffiliated with a faith (atheist, agnostic, and nothing in particular) (Pew Research Center, 2015a). Adults who describe themselves as "Christian" have dropped almost 8 points since 2007, according to findings by the Pew Research survey. Furthermore, about 66% note that they are members of a church, synagogue, or mosque. The largest religious groups are Protestant, 46.5%; Catholic, 20.8%; Jewish, 1.9%; and Mormon, 1.6% (Pew Research Center, 2015a). The largest specific Protestant denominations are the United Methodist Church, American Baptist Church, Evangelical Lutheran Church, Presbyterian Church, and Episcopal Church.

Although the nurse cannot be an expert on each of the estimated 1200 religions practiced in the United States, knowledge of health-related beliefs and practices and general information about religious observances are important in providing culturally competent nursing care. For example, when planning home visits or scheduling clinic visits for members of a specific religious group, the nurse should consult the group's religious calendar and work around designated holy days. The nurse should also know the customary days of religious worship observed by members of the religion. Most Protestants worship on Sundays, whereas Muslims' holy day of worship extends from sunset on Thursday to sunset on Friday, and Jews and Seventh-Day Adventists' holy day extends from sunset on Friday to sunset on Saturday. Roman Catholics may worship in the late afternoon or evening of Saturday or all day Sunday. Some religions may meet more than once weekly.

As an integral component of the individual's culture, religious beliefs may influence the client's explanation of the cause of illness, perception of its severity, and choice of healer. In times of crisis, such as serious illness and impending death, religion may be a source of consolation for the client and family and may influence the course of action believed to be appropriate.

Religion and Spirituality

Religious concerns evolve from, and respond to, the mysteries of life and death, good and evil, and pain and suffering. Nurses frequently encounter clients who find themselves searching for a spiritual meaning to help explain illness or disability. Some nurses find spiritual assessment difficult because the topic is abstract and personal, whereas others feel comfortable discussing spiritual matters. Comfort with personal spiritual beliefs is the foundation for effective assessment of spiritual needs in clients.

Although religions offer various interpretations of many of life's mysteries, most people seek a personal understanding and interpretation at some time in their lives. Ultimately, this personal search becomes a pursuit to discover a supreme being (e.g., Allah, God, Yahweh, or Jehovah) or some unifying truth that will render meaning, purpose, and integrity to existence.

An important distinction must be made between religion and spirituality. **Religion** refers to an organized system of beliefs concerning the cause, nature, and purpose of the universe, especially belief in or the worship of a god or gods. As already stated, more than 1200 religions are practiced in the United States. **Spirituality**, in contrast, is born out of the individual's unique life experience and personal effort to find purpose and meaning in life. Box 13.1 provides suggested guidelines for assessing the spiritual needs of culturally diverse clients. Table 13.3 illustrates a shared belief among various religions.

Religion may influence decisions regarding prolongation of life, euthanasia, autopsy, donation of a body for research, disposal of a body and body parts including fetus, and type of burial. The nurse should use discretion in asking clients and their families about these issues and gather data only when the clinical situation necessitates that the information be obtained. The nurse should encourage clients and families to discuss these issues with their religious representative when necessary. Before

---

BOX 13.1 Methods of Assessing Spiritual Needs in Culturally Diverse Clients

Environment
- Does the client have religious objects in the environment?
- Does the client wear outer garments or undergarments that have religious significance?
- Are get-well greeting cards religious in nature or from a representative of the client's religious institution?
- Does the client receive flowers or bulletins from a church or other religious institution?

Behavior
- Does the client appear to pray at certain times of the day or before meals?
- Does the client make special dietary requests (e.g., kosher diet; vegetarian diet; or diet free from caffeine, pork, shellfish, or other specific food items)?
- Does the client read religious magazines or books?

Verbalization
- Does the client mention a Supreme Being (e.g., God, Allah, Buddha, or Yahweh), prayer, faith, church, or religious topics?
- Does the client request a visit by a clergy member or other religious representative?
- Does the client express anxiety or fear about pain, suffering, or death?

Interpersonal Relationships
- Who visits the client? How does the client respond to visitors?
- Does a church representative visit?
- How does the client relate to nursing staff and roommates?
- Does the client prefer to interact with others or remain alone?

Data from Andrews MM, Boyle JS, editors: *Transcultural concepts in nursing care*, ed 7, Philadelphia, PA, 2016, Wolters Kluwer.

TABLE 13.3 Shared Beliefs Among Various Religions: The "Golden Rule"

Religion	Scripture	Source
Buddhism	"Hurt not others in ways that you yourself would find hurtful."	Udana-varga 5:18
Christianity	"Whatsoever you would that men should do to you, do you even so to them."	Matthew 7:12
Confucianism	"Do not do to others what you do not want them to do to you."	Analects 15:23
Hinduism	"One should not behave towards others in a way which is disagreeable to oneself."	Mahabharata 5:1517; Mencius Vii.A.4
Islam	"Not one of you is a believer until he loves for his brother what he loves for himself."	Number 13 of Al-Nawawi's Forty Hadiths
Judaism	"Thou shalt love thy neighbor as thyself."	Leviticus 19:18
Taoism	"Regard your neighbor's gain as your own gain and your neighbor's loss as your own loss."	T'ai Shang Kan Ying P'ien

dealing with potentially sensitive issues, the nurse should establish rapport with the client and family by gaining their trust and confidence in less sensitive areas.

Childhood and Spirituality

Serious illness during childhood is especially difficult. Children have spiritual needs that vary according to the child's developmental level and the religious climate that exists in the family. Parental perceptions about the illness of their child may be partially influenced by religious beliefs. For example, some parents may believe that a transgression against a religious law is responsible for a congenital anomaly in their offspring. Other parents may delay seeking medical care because they believe that prayer should be tried first. Certain types of treatment (e.g., administration of blood or medications containing caffeine or other prohibited substances and selected procedures) may be perceived as cultural taboos, which are to be avoided by children and adults.

> ### ❓ ACTIVE LEARNING
>
> 1. Attend religious services at a church, temple, synagogue, or place of worship for a religion unfamiliar to you.
> 2. Interview an official representative (e.g., priest, elder, monk, or bishop) of a religion unfamiliar to you. Ask about health-related beliefs and practices, healing rituals, support network for the sick, and dietary practices.

CULTURE AND AGING

Values held by the dominant U.S. culture, such as emphasis on independence, self-reliance, and productivity, influence aging members of society. Americans define people 65 years and older as "old" and limit their work. In some other cultures, people are first recognized as being unable to work and then identified as being old. In some cultures the wisdom, not the productivity, of the older adult is valued; the diminution of one's activity level and the reduction of physical stamina associated with growing old are accepted more readily without loss of status among culture members. Retirement is also culturally defined, with some older adults working as long as physical health continues and others continuing to be active but assuming less physically demanding jobs.

The main task of older adults in the dominant culture is to achieve a sense of integrity in accepting responsibility for their own lives and having a sense of accomplishment. Individuals who achieve integrity consider aging a positive experience, make adjustments in their personal space and social relationships, maintain a sense of usefulness, and begin closure and life review. Not all cultures value accepting responsibility for an individual's own life. For example, among Hispanics, Asians, Arabs, and other groups, older adults are often cared for by family members who welcome them into their homes when they are no longer able to live alone. The concept of placing an older family member in an institutional setting to be cared for by strangers is perceived as an uncaring, impersonal, and culturally unacceptable practice by many cultural groups (Andrews and Boyle, 2016; Giger, 2017).

Older adults may develop their own means of coping with illness through self-care, assistance from family members, and social group support systems. Some cultures have developed attitudes and specific behaviors for older adults that include humanistic care and identification of family members as care providers. Older adults may have special family responsibilities (e.g., the older Amish adults provide hospitality to visitors, and older Filipino adults spend considerable time teaching the youth skills learned during a lifetime of experience).

Older adult immigrants who have made major lifestyle adjustments in the move from their homeland to the United States or from a rural to an urban area, or vice versa, may need information about health care alternatives, preventive programs, health care benefits, and screening programs for which they are eligible. These individuals may also be in various stages of **culture shock**, the state of disorientation or inability to respond to the behavior of a different cultural group because it holds sudden strangeness, unfamiliarity, and incompatibility for the newcomer's perceptions and expectations (Leininger and McFarland, 2002).

Several examples of how being an elderly immigrant influences health can be found in the nursing literature. Wilmoth and Chen (2003) studied living arrangements and symptoms of depression among middle-aged and older immigrants and concluded that immigrants had significantly more depressive symptoms than nonimmigrants. Furthermore, immigrants who lived alone or with family had more depressive symptoms than those who lived with a spouse.

CROSS-CULTURAL COMMUNICATION

Verbal communication and nonverbal communication are important in community health nursing and are influenced by the cultural background of the nurse and client. *Cross-cultural, or intercultural, communication* refers to the communication process between a nurse and a client with different cultural backgrounds as each attempts to understand the other's point of view from a cultural perspective.

Nurse–Client Relationship

From the introduction of the nurse to the client through termination of the relationship, communication is a continuous process for the community health nurse. First impressions are important in all human relationships; therefore cross-cultural considerations concerning introductions warrant a few brief remarks. To ensure a mutually respectful and trusting relationship, the nurse should introduce himself or herself and indicate how the client should refer to the nurse (i.e., by first name, last name, or title). Having done so, the nurse should ask the client to do the same. This enables the nurse to address the client in a manner that is culturally appropriate, thereby avoiding potential embarrassment. For example, some Asian and European cultures write the last name first; confusion can be avoided in an area of sensitivity (i.e., the client's name).

Space, Distance, and Intimacy

Sense of spatial distance is significant because culturally appropriate distance zones vary widely. For example, the nurse may back away from clients of Hispanic, East Indian, or Middle Eastern origin who invade personal space with regularity in an attempt to bring the nurse closer into the space that is comfortable to them. Although the nurse is uncomfortable with clients' close physical proximity, clients are perplexed by the nurse's distancing behaviors and may perceive the community health nurse as aloof and unfriendly. Table 13.4 summarizes the four distance zones identified for the functional use of space that are embraced by the dominant cultural group in the United States, including most nurses.

Overcoming Communication Barriers

Nurses tend to have stereotypical expectations of the client's behavior. In general, nurses expect behavior to consist of undemanding compliance, an attitude of respect for the health care provider, and cooperation with requested behavior throughout the examination. Although clients may ask a few questions for clarification, slight deference to recognized authority figures (e.g., health care providers) is expected. However, individuals from culturally diverse backgrounds may have significantly different perceptions about the appropriate role of the individual and family when seeking health care. If nurses find themselves becoming annoyed that a client is asking too many questions, assuming a defensive posture, or otherwise feeling uncomfortable, they may pause for a moment to examine the source of the conflict from a cross-cultural perspective.

During illness, culturally acceptable "sick-role" behavior may range from aggressive, demanding behavior to silent passivity (Cockerham, 2009). Complaining, demanding behavior during illness is may be rewarded with attention in some cultures, whereas others may promote quiet and compliance in clients during illness (Andrews and Boyle, 2016). Furthermore, during an interview, Asian clients may provide the nurse with the answers they think the nurse wants to hear, behavior that is consistent within their cultural value for harmonious relationships with others. The nurse should attempt to phrase questions or statements in a neutral manner that avoids

TABLE 13.4	Functional Use of Space
Zone	**Remarks**
Intimate zone (0 to 1.5 feet)	Visual distortion occurs.
	Best for assessing breath and other body odors.
Personal distance (1.5 to 4 feet)	Perceived as an extension of the self, similar (1.5 to 4 feet) to a "bubble."
	Voice is moderate.
	Body odors are inapparent.
	Visual distortion does not occur.
	Much of the physical assessment will occur at this distance.
Social distance (4 to 12 feet)	Used for impersonal business transactions.
	Perceptual information is much less detailed.
	Much of the interview will occur at this distance.
Public distance (>12 feet)	Interaction with others is impersonal.
	Speaker's voice must be projected.
	Subtle facial expressions are imperceptible.

Data from Hall E: Proxemics: The study of man's spatial relations. In Galdston I, editor, *Man's image in medicine and anthropology*, New York, 1963, International Universities Press.

foreshadowing an expected response. Appalachian clients may reject a community health nurse whom they perceive as prying or nosy because a cultural ethic of neutrality mandates that people mind their own business and avoid assertive or argumentative behavior (Giger, 2017).

Nonverbal Communication

Unless the nurse makes an effort to understand the client's nonverbal behavior, he or she may overlook important information such as that conveyed by facial expressions, silence, eye contact, touch, and other body language. Communication patterns vary widely cross-culturally, even for seemingly "innocent" behaviors such as smiling and shaking hands. For example, among many Hispanic clients, smiling and shaking hands are considered an integral part of sincere interaction and essential to establishing trust, whereas a Russian client may perceive the same behavior from the nurse as insolent and frivolous (Giger, 2017).

Gender issues also become significant. For example, among some groups of Middle Eastern origin, men and women do not shake hands or touch each other in any manner outside the marital relationship. However, if the nurse and client are both female, a handshake is usually acceptable (Andrews and Boyle, 2016).

Wide cultural variation exists in the interpretation of silence. Some individuals find silence extremely uncomfortable and make every effort to fill conversational lags with words. In contrast, Native Americans consider silence essential to understanding and respecting the other person. A pause after a question signifies that what the speaker has asked is important enough to be given thoughtful consideration. In traditional Chinese and Japanese cultures, silence may mean that the speaker wishes the listener to consider the content of what has been said before continuing. The English and Arabs may use silence out of respect for another person's privacy, whereas the French, Spanish, and Russians may interpret it as a sign of agreement. Asian cultures often use silence to demonstrate respect for elders (Giger, 2017).

Eye contact is among the most culturally variable nonverbal behaviors. Although most nurses have been taught to maintain eye contact while talking with clients, individuals from culturally diverse backgrounds may misconstrue this behavior. Asian, Native American, Indochinese, Arab, and Appalachian clients may consider direct eye contact impolite or aggressive, and they may avert their own eyes during the conversation. Native American clients often stare at the floor when the nurse is talking. This culturally appropriate behavior indicates that the listener is paying close attention to the speaker (Giger, 2017; Andrews and Boyle, 2016).

In some cultures, modesty for women is interrelated with eye contact. For a Muslim woman, modesty is achieved in part by avoiding eye contact with men, except for her husband, and keeping the eyes downcast when encountering members of the opposite sex in public situations. In many cultures, the only women who smile and establish eye contact with men in public are prostitutes (Giger, 2017). Hasidic Jewish men also have culturally based norms concerning eye contact with women. Such a man may avoid direct eye contact and turn his head in the opposite direction when walking past or speaking to a woman. It is important to understand that the preceding examples are intended to be illustrative and are not exhaustive, nor do they represent values, actions, and beliefs of all members of the cultural groups described.

Language

To assess non–English-speaking clients, the nurse may need the help of an interpreter. Interviewing a non–English-speaking person requires a bilingual interpreter for full communication. Even the person from another culture or country who has a basic command of English may need an interpreter when faced with the anxiety-provoking situation of becoming ill; encountering a strange symptom; or discussing sensitive topics such as birth control, gynecological concerns, and urological problems. The nurse may be tempted to ask a relative or friend of another client to interpret because this person is readily available and is anxious to help. However, doing so is disadvantageous because it violates confidentiality for the client, who may not want personal information shared with another. Furthermore, the friend or relative, although fluent in ordinary language, is likely to be unfamiliar with medical terminology, clinical procedures, and medical ethics.

Whenever possible, the nurse should use a bilingual team member or trained medical interpreter. This person knows interpreting techniques, has a health care background, and understands clients' rights. The trained interpreter is also knowledgeable about cultural beliefs and health practices, can help bridge the cultural gap, and can provide advice concerning the cultural appropriateness of recommendations.

Although the nurse is in charge of the client–nurse interaction, the interpreter is an important member of the health care team. Whenever feasible, the nurse should ask the interpreter to meet the client before the visit to establish rapport and learn about the client's age, occupation, educational level, and attitude toward health care. This knowledge enables the interpreter to communicate on the client's level.

The nurse should allow more time for visits with culturally diverse clients who require an interpreter. With the third person repeating everything, it can take considerably longer than interviewing English-speaking clients. The nurse will need to focus on the major points and prioritize data.

Line by line and summarization are interpretation styles. Translation line by line ensures accuracy, but it takes more time. The nurse and client should speak only a sentence or two and then allow the interpreter time to interpret. The nurse should use simple language, not medical jargon that the interpreter must simplify before translating. Summary translation is faster and useful for teaching relatively simple health techniques with which the interpreter is already familiar. The nurse should be alert for nonverbal cues as the client talks because they can give valuable data. A good interpreter will also note nonverbal messages and communicate those to the community health nurse. Box 13.2 summarizes suggestions for the selection and use of an interpreter.

Although use of an interpreter is ideal, the nurse may find himself or herself in a situation with a non–English-speaking client in which no interpreter is available. Box 13.3 provides some suggestions for overcoming language barriers when an interpreter is not available.

BOX 13.2 Overcoming Language Barriers: Use of an Interpreter

- Before locating an interpreter, the nurse should know what language the client speaks at home because it may be different from the language spoken publicly (e.g., French is sometimes spoken by aristocratic or well-educated people from certain Asian or Middle Eastern cultures).
- The nurse should avoid interpreters from a rival tribe, state, region, or nation (e.g., a Palestinian who knows Hebrew may not be the best interpreter for a Jewish client).
- The nurse should be aware of the gender difference between the interpreter and client to avoid violation of cultural mores related to modesty.
- The nurse should be aware of the age difference between the interpreter and client.
- The nurse should be aware of socioeconomic differences between the interpreter and client.
- The nurse should ask the interpreter to translate as closely to verbatim as possible.
- An interpreter who is not a relative may seek compensation for services rendered.

BOX 13.3 Overcoming Language Barriers when an Interpreter is not Available

- The nurse should be polite and formal.
- The nurse should greet the client using his or her last or complete name. The nurse should gesture to himself or herself and say his or her name. The nurse should offer a handshake, nod, or smile.
- The nurse should proceed in an unhurried manner. The nurse should pay attention to efforts by the client or family to communicate.
- The nurse should speak in a low, moderate voice. The nurse should remember that he or she may have a tendency to raise the volume and pitch of his or her voice when the listener appears not to understand, and the listener may perceive that the nurse is shouting or angry.
- The nurse should use words that he or she may know in the client's language. Doing so indicates that the nurse is aware of and respects the client's culture.
- The nurse should use simple words, such as "pain" instead of "discomfort." The nurse should avoid medical jargon and slang. He or she should avoid using contractions such as "don't," "can't," and "won't." The nurse should use nouns repeatedly instead of pronouns. For example, the nurse should say, "Do you take medicine?" instead of "You have been taking your medicine, haven't you?"
- The nurse should pantomime words and simple actions while verbalizing them.
- The nurse should give instructions in the proper sequence. For example, he or she should say, "First, wash the bottle. Second, rinse the bottle," instead of "Before you rinse the bottle, sterilize it."
- The nurse should discuss one topic at a time. He or she should avoid use of conjunctions. For example, the nurse should ask, "Are you cold [while pantomiming]?" and then "Are you in pain?" instead of, "Are you cold and in pain?"
- The nurse should determine whether the client understands by having the client repeat instructions, demonstrate the procedure, or act out the meaning.
- The nurse should write out several short sentences in English and determine the client's ability to read them.
- The nurse should try a third language. Many Indo-Chinese people speak French. Europeans often know three or four languages. The nurse should try Latin words or phrases.
- The nurse should ask who among the client's family and friends could serve as an interpreter.
- The nurse should obtain phrase books from a library or bookstore, make or purchase flash cards, contact hospitals for a list of interpreters, and use both formal and informal networking to locate suitable interpreters.

Touch

Touching the client is a necessary component of a comprehensive assessment. Although benefits exist in establishing rapport with clients through touch, including the promotion of healing through therapeutic touch, physical contact with clients conveys various meanings cross-culturally. In many cultures (e.g., Arab and Hispanic), male health care providers may be prohibited from touching or examining all or certain parts of the female body. During pregnancy, the client may prefer female health care providers and may refuse to be examined by a man. The nurse should be aware that the client's significant other also might exert pressure on health care providers by enforcing these culturally meaningful norms in the health care setting.

Touching children may also have variable meanings cross-culturally. For example, Hispanic clients may believe in *mal ojo* (evil eye), in which an individual becomes ill as a result of excessive admiration by another. Many Asians believe that personal strength resides in the head and consider touching the head disrespectful. The nurse should approach palpation of the fontanelle of an infant of Southeast Asian descent with sensitivity. The nurse may need to rely on alternative sources of information (e.g., assessing for clinical manifestations of increased intracranial pressure or signs of premature fontanelle closure). Although it is the least desirable option, the nurse may need to omit this part of the assessment (Giger, 2017).

Gender

Violating norms related to appropriate male–female relationships among various cultures may jeopardize the therapeutic nurse–client relationship. Among Arab Americans, a man is never alone with a woman, except his wife, and is usually accompanied by one or more other men when interacting with women. This behavior is culturally significant, and failure to adhere to the cultural code (i.e., set of rules or norms of behavior used by a cultural group to guide their behavior and interpret situations) is viewed as a serious transgression, often one in which the lone male will be accused of sexual impropriety. The best way to ensure that cultural variables have been considered is to ask the client about culturally relevant aspects of male–female relationships, preferably at the beginning of the interaction before an opportunity arises to violate culturally based practices.

HEALTH-RELATED BELIEFS AND PRACTICES

One of the major aspects of a comprehensive cultural assessment concerns the collection of data related to culturally based beliefs and practices about health and illness. Before determining whether cultural practices are helpful, harmful, or neutral, the nurse must first understand the logic of the belief system underlying the practice and then be sure to grasp fully the nature and meaning of the practice from the client's cultural perspective.

Health and Culture

The first step in understanding the health care needs of clients is to understand personal culturally based values, beliefs, attitudes, and practices. Sometimes this step requires considerable introspection and may necessitate that the nurse confront his or her own biases, preconceptions, and prejudices about specific racial, ethnic, religious, sexual, or socioeconomic groups. The next step is to identify the meaning of health to the client, remembering that concepts are derived, in part, from the way in which members of their cultural group define health.

Considerable research has been conducted on the various definitions of health that may be held by various groups. For example, Jamaicans define health as having a good appetite, feeling strong and energetic, performing activities of daily living without difficulty, and being sexually active and fertile. For traditional Italian women, health means the ability to interact socially and perform routine tasks such as cooking, cleaning, and caring for oneself and others. Individuals may define themselves or others in their group as healthy even though the nurse identifies symptoms of disease (Spector, 2017).

Cross-Cultural Perspectives on Causes of Illness

For clients, symptom labeling and diagnosis depend on the extent of the difference between the individual's behaviors and those the group defines as normal. Other issues that the nurse should consider include the client's beliefs about the causation of illness, level of stigma attached to a particular set of symptoms, prevalence of the disease, and meaning of the illness to the individual and family.

Throughout history, humankind has attempted to understand the cause of illness and disease. Theories of causation have been formulated on the basis of religious beliefs, social circumstances, philosophical perspectives, and level of knowledge. Disease causation may be viewed from the following three major perspectives: biomedical (i.e., sometimes used synonymously with the term *scientific*), naturalistic (i.e., sometimes used synonymously with the term *holistic*), and magicoreligious (i.e., metaphysical or supernatural belief).

Biomedical Perspective

The **biomedical** (i.e., scientific) theory of illness causation is based on the following beliefs:

1. All events in life have a cause and effect.
2. The human body functions more or less mechanically (i.e., the functioning of the human body is analogous to the functioning of an automobile).
3. All life can be reduced or divided into smaller parts (e.g., the human person can be reduced into body, mind, and spirit).
4. All of reality can be observed and measured (e.g., with intelligence tests and psychometric measures of behavior).

Among the biomedical explanations for disease is the germ theory, which posits that microscopic organisms such as bacteria and viruses are responsible for many specific disease conditions. Most educational programs for nurses and other health care providers embrace biomedical, or scientific, theories that explain the causes of physical and psychological illnesses.

Naturalistic Perspective

Another way in which clients may explain the cause of illness is from the **naturalistic** (i.e., holistic) perspective. This viewpoint is found most frequently among Native Americans, Asians, and others who believe that human life is only one aspect of nature and a part of the general order of the cosmos. Individuals from these groups believe that the forces of nature must be kept in natural balance or harmony to maintain health and well-being. A combination of worldviews is possible, and many clients are likely to offer more than one explanation for the cause of their illness. As a profession, nursing largely embraces the biomedical-scientific worldview, but some aspects of holism have begun to gain popularity. These include a wide variety of techniques for management of chronic pain (e.g., hypnosis, therapeutic touch, and biofeedback). Many nurses hold a belief in spiritual power and readily credit supernatural forces with various unexplained phenomena related to clients' health and illness states.

Numerous Asians subscribe to the yin-yang theory, in which health is believed to exist when all aspects of the person are in perfect balance. Rooted in the ancient Chinese philosophy of Tao, the yin-yang theory states that all organisms and objects in the universe consist of yin or yang energy forces. The origin of the energy forces is within the autonomic nervous system, where balance between the opposing forces is maintained during health. Yin energy represents the female and negative forces (e.g., emptiness, darkness, and cold), whereas yang forces are male and positive, emitting fullness, light, and warmth. Foods are classified as hot and cold in this theory and are transformed into yin and yang energy when metabolized by the body. Yin foods are cold, and yang foods are hot. Cold foods are eaten when one has a hot illness, and hot foods are eaten when one has a cold illness. The yin-yang theory is the basis for Eastern or Chinese medicine.

The naturalistic perspective posits that the laws of nature create imbalance, chaos, and disease. Individuals embracing the naturalistic view use metaphors such as the healing power of nature, and they may call the earth "Mother." For example, from the perspective of the Chinese, illness is seen not as an intruding agent but rather as a part of life's rhythmic course and an outward sign of the disharmony that exists within.

Many Hispanic, Arab, African American, and Asian groups embrace a hot-cold theory of health and illness, an explanatory model with its origin in the ancient Greek humoral theory. Blood, phlegm, black bile, and yellow bile, the four humors of the body, regulate basic bodily functions and are described in terms of temperature, dryness, and moisture. The treatment of disease consists of adding or subtracting cold, heat, dryness, or wetness to restore the balance of the humors.

Beverages, foods, herbs, medicines, and diseases are classified as hot or cold according to their perceived effects on the body, not on their physical characteristics. Illnesses believed to be caused by cold entering the body include earache, chest cramps, paralysis, gastrointestinal discomfort, rheumatism, and tuberculosis. Illnesses believed to be caused by overheating include abscessed teeth, sore throats, rashes, and kidney disorders.

According to the hot-cold theory, the individual as a whole, rather than a specific ailment, is significant. Those who embrace the hot-cold theory maintain that health consists of a positive state of total well-being, including physical, psychological, spiritual, and social aspects of the person. Paradoxically, the language used to describe this artificial dissection of the body into parts is a reflection of the biomedical-scientific perspective, not a naturalistic or holistic one.

Magicoreligious Perspective

Another way in which people explain the causation of illness is from a magicoreligious perspective. The basic premise of this explanatory model is that the world is seen as an arena in which supernatural forces dominate. The fate of the world and those in it depends on the action of supernatural forces for good or evil. Examples of magical causes of illness include the belief in voodoo or witchcraft among some African Americans and others from circum-Caribbean countries. Faith healing is based on religious beliefs and is most prevalent among selected Christian religions, including Christian Scientists. Various healing rituals (prayer, anointing, exorcism, laying of hands, etc.) may be found in many religions—Roman Catholicism, Mormonism (i.e., Church of Jesus Christ of Latter-day Saints), and others (Hanson and Andrews, 2016).

Folk Healers

All cultures have their own recognized symptoms of ill health, acceptable sick-role behavior, and treatments. In addition to seeking help from the nurse as a biomedical-scientific health care provider, clients from many groups may seek help from folk or religious healers.

Numerous types of folk healers exist, each with a unique scope of practice. Hispanic clients may turn to a *curandero* (male folk healer) or *curandera* (female folk healer), spiritualist, *yerbo* (herbalist), or *sabador* (healer who manipulates muscles and bones). In many instances, people from diverse cultures combine folk healing and biomedicine. Among the main reasons for seeking care from folk healers is the perception that biomedical practitioners (e.g., physicians and nurses) fail to provide holistic care and use medicines that are not natural (Andrews and Boyle 2016).

Some African American clients may mention having received assistance from a *hougan* (voodoo priest or priestess), spiritualist, or "old lady" (an older woman who has successfully raised a family and specializes in child care and folk remedies). Likewise, Native American clients may seek assistance from a shaman or a medicine man or woman. Clients of Asian descent may mention that they have visited herbalists, acupuncturists, or bone setters (Giger, 2017).

Each culture has its own healers, most of whom speak the native tongue of the client, make house calls, and cost significantly less than healers practicing in the biomedical-scientific health care system. In addition to folk healers, many cultures rely on lay midwives (e.g., *parteras* for Hispanic women) or other health care providers to meet the needs of pregnant women.

In some religions, spiritual healers may be found among the ranks of the ordained or official religious hierarchy ranks and are called *priest, bishop, elder, deacon, rabbi, brother,* or *sister.* Other religions have a separate category of healer (e.g., Christian Science "nurses" [not licensed by states] or practitioners) (Hanson and Andrews, 2016).

A comprehensive discussion of the variety of healing beliefs and practices used by the numerous cultural groups is beyond the scope of this chapter. However, the nurse should be aware of alternative practices and folk healers that are used by the groups for which they care. The nurse should also be aware that most indigenous healing practices are innocuous, regardless of whether they are effective.

Cultural Expressions of Illness

A wide cultural variation exists in the manner in which certain symptoms and disease conditions are perceived, diagnosed, labeled, and treated. The disease that is grounds for social ostracism in one culture may be reason for increased status in another.

Bodily symptoms are also perceived and reported in a variety of ways. For example, individuals of Mediterranean descent tend to report common physical symptoms more often than people of Northern European or Asian heritage. To express emotion, East Asian clients sometimes somaticize their symptoms. For example, a client may complain of cardiac symptoms because the center of emotion in the Chinese culture is the heart. If the client has experienced a loss through death or divorce and is grieving, he or she may describe the loss in terms of a pain in the heart. Although some biomedical-scientific clinicians may refer to this pain as a psychosomatic illness, others will recognize it as a culturally acceptable somatic expression of emotional disharmony (Andrews and Boyle, 2016; Giger, 2017).

Cultural Expression of Pain

Pain, an extensively studied symptom, is used here to illustrate the manner in which symptom expression may reflect the client's cultural background. Pain is a universally recognized phenomenon and an important aspect of assessment for clients of various ages. It is also a private, subjective experience that is greatly influenced by cultural heritage. Expectations, manifestations, and pain management are all embedded in a cultural context. The definition of pain, like that of health or illness, is culturally determined.

The term *pain* is derived from the Greek word for penalty, a fact that helps explain the long association between pain and punishment in Judeo-Christian thought. The meaning of painful stimuli for individuals, the way people define their situation, and the influence of personal experience combine to determine the experience of pain.

Much cross-cultural research has been conducted on pain (Campbell and Edwards, 2012; Ludwig-Beymer, 2008; Zborowski, 1969). Pain has been found to be a highly personal experience that depends on cultural learning, the meaning of the situation, and other factors unique to the individual (Campbell and Edwards, 2012). Health care professionals have identified silent suffering as the most valued response to pain. The majority of nurses have been socialized to believe that in virtually any situation, self-control is better than open displays of strong feelings.

Studies of health care providers' attitudes toward pain reveal that the ethnic background of clients is relevant to the assessment of physical and psychological pain (Campbell and Edwards, 2012). Nurses view Jewish and Spanish clients as experiencing suffering the most and Anglo-Saxon Germanic clients as experiencing suffering the least. In addition, nurses who infer relatively greater client pain tended to report their own experiences as more painful. In general, nurses with an Eastern or Southern European or African background tend to infer greater suffering than do nurses of Northern European background. Years of experience, current position, and area of clinical practice are unrelated to inferences of suffering (Ludwig-Beymer, 2008).

In addition to expecting variations in pain perception and tolerance, a nurse should expect variations in the expression of pain. Individuals turn to their social environments for validation and comparison. A first important comparison group is the family, which transmits cultural norms to its children.

Culture-Bound Syndromes

Clients may have a condition that is culturally defined, known as a **culture-bound syndrome**. Some of these conditions have no equal from a biomedical or scientific perspective, but others, such as anorexia nervosa and bulimia, are examples of health problems found primarily among members of the dominant U.S. cultural group. Table 13.5 presents selected examples from among more than 150 culture-bound syndromes that have been documented by medical anthropologists.

MANAGEMENT OF HEALTH PROBLEMS: A CULTURAL PERSPECTIVE

After a symptom is identified, the first effort at treatment is often self-care. In the United States, an estimated 70% to 90% of all illness episodes are treated first, or exclusively, through self-care, often with significant success. The availability of over-the-counter medications, a relatively high literacy level, and influence of the mass media/technology in communicating health-related information to the general population have contributed to the high percentage of self-treatment. Home treatments are attractive because of their accessibility in comparison with the inconvenience associated with traveling to a physician, nurse practitioner, and pharmacist, particularly for clients from rural or sparsely populated areas. Furthermore, home treatment may mobilize the client's social support network and provide the sick individual with a caring environment in which to convalesce.

However, the nurse should be aware that not all home remedies are inexpensive. For example, urban African American populations in the Southeast sometimes use medicinal potions that cost much more than an equivalent treatment with a biomedical intervention.

Various nontraditional interventions are gaining the recognition of health care professionals in the biomedical-scientific health care system. Acupuncture, acupressure, therapeutic touch, massage, cupping, biofeedback, relaxation techniques, meditation, hypnosis, distraction, imagery, and herbal remedies are interventions that clients may use alone or in combination with other treatments.

Cultural Negotiation

Cultural negotiation refers to the process in which messages, instructions, and belief systems are manipulated, linked, or

TABLE 13.5	Selected Culture-Bound Syndromes	
Group	**Disorder(S)**	**Remarks**
Whites	Anorexia nervosa	Excessive preoccupation with thinness, self-imposed starvation
	Bulimia	Gross overeating, then vomiting or fasting
African Americans	Blackout	Collapse, dizziness, or inability to move
	Low blood	Not enough blood or weakness of the blood that is often treated with diet
	High blood	Blood that is too rich in certain components from ingesting too much red meat or rich foods
	Thin blood	In women, children, and the elderly; renders the individual more susceptible to illness in general
	Diseases of hex, witchcraft, or conjuring	Sense of being doomed by a spell, part of voodoo beliefs
Chinese or Southeast Asians	Koro	Intense anxiety that the penis is retracting into the body
Greeks	Hysteria	Bizarre complaints and behavior because the uterus leaves the pelvis and goes to another part of the body
Hispanics	Empacho	Food forms into a ball and clings to the stomach or intestines, causing pain and cramping
	Fatigue	Asthmalike symptoms
	Mal ojo (evil eye)	Fitful sleep, crying, and diarrhea in children caused by a stranger's attention; sudden onset
	Susto	Anxiety, trembling, and phobias from sudden fright
Native Americans	Ghost	Terror, hallucinations, and sense of danger
Japanese	Wagamama	Apathetic childish behavior with emotional outbursts

processed between the professional and lay models of health problems and preferred treatment. In each act, the nurse gives attention to eliciting the client's views regarding a health-related experience (e.g., pregnancy, complications of pregnancy, or illness of an infant).

Katon and Kleinman (1981) describe negotiation as a bilateral arrangement in which two principal parties attempt to work out a solution. The goal of negotiation is to reduce conflict in a way that promotes cooperation. Cultural negotiation is used when conceptual differences exist between the client and the nurse, a situation that may occur for one or more of the following reasons:

- The nurse and client may be using the same words but applying different meanings to them.
- The nurse and client may apply the same term to the same phenomenon but have different notions of its causation.
- The nurse and client may have different memories or emotions associated with the term and its use.

In cultural negotiation, the nurse provides scientific information while acknowledging that the client may hold different views. If the client's perspective indicates that behaviors would be helpful, positive, adaptive, or neutral in effect, the nurse should include them in the plan of care. However, if the client's perspective would result in behaviors that may be harmful, negative, or nonadaptive, the nurse should attempt to shift the client's perspective to that of the practitioner (Spector, 2008).

Pregnancy and childbirth are social, cultural, and physiological experiences; therefore an approach to culturally sensitive nursing care of childbearing women and their families must focus on the interaction between cultural meaning and biological functions. Childbirth is a time of transition and social celebration that is of central importance in any society; it signals realignment of existing cultural roles and responsibilities, psychological and biological states, and social relationships. Child rearing is also a period during which culturally bound values, attitudes, beliefs, and practices permeate virtually all aspects of

life for the parents and child (Andrews and Boyle, 2016). Careful assessment and attention to culturally based practices are particularly important during these occasions.

MANAGEMENT OF HEALTH PROBLEMS IN CULTURALLY DIVERSE POPULATIONS

The factors responsible for the health disparity between minority and white populations are complex and defy simplistic solutions. Health status is influenced by the interaction of physiological, cultural, psychological, and societal factors that are poorly understood for the general population and even less so for minorities. Despite the shared characteristic of economic disadvantage among minorities, common approaches for improving health are not recommended because of the variations in cultural beliefs and practices that exist among the different minority populations. Rather, solving problems among minorities necessitates activities, programs, and data collection that are tailored to meet the unique health care needs of many different subgroups. Solutions to health care problems among culturally diverse populations include the following recommendations that are the cornerstone of public health nursing (Keller et al., 2011):

- Focus on the health of entire populations
- Reflect community priorities and needs
- Establish caring relationships with the communities, families, and individuals that make up the population
- Remain grounded in social justice, having compassion and respect for the worth of all people, especially the vulnerable
- Provide care for the whole person: mental, physical, emotional, social, spiritual, and environmental aspects
- Promote health through strategies based on epidemiological evidence (evidence-based practice)
- Collaborate with community resources to reach health care goals

Providing Health Information and Education

Minority populations need more information about their health risks and treatment options. This is demonstrated by the following facts (American Cancer Society, 2016; CDC, 2016):

- African Americans have the highest mortality rate and shortest survival rate for many cancers.
- African Americans receive less information about cancer and heart disease than nonminority groups.
- African Americans tend to underestimate the prevalence of cancer, give less credence to the warning signs, obtain fewer screening tests, and receive a diagnosis at later stages of cancer than whites.
- Mexican Americans have a higher incidence of overweight and obesity than non-Hispanic whites, but non-Hispanic Blacks have the highest rates of obesity.

Programs to increase public awareness about health problems have been well received in several areas. For example, the Healthy Mothers, Healthy Babies Coalition, which provides an education program in both English and Spanish, has contributed to greater awareness of measures to improve the health status of mothers and infants. In addition, increased knowledge among African Americans of hypertension as a serious health problem is one of the accomplishments of the National High Blood Pressure Education program. The success of these efforts indicates that carefully planned programs have a beneficial effect, but efforts must continue and must expand to reach even more of the target population and focus on additional health problems.

Planning Health Information Campaigns

Sensitivity to cultural factors is often lacking in the health care of minorities. Key concepts for the nurse to consider in designing a health information campaign include meeting the language and cultural needs of each identified minority group, using minority-specific community resources to tailor educational approaches, and developing materials and methods of presentation that are commensurate with the educational level of the target population. Furthermore, the powerful influences of cultural factors over a lifetime in shaping people's attitudes, values, beliefs, and practices concerning health require health information programs to be sustained over a long period. The following are examples of ways in which the nurse can interweave these concepts into health promotion efforts:

- The nurse should involve local community leaders who are members of the targeted cultural group to promote acceptance and reinforcement of the central themes of health promotion messages.
- Health messages are more readily accepted if they do not conflict with existing cultural beliefs and practices. Where appropriate, messages should acknowledge existing cultural beliefs.
- The nurse should involve families, churches, employers, and community organizations as a support system to facilitate and sustain behavioral change to a more healthful lifestyle. For example, although hypertension control in African Americans depends on appropriate treatment (e.g., medication), blood pressure can be improved and maintained by family and community support of activities such as proper diet and exercise.
- Language barriers, cultural differences, and lack of adequate information on access to care complicate prenatal care for Hispanic and Asian women who have recently arrived in the United States. Through the use of lay volunteers to organize community support networks, programs have been developed to disseminate culturally appropriate health information.

Health Education

Although printed materials and other audiovisual aids contribute to the educational process, client education is inherently interpersonal. The success of educational efforts is often determined by the credibility of the source and is highly dependent on the skill and sensitivity of the nurse in communicating information in a culturally appropriate manner. Education programs are particularly critical and necessary for several health problems with the greatest influence on minority health, such as hypertension, obesity, and diabetes. For example, if patients with diabetes could improve their self-management skills through education, a significant number of complications (e.g., ketoacidosis, blindness, and amputations) could be avoided, saving human misery and health care dollars.

Delivering and Financing Health Services

Innovative models for delivering and financing health services for minority populations are needed. According to community health experts, models should increase flexibility of health care delivery, facilitate minorities' access to services, and improve efficiency of service and payment systems. One of the most commonly used indicators of the adequacy of health services for a population is the distribution of health care providers; however, this is an inadequate measurement. The following observations exemplify the problems associated with health services for minorities:

- The disparities in death rates between minorities and whites remain despite overall increases in health care access and use (AHRQ, 2014).
- Language problems hinder refugees and immigrants when they seek health care.
- African Americans with cancer postpone seeking diagnosis of their symptoms longer than whites and delay initiation of treatment once diagnosed (American Cancer Society, 2016).
- The infant mortality rate among African American women is more than twice as high as the infant mortality rate among white women (CDC, 2015).

Models of Health Promotion

In most health models, SES is assumed to affect health status through environmental or behavioral factors. These models posit that poor families may not have the economic, social, or community resources needed to remain in good health. For example, poverty is thought to affect children's well-being by affecting health and nutrition, the home environment, caregiver interactions with children, caregiver mental health, and neighborhood conditions. The deficits associated with poverty may lead to an inadequate diet, which results in poor growth and delayed development. Likewise, poor housing raises the risk for exposure to many illnesses and infections; overcrowding results in increased risk for infectious diseases such as tuberculosis, meningitis, influenza, and related conditions; and community violence threatens the safety and well-being of children. The combined effect of these stressors is thought to provide the foundation for a cycle of hopelessness and depression among family members, who in turn may engage in risky health behaviors (e.g., smoking, substance abuse, and poor dietary habits resulting in obesity and high cholesterol levels) and unfavorable family interactions.

Although many Latino children live in poverty, they enjoy relatively good health in comparison with children in other low socioeconomic groups. This finding has been called an epidemiological paradox. The assumption is that if the family promotes beneficial health behaviors among its members, these behaviors will become integrated into the culture. Healthy lifestyle behaviors become an integral component of the family identity, traditions, and history.

Continuity of Care

Continuity of care is associated with improved health outcomes and is presumably greater when a client is able to establish an ongoing relationship with a care provider. Many of the leading causes of death among minorities (e.g., cancer, cardiovascular disease, and diabetes) are chronic rather than acute problems; therefore they require extended treatment regimens. Consider the following:

- Refugees are eligible for special medical assistance during their first 18 months in the United States. However, after this period, refugees who cannot afford private health insurance and are ineligible for Medicaid or state medical assistance may become medically indigent.
- Illegal immigrants are ineligible for Medicare and Medicaid. They are medically indigent.
- Many Native Americans and Alaska Natives live in areas where the availability of health care providers is half the national average.

Health Care Financing Problems

As mentioned previously, problems associated with financing health care tend to be more common in minority groups than in the dominant cultural group. Consider the following (National Center for Health Statistics, 2008):

- Economic inequalities cause members of minority groups to rely disproportionately on Medicaid for their health care needs.
- Older minority people are less likely than whites to supplement Medicare with additional private insurance.
- Proportionately, three times as many Native Americans, African Americans, Hispanics, and certain Asian and Pacific Islander groups as whites live in poverty.
- In 2015, 19.4% of Hispanics lacked insurance coverage, compared with 9.9% of African Americans and 6.2% of whites (Ward et al., 2016).

To better manage health problems and reduce the disparity in health indicators, these issues of financing must be addressed. Failure to address them will result not only in continued inequity in access to services but also in continued poor health among minority groups.

Developing Health Professionals from Minority Groups

The need to increase the number of health professionals from minority groups has been recognized for decades. With few exceptions, minorities are underrepresented as students and practitioners of the health professions. Although the number of minority nursing students has been steadily increasing, there still are proportionately more white nursing students.

Differences in the availability of health personnel resources in minority communities are apparent, regardless of the minority group being considered. Communities located in urban-metropolitan areas have significantly more professional resources. Among the factors that contribute to the imbalances in minority representation in health professions are the size of a minority population, number of cultural subgroups, and demographic features. Efforts to encourage more students from minority groups are ongoing, and government and private foundations offer grants, scholarships, and low-cost loans to recruit and retain students from underserved minority groups in nursing and other health care professions. Minority and nonminority health professional organizations, academic institutions, state governments, health departments, and other organizations from the public and private sectors should work together to develop strategies to improve the availability and accessibility of health care professionals to minority communities (Sullivan Commission, 2014).

Enhancing Cooperative Efforts with the Nonfederal Sector

Activities to improve minority health should involve participation of organizations at all levels (i.e., community, municipal, state, and national). Community involvement in developing health promotion activities can contribute to their success by providing credibility and visibility to the activities and facilitating their acceptance. Changes in health behavior frequently depend on personal initiative and are most likely to be triggered by efforts from locally based sources.

However, not all minority communities have the ability to identify their own health problems and initiate activities to address them. Support from the state and federal governments and private-sector assistance are needed to assist with identifying and solving health-related problems afflicting the minority community. Assistance may be provided to minority communities in the following ways:

1. The use of technical assistance to identify high-risk groups
2. Assistance with planning, implementing, and evaluating programs to address identified needs
3. Specialized community services (e.g., federally funded projects for infants and frail older adults)
4. Programs supported by businesses and industries (e.g., health promotion programs organized by unions)

The private sector can also serve as an effective channel for programs targeted to minority health projects. National organizations concerned with minorities, such as the National Urban League and the National Alliance for Hispanic Health, include health-related issues in their national agendas and are actively seeking effective ways to improve the health of minorities. Organizations such as these have a powerful potential for effecting change among their constituencies because they have strong community-level, grassroots support.

Promoting a Research Agenda on Minority Health Issues

The National Center on Minority Health and Health Disparities was developed in 2000 and redesignated in 2010 as the National Institute on Minority Health and Health Disparities (NIMHD) (http://www.nimhd.nih.gov) to assist in the investigation of factors affecting minority health (NIMHD, 2016). Its mission is to lead scientific research to improve minority health and to ultimately eliminate health disparities (NIMHD, 2016). The NIMHD conducts and supports research that examines risk factor prevalence and treatment services. It also reviews health education interventions, preventive services interventions, and sociocultural factors that influence health and outcomes of care.

For further information on current research related to culture and community health nursing, the reader should search library databases for reports of completed studies. Electronic bulletin boards also may be valuable when one is searching for research in progress and for communicating with researchers studying a particular phenomenon of interest. An example of recent nursing research related to culturally competent care is described in the Research Highlights box.

RESEARCH HIGHLIGHTS

Nutritional Patterns of Recent Immigrants

Edmonds (2005) examined the nutritional patterns of 23 women who had recently emigrated from Honduras to assist in understanding health-related nutritional issues in this Hispanic subgroup. She determined that the Honduran women had made both positive and negative changes in their diets since coming to the United States. Rice, beans, natural fruit juices, tortillas, bananas, beef, and eggs were reported as the typical foods eaten every day in Honduras. Positive changes in diets included eating a greater variety of fruits and vegetables, cooking with less grease, baking more frequently than frying, and using vegetable oil rather than lard. The women also ate more meat and dairy products. Negative changes noted were more skipped meals and eating foods high in fat and calories (e.g., fast foods). Research suggests that classes be taught in Women, Infants, and Children programs and other venues that would support the Hondurans' traditional diet and focus on how to eat nutritionally in fast-food restaurants, eat a balanced diet, plan meals and cook ahead, and read food labels.

Data from Edmonds VM: The nutritional patterns of recently immigrated Honduran women, *Journal of Transcultural Nursing*, 16(3): 226–235, 2005.

ROLE OF THE COMMUNITY HEALTH NURSE IN IMPROVING HEALTH FOR CULTURALLY DIVERSE PEOPLE

This chapter provides data detailing the health care problems of culturally diverse individuals, families, groups, and communities. Given the complexity of the problems and the wide variation in incidence and distribution of these problems within specific subgroups, no simple method exists for providing culturally sensitive community health nursing care to all clients. However, the following strategies may assist the community health nurse when working with culturally diverse clients:

- Conduct a "culturological" assessment.
- Conduct a cultural self-assessment.
- Seek knowledge about local cultures.
- Recognize the political issues of culturally diverse groups.
- Provide culturally competent care.
- Recognize culturally based health problems.

Culturological Assessment

All nursing care is based on a systematic, comprehensive assessment of the client; therefore the community health nurse must gather cultural data on clients from racially and ethnically diverse backgrounds. A **culturological assessment** refers to a systematic appraisal or examination of individuals, groups, and communities regarding their cultural beliefs, values, and practices to determine explicit nursing needs and intervention practices within the cultural context of the people being evaluated (Leininger, 1995). The term *culturological* is a descriptive reference to cultural phenomena in their broadest sense.

Culturological assessments are as vital as physical and psychological assessments. Culturological assessments tend to be broad and comprehensive because they deal with cultural values, belief systems, and ways of living now and in the recent past. In conducting a culturological assessment, the community health nurse should be involved in determining and appraising the traits, characteristics, or smallest units of cultural behavior as a guide to nursing care. The following sections summarize major data categories pertaining to the culture of clients and offer suggested questions that the nurse may ask to elicit needed information.

Brief History of Ethnic and Racial Origins of the Cultural Group with Which the Client Identifies

- With what ethnic group or groups does the client report affiliation (e.g., Hispanic, Polish, Navajo, or a combination)? To what degree does the client identify with the cultural group (e.g., "we" concept of solidarity or a fringe member)?
- Where has the client lived (i.e., country and city) and when (i.e., during what years)? If the client has recently relocated to the United States, knowledge of prevalent diseases in the country of origin may be helpful.

Values Orientation

- What are the client's attitudes, values, and beliefs about birth, death, health, illness, and health care providers?
- Does culture influence the manner in which the client relates to body image change resulting from illness or surgery (e.g., importance of appearance, beauty, strength, and roles in the cultural group)?
- How does the client view work, leisure, and education?
- How does the client perceive change?
- How does the client value privacy; courtesy; touch; and relationships with individuals of different ages, of different social class, or caste, and of the opposite sex?
- How does the client relate to people in a different cultural group (e.g., withdrawal, verbal or nonverbal expression, or negative or positive attitude)?

Cultural Sanctions and Restrictions

- How does the client's cultural group regard expression of emotion and feelings, spirituality, and religious beliefs? How are dying, death, and grieving expressed in a culturally appropriate manner?
- How is modesty expressed by men and women in the client's cultural group? Does the client's cultural group have culturally defined expectations about male–female relationships, including the nurse–client relationship?
- Does the client have restrictions related to sexuality, exposure of body parts, or certain types of surgery (e.g., amputation, vasectomy, or hysterectomy)?
- Does the client have restrictions against discussion of dead relatives or fears related to the unknown?

Communication

- What language does the client speak at home? What other language does the client speak or read? In what language would the client prefer to communicate with you?
- What is the written and spoken English fluency level of the client? Remember that the stress of illness may cause clients to use a more familiar language and temporarily forget some English.
- Does the client need an interpreter? If so, make sure to use an interpreter who is fluent in medical language and is not a relative or friend of the client.
- What are the rules (i.e., linguistics) and modes (i.e., style) of communication?
- Is it necessary to vary the technique of communication during the interview and examination to accommodate the client's cultural background (e.g., tempo of conversation, eye contact, sensitivity to topical taboos, norms of confidentiality, and style of explanation)?
- How does the client's nonverbal communication compare with that of individuals from other cultural backgrounds? How does it affect the client's relationship with the nurse and with other members of the health care team?
- How does the client feel about health care providers who are not of the same cultural background (e.g., African American, middle-class nurse, or Hispanic of a different social class)? Does the client prefer to receive care from a nurse of the same cultural background, sex, or age?

ETHICAL INSIGHTS

Disclosure of HIV/AIDS Status

Ortiz (2005) examined the experiences of 19 Latinas who disclosed they were living with HIV/AIDS. She described how the women decided to disclose their HIV status to partners, family members, friends, and employers. Four categories emerged: timing of the disclosure, the need to disclose, controlling disclosure, and supportive disclosing. These factors were influenced by the Latinas' relationship with others, the perceived risks to the women and others, the need to disclose, the wish to give support to themselves or others, and the desire to control who should know and when. Ortiz concluded that nurses should be knowledgeable of the realities of Latinas' lives and be able to incorporate that knowledge into comprehensive care plans that will help them maximize the utilization of appropriate resources.

Data from Ortiz CE: Disclosing concerns of Latinas living with HIV/AIDS. *Journal of Transcultural Nursing*, 16(3):210–217, 2005.

Health-Related Beliefs and Practices

- To what cause(s) does the client attribute illness and disease (e.g., divine wrath, imbalance in hot-cold or yin-yang, punishment for moral transgressions, hex, or soul loss)?
- What does the client believe promotes health (e.g., eating certain foods, wearing amulets to bring good luck, exercise, prayer, ancestors, saints, or intermediate deities)?
- What is the client's religious affiliation (e.g., Judaism, Islam, Pentecostalism, West African voodooism, Seventh-Day Adventism, Catholicism, or Mormonism)?
- Does the client rely on cultural healers (e.g., *curandero,* shaman, spiritualist, priest, minister, or monk)? Who determines when the client is sick and when the client is healthy? Who determines the type of healer and treatment that should be sought?
- In what types of cultural healing practices does the client engage (e.g., herbal remedies, potions, massage, wearing talismans or charms to discourage evil spirits, healing rituals, incantations, or prayers)?
- How does the client perceive biomedical-scientific health care providers? How do the client and family perceive nurses? What are the expectations of nurses and nursing care?
- What constitutes appropriate "sick-role" behavior? Who determines what symptoms constitute disease and illness? Who decides when the client is no longer sick? Who cares for the client at home?
- How does the client's cultural group view mental disorders? Do they show differences in acceptable behaviors for physical versus psychological illnesses?

Nutrition

- What nutritional factors are influenced by the client's cultural background?
- What meanings does the client attach to food and eating? With whom does the client usually eat? What types of foods does the client usually eat? What does the client define as food? What does the client believe defines a "healthy" versus an "unhealthy" diet?
- How does the client prepare foods at home (e.g., type of food preparation; cooking oils used; length of time foods, especially vegetables, are cooked; amount and type of seasoning added to various foods during preparation)?
- Do religious beliefs and practices influence the client's diet (e.g., amount, type, preparation, or delineation of acceptable food combinations, such as kosher diets)? Does the client abstain from certain foods at regular intervals, on specific dates determined by the religious calendar, or at other times?
- If the client's religion mandates or encourages fasting, what does the term *fast* mean to the client (e.g., refraining from certain types or quantities of foods, eating only during certain times of the day)? For what period of time is the client expected to fast? Does the religion allow exemption from fasting during illness, and, if so, is the client believed to have an exemption?

Socioeconomic Considerations

- Who constitutes the client's social network (i.e., family, peers, and healers)? How do they influence the client's health or illness status?

- How do members of the client's social support network define caring (e.g., being continuously present, doing things for the client, or looking after the client's family)? What are the roles of various family members during health and illness?
- How does the client's family participate in the client's nursing care (e.g., bathing, feeding, touching, and being present)?
- Does the cultural family structure influence the client's response to health or illness (e.g., beliefs, strengths, weaknesses, and social class)? Does a key family member have a role that is significant in health-related decisions (e.g., grandmother in many African American families or eldest adult son in Asian families)?
- Who is the principal wage earner in the client's family? What is the total annual income? This is a potentially sensitive question that should be asked only if necessary. Does the family have more than one wage earner? Does the family have other sources of financial support (e.g., extended family or investments)?
- What influence does economic status have on lifestyle, place of residence, living conditions, ability to obtain health care, and discharge planning?

Organizations Providing Cultural Support

- What influence do ethnic and cultural organizations have on the client's receiving health care (e.g., National Association for the Advancement of Colored People, African American Political Caucus, churches, schools, Urban League, and community-based health care programs and clinics)?

Educational Background

- What is the highest educational level the client has obtained? Does the client's educational background affect the client's knowledge level concerning the health care delivery system, how to obtain the care needed, teaching and learning skills, and written material that is distributed in the health care setting (e.g., insurance forms, educational literature, information about diagnostic procedures and laboratory tests, and admissions forms)?
- Can the client read and write English, or does he or she prefer another language? If English is the client's second language, are materials available in the client's primary language?
- What learning style is most comfortable or familiar? Does the client prefer to learn through written materials, oral explanation, or demonstration?

Religious Affiliation

- How does the client's religious affiliation influence health and illness (e.g., death, chronic illness, body image alteration, and cause and effect of illness)?
- What is the role of the client's religious beliefs and practices during health and illness?
- What is the role of significant religious representatives during health and illness? Does the client have recognized religious healers (e.g., Islamic imams, Christian Scientist practitioners or nurses, Catholic priests, Mormon elders, and Buddhist monks)?

Cultural Aspects of Disease Incidence

- Does the client have specific genetic or acquired conditions that are more prevalent in a specific cultural group (e.g., hypertension, sickle cell anemia, Tay-Sachs disease, or lactose intolerance)?
- Are any socioenvironmental diseases more prevalent among the client's specific cultural group (e.g., lead poisoning, alcoholism, AIDS, drug abuse, or ear infections)?
- Do diseases exist against which the client has an increased resistance (e.g., skin cancer in a darkly pigmented individual)?

Biocultural Variations

- Does the client have distinctive physical features that are characteristic of a particular racial group (e.g., skin color or hair texture)? Does the client have variations in anatomy that are characteristic of a particular racial or ethnic group (e.g., body structure, height, weight, facial shape and structure [nose, eye shape, and facial contour], or upper and lower extremity shape)?
- How do anatomical and racial variations affect the assessment?

Developmental Considerations

- Does the client have distinct growth and development characteristics that vary with his or her cultural background (e.g., bone density, psychomotor patterns of development, or fat folds)?
- What factors are significant in assessing children from the newborn period through adolescence (e.g., expected growth on standard grid, culturally acceptable age for toilet training, introduction of various types of foods, sex differences, discipline, and socialization to adult roles)?
- What is the cultural perception of aging (e.g., is youthfulness or the wisdom of old age more highly valued)?
- How are older people handled culturally (e.g., cared for in the home of adult children or placed in institutions for care)? What are culturally acceptable roles for older adults?
- Does the older adult expect family members to provide care, including nurturance and other humanistic aspects of care?
- Is the older adult isolated from culturally relevant supportive people or enmeshed in a caring network of relatives and friends?
- Has a culturally appropriate network replaced family members in performing some caring functions for older adults?

Cultural Self-Assessment

Community health nurses can engage in a cultural self-assessment. Through identification of health-related attitudes, values, beliefs, and practices that are part of the personal cultural meaning brought to the nurse–client interaction, the nurse can better understand the cultural aspects of health care from the perspective of the client, family, group, or community. Everyone has ethnocentric tendencies that must be brought to a level of conscious awareness so that efforts can be made to temper ethnocentrism and view reality from the perspective of the client.

Knowledge About Local Cultures

Community health nurses can learn about the cultural diversity characteristics of the subgroup or subgroups that are most prevalent within their communities. The nurse cannot know about all health-related beliefs and practices of the diverse groups served, but he or she can study select ones. The nurse can accomplish this cultural study through a review of nursing, anthropology, sociology, and related literature on culturally diverse groups; in-service programs held at community health agencies, educational institutions in the community, or organizations serving minority groups; enrollment in courses on transcultural or cross-cultural nursing and medical anthropology; and interviews with key members of the subgroups of interest, such as clergy members, nurses, and physicians, to obtain information about the influence of culture on health-related beliefs and practices.

Recognition of Political Issues of Culturally Diverse Groups

Awareness of the political aspects of health care for culturally diverse groups and communities can help community health nurses influence legislation and funding priorities aimed at improving health care for specific populations. Recognized for their leadership role in community health matters involving culturally diverse groups, community health nurses may be invited by political leaders to participate in political decision making that affects the health of a targeted subgroup. Community health nurses should also be active politically, both individually and collectively, to influence legislation affecting culturally diverse individuals, groups, and communities, and they should offer to serve on key community committees, boards, and advisory councils that affect the health of culturally diverse groups.

Providing Culturally Competent Care

When caring for individuals and families from culturally diverse backgrounds, the community health nurse can assess, diagnose, implement, and evaluate nursing care in a manner that is culturally congruent, competent, relevant, and appropriate. To provide this culturally appropriate nursing care, the nurse must create a relationship of mutual respect by becoming aware of the cultural similarities and differences between herself or himself and the client. A guideline for gathering cultural data has been presented, and the nurse may use this guideline or a similar one to identify significant areas in which the nurse and client differ. Knowledge about biocultural variations in health and illness is particularly important when the nurse is conducting cultural assessments.

Recognition of Culturally Based Health Practices

As discussed previously, the community health nurse should attempt to understand the nature and meaning of culturally based health practices of clients, groups, and communities. Once the practices are understood, the nurse can make a determination

regarding their appropriateness in a particular context. Generally, the nurse should decide whether a cultural practice is useful, neutral, or harmful to the client, group, or community. The nurse should encourage or "tolerate" helpful and neutral practices, whereas he or she should discourage harmful practices.

However, the classification of some cultural healing practices is not so easily determined. For example, many Southeast Asians practice coining, which is the rubbing of a coin over body surfaces to expel "bad winds" that are believed to cause illness (Berg, Morphew and Tran, 2016; Vitale and Prashad, 2017). Community health nurses are faced with an ethical dilemma when coining is practiced on young children, because it leaves abrasions on the skin and may be viewed by some as child abuse. This practice is not useful, so the nurse must make the decision whether it is neutral or harmful. An argument for the practice's being neutral is that abrasions usually heal quickly, so no harm is done to the child as a result. Furthermore, the practice is meaningful to parents who have much confidence in the healing powers associated with coining (Giger, 2017; Vitale and Prashad, 2017).

The argument can also be made that the practice is harmful. The red marks and skin abrasions caused by the coining place the child at increased risk for skin infection. Given that the child may require antibiotics or other medication for a respiratory disorder, encouragement of coining as the only treatment may prevent the child from receiving needed medical intervention and may delay medical treatment. As a solution, the community health nurse may suggest that parents combine traditional treatment with Western biomedicine (i.e., they can use coining in conjunction with a biomedical intervention). Therefore the healing will occur in a manner that has involved the use of both folk and professional health care systems (Giger, 2017; Vitale and Prashad, 2017).

> ### ❓ ACTIVE LEARNING
>
> 1. Select a client from a racially or ethnically diverse background, and conduct a cultural assessment.
> 2. Interview someone from a racial or ethnic background different from your own to determine beliefs about illness causation, use of the lay and professional health care delivery systems, and culturally based treatments.

RESOURCES FOR MINORITY HEALTH

Community health nurses will find federal resources for improving the health care of the federally defined minority populations through the USDHHS. Within the USDHHS, the Office of Minority Health (OMH) and the Indian Health Service (IHS) divisions are concerned with health promotion, disease prevention, service delivery, and research for minority groups.

Office of Minority Health

The OMH coordinates federal efforts to improve the health status of racial and ethnic minority populations (i.e., African Americans, Hispanics, Native Americans and Alaska Natives, and Asians and Pacific Islanders). Directed by the deputy assistant secretary for minority health, the OMH was established by the Disadvantaged Minority Health Improvement Act of 1990 (PL 101-527), which was signed by President George H. W.

TABLE 13.6 Federally Sponsored Initiatives to Improve the Health of Minority Groups

Initiative	Description
Racial and Ethnic Approaches to Community Health (REACH 2010)	This program was launched in 1999 to eliminate health disparities in six priority areas: cardiovascular diseases, immunizations, breast and cervical cancer screening and management, diabetes, HIV/AIDS, and infant mortality. REACH 2010 supports community coalitions in designing, implementing, and evaluating community-driven strategies to eliminate health disparities.
National Breast and Cervical Cancer Early Detection Program (NBCCEDP)	NBCCEDP provides breast and cervical cancer screening, diagnosis, and treatment to low-income, medically underserved, and uninsured women (emphasizing recruitment of minority women).
Ryan White Comprehensive AIDS Resources Emergency (CARE) Act B	Ryan White CARE Act provides services to persons living with HIV disease, primarily racial and ethnic minorities.
National Institute on Minority Health and Health Disparities (NIMHD)	NIMHD mission is to lead scientific research to improve minority health and reduce disparity.

Bush on November 6, 1990. Under the directives of the act, the OMH is charged with duties to:

- Establish short- and long-range goals and objectives relating to disease prevention, health promotion, service delivery, and research on the health of minority people
- Promote increased participation of disadvantaged people, including minorities, in health service and health promotion programs
- Create a national minority health resource center
- Support research, demonstrations, and evaluations of new and innovative models that increase understanding of disease risk factors and support better information dissemination, education, prevention, and service delivery to minority communities
- Promote minority health–related activities in the corporate and voluntary sectors
- Develop minority-focused health information and health promotion materials and teaching programs
- Assist providers of primary care and preventive services in obtaining assistance of bilingual health professionals when appropriate

As the focal point for minority health efforts, the OMH plays a key role in major initiatives launched by the secretary of the USDHHS. Table 13.6 lists some of these initiatives.

Indian Health Service

The IHS is responsible for providing federal health services to Native Americans and Alaska Natives. Federal Indian health services are based on a special government-to-government relationship and laws that Congress has passed pursuant to its authority to regulate commerce with the Indian Nations as specified in the Constitution and other documents.

The primary responsibility of the IHS is to elevate the health status of Native Americans and Alaska Natives to the highest level possible. The mission is to ensure quality, availability, and accessibility of a comprehensive, high-quality health care delivery system, providing maximum involvement of Native Americans and Alaska Natives in defining their health needs, setting health priorities for their local areas, and managing and controlling their health programs.

The IHS also acts as the principal federal health advocate for Native Americans by ensuring that they have knowledge of, and access to, all federal, state, and local health programs to which they are entitled as American citizens. The IHS carried out its responsibilities through development and operation of a health services delivery system designed to provide a broad-spectrum program of preventive, curative, rehabilitative, and environmental services. This system integrates health services delivered directly through IHS facilities and staff with those purchased by IHS through contractual arrangements. Tribes are also actively involved in program implementation.

The 1975 Indian Self-Determination Act (PL 93-638), as amended, builds on IHS policy by giving tribes the option of staffing and managing IHS programs in their communities and provides funding for improvement of tribal capability to contract under the act. The 1976 Indian Health Care Improvement Act (PL 94-437), as amended, was intended to elevate the health care status of Native Americans and Alaska Natives to a level equal to that of the general population through a program of authorized, higher-resource levels in the IHS budget. Appropriated resources were used to expand health services, build and renovate medical facilities, and step up the construction of safe drinking water and sanitary disposal facilities. It also established programs designed to increase the number of Native American health professionals for Native American needs and to improve health care access for Native Americans living in urban areas.

The operation of the IHS health care delivery system is managed through local administrative units called *service units*. A service unit is the basic health organization for a geographic area served by the IHS program, just as a county or city health department is the basic health organization in a state health department. These are defined areas usually centered on a single federal reservation in the continental United States or a population concentration in Alaska. The IHS serves approximately 50% of the total Native American and Alaska Native population in the United States, primarily those residing on reservations.

CASE STUDY   Application of the Nursing Process

Asian Family and Cultural Practices

Community health nurse Maria Gonzales visited the home of 5-year-old Nguyen Van Nghi, who was discharged from the hospital on the previous day. The pediatrician had diagnosed pneumonia and "suspected failure to thrive" in the child because the child's growth fell below the third percentile on a standard growth chart for height and weight, and he performed poorly on a screening test used to identify developmental delays for a 5-year-old child.

Residing in the home were the child's parents, four siblings, grandmother, aunt, uncle, and three cousins. Although the child's father and uncle spoke some English, other members of the household communicated in a language unfamiliar to Maria, which "sounded like Chinese." When Maria approached the child, he did not look at her or speak to her, even when she called him Nguyen (pronounced "we'en").

Assessment

In a brief survey of the Nguyens' home, Maria noted that the home and furnishings were modest but very clean. The pantry held a considerable amount of food, including rice and dried noodles. The small refrigerator smelled of fish and contained some vegetables that Maria did not recognize. She did not see any green vegetables, milk, or other dairy products.

During her initial assessment of Nghi, Maria observed multiple tender, ecchymotic areas with petechiae between the ribs on the front and back of the body, resembling strap marks. Suspecting child abuse, Maria told the family that she would return later in the day with an interpreter. She located an interpreter who spoke Mandarin Chinese and briefed him about her concerns with child abuse. When Maria and the interpreter returned to the client's home, she instructed the interpreter to ask the parents for an explanation of the bruises. The interpreter told Maria that the family was Vietnamese and could not understand his Chinese dialect. Both the interpreter and the child's father knew a little French and awkwardly managed to communicate.

The interpreter advised the nurse that in the Vietnamese culture, the person's family name is given first, followed by the middle name and then the first name. Only a few different family names exist among the Vietnamese; therefore it is common practice to call people by their given first name. At this point, Maria also learned that the child was actually 4 years old, because the Vietnamese consider a newborn to be 1 year old at birth.

The interpreter explained that a Vietnamese healer performed cao gio, or coining, to exude the "bad wind" from Nghi. Cao gio is performed by applying a special menthol oil to the painful or symptomatic part of the body and then rubbing a coin over the area with firm, downward strokes. When Nghi's condition seemed to worsen after his hospital discharge, his grandmother persuaded his parents that Western biomedicine had failed and that their son required the stronger power of folk healing.

Diagnosis

- Maria must set priorities and focus on selected cultural data categories because they seem most relevant for the Nguyen family at present.

Individual

- High risk for Nghi's pneumonia to worsen
- Potential for child abuse/neglect
- Possible physical and/or developmental delay (low weight/height for age)

Family

- Increased risk for poor health outcomes related to distrust of Western health care practices
- Increased risk for nutritional deficits

Community

- Potential for poor health of area Vietnamese immigrants related to limited knowledge of good nutritional practices and general health promotion

Planning
Individual
Short-Term Goals

- Nghi's pneumonia will resolve.
- Nghi will show no more evidence of the practice of "coining."

Long-Term Goal

- Nghi's height and weight will increase proportionally to at least the 50th percentile for age.

Family

Short-Term Goals

- Family members will cease the practice of "coining."
- Caregivers will recognize the importance of completing the antibiotic therapy as prescribed.

Long-Term Goal

- A family nutritional assessment will be completed, and adjustments will be made to their diet to provide needed nutrients.

Community

Long-Term Goal

- Leaders of the area's Vietnamese community will work with area health care providers to promote good nutritional practices.

Intervention
Individual

Through the interpreter, Maria was able to communicate with the Nguyen family that it was vital for Nghi to take all of the prescribed antibiotics. She also attempted to convey the potentially harmful effect of the practice of coining and suggested that that procedure be stopped. She set a follow-up appointment for the next day.

Family

Maria was able to bring a Vietnamese interpreter for the follow-up appointment. So in addition to reiterating the importance of taking the medications, she was able to teach about basic nutritional principles and perform additional nutritional assessments. Although Nghi was not as small as initially thought, he was still below the 50th percentile for his age. Maria gave nutritional pamphlets written in Vietnamese to the parents and provided them with information on where to find low-cost foods in the neighborhood.

Community

Working with the health department's social worker and the Vietnamese interpreter, Maria visited several area markets to gather information on diet and nutritional practices of Vietnamese immigrants. They decided that they would seek a small grant to develop more teaching materials on nutrition for this population.

Evaluation
Individual

By the third follow-up visit, Maria determined that although Nghi still had a residual cough, his chest was clearing. In addition, there was no evidence of coining. Furthermore, Maria was shown that the family's refrigerator now

continued

CASE STUDY **Application of the Nursing Process—cont'd**

Asian Family and Cultural Practices

contained whole milk and some leafy green vegetables. It was decided that she would return in 6 weeks for a follow-up visit to weigh and measure Nghi.

Family

The presence of the interpreter who spoke Vietnamese and who was familiar with the culture was vital. And by the third visit, most of the family members appeared to be at ease with Maria. Mrs. Nguyen asked a number of questions about nutrition and other health issues and requested that Maria monitor the heights and weights of the other children.

Community

The health department's social worker was able to identify a small grant to develop and purchase teaching materials for the Vietnamese population. The nurse and social worker applied for the funds and are eagerly waiting to hear the outcome.

Levels of Prevention

The following are examples of three levels of prevention as applied to the case study.

Primary Prevention

- Nutritional education for the Nguyen family
- Health education targeted at developing comfort with the U.S. health care system and Western medicine
- Education related to potentially harmful practices (e.g., coining)

Secondary Prevention

Monitoring the height and weight of Nghi and his siblings

Tertiary Prevention

Evaluation of resolution of pneumonia

SUMMARY

To provide community health nursing for individuals, groups, and communities representing the hundreds of different cultures and subcultures found in the United States, the nurse should include cultural considerations in nursing care. Guidelines for gathering data from clients of culturally diverse backgrounds have been suggested in this chapter and are interwoven throughout the text. Knowledge about culture-specific and culture-universal nursing care is foundational and is an integral component of community health nursing.

ⓔ EVOLVE WEBSITE

http://evolve.elsevier.com/Nies/community

- NCLEX Review Questions
- Case Studies

BIBLIOGRAPHY

Agency for Healthcare Research and Quality: *2016 National health quality and disparities report*, 2017. Available from: https://www.ahrq.gov/sites/default/files/wysiwyg/research/findings/nhqrdr/nhqdr16/final2016qdr.pdf.

American Association of Colleges of Nursing: *Fact sheet: enhancing diversity in the nursing workforce*, 2016. Available from: http://www.aacn.nche.edu/media-relations/diversityFS.pdf.

American Cancer Society: *Cancer facts & figures for African Americans*, 2016. Available from: https://www.cancer.org/content/dam/cancer-org/research/cancer-facts-and-statistics/cancer-facts-and-figures-for-african-americans/cancer-facts-and-figures-for-african-americans-2016-2018.pdf.

Andrews MM, Boyle JS: *Transcultural concepts in nursing care*, ed 7, Philadelphia, 2016, Wolters Kluwer.

Baker B, Rytina N: *Estimates of unauthorized immigrant population residing in the United States: January 2012*, 2013. Available from: https://www.dhs.gov/sites/default/files/publications/Unautho rized%20Immigrant%20Population%20Estimates%20in%20the%20US%20January%202012_0.pdf.

Berg J, Morphew T, Tran J: Prevalence of complimentary and alternative medicine usage in Vietnamese American asthmatic children, *Clinical Pediatrics* 55(2):157–164, 2015.

Campbell CM, Edwards RR: Ethnic differences in pain and pain management, *Pain Manag* 2(3):219–230, 2012. Available from: https://www.ncbi.nlm.nih.gov/pmc/articles/PMC3654683/.

Centers for Disease Control: *Adult obesity facts*, 2016. Available from: https://www.cdc.gov/obesity/data/adult.html.

Centers for Disease Control: Infant mortality statistics from the 2013 period linked birth/infant death data set, *Natl Vital Stat Rep*, 2015. Table 1. Available from: Cockerham WC: *Medical sociology* https://minorityhealth.hhs.gov/omh/browse.aspx?lvl=4&lvlid=23.

Cockerham WC: *Medical sociology*, ed 11, Upper Saddle River, NJ, 2009, Prentice Hall.

The Commonwealth Fund: *Closing the divide: how medical homes promote equity in health care: results from the Commonwealth Fund 2006 healthcare quality survey*, 2006. Available from: www.commonwealthfund.org/Content/Publications/Fund-Reports/2007/Jun/Closing-the-Divide-How-Medical-Homes-Promote-Equity-in-Health-Care-Results-From-The-Commonwealth-F.aspx.

Colby SL, Ortman JM: *Projections of the size and composition of the U.S. Population: 2014 to 2060, Current Population Reports, P25-1143*, Washington, DC, 2015, U.S. Census Bureau.

Edmonds VM: The nutritional patterns of recently immigrated Honduran women, *J Transcult Nurs* 16(3):226–235, 2005.

Expert Panel on Global Nursing & Health: *Standards of practice for culturally competent nursing care*, 2010. Available from: http://www.tcns.org/files/Standards_of_Practice_for_Culturally_Compt_Nsg_Care-Revised_.pdf.

Fry Richard: *U.S. high school dropout rate reaches record low, driven by improvements among Hispanics, blacks*, Pew Research Center, 2014. Available from: http://www.pewresearch.org/fact-tank/2014/10/02/u-s-high-school-dropout-rate-reaches-record-low-driven-by-improvements-among-hispanics-blacks/.

Giger JN: *Transcultural nursing: Assessment and intervention*, ed 7, St Louis, 2017, Elsevier.

Hanson PA, Andrews MM: Religion, culture and nursing. In Andrews MM, Boyle JS, editors: *Transcultural concepts in nursing care*, ed 7, Philadelphia, 2016, Wolters Kluwer.

Kaiser Family Foundation (KFF): *Health coverage of immigrants,* 2017. http://files.kff.org/attachment/Fact-Sheet-Health-Coverage-for-Immigrants.

Kaiser Family Foundation: Percent of Adults Reporting Fair or Poor Health Status, by Race/Ethnicity 2016, 2016. Available from: https://www.kff.org/other/state-indicator/percent-of-adults-reporting-fair-or-poor-health-status-by-raceethnicity/?current Timeframe=0&sortModel=%7B%22colId%22:%22Location%22,%22sort%22:%22asc%22%7D.

Katon W, Kleinman A: Doctor-patient negotiation and other social science strategies in patient care. In Eisenberg L, Kleinman A, editors: *The relevance of social science for medicine,* Boston, 1981, D. Reidel.

Keller L, Strohschein S, Schaffer M: Cornerstones of public health nursing, *Public Health Nurs* 28(3):249–260, 2011.

Kluckhohn F, Strodtbeck F: *Variations in value orientations,* Evanston, IL, 1961, Row, Peterson.

Kohls LR: *Survival kit for overseas living,* Yarmouth, ME, 1984, Intercultural Press.

Leininger MM: *Nursing and anthropology: two worlds to blend,* New York, 1970, Wiley.

Leininger MM: *Transcultural nursing: concepts, theories, and practice,* New York, 1978, Wiley.

Leininger MM: *Culture, care, diversity, and universality: a theory of nursing,* New York, 1991, National League for Nursing Press.

Leininger MM: *Transcultural nursing: concepts, theories, research and practice,* ed 2, New York, 1995, McGraw-Hill.

Leininger MM, McFarland MR: *Transcultural nursing: concepts, theories, research and practice,* ed 3, New York, 2002, McGraw-Hill.

Ludwig-Beymer PA: Transcultural aspects of pain. In Andrews M, Boyle JS, editors: *Transcultural concepts in nursing care,* ed 5, Philadelphia, 2008, Lippincott Williams & Wilkins.

National Center for Health Statistics: *People without health insurance coverage by race and ethnicity,* 2008. Available from: www.cdc.gov/Features/dsHealthInsurance/.

National Institute on Minority Health and Health Disparities: *National Institute on Minority Health and Health Disparities Fact Sheet,* 2016. Available from: https://www.nimhd.nih.gov/docs/about-nimhd-factsheet.pdf.

Ortiz CE: Disclosing concerns of Latinas living with HIV/AIDS, *J Transcult Nurs* 16(3):210–217, 2005.

Pew Research Center: *America's changing religious landscape,* 2015a. Available from: http://www.pewforum.org/2015/05/12/americas-changing-religious-landscape/.

Pew Research Center: *Chapter 5: Foreign born population trends,* 2015b. Available from: http://www.pewhispanic.org/2015/09/28/chapter-5-u-s-foreign-born-population-trends/.

Spector RE: *Cultural diversity in health and illness,* ed 9, New York, 2017, Pearson.

Spector R: *Cultural diversity in health and illness,* ed 7, Upper Saddle River, NJ, 2008, Prentice Hall.

Sullivan Commission: *Missing persons: minorities in the health professions,* 2014. Available from: http://campaignforaction.org/wp-content/uploads/2016/04/SullivanReport-Diversity-in-Healthcare-Workforce1.pdf.

Tylor EB: *Primitive culture,* London, 1871, Murray.

U.S. Census Bureau: *Current Population Estimates,* 2017. Accessed from: https://www.census.gov/quickfacts/fact/table/US/PST045217.

U.S. Census Bureau: *Projections of the Size and Composition of the U.S. Population: 2014 to 2060,* 2015. Accessed from: https://census.gov/content/dam/Census/library/publications/2015/demo/p25-1143.pdf.

U.S. Census Bureau: *Current Population Reports, P60-256(RV), Income and Poverty in the United States: 2015,* Washington, DC, 2016, U.S. Government Printing Office.

U.S. Department of Health and Human Services: *Healthy People 2020: topics and objectives,* 2018. Available from: http://www.healthy-people.gov/2020/topicsobjectives2020/default.aspx.

U.S. Department of Homeland Security: *2015 Yearbook of Immigration Statistics,* 2016. Available from: https://www.dhs.gov/immigration-statistics/yearbook/2015/table1.

Vitale SA, Prashad T: Cultural awareness: Coining and cupping. International archives of nursing and health care, *Int Arch Nurs Health Care* 3:3, 2017, open access. https://doi.org/10.23937/2469-5823/1510080.

Ward BW, Clarke TC, Nugent CN, Schiller JS: *Early release of selected estimates based on data from the 2015 National Health Interview Survey,* National Center for Health Statistics, May 2016. Available from: https://www.cdc.gov/nchs/data/nhis/earlyrelease/earlyrelease201605.pdf.

Wilmoth JM, Chen PC: Immigrant status, living arrangements, and depressive symptoms among middle-aged and older adults, *J Gerontol B Psychol Sci Soc Sci* 58B(5):S305–S313, 2003.

Zborowski M: *People in pain,* San Francisco, 1969, Jossey-Bass.

Environmental Health

Tamara Rose*

OBJECTIVES

Upon completion of this chapter, the reader will be able to do the following:

1. Describe areas of environmental health, environmental health problems, and related human health risks.
2. Apply the basic concepts of critical theory to environmental health nursing problems.
3. Describe the importance of air, water, and food quality as a determinant of health.
4. Identify social, cultural, economic, and political factors that contribute to pollution and affect environmental problems.
5. Develop an understanding of the risk assessment and risk management role of nurses.
6. Explain laws and regulations relevant to environmental health and how government agencies use them to address environmental issues.

KEY TERMS

air quality index
biosolids
built environment
climate change
critical theory
environmental health
environmental justice

environmental risks to health
food desert
food safety
global warming
Healthy Home
outdoor air quality
participatory action research

population
sick building syndrome
social capital
waste management
water quality
work-related exposures

The World Health Organization (WHO) (2016) defines environmental health as "all the physical, chemical, and biological factors external to a person, and all related behavior, but excluding those natural environments that cannot reasonably be modified." "As a fundamental component of a comprehensive public health system, environmental health works to advance policies and programs to reduce chemical and other environmental exposures in air, water, soil, and food to protect residents and provide communities with healthier environments" (National Environmental Health Association, 2016). Fig. 14.1, from the U.S. Department of Health and Human Services *Healthy People 2020* program, demonstrates these factors.

Environmental health experts believe that the purpose of environmental health is to assure the conditions of human health and provide healthy environments for people to live,

* The author would like to acknowledge the contribution of Diane Santa Maria, who wrote this chapter for the previous edition.

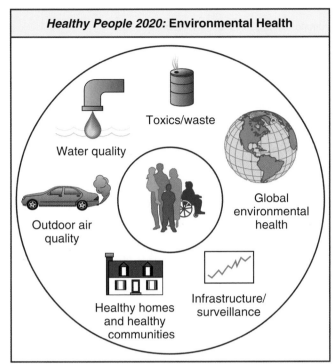

FIG. 14.1 *Healthy People 2020:* Elements of environmental health. (From U.S. Department of Health and Human Services: *Healthy People 2010*, ed 2, Washington, DC, 2000, U.S. Government Printing Office.)

work, and play. This can be accomplished through risk assessment, prevention, and intervention.

Efforts are made to reduce and eliminate contaminant and contagion threats to human health from air, water, food, and the built environment (Lindland and Kendall-Taylor, 2011). Maintaining a healthy environment is vitally important to promoting the health of **populations**—particular groups or types of people. A healthy environment improves quality of life and increases years of healthy living. Accumulated evidence shows that the environmental changes of the past few decades have profoundly influenced the status of public health. Globally, environmental risk factors, including air, water and soil pollution, exposure to chemicals, radiation, and climate changes, contribute to nearly 25% of all deaths and increase disease burden (WHO, 2016). The safety, beauty, and life-sustaining capacity of the physical environment are unquestionably of global consequence. Since the beginning of the twenty-first century, it has become apparent that the world must address urgent environmental difficulties, including extinction of some species, diminishing rainforests, proliferation of toxic waste dumps, progressive destruction of the ozone layer, shortage of landfill sites, consequences of climate change, threats of terrorism, development of deadly chemical and ballistic weapons, adulteration of food by pesticides and herbicides, oceanic contamination through toxic dumping and petroleum spills, overcrowding of urban areas, and traffic congestion.

This chapter uses critical theory to explore the health of communities in relation to the environment. Critical theory is particularly useful in examining environmental health because it offers a framework for discussion and a basis for describing community

health nursing practice (Martins and Burbank, 2011; Stevens and Hall, 1992). Applying critical theory is a way of thinking upstream (see Chapter 3). **Critical theory** is an approach that raises questions about oppressive situations, involves community members in the definition and solution of problems, and facilitates interventions that reduce health-damaging effects of environments. By applying the nursing process in a critical fashion, nurses can be dynamically involved in the design of interventions that alter the precursors of poor health.

Recognition of the gravity and pervasiveness of environmental hazards can be overwhelming. Looking beyond the individual to recognize the environmental determinants of health can be complicated and alarming. Intervening to improve the quality of air, water, housing, food, and waste disposal and reducing the risks of harmful exposures to environmental toxins require individual, social, economic, and political changes. Nurses are powerful change agents who use their assessment, management, and communication skills to promote environmental health locally and nationally. Nurses are becoming increasingly active in efforts to address environmental health issues and to increase awareness of the effects of the environment on well-being.

A CRITICAL THEORY APPROACH TO ENVIRONMENTAL HEALTH

Critical theory suggests that nurses must be aware of environmental threats or factors that might detrimentally affect the safety and well-being of particular populations or deprive them of access to resources necessary in the pursuit of health. This awareness may include recognizing, supporting, and maintaining positive environmental influences. For instance, a nurse must consider the effects of having access to a safe place to walk on one's ability to maintain healthy levels of physical activity. Research studies indicate that access to recreation facilities is an important correlate of physical activity (Troped et al., 2011; Tsunoda et al., 2012). Nurses can help individuals adopt healthy behaviors by considering not only individual-level issues but also those issues in the environment that facilitate or create barriers to healthy living.

Nurses need to ask critical questions about their clients' environments to help discern the contributions of specific hazards to their health. Occupational exposure to environmental hazardous can cause harm to workers as well as their families. For example, farm workers and pesticide applicators who accumulate agricultural chemicals on their skin and clothing take these substances home with them, increasing their children's exposure to toxicants (Thompson et al., 2008). Nurses must provide answers to farm workers who ask questions such as "What do I do if I'm exposed to a pesticide? How long should I wait until after a pesticide application to go back into the field? How do I find out how toxic a certain pesticide is? Where can I get information on a specific pesticide?" Nurses can take an environmental health history. An environmental health history can benefit the client in the following ways:

- Increase awareness of environmental health concerns
- Improve timelines and accuracy of diagnosis
- Prevent disease and aggravation of conditions
- Identify potential environmental hazards

1. Do you live next to or near an industrial plant, commercial business, dump site, or nonresidential property?

2. Have you been exposed to hazardous materials at work now or in the past?

3. Which of the following do you have in your home?

    ___ air conditioner   ___ air purifier   ___ central heating (_ gas _ oil)

    ___ gas stove   ___ fireplace   ___ wood stove

    ___ humidifier

4. Have you recently acquired new furniture or carpet, refinished furniture, or remodeled your home?

5. Have you weatherized your home recently?

6. Are pesticides or herbicides (bug or weed killers; flea and tick sprays; collars, powders, shampoos) used in your home, garden, or on your pets?

7. Do you (or any household member) have a hobby or craft?

8. Have you ever changed your residence because of a health problem?

9. Does your drinking water come from a private well?

10. Approximately what year was your home built?

11. Has your routine changed recently?

12. Does anyone in your household smoke?

13. Has your home been tested for radon?

FIG. 14.2 Environmental history assessment.

Environmental health histories should be obtained for both adults and children, although the relationship between the environment and children's health is frequently overlooked. Fig. 14.2 demonstrates common assessment items of an environmental history. When looking at the community from a critical perspective, nurses have the opportunity to promote population health. In identifying environmental sources of health problems, nurses must be involved with the affected communities. Rather than impose their views of the problem, nurses should share their ideas and dialogue with community members. For example, nurses should listen to what the community believes is problematic, help raise consciousness about environmental dangers, and help bring about change. If nurses become involved in conducting community assessments and analyses, they can learn how the community members perceive themselves, their health, and their environmental influences.

From a critical standpoint, helping communities become more aware of the environmental effects on health and helping them make needed changes in their environment are legitimate nursing actions. Collective actions have been instrumental in accomplishing positive environmental changes since the 1980s. Some of the mechanisms have included strategic organization, litigation, public hearing testimony, letter-writing campaigns, legislative lobbying, mass demonstrations, and fundraising.

Fundraising for environmental causes such as the 2012 storms that devastated the Northeast United States and the 2010 earthquake in Haiti facilitated rapid availability of resources, minimized loss of life, and helped restore basic necessities such as clean water and shelter. Public response to "acute" environmental disasters needs to be extended to an ongoing, consistent pressure to ensure day-to-day environmental integrity; hence "chronic" environmental problems need to be addressed more effectively.

A critical perspective can help nurses plan and implement population-level interventions by emphasizing collective strategies for change. Acting collectively can empower nurses to affect environmental health. Assessing environmental health problems, planning and implementing interventions, and evaluating the effectiveness of community-based actions need to be based on a wide lens. Community health nurses should be familiar with physical surroundings and their mutual interaction with cultural realities, social relations, economic circumstances, and political conditions of communities, applying a critical perspective to community health.

AREAS OF ENVIRONMENTAL HEALTH

Environmental health hazards are ubiquitous in communities across the United States and place people at risk for disease

TABLE 14.1	Areas of Environmental Health
Area	Definition
Built environment	Buildings, spaces, and products that are created or modified by people, including homes, schools, workplaces, parks/recreation areas, greenways, business areas, and transportation systems.
Work-related exposure	Occupational exposure to environmental hazards that can cause illness or injury.
Outdoor air quality	The protectiveness of the atmospheric layers, the risks of severe weather, and the purity of the air for breathing purposes.
Healthy home	The availability, safety, structural strength, cleanliness, and location of shelter, including public facilities and family dwellings. This includes indoor air quality.
Water quality	The availability of and accessibility to a clean water supply, the mineral content levels, pollution by toxic chemicals, and the presence of pathogenic microorganisms.
Food safety	The availability, relative costs, variety, safety, and health of animal and plant food sources.
Waste management	The management of waste materials resulting from industrial and municipal processes, human consumption, and efforts to minimize waste production.

TABLE 14.2	Examples of Environmental Health Problems
Area	Problems
Built environment	Drunk driving
	Secondhand smoke
	Noise exposure
	Urban crowding
	Technological hazards
Work-related exposure	Asbestos exposure
	Agricultural accidents
	Excessive exposure to x-rays
Outdoor air quality	Gaseous pollutants
	Greenhouse effect
	Destruction of the ozone layer
	Aerial spraying of herbicides and pesticides
	Acid rain
	Nuclear facility emissions
Healthy home	Homelessness
	Rodent and insect infestation
	Presence of lead-based paint
	Sick building syndrome
	Unsafe neighborhoods
	Radon gas seepage in homes and schools
Water quality	Contamination of drinking supply by human waste
	Oil spills in the world's waterways
	Pesticide or herbicide infiltration of groundwater
	Aquifer contamination by industrial pollutants
	Heavy metal poisoning of fish
Food safety	Malnutrition
	Bacterial food poisoning
	Food adulteration
	Disruption of food chains by ecosystem destruction
	Carcinogenic chemical food additives
Waste management	Use of nonbiodegradable plastics
	Poorly designed solid-waste dumps
	Inadequate sewage systems
	Transport and storage of hazardous waste
	Illegal industrial dumping
	Radioactive hazardous wastes

or injury. This chapter divides the vast field of environmental health into the following subcategories: the built environment, work-related exposures, outdoor air quality, healthy homes, water quality, food safety, and waste management (Table 14.1). A brief discussion introduces nurses to these seven areas of environmental health, describes how they affect health, and demonstrates basic strategies nurses can use to address them. Table 14.2 provides examples of health problems within each area of environmental health.

It should be noted that a critical perspective does not separate the idea of a safe social environment from a safe physical environment. For example, interpersonal violence is a significant and growing risk, with consequences ranging from bodily injury to psychiatric aftereffects that may last for decades in some individuals. Intergenerational patterns of abuse, hate crimes toward marginalized groups, sexual predators, and hazards of combat might be considered from an environmental health perspective. Issues of violence are discussed in more depth in Chapter 27.

Finally, we must be prepared for the public health effects of terrorism. Terrorism is a word that evokes many images and a range of reactions from rage to grief and loss. Acts of terrorism have drawn the public and political focus to establishing environmental security. Bioterrorism and homeland security are new areas where nurses will have an impact. A critical perspective is needed now more than ever, because security issues are linked to religious imperatives, moral stances, values, profit motives, health care systems and information, and cultural differences. These issues are also clearly within the scope of community health nursing and are discussed in more detail in Chapter 28.

The Built Environment

The **built environment** consists of the connections among people, communities, and their surrounding environments that affect health behaviors and habits, interpersonal relationships, cultural values, and customs. There is growing evidence that the built environment directly and indirectly affects health outcomes and disease rates (Table 14.3). One review of the literature found that neighborhoods that are more walkable are associated with increased physical activity, increased social capital, lower overweight, lower reports of depression, and less reported alcohol abuse (Renalds et al., 2009). **Social capital** refers to networks and the associated norms and expected collective benefits derived from cooperation between individuals and groups. Structural characteristics of the built environment, such as street condition, neighborhood deterioration, and the proportion of parks and playgrounds, affect levels of physical activity and obesity (Schulz et al., 2013; Kerr et al. 2010) found that women are more likely to increase physical activity if they

TABLE 14.3   A Conceptual Model of How the Built Environment Affects Health

The Built Environment (Underlying Context)	Mediating Factors (Exposure Media)	Downstream Pathways (Human Response)	Health Status (Outcome Indicators)
• Land use patterns • Transportation networks • Infrastructure systems • Public facilities • Buildings	• Environmental toxins • Local climate • Noise level • Crime level • Disasters and accidents • Access to services	• Behavioral (e.g., physical activity, diet behavior, smoking, drinking, taking drugs) • Psychological (e.g., satisfaction, depression/distress, social cohesion) • Physiological (e.g., infection, immune system activation, hormonal response)	• Individual level (e.g., body mass index [BMI], perceived health status, well-being) • Population level (e.g., cause-specific mortality rates, morbidity rates)

Developed by Fan Y, Song Y: Is sprawl associated with a widening urban–suburban mortality gap? *J Urban Health* 86(5):708–728, 2009; adapted from a conceptual model by Klitzman S., Matte TD, Kass DE: The urban physical environment and its effects on health. In Freudenberg N, Galea S, Vlahov D, editors: *Cities and the health of the public,* Nashville, TN, 2006, Vanderbilt University Press, p 364.

live in a walkable community compared with men, indicating safety to be an attributing factor. Simply put, having a safe, intact place to walk may encourage exercise among adults.

Many people live within areas that require almost daily contact with potential health risks and threats. These include intoxicated or impaired drivers, secondhand smoke, urban crowding, noise exposure, unabated traffic, and the stress of increased mechanization. The type of area one lives in can greatly affect one's health. For example, a research study found that adolescents living in rural working-class or mixed-race urban neighborhoods were more likely to be overweight than peers in newer suburbs, regardless of their socioeconomic status, age, or race/ethnicity (Nelson et al., 2006). In another study investigating the role of neighborhood characteristics and childhood obesity, neighborhood socioeconomic status (SES) was found to be a greater mediator of childhood obesity than racial or ethnic disparities (Sharifi et al., 2016). Access to equipment and facilities, neighborhood pattern (e.g. rural, exurban, suburban), walkability, and urban sprawl are also associated with obesity outcomes in adolescents (Ding et al., 2011; Dunton et al., 2009).

Urban sprawl has been defined as the conversion of land to nonagricultural or nonnatural uses at a faster rate than the population growth (Environmental Protection Agency [EPA], 2002). The sprawling development often occurs more rapidly than the expansion of the infrastructure (e.g., schools, sewer systems, water lines) needed for support. The urban sprawl is characterized by four dimensions: "low residential density; rigidly separated homes, shops, and workplaces; roads with large blocks and poor access; and lack of well-defined activity centers" (James et al., 2016, p. 369). Consequences of sprawl include air and water pollution, floods, infrastructure expenses, and a decrease in natural areas and forests (EPA, 2002).

One unfortunately common problem associated with living patterns relates to residing near hazardous facilities (e.g., waste incinerators, sewage treatment plants, landfills, refineries, and some correctional facilities). Molitor and colleagues (2011) found that higher levels of pollutants are generally associated with higher poverty. Discriminatory land use ensures that many impoverished and marginalized groups, especially minorities, live in close proximity to industrial contamination (Collins, 2011; Nweke, 2011). People who live near such environmental hazards are in danger of becoming victims of illness and injury related to violence, poisonings and exposures, fires, and malignant and nonmalignant diseases. Clinical Example 14.1 provides an example. Though historically outdoor pollution and hazards have been considered the major contributors affecting environmental quality, one must also consider the influence of indoor residential environmental hazards, such as radon, asbestos, lead, insect and pet allergens, chemicals, and other consumer products, as well as secondhand smoke and fungi (Adamkiewicz et al., 2011).

Many communities lack sufficient resources to respond when urban development and technological advances jeopardize the health and well-being of families in affected areas. The environmental movement of the 1960s and 1970s succeeded in building political power capable of passing monumental environmental reforms; however, charges that poor and minority communities are dumping grounds for environmental hazards have been substantiated by governmental agencies (EPA, 2004, 2013c).

Difficulties in alerting state and federal officials about environmental health dangers, as well as in obtaining compensation for environmental toxin–causing disease and death, often result in resident revictimization. Tightly knit social structures and a lack of low-cost housing may hinder the mobility of residents and perpetuate the exposure to health hazards. Residents may be unwilling to disrupt family ties and cultural roots to start over elsewhere, or they may be unable to afford a move. These residents may live with uncertainty and conflict. Long-term, community-wide effects of division, animosity, distrust, cynicism, and despair can abound in these situations, negatively affecting social capital.

In the 1990s, the central issues of equity and justice emerged in environmental health policy. In 1994, President Clinton signed Executive Order (EO) 12898, which required all federal agencies to develop comprehensive strategies for achieving **environmental justice**. This directive has served to increase public participation and access to information as well as provision of education about multiple risks and cumulative exposures (EPA, 2005, 2013c) (Box 14.1). A recent investigation of the impact of EO 12898 determined the order failed to address an important contributor to environmental justice: poor economic growth in low-income minority communities. In 2008, President Obama signed a memorandum of understanding in regard to EO 12898 to identify and address environmental justice at the program, policy, and initiative level (Geltman et al., 2016). Nurses are part of the interdisciplinary team made up of urban planners, public health practitioners, and policy makers needed to understand and address issues of the built environment that are critical to establishing health equity.

EXAMPLES OF ENVIRONMENTAL HEALTH ISSUES AFFECTING COMMUNITIES

Water pollution from local industry.

Sidewalks in disrepair.

Motor vehicle emissions (primary mobile source of air pollutants).

Food safety meat inspection.

Air pollution from local industry.

Clinical Example 14.1

In an urban city in the south, the health department is becoming increasingly concerned about the overweight and obesity rates of young school-age children. At health fairs held around the city, nurses are seeing more children with acanthosis nigricans, elevated blood pressure, high body mass index (BMI), and hypercholesterolemia. Though the public health nurse diligently counsels patients on the benefits of exercise, his patients do not increase their physical activity. When the nurse drives around the neighborhood where many of his patients reside, he realizes there are no recreational parks nearby, the sidewalks are in disrepair, the smokestacks cloud the air, and there appears to be gang-related activity. The nurse considers the impact of the built environment on the ability of his patients to be physically active. In partnership with the school board and neighborhood watch group, the nurse and community members successfully petition

BOX 14.1 Landmark Federal Environmental Legislation

Year	Legislation
1970	Clean Air Act
	Poison Prevention Packaging Act
	National Environmental Policy Act
1971	Lead-Based Paint Poisoning Prevention Act
1972	Federal Water Pollution Control Act Amendments
	Noise Control Act
	Clean Water Act
1973	Endangered Species Act
1974	Safe Drinking Water Act
1975	Hazardous Materials Transportation Act
1976	Resource Conservation and Recovery Act
	Toxic Substances Control Act
	Surface Mining Control and Reclamation Act
1980	Low-Level Radiation Waste Policy Act
	Comprehensive Environmental Response, Compensation, and Liability Act (i.e., Superfund)
1990	Oil Pollution Act
	Clean Air Act
2003	Healthy Forests Restoration Act
2016	Fuel Economy Standards raised (original legislation: 1975)

for a park to be built within walking distance of the school. Additionally, the partnership is able to establish a "walking school bus," a program where students walk in a group to or from school, as a way for children to increase their physical activity.

Work-Related Exposures

Work-related exposures can happen as a result of poor working conditions and can lead to potential injury or illness. Environmental health problems posed by work-related exposures include such issues as occupational toxic poisoning, machine-operation hazards (e.g., falls, crushing injuries, burns), electrical hazards, repetitive motion injuries, carcinogenic particulate inhalation (e.g., of asbestos, coal dust), and heavy metal poisoning (Centers for Disease Control and Prevention [CDC], 2013; Krieger et al., 2008). Prevention of work-related health problems requires integrated action to improve job safety and the working environment. Occupational and environmental health nurses often collaborate on initiatives to reduce and eliminate work-related exposures, illnesses, and injuries. Nurses can be sure that workers are aware of and know where to access the safety data sheets relevant to their workplace. The U.S. Department of Labor's Occupational Safety and Health Administration (OSHA) (2013) requires chemical manufacturers, distributors, and importers to provide safety data sheets that communicate the hazards of chemical products.

According to the Bureau of Labor Statistics (2016) approximately 2.9 million nonfatal workplace injuries and illnesses were reported by private industry employers in 2015. This rate continues a pattern of decline annually for the past 13 years,

apart from 2012, where there was either equal or more days away from work because of injury compared with the previous year (Bureau of Labor and Statistics, 2016). The EPA estimates that 10,000 to 20,000 physician-diagnosed pesticide poisonings occur each year among the approximately 2 million U.S. agricultural workers (EPA, 2013). In one year (2010), 476 farm workers died from work-related injuries, with tractor overturns being the leading cause of death (CDC, 2013).

These statistics do not reflect unreported health problems. For example, a clerical worker leaves the office every day with back strain and a headache because of ventilation problems in the building. After 5 years on a repetitive hand-movement job task, an employee is diagnosed with carpal tunnel syndrome. An operating room nurse has a miscarriage and recalls that many of her coworkers have also been unable to carry their babies to term. A dry cleaner often leaves work feeling light-headed and dizzy from inhaling solvents at the shop, and one day she has a car accident on her way home. Collective problems related to employment or occupation are often perceived as individualized injuries, and no one "connects the dots." Research is ongoing to determine the outcomes of work-related environmental exposures. For example, the GuLF STUDY (Gulf Long Term Follow-Up Study) is a health study, sponsored by the National Institutes of Health (NIH), for individuals who helped with oil spill clean-up after the 2010 Deepwater Horizon disaster in the Gulf of Mexico (NIH, 2014). Clinical Example 14.2 illustrates another case of work-related exposure.

Clinical Example 14.2

Sanitation workers in an urban area experienced a rising incidence of puncture injuries while transporting hazardous wastes from the public medical center; these puncture injuries caused several cases of hepatitis. When the story became public, members of the city health commission contacted community health nurses and instructed them to politically support the interests of the city and the medical center "at all costs." Subsequently, the sanitation workers' union contacted the community health nursing office and requested information about procedures for safely packaging medical wastes. They also requested that a nurse speak to their membership about immediate measures for preventing further injuries on the job.

The nurses met to resolve the conflict. Most agreed that the sanitation workers had pressing needs for education and support. Despite the city's demand for loyalty, they decided to "choose sides" with the workers and respond to their requests. They collectively drafted a letter to the city health commission and arranged a meeting with the commissioners to discuss their plan to assist the sanitation workers. The health commission held a press conference, which depicted the nurses' actions as mediational efforts that benefited the union and the city. Eventually, the nurses and the commission developed a new medical waste disposal plan, and injured workers received reasonable compensation through an out-of-court settlement.

Outdoor Air Quality

Outdoor air quality refers to the purity of the air and the presence of air pollution. The EPA (2012b) has classified six common

TABLE 14.4 Major Air Pollutants

Pollutant	Sources	Effects
Ozone: A colorless gas that is the major constituent of smog at the earth's surface	Ozone is formed in the lower atmosphere as the result of chemical reactions among oxygen, volatile organic compounds, and nitrogen oxides in the presence of sunlight, particularly during hot weather. Sources of this harmful pollutant include vehicles, factories, landfills, lawn equipment, farm equipment, and industrial solvents.	Ozone can irritate the respiratory tract; impair lung function; and cause throat irritation, chest pain, cough, and susceptibility to lung infection. Individuals with asthma and other existing respiratory conditions are particularly vulnerable. Ozone can also reduce agricultural yields and injure forests and other vegetation.
Carbon monoxide: A colorless and odorless gas that is emitted in the exhaust of motor vehicles and other kinds of engines during combustion of fossil fuels	Carbon monoxide is emitted from the engines of cars, buses, trucks, and other small engines and from some industrial processes. High concentrations can be found in confined spaces (e.g., parking garages, poorly ventilated tunnels, or along roadsides during periods of heavy traffic).	Carbon monoxide reduces the ability of the blood to deliver oxygen to vital tissues, affecting primarily the cardiovascular and nervous systems. Lower concentrations have been shown to adversely affect individuals with heart disease and to affect exercise performance. Higher concentrations can cause symptoms such as dizziness, headaches, and fatigue.
Nitrogen dioxides: A light-brown gas at lower concentrations; in higher concentrations, a significant component of brown urban haze	Nitrogen dioxide forms from the burning of fuels in utilities, industrial boilers, and the engines of cars and trucks.	Nitrogen dioxide is a major component of smog and acid rain. When concentrations are high, it can increase respiratory illnesses (e.g., chest colds and coughing) in children. For asthmatic people, it may exacerbate breathing difficulty.
Sulfur dioxide: A colorless gas, odorless at low concentrations but pungent at very high concentrations	Sulfur dioxide is emitted from industrial, institutional, utility, and apartment-house furnaces and boilers as well as petroleum refineries, smelters, paper mills, and chemical plants.	Sulfur dioxide is one of the major components of smog. At high concentrations, it can harm humans; asthmatic people are particularly vulnerable. It can also harm vegetation and metals and acidify lakes and streams.
Particulate matter: Droplets from smoke, dust, ash, and condensing vapors that can be suspended in the air for long periods	Particulates are emitted from industrial processes, vehicles, wood smoke, dust from paved and unpaved roads, construction, and agriculture.	Particulates can affect breathing and elicit respiratory symptoms, causing increased respiratory disease and lung damage. Children, elders, and people with heart or lung disease are especially at risk. They can also damage paint, soil, and clothing and reduce visibility.
Lead: A metal found in nature as well as a by-product of industry; can contaminate substances (e.g., soil, dust) that can be directly inhaled	Metals processing is the major source of lead emissions into the air today. Lead is generally found near lead smelters, waste incinerators, utilities, and lead-acid battery manufacturers.	Lead can adversely affect mental development and performance, kidney function, and blood chemistry. Young children are particularly at risk to its effects.

From Environmental Protection Agency: *What are the six common air pollutants?* Retrieved January 26, 2018 from https://www.epa.gov/criteria-air-pollutants /

air pollutants (Table 14.4). WHO estimates that air pollution is the thirteenth leading cause of mortality worldwide, contributing to approximately 800,000 premature deaths annually. Particulate matter, one common pollutant, causes worsening respiratory symptoms, more frequent asthma-related medication use, decreased lung function, recurrent health care utilization, and increased mortality (Anderson et al., 2012).

Air pollution originates from industry (dry cleaning, factories, oil refineries, coal-burning power plants), modes of transportation (cars, buses, trucks, and planes), and naturally occurring events (volcanic eruptions and windstorms). Tornadoes, electrical storms, smog, gaseous pollutants (e.g., carbon monoxide), excessive hydrocarbon levels, aerial herbicide spraying, and acid rain all contribute to air pollution. Under provisions of the Clean Air Act, the EPA sets the national ambient air quality standards for pollutants considered harmful to humans or the environment.

Ozone is the most common pollutant in the United States and is the primary component of smog. Ozone is formed when nitrogen oxides (created by the burning of fossil fuels in power plants, automobiles, and factories) react with oxygen and sunlight (EPA, 2013f). Ozone, along with other hazardous

atmospheric pollutants, causes and/or contributes to asthma, allergic reactions, bronchitis, lung cancer, chronic respiratory disease, and death and harms animal and plant species (Ciencewicki et al., 2008; Sheffield et al., 2011). Furthermore, sulfur dioxide, a by-product of burning coal and other fossil fuels, contributes to acid rain, which affects terrestrial ecosystems by increasing soil acidity, reducing nutrient availability, mobilizing toxic metals, leaching soil chemicals, and altering species composition (EPA, 2012c).Two significant issues related to outdoor air quality are of global concern. First, the amount of protection in the atmospheric layers is diminishing (EPA, 2013e). Chemicals such as chlorofluorocarbons, halons, and carbon tetrachloride, which have been in widespread use for refrigeration, air conditioning, and aerosol propellants, remain in the atmosphere. These molecules cause depletion of the atmosphere's protective ozone layer. The resulting "holes" in the ozone layer allow excess ultraviolet radiation to penetrate, which has harmful effects on many organisms. Long-term problems include increases in rates of skin cancer and cataracts, suppression of immune response, and environmental damage.

Second, there is a disruption in the key processes that break down atmospheric carbon dioxide. The ongoing deforestation

Air Quality Guide for Particle Pollution		
Good	0-50	None
Moderate	51-100	Unusually sensitive people should consider reducing prolonged or heavy exertion
Unhealthy for Sensitive Groups	101-150	People with heart or lung disease, older adults, and children should reduce prolonged or heavy exertion.
Unhealthy	151 to 200	People with heart or lung disease, older adults, and children should avoid prolonged or heavy exertion. Everyone else should reduce prolonged or heavy exertion.
Very Unhealthy Alert	201 to 300	People with heart or lung disease, older adults, and children should avoid all physical activity outdoors. Everyone else should avoid prolonged or heavy exertion.

FIG. 14.3 Environmental Protection Agency air quality index. (From AirNow: *Local air conditions and forecasts,* n.d. Retrieved from www.airnow.gov)

of the earth's surface, especially the diminishing of tropical rainforests, not only releases the carbon stored in the biomass but also eliminates sources of photosynthesis (i.e., the process by which plants absorb carbon dioxide and release oxygen). The loss of carbon dioxide–consuming resources increases carbon dioxide and traps part of the heat reemitted by the earth. As a result, the earth's surface temperature is rising (i.e., the "greenhouse effect"), with potentially catastrophic ecological consequences. Global climate change, including evidence that glaciers are shrinking, ice on rivers and lakes is breaking up earlier than usual, and a shift in plant and animal ranges, has already been observed (NASA, 2014).

In 1968, the National Air Pollution Control Administration developed the **air quality index** (AQI) to increase public awareness of air pollution (Fig. 14.3). The AQI is a number used by government agencies to communicate current and forecasted air pollution conditions to the public. As the AQI rises, a larger percentage of the population, particularly vulnerable populations, may experience adverse health effects. The AQI fluctuates on the basis of the dilution of air pollutants. Air stagnation can lead to high concentrations of pollutants and haze. Although most air contaminants do not have an associated AQI, many countries monitor ground-level ozone, particulates, sulfur dioxide, carbon monoxide, and nitrogen dioxide to calculate the air quality index (EPA, 2013g). Nurses need to be aware of the AQI and the corresponding recommendations for the public to limit exposure to outdoor air during peak times of high AQI (Clinical Example 14.3). Additionally, nurses must consider the AQI when making recommendations for physical activity, particularly for asthmatic patients. One study suggests that population-level health benefits from increased physical activity in high-walkability neighborhoods may be offset by the adverse effects of exposure to air pollution (Hankey et al., 2012). A recent study on the effects of particulate matter for individuals who walk or cycle to work found that the health benefits of active travel far outweighed the health risks from air pollution (Tainio et al., 2016).

Clinical Example 14.3

During a recent summer, a sudden increase occurred in the number of clinic visits from residents of a particular urban neighborhood. The patients were elderly men and women who felt ill after going for a walk and asthmatic children with worsening respiratory symptoms. A nurse at the federally qualified health clinic in the neighborhood suspected that air pollution might be contributing to the increase in health concerns.

The nurse went online to the site www.airnow.gov and searched for the air quality index for the region. She discovered that the region was experiencing a very unhealthy level of outdoor air pollution. She immediately alerted the health care staff that people with heart or lung disease, older adults, and children should avoid all physical activity outdoors and that everyone should avoid prolonged or heavy exertion outdoors. The nurse contacted the local summer camps and nursing homes in the area to alert them of the recommendation. The clinic quickly decided to move their regularly scheduled outdoor picnic to an indoor venue. One week later, the nurse noticed a drop in the number of patients complaining of respiratory distress.

Healthy Homes

A **Healthy Home** refers to the availability, safety, structural strength, cleanliness, location, and indoor air quality of shelter. According to the EPA (2017), many of the health concerns related to indoor living are a result of exposure to radon, carbon monoxide, molds and dust, secondhand smoke, cooking vapors, lead paint, and rodents. The CDC and surgeon general have developed a Healthy Home checklist that nurses can use with patients to guide a thorough assessment and develop a care plan to help patients improve the quality of their homes and their indoor air quality (CDC, 2011).

Radon causes an estimated 21,000 lung cancer deaths in the United States every year. It is the second leading cause of lung cancer, after active smoking, and the leading cause among nonsmokers (EPA, 2013f). Nine federal agencies are currently working on an initiative to reduce radon exposures and illnesses (EPA, 2013d). Carbon monoxide is an odorless, colorless, toxic gas. It can cause mild flulike effects such as headaches, dizziness, disorientation, nausea, and fatigue at lower levels of exposure and death at higher levels (EPA, 2012d). Molds, dust, and secondhand smoke exposure can often exacerbate asthma symptoms.

Other health problems related to housing include fire hazards; lack of accommodations for people with disabilities; illnesses caused by overcrowding; psychological effects of architectural design (e.g., low-cost, high-rise housing projects); injuries sustained from collapsed building structures; and exposure deaths from inadequate indoor heating or cooling (Clinical Example 14.4). Poor housing conditions can contribute to the spread of infectious disease (EPA, 2012e) as well as cardiovascular and respiratory disorders, cancers, allergies, and mental illnesses (Barton et al., 2007; Jones-Rounds et al., 2013; Rauh et al., 2008). The term **sick building syndrome** describes a phenomenon in which public structures and homes cause occupants to experience a variety of symptoms, such as headache, fatigue, and exacerbation of allergies. It typically results from poor ventilation and building operations, hazardous building materials, furniture and carpeting substances, and cleaning agents (EPA, 1991). Additionally, volatile organic compounds (VOCs) have been found in soil and soil vapor as a result of industrial spills that contaminate indoor air. One such spill in Endicott, New York, has been linked to congenital cardiac defects, low birth weight, and fetal growth restriction (Farand et al., 2012).

Other problems may arise related to building structures, composition, and settings. For example, commercial buildings with offices near underground parking garages may cause workers to have carbon monoxide intoxication. Formaldehyde, asbestos, and VOCs—which are common components of thermal insulation, cement, flooring, furnishings, and household consumer products—have carcinogenic properties. Additionally, "toxic mold" arising from chronically damp wood and improperly sealed areas in homes and offices has been recognized as contributing to respiratory irritation, allergies, and infections in susceptible individuals (EPA, 2012e).

Clinical Example 14.4

In a large, northeastern U.S. city, an economic recession led to large company layoffs, leaving many unemployed or underemployed. Because of the loss of income, many families faced tough decisions during the upcoming winter months. Temperatures often went below zero, requiring constant heating. Unfortunately, many people did not have the money to continue to pay their heating bill, fix leaky windows and doors, or buy warm clothes. Some families began to use space heaters and burned scraps of wood that were discarded. Often, this wood came from old abandoned buildings and homes. Other families took to sleeping in their cars.

Soon, hospitals began to see an uptick in patients presenting with respiratory illnesses, carbon monoxide exposure, and burns. The community health nurses in the area met with struggling families to assess their needs and determine a plan to meet their immediate needs. The nurses met with local politicians and church groups to find ways to supply healthy wood for heating, help financially with home utility bills, provide warm clothes for families, and find shelters for homeless families. Within a few months, the local hospitals began to see a decline in home-related injuries and illnesses.

Water Quality

Water quality refers to the water supply's availability, volume, mineral content levels, toxic chemical pollution, and pathogenic microorganism levels. Water quality consists of the balance between water contaminants and the existing capabilities to purify water for human use and plant and wildlife sustenance. Water quality problems include experiencing droughts, dousing reservoirs with chemicals to reduce algae, contaminating aquifers with pesticides and fertilizers (Clinical Example 14.5), leaching lead from water pipes, and oil spilling from

transport tankers or leaking offshore wells. Other sources of water pollution are microbial contamination from poorly managed or maintained septic or sewage systems and animal feedlot wastes (EPA, 2013b). Water pollution can be from point sources (a well-defined source, e.g., factory wastewater discharge) or nonpoint sources (urban runoff, domestic lawn care, and air-to-water transfer).

Advances in water treatment technologies in industrialized countries have controlled many water-related diseases, such as cholera, typhoid, dysentery, and hepatitis A. Nevertheless, disease outbreaks resulting from contamination by untreated groundwater and inadequate chlorination are increasing in both urban and rural areas. In addition, more than 45 million Americans (15%) obtain their drinking water from private water supplies (e.g., wells) that have no treatment or monitoring guidelines (CDC, 2011). Other potential water contaminants include accelerated soil erosion caused by construction, agriculture, and deforestation, which can contribute to high sediment levels in drinking water supplies.

Heavy metal and toxic chemical pollution may also occur during the water treatment process or in the drinking water distribution system. The EPA monitors drinking water for more than 90 organic and inorganic pollutants that have potential health effects in humans, including those who are most vulnerable, such as children and people with weakened immune systems (EPA, 2016). Pesticides, herbicides, and carcinogenic industrial waste infiltrate an increasing amount of groundwater, the underground source of half the U.S. population's drinking water (U.S. Geological Survey, 2005). Additionally, commonly used medications and personal care products that contain endocrine disruptors have been found in water supplies (Wu et al., 2012). This development is particularly tragic because groundwater is uniquely susceptible to long-term contamination. Unlike river or lake water, once groundwater becomes contaminated, it is impossible to cleanse.

Clinical Example 14.5

In a Midwestern farm community, there is growing concern about seepage of agricultural pesticides and herbicides into groundwater. Families obtain water from private wells rather than a central municipal source. The families had heard about potential long-term carcinogenic effects of the chemicals, such as pesticides and herbicides, commonly used on the farms in the community. Although family farmers decreased their use of these chemicals, the large-scale agribusiness companies continued to use large amounts of these chemicals.

A community health nurse from the county health department lobbied local officials to begin a comprehensive program to monitor groundwater pollutants and enforce standards for herbicide and pesticide use. However, the powerful agribusiness companies pressured these officials to stand back. Together, some county farmers and nurses organized grassroots information and support groups for the rural families. The families and nurses, in coalition with environmental activist groups in the state, established several projects. These projects included collecting and testing samples from each family well, forming a local organization called

"Water Watch" to coordinate actions and communications, and implementing a research project with a local university to track water contamination and health problems of local residents. The organization also disseminated an emergency plan to families whose wells were found to have toxic levels of pesticides, herbicides, or other pollutants.

CLEAN   SEPARATE   COOK   CHILL

FIG. 14.4 Steps to food safety. (From FoodSafety.gov: *Keep food safe,* n.d. Retrieved from http://www.foodsafety.gov/keep/basics/index.html)

Food Safety

Food safety refers to availability, accessibility, and relative cost of healthy food free of contamination by harmful herbicides, pesticides, and bacteria. Food safety concerns include malnutrition, bacterial food poisoning (Clinical Example 14.6), carcinogenic chemical additives (e.g., nitrites, dyes, and cyclamate), improper or fraudulent meat inspection or food labeling, microbial epidemics among livestock (e.g., *Escherichia coli*), food products from diseased animal sources, and disruption of vital natural food chains by ecosystem destruction. Increased mobility and globalized trade also contribute to global contamination of the food supply. Finally, there are significant disparities in access to healthy and fresh food supplies, with poor minority families being more likely to live in a food desert—a neighborhood with little to no access to healthy foods (Institute of Medicine [IOM], 2009).

Annually, nearly 60 to 70 million Americans contract gastrointestinal illnesses, accounting for about 10% of all hospitalizations and 15% of in-patient hospital procedures for the treatment of digestive diseases (National Institute of Health [NIH], 2009). Potential microbial contaminants of foods include bacteria (e.g., *Shigella salmonella, E. coli, Campylobacter, Listeria*), parasites (e.g., *Balantidium coli, Cryptosporidium parvum, Entamoeba histolytica Giardia intestinalis*), and viruses (e.g., calicivirus, rotavirus, hepatitis A virus, enterovirus) (FoodSafety.gov, 2016). The federal government utilizes meat inspectors to prevent misbranded meat and meat products from being sold as food and ensure that meat animals are slaughtered and meat products processed under sanitary and humane conditions. The United States currently depends on the Foodborne Diseases Active Surveillance Network (FoodNet) of the CDC's Emerging Infections Program to collect data on diseases caused by enteric pathogens transmitted through food (CDC, 2010). Public health nurses play a key role in foodborne illness investigations.

Food can also be contaminated by agrichemicals, such as pesticides and fertilizers; materials from mechanical handling devices; detergents; and organic packaging materials. Toxic chemicals from farming and ranching may be introduced into the food chain, increasing risk of reproductive and mutagenic effects in humans (Driehuis et al., 2008; Knobeloch et al., 2009). For instance, farmers spray dioxin-containing weed killers on rangeland. Beef cattle graze on the land, herbicide accumulates in their fatty tissue, and the contaminated meat is sold in markets. The complexity of transfer of these contaminants makes for difficulty in establishing causality and tracing accountability for these health risks.

Unsuitable handling, storage, processing, and transport techniques can damage food and make it unsuitable for consumption. Nurses can council patients on the proper handling of food (Fig. 14.4). Furthermore, additives are often used to improve food properties. For example, vitamins and minerals are used to enhance nutritional content; salt, sugars, and monosodium glutamate are used to improve flavor; dyes are used to enhance color; leavening agents, gums, or thickening agents are used to improve consistency; and various preservatives are used to increase shelf life. Many of these additives are not nutritious, and some may be harmful. Additionally, residues from the overuse of antibiotics in animal husbandry remain in meat and milk products, causing consumers to develop resistance, thus rendering these antibiotics ineffective in treating human infections (Hurd and Malladi, 2008).

Another potential threat related to food quality involves "genetically modified" (GM) or genetically engineered foods. GM foods, which have been in existence since the early 1970s, are created by a process in which scientists splice plant or animal genes with particular traits into the DNA of other organisms. This technology has contributed to crops and livestock that grow faster, are more resistant to disease and insects, and produce higher yields and greater nutritive value. Often GM crops require less water and fertilizer. There is concern that genetic alteration of food is growing despite the fact that the long-term health effects of eating GM food are unknown. Some believe that allergies and other immunity problems may proliferate because unique antigens are present on GM proteins, and GM foods have unpredictable metabolic processes in animals, humans, and plants (Whitney et al., 2004). Although the U.S. Department of Agriculture and the U.S. Food and Drug Administration set policy for foods produced from new plant varieties and breeding, a number of groups and organizations have called for greater public awareness of the potential risks of genetically engineered foods and are working to require more stringent testing of them. The American Nurses Association was among several professional groups that developed principles of a healthy and sustainable food system (Box 14.2) (American Planning Association, 2010).

Clinical Example 14.6

A southwestern U.S. town with a population of 10,000 has three elementary schools. School nurses at all three schools had an influx of children into their offices one afternoon with complaints of gastrointestinal symptoms. After verifying that this was happening at all three schools, the nurses called the county health department to report possible foodborne

BOX 14.2 Healthy and Sustainable Food Systems

Health-Promoting

- Supports the physical and mental health of all farmers, workers, and eaters
- Accounts for the public health impacts throughout the entire lifecycle of how food is produced, processed, packaged, labeled, distributed, marketed, consumed, and disposed

Sustainable

- Conserves, protects, and regenerates natural resources, landscapes, and biodiversity
- Meets our current food and nutrition needs without compromising the ability of the system to meet the needs of future generations

Resilient

- Thrives in the face of challenges, such as unpredictable climate, increased pest resistance, and declining, increasingly expensive water and energy supplies

Diverse In

- Size and scale—includes a variable range of food production, transformation, distribution, marketing, consumption, and disposal practices, occurring at different scales, from local and regional to national and global
- Geography—considers geographic differences in natural resources, climate, customs, and heritage

Culture—appreciates and supports a diversity of cultures, sociodemographics, and lifestyles

- Choice—provides a variety of health-promoting food choices for all

Fair

- Supports fair and just communities and conditions for all farmers, workers, and eaters
- Provides equitable physical access to affordable food that is health promoting and culturally appropriate

Economically Balanced

- Provides economic opportunities that are balanced across geographic regions of the country and at different scales of activity, from local to global, for a diverse range of food system stakeholders
- Affords farmers and workers in all sectors of the system a living wage

Transparent

- Provides opportunities for farmers, workers, and eaters to gain the knowledge necessary to understand how food is produced, transformed, distributed, marketed, consumed, and disposed
- Empowers farmers, workers, and eaters to actively participate in decision making in all sectors of the system

---

illness outbreak. The county health nurse came out to the schools that afternoon to investigate the foodborne outbreak. She interviewed the school nurses, the affected and unaffected students, and the cafeteria staff.

After having all students in the school fill out a form describing what they had eaten for lunch, the county nurse was able to determine that the chicken salad was the likely source of contamination. The nurses sent the chicken salad as well as samples of all the ingredients in the salad for laboratory testing. Within 2 days, the nurse received confirmation that the chicken salad had been the source of the illness, related to the use of contaminated celery. The nurse then alerted federal officials. A warning was issued on www.foodsafety.gov to alert officials across the nation. Food inspectors were sent to the factory that prepared and sold the celery. The source of contamination was isolated to three of the five machines used to slice the prepackaged celery. The factory was temporarily shut down for thorough disinfection. The school and county nurses worked together to assess the outbreak, alert the appropriate officials, and stop the outbreak from spreading. They undoubtedly saved thousands from illness and possibly death.

Waste Management

Waste management entails the handling of waste materials resulting from industry, municipal processes, and human consumption as well as efforts to minimize waste production. Environmental health problems related to waste management include nonbiodegradable plastics, inefficient recycling programs, unlicensed waste dumps, inadequate sewage systems for growing populations, unsafe dumping of industrial toxins, exportation of radioactive medical wastes, illicit dumping

(Clinical Example 14.7), and nonenforcement of environmental regulations.

American consumers' increasing trash production and the improper treatment, storage, transport, and disposal of waste are a significant concern. Routinely, commercial and institutional wastes are dumped with household waste in the same municipal incinerator, landfill, or sewer system. These commercial enterprises are generally exempt from the strict waste regulation applied to industry, although they often generate the same hazardous materials. Small businesses such as dry cleaners, photography laboratories, pesticide formulators, construction sites, and car repair shops discard a variety of substances that can cause serious public health problems.

Traditionally, U.S. economic development has produced optimal wealth with the assumption that the environmental health consequences would be minor. This notion of sustainable development has proved inadequate, and cumulative hazardous episodes necessitate tough pollution control technologies. The sustainability paradigm has led to a shift from disposing to recycling of biosolids. **Biosolids** refers to sewage sludge that has been treated for pathogens to meet the regulatory requirements for land application. This has been a cost-effective practice, but more research needs to be conducted on human health risks of biosolid distribution in the ecosystem.

A number of potential health problems are associated with waste management. For example, solid waste landfills accumulate methane gas, a by-product of decomposing organic wastes. Without proper venting, this volatile gas can move through soil and cause fires and explosions in nearby areas. Waste incineration causes particulate air pollution and is ineffective in the combustion of many materials. Improper design, operation, or location of a waste site causes hazardous substances to spread through air, soil, and water to poison humans, animals, and plant life. Alarmingly, only a small percentage of hazardous waste actually reaches the designated waste sites; much is disposed of in open pits and in bodies of water, with dangerously uncertain long-term effects. New methods are being developed to estimate long-term rates of leaching of materials in various types of waste sites, based on probability principles (Sanchez and Kosson, 2005).

In 1980, Congress passed the Environmental Response Compensation and Liability Act, which established a revolving fund called the *Superfund* to clean up several hundred of the worst abandoned chemical waste disposal sites. One of the most notorious sites is the Love Canal in Niagara Falls, New York. For 40 years before the 1960s, more than 80 different types of chemicals, including benzene, dioxin, trichloroethylene, toluene, and chloroform, were dumped in an abandoned canal. Afterward, the covered area became the site for a school and several hundred homes. In the winters of 1976 and 1977, heavy snowfall and rain caused toxic wastes to reach the surface. Subsequently, the inhabitants experienced elevated miscarriage rates, blood and liver abnormalities, birth defects, and chromosome damage.

Clinical Example 14.7

In a city on the Mississippi River, an outbreak of shigellosis was traced to a group of high school students who had been swimming in a particular area of the river. The local meatpacking plant was releasing waste material, including human and animal feces, directly into the river. After intervening to contain the *Shigella* outbreak, the local community health nurses began to assess the situation. Their research indicated that the meatpacking facility had been in violation of waste control laws for some time. City officials imposed fines, which the company paid, but the dumping continued. Signage placed along the riverbanks prohibited swimming. Frustrated by their attempts to negotiate with the city and the plant, the nurses wrote a letter to the state capital newspaper, which had a large state readership. In the letter, they voiced concern about the community's health and the river's ecological integrity. The paper published their commentary, prompting responses from two local environmental groups, several activist groups, and a national organization concerned with clean water. These groups provided legal support and brought a collective suit against the meatpacking company. Subsequently, the company improved its waste treatment process to avoid legal ramifications.

GENETICS IN PUBLIC HEALTH
The Built Environment

Obesity is a preventable condition yet worldwide has nearly tripled in the past four decades (World Health Organization, 2017). Obesity and weight gain is linked to genetic disposition but not as an isolated factor (Trasande et al., 2009). Lifestyle interactions with the built and natural environments are implicated in obesity risk where access to safe and walkable surroundings is not available (Hruby et al., 2016). Integrating environmental information with genetic characteristics allows for developing better understanding about health outcomes and health behavior (Population Reference Bureau) and identifying risk predictors for obesity and other human conditions (Liu et al., 2012).

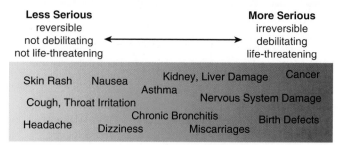

Which Risks are of Greatest Concern?

FIG. 14.5 Degrees of health effects from environmental exposures. (From Environmental Protection Agency: *Air pollution and health risk,* 1991. Retrieved from http://www.epa.gov/ttnat w01/3_90_022.html)

EFFECTS OF ENVIRONMENTAL HAZARDS

Environmental hazards are ubiquitous, and their effects on the public's health are complex and generally interconnected. Nurses must understand the multiple and complex sequences leading to health concerns (Fig. 14.5). For example, nuclear power plant emissions may contaminate water and air supplies, affecting water quality, atmospheric quality, and radiation risk. Overcrowded housing may exacerbate problems in managing human waste, which may taint foodstuffs and contribute to the spread of communicable disease. Climate change continues to affect humans, the food chain, vegetation, and wildlife.

Effects of environmental hazards may be general or specific. For example, the ramifications of high unemployment, drought, and extensive smog cover affect the public generally. Other environmental health concerns, such as the housing needs of elderly people who use walkers or canes, the occupational risks of electrical line repair workers, and the mentally incapacitating effects of elevated blood lead values in children, affect the public more specifically.

Environmental health effects can be immediate, long-term, or intergenerational. Burns, gunshot wounds, hurricane damage, and outbreaks of gastrointestinal distress among cafeteria customers are examples of immediate effects from health-damaging environments. Examples of long-term health effects include gradual occupational hearing loss, "black lung" in coal miners, and increased rates of thyroid cancer among young victims of the Chernobyl nuclear reactor accident (Ron, 2007). Intergenerational effects will likely occur with climate change by affecting women of childbearing age.

Certain environmental exposures have been found to have a direct relationship with the development of some cancers, chronic diseases, and other health-related problems (Boyd and Genuis, 2008; Crouse et al., 2015). Furthermore, oppressive environments may affect health directly. In one case, an American company dumped dangerous waste material in Mexico rather than pay for proper disposal (Schrieberg, 1991). Poor children who lived nearby and scavenged for food in the dump picked up and played with the shiny, brightly colored radioactive medical waste. The severe burns they suffered and the wine-colored spots on their skin were direct effects of the illegally dumped toxic waste.

Effects of environmental risks may also be indirect, such as in the case of global warming (Akhtar et al., 2009; Pan and

Kao, 2009). **Global warming** is the gradual increase in the average temperature of Earth's near-surface air and oceans since the mid-twentieth century and its projected continuation (Easterling, 2011). Rising global temperatures may enhance the quantity and distribution of parasites, insects, and other disease vectors, potentially increasing the prevalence of a variety of infectious diseases. For example, global warming contributed to the entry and propagation of the West Nile virus in the United States (Epstein, 2001) and is suspected in facilitating the rapid spread of the Zika virus (Chan et al., 2016). Higher air and water temperatures facilitate the spread of vectorborne diseases transmitted by mosquitoes (e.g., West Nile virus). As a result, 2012 saw more cases of West Nile virus infection (5387) than any year since 2003, with a higher proportion of deaths (243) (CDC, 2012); however, between 2012 and 2015 there has been an annual consecutive reduction in both the number of cases and deaths related to West Nile Virus (CDC, 2016).

EFFORTS TO CONTROL ENVIRONMENTAL HEALTH PROBLEMS

The 1970s were the decade of environmental concern. Cynicism toward institutions grew during the years of U.S. involvement in Vietnam, and legislative activism for environmental preservation exploded (Burger, 1989). During the 1970s, Congress created new agencies to regulate environmental conditions on a national level, including the EPA, the Occupational Safety and Health Administration, and the Nuclear Regulatory Commission. The EPA has enormous responsibilities for protecting the environment and minimizing risks to human health. Among its roles are health surveillance and monitoring; setting standards for air and water quality; evaluating environmental risks; acquiring information; screening new chemicals; performing basic research and training; and establishing, evaluating, and enforcing regulatory efforts.

The legislative activism of the 1970s was aimed toward a comprehensive national environmental policy. For example, stricter automobile fuel and emissions standards created improvements in air quality, which caused lead levels in urban air to decrease dramatically over the next decade. The momentum to control environmental pollution in the United States slowed in the 1980s and 1990s, with several policy reversals and the defunding of regulatory mechanisms. In recent years, administrative and legislative activity related to the environment has focused on such issues as climate change, oil spills, hazardous waste, and toxic exposures.

Frequently, laws and regulatory structures are weak or nonexistent with regard to environmental health problems. For example, federal mandates for recycling do not exist, although local communities have made great strides in this area. Comprehensive groundwater legislation, similar to adopted measures to preserve marine and surface waters, also does not exist. Additionally, the EPA tends to set priorities for the reduction of environmental problems but does not allocate the resources necessary to accomplish these goals.

RESEARCH HIGHLIGHTS

I PREPARE: Development and Clinical Utility of an Environmental Exposure History Mnemonic

The I PREPARE environmental exposure history mnemonic is a quick reference tool created by Paranzino and colleagues (2005) for primary care providers. A total of 159 health care providers, both students and professionals, were asked to evaluate a prototype of the mnemonic, to suggest new health history questions, and to propose the deletion of less relevant questions. The prototype was formatted as a pocket guide. The goal of this evaluation was to create a practical and clinically relevant mnemonic rather than to obtain quantitative estimates of its validity. This mnemonic is meant to serve as a mental cue to facilitate the collection and documentation of health information in a systematic manner:

I—Investigate Potential Exposures
P—Present Work
R—Residence
E—Environmental Concerns
P—Past Work
A—Activities
R—Referrals and Resources
E—Educate

Questions to ask are presented for each letter in the mnemonic, except for Referrals and Resources, which provides sources of additional information. A checklist of strategies to prevent or minimize exposures can be used by the health care provider to help clients identify potential exposures. The sequence of I PREPARE makes intuitive sense by cueing the provider to ask specific questions and then provide educational materials to the client. The final version was reprinted on heavy laminated material. The I PREPARE mnemonic increases the repertoire of tools clinicians have available to elicit an appropriate health history. The national improvements in the quality of environmental exposure history are predicated, in part, on the creation of simple and convenient tools for use in clinical practice.

Data from Paranzino GK, Butterfield P, Nastoff T, Ranger C: I PREPARE: Development and clinical utility of an environmental exposure history mnemonic, *J American Association Occupational Health Nurses* 53(1):37–42, 2005.

Most of the U.S. environmental health efforts have aimed for short-term results rather than anticipating future issues and problems. A crucial need exists in the development of human resources in the area of environmental health. Nurses in all areas of practice should be aware of the implications of the environment for their clients and their health. It is for this reason that nurses need to take and record an environmental health history for every client.

EMERGING ISSUES IN ENVIRONMENTAL HEALTH

Within the past decade, we are beginning to recognize that our environmental public health infrastructure is quite weak and that the United States is susceptible to many of the same problems that burden the rest of the world. For example, the illegal use of pesticides, medical waste incineration, and the increased incidence of asthma related to air pollution are just a few of the challenges facing the United States today. The manufacturing of methamphetamine in home-based and mobile laboratories continues to rise, and the "cooking process" emits dangerous levels of toxic chemicals into the air.

Similarly, the abandoned labs also pose a threat (Grant et al., 2010). Finally, natural disasters and climate change affect the entire world.

Natural disasters can disrupt and oftentimes overwhelm private and public health systems. Natural disasters, such as the tsunami that struck the coast of Indonesia in December 2004, Hurricane Katrina in August 2005, the devastating earthquakes in the Sichuan Province of China in 2008 and in Haiti in 2010, and superstorm Sandy in 2012, require mobilization of disaster relief units that offer substantial assistance and expertise. Natural disasters such as hurricanes, tornados, and earthquakes frequently receive notable publicity, but other, more insidious disasters, such as droughts, floods, heat waves, and extreme cold, also pose major public health concerns. All of the aforementioned threats can cause significant mortality and morbidity and therefore have the potential to burden the health care delivery system.

Global warming is part of a larger issue called *climate change* that poses significant health hazards. **Climate change** is the change in weather over a certain period. Weather patterns are greatly affected by atmospheric and oceanic temperature rises. Climate change projections suggest that heat waves and hot weather are likely to increase in frequency, with the overall temperature distribution shifting away from extreme cold (O'Neill and Ebi, 2009). Climate change can have severe adverse health effects, such as health-related illness and death; increases in air pollution; water-, food-, vector-, and rodent-borne diseases; malnutrition; contaminated water supply; and injuries and deaths related to extreme weather and storm surges (Balbus, 2011; Sheffield et al., 2011). There are regional differences in the effects of climate change, although vulnerable populations will be affected the most. For instance, climate change will raise the risks of infant and maternal mortality, birth complications, and poorer reproductive health, especially in developing countries (Rylander et al., 2013).

Nursing Actions

Nurses must work with the public to promote more stringent and actively enforced environmental legislation and regulations. In the twenty-first century, actions must include not only national but also worldwide environmental policies. Ozone depletion, climate change, fossil fuel burning, marine dumping, abandonment of active land mines in war-torn areas, and destruction of tropical rainforests are among the key global environmental health concerns.

Environmental concerns for clean air, clean water, and freedom from noxious chemicals must become nursing concerns. Community health nurses can be catalysts to neighborhood efforts to produce safe living environments. Community health nursing must expand its theory and practice to incorporate the fact that individual and community health ultimately depends on global environmental integrity. Many organizations work to preserve and protect the environment and could benefit from the active involvement and support of nurses. Box 14.3 lists some of these organizations. Nursing must include an environmental perspective by committing to environmental health

---

BOX 14.3 Nongovernmental Environmental Organizations

- Alliance of Nurses for Healthy Environments (http://envirn.org/)
- American Farmland Trust (http://www.farmland.org/)
- Citizens for a Better Environment (http://www.cbezambia.org/)
- Clean Water Action (http://www.cleanwateraction.org/)
- Green America (http://www.greenamerica.org/)
- Environmental Defense Fund (http://www.edf.org/)
- Environmental Working Group (http://www.ewg.org/)
- Greenpeace (http://www.greenpeace.org/usa/en/)
- International Rivers Network (http://www.internationalrivers.org/)
- National Audubon Society (http://www.audubon.org/)
- National Environmental Law Center (http://www.nelconline.org/)
- National Geographic Society (http://www.nationalgeographic.com/about/)
- Natural Resources Defense Council (http://www.nrdc.org/)
- National Wildlife Federation (http://www.nwf.org/)
- Ocean Alliance (http://www.oceanalliance.org/)
- Pesticide Action Network (http://www.panna.org/)
- Rainforest Action Network (http://ran.org/)
- Sierra Club (http://www.sierraclub.org/)
- The Nature Conservatory (http://www.nature.org/)
- Trust for Public Land (http://www.tpl.org/)
- Wilderness Society (http://wilderness.org/)
- World Wildlife Fund (http://worldwildlife.org/)

For further information, see the report by the Institute of Medicine Committee on Enhancing Environmental Health Content in Nursing Practice: *Nursing, health, and the environment*, Washington, DC, 1995, National Academies Press.

---

promotion initiatives that promote social justice and environmental responsibility.

APPROACHING ENVIRONMENTAL HEALTH AT THE POPULATION LEVEL

In the United States, personal independence and individual responsibility for success and failure are valued. These values can lead nurses to overlook environmental hazards and instead blame individual clients for their health problems. Placing responsibility for the cause and cure of health problems exclusively on the individual reinforces the belief that all individuals are free to exert meaningful control over the quality and length of their lives. Such a perspective absolves society, government, industry, and business from accountability.

Research suggests that changing individual behaviors does not lead to significant reductions in overall morbidity and mortality in the absence of basic social, economic, and political changes (Bhatia and Wernham, 2008). Emphasizing only interventions that address deleterious personal habits through exercise programs, weight loss regimens, smoking cessation classes, and stress reduction tactics fails to take into account the broader environmental origins of disease, injury, and ecological degradation. An attempt to approach health at the aggregate level is the *Healthy People 2020* initiative (USDHHS, 2013). The *Healthy People 2020* box lists selected environmental health objectives of the *Healthy People 2020* initiative.

Selected Objectives for Environmental Health

EH–2: Increase use of alternative modes of transportation for work

EH–3: Reduce air toxic emissions to decrease the risk of adverse health effects caused by mobile, area, and major sources of airborne toxins

EH–4: Increase the proportion of persons served by community water systems who receive a supply that meets the regulations of the Safe Drinking Water Act

EH–5: Reduce waterborne disease outbreaks arising from water intended for drinking among persons served by community water systems

EH–8.1: Eliminate elevated blood lead levels in children

EH–12: Increase recycling of municipal solid waste

EH–14: Increase the proportion of persons living in homes at risk that have an operating radon mitigation system

From U.S. Department of Health and Human Services. (n.d.) *Environmental health.* Retrieved from http://www.healthypeople.gov/2020/topicsobjectives2020/objectiveslist.aspx?topicId=12

ETHICAL INSIGHTS

Protecting Vulnerable Aggregates

Community health nurses have a mandate to assist vulnerable aggregates who have fewer options in protecting themselves from pollution, inadequate housing, toxic poisoning, unsafe products, and other hazards. Non–English-speaking individuals, children, very low-income women and families, undocumented manual laborers, and people from racial and ethnic minorities are just some of the groups in the United States who hold minimal influence with industry, government, business, and other large institutions for environmental changes and compensations for harm from environmental hazards.

Interventions designed for individuals must consider the environmental determinants of behavior and health outcomes (Bartholomew et al., 2011; Coughenour et al., 2014). Community health nurses who base their practices on theory and evidence are better prepared to respond to collective challenges. These nurses can facilitate community participation in identifying and solving environmental health problems and bringing about changes that improve environments and eliminate hazards.

CRITICAL ENVIRONMENTAL HEALTH NURSING PRACTICE

The National Center for Environmental Health, the CDC, and the American Public Health Association has established three core competencies for environmental health professionals: assessment, management, and communication (Box 14.4). Several clinical examples throughout the chapter illustrate how nurses can focus their efforts by organizing groups of people, taking a stand, and acting as advocates for change. The nurses ask critical questions, stay engaged with the communities they serve, form coalitions, and use various collective strategies. The American Nurses Association highlights 10 critical environmental health principles. In the interest of educating future practitioners about the critical practice of environmental community health nursing, the following sections discuss each of these interventions.

Taking a Stand: Advocating for Change

Nurses must make individual and collective decisions about which interests they want to serve with their specialized knowledge and skills. Nurses may choose to work with

---

BOX 14.4 Core Environmental Health Competencies

Assessment

Research: The capacity to identify and compile relevant information to solve a problem and the knowledge of where to go to obtain the relevant information

Data analysis and interpretation: The capacity to analyze data, recognize meaningful test results, interpret findings, and present the results in a meaningful way to different types of audiences

Evaluation: The capacity to evaluate the effectiveness or performance of procedures, interventions, and programs

Management

Problem solving: The capacity to understand and solve problems.

Economic and political issues: The capacity to understand and appropriately utilize information concerning the economic and political implications of decisions.

Organizational knowledge and behavior: The capacity to function effectively within the culture of the organization and to be an effective team player.

Managing work: The capacity to plan, implement, and maintain fiscally responsible programs/projects using appropriate skills and to prioritize projects across the employee's entire workload.

Computer/information technology (IT): The capacity to utilize information technology as needed to produce work products.

Reporting, documentation, and record keeping: The capacity to produce reports that document actions, keep records, and inform appropriate parties.

Partnering: The capacity to form partnerships and alliances with other individuals and organizations in order to enhance performance on the job.

Communication

Education: The capacity to use the environmental health practitioner's frontline role to effectively educate the public on environmental health issues.

Communication: The capacity to effectively communicate risk and exchange information with colleagues, other practitioners, clients, policy makers, interest groups, media, and the public through public speaking, print and electronic media, and interpersonal relations.

Conflict resolution: The capacity to facilitate the resolution of conflicts within the agency, in the community, and with regulated parties.

Marketing environmental/public health as a service: The ability to articulate basic concepts of environmental health and public health and convey an understanding of their value and importance to clients and the public.

Data from American Public Health Association: *Environmental Health Competency Project: Draft recommendations for non-technical competencies at the local level,* 2013. Retrieved from http://www.apha.org/programs/standards/healthcompproject/corenontechnicalcompetencies.htm.

---

vulnerable people or those disproportionally experiencing the consequences of environmental hazards. Vulnerable groups are exposed to more health-damaging effects than less vulnerable groups (Chakraborty and Zandbergen, 2007; EPA, 2013c). Nurses can work toward health equity through the decisions they make, the positions they accept, and the interventions they undertake. Environmental problems are clearly intertwined with social, political, and economic policies; resource barriers; and the interests of those in positions of control. Nurses need to connect the immediate and long-term health problems experienced by particular communities to this larger sphere of influence.

BOX 14.5 Critical Questions About Environmental Health Problems

- What is the problem?
- Who is defining the problem?
- In what terms is the problem described?
- How are others in the situation viewing the problem?
- What is the history of the problem?
- How did things get the way they are?
- What other situations does this problem directly affect?
- Who does the problem affect?
- Whose health is damaged because things are this way?
- Who benefits from the way things are?
- Whose interests do current solutions serve?
- What are the economic inequities in the situation?
- Who has political power in the situation?
- Who knows about the problem?
- Who needs to know more about the problem?
- How effective are current programs, strategies, and policies?
- What are the barriers to solving the problem?
- What strategies may alleviate the problem?
- How successful have these strategies been?
- What existing groups might deal with this problem?
- What resources are needed to solve the problem?
- How accessible are the resources?
- How can nurses evaluate potential solutions?

Asking Critical Questions

Community health nurses must also consider the relationships between nonhealth policies and health policies. They should ask how policies concerning ecological preservation, energy, housing, immigration, civil rights, crime, nutrition, minimum wage, occupational safety, and defense might affect the health and well-being of people. Addressing critical questions such as who has access to resources in this country and whose interests are served in the existing system provides a way to include social, political, and economic factors in environmental nursing assessments. Box 14.5 provides a sample set of questions that are useful in this endeavor. Nurses can ask these critical questions when approaching environmental health problems.

Facilitating Community Involvement

Approaching community health from a critical perspective requires working to improve health conditions and creating the context in which people can identify health-damaging problems in their environments. One important nursing goal is to help people learn from their own experiences and analyze the world with an intention to change it. It is essential that the affected people participate in the process of identifying and working to solve environmental problems (White et al., 2014). To foster community-based, active participation, nurses must be prepared to take leadership positions and join in mutual exchanges with community members that consider each person's experience. The nurse's role changes from presenting solutions and directing lifestyle changes to providing support, information, and expertise to assist in meeting the group goals. Using critical questions, community health nurses can help community members look beyond immediate environmental problems and

explore social, cultural, economic, and political circumstances that contribute to them. Nurses can share their knowledge about the scientific basis for health problems, their insights about the historical origins of particular environmental hazards, their technical skills, and their expertise in communicating and organizing. By addressing people's everyday concerns and targeting the problems they identify, nurses situate their efforts in community struggles.

Forming Coalitions

Another very important nursing task that arises from approaching environmental health from a critical perspective involves forming coalitions to produce social change. By initiating dialogue and building a strong base of collective support, nurses join with communities to eliminate hazards and improve public health. Nurses can approach existing community organizations, churches, and family and friendship networks to help mobilize aggregate members who have not previously socialized or acted together. Nurses can then discuss environmental concerns, assess needs, plan actions, secure appropriate resources, and advocate for legislative changes.

Nurses can be instrumental in these efforts by helping community groups make connections with larger, more powerful organizations. Nurses can organize forums whereby community groups meet with scientific experts who can help them gather evidence about health threats, with business managers whose actions impinge on the economic life of the community, with industry leaders whose companies create ecological hazards, and with legislators who can bring community concerns to lawmaking bodies. Using available institutional resources, skills, and knowledge, nurses can also explore what is happening elsewhere. Making connections with groups in other locales who are struggling for similar environmental changes can enhance collective strength and solidarity. Press releases, media events, interviews, television spots, speeches, newsletters, and leaflets are important means of calling attention to a situation and raising awareness among communities.

Using Collective Strategies

Nurses can use a variety of strategies to intervene at the population level and facilitate improvement in a community's health. Nurses can organize people to change health-damaging environments through combinations of strategies, including building coalitions, providing educational forums, facilitating a community needs assessment, disseminating research, and lobbying for legislative changes.

One collective strategy that is an effective population-level community health nursing intervention is **participatory action research**. This form of research calls for nurses, community members, and other resource people to work together in identifying health problems, designing the studies, collecting and analyzing the data, disseminating the results, and posing solutions to the problems (Garwick et al., 2010; Li et al., 2011). In PAR applied to environmental health, community health nurses and community members would gather information on suspected environmental hazards, determine their effects on health, and devise a plan of action to mitigate the threat.

Although nurses have not traditionally used all of these collective strategies to intervene in community health matters, environmental hazards are multiplying geometrically, pushing nurses to expand their skills repertoire. Pioneers such as Hollie Shaner, RN, have embraced that concept and are blazing the path to environmental awareness (Sattler, 2003). In the 1990s, Shaner frequently left her home, where she avidly separated and recycled, to work at a Vermont hospital, where none of the waste was recycled. Shaner was not comfortable throwing everything into a "red bag" and decided that there must be a way to change the environmental unfriendliness of her place of employment. She began voluntarily recycling the hospital's cardboard and then began to recycle the newspapers, glass, and plastics. In addition, she received a grant from the state of Vermont to maximize her efforts in medical waste reduction. The efforts and savings did not go unnoticed by the hospital, as Shaner received a new job title of clinical waste reduction coordinator and saved the hospital $175,000 per year.

Shaner also wrote a book for the American Hospital Association on medical waste management. She quickly realized the negative impact the health care industry was having on the environmental health of the communities served. Mercury was being released into the streams from medical waste, and dioxins were being released into the air from medical waste incineration. From this realization, in 1996, Shaner and a small group of other health professionals launched a campaign to lead the health care industry toward environmental stewardship. This campaign, supported by the American Nurses Association, was named Health Care Without Harm. "The goal of the campaign was to reduce the environmental health risks that were being created by the health care industry" (Sattler, 2003, p. 8). The campaign still exists and is building momentum; today there are 433 participating organizations in 52 different countries (Health Care Without Harm, 2013). In 2015 the 2020 Health Care Climate Challenge was launched, aiming to reduce the health care carbon footprint, respond with resiliency to the changing patterns of disease, and lead the way for creating a healthier climate (Global Green and Healthy Hospitals, 2015).

◢ RESEARCH HIGHLIGHTS
Participatory Action Research

Asthma is a significant public health problem that disproportionately affects preschool-age, low-income children. Indeed, children from low-income families have significantly higher asthma prevalence rates, hospitalization rates, and emergency department visits than children from middle-income and wealthier families. This problem is even more pronounced among children in urban areas.

A team of public health nurses led by Garwick (2010) used participatory action research (PAR) techniques in working with teachers in an urban Head Start program with multiple sites to address asthma management among the children at their sites. In this project, teachers and managers from 16 Head Start centers were identified to participate in three focus groups. During the focus groups, participants identified asthma management issues and challenges, including undiagnosed and unreported asthma, coordination of asthma care with parents, medication administration issues, and variability among asthma action plans. As a result of the PAR, a standardized, comprehensive Head Start asthma action plan was developed that outlined strategies the teachers could use to better manage the problem of asthma among children.

Data from Garwick AW, Seppelt A, Riesgraf M: Addressing asthma management challenges in a multisite, urban Head Start Program, *Public Health Nurs*, 27(4): 329–336, 2010.

CASE STUDY   Application of the Nursing Process
Air Pollution

In July 2001, the *Metro Pulse* newspaper reported an extensive air pollution problem in the city of Knoxville, Tennessee (Tarr, 2001). The American Lung Association had recently named Knoxville the ninth most polluted city in the country on the basis of the ozone contamination in the air. The following case study expands on some of the reported facts of the situation to construct hypothetical nursing interventions.

Knoxville's community health nurses and the public health department were aware of increasing rates of asthma in particular neighborhoods. In the wake of alarming newspaper and research articles about the dangerous incidence of air pollution and related asthma, the nurses decided to make the health issues a priority. The community health nurses and several nursing students assigned to their department researched the topics and uncovered the following information.

Asthma has long been recognized as a condition in which an acute respiratory response may follow inhalation of a material to which a person is sensitized. Scientists now know that air pollution can lead to nonspecific generalized inflammation. One study found strong evidence that ozone can *cause*, as well as exacerbate, asthma (Sheffield, et.al, 2011). The study found that days with worse AQI values resulted in significantly higher school absences due to respiratory illness, and asthma was more likely to develop in children living in high-ozone communities who actively participated in several outdoor sports than in children in communities not participating in sports.

Indeed, the nation's leading group of pediatricians, the American Academy of Pediatrics (AAP), revised its policy statement on outdoor air pollution and the health hazards to children (Schwartz, 2004). The AAP's Committee on Environmental Health strengthened its warning about the dangers that air pollution poses to children because of the recent studies correlating air pollution with asthma and negative lung growth and function. Estimates are that more than 25 million Americans have asthma (Asthma and Allergy Foundation, 2013).

An economically depressed neighborhood in Knoxville, hypothetically called Trent Park, is situated near numerous railways, freeways, and industrial yards. High numbers of African American, Latino, and Southeast Asian residents live in the older homes that line the streets of Trent Park. Isolated by language and economic circumstances, many Trent Park residents do not know they are exposed to these environmental health hazards.

Assessment

Elena Garcia, an 8-year-old girl who lives in Trent Park, presented to the pediatric primary clinic at the health department at 8 AM in November. Elena had been diagnosed with asthma 2 months ago and was now in mild respiratory distress. Elena explained to the nurse that she had gone trick-or-treating the night before in her neighborhood. It had turned cold that weekend, and she had also played outside in her neighborhood with friends the day before. In addition, the child's mother explained that Elena had recently had a respiratory virus. The nurse realized that Elena and her mother both mentioned several factors, such as her playing outside on a cold afternoon/evening in a polluted neighborhood and a respiratory virus, that could have exacerbated her asthma.

At the clinic visit, the nurse assessed the following:
- Elena's heart rate and cardiovascular status
- Elena's pattern of breathing, which includes rate, rhythm, and effort
- Elena's asthma medication history
- Evidence of diaphoresis, papillary dilation, and fear, which are all features of the adrenergic response to hypoxia

continued

Air Pollution

- Elena's global central nervous system function, such as alertness, cooperation, and motor activity
- Elena's environmental health assessment

Diagnosis
Individual
- Ineffective respirations related to environmental exposure to air pollution
- Insufficient knowledge related to precipitating factors that can cause/worsen an asthma attack
- Stress related to ongoing fear of daughter's illness

Family
- Risk for family crisis related to instability caused by the illness
- Insufficient knowledge related to factors that can cause/worsen an asthma attack

Community
- Risk for increased incidence of asthma due to air pollution
- Inadequate programs for asthma screening

Planning
A plan of care was developed at the individual, family, and community levels. Mutual goal setting and contracting are essential if the outcome is to be optimal.

Individual
Long-Term Goals
- Client will modify outdoor time daily according to the AQI
- Client will reduce exposure to allergy triggers
- Client will avoid secondhand tobacco smoke
- Client will keep pets out of the bedroom
- Client will experience successful maintenance of asthma

Short-Term Goals
- Client will report reduced outdoor time on days with poor AQI values
- Client will keep an asthma diary and identify which allergy triggers are problematic
- Client will remain free of acute asthma attacks

Family
Long-Term Goals
- Family will follow the city's daily AQI
- Family will encourage child to stay indoors on days with high pollution levels
- Family will remove as many allergy triggers from home as possible
- Family will enforce the pets-out-of-the-bedroom policy
- Family will cope effectively with daughter's asthma

Short-Term Goals
- Family will provide encouragement for client to keep an asthma diary

Community
Long-Term Goals
- Citizens will be involved in decision-making process about proposed activities that could pose an environmental hazard
- Citizens will encourage utility companies, government, and industries to reduce air pollution
- Citizens will be encouraged to use mass transit and carpools to reduce vehicle emissions

Short-Term Goals
- Citizens will be alerted about the air pollution problem in the area
- Citizens will be educated about the AQI and its implications for outdoor activity

Intervention
Individual
- Identify Trent Park children with asthma and plan follow-up home visits to provide education on basic pathophysiology, symptoms of distress, and environmental controls needed for successful asthma management

- Add environmental health assessments to child health assessment protocol
- Coordinate with school nurses to ensure they incorporate similar changes into their health assessment protocols
- Prepare and distribute an educational pamphlet with members of Trent Park that details Trent Park residents' air pollution and asthma risks
- Prepare translations of the pamphlet in languages and reading levels appropriate for Trent Park residents, and mail it to individual households.

Family
- Facilitate the formation of a support group for families with children who have asthma

Community
- Initiate an asthma awareness program for Trent Park community members.
- Coordinate with school nurses to implement an asthma awareness program in Trent Park schools.
- Develop an asthma action team consisting of Trent Park community members.
- Participate in the action team's development of an intervention to reduce asthma-related illness in Trent Park.
- Encourage nursing students and community health nursing faculty from the local university and college programs to participate.
- Lobby state legislatures, municipal officials, local medical associations, local hospitals, and city clinics regarding the project.
- Form broader coalitions with Knoxville churches, the local nurses association, several preschool and day care centers, and the Knoxville School Board to design a comprehensive, nonduplicative, cost-effective asthma screening program.
- Train action team members on how to conduct Healthy Home assessments.
- Contact state environmental groups for advice on local efforts, and join in their fight for stricter regulation of air pollutants and toxic wastes.
- Contact local media (e.g., television, radio, and newspaper) about running a series of stories about Knoxville air pollutants and related asthma risks; supply information and contacts for interviews and photographs.

Evaluation
Individual
- Evaluate the child's and mother's understanding of asthma treatments at follow-up home visits.
- Facilitate the evaluation of ongoing interventions.
- Track the number of asthma screening tests that Trent Park children receive and their rates of asthma to determine the effectiveness of their efforts in these areas.
- Keep close contact with the school nurses, and organize an after-school educational and screening program at schools that are understaffed.
- Ask school nurses to report on the educational sessions' success.

Family
- Document participation levels at educational programs and family training sessions.
- Document ongoing participation in referrals and support groups.

Community
The action team was able to get funding to provide Healthy Home assessments and asthma screening to at-risk youth in Trent Park.

Levels of Prevention
Primary Prevention
Educating the community regarding air pollution and its relationship to asthma

Secondary Prevention
Screening at-risk populations for asthma

Tertiary Prevention
Follow-up treatment for people with asthma and reduction of air pollutants in the community environment

? ACTIVE LEARNING

1. Identify a health-related problem associated with some aspect of the environment. It may be a problem in a nearby community, a problem publicized in the media, or a difficulty experienced by a family. Examine the problem using the sample series of critical questions listed in Box 14.5. Without sharing the results, present the problem to the group and ask them to discuss it by responding to the same questions. Were there differences or similarities in the initial results and the group's answers? On what points did everyone agree? Why? What questions caused the most disagreement? Why? Now repeat the entire activity by involving people other than nursing students in the group discussion. How did this discussion compare with the previous discussion and responses?

2. Attend meetings that hold environmental hazard discussions. If meetings or public forums are not available in the vicinity, write for information about the state's actions to fight environmental hazards. The reference librarians at colleges or public libraries can suggest ways of contacting sources and will supply addresses. Organizations that are likely to sponsor forums and provide information include those listed in Box 14.3, the Environmental Protection Agency, the National Institute for Occupational Safety and Health, state and municipal agencies for environmental protection and occupational health, environmental caucuses of political parties, the American Public Health Association, the local public health department, farmers' organizations, and labor unions.

3. This chapter described how to use participatory research as an intervention in dealing with ecological hazards. In a group, brainstorm about possibilities for participatory action research projects in the area. Try to identify examples from a variety of environmental health areas. Be creative in planning. How might a nurse mobilize community support and participation in the research? What groups would be approachable? What critical questions might facilitate dialogue about the problem? What kinds of data could be collected, and how could they be used? How could research results be publicized? What ramifications could the completed study have for community members, other communities in the state, and community health nurses in other locales?

4. Nurses may have to supplement their knowledge of collective strategies by reading books about political action and by learning from community members who are experienced in political organizing. Visit a college or public library to investigate books and journal articles outside the nursing literature. Compile a list of references related to one of these political strategies (e.g., grassroots organizing, legislative lobbying, community education, policy analysis, use of the media, coalition building, citizen surveys, public protest, letter-writing campaigns, or consciousness-raising groups). Exchange reference lists with peers to benefit from their efforts. Then choose one or two books of interest and read them.

SUMMARY

This chapter provided a glimpse into the complex world of environmental health from a critical community health nursing perspective. The case study and clinical examples illustrate that nurses must evaluate the broader picture in assessing the environmental health status of communities and the vulnerable aggregates within them. In preventing, minimizing, and resolving environmental health problems, nurses must recognize patterns, detect subtle changes, identify underlying issues, and work collaboratively with a variety of individuals and groups. In the past, environmental threats to health were usually suspected only when other possible causes of illness were ruled out. Nurses can expect this pattern to change dramatically in the twenty-first century as environmental health moves increasingly to the forefront of the public health agenda.

ⓔ EVOLVE WEBSITE

http://evolve.elsevier.com/Nies/community

- NCLEX Review Questions
- Case Studies

BIBLIOGRAPHY

Adamkiewicz G, Zota AR, Fabian MP: Moving environmental justice indoors: understanding structural influences on residential exposure patterns in low-income communities, *Am J Public Health* 101(1):238–245, 2011.

Akhtar AZ, Greger M, Ferdowsian H, et al.: Health professionals' roles in animal agriculture, climate change, and human health, *Am J Prev Med* 36(2):182–187, 2009.

American Planning Association: *Principles of a healthy sustainable food system.* Available from: <http://www.planning.org/national-centers/health/foodprinciples.htm>.

Anderson JO, Thundiyil JG, Stolbach A: Clearing the air: a review of the effects of particulate matter air pollution on human health, *J Med Toxicol* 8(2):166–175, 2012.

Asthma and Allergy Foundation: *Asthma facts and figures.* Available from: <http://aafa.org/display.cfm?id=8&sub=42>.

Balbus JM: Health implications. In: *Climate change: mastering the public health role, a practical guidebook.* American Public Health Association: Washington, DC, 2011, pp 15–30.

Bartholomew LK, Parcel GS, Kok G, et al.: *Planning health promotion programs: an intervention mapping approach.* Jossey-Bass/Wiley: Hoboken, NJ.

Barton A, Basham M, Foy C, et al.: The Watcombe housing study: the short term effect of improving housing conditions on the health of residents, *J Epidemiol Community Health* 61:771–777, 2007.

Bhatia R, Wernham A: Integrating human health into environmental impact assessment: an unrealized opportunity for environmental health and justice, *Environ Health Perspect* 116(8):991–1000, 2008.

Boyd DR, Genuis SJ: The environmental burden of disease in Canada: respiratory disease, cardiovascular disease, cancer and congenital affliction, *Environ Res* 106(2):240–249, 2008.

Bureau of Labor Statistics: *Current injury, illness, and fatality data.* Available from: <http://data.bls.gov/search/query/results?cx=013738036195919377644%3A6ih0hfrgl50&q=2008+inurl%3Abls.gov%2Fiif>.

Bureau of Labor Statistics: *Employer reported workplace injuries and illnesses - 2015.* Available from: https://www.bls.gov/news.release/pdf/osh.pdf. Accessed March 2017.

Bureau of Labor Statistics: *Workplace injuries and illnesses—2011*. Available from: <http://www.bls.gov/news.release/archives/osh_10252012.pdf>

Burger EJ: Human health: a surrogate for the environment: the evolution of environmental legislation and regulation during the 1970s, *Regul Toxicol Pharmacol* 9:196–206, 1989.

Centers for Disease Control and Prevention: *Novel influenza A (H1N1) virus infection—Mexico*, March-May 2009, *MMWR Morb Mortal Wkly Rep* 58(21):585–589, 2009.

Centers for Disease Control and Prevention: Preliminary FoodNet data on the incident of infection with pathogens transmitted commonly through food: 10 sites—United States, 2009, *MMWR Surveill Summ* 59(14):418–422, 2010.

Centers for Disease Control and Prevention: *Drinking water*. Available from: <http://www.cdc.gov/healthywater/drinking/private/wells/>.

Centers for Disease Control and Prevention: *Healthy homes*. Available from: <http://www.cdc.gov/healthyhomes>.

Centers for Disease Control and Prevention: *West Nile Virus*. Available from: <http://www.cdc.gov/ncidod/dvbid/westnile/index.htm>.

Centers for Disease Control and Prevention: *West nile virus disease cases and presumptive viremicblood donors by state – United States 2015*. Available from: https://www.cdc.gov/westnile/.../wnv-disease-cases-and-pvds-by-state-2015_0707201. Accessed March 2017.

Centers for Disease Control and Prevention: *Workplace safety and health topics: agricultural safety*. Available from: <http://www.cdc.gov/niosh/topics/aginjury/>

Chakraborty C, Zandbergen PA: Children at risk: racial/ethnic disparities in potential exposure to air pollution at school and home, *J Epidemiol Community Health* 61:1074–1079, 2007.

Chan JFW, Choi GKY, Yip CCY, et al.: Zika fever and congenital zika syndrome: an unexpected emerging arboviral disease, *J Infect* 72:507–524, 2016.

Ciencewicki J, Trivedi S, Kleeberger SJ: Oxidants and the pathogenesis of lung disease, *J Allergy and Clin Immunol* 3(122):456–468, 2008.

Collins MB: Risk-based targeting: identifying disproportionalities in the sources and effects of industrial pollution, *Am J Public Health* 101(S1):S231–S237, 2011.

Coughenour C, Coker L, Bungum TJ: Environmental and social determinants of youth physical activity intensity levels at neighborhood parks in Las Vegas, NV. *J Community Health* 39:1092–1096, 2014.

Crouse DL, Peters PA, Hystad P, et al.: Ambient pm 2.5 O 3 and NO2 exposures an associations with mortality over 16 years of follow-up in the Canadian census health and environment (CanCHEC), *Environ Health Perspect* 123(11):1180–1186, 2015.

Ding D, Sallis JF, Kerr J, et al.: Neighborhood environment and physical activity among youth: a review, *Am J Prev Med* 41(4):442–455, 2011.

Driehuis F, Spanjer MC, Scholten JM, et al.: Occurrence of mycotoxins in feedstuffs of dairy cows and estimation of total dietary intakes, *J Dairy Sci* 91(11):4261–4271, 2008.

Dunton GF, Kaplan J, Wolch J, et al.: Physical environmental correlate of childhood obesity: a systematic review, *Obesity Rev* 10 393–402, 2009.

Environmental Protection Agency: *Indoors air facts No. 4 (revised): sick building syndrome*. Available from: <http://www.epa.gov/iaq/pdfs/sick_building_factsheet.pdf>.

Environmental Protection Agency: *Urban sprawl modeling, air quality monitoring and risk communication*: *The Northeast Ohio Project*, EPA/625/R-02/016. Author: Washington, DC.

Environmental Protection Agency: *Ensuring risk reduction in communities with multiple stressors: environmental justice and cumulative risks/impacts*. Author: Washington, DC.

Environmental Protection Agency: *Highlighting success: the region 9 environmental justice small grant program, fiscal years* 1994–99, EPA 909-R99–002. Author: Washington, DC.

Environmental Protection Agency: *Air quality index (AQI): a guide to air quality and your health*. Available from: <http://www.airnow.gov/index.cfm?action=aqibasics.aqi>.

Environmental Protection Agency: *Food safety*. Available from: <http://www2.epa.gov/safepestcontrol>.

Environmental Protection Agency: *Public water systems: laboratories and monitoring*. Available from: <http://water.epa.gov/infrastructure/drinkingwater/pws/labmon.cfm>.

Environmental Protection Agency: *The effects of acid rain*. Available from: <http://www.epa.gov/acidrain/effects/>.

Environmental Protection Agency: *What are the six common air pollutants?* Available from: <http://www.epa.gov/airquality/urbanair/>.

Environmental Protection Agency: *You're your house and healthy home*. Available from: <http://yosemite.epa.gov/ochp/ochp-web.nsf/content/Healthy_Homes_Action_Card_English.htm/$-File/Healthy_Homes_Action_Card_English.pdf>.

Environmental Protection Agency: *An introduction to indoor air quality*. Available from: <http://www.epa.gov/iaq/co.html>.

Environmental Protection Agency: *Drinking water contaminants*. Available from: <http://water.epa.gov/drink/contaminants/>.

Environmental Protection Agency: *Environmental justice*. Available from: <http://www.epa.gov/environmentaljustice/>.

Environmental Protection Agency: *Federal radon action plan: celebrating success, looking to the future*. Available from: <http://www.epa.gov/radon/pdfs/FRAP_2013Accomplishments.pdf>

Environmental Protection Agency: *Ozone layer protection*. Available from: http://www.epa.gov/ozone/strathome.html.

Environmental Protection Agency: *Radon: health risks*. Available from: <http://www.epa.gov/radon/healthrisks.html>.

Epstein PR: West Nile virus and the climate, *J Urban Health* 78:367–371, 2001.

Easterling D: Basic Climate change science. In: *Climate change: mastering the public health role, a practical guidebook*. American Public Health Association: Washington, DC, pp 7–14.

Fan Y, Song Y: Is sprawl associated with a widening urban–suburban mortality gap? *J Urban Health* 86(5):708–728, 2009.

Farand SP, Lewis-Michl EL, Gomex MI: Adverse birth outcomes and maternal exposure to trichloroethylene and tetrachloroethylene through soil vapor intrusion in New York State, *Environ Health Persp* 120(4), 2012.

Food Safety.gov. *Causes of food poisoning*. Available from: <http://www.foodsafety.gov/poisoning/causes/index.html>.

Garwick AW, Seppelt A, Riesgraf M: Addressing asthma management challenges in multisite, urban Head Start Program, *Public Health Nurs* 27(4):329–336, 2010.

Geltman EG, Gill G, Jovanovic M: Beyond baby steps: an empirical study of the impact on environmental justice executive order 12898, *Fam Community Health* 39(3):143–150, 2016.

Global Green and Healthy Hospitals: *2020 health care climate change challenge*. Available from: https://noharm-global.org/issues/global/2020-health-care-climate-challenge. Accessed March 2017.

Grant P, Bell K, Stewart D, et al.: Evidence of methamphetamine exposure in children removed from clandestine methamphetamine laboratories, *Pedi emerg care* 26(1):10–14, 2010.

Hankey S, Marshall JD, Brauer M: Health impacts of the built environment: within-urban variability in physical inactivity, air pollution, and ischemic heart disease mortality, *Environ health persp* 120(2):247, 2012.

Health Care Without Harm: *About us*. Available from: <http://noharm.org/us_canada/about/>.

Hurd HS, Malladi S: A stochastic assessment of the public health risks of the use of macrolide antibiotics in food animals, *Risk Anal* 28(3):695–710, 2008.

Hruby A, Manson JE, Qi L, et al.: Determinants and consequences of obesity, *Am J Public Health* 106(9), 2016.

Institute of Medicine: *Committee on enhancing environmental health content in nursing practice: nursing, health, and the environment.* National Academies Press: Washington, DC.

Institute of Medicine: *The public health effects of food deserts*: workshop summary. Available from: <http://www.iom.edu/Reports/2009/FoodDeserts.aspx>.

James P, Troped PJ, Hart JE, et al.: Urban sprawl, physical activity, and body mass index: nurses' health study and nurses' health study II, *Am J Public Health* 103(2):369–375, 2013.

Jones-Rounds ML, Evans GW, Braubach, M: The interactive effects of housing and neighborhood quality on psychological well-being, *J Epidemiol Community Health* 68:171–175, 2014.

Kerr J, Norman GJ, Adams MA, et al.: Do neighborhood environments moderate the effect of physical activity lifestyle interventions in adults? *Health Place* 16:903–908, 2010.

Klitzman S, Matte TD, Kass DE: The urban physical environment and its effects on health. In: (editors: Freudenberg Nicholas; Galea Sandro; Vlahov David.) *Cities and the health of the public.* Vanderbilt University Press: Nashville, TN, pp 61–84.

Knobeloch L, Turyk M, Imm P, et al.: Temporal changes in PCB and DDE levels among a cohort of frequent and infrequent consumers of Great Lakes sportfish, *Environ Res* 109:66–72, 2009.

Krieger N, Chen JT, Waterman PD, et al.: The inverse hazard law: blood pressure, sexual harassment, racial discrimination, workplace abuse and occupational exposures in US low-income black, white, and Latino workers, *Soc Sci Med* 67:1970–1981, 2008.

Li IC, Chen YC, Hsu LL, et al.: The effects of an educational training workshop for community leaders on self-efficacy of program planning skills and partnerships, *J of Adv Nursing* 68(3): 600–613, 2011.

Lindland EH, Kendall-Taylor N: *People, polar bears, and the potato salad: mapping the gaps between expert and public understandings of environmental health.* Frame Works Institute: Washington, DC.

Liu C, Maity A, Lin X, Wright RO, Christiani DC: Design and analysis issues in gene and environment studies, *Environ Health* 11(93), 2012.

Martins DC, Burbank PM: Critical interactionism: an upstream-downstream approach to health care reform, *Adv in Nurs Sci* 34(4):315–329, 2011.

Molitor J, Su JG, Molitor NT, et al.: Identifying vulnerable populations through an examination of the association between multipollutant profiles and poverty, *Environ Sci Technol* 45(18):7754–7760, 2011. Available from: <https://doi.org/10.1021/es104017x>.

National Aeronautics and Space Administration (NASA): *Global climate change: Vital signs of the planet.* Available from: https://climate.nasa.gov/. Accessed March 2017.

National Environmental Health Association. Annual Report. Available from: <https://www.neha.org/. Accessed March 2017.

National Institute of Health: *National Institute of Environmental Health Sciences.* GuLF Study. Available from: <https://gulfstudy.nih.gov/en/index.html>. Accessed Jan 2014.

National Institute of Health (NIH): *Opportunities and challenges in digestive diseases research: recommendations of the national commission on digestive diseases.* Available from: https://www.niddk.nih.gov/.../NCDD%20Research%20Plan/NCDD_04272009_Research. Accessed March 2017.

Nelson MC, Gordon-Larsen P, Song Y, et al.: Built and social environments: associations with adolescent overweight and activity, *Amer J Prev Med* 31(2), 2006.

Northridge ME, et al.: Environmental equity and health: understanding completely and moving forward, *Am J Public Health* 93(2):209–213, 2003.

Nweke OC: Achieving environmental justice: perspectives on the path forward through collective action to eliminate health disparities, *Am J Public Health* 101(S1):S6–S8, 2011.

O'Neill MS, Ebi KL: Temperature extremes and health: impacts of climate variability and change in the United States, *J Occup Environ Med* 51(1):13–25, 2009.

Pan TC, Kao JJ: Inter-generational equity index for assessing environmental sustainability: an example of global warming, *Ecol Indic* 9(4):725–1721, 2009.

Rauh VA, Landrigan PJ, Claudio L: Housing and health: intersection of poverty and environmental exposures, *Ann N Y Acad Sci* 1136:276–288, 2008.

Renalds A, Smith T, Hale P: A systematic review of built environment and health, *Fam and Comm Health* 33(1):68–78, 2009.

Ron E: Thyroid cancer incidence among people living in areas contaminated by radiation from the Chernobyl accident, *Health Phys* 93(5):502–511, 2007.

Rylander C, Odland JO, Sandanger TM: Climate change and the potential effects on maternal and pregnancy outcomes: an assessment of the most vulnerable—the mother, fetus, and newborn child, *Glob Health Action* 11(6):1–9, 2013.

Sanchez F, Kosson DS: Probabilistic approach for estimating the release of contaminants under field management scenarios, *Waste Manag* 25(4):463–472, 2005.

Sattler B: The greening of health care: environmental policy and advocacy in the health care industry, *Policy Polit Nurs Pract* 4(1):6–13, 2003.

Schrieberg D: Death from a healing machine: radioactive waste goes on Mexican odyssey after sale of medical device, *San Francisco Examiner* 1:12, 1991.

Schwartz J: Air pollution and children's health, *Pediatrics* 113:1037–1046, 2004.

Sharifi M, Sequist TD, Rifas-Shiman SL: The role of neighborhood characteristics and the built environment in understanding racial/ethnic disparities in childhood obesity. *Prev Med*, 91, 103–109.

Sheffield PE, Knowlton K, Carr JL, et al.: Modeling of regional climate change effects on ground-level ozone and childhood asthma, *Am J Prev Med* 41(3):251–257, 2011.

Schulz A, Mentz G, Johnson-Lawrence V, et al.: Independent and joint associations between multiple measures of the built and social environment and physical activity in a multi-ethnic urban community, *J Urban Health*, 2013.

Stevens PE, Hall JM: Applying critical theories to nursing in communities, *Public Health Nurs* 9:2–9, 1992.

Tainio M, Nazelle AJ, Gotschi T: Can air pollution negate the health benefits of cycling and walking? *Prev Med* 87:233–236, 2016.

Tarr J: Knoxville's pollution rivals that of Los Angeles, Houston and Atlanta, but Green Power might help clear the air, *Metro Pulse* 11(18), 2001.

Thompson B, et al.: Para Ninos Saludables: a community intervention trial to reduce organophosphate pesticide exposure in children of farmworkers, *Environ Health Perspect* 116(5):687–694, 2008.

Trasande L, Cronk C, Durkin M, et al.: Environment and obesity in the national children's study, *Environ Health Perspect* 117(2), 2009.

Troped PJ, Tamura K, Whitcomb HA, et al.: Perceived built environment and physical activity in U.S. women by sprawl and region, *Am J Prev Med* 41(5):473–479, 2011.

U.S. Department of Health and Human Services: *Office of Disease Prevention and Health Promotion: Healthy People 2020*, n.d. Available from: <http://www.healthypeople.gov/2020/>. Accessed March 6, 2013.

Tsunoda K, Tsuji T, Kitano N: Associations of physical activity with neighborhood environments and transportation modes in older Japanese adults, *Prev Med* 55:113–118, 2012.

U.S. Department of Labor: *Occupational Safety and Health Administration*. OSHA QUICKCARD: Hazard communication safety data sheets. Available from: <http://www.osha.gov/Publications/HazComm_QuickCard_SafetyData.html>.

U.S. Food and Drug Administration: *Food safety for moms-to-be: Medical professionals fast facts*. Available from: <http://www.fda.gov/Food/FoodborneIllnessContaminants/PeopleAtRisk/ucm091671.htm>.

U.S. Geological Survey: *What is ground water?* Available from: <http://pubs.usgs.gov/of/1993/ofr93-643/>.

White BM, Hall ES, Johnson C: Environmental health literacy in support of social action: an environmental justice perspective, *J Environ Health* 77(1):24–29, 2014.

Whitney SL, Maltby HJ, Carr JM: "This food may contain...." What nurses should know about genetically engineered foods, *Nurs Outlook* 52:262–266, 2004.

World Health Organization: *World day for safety and health at work 2005: a background paper*. International Labour Office: Geneva.

Worls Health Organizaiton: *Obesity and overweight*, 2017. Available from: http://www.who.int/mediacentre/factsheets/fs311/en/.

World Health Organization: *Preventing disease through healthy environments.* Author: Geneva.

World Health Organization: *Influenza A (H1N1) update 46.* Available from: <http://www.who.int/csr/disease/swineflu/en/index.html>.

World Health Organization: *Preventing disease through healthy environments: A global assessment of the burden of disease from environmental risks.* Author: Prus-Ustun, A., Wolf, J., Corvalan, C., Bos, R., & Neira, M. Available from: www.who.int/quantifying_ehimpacts/publications/preventing-disease/en/. Accessed March 2017.

World Health Organization: Ionizing radiation in our environment. Available from: <http://www.who.int/ionizing_radiation/env/en/>.

World Health Organization: *Global alert and response (GAR): Severe acute respiratory syndrome (SARS).* Available from: <www.who.int/csr/sars/guidelines/en/index.html>.

World Health Organization: *Environmental health.* Available from: <http://www.who.int/topics/environmental_health/en/>.

Wu Q, Shi H, Adams CD, et al.: Oxidative removal of selected endocrine-disruptors and pharmaceuticals in drinking water treatment systems, and identification of degradation products of triclosan, *Sci Total Environ* 439:18–25, 2012.

Health in the Global Community

Julie Cowan Novak

OUTLINE

OBJECTIVES

Upon completion of this chapter, the reader will be able to do the following:

1. Describe globalization and international patterns of health and disease.
2. Discuss the World Health Organization's concepts of "health for all" and primary health care.
3. Identify international health care organizations and how they collaborate to improve global nursing and health care.

4. Describe the role of the community or public health nurse in international health.
5. Discuss key elements and effective models for successful international service learning community health projects, including the International Community Assessment Model, the Furco service learning framework, and the Integrated Model of Sustainability and Innovation

KEY TERMS

Bill & Melinda Gates Foundation
Carter Center
Centers for Disease Control and Prevention
Declaration of Alma-Ata
globalization
health for all by the year 2000
Integrated Model of Sustainability and Innovation

International Council of Nurses (ICN)
Millennium Development Goals
nongovernmental organizations
Pan American Health Organization
primary care
primary health care
United Nations

United Nations International Children's Emergency Fund (UNICEF)
U.S. Department of Health and Human Services
World Bank
World Health Organization

Health care and health care reform are subjects of critical political, social, moral, and ethical debate throughout the world. Human health and its influence on every aspect of life are central to the global agenda. Nurses, as first responders; expert care providers; and leaders in international health care assessment, planning, evaluation, and policy development promote and restore health to individuals, families, and communities across settings and geographic boundaries. Nurses must study models of health promotion, community assessment, community empowerment, service learning, and sustainability to improve health care access and efficient and effective delivery. Community public health nurses must also be aware of forces that threaten health in the global community. Our global society, the Internet, and reduction in travel time provide access that was unimaginable even a decade ago. Globalization—the process of increasing social and economic dependence and integration as capital, goods, persons, concepts, images, ideas, and values cross state boundaries—is inextricably linked to the benefits and challenges of our time.

This chapter highlights population characteristics; international patterns of health and disease; social, cultural, and economic factors; international health care agencies and organizations; health care providers; health care delivery systems and models; and the community public health nurse's role as a leader in the global community. The chapter presents an International Community Assessment Model (ICAM; see Case Study 15.1 later in chapter); the Furco service learning framework (Furco, 2002) for faculty and student discovery, learning, reflection, engagement, policy, and system design; and the Integrated Model of Sustainability and Innovation (IMSI).

Population characteristics, including patterns of growth, demographics, and pandemics, are among the many health issues that merit attention and study because they have global effects that threaten human life. This chapter explores these issues and other environmental factors, including identified stressors and patterns of health and disease.

POPULATION CHARACTERISTICS

More than 1 billion people entered the twenty-first century without benefiting from the health care revolution. Population growth presents a threat to the health and the economy of many nations. The exponential nature of world population growth is evident. In 1804, after 2 to 5 million years of human existence, the world population exceeded 1 billion. Between 1804 and 1927, the population reached 2 billion, and between 1927 and 1960, 3 billion. The population soared to 4 billion between 1960 and 1974 and to 5 billion between 1974 and 1987. In 1999, the world population was about 6 billion; by 2016 it had grown to 7.4 billion. The population is projected to reach 8 billion by 2025, 9.8 billion by 2050, and 11.2 billion by 2100 (United Nations, 2017). One concern is that 99% of the growth is expected to occur in resource-poor countries (Population Reference Bureau [PRB], 2015).

In any society, large populations create pressure. For example, feeding a population becomes problematic in developing countries when famine, international trade problems, and war occur. Malnutrition, disease, or death may be the outcome. Pressures from population growth are also felt in industrialized nations. Although food may be plentiful, overcrowding leads to pollution, stress, disease, and violence. Each of these challenges represents a major barrier to economic growth. The poor suffer this burden of excess mortality and morbidity disproportionately. Thus health promotion, effective health care delivery systems, and the enhancement of the environmental infrastructure will address the origins of poverty and ultimately increase productivity and improve quality of life (QOL).

World population distribution is uneven. More than 50% of the population lives in just four countries: China (1.38 billion), India (1.32 billion), the United States (324 million), and Indonesia (261 million) (World Bank, 2016). In 2013, 26.1% of the world's population consisted of children 0 to 14 and only 8.3% over 65 years of age (World Bank, 2016). In developed countries, life expectancy is increasing; however, in countries severely affected by the HIV/AIDS epidemic, life expectancy dropped to 35 to 40 years, although it has significantly improved over the last decade. Today, a girl born in Zambia can expect to live 64.7 years, whereas a girl born in Japan can expect to live 86.8 years (WHO, 2015.) Of note, 56% of the deaths in Africa are due to communicable, maternal, perinatal or nutritional conditions (WHO, 2015). Malcolm Potts (1994), a world-renowned population theorist, predicted that "the world may end up divided not into political or economic groups but by demographic structure," in which countries will be classified into slow-growth or fast-growth countries instead of rich or poor countries. This will eventually further divide the rich and poor.

 ACTIVE LEARNING

Discuss population characteristics and the threat of population growth to health and health care systems.

ENVIRONMENTAL FACTORS

The relationship between humans and their environment is an important component of individual, family, and global health. The fields of environmental health and sustainable resource development have exploded over the past three decades. Environmental stressors are categorized into five types. First, stressors such as lead poisoning and air pollution directly assault human health. Second, stressors such as the effects of air pollution on products and structures damage society's goods and services. Third, stressors such as noise and litter affect QOL. Fourth, stressors such as global warming interfere with the ecological balance. Finally, natural disasters, terrorism, and war affect all aspects of life.

Air pollution, water pollution, and land pollution are among the consequences of environmental stressors. For example, 50% of the worldwide air pollution problem is attributable to the chemical carbon monoxide. Other primary pollutants, such as nitrogen monoxide, sulfur oxides, particulate matter, and hydrocarbons, combine with carbon monoxide to create 90% of the world's pollution. According to joint WHO and United Nations Children's' Fund (UNICEF) data, 36% of the world's population lack access to basic sanitation facilities, and 768 million people regularly go without clean drinking water. Inadequate access to sanitation and clean water contributes to the deaths of 4000 vulnerable children each day. Without clean water sanitation and hygiene, efficient and sustainable development is unattainable (Borgen Project, 2014).

Agricultural, industrial, residential, and commercial wastes increase land pollution. For example, chemical fertilizers have displaced natural fertilizers; synthetic pesticides have displaced natural means of pest control; and petrochemical products, such as detergents, synthetic fiber, and plastics, have replaced soap, cotton, and paper. Disposable goods have replaced reusable goods, resulting in increased waste. Production technologies are contributing to worldwide environmental and ecological stress.

PATTERNS OF HEALTH AND DISEASE

Lifestyles, health and cultural beliefs, infrastructure, economics, and politics affect existing illnesses and society's commitment to prevention. Disease patterns vary throughout the world; therefore primary causes of death differ in developed and developing countries. Racial, ethnic, and access disparities exist within and between countries. For example, of the 56.4 million deaths worldwide in 2015, 54% were due to ischemic heart disease and stroke. This was followed by pneumonia, chronic obstructive pulmonary disease, lung tracheal and bronchial cancers, and diabetes. Deaths from Alzheimer and other dementias doubled between 2000 and 2015, making dementias the seventh leading cause of death globally. In contrast, deaths from diarrheal diseases halved between 2000 and 2015. Finally, deaths from tuberculosis rounded out the top 10, and notably, HIV/AIDS is no longer among the world's top 10 causes of death (WHO, 2017). Once plagued with high rates of infectious disease, developed countries significantly reduced such rates through improved sanitation, nutrition, immunization, and improved health care. Most developed countries have a more stable economy and a wide range of industrial and technological development. These countries experience an epidemiological transition. For example, the morbidity and mortality profile of a country changes from a lesser developed one to a developed one. Many developed countries experienced an epidemiological transition from having an infectious disease profile to having a chronic disease profile and are now plagued by chronic diseases such as cardiovascular disease, respiratory disease, and cancer secondary to air pollution and the tobacco use pandemic. This altered profile has created a demographic transition from traditional societies, in which almost everyone is young, to societies with rapidly growing numbers of middle-aged and elderly people.

Among the infectious diseases that contribute to higher mortality rates in developing countries are AIDS, tuberculosis (TB), malaria, hepatitis B, rheumatic heart disease, parasitic infection, and dengue fever. Although these diseases claim the lives of millions, it is estimated they could be reduced by up to 50% through effective public health interventions. It is hoped that many of these diseases could join smallpox as a disease known only to history through the development and implementation of immunization programs. Immunization is the most powerful and cost-effective strategy at our disposal for many infectious diseases. Efforts to reduce the incidence of TB were included in the "Commission for Africa" report, which called for wealthy nations to double their aid to Africa in order to rebuild systems to deliver public health services, provide staff training, develop new medicines, and provide better sexual and reproductive health services. The bacille Calmette-Guérin vaccine series, for example, induces active immunity to TB, but it does not reduce the transmission of infectious types of TB. At least one third of the world's population harbors the TB pathogen, *Mycobacterium tuberculosis*. Other WHO programs, including Zika: Then, Today, Tomorrow; Roll Back Malaria; Unite to End TB; HIV/AIDS Control; Tobacco Free Initiative; and Avian Influenza Pandemic Preparedness, target key infectious and chronic disease issues of the twenty-first century.

Although significant progress has been made, AIDS continues to be a global concern. In 2015, 1 in 25 adults was estimated to be living with HIV in sub-Saharan Africa and 36.7 million adults and children were thought to be doing so worldwide. Sadly, the total number of AIDS deaths from 1981 to 2015 exceeds 35 million (WHO, 2015).

Rates of HIV infection vary demographically in different parts of the world. For example, the estimated male-to-female ratio of HIV infections in North America is 5:2, whereas in Africa the ratio is 1:1 (WHO, 2015). Urbanization and within-country migration play a role in the spread of AIDS. For instance, in Rwanda the HIV seroprevalence is 14 to 20 times higher in urban areas than in rural areas. Annually, HIV threatens more lives as more people migrate to the world's largest cities. In 2015, 50% of the developing world lived in cities. This is an increase from 25% in 1970. Over the past three decades, significant progress has been made in HIV education, prevention, treatment, social policy, and legislation; however, stigma against people living with HIV persists.

Malaria is a life-threatening parasitic disease transmitted by mosquitoes. Today approximately 40% of the world's population is at risk for malaria; however, because of improved public health efforts, malaria rates fell 21% between 2010 and 2015. Malaria is found throughout the tropical and subtropical regions of the world and causes more than 212 million acute illnesses and at least 429,000 deaths annually (WHO, 2015). Effective low-cost strategies are available for its prevention, treatment, and control, including insecticide-treated nets and new-generation medications. Successful administration of antimalarial medications has included a challenge of evolving drug-resistant parasites and the search for new drug formulations. Indeed, resistance to chloroquine has rendered the drug ineffective in many regions (CDC, 2016; Mayo Clinic, 2016). Of note, the first malaria vaccine was approved in 2015 and reports an efficacy of 25% to 50%.

With approximately 5 million deaths annually worldwide due to the use of tobacco, tobacco control is a critical component of the international health care agenda. Including deaths from secondhand smoke, by 2020, an estimated one in seven deaths will be tobacco related. Since 1990, tobacco control and secondhand smoke policies have been implemented at various political levels in the United States and abroad. The magnitude and consequences of the tobacco pandemic were unexpected. Smoking prevention and cessation programs, state and federal mandates, tobacco taxation, the 1998 Tobacco Master Settlement Agreement, antitobacco media campaigns, strict licensing of tobacco retailers, the elimination of tobacco vending machines and point-of-sale advertising, and the elimination of tobacco sales by pharmacies have had an impact on tobacco sales in the United States. Because of health concerns and cost, 29 countries, from Ireland to New Zealand, have developed tobacco-free policies and banned all forms of tobacco advertising, promotion, and sponsorship. Although American adults have enrolled in cessation programs, the tobacco industry has targeted youth and dramatically increased international exports. A global commitment to tobacco control can avert millions of premature deaths in the next half-century.

In 2003, the first global public health treaty was adopted at the World Framework Convention on Tobacco Control. The treaty was designed to reduce tobacco-related deaths and diseases around the world. In 2008, the WHO introduced MPower, which stands for **M**onitor tobacco use and prevention policies; **P**rotect people from tobacco use; **O**ffer help to quit tobacco use; **W**arn about the dangers of tobacco; **E**nforce bans on tobacco advertising, promotion and sponsorship; and **R**aise taxes on tobacco (WHO, 2018).

The global approach to tobacco control can guide the development of effective interventions based on best evidence and best practice. Countering potential threats to health resulting from economic crises, unhealthful environments, or risky behavior is critical. Promotion of a healthy lifestyle underpins a proactive strategy for risk reduction, tobacco use prevention and cessation, immunization provision, cleaner air and water, adequate sanitation, healthful diets, fitness and exercise programs, and safe transportation.

INTERNATIONAL AGENCIES AND ORGANIZATIONS

Promoting worldwide health is humankind's greatest challenge. Several global agencies, such as the WHO, the Pan American Health Organization (PAHO), the United Nations, UNICEF, the World Bank, the Centers for Disease Control (CDC), and nongovernmental organizations such as foundations, play important roles in improving the health of all nations. Founded on April 7, 1948 (now celebrated as World Health Day), the World Health Organization is an international health agency of the United Nations. With six regional offices in the United States, Congo, Denmark, Egypt, India, and the Philippines, the WHO's primary role is to direct and coordinate international health efforts, disseminate global health standards and guidelines, and help countries address public health concerns within the United Nations system. The main areas of work include health systems, promoting health through the life course, noncommunicable diseases, communicable diseases, corporate services, preparedness, surveillance, and response. The WHO's goal of "health for all by the year 2000" was framed at the conference in Alma-Ata, the former USSR (now known as Almaty, Kazakhstan), in 1978. The conference defined "health for all" as "the attainment by all citizens of the world by the year 2000 of a level of health that will permit them to lead a socially and economically productive life" (WHO, 1999, p. 65). Not being met, the target year for achievement was extended first to 2010 and now to 2020.

The Alma-Ata conference on primary health care expressed the need for urgent action by all governments. The WHO's statement of beliefs, goals, and objectives is outlined in the Declaration of Alma-Ata, which is presented in Box 15.1. The concept of primary health care stresses health as a fundamental human right for individuals, families, and communities; the unacceptability of the gross inequalities and disparities in health status; the importance of community involvement; and the active role of all sectors.

Primary health care seeks to obtain the highest level of health care for all people. The program promotes seven elements of primary health care: health education regarding disease prevention and cure, proper food supply and nutrition, adequate supply of safe drinking water and sanitation, maternal and child health care, immunizations, control of endemic diseases, and the provision of essential drugs. According to the declaration, a primary health care system should provide the entire population with universal coverage; relevant, acceptable, affordable, and effective services; a spectrum of comprehensive services

that provide for primary, secondary, and tertiary care and prevention; active community involvement in the planning and delivery of services; and integration of health services with development activities to ensure that complete nutritional, educational, occupational, environmental, and safe housing needs are met.

The year 2010, the tenth anniversary of the adoption of the WHO Global Strategy on Diet, Physical Activity, and Health, presented a time for reflection and evaluation of progress. The WHO created an action plan depicting 2020 targets related to the prevalence of unhealthy diets, inactivity, tobacco use, and alcohol. Soft drink and candy taxes were promoted and have been implemented in some areas.

The Pan American Health Organization (PAHO) is an international public health agency with nearly a century of experience in working to improve the health and living standards of the Americas. It serves as the regional office of WHO and is recognized as part of the United Nations system.

Founded in 1945 after World War II, the United Nations (UN) now comprises 193 member nations committed to world peace and security through international cooperation. The UN attempts to resolve global conflicts and formulates policies that affect all nations. Regardless of size, wealth, or political system, all member nations have an equal vote in the decision-making process. UN decisions seek to reflect world opinion and the moral authority of the community of nations (United Nations, 2018). In 2000, the Millennium Development Goals were developed to coordinate and strengthen global efforts to meet the needs of the poorest of the poor. Governments throughout the world and leading global development agencies agreed on the following goals (United Nations, 2000):

1. Eradicate extreme hunger and poverty.
2. Achieve universal primary education.
3. Promote gender equality and empower women.
4. Reduce child mortality.
5. Improve maternal health.
6. Combat HIV/AIDS, malaria, and other infectious diseases.
7. Ensure environmental sustainability.
8. Develop global partnerships.

Collaborating with the UN are nongovernmental organizations (NGOs) such as the Carter Center and the Bill & Melinda Gates Foundation. Founded in 1982, the Carter Center is a nonprofit NGO founded by former President Jimmy Carter and First Lady Rosalynn Carter and based in Atlanta, Georgia. The Carter Center's objectives include (1) to prevent and resolve conflicts, (2) to enhance freedom and democracy, and (3) to improve health and quality of life.

The bond of our common humanity is stronger than the divisiveness of our fears and prejudices. God gives us the capacity for choice. We can choose to alleviate suffering. We can choose to work together for peace. We can make these changes—and we must.

(Jimmy Carter, Nobel Laureate, Carter Center, 2016)

Founded in 2000, the Bill & Melinda Gates Foundation has local, national, and global objectives. Globally, the foundation focuses on reducing hunger and poverty, improving health

BOX 15.1 Declaration of Alma-Ata

The International Conference on Primary Health Care, meeting in Alma-Ata this twelfth day of September in the year Nineteen hundred and seventy-eight, expressing the need for urgent action by all governments, all health and development workers, and the world community to protect and promote the health of all the people of the world, hereby makes the following Declaration:

- The Conference strongly reaffirms that health, which is a state of complete physical, mental, and social well-being and not merely the absence of disease or infirmity, is a fundamental human right and that the attainment of the highest possible level of health is a most important worldwide social goal, whose realization requires the action of many other social and economic sectors in addition to the health sector.
- The existing gross inequality in the health status of the people, particularly between developed and developing countries and within countries, is politically, socially, and economically unacceptable and is therefore of common concern to all countries.
- Economic and social development, based on a New International Economic Order, is of basic importance to the fullest attainment of health for all and to the reduction of the gap between the health status of developing and developed countries. The promotion and protection of the health of the people are essential to sustained economic and social development and contribute to a better quality of life and to world peace.
- The people have the right and duty to participate individually and collectively in the planning and implementation of their health care.
- Governments have a responsibility for the health of their people which can be fulfilled only by the provision of adequate health and social measures. In the coming decades, a main social target of governments, international organizations, and the whole world community should be the attainment by all peoples of the world by the year 2000 of a level of health that will permit them to lead a socially and economically productive life. Primary health care is the key to attaining this target as part of development in the spirit of social justice.
- Primary health care is essential health care based on practical, scientifically sound, and socially acceptable methods and technology made universally accessible to individuals and families in the community through their full participation and at a cost that the community and country can afford to maintain at every stage of their development in the spirit of self-reliance and self-determination. It forms an integral part both of the country's health system, of which primary health care is the central function and main focus, and of the overall social and economic development of the community. It is the first level of contact for individuals, the family, and the community with the national health system bringing health care as close as possible to where people live and work and it constitutes the first element of a continuing health care process.
- Primary health care:
  - reflects and evolves from the economic conditions and sociocultural and political characteristics of the country and its communities and is based on the application of the relevant results of social, biomedical, and health services research and public health experience;
  - addresses the main health problems in the community, providing promotive, preventive, curative, and rehabilitative services accordingly;
  - includes at least: education concerning prevailing health problems and the methods of preventing and controlling them; promotion of food supply and proper nutrition; an adequate supply of safe water and basic sanitation;

maternal and child health care, including family planning; immunization against the major infectious diseases; prevention and control of locally endemic diseases; appropriate treatment of common diseases and injuries; and provision of essential drugs;
  - involves, in addition to health sector, all related sectors and aspects of national and community development, in particular agriculture, animal husbandry, food industry, education, housing, public works, communication, and other sectors; and demands the coordinated efforts of all those sectors;
  - requires and promotes maximum community and individual self-reliance and participation in the planning, organization, operation, and control of primary health care making fullest use of local, national, and other available resources; and to this end, develops through appropriate education the ability of communities to participate;
  - should be sustained by integrated, functional, and mutually supportive systems, leading to the progressive improvement of comprehensive health care for all, and giving priority to those most in need;
  - relies, at local and referral levels, on health workers, including physicians, nurses, midwives, auxiliaries, and community workers, as applicable, and on traditional practitioners as needed, suitably trained socially and technically to work as a health team and to respond to the expressed health needs of the community.
- All governments should formulate national policies, strategies, and plans of action to launch and sustain primary health care as part of a comprehensive national health system and in coordination with other sectors. To this end, it will be necessary to exercise political will, to mobilize the country's resources, and to use available external resources rationally.
- All countries should cooperate in a spirit of partnership and service to ensure primary health care for all people because the attainment of health by people in any one country directly concerns and benefits every other country. In this context the joint WHO-UNICEF report on primary health care constitutes a solid basis for the further development and operation of primary health care through the world.
- An acceptable level of health for all the people of the world by the year 2000 can be attained through a fuller and better use of the world's resources, a considerable part of which is now spent on armaments and military conflicts. A genuine policy of independence, peace, détente, and disarmament could and should release additional resources that could well be devoted to peaceful aims and in particular to the acceleration of social and economic development of which primary health care, as an essential part, should be allotted its proper share.

The International Conference on Primary Health Care calls for urgent and effective national and international action to develop and implement primary health care throughout the world and particularly in developing countries in a spirit of technical cooperation and in keeping with a New International Economic Order. It urges governments, WHO and UNICEF, and other international organizations, and multilateral and bilateral agencies, nongovernmental organizations, funding agencies, all health workers and the whole world community to support national and international commitment to primary health care and to channel increased technical and financial support to it, particularly in developing countries. The Conference calls on all the to collaborate in introducing, developing and maintaining primary health care in accordance with the spirit and content of this Declaration.

Reprinted by permission from Alma-Ata 1978: *Primary health care, report of the international conference on primary health care,* Alma Ata, USSR, 6–12 September, 1978 (Health for All Series, 1, 2–6), Geneva, 1978, World Health Organization.
UNICEF, United Nations International Children's Emergency Fund; *WHO,* World Health Organization.

through harnessing advances in science and technology to save lives in developing countries, and to improve U.S. high school and postsecondary education and support vulnerable children and families (Gates Foundation, 2017). Within Africa, the foundation has had a profound effect on improving access to antiretroviral medications and prevention and treatment for HIV, TB, and malaria.

Created in 1946, the **United Nations International Children's Emergency Fund (UNICEF)** was founded to assist millions of sick and hungry children in war-ravaged Europe and China. In 1950, the UNICEF mandate was expanded to address the needs of children and women throughout the world. UNICEF works for children's survival, development, and protection by developing and implementing community-based programs with well-documented achievements in child health, nutrition, education, water, sanitation, and women's rights. In 1953 the name was shortened to the UN Children's Fund; however, the UNICEF acronym was retained (WHO, 2015).

Within a dramatically changing world economy, the major goal of the **World Bank** is to improve the health status of individuals living in areas that lack economic development. The World Bank was established in 1945 to provide low-interest loans and grants to developing countries for education, health initiatives such as education of health care providers, disease prevention and control, infrastructure, agriculture, communications, environmental protection, and economic and institutional development (World Bank, 2017). Since 1970, the World Bank has become more focused on health-related initiatives to promote sustainable economic growth. Projects range from alleviation of poverty to safe water to effective sanitation to affordable housing The largest shareholder countries are the United States (17.25%), Japan (7.42%), China (4.78%), Germany (4.33%), France (4.06%), and the United Kingdom(4.06%) (World Bank, 2016). Since 1963, the World Bank has provided $61 billion in loans and credits, and funds educational, health, nutrition, and population projects (World Bank, 2017).

The **Centers for Disease Control and Prevention**, located in Atlanta, Georgia, is one of the 13 major operating components of the U.S. Department of Health and Human Services (USDHHS, also called HHS). The principal agency in the U.S. government for protecting the health and safety of all Americans and for providing essential human services, the CDC was founded in 1946 to help control malaria. The agency has remained at the forefront of public health efforts to prevent and control infectious and chronic diseases, injuries, workplace hazards, disabilities, and environmental health threats and to protect the health of international travelers through advisories and immunization and vaccine recommendations. The CDC is globally recognized for conducting research and investigations and for its action-oriented approach. It applies research and findings to improve people's daily lives and responds to health emergencies—a feature that distinguishes the CDC from many of its peer agencies. The CDC is committed to achieving evidence-based health improvements. The agency is defining specific health-impact goals to prioritize and focus its work and investments, to measure progress, and to work toward attainment of its National Public Health Performance Standards

(CDC, 2017). In one example of their efforts, over the past three years the CDC has broadened its focus on the Zika virus. Zika was first discovered in 1947. In 1952 the first human cases were detected. Before 2007, 14 cases were documented. Zika spreads primarily through the bite of an infected mosquito, through sexual contact with an infected partner, and from an infected pregnant woman to her fetus. Most cases of microcephaly, other fetal malformations, and Guillain-Barré syndrome have been reported in Brazil (1046 cases). Cabo Verde, Colombia, French Polynesia, Martinique, and Panama have also reported cases. Other cases have been linked to a stay in Brazil (WHO, 2016).

Founded in 1899 and representing 16 million nurses in 130 national nurses associations, the **International Council of Nurses (ICN)** works to ensure quality nursing care for all; sound health policies; the advancement of nursing knowledge; and the presence of a respected, competent, and satisfied nursing workforce worldwide. Nursing research, advanced practice registered nursing (APRN), doctoral education, socioeconomic welfare, first responders, disaster preparedness, mass casualties, policy, and advocacy have received increased emphasis over the past three decades. The ICN has five core values: visionary leadership, inclusiveness, flexibility, partnership, and achievement. The ICN Code for Nurses is the foundation for ethical nursing practice throughout the world (ICN, 2015). ICN, WHO, the UN, the World Bank, the International Labor Organization, and a wide range of NGOs are attempting to address the global shortage of nurses and other health care providers and complex global health care challenges.

The **U.S. Department of Health and Human Services** (USDHHS) created a program titled *Healthy People* that serves as the foundation for efforts throughout the HHS to create a healthier Nation. *Healthy People 2020* is based on the accomplishments of the following four previous *Healthy People* initiatives: (1) 1979 Surgeon General's Report, *Healthy People: The Surgeon General's Report on Health Promotion and Disease Prevention;* (2) *Healthy People 1990: Promoting Health/ Preventing Disease: Objectives for the Nation;* (3) *Healthy People 2000: National Health Promotion and Disease Prevention Objectives;* and (4) *Healthy People 2010: Objectives for Improving Health. Healthy People* provides science-based, 10-year national objectives for improving the health of all Americans. *Healthy People 2020* is the result of a multiyear process that reflects input from a diverse group of individuals and organizations. The vision of *Healthy People* is a society in which all people live long, healthy lives. The overarching goals of *Healthy People* are to:

- Attain high-quality, longer lives free of preventable disease, disability, injury, and premature death; achieve health equity; eliminate disparities; and improve the health of all groups
- Create social and physical environments that promote good health for all
- Promote quality of life, healthy development, and healthy behaviors across all life stages

Four foundation health measures that serve as an indicator of progress toward achieving these goals are general health status, health-related QOL and well-being, determinants of health, and disparities.

INTERNATIONAL HEALTH CARE DELIVERY SYSTEMS

In the comparison of health care systems, developed and developing countries can learn much from one another. Although transferring specialized medical technologies from developed to developing countries may not always be appropriate, developing countries are currently learning from health care reform policies and the technological revolution in developed countries. Likewise, developed countries have much to learn about low-technology initiatives, such as oral rehydration therapy for the treatment of diarrhea and the delivery of primary health care as defined by the WHO. Participatory approaches to health care delivery, such as community involvement in health and education and maternal-newborn interventions such as delayed cord clamping, are also essential. This exchange is important given the state of the current health care policy in developed countries, many of which have made health care inaccessible to portions of their general public.

Even in countries with socialized medicine, medical costs rise annually and citizens are faced with paying supplemental medical fees or copayment. There is a need to expand the knowledge base that made the twentieth-century health care revolution possible. In the twenty-first century, it is critical to provide research and development that are relevant to the infectious diseases that overwhelmingly affect the poor. In addition, it is necessary to systematically generate an information base that countries can use to shape the future of their health care systems (WHO, 2015).

The Lalonde Report (1974) on the health of Canadian citizens proposed the "health field concept" as a useful way to consider the determinants of health such as biology, lifestyle, environment, and health services. This report emphasized lifestyle and environment as determinants of health outside the traditional medical sphere. It became the basis for rethinking new paradigms for health care delivery. The report signified the early beginnings of a health care paradigm shift from the traditional medical model to a more holistic system–environment perspective (Boothroyd and Eberle, 1990).

In the 1980s, 1990s, and early 2000s, the rising costs of health care were a major catalyst for change, focusing attention on the need to provide alternative models of care. Over the past three decades, population-based approaches to health promotion and disease prevention and new nursing degrees such as the doctor of nursing practice (DNP) have been developed to address system access, quality, efficiency, effectiveness, and value-based care (Porter, 2016; Wall et al., 2005). Birthing centers, same-day surgery, outpatient and ambulatory services, home care, nurse-managed clinics, and wellness centers provide alternatives to hospital-based care. In each of these areas, the nurse plays a prominent role and has the potential to bring a needed dimension of health promotion and disease prevention to individuals, families, and communities attempting to navigate a complex health care system. An emphasis of the integration of research/discovery, teaching/learning, and practice/service/engagement with nurse-led innovation led to the development of the Integrated Model of Sustainability and Innovation (IMSI) presented in Fig. 15.1.

The key components of the IMSI include effective communication, collaboration, community partnership, and a mosaic of support or a diverse portfolio of funding sources to promote long-term sustainability of local to global community-based projects. Conversely, unsustainable projects lack clear communication, mutual respect, and community and administrative partnership and are often dependent on only one or two sources of support (Novak, 2016).

Nurses must think more broadly about potential collaborators in solving the problems of the health care delivery system. Disciplines such as industrial engineering have much to offer nursing and other health care professionals, because engineering principles are applied to information technology; system design; patient safety; medication administration and reconciliation; simulation; chronic disease management; and hospital and clinic development, design, and renovation. The DNP was developed by nursing leaders and endorsed by the American Association of Colleges of Nursing to reengineer health care (Wall et al., 2005). Since 2000 this revolution in nursing education has grown to more than 289 programs, with many more programs in the developmental phase (AACN, 2016).

In 2015, U.S. expenditures for health care were 17.8% of the gross domestic product (GDP) and are expected to grow to 19.9% GDP by 2025 (Centers for Medicaid and Medicare Services [CMS], 2016). A market-based, developed country such as the United States treats health care as a market commodity; therefore it focuses on curative medicine rather than preventive medicine because doing so creates more capital. A market-based health care system could lead to a goal opposite that of health for all. Theoretically, the advent of the managed care system in the United States proposed a capitated model to cut health care costs. The Affordable Care Act was to address the problem of the large number of uninsured Americans, but since its implementation in 2010 is slowly being unraveled by both states and insurers, leaving a gap that will need to be filled. This may be accomplished through changes as moving to a single-payer system, expanding Medicare, removing barriers to APRN practice, and other diverse proposals.

Given the two basic health care systems, market based and population based, and the fact that countries at different levels of development need to learn from one another, it is evident that a single model of health care delivery is not appropriate for every country. For example, in 1985, Cuba was recognized for reaching WHO's goal of "health for all." Cuba began to demonstrate to the world that health care could be provided as a basic human right rather than a privilege. In another example, Canada developed a universal health care system, and Canadian community health nurses (CHNs) created innovative models for practice. A 1986 report by the Canadian Minister of National Health and Welfare, entitled *Achieving Health*

FIG. 15.1 Integrated Model of Sustainability and Innovation (IMSI) (Novak JC: Interdisciplinary and interprofessional collaboration. In Dreher HM and Glasgow EMS, editors, *Role development for doctoral advanced nursing practice,* New York, 2016, Springer, pp 397–414)

for All, offered a health promotion framework that involves fostering public participation in decisions that affect health, strengthening community health service networks with the disadvantaged communities they serve, and coordinating public health policy efforts (Epp, 1986).

The pressure for change provides the opportunity for reform, and the broad goal of health for all should guide this reform. Effective health care delivery systems must increase access and efficiency, improve health status through health promotion and disease prevention, eliminate health disparities, and protect individuals and families from financial loss due to catastrophic illness. One lesson learned from Canada's experience is that a narrow focus on individual responsibility and biology with acute interventions does not ensure the overall health of a country. Thirty years after the start of the "Health for All" programs, inequity in health in Canada is still linked to socioeconomic status. This suggests that a collective responsibility or population-based focus must be established with less emphasis on the individual. Collective mandates, such as required physical education classes in elementary and middle schools, may be instrumental in changing the social and economic environments in which people live. Health promotion and wellness programs are the first line in reducing disease by providing education on healthy lifestyle (Low, 2008).

McKinley argued that treatment of disease is akin to standing downstream and pulling people out of the river after they have fallen in (Low, 2008). In contrast, health promotion stresses prevention, taking into account how social structure produces ill health and the economic framework of a society shapes lifestyle decisions. They are thus analogous to upstream activities by which people are prevented from falling into the river in the first place (Low, 2008).

The Role of the Community Health Nurse in International Health Care

In a rapidly changing health care environment, the nursing role is becoming less traditional. The traditional structure of provider roles is challenged as professional disciplines are recruited to provide expanded and diverse health care services. The nursing role is reciprocal and interdependent with clients and families, physicians, and other health care professionals. The nurse's role expectations and societal expectations influence the formation of behavior patterns specific to the professional nursing role. These expectations provide the basis for the role of the community and public health nurse in global health care.

HEALTH INITIATIVES TAKING PLACE THROUGHOUT THE WORLD

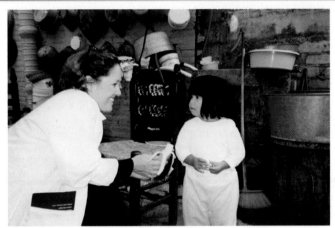

Home health visit, San Luis, Xochimilco, Mexico. (Courtesy Dr. Julie Novak.)

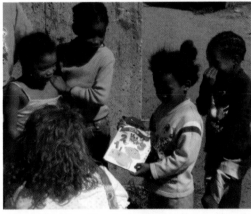

Community home health visits, Cape Town, South Africa. (Courtesy Dr. Julie Novak.)

Nurse-managed clinics in San Luis, Xochimilco, and Mexico City. (Courtesy Dr. Julie Novak.)

Nurse-managed public health clinic, Universidad Nacional Autonomo de Mexico, San Luis, Xochimilco, Mexico. (Courtesy Dr. Julie Novak.)

Cape Town, South Africa, school inauguration and health fair. (Courtesy Dr. Julie Novak.)

Florence Nightingale was the first nurse to establish international linkages and networks that moved from her own country of England to nurses throughout the world. As the first woman and first nurse inducted into the Royal Statistics Society, she recognized the importance of evidence-based nursing and health care. Every obstacle to health and wellness confronted her. She overcame obstacles systematically, developing the foundation and legacy for modern nursing and for community and public health nursing. Nightingale channeled her energies into all aspects of health from the care of wounded soldiers at Scutari in the Crimea to the broad public policies that affected health in her time.

CHNs seek to ensure the attainment of health for all in a cost-effective, efficient, accessible health care system. They must be involved in research, community assessment, planning, implementation, management, evaluation, health services delivery, disaster preparedness and emergency response, health policy, advocacy, and legislation. Nurses in all countries coordinate their work with other health care personnel, as well as informal and formal community leaders. Health for all requires attitudes, levels of competence, knowledge, and skills that differ substantially from those required in traditional nursing or medicine. The changes in the health environment, such as technological advancements, changes in the morbidity and mortality patterns of the population, and social and political changes, all form the basis for the nursing role and system redesign.

With the development of the nurse practitioner (NP) role over the past 50 years in the United States and over the past 30 years abroad, nurses with advanced degrees and areas of specialization have strengthened the community-based health care system. The development of the DNP degree in the United States and PhDs in nursing in many countries further elevates the knowledge and skill base for nursing's role in reengineering health care (Wall et al., 2005).

Because primary health care and primary care may be practiced differently in other countries, the NP and the CHN face multiple challenges. **Primary health care** refers to essential services that support a healthy life. It involves access, availability, service delivery, community participation, and the citizen's right to health care. In contrast, **primary care** refers to first-line or point-of-access medical and nursing care controlled by providers and focused on the individual. Primary care may not be the norm, particularly in communities in developing or less developed countries that have overwhelming needs for basic necessities such as safe drinking water, sanitation, and basic hygiene. The needs of the group outweigh the needs of the individual.

Nurses can make a difference in helping solve the existing and emerging health problems in countries throughout the world. The advent of technology has enhanced global communication and facilitated travel. It is important that nurses throughout the world understand and learn from one another. With 3.3 million nurses in the United States and over 25 million worldwide, nurses are the largest cadre of health care professional. Community public health nurses

improve access to care for the most vulnerable and hard-to-reach groups. The future demands evidence-based education, practice, engagement, service, growth in information technology/health informatics, and local to global health policy and advocacy. Population-based nursing experts are critical to solving the challenges of the fragmented, mismanaged, expensive, ineffective, inefficient health care delivery system that exists in many parts of our global community.

? ACTIVE LEARNING

1. Compare and contrast the scientific progress for HIV, TB, and malaria over the past two decades. Discuss methods of prevention.
2. Describe the status of Zika in the Americas. What are the best methods of prevention?
3. Conduct research and compare the rates of infant mortality and life expectancy in Africa, Mexico, Japan, and the United States. What factors might account for the similarities and differences in rates between the developing and the developed countries?

RESEARCH IN INTERNATIONAL HEALTH

Since 1990, international nursing research has focused predominantly on the following areas: (1) multiple aspects of student and faculty educational exchange programs, (2) diverse clinical conditions and experiences, (3) maternal-child health, and (4) the global development of home care or transition from hospital to home.

WHO collaborating centers in nursing and midwifery development provide a framework for research, education, practice, and service delivery partnerships in 44 institutions from the six WHO regions. Purdue University and the University of Virginia, both affiliates of Case Western Reserve University and the University of Mexico WHO Collaborating Centers, contributed to a partnership for educational programming, clinical practice, and research for graduate students in primary health care nursing and community health. Team Reach Out South Africa, one of the resulting programs, is presented in Case Study 15.2.

U.S. models of home health care are developing in many countries. These models provide a variety of services to bridge the gap between the hospital and community-based care. Sources of home care include home visits by nurses from official government public health agencies, nonprofit voluntary agencies, and for-profit home care agencies. Examples of home care services include assistance with activities of daily living, treatment, rehabilitation, transportation, and respite for caregivers. Home care service providers in the United States and abroad face many challenges. Estimating financial implications and calculating potential caseloads are complex factors in the design of effective delivery systems.

CASE STUDY Application of the International Community Assessment

A Collaborative Model for Community Assessment, Education, and Health Care Delivery

In Mexico and South Africa, the provision of equitable health care services to populations that are geographically and educationally disparate is both economically and logistically challenging. Both countries are further challenged by a lack of infrastructure necessary for health promotion, protection, and maintenance. South Africa is challenged by extreme poverty and staggering rates of HIV and TB. In planning interventions, nurses need a globally diverse assessment tool and methodology to empower communities to achieve health care goals and reduce health care costs. U.S. nursing students gaining international health care experience in a community in rural Mexico and urban South Africa can implement the International Community Assessment Model (ICAM) (Fig. 15.2) before planning targeted programs with local community leaders. The ICAM, tested in rural Mexico and as a component of Team Reach Out South Africa (see Case Study 15.2), is part of an ongoing project. U.S. nursing students compare and contrast practices in various countries using the ICAM and Furco Service Learning Model (Fig. 15.3). Service learning is discipline specific, experiential, and embedded in course objectives and relies heavily on reflection and journaling.

The Model
Community Empowerment

A critical element of designing and implementing global health care projects is community empowerment. If a community is not fully engaged, the project will be unsustainable. In community empowerment, the community identifies its problems and a plan of action, and nurses remain as partners, consultants, and team members. Working with communities is a dance, and the community leads the dance. This mutually respectful, shared decision-making process helps the community develop interventions that are culturally acceptable, breaking down cultural barriers. In developing countries, health promotion programs that do not involve community participation and education often fail after the so-called experts leave the community.

Assessment

During the assessment phase, the nurse identifies key influential community members and leaders and encourages them to join a board of community partners with the goal of assessing community health. The community partners may choose to use the ICAM for the purpose of providing a globally diverse assessment framework and for data gathering. Assessment of community culture helps identify potential cultural barriers to nursing interventions. The center of the model assesses the heart of the community's culture by identifying individual, family, and community characteristics, including their history, demographics, values, beliefs, rituals, and the effect of these characteristics on social and economic conditions.

The ICAM assesses the following:

Recreation: Community cardiovascular fitness; stress management; energy renewal; and relaxation through sports, hobbies, games, fun run walks, 5Ks, yoga, and tai chi.

Perceptions: Community perceptions of health, including community members' physical, social, and mental balance and lifestyle choices.

Spirituality: The community's religious beliefs and practices.

Support systems: Family support systems, including parental support of children and adult children, adult children's support of their parents, and support among extended family members. (*Family* is defined as a group of individuals who have common experiences and goals and are often linked together by genetics, marriage, living situation, or a common emotional bond.)

The physical environment encompasses the community's infrastructure, including homes, water sources, waste disposal sites, roadways, buildings for businesses and shops, factories, power lines, and considerations related to occupational health (e.g., nurses must seek new collaborators in solving the complex problems of the health care delivery system).

The ICAM also assesses the following:

Education: The concept of education reflects the community's knowledge, skills, level of schooling or training, and literacy rate.

Transportation: Defined as how community members travel from point A to point B.

Safety: Evaluation of the community's safety includes examining both the potential dangers in the community that could lead to injury or death and the safety measures and plans developed by the community to prevent these problems.

Government and politics: How the community is governed or ruled.

Economy: The efficacy of economic resources is analyzed in terms of production, dispersal, and expenditure of resources.

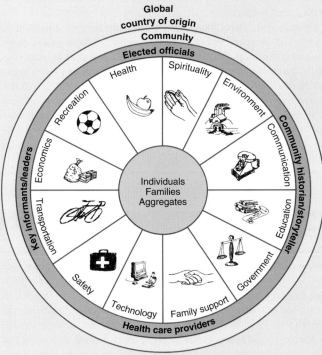

FIG. 15.2 International Community Assessment Model. (Courtesy J. C. Novak.)

Recipient	BENEFICIARY	Provider
Service	FOCUS	Learning

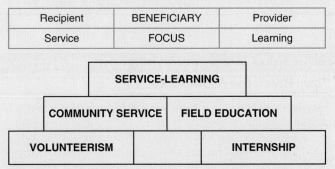

FIG. 15.3 Distinction among service programs. (Furco A: Service learning: A balanced approach to experiential education. In *Expanding boundaries: Service and learning,* Washington, DC, 1996, Corporation for National Service, pp 2–6.)

continued

CASE STUDY   Application of the International Community Assessment—cont'd

A Collaborative Model for Community Assessment, Education, and Health Care Delivery

Communication: Communication is evaluated by examining face-to-face and community-wide information exchange through speech, body language, writing, and drawings. Key components of the community's communication are native languages and forms of communication, such as letters, telephone, computer networks, electronic health records, the Internet, fax machines, television, billboards, signs, magazines, newspapers, and telegrams.

Access: Electricity, public sanitation, public water systems, radio, television, technology, computers, the Internet, fax machines, libraries, industrial machinery, and agricultural practices must be examined.

The ICAM encourages the partners to examine all the public health threats to the community and additional barriers to an effective cultural awareness, sensitivity, proficiency, and humility. It also reflects the importance of assessing the country of origin and global effects on the community. When assessing a community, the nurse must consider the external factors affecting the community. For example, the economy depends on vendors and international purchasing of their main exports.

After the community assessment, the collaborative team should develop an educational program that identifies potential challenges to an educational program or intervention. This program should motivate community partners to identify these problems and then search for effective solutions. As partners become further aware of the health care barriers or health hazards, resources should be provided that will aid in their response.

Next, partners should be assisted in completing a survey and offering focus groups related to needs assessment and attitudes.

The nursing team, local experts, key community informants, and partners need to establish the root cause of problems in a collaborative manner in order to develop effective interventions.

Planning and Intervention

The board and community identify central issues, challenges, and barriers. The board then enters the planning phase of the intervention campaign. Community board members can collaborate with environmental experts and the nurse to identify individual, family, and community educational and service learning goals, strategies, and interventions based on best evidence and practice.

The collaborative team subsequently analyzes possible interventions. This body of knowledge allows the community partners to determine which, if any, of the proposed interventions would be relevant and appropriate for their community. In addition, they may be able to apply these ideas in creating their own interventions. When the community partners have selected or developed an intervention for their project, they can be encouraged to create strategies to educate the community.

Implementation

Before the project is implemented, the outcome of the community-needs assessment must be clarified. The community must be given the opportunity to provide feedback to all collaborators regarding proposed interventions. The partners must be willing to compromise to meet the community's needs. After community-wide education has occurred and necessary consensus and compromise have been achieved, the project can be implemented. At this point, the community members understand ways to sustain the project. Once the implementation is completed, evaluation of the project can begin to ensure that the goals and objectives of the board and the community are met.

Evaluation

The collaborative team should evaluate the project in a formative and summative manner. In addition, the nurse should conduct community surveys to determine whether members continue to recognize the need to maintain the project; to provide feedback related to progress, facilitators, and barriers; and to identify necessary modifications or innovations.

Applications

The ICAM was tested in rural Mexico and South Africa as part of the Team Reach Out project. The targeted communities have a high incidence of poverty. As a result, 80% of the communities reside in crowded living conditions. Many factors in the community pose serious health threats, including infectious disease, chronic conditions, tobacco use, secondhand smoke, farm chemicals, and air pollution. Field workers are often powerless and have minimal recourse when exposed to unhealthy environmental contaminants causing increased morbidity and mortality.

In rural Mexico, the top causes of mortality in the communities are cardiac disorders, diabetes, automobile accidents, and dramatic increases in violence, particularly in urban Mexico and border communities. The leading causes of morbidity are respiratory infections, diabetes, hypertension, and gastrointestinal illnesses. The community's high rate of gastrointestinal illness is related to limited access to potable water. The community historians, community political leaders, key employers, full-time staff at nurse-run public health clinics, local community health faculty, and the *pasantes* (nursing graduates who have completed 1 year of community service at nurse-run clinics and public health agencies) are critical to the success of the project.

A multidisciplinary team of key influential community members, environmental experts, and nurses will further assess the community using the ICAM model. The goal of this assessment is to assist the community members in further diagnosing the community's health care needs and other issues as they are identified. Nurses collaborate with community partners to develop culturally proficient interventions. After the interventions are developed, the local partners, clinic staff, and *pasantes* continue to evaluate the effectiveness of these interventions, promoting a sense of ownership of the project in the community and helping ensure improvements in health care long after the multidisciplinary team leaves the community (see Case Study 15.2).

CASE STUDY   Application of the International Community Assessment

Team Reach Out South Africa

Team Reach Out started as a student-initiated service learning project with the goal of providing ongoing assistance to the victims of Hurricane Katrina. Four years after Hurricane Katrina, Team Reach Out refocused its efforts in Cape Town, South Africa. Four senior nursing students and one premed science student integrated their leadership skills with the application of public health knowledge, compassion, and concern as they worked in partnership with several international health agencies. This case reviews the service learning framework (Furco, 1996, course planning, implementation, and evaluation.

Service learning is a reciprocal partnership that bridges the gap between professional education and society. It is a powerful teaching and learning strategy that engages students in learning while helping communities help themselves (Poirrier, 2001). Service learning provides an experiential, collaborative, discipline-based relationship between students and community members for a reciprocal learning experience and allows an opportunity for reflection. Service learning sets the stage for a lifelong commitment to the development of civic duty, social awareness, and engagement while providing unique learning experiences that focus on building citizenship, cultural diversity, community partnerships, knowledge of community resources, critical thinking skills, and mutual respect .

Both students and the community benefit from service learning. Students benefit from the exposure to real-life dilemmas and firsthand experience of joint

CASE STUDY   Application of the International Community Assessment—cont'd

Team Reach Out South Africa

team efforts. Communities benefit from the knowledge and creativity available from academia (Richards et al., 2009).

The faculty team leader/advisor completed an exploratory trip to Johannesburg and Cape Town, South Africa, meeting with prospective community partners. Each of the local health care leaders invited the development of a collaboration. Because of the richness of each setting and the overwhelming need for human and financial resources, the choice was extremely difficult. Cape Town was selected as the city site through a comprehensive assessment using the ICAM (Richards, et al., 2009; Richards and Novak, 2010). Health care and educational partners within the city were selected in collaboration with the school nurse, faculty, and staff of Christel House Academy in Cape Town. Subsequently, students from the School of Nursing and College of Science were invited to apply through notification in their respective student newsletters. Selection was based on the clarity of the student's goals and understanding of cultural humility and service learning. After selection, each student wrote an additional travel grant application to the university's Office of Engagement. Following is a description of the partners involved in this project and the experiences each provided.

Partners

Christel House International is a 501(c)(3) public charity that operates learning centers in impoverished neighborhoods with the goal of creating sustainable social and educational impact, breaking the cycle of poverty through a comprehensive holistic approach that transforms the child, family, and community. Between 1999 and 2015, Christel House opened nine learning centers in Mexico, South Africa, India, Venezuela, and the United States. Currently, Christel House serves more than 5000 students, their families, and communities. Christel House K-12 Academy in Cape Town helps children around the world break the cycle of poverty, realize their hopes and dreams, and become self-sufficient, contributing members of society. The academy invited the students to participate in the inaugural celebration of a new school facility and campus. Weekend cultural experiences included a trip to Robben Island, an ecological and historical heritage site where Nelson Mandela was imprisoned from 1963 to 1990; Table Mountain, a protected natural habitat with 1500 plant species; and a game and nature preserve.

The Themba Care Orphanage provides a safe and compassionate environment for approximately 20 children who are HIV positive. In the majority of cases their parents have died of AIDS; however, some children are placed in the setting by their parents to avoid stigma within their respective communities. The orphanage is run by an executive director, two registered nurses/"sisters," a teacher, a staff of five nursing assistants, and local volunteers. Team Reach Out worked with volunteers from three different U.S. universities on site. In addition to one older child, 95% of the children at the orphanage ranged in age from 18 months to 4 years. Students were able to complete Denver Developmental Screenings and health assessments and to work with

the sisters in medication dispensation and reconciliation. The majority of the children demonstrated global developmental delay on the screenings. Students played with, fed, and cared for the children in this warm, caring, inviting preschool environment. The students reflected on their difficulty in saying goodbye to the children.

The Gatesville Medical Center is a multispecialty large private Indian hospital located in Cape Town. Team Reach Out students were able to care for pediatric patients and effectively compare and contrast this South African state-of-the-art private hospital with other health care settings. Diagnoses included respiratory syncytial virus, pneumonia, asthma, gastroenteritis/dehydration, and meningitis.

The Tafelsig Community Health Center provides care to approximately 9000 low-income patients each month. Patients receive health promotion visits throughout the lifespan. Tafelsig treats one of the largest TB and HIV patient populations in Cape Town. Students were able to complete health assessments and immunize patients under the supervision of South African RN specialty clinic coordinators and their faculty advisor.

The students' week of clinical experiences culminated with a presentation of a health fair at the Christel House Academy. The health fair focused on school and family health promotion; prenatal and newborn care and parenting; prevention of TB, HIV, and malaria; health care careers; science experiments (with the premed student); and health screenings, including measurements of height, weight, blood pressure, glucose, and cholesterol. The academy ran special bus routes from the school to and from area informal settlements to bring parents and other community members to the school health fair. The students worked with the WHO, the CDC, Johnson & Johnson, and local Cape Town universities to ensure culturally appropriate materials for the health fair. The Christel House Academy Health Fair was attended by 600 children and 200 parents.

Student Responses

Team Reach Out South Africa students provided poignant and insightful reflections about their experiences. Community partners indicated that the students were very professional and were able to provide much-needed support.

Summary

Students felt strongly that service learning enhanced their community public health experience while building relationships with community service organizations. Students reported encountering minimal barriers to the implementation of this project and also were not reluctant to participate in these activities. Students also agreed that they would continue to participate in service-learning activities in the near future. Table 15.1 includes more student reflections on their experiences. Table 15.2 and Box 15.2 highlight students' feelings about service learning in general (Richards and Novak, 2010).

TABLE 15.1   Student Reflections on Team Reach Out Projects

Reflections from Team Reach Out Biloxi

"It was a wonderful experience to be able to meet so many interesting people and use our knowledge of health care to provide support to this community."
"Every student was thinking about their neighbor in terms of their needs."
"Everyone expressed appreciation and hope."
"My most meaningful memory is the incredible impression each patient made on me. It was amazing to me that through all of the tragedy, devastation, and loss, their hospitality and gentleness was still very much alive."

Reflections from Team Reach Out South Africa

"We were so fortunate to see the health care extremes, from the poorest of the poor clinics to the private hospitals. It was such a diverse spectrum to work in."
"Traveling to South Africa was an eye-opening experience in so many ways. I'll never forget the striking beauty of the country contrasted with the devastating poverty that runs rampant; I was both impressed and surprised by the resourcefulness of their health care system."
"The trip was incredible. So much poverty and beauty and riches in the same area. The people touched my life and I hope that I did the same for some of them."

TABLE 15.2 **Student and Provider Responses to Service Learning Questionnaire**	
Purdue University School of Nursing Service-Learning Questionnaire: Strongly Agree (5), Agree (4), Undecided (3), Disagree (2), Strongly Disagree (1)	**Student Average (N = 5)**
Service learning at Purdue University School of Nursing may be a catalyst for	
Assisting societal needs	4.75
b. Student learning	4.8
c. Building relationships with community service organizations	4.6
d. Engagement opportunities	4.8
2. I encountered significant barriers to completing this service-learning activity.	1.8
3. Service learning should only be integrated into senior course leadership.	2.4
4. Service learning enables a positive change through leadership.	4.4
5. I was reluctant to participate in community and civic service-learning activities.	1.2
6. Service learning is a community-building and democracy-building activity.	4
7. I plan to continue service-learning activities in the immediate future.	4.2
8. This experience embraced the concepts of reciprocity between learning and the community being served.	4.2
9. This experience allowed students to engage in activities that addressed community needs.	4.8

BOX 15.2   **Student Responses: What is the Definition of Service Learning?**

Service learning is:

- Providing services to those in need while at the same time learning in your field of interest and having the ability to work with those less fortunate. It is a hands-on learning experience that, for me, was life changing and eye opening.
- Volunteering with doing something that you are in the field of doing or obtaining a degree in.
- A unique way of learning in and about a community and providing services for the betterment of a community. Service projects provide communities with

people who are able to use their time, resources, and expertise in order to improve or help the community in which they are serving. At the same time, the people involved in the service project are learning from their experiences with the project.

- A volunteering project that is done to help the community in some positive way while the volunteer has the opportunity to broaden their own horizons by learning something new.
- Utilizing skills and knowledge acquired in the classroom as a means to enhance the community.

Modified from Richards E, Novak J: From Biloxi to Cape Town: Curricular integration of service learning. *Journal of Community Health Nursing,* 27(1):46–50, 2010.

⁇ ACTIVE LEARNING

1. Compare population-focused nursing in a developing country with community health nursing in the community. How are they the same, and how do they differ?
2. Test the ICAM in a community. Evaluate its effectiveness.
3. Describe the Furco Service Learning Model and its potential application in local to global projects in your university.
4. Describe the key elements of an effective health care delivery system. Will the focus of future health care services reflect downstream thinking, or will the team create innovative, sustainable models of health promotion, disease prevention, and early intervention?

▌SUMMARY

Community public health nurses face many exciting challenges in health care reform and the design of effective systems of health care delivery. These include being responsive to emerging needs and health issues in the population, developing multidisciplinary practice models that adhere to the principles of primary health care in the context of a reengineered health care system, and mobilizing research dissemination and practice implementation strategies to ensure evidence-based practice as the norm rather than the exception. Using evidence-based models as a framework for local to global community public health partnerships and projects should be tested and evaluated. There is still much to be done to meet the challenge of WHO's goal of "health for all." Studying the progress achieved in other countries is critical; however, success will ultimately depend on societal commitment to addressing complex issues of poverty, disparity, and health care inaccessibility.

ⓔ EVOLVE WEBSITE

http://evolve.elsevier.com/Nies/community

- NCLEX Review Questions
- Case Studies

BIBLIOGRAPHY

American Association of Colleges of Nursing (AACN). www.aacn.org/ DNP fact sheet, 2016.

Boothroyd P, Eberle M: *Healthy communities: what they are, how they're made, CHS Research Bulletin, UBC Centre for Human Settlements*, Vancouver, 1990, University of British Columbia.

Carter Center: *About the center.* Available from: <www.cartercenter. org/about/index.html>, 2016.

Centers for Disease Control and Prevention. Available from: <www. cdc.gov/malaria >, 2016.

Centers for Disease Control and Prevention. Available from: www. cdc.gov/zika, 2017.

Christel House: *About us, 2016 Annual Report.* Available from: <http://www.christelhouse.org/about-us>.

Epp J: *Achieving health for all: a framework for health promotion*, Ottawa, 1986, Health and Welfare Canada.

Furco A: Service learning: a balanced approach to experiential education. In Raybuck J, Taylor B, editors: *Expanding boundaries: serving and learning*, Washington, DC, 1996, Corporation for National Service. Accessed from: https://digitalcommons.unomaha.edu/cgi/ viewcontent.cgi?article=1104&context=slceslgen.

Gates Foundation: who we are. www.gates foundation.org, 2017.

International Council of Nurses: *About ICN.* Available from: <www. icn.ch/abouticn.htm>, 2016.

Lalonde M: *A new perspective on the health of Canadians*, Ottawa, 1974, Minister of Supply and Services.

Low J, Theriault L: Health promotion policy in Canada: lessons forgotten, lessons still to learn, *Health Promot Int* 23(2):200–206, 2008.

Novak JC: Interdisciplinary and interprofessional collaboration. In *Dreyer and Glasgow: Role development for doctoral advanced practice nursing*, New York, 2016, Springer.

Population Reference Bureau: *World population data sheet.* Available from: http://www.prb.org/Publications/Datasheets/201506/201506 WorldPopulationDataSheet.aspx, 2015 >.

Poirrier G: *Service learning: curricular applications in nursing*, New York, 2001, National League for Nursing.

Porter ME: *Value based healthcare delivery*, Harvard University School of Business, 2016.

Potts M: Common sense prevailing at population conference, *Lancet* 344:809, 1994.

Richards E, Novak J: From Biloxi to Cape Town: curricular integration of service learning, *J Community Health Nurs* 27(1):46–50, 2010.

Richards E, Novak J, Davis L: Disaster response after Hurricane Katrina: a model for an academic-community partnership in Mississippi, *J Community Health Nurs* 26(3):114–120, 2009.

United Nations: *News: World Population.* Available from: https://www. un.org/development/desa/en/news/population/world-population-prospects-2017.html, 2017.

United Nations: *Resolution adopted by the general assembly: United Nations millennium declaration*, New York, 2000, The Author.

United Nations: About the UN; 2018. Available from: http://www. un.org/en/about-un/index.html, 2018.

Wall B, Novak J, Wilkerson S: The doctor of nursing practice: reengineering healthcare, *J Nurs Educ* 44(9):396–403, 2005.

World Bank: *What We Do.* Available from: <http://www.worldbank. org/en/about>, http://www.worldbank.org/en/about/what-we-do, 2017.

World Bank. <http://www.worldbank.org/data>, 2016.

World Health Organization: *Roll back malaria info sheet*, Geneva, 2005, Author. <www.who.int/malaria/docs/Basicfacts.pdf>.

World Health Organization: *Unite to End TB*, Author, 2016.

World Health Organization: *Tobacco free initiative.* Available from: <http://www.who.int/tobacco/en/>, 2018.

World Health Organization: *Global health atlas database*, Author, 2015.

World Health Organization: *The top 10 causes of death worldwide*, Author, 2017.

16

Child and Adolescent Health

Melissa Domingeaux Ethington*

OUTLINE

OBJECTIVES

Upon completion of this chapter, the reader will be able to do the following:
1. Identify major indicators of child and adolescent health status.
2. Describe social determinants of child and adolescent health.
3. Discuss the individual and societal costs of poor child health status.

4. Discuss public programs and prevention strategies targeted to children's health.
5. Apply knowledge of child and adolescent health needs in planning appropriate, comprehensive care at the individual, family, and community levels.

KEY TERMS

child maltreatment
childbirth educator
childhood immunization

Children's Health Insurance Program (CHIP)
Early and Periodic Screening,

Diagnosis, and Treatment (EPSDT)
fetal alcohol spectrum disorders (FASD)

* The author would like to acknowledge the contribution of Susan Rumsey Givens, who wrote this chapter for the previous edition.

infant mortality
lactation consultant
late preterm birth
lead poisoning
low birth weight
Medicaid
preconception health

prenatal care
preterm birth
Safe to Sleep
Special Supplemental Nutrition
   Program for Women, Infants, and
   Children (WIC)

teen childbearing
teen dating violence
WIC

A nation's destiny lies with the health, education, and well-being of its children. The United States has made tremendous progress over the past century toward improving children's lives. Advancements in public health measures—such as sanitation, infectious disease control, environmental regulation, health screening, and education—and remarkable strides in medical care have all contributed to the good health status that most children enjoy. However, these improvements have not equally benefited children of all races and ethnic groups, children at all income levels, or children in all geographic areas of the country. For example, significant disparities persist in the health status of white children versus children of color. Children living in suburban areas and most outer urban areas experience access to health care services superior to that of children living in rural areas and inner cities, especially if they are poor.

Although most of the nation's children are healthy and succeed in school, many are not enjoying optimal health and well-being and are not reaching their full potential as contributing members of society. Despite improvements, the mortality and morbidity rates for U.S. children in all age groups are unacceptably high. Consider the following facts (Jiang, Granja, and Koball, 2017; Khan et al., 2016; Kochanek et al., 2016):

- Each year about 23,000 to 25,000 infants die before reaching their first birthday. Black infants are more than twice as likely to die as white infants.
- Nearly one-half million babies are born prematurely each year. Prematurity is the leading cause of infant death and long-term neurological disabilities.
- Twenty-two percent of children aged 0 to 18 years live in poverty.
- Every day, five children die as the result of child abuse; most are younger than 4 years.
- More than 249,000 girls aged 15 to 19 years give birth each year.
- An average of 22% of twelfth graders are cigarette smokers and nearly 28% smoke marijuana.
- Well over half of children currently residing in the United States will be affected by violence, crime, abuse, or psychological trauma this year.

The health of a child has long-term implications. Health habits adopted by children and youth will profoundly influence their potential to lead healthy, productive lives. The physical and emotional health experienced by a child plays a pivotal role in his or her overall development and the well-being of the entire family. Children who go to school sick or hungry, who cannot see well enough to read, who cannot hear the teacher, who have learning disabilities, who are troubled by abusive parents or disruptive living circumstances, or who fear for their safety at home or in school often do not perform on the level of their counterparts who are healthy, well nourished, well cared for at home, and safe and secure in their world. From fetal life onward, the health and well-being of individuals has a substantial impact on their futures.

In 2015 there were 73.7 million U.S. children younger than 18 years. Children represent about 24% of the country's population, down from a peak of 36% at the end of the mid-1960s baby boom. The birth rate for children of all races has declined in recent years, and the racial and ethnic diversity of children is changing rapidly. For example, by 2050, Hispanic children are expected to account for 32% of the population, up from 25% in 2015. The percentage of children who are Hispanic has increased faster than that of any other racial or ethnic group (Federal Interagency Forum on Child and Family Statistics, 2016) (Fig. 16.1).

Children are a dependent population and rely primarily on parents or other adults to protect and promote their health and well-being. Community health nurses can learn more about this important population group and the positive and negative factors that influence their health. Nurses can use this information to help improve the chances that children will grow up to be healthy, both physically and emotionally.

This chapter focuses on the health status of children and adolescents and the medical, socioeconomic, cultural, environmental, educational, safety, and public health factors that community health nurses must address to improve child and adolescent health. The chapter also discusses the individual and societal costs of poor child health, public programs targeted to children's health, and strategies to improve child and adolescent health at the individual, family, and community levels.

ISSUES OF PREGNANCY AND INFANCY

The health of the mother before, during, and after pregnancy has a direct impact on the health and well-being of her child. The conditions that surround a child's fetal development and early years shape his or her life. Adapting healthy lifestyles and obtaining regular medical care before becoming pregnant can help ensure a healthy pregnancy. Unfortunately, many women face barriers to good health throughout their lives, including racism, violence, poverty, and lack of access to health care.

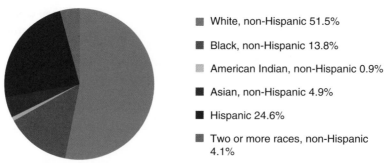

FIG. 16.1 Percentage distribution of U.S. children by race/ethnicity, 2016. (From Federal Interagency Forum on Child and Family Statistics: *America's children in brief: Key national indicators of well-being,* 2016. Retrieved from https://www.childstats.gov/pdf/ac2016/ac_16.pdf)

A comprehensive approach that helps women identify and treat potential risks and overcome barriers to good health before, between, and beyond their pregnancies will help protect and promote the health of women and children and can help ensure the health of future generations (Moos, 2010; Moos et al., 2010). Consider the following findings:

1. Women who are not in optimal health before becoming pregnant are at increased risk for poor pregnancy outcomes.
2. Babies whose mothers have uncontrolled medical conditions, such as infections, diabetes, hypertension, and obesity, are more likely to be born at low birth weights and with serious medical conditions.
3. A fetus exposed to maternal drug, alcohol, or tobacco exposure or poor nutrition is more likely to have chronic conditions that affect health and well-being.
4. Infants exposed to unsafe environmental conditions, such as secondhand smoke and lead-based paint, are more likely to have chronic conditions throughout childhood and, in some cases, through adolescence and adulthood.
5. Children who do not receive preventive health care and do not obtain all necessary immunizations are more likely to have preventable diseases or chronic conditions that could have been prevented or minimized and controlled.

Infant Mortality

Infant mortality, the deaths of children during the first year of life, is a critical gauge of children's health status. It is an important marker because it is related to several factors, including maternal health, medical care quality and access, socioeconomic conditions, and public health practices. Infant mortality reflects the health and welfare of an entire community and is used as a broad indicator of health care and health status. Box 16.1 lists some terms and definitions associated with infant health and mortality. The five leading causes of infant death are congenital defects; disorders related to short gestation or low birth weight; maternal complications of pregnancy; sudden infant death syndrome (SIDS; see later in the chapter); and accidents such as suffocation. These five factors account for close to 60% of all infant deaths. The order of the top five leading causes changed slightly from 2012 to 2013. In 2012, SIDS was the third leading cause, followed by maternal complications, whereas in 2013, maternal complications was third and SIDS was fourth (Mathews et al., 2015). Box 16.2 lists sources of vital statistics birth data.

BOX 16.1   Infant Health Definitions

Infant death: Death of an infant before his or her first birthday.
Infant mortality rate: Number of infant deaths per 1000 live births.
Preterm birth: Birth before 37 completed weeks of gestation.
Very preterm birth: Birth before 32 completed weeks of gestation.
Late preterm birth: Birth from 34 to 36 completed weeks of gestation.
Term birth: Birth from 37 to 41 completed weeks of gestation.

From MacDorman MF, Mathews TJ: *Understanding racial and ethnic disparities in U.S. infant mortality rates,* NCHS data brief, no 74. Hyattsville, MD, 2011, National Center for Health Statistics. Retrieved from https://www.cdc.gov/nchs/data/databriefs/db74.pdf

---

BOX 16.2   Sources of Vital Statistics Data for Children

In the United States, laws require birth certificates to be completed for all babies born. Information concerning an infant's birth, including the total number of the mother's prenatal care visits; the mother's and father's ages and race; mother's marital status and education; and the infant's weight, gestational age, and birth date, appears on a baby's birth certificate.

Information concerning an infant's death, such as the cause(s), date, and other details, appears on the death certificate. In each state, the vital statistics office in the state health department stores these certificates. This agency collects and regularly reports the aggregated data and forwards them to the National Center for Health Statistics.

The National Center for Health Statistics collects, analyzes, and publishes numerous reports on the health and well-being of the nation's infants. These data sources are very important in tracking the health of infants as well as of other population groups; they help determine necessary interventions from various perspectives (e.g., clinical, public health, public policy, and environmental).

From National Institute of Child Health & Human Development: *Safe to sleep public education campaign, 2012.* https://www1.nichd.nih.gov/sts/Pages/default.aspx

---

Surprisingly, the United States ranks a dismal nineteenth in infant mortality, behind most other industrialized nations, including South Korea, Sweden, Spain, Israel, Italy, France, and Australia (Table 16.1). Fifty years ago, the United States ranked twelfth (Organisation for Economic Co-operation and Development [OECD], 2012). The gap in infant mortality between the United States and other nations has occurred in spite of the United States' comparatively high per capita spending on health care and technological advancements.

Despite a poor ranking among other nations in the world, the infant mortality rate in the United States has declined every year

TABLE 16.1 International Comparisons of Infant Mortality Rates* for Selected Countries and Territories (2015)

World Rank	Country	1960	2015
1	Slovenia	N/A	1.6
2	Finland	21.0	1.7
3	Iceland	13.0	2.2
4	Norway	16.0	2.3
5	Czech Republic	20.0	2.5
5	Sweden	16.6	2.5
5	Estonia	N/A	2.5
6	South Korea	N/A	2.7
6	Spain	43.7	2.7
7	Luxembourg	N/A	2.8
8	Italy		2.9
8	Portugal	77.5	2.9
9	Austria	37.5	3.1
9	Israel	N/A	3.1
10	Australia	20.2	3.2
11	Belgium	31.4	3.3
11	Germany	35.0	3.3
11	Netherlands	16.5	3.3
12	Ireland	29.3	3.4
13	Denmark	21.5	3.7
13	France	27.7	3.7
14	Switzerland	21.1	3.9
14	United Kingdom	22.5	3.9
15	Greece	40.1	4.0
15	Poland	54.8	4.0
16	Latvia	N/A	4.1
17	Hungary	47.6	4.2
17	Lithuania	N/A	4.2
18	Slovak Republic	28.6	5.1
19	United States	26.0	5.9
19	Russia	N/A	6.5
20	Costa Rica	N/A	8.5
21	China	N/A	9.2
22	Turkey	189.5	10.7
23	Mexico	92.3	12.5
24	Columbia	89.3	13.6
25	Brazil	129.4	14.6
26	Indonesia	148.4	22.8
27	South Africa	N/A	33.6
28	India	165.1	37.9

*Infant mortality rate represents infant deaths per 1000 live births.
From Organisation for Economic Co-operation and Development: *Health: Key tables from OECD, No. 14: Infant mortality,* 2015. Retrieved from https://data.oecd.org/healthstat/infant-mortality-rates. htm; Centers for Disease Control and Prevention: Deaths final data 2015, 2016. Retrieved from https://www.cdc.gov/nchs/data/nvsr/nvsr65/nvsr65_04.pdf

since 1940 with the exception of 2002 (Fig. 16.2). The 2016 figure, 5.8 deaths per 1000 live births (Central Intelligence Agency, 2017), was the lowest infant mortality rate ever recorded in this country. This drop can be attributed largely to public health measures and improved standard of living (e.g., better sanitation, a clean milk supply, immunizations against deadly childhood diseases, the increased availability of nutritious food, and enhanced access to maternal health care). Technological advances in neonatal care—for example, the introduction of synthetic lung surfactant—have also contributed to reductions in infant mortality.

Declines in infant mortality have stagnated during the past decade, however, and the gap between black and white infant mortality rates remains stubbornly high, with black infants dying at a rate of approximately 2.2 times higher than that of white infants. Identifying and remedying the causes of higher infant mortality rates among certain population subgroups remains a vexing societal problem that must be addressed (Fig. 16.3).

The first year of life is the most hazardous a person faces until he or she reaches 65 years. Therefore it is particularly important for women to be as healthy as possible before becoming pregnant and to receive prenatal care and adopt healthy lifestyle choices, and for infants to receive primary health care to maintain health and prevent or minimize serious, long-lasting health problems.

Preterm Birth and Low Birth Weight

Preterm birth (birth before 37 completed weeks of gestation) and low birth weight (weighing less than 5.5 pounds at birth) are the most important predictors of infant health. In 2014, 9.57% of babies in the United States were born preterm; the percentage of low-birth-weight babies was essentially unchanged in 2014 over the previous year. Black women are more likely than white women to have a preterm birth and about twice as likely to have babies born at low birth weight (Hamilton et al., 2017).

Infants born preterm or at a low birth weight have a far greater risk of death as well as of mental and physical disabilities such as cerebral palsy, visual problems such as retinopathy of prematurity, feeding problems, and hearing loss than infants born at term with normal weight. Even babies born late preterm (34 to 36 completed weeks of gestation) carry a risk for physical problems and developmental delay that is much higher than for babies born at full term. Important growth and development occur even in the last few days of a pregnancy. Factors associated with preterm birth and low birth weight include the following:

1. Minority status
2. Chronic stress
3. Maternal age less than 17 years or more than 35 years
4. Chronic health problems such as diabetes mellitus, hypertension, and some infections
5. Lack of prenatal care
6. Multiple births
7. Certain problems with the uterus or cervix
8. Low socioeconomic status
9. Unhealthy maternal habits (e.g., poor nutrition, obesity, alcohol and drug use, and cigarette smoking)
10. Induced labor before 39 weeks of pregnancy without a medical indication
11. Elective cesarean birth

One reason that infant mortality has declined so slowly in recent years is that the preterm rate rose very quickly from 1990 to 2006. A portion of this rise was due to increases in multiple births, which in turn was due in part to childbearing in later years, which increases the likelihood of multiple

FIG. 16.2 Infant, neonatal, and postneonatal mortality rates: United States, 1940–2014. Rates are infant (under 1 year), neonatal (under 28 days), and postneonatal (28 days–11 months) deaths per 1000 live births in specified group. (From National Center for Health Statistics: Deaths: *Final data for 2014.* National Vital Statistics Report, 65[4], 2016. Retrieved from https://www.cdc.gov/nchs/data/nvsr/nvsr65/nvsr65_04.pdf.)

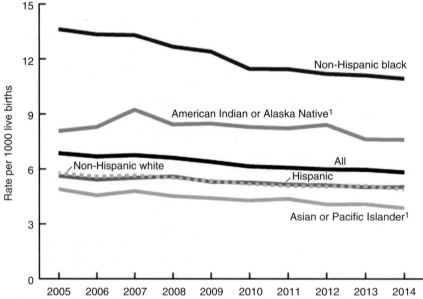

FIG. 16.3 Infant mortality rates by race and ethnicity of mother, 2005–2014. (From National Center for Health Statistics: *Trends in infant mortality in the United States, 2005–2014,* 2017. Retrieved from https://www.cdc.gov/nchs/products/databriefs/db279.htm)

conceptions. Also there was an increase in the rate of multiples that resulted from assisted reproductive technology. Yet the rate of preterm births among singleton births also rose during this time. Further, medical management of pregnancy has increased the numbers of labor inductions and elective cesarean births and has helped push the rate of late preterm births upward (Martin et al., 2017). Success stories of tiny survivors are sensationalized in the news, but the long-term consequences of babies born even a few weeks early are not well publicized. Consequences of preterm and late preterm birth can be long-lasting and costly (Engle and Kominiarek, 2008; Morse et al., 2009; Petrini et al., 2009; Ramachandrappa and Jain, 2009). Because late preterm births account for the majority of preterm births, it is imperative that all possible measures are taken to decrease elective births before 39 weeks of gestation (Oshiro et al., 2009).

Preventing the occurrence of prematurity and low birth weight is a high priority for clinical and public health research and policy. Nurses can play important roles in preventing prematurity through the provision of evidence-based primary care, research, screening, counseling, education, advocacy, referral, and implementation of interventions to reduce risk among target population groups.

Preconception Health

Developing fetal organ systems are highly vulnerable to the effects of poor maternal nutrition, drugs, alcohol, tobacco, chronic maternal diseases, environmental toxins, and other exposures. The fetus can suffer damage very early in pregnancy (3 days after a missed period), even before a woman knows she is pregnant. Because approximately half of the pregnancies in the United States are unintended (Finer and Zolna, 2011), achieving good health for all women throughout their reproductive years—preconception health—can help ensure optimal fetal health and development should pregnancy occur. Healthy lifestyle measures for women (regardless of their intent to become pregnant) include maintaining a healthy weight and good nutrition; tending to chronic medical problems such as diabetes and hypertension; being up to date on vaccinations; avoiding environmental toxins; decreasing stress and eliminating abusive relationships; and avoiding illicit drugs, tobacco, and alcohol. Effective contraception can help women avoid unintended pregnancies and lengthen pregnancy spacing. Close pregnancy spacing (less than 18 months apart) may increase the likelihood of low birth weight, preterm birth, and placental problems (Conde-Agudelo et al., 2006). Preconception health focuses on taking steps in the present to ensure the health of future children and considering effective contraception if pregnancy is not desired.

Simple measures such as consuming 400 micrograms of the B vitamin folic acid every day for at least a month before becoming pregnant and during pregnancy can help decrease the likelihood of defects of the brain and spine, known as *neural tube defects,* by 50% to 70% (Wolff et al., 2009). Some foods, such as leafy vegetables, bananas, and beans, are naturally high in folic acid. Other foods, including breads, cereals, flours, cornmeal, pastas, rice, and select grain products, are enriched with folic acid as required by the U.S. Food and Drug Administration.

Prenatal Care

Obtaining early and regular prenatal care enhances a woman's chance of delivering a healthy, term baby. **Prenatal care** includes client education, risk identification, and monitoring and treatment of symptoms. It also includes referral to health, nutrition, childbirth education, and social service programs that can help a woman optimize her chances for a healthy pregnancy. Until the late twentieth century, prenatal care was seen as the best solution for improving birth outcomes. But even with expansions in the Medicaid program to cover health care for increasing numbers of low-income pregnant women and infants and significant federal, state, and local investments, poor pregnancy outcomes have persisted, especially for non-Hispanic black, American Indian, and Puerto Rican women.

Although prenatal care is not the *only* solution to reducing infant mortality, comprehensive prenatal care can improve the identification of specific and treatable causes of infant morbidity and mortality, such as maternal anemia, diabetes, hypertension, urinary tract infections, sexually transmitted infections, and poor nutrition. Ideally, such counseling and treatment of chronic health conditions should begin before a woman becomes pregnant. Optimal health throughout her life, including treatment of chronic health conditions and the adaptation of a healthy lifestyle, will have far more of an impact on healthy pregnancy than prenatal care alone.

Prenatal Substance Use

Tobacco, alcohol, and illicit drug use are social factors that affect the health of women and their children. During pregnancy, substance use profoundly affects the neurological and physical development of the fetus. The use of these substances, in any combination, is dangerous to a woman's health and worsens infant health and development outcomes.

Tobacco

Smoking tobacco during pregnancy is one of the most preventable causes of infant morbidity and mortality. The adverse health effects of tobacco use during pregnancy are well documented; they include low birth weight, prematurity, stillbirth, intrauterine growth retardation, premature rupture of membranes, placenta previa, placental abruption, neurodevelopmental impairment, and SIDS (USDHHS, 2010). Cigarette smoke contains more than 2500 chemicals. The fetal effects of most of these chemicals are unknown. What is known, however, is that when a pregnant woman inhales cigarette smoke, the oxygen supply to her fetus is disrupted by nicotine and carbon monoxide. Nicotine crosses the placenta and becomes concentrated in fetal blood and amniotic fluid. Nicotine concentrations in the fetus of a smoking woman can be as much as 15% higher than maternal levels. Secondhand smoke exposure also is dangerous to the fetus and newborn. It is linked to SIDS, decreased respiratory functioning, and childhood asthma. Pregnant women who are exposed to secondhand smoke have higher odds of giving birth to low-birth-weight babies than women who are not exposed to secondhand smoke during pregnancy (CDC, 2016a).

An estimated 10% of women report smoking during the last 3 months of pregnancy. Teenagers and young women have the highest rates of maternal smoking (Curtin and Mathews, 2016). The elimination of tobacco use among pregnant women would significantly reduce the rates of low-birth-weight infants, preterm delivery, intrauterine growth restriction, and infant mortality. Quitting is very difficult because the nicotine in tobacco is addictive, but quitting is best. Merely reducing cigarette use during pregnancy may not be enough to benefit the fetus because women who cut back tend to inhale more deeply or take more puffs to get an equivalent amount of nicotine.

The need for widespread implementation of smoking cessation programs for women in the childbearing years is clear. Many smoking cessation programs have been developed and implemented by national, state, and local governments and organizations. Because pregnant women who have received even brief smoking cessation counseling are more likely to quit smoking, the nurse should offer evidence-based smoking cessation interventions to the pregnant smoker at the first prenatal visit and throughout the pregnancy (Lumley et al., 2009; Tong et al., 2008).

Alcohol and Illicit Drugs

The use of alcohol and illicit drugs is a major risk factor for poor infant outcomes. Alcohol exposure during pregnancy can lead to fetal alcohol syndrome and other **fetal alcohol spectrum disorders (FASDs).** FASDs range from mild, subtle learning disabilities to severe learning disabilities. Children with FASDs are at risk for psychiatric problems, criminal behavior, unemployment, and incomplete education. Many children with FASDs also have physical abnormalities, growth deficiencies, and central nervous system disorders. *No level of alcohol intake has been determined to be safe during pregnancy, and there is no safe time to drink during pregnancy.* Women who are pregnant or who may become pregnant should abstain from drinking alcohol (CDC, 2018).

An estimated 10.2% of pregnant women drink during their pregnancies. Binge drinking, which is defined for women as four or more drinks on an occasion in the past 30 days, is especially harmful to fetal development. About 3.1% of pregnant women report binge drinking (CDC, 2015a). There is a compelling need for research on intervention strategies that can help prevent alcohol-exposed pregnancies.

Like alcohol, illicit drugs can cause permanent harm to an unborn baby. Current illicit drug use, including marijuana/hashish, cocaine (including crack), heroin, hallucinogens, and inhalants or prescription-type psychotherapeutics used non-medically among pregnant women has remained constant at 5.9% despite efforts of prevention and education programs (Substance Abuse and Mental Health Services Administration [SAMHSA], 2013). Risks to the baby include prematurity, low birth weight, birth defects, newborn withdrawal symptoms, and learning and behavioral problems. Substance use is often a sign of more complex psychosocial problems, such as depression, poverty, abuse, and violence. Illicit drug use often goes hand in hand with other maternal risks, including tobacco and alcohol use, poor nutrition, intimate partner violence, and risk of sexually transmitted infections. Surveys now indicate that many pregnant women *do* understand the negative impact of substance use during pregnancy and cut back or stop use but then rapidly resume use after pregnancy. Evidence-based public health measures are needed to further reduce substance use during pregnancy and to prevent postpartum resumption.

Because of serious potential risks to the developing fetus, women who are pregnant or who could become pregnant should be asked about substance use and counseled to abstain from alcohol, tobacco, and the use of illicit drugs, through the use of evidence-based practices. For women who already use alcohol, tobacco, and illicit drugs, a comprehensive and long-lasting approach to treatment is required.

Breast-feeding

Breastfeeding is a natural and beneficial source of nutrition and provides the healthiest start for an infant. In addition to the nutritional benefits, breastfeeding promotes a unique and emotional connection between mother and baby.
(American Academy of Pediatrics, 2012)

The American Academy of Pediatrics (AAP) recommends exclusive breast-feeding for about the first 6 months of a baby's life, followed by breast-feeding in combination with the introduction of complementary foods until at least 12 months of age, and continuation of breast-feeding for as long as mutually desired by mother and baby. Breast-feeding has many advantages for the mother, for the baby, and for society. The cells, hormones, and antibodies in breast milk protect babies from illness such as infections and lower the childhood risk of asthma, obesity, diabetes, and SIDS. For mothers, breast-feeding is linked to a lower risk of breast and ovarian cancer and type 2 diabetes (Chowdhury et al., 2015). Breast-feeding can save more than $1500 per year in formula and supplies, and even more in the costs of infant illness (Womenshealth.gov, n.d.).

Initiation of breast-feeding occurs in about 77% of hospital births. Maternity practices that discourage separation of mothers and their babies have helped boost these rates, but more attention is required to meet AAP recommendations. The breast-feeding initiation rate for Hispanic infants is 80% compared with 75% for white infants and 60% for black infants. Only about 24% of infants are being breast-fed by 12 months. The prevalence is 12% for black infants. Black infants have the lowest rates of breast-feeding initiation and duration (CDC, 2013). This gap points to the need to understand and act upon barriers to breast-feeding that are unique to black women.

The *2011 Surgeon General's Call to Action to Support Breastfeeding* suggests actions aimed at increasing societal support for breast-feeding women. These suggestions call on communities, employers, health care providers, governments, and nonprofit organizations to implement strategies to support breast-feeding (U.S. Department of Health and Human Services [USDHHS], Office of the Surgeon General, 2011). There are many community sources of support for breast-feeding mothers, and nurses can play a key role in linking breast-feeding mothers with help if it is needed. In addition to nurses, health professionals such as **lactation consultants, childbirth educators,** physicians, trained home visitors, and doulas can provide assistance. Peer support groups such as La Leche League and breast-feeding centers can also be helpful. The federally supported Women, Infants, and Children (WIC) program also provides counseling and support for breast-feeding mothers.

Sudden Unexplained Infant Death

Sudden unexplained infant death (SUID) is defined as death in an infant less than 1 year of age that occurs suddenly and unexpectedly, the cause of which is not immediately obvious before investigation. About 4500 infants die each year from SUID. Later investigation may reveal death in infants with SUID to be from poisoning, metabolic disorders, hyperthermia or hypothermia, neglect and homicide, and suffocation. About half of the infants who die from SUID die from SIDS, defined as the sudden death of an infant less than 1 year of age that cannot be explained after a thorough investigation is conducted, including a complete autopsy, examination of the death scene, and review of the clinical history. SIDS is the third leading cause of infant mortality. Non-Hispanic black and American Indian/Alaska Native infants are far more likely to die from SIDS than infants of other races (CDC, 2017a).

In 1994, with the recognition that placing infants on their backs for sleep lowered SIDS rates, the federal government, along with private entities, launched the successful Back to Sleep Campaign to heighten awareness of the safety of positioning infants on their backs for sleep. Since 1994, SIDS deaths have declined by more than 50% (CDC, 2017a) (Box 16.3). More has been learned about other factors that can lower the risk of SIDS. In 2012, the AAP released new guidelines for safe sleeping environments (AAP, 2011). Drawing from the success of Back to Sleep, the Safe to Sleep campaign was launched to educate parents, caregivers, and health care providers about ways to reduce the risk of infant death from SIDS as well as death from known sleep-related causes, such as suffocation.

BOX 16.3   "Safe to Sleep" Public Education Campaign

Recommendations to reduce the risk of sudden infant death syndrome (SIDS) and sleep-related causes of infant death: Always place a baby on his or her back to sleep, both for naps and at night.

- Use a firm sleep surface, covered by a fitted sheet.
- Your baby should not sleep in an adult bed, on a couch, or on a chair alone, with you, or with anyone else.
- Keep soft objects, toys, and loose bedding out of your baby's sleep area.
- Do not smoke during pregnancy, and do not smoke or allow smoking around your baby.
- Breast-feed your baby.
- Do not let your baby get too hot during sleep.
- Follow health care provider guidance on your baby's vaccines and regular health checkups.
- Avoid products that claim to reduce the risk of SIDS and other sleep-related causes of infant death.
- Get regular health care during pregnancy, and do not smoke, drink alcohol, or use illegal drugs during pregnancy or after the baby is born.

From National Institute of Child Health & Human Development: *Safe sleep for your baby* (NIH Pub. No. 12-7040), 2013. Retrieved from https://www.nichd.nih.gov/publications/pubs/Documents/STS_SafeSleepForYourBaby_General_2013.pdf

---

? ACTIVE LEARNING

1. Examine infant mortality statistics in the community, and compare the rates with state and national averages. Is infant mortality higher for any particular racial or ethnic group within the community?
2. Determine how a non–English-speaking immigrant without finances or available transportation would obtain prenatal care.
3. Accompany a pregnant woman to a local department of social services and observe as she tries to establish Medicaid eligibility for herself and her unborn child.
4. Survey businesses in the community to determine whether they offer maternity health insurance benefits, paid or unpaid maternity or paternity leave, and leave for prenatal care appointments. Is there a location within each worksite where women can pump breast milk? Use this information to develop a strategy to encourage family-friendly policies and practices in the business community.

CHILDHOOD HEALTH ISSUES

At all ages, appropriate and timely medical care plays an important role in children's health status. However, other factors, including parental influences, nutrition, environment, community safety, and the overall quality of home life, exert even stronger influences over a child's well-being. Childhood is generally a healthy time of life, as evidenced by the improvement in many indicators of child health status over the past century. For example, the incidence of childhood disease has diminished because the majority of children receive a full complement of immunizations during infancy and toddlerhood.

The causes of childhood death vary with age. Parents and the community have important responsibilities in promoting healthy lifestyles, creating safe environments, and ensuring access to medical care. They must take steps to protect children from the leading threats to children's health (i.e., accidental injury and exposure to environmental toxins, abuse, and violence).

🧬 NEWBORN SCREENING

Newborn screening checks for rare but serious health conditions shortly after birth. Often babies with certain health disorders appear healthy at birth; thus all babies are tested for selected conditions that can be treated if they are identified early. Babies can be screened for blood, heart, and hearing conditions.

Screening can be conducted in three ways. Blood screening is conducted by collecting a few drops of blood from the newborn's heel. This sample is tested at a laboratory, and parents are notified of abnormalities. Hearing screening requires that a tiny, soft speaker be placed in the baby's ear to see how the baby responds to sound. Heart screening uses pulse oximetry to evaluate the baby for congenital heart disease.

Newborn screening is state based, and the number of conditions that babies are screened for varies from state to state. All U.S. states and territories currently test for 26 health conditions, including phenylketonuria, galactosemia, congenital hypothyroidism, and sickle cell disease.

Modified from March of Dimes: *Newborn screening*, n.d. Retrieved from https://www.marchofdimes.org/baby/newborn-screening-tests-for-your-baby.aspx http://www.marchofdimes.com/baby/newborn-screening.aspx.

This clinic provides services through the Early and Periodic Screening, Diagnosis, and Treatment (EPSDT) Program, which was developed to provide health care for children in low-income families receiving Medicaid.

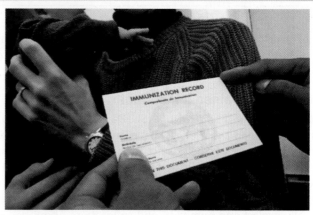

Reviewing immunization records is an important primary prevention role for the community health nurse. This is a teachable opportunity for the nurse to stress the importance of maintaining immunizations for the child. In California parents are provided with a yellow state immunization record for the child, which they should use to record all immunizations and to show proof of immunizations when needed.

The nurse has an opportunity to observe the client and the family as they register and wait for their appointment. The parent registers the 5-year-old daughter for a school entry health physical examination. Medicaid insurance is verified for the physical.

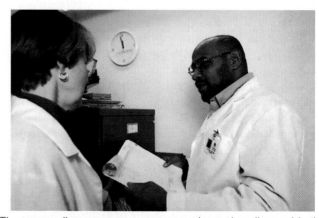

The nurse discusses any concerns about the client with the practitioner before the examination.

Trust can be established in a short time. The nurse can begin by explaining the steps in the clinic process so that the client knows what is expected. The nurse should always listen to the client attentively and should allow enough time for the client to reflect and respond to questions.

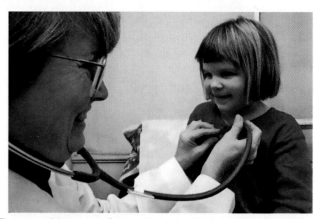

The practitioner performs the physical examination of the child with the help of the parent. The practitioner discusses the result of the vision test with the parent and the need for a follow-up appointment with an ophthalmologist. The child has not undergone a blood lead measurement and requires booster immunizations. The practitioner orders laboratory tests, immunizations, and a referral to an ophthalmologist.

COMMUNITY HEALTH VISIT—cont'd

The clinic staff performs the laboratory work: hematocrit, urinary analysis, and lead measurement. The immunization consent forms have been signed by the parent. The nurse administers the immunizations and takes this opportunity to reinforce the importance of immunizations for both children.

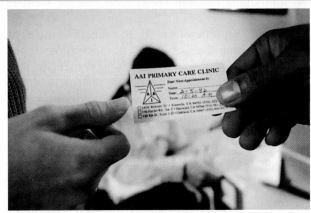

The community health nurse gives the parent a business card with the nurse's name and the agency's address and phone number. The nurse advises the parent to call the nurse if there is anything else that the family may need.

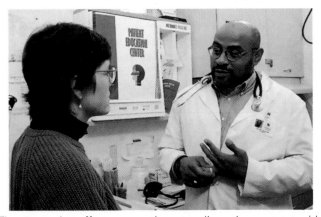

The nurse also offers suggestions to relieve the common side effects of immunizations.

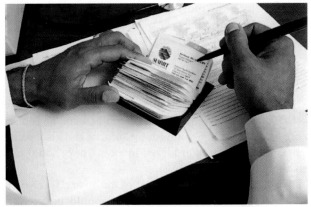

The nurse searches for resources for an ophthalmologist and a family planning clinic that accept Medicaid and a resource for day care providers. The nurse obtains phone numbers for a couple of ophthalmologists, a family planning clinic, and a day care consortium service.

The parent asks about an ophthalmologist who takes Medicaid and about day care facilities in the area for the younger child. The parent also asks about family planning services in the community.

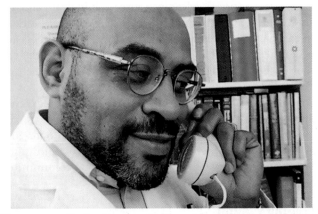

The nurse calls the family with the referrals for an ophthalmologist and a phone number to obtain a list of day care providers.

Story by Leonard Kaku, RN, MSN. Photography by George Draper.

Accidental Injuries

Infants and young children are at great risk for accidental injuries. They are curious and eager to explore their environments, but they often lack the coordination and cognitive abilities to keep themselves safe from harm. Their small size and developing bones and muscles make them especially susceptible to injury. The leading cause of injury death for children younger than 1 year is accidental suffocation due to choking or strangulation. Unintentional injury is the leading cause of death for children ages 1 to 14. For children younger than 5, drowning is the leading cause of death. From 5 to 14 years, motor vehicle–related injuries are the cause of most deaths. Low-income and minority children suffer disproportionately from accidental injuries. They are more likely to sustain injuries and more likely to die from their injuries. For example, Native American children are more than twice as likely to experience accidental injury as their white counterparts (Safe Kids USA, 2013).

Many accidents can be avoided by improving the safety of a child's environment. Ensuring a child's safety in a motor vehicle is critical. The most important steps that a parent can take to ensure a child's safety in a motor vehicle is to correctly secure the child into a car seat based on the child's age and size. The safest place for all children younger than 13 years to ride is in the back seat, regardless of weight and height (National Highway Traffic Safety Administration, 2013). Leaving children unattended in a motor vehicle is another safety concern. In only a few minutes a car can become hot enough to cause heat stroke in a youngster. Children can also become entrapped in a car trunk or locked in a car. They should never be left alone in a car.

Smoke alarms should be installed on every level of the home and in bedrooms. Escape plans should be practiced often. Small children can drown in as little as an inch of water. Toilets, buckets, bathtubs, and pools are all potential drowning hazards. Storage of medications and hazardous substances and playground safety are also important safety education topics.

Finally, head injury from cycling and other wheeled sports, such as skateboarding, is a leading cause of child death and disability. Without proper head protection, a fall from as little as 2 feet can cause traumatic brain injury. The use of helmets and proper protective equipment can substantially reduce the risk of injuries. Box 16.4 discusses how toys can be another threat to small children.

Low-income parents may have difficulty affording safety equipment such as safety latches for cabinets, smoke alarms, car seats, and helmets. The grassroots coalition Safe Kids USA can help link parents and professionals to child injury prevention advocacy and events in local communities (Safe Kids USA, 2013).

Unhealthy Weight

Childhood obesity has become a health crisis in the United States. The rate of obesity has more than doubled in children and tripled in adolescents since the 1970s, but has leveled off in the past decade. An estimated one-third of children are

---

BOX 16.4 Toy-Related Injuries

Although most toys are safe, children are at risk for toy-related injuries and death. Approximately 168,000 children younger than 14 years are treated in hospital emergency departments for toy-related injuries. Though the majority of toy-related injuries are minor, permanent disability can occur. Riding toys, such as nonmotorized scooters and tricycles, are associated with more injuries than any other toy group.

Laws and regulations have been put into place to protect children from toy injuries. An example is the Federal Hazardous Substances Act, which bans children's toys that contain any hazardous substance, such as lead. The Child Safety Protection Act of 1994 was designed to reduce toy-related choking and requires manufacturers to place choking hazard warning labels on balloons, marbles, small balls, and games with small parts intended for use only by children 3 years and older. The act also requires manufacturers, importers, distributors, and retailers to report choking incidents involving such products to the Consumer Product Safety Commission. The U.S. Department of Commerce requires toy guns to be distinguished from real guns. In addition, the toy industry has established voluntary safety standards to minimize risk of injury.

Although regulations and laws are helpful, parents and caretakers must also provide adequate supervision of children and must adopt strategies recommended to prevent toy-related injuries, as follows: use only age-appropriate toys; use Mylar balloons instead of latex (which can cause children to choke or suffocate); purchase a "small parts" tester to determine whether small toys pose choking hazards; check the website of the U.S. Consumer Product Safety Commission (www.cpsc.gov) to obtain information on toy recalls; follow age and safety recommendations on toy labels; and ensure that toys are used in a safe and proper environment.

Data from Safe Kids USA: *Preventing accidental injury: Toy safety.* Retrieved from https://www.safekids.org/safetytips/field_risks/toy-safety?gclid=EAIaIQobChMI16TRze7I2AIVVyOBCh1HPQyXEAAYAiAAEgIWQfD_BwE /

---

overweight or obese Ogden et al., 2014). Children who are overweight are more likely to experience cardiovascular disease, diabetes, bone and joint disease, and sleep apnea and to face social discrimination that can lead to poor self-esteem and depression.

Obesity prevalence is higher among Hispanic (21.9%) and non-Hispanic black (19.5%) children and adolescents than among non-Hispanic white children (14.7%) (Ogden et al., 2015). Minority groups, those with less income, and those with lower education levels are more likely to be overweight. The higher cost and unavailability of healthy foods, food insecurity, and the lack of access to safe places to exercise contribute to obesity in lower-income communities (Widome et al., 2009).

The *body mass index* (BMI) is a screening tool calculated from a person's weight and height that can be used to determine whether the person is underweight, of normal weight, overweight, or obese. BMI can be calculated in children from as young as 2 years to teenage with the use of age- and sex-specific growth charts. BMI does not calculate actual body fat percentage, but it is an easy and inexpensive method that can identify weight problems (CDC, 2015c).

A number of factors contribute to childhood obesity. The typical American diet, which is both high in fat and calories and low in nutrients, has resulted in an increase in obesity. Widely available fast food, increasing portion sizes, the presence of vending machines in schools, availability of sugar-sweetened drinks, and the eating of fewer meals at home have contributed to the trend. Modern technologies such as electronic games and television, a lack of safe convenient outdoor exercise areas, and readily accessible transportation have also led to more sedentary lifestyles.

In some urban neighborhoods where high concentrations of people living in poverty are prevalent, there may be little to no access to fresh, nutritious, affordable foods, which also contributes to obesity. Such neighborhoods are called *food deserts*. Residents are limited to obtaining food from convenience stores and fast-food restaurants rather than from grocery stores and fresh food markets; nutritious foods are not available.

Nurses can play a leading role in generating public awareness of factors that contribute to obesity and can focus on preventive measures such as healthy lifestyles and physical activity. For example, breast-feeding provides some protection against later obesity. At least 60 minutes of moderately strenuous exercise is recommended for children most days of the week. Nurses can design and implement nutrition, healthy eating, and physical activities policies and standards in schools; take part in initiatives that make fresh, healthy foods available to all; and challenge policy makers and industry leaders such as fast-food restaurants to mobilize resources for good nutrition and fitness.

Immunization

Childhood immunization is a benchmark of child health. Maintaining appropriate immunization protects all members of the community, especially immune-compromised individuals and pregnant women, who are particularly vulnerable to certain infectious diseases. Adequate immunization protects children against several diseases that kill or disable many children. Poliomyelitis, a crippling disease of the past, has been eliminated in the United States thanks to the public health effort that made the polio vaccine accessible and affordable. Over the ensuing decades, new vaccines have been developed, and children can now be protected from more than 14 vaccine-preventable diseases. State laws requiring proof of vaccination before entry to school or child care have helped ensure high vaccination levels in the population.

Vaccine-preventable disease levels are at or near record lows, but many children and adolescents remain underimmunized. Concerns about the frequency and timing of vaccines and widespread fears that childhood vaccines are linked to autism have prevented some parents from vaccinating their children (Institute of Medicine, 2013). In 2009, however, the U.S. Court of Federal Claims ruled that childhood vaccines do not cause autism. This ruling was consistent with 18 major scientific studies that failed to show a link between vaccines and autism (U.S. Court of Federal Claims, n.d.). Nurses can help educate community members about the safety of vaccines and recommended vaccination schedules and about the consequences of undervaccination. The following vaccines are recommended for children and adolescents (CDC, 2017b):

- Tetanus, diphtheria, acellular pertussis
- Inactivated polio
- Rotavirus
- Influenza
- Measles, mumps, and rubella vaccine
- Hepatitis A vaccine
- Hepatitis B vaccine
- Varicella (chickenpox) vaccine
- *Haemophilus influenzae* type b (Hib)
- Pneumococcal conjugate
- Human papillomavirus vaccine (males and females)
- Meningococcal conjugate

Most insurance plans cover the cost of childhood vaccines, and the Affordable Care Act (ACA) required new insurance plans to eliminate copays and deductibles for preventive services such as vaccinations. Another source of assistance is the Vaccines For Children program, a federally funded program that provides vaccines at no cost to children who might not otherwise be vaccinated because of inability to pay.

Environmental Concerns

Potential threats to the health of children sometimes exist in their living environments. Threats can be found in the air, in the water, and from toxic exposures to chemicals. For example, air pollution, poor indoor air quality, and secondhand smoke can cause or trigger childhood asthma. Asthma is one of the most common chronic childhood disorders, affecting an estimated 6.3 million (8.6%) children in 2014 (CDC, 2017). Lead—a neurotoxin that can sometimes be found in drinking water (often from lead pipes and fittings), in old paint dust or chips that crumble from walls on older housing units, and in contaminated soil—is a cause of cognitive and behavioral problems, decreased growth, and neurological disabilities. The reduction of childhood blood lead levels is among the greatest public health stories of the latter half of the twentieth century, but unfortunately lead is still a threat. Although lead is banned from the manufacture of paint, many millions of housing units in the United States still contain lead-based paint. Most of these units are located in poor, inner-city neighborhoods. Despite dramatic declines in blood lead levels for most U.S. populations, levels remain high among children in low-income families who live in older housing with lead-based paint. Treatment for children with elevated blood lead values is long and difficult and carries risks. Better prevention, elimination of risks in the environment (particularly in older housing units), more efficient tracking, and education of the public are essential to further reduce the menace of **lead poisoning**.

Exposure to toxic cleaning products, pesticides, medicines, and herbicides is another area of concern. Simple steps can help protect children from accidental exposures, including child-resistant packaging, cabinet safety latches, and careful supervision.

Child Maltreatment

Child maltreatment refers to all types of abuse and neglect of a child under age 18 by a parent, caregiver, or another person in a custodial role (Leeb et al., 2008), and is another indicator of children's physical and emotional health status. Almost five children die every day in the United States from child abuse and neglect. The reported number of child deaths from abuse and neglect increased to 1670 in 2017 from 1580 in 2014. Of note, nearly 50% of child abuse victims are under 1 year of age (USDHHS Administration for Children and Families, 2017).

Child abuse may be physical, sexual, or emotional. Neglect is by far the most prevalent form of child maltreatment. *Child neglect* is the failure to provide for a child's basic physical, medical, emotional, or educational needs or to protect a child from harm or potential harm. It may include failure to provide affection, warmth, understanding, and supervision adequate for healthy development (USDHHS, Administration for Children and Families, Administration on Children, Youth and Families, Children's Bureau, 2017).

Child maltreatment affects children of all races, ages, and ethnicities. Factors that place children at a higher risk for maltreatment include living in a family that is stressed by drug and alcohol abuse, poverty, chronic health problems, violence in the community or at home, and social isolation (USDHHS Administration for Children and Families, 2017).

There are many long-term effects of child abuse and neglect. The effects may be physical, such as brain damage in shaken baby syndrome; emotional, such as depression and low self-esteem; and behavioral, such as delinquency, promiscuity, eating disorders, poor academic achievement, and drug abuse. Extreme stress caused by abuse and neglect interferes with normal brain development, harming the basic architecture of the brain. Healthy brain development relies on consistent, reciprocal, and appropriate interactions between young children and their caretakers. Chronic deprivation of healthy, reciprocal interactions can lead to the persistent activation of the stress response, leading to poor academic achievement, low self-esteem, depression, promiscuity, drug abuse, and chronic health problems (Center on the Developing Child at Harvard University, 2012).

Often, the perpetrators of maltreatment are parents, who themselves were victims, forming a cycle of abuse. The two dominant characteristics of abusive parents are a history of substance abuse and abuse from their own parents. Often, caretakers do not intend to hurt their children. They may be stressed by poverty, illness, or disability, and they may lack social support systems or coping skills. Young and inexperienced parents may not understand the physical, emotional, and behavioral needs of their children.

Children are never responsible for the harm done to them by others, and yet they may feel guilty for causing it. Many professionals, including nurses, social service workers, and teachers, are required by law to report child abuse. Nurses in the community must understand their ethical and legal obligations to report child maltreatment. They can also help create a climate that supports families and provides parents with alternatives to abusive behavior. Programs for parents can take many different forms. Positive parenting skills are at the core of such programs. Positive parenting skills include responsiveness to the emotional and physical needs of children, good communication, and appropriate discipline. This education may occur in parents' homes, in schools, in medical or mental health clinics, or in other community settings. Nurse home visitors can be key in providing education. The ultimate goal is to prevent child maltreatment before it starts.

Children With Special Health Care Needs

Children and youth with special health care needs are those who are at risk or have chronic physical, developmental, behavioral, or emotional conditions that necessitate health and related services beyond those required by children generally. These conditions include developmental disorders such as Down syndrome and autism spectrum disorder, mental health disorders such as depression and anxiety, seizures, allergies, asthma, and attention-deficit/hyperactivity disorder (Child and Adolescent Health Measurement Initiative, 2012). Chronic conditions are those expected to last 12 months or more. Often children with special health care needs experience two or more chronic conditions (USDHHS, Health Resources and Services Administration, 2015).

Children with special health care needs frequently have multiple service needs, including public health; physical and mental health care; specialized diagnostic services; social services; and educational, vocational, and sometimes corrective services. Families trying to obtain care for children with special needs face challenges in dealing with differing eligibility criteria; duplication and gaps in services; inflexible funding sources; geographic, cultural, and financial barriers; and poor coordination of care. Children with special needs can benefit from a coordinated, comprehensive, integrated system of care—often called a medical home. A *medical home* is not a place, but, rather, an approach to providing care. Having a medical home strengthens the ability of children with multiple service needs to receive comprehensive care for complex conditions (Box 16.5).

The Individuals with Disabilities Education Act (IDEA), enacted by Congress in 1975, is intended to ensure that children with disabilities receive a free, appropriate public education. The law has been amended many times and addresses the needs of babies through school-age children. IDEA is known as the nation's "special education law" and is administered through the U.S. Department of Education (n.d.).

ADOLESCENT HEALTH ISSUES

Adolescence is a time of generally good health. It is a period when preteens and teens form lifelong health habits, including dietary and exercise habits and emotional health skills such as problem solving and coping strategies. Typically, adolescents do not use health services unless they have an underlying chronic condition or an acute illness. They rarely use preventive health services.

BOX 16.5 The Patient-Centered Medical Home

The American Academy of Family Physicians (AAFP), American Academy of Pediatrics (AAP), American College of Physicians (ACP), and the American Osteopathic Association have long endorsed the concept of a "medical home." This ideal suggests that every child, including special needs children, should have "accessible, continuous, comprehensive, family-centered, coordinated, culturally effective and compassionate" health care (AAP, 1992).

A medical home should be within a community-based system that has coordinated networks designed to promote the healthy development and well-being of children as they move from adolescence to adulthood. Such a system requires appropriate financing to support and sustain quality care, optimal outcomes, family satisfaction, and cost-efficiency (AAP, 1992, n.d.).

In their struggle to gain independence, many adolescents engage in risk-taking behaviors, including alcohol and drug abuse, tobacco use, early and unprotected sexual activity, unsafe driving, and participation in delinquent and violent activities that threaten their health. Such behaviors are influenced by peers, the family, and characteristics of communities in which they live. Risk taking among adolescents is greatly influenced by their ability to control their impulses at this stage of brain development. The part of the brain that is responsible for executive functioning, the prefrontal cortex, is not fully mature until near age 25. Even though a teen may understand that a behavior is risky, he or she may have difficulty "putting on the brakes" because of the immaturity of brain development and connections (USDHHS, Office of Population Affairs, 2013).

Traditional approaches to improving adolescent health have focused on specific risks; however, a collaborative, multipartner approach that centers on the strengths of the whole person in the community, rather than focusing on individual risks, may be more effective in helping adolescents avoid risks and develop social competence. The community health nurse can help parents and communities understand the nonmedical, public health nature of risky behaviors and can assist in the development of community-wide strategies to effectively deal with them. The Youth Risk Behavior Surveillance System (YRBSS), administered by the CDC's Division of Adolescent and School Health, monitors health risk behaviors in ninth through twelfth graders that lead to morbidity and mortality (Khann et al., 2016).

Sexual Risk Behavior

One of many risk-taking adolescent behaviors is sexual intercourse. Adolescent sexual activity is often unprotected and can result in unintended pregnancy, infection with HIV, and other sexually transmitted infections (STIs).

Among students surveyed in 2015, about 41.2% had ever had sexual intercourse. Nearly 30.1% had engaged in sexual intercourse during the 3 months preceding the survey. Of these, 56.9% reported that either they or their partner had used a condom during last sexual intercourse. Another 26.8% used another form of birth control, such as birth control pills, an injectable form of birth control, a birth control ring, an implant, or an intrauterine device to prevent pregnancy. Nearly 14% used

no method of birth control during the last sexual intercourse. Of consequence, 20.6% had used alcohol or drugs before last sexual intercourse (Khann et al., 2016).

🔲 RESEARCH HIGHLIGHTS

Does a Satisfactory Relationship With Her Mother Influence When a 16-Year-Old Female Begins to Have Sex?

A prospective panel study of more than 1500 female adolescents (not randomly selected) examined whether the dimensions within the mother–daughter relationship during young adolescence influenced sexual initiation prior to age 16 years. Researchers found that three dimensions within the relationship were associated with delayed sexual initiation: positive cohesion, communication, and satisfaction with time spent together. The researchers concluded that efforts in delaying sexual initiation in young adolescents need to be directed toward promoting positive mother–daughter relationships.

Data from Kovar C, Salsberry P: Does a satisfactory relationship with her mother influence when a 16-year-old begins to have sex? *MCN Am J Matern Child Nurs* 37(2):122–129, 2012.

Teen childbearing has been on the decline since the late 1950s, reaching a historic low at 22.3 births per 1000 women aged 15 to 19 years (Martin et al., 2017). In recent years, teens seem to be less sexually active, and more of those who are sexually active seem to be using birth control than in previous years (Martinez and Abma, 2015). Despite the declines in teen childbearing, the U.S. adolescent birth rate remains one of the highest among industrialized nations (Ventura et al., 2014). Large disparities exist among racial and ethnic groups. The teen pregnancy rate is lowest among Asian and Pacific Islanders and highest among Hispanic teenagers (Hamilton et al., 2015).

The consequences of early childbearing on mothers, children, and society are significant. Teen childbearing contributes greatly to high school dropout rates. Only half of teen mothers receive a high school diploma by 22 years of age, compared with approximately 90% of girls who did not give birth during adolescence (Perper et al., 2010). For the infant, having a teenage mother poses serious health risks, including death, prematurity, low birth weight, and social risks, such as lower school achievement, incarceration, teen pregnancy, and adult unemployment. Children born to teenage parents have lower school achievement and are more likely to drop out of high school. They are more likely to be incarcerated at some time during adolescence, father children as teenagers, require public assistance, and face unemployment as young adults. According to an analysis by the National Campaign to Prevent Teen Pregnancy, the estimated national cost of teen childbearing in the United States for taxpayers (federal, state, and local) is at least $9.4 billion per year (National Campaign to Prevent Teen and Unplanned Pregnancy, 2015).

STIs are another consequence of sexual risk behavior. These include human papillomavirus (HPV), *Chlamydia trachomatis*, herpes simplex virus type 2, HIV/AIDS, hepatitis B, gonorrhea, syphilis, and vaginal trichomoniasis. Teenagers are more likely than adults to acquire STIs (CDC, 2016b). For some infections, such as *C. trachomatis*, the difference may be due to a physiological susceptibility. Barriers to health care such as lack of transportation, concerns about confidentiality, and lack of access to preventive health services also contribute to a higher prevalence of STIs among teens. STIs may be asymptomatic in both males and females. Although many STIs clear on their own, others can persist over time, putting women at high risk for cervical cancer, pelvic inflammatory disease, ectopic pregnancy, and infertility. Not only is a woman's health affected, especially if the infections go untreated, but the infant born to a woman with an STI is at risk of infection and can suffer long-term consequences. Routine counseling and voluntary testing for sexually active teens and pregnant women is recommended. The HPV vaccination can protect against related disease and is the best way to prevent many types of cancer. The HPV vaccine is recommended for preteen girls and boys at age 11 or 12 years (CDC, 2015b).

The causes and effects of risky sexual behaviors are complex, and the solutions are multifaceted. One survey found that most parents feel they play an important role in providing guidance to their children about healthy sexual behavior, yet half of children are uncomfortable with these conversations. Parents who were surveyed overwhelmingly support school-based sex education programs, including information about birth control (Planned Parenthood, 2012).

Abstinence from vaginal, anal, and oral intercourse is the only 100% effective way to prevent HIV, other STIs, and pregnancy. Primary prevention models are most successful when they are evidence based and tailored to the community's individual needs. Components of such programs can include the following:

- Abstinence promotion
- Education about contraception and its availability
- Sex education
- Character development
- Problem-solving skill development
- Peer counseling programs
- Strategies for ensuring teenagers' school success
- Job training

Such efforts are more likely to succeed when there are partnerships among parents, adolescents, and agencies for health, education, religion, social service, and government. Nurses working within such organizations can play leadership roles in developing community programs for prevention of adolescent sexual risk behaviors.

Violence

Youth violence can be seen as a reflection of how well parents, schools, and the community are able to supervise and channel youth behavior in positive ways. Children and adolescents can be victims of, aggressors in, or witnesses to violence. For the victims, violence can cause both emotional and physical harm. For too many of the nation's youth, violence is a way of life, a way of coping with challenging and difficult situations, and a significant public health problem.

The rate of serious violent crime against youth ages 12 to 17 years declined 77% between 1994 and 2010. In 2010,

male (14.3 victimizations per 1000) and female (13.7 per 1000) youth were equally likely to experience serious violent crime—rape or sexual assault, robbery, and aggravated assault. Black males are the racial group most likely to be victimized (White and Lauritsen, 2012). Homicide is the third leading cause of death for young people ages 15 to 24 years. Of victims in 2014, 86% were killed with a firearm (CDC, 2016c). Handguns are readily accessible to America's youth. Federal law prohibits anyone under age 21 years from purchasing a handgun from a licensed dealer, but it does not prohibit anyone under age 21 years from purchasing a handgun from a nonlicensed dealer (Law Center to Prevent Gun Violence, n.d.).

Teen dating violence consists of physical, sexual, or psychological/emotional violence (including stalking) within a dating relationship. In the 2015 Youth Risk Behavior Survey, 9.6% of high school students reported having been hit, slapped, or physically hurt on purpose by their boyfriend or girlfriend in the preceding 12 months (Khann et al., 2016). Teen dating violence can be emotionally and physically traumatizing and can lead to victimization and unhealthy relationships in the future.

Violence among youth is a complex public health problem with multifaceted risk factors. Risk factors include individual factors; influences by families and peers; and social, political, and cultural factors. The home environment is a key to the development of violent behavior in young people. Poor supervision of children and harsh physical punishment are associated with youth violence. Also linked to youth violence is associating with delinquent peers. At the social level, gang involvement, access to firearms, and drug use are more likely to increase youth violence (World Health Organization, 2016).

Teen violence does not have simple remedies. Solutions require community and neighborhood efforts to help young people diffuse anger and frustration before they escalate; to help parents, religious organizations, and schools assist their youth in managing anger and resolving conflicts; and to work with children and teenagers to assure them that they are loved, appreciated, and accepted for who they are. Reducing children's unsupervised exposure to guns, engaging communities in strengthening law enforcement, modifying the design of guns, and limiting the flow of illegal guns to youth are also strategies to reduce youth gun violence (Reich, 2002).

Tobacco, Alcohol, and Drug Use

The use of tobacco, alcohol, and illicit drugs has serious and long-lasting consequences for adolescents and for society. The YRBSS (Khann et al., 2016) provides a snapshot of behavioral trends. In 2015, the survey revealed the following:

- 10.8% of students had smoked cigarettes in the 30 days before the survey.
- 32.3% of students had ever tried cigarette smoking.
- 24.1% of students had used electronic vapor products in the 30 days before the survey.
- 44.9% of students had ever used electronic vapor products.
- 32.8% of students had had at least one drink of alcohol in the 30 days before the survey.

- 17.7% of students had had five or more drinks of alcohol in a row (i.e., within a couple of hours—also known as binge drinking) in the 30 days before the survey.
- 63.2% of students had had at least one drink of alcohol on at least 1 day during their lives (i.e., had ever drunk alcohol).
- 20.7% of students had taken prescription drugs (e.g., Oxy-Contin, Percocet, Vicodin, codeine, Adderall, Ritalin, or Xanax) without a doctor's prescription one or more times during their lives (i.e., had ever taken prescription drugs without a doctor's prescription).
- 38.6% of students had used marijuana one or more times during their lives (i.e., had ever used marijuana).
- 21.7% of students had used marijuana one or more times during the 30 days before the survey (i.e., current marijuana use).
- 9.2% of students had used synthetic marijuana one or more times during their lives.
- 21.7% of students had been offered, sold, or given an illegal drug by someone on school property during the 12 months before the survey.

Among the findings of the latest YRBSS survey are that smoking rates among teens have continued to decline since peaking in the mid-1990s. In contrast, illicit drug use by youths is constantly evolving as new drugs in new forms are introduced. "Designer drugs" or synthetic cannabinoids (aka "Spice" or "K2") have been banned in most states, but minor changes to the chemical makeup of these substances result in new substances that allow law breakers to circumvent existing drug laws (National Conference of State Legislatures, 2012; Sacco and Finklea, 2016). Also, prescription drugs used outside of medical supervision—for example, OxyContin, Ritalin, and steroids—have become more popular. Vaping prevalence grew rapidly from near-zero prevalence in 2011 to one of the most common forms of adolescent substance use. Despite a decline in 2016, the prevalence of vaping remains substantially higher than the use of any other tobacco product, including cigarettes (Johnston et al., 2017).

According to the Monitoring the Future Project of the University of Michigan, rumors of the supposed benefits of using a drug usually spread much faster than information about the adverse consequences. It generally takes much longer for evidence of adverse consequences, such as death, disease, overdose, and addictive potential, to become widely known, thus contributing to the widespread use of both legal and illegal drugs (Johnston et al, 2010).

Adolescence is a critical time to prevent substance addiction. Drugs change brains, and early use of drugs increases a person's chances of more serious drug abuse and addiction (National Institute on Drug Abuse, 2014). Broad evidence-based prevention efforts, including addressing the issues of housing, poverty, and crime, are needed.

FACTORS AFFECTING CHILD AND ADOLESCENT HEALTH

As in other age groups, social, nonmedical factors largely determine children's health. Children depend on their families or caregivers for their health and well-being; therefore the following factors significantly affect children's physical health, mental health, and overall well-being:

- Parents' or caregivers' income, education, and stability
- Security and safety of the home
- Nutritional and environmental issues
- Health care access and use

Poverty

Poverty is the greatest threat to child health. Child poverty in the United States is higher than in most other industrialized countries, and the rate is rising (National Center for Children in Poverty, 2017). About 15 million (21%) of the nation's children live below the federal poverty level (Jiang et al., 2017). The official poverty level is calculated by using poverty thresholds that are issued each year by the U.S. Census Bureau. The thresholds represent the annual amount of cash income minimally required to support families of various sizes. The 2017 poverty guideline for a family of three in the 48 contiguous states and the District of Columbia was $24,600 (USDHHS, 2017b). Many more children (about 43%) live in low-income families that are close to the poverty level and unable to meet basic living expenses. Children are far more likely than adults to live in poverty. Poverty rates are highest for black, Hispanic, and American Indian children (Jiang et al., 2017).

Factors associated with poverty include parental education, employment, and single parenting. Eighty-five percent of children whose parents do not have a high school education live in low-income families. Even if parents have full-time employment, low education levels make their children susceptible to poverty. Likewise, children in households headed by a single parent (usually the mother) are far more likely to live in poverty and thus to have more health risks; 68% of all children with single parents live in low-income families (Jiang et al., 2017).

Poverty by itself does not always put a child at risk; however, poor children face the following health and socioeconomic risks that can compound the burdensome influence of poverty (Federal Interagency Forum on Child and Family Statistics, 2016):

- Children in poverty have less access to nutritious food, shelter, and health care.
- Poor children are often deprived of advantages such as good schools, libraries, and other community resources.
- Deaths from unintended injuries, child maltreatment, homicide, STIs, and infectious diseases are more common among poor children.
- Many poor children live in substandard housing, have stressful home lives, may live surrounded by drugs and crime, and lack positive and nurturing adult role models.
- Poor children may feel hopeless about the future.
- Poor children often suffer from low birth weight, asthma, dental decay, high blood lead levels, learning disabilities, and teenage unmarried childbearing.
- Poor children are more likely to move frequently. Residential instability and extreme living conditions of poor children who are homeless or migrants usually compound their health problems.

These social and economic burdens can be overwhelming to parents or caregivers and may cause them to neglect other

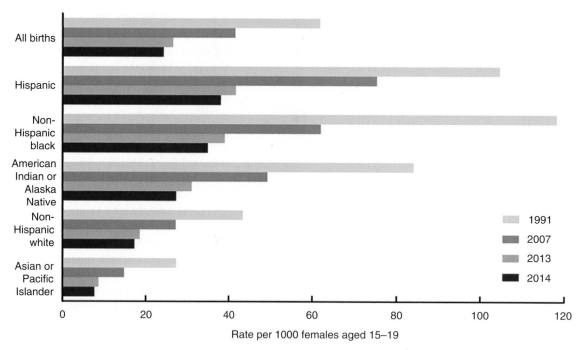

NOTE: Rates for 1991 for non-Hispanic white, non-Hispanic black, and Hispanic females exclude data for New Hampshire, which did not report Hispanic origin.

FIG. 16.4 Birth rates for women aged 15 to 19 years by race and Hispanic origin: United States, 1991, 2007, 2013, and 2014. (From National Center for Health Statistics: *Births United States, 2014,* 2015. Retrieved from https://www.cdc.gov/nchs/products/databriefs/db216.htm)

matters, such as providing a nutritious breakfast before school, taking a child for a well-child appointment, and getting his or her immunizations completed on schedule. They can create a sense of despair and hopelessness among parents and children, which greatly hinders healthy behavior. These factors clearly increase a child's physical and emotional health risks.

Racial and Ethnic Disparities

Although children in the United States are healthier now than in any other time in our nation's history, overall improvements in health mask the poor health of some racial and ethnic subgroups (Fig. 16.4). For example, as mentioned previously, the infant mortality rate has plunged over the past century, yet infants born to non-Hispanic black women are 2.5 times more likely to die in the first year of life than babies born to non-Hispanic white mothers. Native Americans and African Americans account for a disproportionate share of disabilities and deaths due to fetal alcohol exposure. African American youth are at higher risk for gun violence than white youth and are more than four times as likely to die from asthma as non-Hispanic white children. Childhood obesity affects racial and ethnic minority children at much higher rates than non-Hispanic whites, driving up rates of associated diabetes.

Eliminating health disparities is an important national health priority. *Healthy People 2020* (USDHHS, 2018; see later) targets persistent differences in health among children of varying racial and ethnic groups and calls for the elimination of disparities in health. Social determinants of health—the circumstances into which children are born—exert a strong and persistent influence over their lifelong health. A child's ability to be healthy and productive in life is negatively affected by poverty, violence, and

a family history of poor health along with systemic inequities such as limited access to quality health care, education, and job opportunities.

Community health nurses can develop an understanding of differences in health based on race, ethnicity, and economic circumstances. They can translate experiences in the field into evidence-based intervention strategies that incorporate social programs such as education, employment, and housing into solutions for addressing health disparities.

Health Care Use

Children grow and develop rapidly between infancy and adolescence; therefore they are extremely vulnerable to the effects of illness and of environmental factors that influence physical and emotional health. Preventive health and dental care offer children and parents a chance to periodically meet with a health care provider to do the following:

- Discuss the child's physical and emotional growth and development.
- Learn about good nutrition.
- Address safety issues, such as the use of car seats and seatbelts.
- Receive immunizations and vision and hearing screening.
- Learn about potential environmental threats to the child's health.
- Begin prompt treatment for a condition discovered during the examination.
- Ask other questions or obtain a referral if necessary.

Access to a regular health care source can facilitate prompt attention to acute medical problems, which can help prevent chronic, disabling conditions. For example, untreated ear infections can cause hearing loss, which can lead to learning disabilities, school problems, and even school dropout. Resulting low self-esteem can increase the likelihood of depression, behavior problems, early sexual activity, STIs, and unplanned pregnancy. Comprehensive, regular health care helps all children achieve their potential.

STRATEGIES TO IMPROVE CHILD AND ADOLESCENT HEALTH

One of the most important ways to ensure the success and well-being of future generations is for each child to start life healthy and maintain his or her physical and emotional health status throughout childhood and adolescence. Since the beginning of the twentieth century, the nation has made remarkable progress in many areas of child and adolescent health, but the results are mixed. Fortunately, scientific, medical, environmental, parenting, and other knowledge can lessen or eliminate many of the problems. It is a matter of making these concerns a priority and taking the necessary steps to elicit change. Box 16.6 lists several resources for monitoring the health and well-being of children.

Monitoring and Tracking

Federal, state, and local governments and many national organizations collect and analyze data to track the well-being of children and adolescents. For example, the Maternal and Child Health Bureau of the USDHHS (2015) generates a yearly report, *Child Health USA,* on child population characteristics, health status, and health care utilization. Such data are readily accessible online to citizens, health professionals, policy makers, and the media. A number of key indicators are tracked on a regular basis by the federal statistical system so that trends are revealed. State and local data also are used to track the well-being of children.

 ### *Healthy People 2020:* Child and Adolescent Health

Many professions establish goals and set measurable objectives. Educators use these techniques to organize their teaching materials, measure their students' progress, and evaluate the effectiveness of their teaching strategies and plans. Health care professionals use them for similar purposes in client care. The individual community health nurse uses them in working with a family to ensure that the nurse and family are organized and are guided by common purposes. Goals and objectives help the nurse and family evaluate progress and make necessary midcourse corrections.

These strategies are also important at the macro level and the programmatic level, where multiple players must collaborate to address complicated statewide or nationwide problems. In 1979, the surgeon general of the United States embarked on an ambitious task of convening hundreds of public health experts, health care researchers, health professional organizations, and others to develop the first health goals and objectives for the nation. At each of the intervening decades, these groups have developed a new set of goals and objectives to help bring clear focus to the health concerns of the nation and to set measurable and attainable goals for different age groups and issues across the country.

Healthy People 2020 (USDHHS, 2018) sets broad national health goals for the first decade of the twenty-first century. This initiative, like its predecessors, helps define the nation's health agenda and guides policy development. *Healthy People 2020* addresses many challenges facing the country and helps the public and private sectors understand the nation's leading health problems, helps the two sectors develop strategic plans for addressing them, and collaborates to reach common goals. The Healthy People box lists selected objectives from *Healthy People 2020* related to child and adolescent health.

Since the inception of the *Healthy People* initiative in 1979, child and adolescent health has improved. For instance, there have been improvements in infant, child, and adolescent mortality; adolescent smoking; pregnancy; and violence.

 HEALTHY PEOPLE 2020

Selected Objectives for Child and Adolescent Health

AH 2020-1: Increase the proportion of adolescents who have had a wellness checkup in the past 12 months.

AH HP2020–2: Increase the percentage of adolescents who participate in extracurricular and out-of-school activities.

EMC HP2020–1: (Developmental) Increase the proportion of children who are ready for school in all five domains of healthy development: physical development, social-emotional development, approaches to learning, language, and cognitive development.

EMC HP2020–3: Increase the proportion of elementary, middle, and senior high schools that require school health education.

EH HP2020-3: Reduce air toxic emissions to decrease the risk of adverse health effects caused by mobile, area, and major sources of airborne toxics.

Health Promotion and Disease Prevention

Health promotion and disease prevention are more significant and cost effective for children than for any other age group. Primary health care and early intervention for children and families can help prevent costly problems, suffering, and lost human potential. The following examples illustrate this point:

1. Preterm birth, the leading cause of infant death and long-term neurological disabilities in children, costs the U.S. health care system more than $26 billion each year (CDC, 2013b).

2. Preventing pregnancy among teenagers can reduce the rates of school dropout, welfare dependency, low birth weight, and infant mortality. It has been estimated that teen childbearing costs taxpayers billions of dollars every year in expenses associated with health and foster care, criminal justice, and public assistance (National Campaign to Prevent Teen and Unplanned Pregnancy, 2015).

Health promotion and disease prevention strategies for improving child and adolescent health come in many forms and originate in research institutions, public agencies, private businesses, and community-based organizations. They can include the following:

1. Clinical interventions

2. Public health efforts that identify trends and develop population-based, community-wide, or individual strategies to affect them

3. Philanthropic endeavors that fund initiatives at the community, state, and regional levels

4. Public policy initiatives that create or improve public programs or provide incentives for nongovernmental entities to address identified problems

PUBLIC HEALTH PROGRAMS TARGETED TO CHILDREN AND ADOLESCENTS

A number of public programs address the health needs of children, and many target medically underserved or low-income individuals and families. In addition, local and state public health and social service agencies aim to protect the health of an entire community or state through programs such as water fluoridation, sanitation, and infectious disease control. Furthermore, broad-based strategies such as lead-based paint elimination, mandatory child safety seats in automobiles, bicycle helmet laws, teen pregnancy prevention programs, comprehensive school health clinics, and drug and violence prevention programs serve to improve the health of children using community-wide approaches.

Health Care Coverage Programs

Approximately 9.4% of American children under 18 years of age do not have health insurance. Hispanic children are far more likely than children of other races to be uninsured (Fig. 16.5). Those who do not have health insurance are more likely to lack a source of health care, to have unmet health needs, and to experience worse health outcomes than children with insurance. Efforts to expand health care coverage for pregnant women and children have been successful, and provisions of the ACA helped further ensure affordable preventive services and health care coverage.

Among other provisions, for pregnant women, the ACA expanded options for health care insurance. Job-based health plans and new insurance plans are not allowed to deny or exclude coverage for pregnant women or children on the basis of a preexisting condition, including a disability. The ACA mandated certain preventive services at no cost, such as vaccinations for children and breast-feeding support. Teens and adults younger than 26 years can stay insured under their parent's insurance plan if the plan allows dependent coverage.

Medicaid and the Children's Health Insurance Program

The ability to pay for health care greatly influences whether a parent takes a child to see a health care provider. **Medicaid** (Title XIX of the Social Security Act) is a health insurance program for poor and low-income people. It is a federal/state entitlement program that plays an important role in providing health coverage for low-income women and children. The federal government sets the minimum guidelines for Medicaid eligibility, and states can chose to expand eligibility through the **Children's Health Insurance Program (CHIP)**. Depending on the state, the average CHIP income eligibility level for children is 200% to 250% of the federal poverty level (FPL). Together, Medicaid and CHIP serve about half of all low-income children (Centers for Medicare and Medicaid Services, 2017).

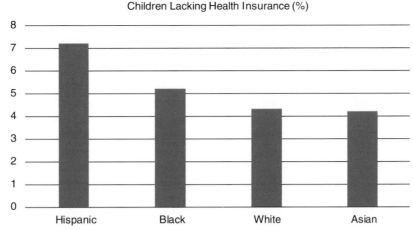

Children Lacking Health Insurance (%)

FIG. 16.5 Children less than 18 years of age and lacking health insurance by race, 2015. (Data from U.S. Census Bureau Current Population Reports: *Health insurance coverage in the United States: 2015 current population reports,* 2016. Retrieved from https://www.census.gov/content/dam/Census/library/publications/2016/demo/p60-257.pdf)

Within broad national guidelines, each state establishes eligibility standards based on a family's income in comparison with the FPL, determines the type and scope of services, and administers its own Medicaid and CHIP programs. States have some discretion in determining which population groups their programs will cover. Thus a pregnant woman or child who is eligible for the program in one state may not be eligible in another.

Through the **Early and Periodic Screening, Diagnosis, and Treatment (EPSDT)** program, a child covered by Medicaid can receive a range of health and health-related services beginning in infancy. The program is designed to assure availability and accessibility of health care resources and to help Medicaid recipients and their parents effectively use them. The program's services far exceed those usually covered by private insurance and include the following:

- Health, developmental, and nutritional screening
- Physical examinations
- Immunizations
- Vision and hearing screening
- Certain laboratory tests
- Dental services

Expansions in public health care insurance programs have helped many children achieve insurance coverage, but many children still lack insurance or other health care coverage like Medicaid or CHIP for many reasons, some of which are as follows:

- Insurance is too expensive.
- Medicaid has a welfare stigma, and parents do not want to be associated with it.
- Medicaid application forms and processes can be complex and burdensome and can intrude on a family's privacy.
- Parents may be concerned that their illegal immigration status may be revealed.
- Parents may not consider the importance of health insurance.

- Parents may not know their child is eligible for programs such as Medicaid and CHIP.
- Applications and other information may not be available in the family's language.

Although insurance gives a child financial access to health care, some children may not obtain the health care they need for other reasons. Numerous health care or family barriers can still stand in the way. They include the following (Angier et al., 2014; World Health Organization, n.d.):

- Lack of transportation
- Language barriers
- Lack of knowledge and awareness
- Inconveniences associated with provider's office (clinic or office hours that conflict with work or school schedules; overcrowded clinics with delays in the waiting room)
- Competing family or personal priorities that reduce the importance of obtaining care
- Providers' unwillingness to see Medicaid or low-income clients
- Parent's concerns that care providers are either unresponsive to their medical needs or interpersonally disrespectful
- Lack of affordability, such as cost of deductibles, copayments, medications

To successfully meet the health needs of children and adolescents, especially those with known risk factors, the community health nurse must be cognizant of health care access issues, family and neighborhood influences, and other social concerns in a child's life. The nurse must be prepared to help the family solve problems, to be their health care system advocate, and to address the child's health needs in a culturally competent manner.

Direct Health Care Delivery Programs

Although Medicaid and CHIP finance health care for their enrollees like private insurance, several other public programs deliver health care services directly to underserved populations. Most underserved aggregates live in inner cities or rural areas with few health care providers and facilities. Some have Medicaid, CHIP, or other insurance coverage, but many are uninsured.

Maternal and Child Health Block Grant

The Maternal and Child Health (MCH) Block Grant program (also called *Title V,* because it is the fifth section, or title, of the Social Security Act) allocates federal funds to the states, and the states must contribute their own funds for maternal and child health services. It is administered by the Maternal and Child Health Bureau as a part of the USDHHS's Health Resources and Services Administration. Established in 1935, the Title V MCH Block Grant has provided a foundation of health care services for mothers, children (including those with special health care needs), and families over the years. States must match every four dollars of federal Title V money with three dollars of state and/or local funding to help ensure the delivery of basic health care to pregnant women and children and help deliver additional services to children with special health care needs. Agencies in state health departments also monitor the health status of mothers and children throughout their respective states and work with other state agencies to develop programs to improve the health of this population.

The Consolidated Health Centers Program, managed by the Health Services Administration (HRSA) within the Department of Health and Human Services (HHS), provides funding to more than 9000 primary health care clinics in geographically isolated and economically distressed areas.

These health centers provide comprehensive, culturally competent, primary, and preventive health care to a diverse population, including individuals who are low income, uninsured, and experiencing homelessness. Services are provided to all residents of the service area without regard to an individual's ability to pay. This successful program provides primary care services, including health, dental, mental health, and pharmacy, as well as services that promote access to health care such as language interpretation, case management, and transportation.

School-Based Health Centers

Adolescents are the least likely aggregate to use health care services, especially preventive services. Their adolescent health care needs are different from their childhood needs, and they may be uncomfortable seeing a pediatrician or their childhood provider. Furthermore, they may or may not be able to discuss sensitive topics such as sexuality, substance use, and peer relationships with their parents. Some may not want their parents to know they have a health problem; therefore they may not want to see the family's health care provider out of concern about privacy and confidentiality. As a result, their health care needs may go unmet.

School-based health centers typically provide a combination of screening and preventive services, primary care, mental health and substance abuse counseling, dental health, nutrition education, and other health promotion activities. State dollars, mostly from general funds and the MCH Block Grant, are the primary sources of funding for school-based health care. A growing number of health centers participate in the Medicaid and CHIP programs, and some provide services within a managed care network. Expansion of school-based health centers has been made possible under the ACA.

Special Supplemental Nutrition Program for Women, Infants, and Children (WIC)

Although it is not a health program exclusively, WIC gives federal grants to states for the purpose of serving nutritionally at-risk, low-income, pregnant and postpartum women, and their children up to 5 years of age. WIC programs provide highly nutritious foods, nutrition education and counseling, and screening and referral to needed services. To be eligible, women and children must meet income guidelines established by each state, and a health professional must determine they are at "nutritional risk." Women and children who participate in Medicaid, the food stamp program, or the Temporary Assistance for Needy Families program are automatically eligible for WIC. Fifty-three percent of all infants born in the United States are served by WIC (U.S. Department of Agriculture Food and Nutrition Service, 2017).

WIC clinics operate in a number of sites, including health clinics, hospitals, schools, public housing sites, and mobile clinics. Women participating in the program are encouraged to obtain prenatal care if they are pregnant. They are also encouraged to maintain healthy diets and obtain preventive health care for themselves and their children, including childhood immunizations.

Established in 1972, WIC is one of the most successful, popular, and cost-effective public health programs. Some of the many benefits attributed to WIC include the following:

- Improvements in birth outcomes and health care cost savings
- Improved infant feeding practices, better low-birth-weight rate, and more regular primary care
- Lower rates of childhood obesity

SHARING RESPONSIBILITY FOR IMPROVING CHILD AND ADOLESCENT HEALTH

Most children in the United States are born healthy and remain healthy throughout childhood. However, the protective factors operating in the lives of healthy children and the interventions they receive are not available to all children. Although public-sector programs have attempted to provide a "safety net" for children, these interventions cannot address all the needs of children. For example, the health care system may provide emergency care to a 9-year-old child injured by gunfire in a drive-by shooting, but it cannot address the community conditions that perpetuate violence.

Child health is affected by many factors; therefore the responsibility for improving children's health rests with the entire community. This responsibility begins with parents and includes health care professionals, community groups, businesses, and the public sector. When a child is older, he or she can be responsible for practicing healthy behaviors and obtaining proper health care.

BOX 16.7 Breast-Feeding: The Feeding Method of Choice

Breast-feeding is uniquely superior for infant feeding. The practice imparts many health benefits for mothers and babies.

Benefits for children include the following:

- Decreased incidence and severity of a wide range of infectious diseases
- Decreased infant mortality
- Decreased risk of sudden infant death syndrome
- Reduction in the incidence of diabetes, respiratory infections, and some cancers
- Lower risk of overweight and obesity
- Enhanced cognitive development

Benefits of breast-feeding for mothers include the following:

- Decreased postpartum bleeding
- Earlier return to prepregnancy weight
- Decreased risk of breast and ovarian cancer

The American Academy of Pediatrics (AAP) and many other health organizations recommend exclusive breast-feeding for the first 6 months of life with continuation of breast-feeding for 1 year or longer as mutually desired by mother and infant (AAP, 2012).

Parents' Role

Even before conception, a woman can help ensure the health of her fetus by practicing healthy behaviors herself. Reproductive life planning can help a woman set personal goals and priorities and design strategies to meet these goals. This planning may entail avoiding unwanted pregnancy and/or learning about specific actions she can take to increase her chances for having a healthy baby should she desire a child in the future. If pregnancy is desired, a woman can learn to manage chronic health conditions and to develop healthy behaviors, including proper nutrition with folic acid supplementation and avoidance of tobacco, alcohol, drugs, and other behaviors that could harm a developing baby. It is also important for the mother to receive prenatal care early in pregnancy.

Starting with breast-feeding, parents must give their children nutritious food and ensure that they are immunized, receive needed health care services, and acquire healthful lifestyles. Breast-feeding provides many health benefits for mothers and their children (Box 16.7).

Another important task for parents is to ensure that their children have a safe environment at home, in the neighborhood, and at school. They must protect their children from injury, violence, abuse, and neglect. Parents must learn how to nurture, guide, and protect their children effectively through the developmental stages of childhood and adolescence.

Community's Role

Families need support from their community and society to fulfill their roles and responsibilities. This is particularly true for families who live in poverty and for parents who are isolated and disenfranchised. Ensuring access to health care is an important community role, but communities are also responsible for promoting well-being, which goes far beyond the provision of traditional medical care.

Communities should work to create safe neighborhoods and support the development of community-based comprehensive health, education, housing, and social service programs. Collaborative, multipartner approaches that concentrate on helping children and adolescents avoid risks and develop social competence are more likely to be effective than fragmented programs focusing on individual risks, such as teen drug use. Communities are well situated to facilitate the integration of health, education, and social services; to eliminate fragmentation and duplication of services; to provide culturally competent care; and to better organize more comprehensive and streamlined systems of care. Although many health and social service programs exist, they can be poorly coordinated with one another, with little collaboration among the professional disciplines.

The media are part of the community at large and should be involved in promoting child and adolescent health. The media significantly influence children's lives, their perceptions of the world, and their self-images. From developing informational campaigns about prenatal care and immunizations to discouraging violence and explicit sex in advertising and popular television programs, the media can have a profound effect on improving children's health and well-being.

Employer's Role

Business and industry have an enormous stake in the health of the nation's children. A strong, productive workforce is ensured only when the health, social, and educational needs of the next generation of workers are met. Furthermore, health risks cost employers in lost productivity and increased health care costs.

The private sector can play a role in improving the health of individual children or the community in general. An employer can make health care more accessible to families with children by offering affordable health insurance that covers employees and dependents. The provision of insurance plans that offer full pregnancy and well-child health care benefits is essential to employee health promotion. Employers can meet the requirements of the U.S. Department of Labor (2015) by supporting nursing mothers in the workplace. This includes providing reasonable break time to express milk and a private space other than a bathroom in which to do so.

Maintaining a workplace that allows flexible leave for prenatal and pediatric health care and allows time off to care for newborn and sick children can also contribute to child health improvements. In 1993, the Family and Medical Leave Act (FMLA) mandated that employers with 50 or more employees must allow a total of 12 work weeks of unpaid leave during any 12-month period for the birth, adoption, or foster care of a child or for the care of a seriously ill family member or the employee himself or herself. The Department of Labor issued a Final Rule on February 25, 2015, revising the definition of spouse under the FMLA of 1993. Revision of the definition ensures same-sex married spouses the same ability as all spouses to fully exercise their FMLA rights (U.S. Department of Labor, 2015).

In addition, employers can sponsor education opportunities for employees about topics such as healthy diets, healthy pregnancies, substance abuse, and stress management. Businesses can also offer onsite child care and can work with community leaders and public officials to initiate community-wide health promotion projects targeted to children. Finally, employers can be catalysts in their communities for linking health, education, and social services for children.

Government's Role

In the United States, government's role in promoting or ensuring children's health is more limited than in many other countries. Other countries often have defined policies on children's health; the United States does not. Such policies not only indicate that children are a priority of the citizenry but also help shape the operation of programs and their funding.

As discussed earlier, U.S. state and federal governments have several public health programs that provide assistance to children, especially to those at risk from poverty or other disadvantages. Monitoring the health of children is also a governmental role. Although these programs are not a substitute for a family or caregiver's care and concern, they are important in protecting and promoting health and delivering services to those who would otherwise go without. Programs with significant funding exist, but many children with health problems do not receive the services they need for reasons previously discussed.

Managers and front-line workers (e.g., community health nurses, social workers, physicians, and caseworkers) in effective community programs should be encouraged to collaborate and thereby assist children with problems that adversely affect their health. "One-stop shopping" (i.e., user-friendly, accessible services for children and families) is an important concept for public and community programs to embrace to ensure that children easily receive needed services. Outreach and referral efforts should be an integral part of health initiatives to provide children with the services they require. Community health nurses are often an essential part of these efforts.

Community/Public Health Nurse's Role

Public health nurses have always played pivotal roles in improving the health status of pregnant women, children, and adolescents. Within the community, the community health nurse is often most aware of children's health status, any barriers that prevent children from receiving necessary care, and other factors that may adversely affect their health. Armed with this information and knowledge about available health resources in the community, the community health nurse is:

- An advocate for improved individual and community responses to children's needs
- A researcher for effective strategies to serve women and children
- A participant in publicly funded programs
- A promoter of social interventions that enhance the living situations of high-risk families
- A partner with other professionals to improve service collaboration and coordination

One important role of the community health nurse is to help link local health and social services with the school system. Children must be healthy to learn; however, children may come to school with vision, hearing, and other health problems that appropriate education, screening, and treatment could have prevented or alleviated. When children pass the preschool years, the school health nurse is sometimes their only connection to the health care system. School health nurses can be important sources of primary health care and health information for students and their families.

Community health nurses can alert the health professional community, business leaders, religious groups, and voluntary organizations to children's and adolescents' needs and to the strategies that can improve their health. Community health nurses can influence the planning and implementation of necessary changes in the health care system to ensure improved children's health and to achieve the national health goals for the year 2020. Also, they can promote commitment within their own institutions for comprehensive, culturally competent care.

Home visiting is a promising strategy that connects community health nurses, paraprofessionals, or lay home visitors to families in order to provide education, support, and referrals (Olds et al., 2010). One home visiting model, administered through the Nurse-Family Partnership, partners low-income, first-time mothers with maternal and child health nurses. Pregnant women develop trusting relationships with their nurse home visitors and receive the care and support needed for healthy pregnancy and parenting. Financial self-sufficiency is encouraged (http://www.nursefamilypartnership.org/).

LEGAL AND ETHICAL ISSUES IN CHILD AND ADOLESCENT HEALTH

Every day, community health nurses are involved in making decisions. In each encounter with a client, the nurse's decisions or the family's choices have the potential to influence the health and well-being of the family or the community at large for better or for worse.

People often assume that health care professionals, particularly nurses, are by nature attuned to the ethical implications of their decisions. In addition, the community trusts that nurses are aware of the legal ramifications of their actions and decisions, of their clients' decisions, and of the health care and legal systems' decisions. In reality, the ever-changing pressures of serving the community's health care needs leave little time to reflect on the ethical and moral implications of a given situation. In some cases, it may seem easier to avoid tough decisions. An ethical approach to decision making allows the community health nurse to evaluate a client's or a population's needs more honestly and completely and take appropriate action. Understanding the legal environment will help the nurse make informed decisions and effectively assist clients with their decision-making processes.

Ethical Issues

The complex nature of public health and health care delivery environments often sets the stage for conflicts of interest and values. Meanwhile, nurses and other health professionals must work within the system to improve child and adolescent health in a country of great differences. Such differences exist between races and cultures, and there are great dichotomies, such as the affluence of some and the poverty of many others. For the perinatal nurse, for example, ethical dilemmas may arise because she is an advocate for two clients: the pregnant woman and her fetus. The scope of ethical and legal dilemmas is broad. The Ethical Insights box lists specific ethical issues related to child and adolescent health.

ETHICAL INSIGHTS

Ethical Issues Related to Child and Adolescent Health

Allocation decisions: Given limited time and resources, what level of care should a nurse offer a child and his or her family?

Maternal-fetal conflict: Sometimes there are opposing ethical concerns for the pregnant woman and her fetus—for example, whether the benefits of prolonging a pregnancy justify the risk of complications for a pregnant woman or whether court-ordered treatment for a substance-abusing pregnant woman overrides the right to autonomy for a pregnant woman.

Client autonomy: In each specific case, who should make health care decisions for a young client, especially when opposing opinions arise? The client? The parents or guardian? The nurse or other health care professional? At what age does a child become mature enough to participate in such decision making? What laws does any given state have that affect adolescent client autonomy? What should the community health nurse do if he or she believes the client's or parent's decisions are not in the best interest of the client?

Privacy and confidentiality: Is an intervention appropriate if the community health nurse identifies gross noncompliance, neglect, or abuse? Is an intervention appropriate if in making it the nurse must break confidentiality? When and how should the nurse take action?

"Gaming the system": When the health care system's rules appear to impede the nurse's ability to serve the client's best interest, is it acceptable to circumvent the system? If so, what are the moral and legal costs?

Cultural competence: The United States will continue to experience huge demographic changes and greater diversity; nurses will face different cultural definitions of what is and what is not acceptable or ethical. How should the community health nurse respond to a client or population group that does not share the same cultural outlook on health? What is the nurse's legal justification, if any, for responding in a certain way?

Health disparities and access to care: What are the nurses' responsibilities in ensuring that women and children have access to health care? How can nurses influence policy decisions that affect community health care?

Prenatal diagnosis and newborn screening: What are potential long-term consequences of identifying genetic conditions? Are parents fully informed of negative consequences of genetic diagnoses, including stigmatization, discrimination, and psychological effects?

These issues invariably involve value judgments and challenge a nurse's bounds of professional and personal duty. They also require the community health nurse to stay abreast of legislative changes at the local, state, and national levels and participate in professional activities that can help him or her stay current in these important matters. By recognizing the ethical implications of the care and advice they give or the actions they take, nurses can embrace their duty to promote the health and well-being of individual clients and the community more completely, protect their clients from harm, and strive for health care fairness and justice for all clients.

Recognizing the value of engaging in a shared dialogue with colleagues regarding ethical decision-making issues and understanding the possible legal implications of their decisions are equally important. The choices can be complex; therefore receiving the guidance of an ethics board or gaining a second opinion can be critical to making the right choices. On a broader scale, a community health nurse's ethical perspective can enhance any discussion about individual client care and overall community health and also can affect the direction of the country's public health policy.

�*ACTIVE LEARNING

1. Develop strategies to inform parents whose children are uninsured about the availability of CHIP.
2. Spend a day with a school health nurse and analyze what could help prevent or address the health problems and issues he or she encountered throughout the day.
3. Communicate with those in policy-making positions by writing letters or holding meetings about children's needs.
4. Identify the public health and advocacy organizations in the community that are working to address children's health needs and identify their strategies for promoting child health within the community.
5. If your community has a lay home visitor program, meet with a home visitor and, if possible, accompany him or her during home visits.

CASE STUDY   Application of the Nursing Process

Pregnant Teenager

By applying the principles of the nursing process to the individual, family, and community, the community health nurse can provide services to children and adolescents more systematically and effectively. Most communities offer a range of preventive services and other important programs that children need. The community health nurse must thoroughly understand the needs of the individual child and family and must be aware of available community resources to help meet the child's health needs, as this case study illustrates.

Maria Martinez, a community health nurse working for the county health department, received a call from the high school nurse informing her that a 16-year-old high school student named Kaylah M. would come in that afternoon for a pregnancy test. Kaylah had already missed three menstrual periods and was afraid to talk about it with her family. She had a long discussion with the school nurse and asked her boyfriend, also aged 16, to take her to the health department clinic after school for the pregnancy test.

continued

Pregnant Teenager

Assessment

Kaylah's pregnancy test result was positive, and she was an estimated 3 months pregnant. She was upset and would not speak with Maria at the health department. With agreement from Kaylah, Maria arranged to make a home visit the next afternoon.

Knowing that she needed to address a number of issues at the first home visit, Maria prepared by developing a list of possible assessment areas that covered individual, family, and community concerns, as follows:

Individual

- Medical risk factors
- Emotional well-being, including concerns about community safety, domestic violence, and sexual abuse
- Cultural beliefs and attitudes toward pregnancy and medical care
- Barriers to communication with providers, such as language, hearing, and sight
- Understanding and acceptance of pregnancy
- Health-promoting and risk-taking behaviors
- Understanding the importance of obtaining preventive care services
- Health insurance status
- Access to transportation

Family

- Adequacy of housing structure
- Safety of neighborhood
- Ability of family members to provide emotional support
- Ability of family to provide financial support
- Ability and willingness of the father of the baby to provide support

Community

- Availability of affordable and culturally sensitive prenatal and pediatric care
- Health and social services coordination
- Emotional guidance and counseling
- Educational opportunities for pregnant and parenting teenagers
- Job training
- Nutrition services such as WIC and food stamps
- Pregnancy and parenting education
- Child care availability

Assessment Data

Individual

- Kaylah was already in the early second trimester of pregnancy and had not received prenatal care. She also engaged in risk-taking behaviors (i.e., smoking, alcohol use, unprotected sex, and poor eating habits) potentially detrimental to her baby.
- During the interview, Kaylah seemed quiet and reserved. She said she was excited to have a baby but feared labor and delivery.
- Her boyfriend wanted her to keep the baby but was not committed to supporting Kaylah or the baby. He did not want to involve his own parents.
- Kaylah said she did not think about prenatal care much but would probably visit a health clinic sometime before her delivery. Her family did not have health insurance, and she said they could not afford prenatal care.
- She wanted to keep the baby and remain in school, yet she did not have a realistic understanding of parental responsibilities.

Family

- When Kaylah told her parents she was pregnant, they expressed disappointment. Her mother voiced a willingness to provide emotional support, but her seemingly emotionally distant father expressed anger.
- Both parents expressed concern about how the family would manage financially.

- After a brief review of the family's financial situation, it appeared that Kaylah was eligible for Medicaid and WIC.
- Her parents wanted her to have no further contact with her boyfriend.

Community

- Maria determined that prenatal services were available, but only during school hours. Although the only clinic that accepted Medicaid clients was on the other side of town, a nearby obstetrical practice with a certified nurse-midwife on staff accepted clients with Medicaid coverage. However, their primary clientele consisted of middle-class, married women.
- Applying for Medicaid and the WIC program required Kaylah to go to the welfare office and apply during school hours. However, the hospital outpatient department could make a preliminary Medicaid eligibility determination, which might be more convenient.
- Although Medicaid would pay for some prenatal classes, those nearby were geared to older, married couples.
- Kaylah's school encouraged her to remain in regular classes until her delivery date and participate in home study for a limited time thereafter.
- No parenting classes geared toward adolescents were available.
- Child care was not available at the high school, making a return to school more difficult for Kaylah.
- Although the community has a lay home visitor program that matches mentors with pregnant and parenting teens and provides health information and encouragement, the project does not serve Kaylah's neighborhood.

Diagnosis

Individual

- Unhealthy lifestyle choices related to the lack of prenatal care and the effect of poor nutrition, smoking, and alcohol use on fetal development
- Parenting issues related to unrealistic expectations about parenting responsibilities
- Lack of knowledge related to infant and child safety issues, such as the use of child safety seats, advantages of breast-feeding, safe sleep for infants, and use of preventive health care, including immunizations

Family

- Disrupted family dynamics related to anger and disappointment over daughter's pregnancy
- Altered financial status resulting from the addition of another dependent to the family

Community

- Lack of coordinated, culturally sensitive, accessible prenatal and parenting services for adolescents
- Existing lay home visitor program not available

Planning

To ensure the action plan is complete, realistic, and successfully implemented, Maria must thoroughly identify the factors affecting Kaylah's health and well-being. In addition, Kaylah, her family, and Maria must set mutual goals.

Individual

Long-Term Goals

- Pregnancy outcome will be healthy for mother and infant.
- Kaylah will demonstrate successful parenting behaviors.
- Kaylah will complete high school.

Short-Term Goals

- Kaylah will obtain prenatal care.
- Kaylah will understand the reasons to change nutrition and substance use habits.

CASE STUDY Application of the Nursing Process—cont'd

Pregnant Teenager

- Kaylah and the nurse will plan actions to change poor health habits.
- Kaylah will remain in school throughout her pregnancy and will use the home study program until she returns to school after her baby is born.
- Kaylah will enroll in parenting class. If classes are not available, she will use age-appropriate reading materials, films, CDs, Internet resources, opportunities for group discussion with other teens, or visits with experienced parents.
- Kaylah will breast-feed her baby.
- Kaylah will speak with the community health educator to determine methods to protect the health and safety of her newborn.

Family
Long-Term Goal

- The family's ability to handle crises will improve with their ability to discuss problems and engage in mutual problem solving.

Short-Term Goal

- Kaylah's parents will display supportive behaviors, such as accompanying her to prenatal care appointments, helping her engage in healthy behaviors, and helping her arrange child care so she can remain in school.

Community
Long-Term Goal

- Accessible, comprehensive, culturally sensitive prenatal and other health care services will be established, including home visiting and parenting classes targeted to adolescents.

Short-Term Goals

- The health department clinic will extend evening hours to accommodate students and working families.
- A child care facility will open in or near the high school.

Intervention

The nurse, family, and individual must address their immediate, mutual goals to help Kaylah achieve a healthy birth outcome and begin successful parenting. Interdisciplinary planning among Kaylah's school health nurse, caseworker, community health nurse, primary pregnancy care provider, childbirth educator, and family planning nurse is critical. In addition, Maria must be an advocate for community-wide change to ensure that the community is meeting individuals' needs.

Individual

Maria worked with the school nurse and other health professionals to help Kaylah obtain Medicaid and WIC; she was referred to an obstetrician who saw her regularly. Kaylah's pregnancy was also monitored by the school nurse, who had her come to the clinic on a weekly basis to check her weight and blood pressure and to talk with her about pregnancy-related issues.

Working with the school nurse, Maria provided Kaylah with information on childbirth classes and nutrition as well as booklets detailing how to promote a healthy pregnancy. She was counseled to avoid tobacco, alcohol, and all drugs. Near the end of the pregnancy, Kaylah was encouraged to attend parenting classes with her boyfriend.

Family

Maria and the social worker referred Kaylah's parents to other social service agencies that might be able to help financially. In particular, they focused on providers who could assist with utilities, job placement, and child care. The family was also referred to a family counselor who specialized in working with families with adolescent children.

Community

Maria worked with the maternal-child health division of the county health department to help facilitate offering parenting classes at an area high school, targeting the learning needs of pregnant teens. She and the school nurse also met with school district officials and community leaders to stimulate dialogue about the consequences of dropping out of high school and to facilitate action in policies such as child care for parenting teenagers to help them remain in school.

Evaluation

Evaluation strategies must involve both process and outcome measures on the individual, family, and community levels.

Individual

The school nurse was able to monitor Kaylah throughout her pregnancy and was aware that she finished classes for the term. Kaylah's pregnancy was unremarkable, and she delivered a healthy boy. Their health care expenses were covered by Medicaid, and the baby was determined to also be eligible for CHIP. A home-based teacher was assigned to work with Kaylah for 1 month after delivery to ensure that she was able to keep up with her coursework. With the assistance of the social worker, Kaylah was able to place the baby in a subsidized day care facility, allowing her to finish school.

Family

Family counseling helped the family resolve some of their issues. Maria observed that Kaylah's parents were proud of their grandson and eager to help with his care.

Community

With the help of the school nurse and other interested parties, Maria was able to initiate a collaborative program in which health department nurses and developmental specialists offered parenting classes in high schools on a regular basis. They were also planning on writing for a Maternal Child Health Block Grant to implement a school-based clinic focusing on the needs of pregnant teens and their infants.

Levels of Prevention
Primary

- Primary prevention depends largely on the child's age. For the youngest children, strategies include encouraging healthy behaviors by girls and women.
- Primary prevention also includes the prevention of unwanted pregnancy, which is especially important for adolescents.

Secondary

- Once pregnant, the woman must receive early and adequate prenatal care, practice healthy behaviors, obtain necessary social and supportive services, and prepare herself for becoming a parent.
- It is incumbent on the community to ensure that adequate preventive health services, such as prenatal care, nutrition and dietary counseling, pregnancy and parent education, and social services, are available.

Tertiary

- Initiate programs and services that prevent future unwanted pregnancy among teenagers and help the parenting teenager provide the best possible care to the child.
- Establish programs such as parenting classes; support services to help adolescents complete their education; coordination of health and social services for the mother and her child; and well-child care, immunizations, and nutrition services.

SUMMARY

Child and adolescent health status remains an important indicator of the nation's health. The health of a child sets the foundation for school readiness and future success. Child and adolescent health problems are reflections of rapidly changing social conditions, not isolated events. Despite generally improving trends in health for most children, community health nurses must address discrepancies that exist between racial and ethnic groups. Poverty is the basis for many continuing health problems among children in this country, and nurses must recognize and treat it as such.

The best way to ensure the success and well-being of future generations is for each child to begin life healthy and maintain that health status throughout childhood. Any health problem (e.g., hunger and poor nutrition, asthma, poor vision or hearing, anemia, dental caries, mental health problems, illicit drug use, or teen pregnancy) can interfere with school attendance, academic success, normal growth and development, learning ability, and life success.

The prevention of health problems is most significant and cost effective for children. Each dollar spent on the prevention of physical and emotional problems in children is a sound investment. Primary health care and early intervention for children and families can help prevent costly problems, suffering, and the loss of human potential. Community health nurses can use their experience and "inside knowledge" of barriers to child health to educate others. Rather than limiting their approach to caring for the individual and family only, community health nurses can maximize their roles to collaborate and forge necessary alliances to solve children's health problems. Nurses are authority figures in the least expected places. Working on health care's front line is a powerful and very real position to members of Congress, state legislators, mayors, and other leaders. By creatively using this kind of power, community health nurses can contribute greatly to improving the health and well-being of all children.

Ⓔ EVOLVE WEBSITE

http://evolve.elsevier.com/Nies/community

- NCLEX Review Questions
- Case Studies

BIBLIOGRAPHY

American Academy of Pediatrics: Ad Hoc task force on definition of the medical home: the medical home, *Pediatrics* 90(5): 774, 1992. Also available from: <http://pediatrics.aappublications. org/content/90/5/774.abstract?sid=655ecdcd-5e4f-47ab-9dad-59ab0865762a>.

American Academy of Pediatrics: Section on breastfeeding: breastfeeding and the use of human milk, *Pediatrics* 129(3):e827–e841, 2012. Also available from: <http://pediatrics.aappublications.org/ content/early/2012/02/22/peds.2011-3552>.

American Academy of Pediatrics National Center for Medical Home Implementation: *National initiatives overview*, n.d. Available from: <http://www.medicalhomeinfo.org/national/>.

American Academy of Pediatrics: Task force on sudden infant death syndrome: SIDS and other sleep-related infant deaths: expansion of recommendations for a safe infant sleeping environment, *Pediatrics* 128(5):e1341–e1367, 2011. Also available from: http:// pediatrics.aappublications.org/content/128/5/e1341.full?sid= bd9574fb-4575-4d35-a46e-a63394e68331.

Angier H, Gregg J, Gold R, et al.: Understanding how low-income families prioritize elements of health care access for their children via the optimal care model, *BCH Health Res* 14:585, 2014.

Center on the Developing Child at Harvard University: *The Science of neglect: the persistent absence of responsive care disrupts the developing brain: working paper 12*, 2012. Available from: <www.developingchild.harvard.edu>.

Centers for Disease Control and Prevention: *About BMI for children and teens*, 2015c. Available from: https://www.cdc.gov/healthyweight/ assessing/bmi/childrens_bmi/about_childrens_bmi.html.

Centers for Disease Control and Prevention: *Sexually transmitted disease surveillance 2015*, Atlanta, 2016b, U.S. Department of Health and Human Services. Available from: https://www.cdc. gov/std/stats15/std-surveillance-2015-print.pdf.

Centers for Disease Control and Prevention: *HPV vaccine for preteens and teens*, 2015b. Available from: https://www.cdc.gov/vaccines/ parents/diseases/teen/hpv-basics-color.pdf.

Centers for Disease Control and Prevention: Alcohol use and binge drinking among women of childbearing age—United States, 2011-2013, *MMWR Morb Mortal Wkly Rep* 64(37):1042–1046, 2015a. Also available from: https://www.cdc.gov/mmwr/preview/mmwrhtml/ mm6437a3.htm.

Centers for Disease Control and Prevention: *Facts about fetal alcohol spectrum disorders*, 2018. Available from: <https://www.cdc.gov/ ncbddd/fasd/facts.html>.

Centers for Disease Control and Prevention: *Youth violence: facts at a glance*, 2016c. Available from: https://www.cdc.gov/ violenceprevention/pdf/yv-datasheet.pdf.

Centers for Disease Control and Prevention: *Immunization schedules*, 2017b. Available from: https://www.cdc.gov/vaccines/schedules/ hcp/child-adolescent.html.

Centers for Disease Control and Prevention: *Preterm birth*, 2103b. Available from: <http://www.cdc.gov/reproductivehealth/ maternalinfanthealth/PretermBirth.htm>.

Centers for Disease Control and Prevention: Progress in increasing breastfeeding and reducing racial/ethnic differences—United States, 2000–2008 births, *Morb Mortal Wkly Rep* 62(05): 77–80, 2013a. Also available from: <http://www.cdc. gov/mmwr/preview/mmwrhtml/mm6205a1.htm?s_cid=govD_ dnpao_260>.

Centers for Disease Control and Prevention: *Health Effects-Smoking during pregnancy*, 2016a. Retrieved April 2, 2017 https://www. cdc.gov/tobacco/basic_information/health_effects/pregnancy/.

Centers for Disease Control and Prevention: *Sudden unexplained infant death and sudden infant death syndrome*, 2017a. Available from: https://www.cdc.gov/sids/data.htm.

Centers for Medicare and Medicaid Services: *Medicaid & CHIP*, 2017. Available from: <https://www.medicaid.gov/medicaid/program-information/downloads/accomplishments-report.pdf>.

Central Intelligence Agency Web site (nd): *The World Factbook*, 2016. Retrieved from: https://www.cia.gov/library/publications/the-world-factbook/rankorder/2091rank.html.

Child and Adolescent Health Measurement Initiative: *"Who are children with special health care needs (CSHCN)."* Data Resource Center, supported by Cooperative Agreement 1-U59-MC06980-01 from the U.S. Department of Health and Human Services, Health Resources and Services Administration (HRSA), Maternal and Child Health Bureau (MCHB), 2012. Available at www.childhealthdata.org.

Chowdhury, et al.: Breastfeeding and maternal health outcomes: a systematic review and meta-analysis, *ACTA Paediatrica* 105:96–113, 2015.

Conde-Agudelo A, Rosas-Bermúdez A, Kafury-Goeta A: Birth spacing and risk of adverse perinatal outcomes: a meta-analysis, *JAMA* 295(15):1809–1823, 2006, https://doi.org/10.1001/jama.295.15.1809.

Curtin SC, Mathews TJ: *Smoking prevalence and cessation before and during pregnancy: data from the birth certificate, 2014*, National vital statistics reports; vol. 65 no 1. Hyattsville, MD, 2016, National Center for Health Statistics.

Engle WA, Kominiarek MA: Late preterm infants, early term infants and timing of elective deliveries, *Clin Perinatol* 35(2):325–341, 2008.

Federal Interagency Forum on Child and Family Statistics: *America's children: key national indicators of well-being*, 2016. Retrieved from March 9, 2017, from https://www.childstats.gov/pdf/ac2016/ac_16.pdf.

Federal Interagency Forum on Child and Family Statistics: *America's children: key national indicators of well-being*, 2015. Retrieved from March 9, 2017, from https://www.childstats.gov/pdf/ac2015/ac_15.pdf.

Federal Interagency Forum on Child and Family Statistics: *America's children: key national indicators of well-being*, 2016. Retrieved from March 9, 2017, from https://www.childstats.gov/pdf/ac2016/ac_16.pdf.

Finer LB, Zolna MR: Unintended pregnancy in the United States: incidence and disparities, 2006, *Contraception* 84(5):478–485, 2011.

Hamilton BE, Martin JA, Osterman MK, et al.: Births: final data for 2014, *Natl Vital Stat Rep* 64(12):1–64, 2015.

Institute of Medicine: *The childhood immunization schedule and safety: stakeholder concerns, scientific evidence, and future studies*, Washington, DC, 2013, National Academies Press, <http://www.iom.edu/Reports/2013/The-Childhood-Immunization-Schedule-and-Safety.aspx>.

Ip S, Chung M, Raman G, et al.: *Breastfeeding and maternal and infant health outcomes in developed countries*. Evidence Report/Technology Assessment No. 153 (Prepared by Tufts-New England Medical Center Evidence-based Practice Center, under Contract No. 290-02-0022). AHRQ Publication No. 07-E007, Rockville, MD, April 2007, Agency for Healthcare Research and Quality.

Jiang Y, Granja MR, Koball H: *Basic facts about low-income children: children under 18 years, 2015*, New York, 2017, National Center for Children in Poverty, Columbia University Mailman School of Public Health.

Johnston LD, O'Malley PM, Bachman JG, Schulenberg JE: *Monitoring the future national results on adolescent drug use: overview of key findings, 2009* (NIH Publication No. 10-7583), Bethesda, MD, 2010, National Institute on Drug Abuse.

Johnston LD, O'Malley PM, Miech RA, et al.: *Monitoring the future national survey results on drug use, 1975-2016: overview, key findings on adolescent drug use*, Ann Arbor, 2017, Institute for Social Research, The University of Michigan.

Khann L, McManus T, Harris W, et al.: Youth risk behavior surveillance—United States, 2015, *MMRW Surveill Summ* 65(6):2016. https://www.cdc.gov/mmwr/volumes/65/ss/ss6506a1.htm?s_cid=ss6506a1_w.

Kochanek KD, Murphy SL, Xu JQ, et al.: *Deaths: final data for 2014. National vital statistics reports*, vol. 65 no 4, Hyattsville, MD, 2016, National Center for Health Statistics.

Kovar C, Salsberry P: Does a satisfactory relationship with her mother influence when a 16-year-old begins to have sex? MCN, *Am J Matern Child Nurs* 37(2):122–129, 2012.

Law Center to Prevent Gun Violence: *Minimum age*, 2016. Accessed April 1, 2017 from http://smartgunlaws.org/gun-laws/policy-areas/consumer-child-safety/minimum-age/.

Leeb RT, Paulozzi L, Melanson C, et al.: Child maltreatment surveillance: uniform definitions for public health and recommended data elements, 2008. Available from: <https://www.cdc.gov/violenceprevention/pdf/CM_Surveillance-a.pdf >.

Leonardi-Bee J, Smyth A, Britton J, et al.: Environmental tobacco smoke and fetal health: systematic review and meta-analysis, *Arch Dis Child Fetal Neonatal Ed* 93:F351–F361, 2008.

Lumley J, Chamberlain C, Dowswell T, et al.: Interventions for promoting smoking cessation during pregnancy, *Cochrane Database Syst Rev* 3:CD001055, 2009, https://doi.org/10.1002/14651858.CD001055.pub3.

MacDorman MF, Mathews TJ: *Understanding racial and ethnic disparities in U.S. infant mortality rates*, NCHS data brief, no 74. Hyattsville, MD, 2011, National Center for Health Statistics.

MacDorman MF, Mathews TJ: *Understanding racial and ethnic disparities in U.S. infant mortality rates (NCHS Data Brief no 74)*. Hyattsville, MD, 2011, National Center for Health Statistics, <http://www.cdc.gov/nchs/data/databriefs/db74.htm>.

Martin JA, Hamilton BE, Osternman MK, et al.: *Births: final data for 2015*, (National Vital Statistics Report vol. 66, no. 1). Hyattsville, MD, 2017, National Center for Health Statistics.

Martinez GM, Abma JC: *Sexual activity, contraceptive use, and childbearing of teenagers aged 15-19 in the United States*, NCHS Data Brief, no 209. Hyattsville, MD, 2015, National Center for Health Statistics.

Mathews TJ, MacDorman MF, Thoma ME: *Infant mortality statistics from the 2013 period linked birth/infant death data set* (National vital statistics reports; vol. 64 no 9). Hyattsville, MD, 2015, National Center for Health Statistics.

Moos MK: From concept to practice: reflections on the preconception health agenda, *J Women's Health* 19(3):561–567, 2010.

Moos MK, Badura M, Posner S, et al.: Quality improvement opportunities in preconception and interconception care. In *March of dimes: toward improving the outcome of pregnancy, III*, White Plains, NY, March of Dimes Foundation.

Morse SB, Zheng H, Tang Y, et al.: Early school-age outcomes of late preterm infants, *Pediatrics* 123(4):e622–e629, 2009.

National Campaign to Prevent Teen and Unplanned Pregnancy: *Annual report-Improving the lives and future prospects of children and families*, 2015. Available https://thenationalcampaign.org/sites/default/files/resource-primary-download/national-campaign-2015-annual-report.pdf.

National Center for Children in Poverty: *Child poverty*, 2017. Available from: http://www.nccp.org/topics/childpoverty.html.

National Conference of State Legislatures: *Synthetic drug threats*, 2012. Available from: <http://www.ncsl.org/issues-research/justice/synthetic-drug-threats.aspx>.

National Highway Traffic Safety Administration: *Child safety: Is your child in the right car seat?*, 2013. Available from: <http://www.nhtsa.gov/Safety/CPS>.

National Institute on Drug Abuse: *Drugs, brains, and behavior- the science of addiction*, 2014. Retrieved April 2, 2017, from https://www.drugabuse.gov/publications/drugs-brains-behavior-science-addiction.

Olds DL, Kitzman HJ, Cole RE, et al.: Enduring effects of prenatal and infancy home visiting by nurses on maternal life course and government spending: follow-up of a randomized trial among children at age 12 years, *Arch Pediatr Adolesc Med* 164(5):419–424, 2010.

Ogden CL, Carroll MD, Fryar CD, et al.: *Prevalence of obesity among adults and youth: United States, 2011–2014*, NCHS data brief, no 219. Hyattsville, MD, 2015, National Center for Health Statistics.

Ogden CL, Carroll MD, Kit BK, Flegal KM: Prevalence of childhood and adult obesity in the United States, 2011-2012, *JAMA* 311(8):806–814, 2014.

Organisation for Economic Co-operation and Development: *Health: key tables from OECD, No. 14: Infant mortality*, 2013. Available from: < http://www.oecd-ilibrary.org/social-issues-migration-health/infant-mortality_20758480-table9>.

Oshiro BT, Henry E, Wilson J, et al.: Decreasing elective deliveries before 39 weeks of gestation in an integrated health care system, *Obstet Gynecol* 113:804–811, 2009.

Perper K, Peterson K, Manlove J: *Diploma attainment among teen mothers (Child Trends, Fact Sheet Publication #2010-01*, Washington, DC, Child Trends.

Petrini JR, Dias T, McCormick MC, et al.: Increased risk of adverse neurological development for late preterm infants, *J Pediatr* 154:169–176, 2009.

Planned Parenthood: Parents and teens talk about sexuality: a national survey 2012. Survey conducted by GfK Custom Research, LLC on behalf of Planned Parenthood, Family Circle magazine, and CLAFH. Available at http://www.plannedparenthood.org/images/LT_2012_Poll_Fact_Sheet_final(2).pdf.

Ramachandrappa A, Jain L: Health issues of the late preterm infant, *Pediatr Clin North Am* 56(3):565–577, 2009.

Reich K, editor: Children, youth, and gun violence, *Future Child* 12(2):1–173, 2002. Available from: <www.futureofchildren.org/pubs-info2825/pubs-info_show.htm? doc_id=154414>.

Sacco LN, Finklea K: *Synthetic drugs: overview and issues for congress*, Congressional Research Service, 2016. Available from: https://fas.org/sgp/crs/misc/R42066.pdf.

Safe Kids USA: *Preventing injuries: at home, at play, and on the way*, 2013. <http://www.safekids.org/search?search_api_views_fulltext=preventing+injuries h. Accessed February 22, 2013.

Substance Abuse and Mental Health Services Administration: *Results from the 2011 national survey on drug use and health: summary of national findings (NSDUH Series H-44, HHS Publication No. [SMA] 12–4713)*, Rockville, MD, 2011, Author. <http://www.samhsa.gov/data/NSDUH/2k11Results/NSDUHresults2011.htm>.

Substance Abuse and Mental Health Services Administration: *Results from the 2012 national survey on drug use and health: summary of national findings*, Rockville, MD, 2013, Administration, S. A. a. M. H. S.

Tong VT, England LJ, Dietz PM, et al.: Smoking patterns and use of cessation interventions during pregnancy, *Am J Prev Med* 35(4):327–333, 2008.

U.S. Court of Federal Claims: *Autism decisions and background information*, n.d. Available from: <http://www.uscfc.uscourts.gov/omnibus-autism-proceeding>.

U.S. Department of Agriculture Food and Nutrition Service: *Women, infants, and children (WIC)*, 2017. Available https://www.fns.usda.gov/wic/women-infants-and-children-wic.

U.S. Department of Education: *Building the legacy: IDEA 2004*, n.d. Available from: <http://idea.ed.gov/explore/home>.

U.S. Department of Health & Human Services, Administration for Children and Families, Administration on Children, Youth and Families, Children's Bureau: *Child maltreatment 2015*, 2017. Available from: http://www.acf.hhs.gov/programs/cb/research-data-technology/statistics-research/child-maltreatment.

U.S. Department of Health and Human Services: *Healthy People 2020*, Washington, DC, 2018, U.S. Government Printing Office. http://www.healthypeople.gov/2020/default.asp.

U.S. Department of Health and Human Services: *A report of the surgeon general: how tobacco smoke causes disease: what it means to you*, U.S. Department of Health and Human Services, Centers for Disease Control and Prevention, National Center for Chronic Disease Prevention and Health Promotion, Office on Smoking and Health, 2010.

U.S. Department of Health and Human Services: 2017 poverty guidelines, *Fed Regist* 82(19):8831–8832, 2017. Also available from Government publishing Office https://www.gpo.gov/fdsys/pkg/FR-2017-01-31/pdf/2017-02076.pdf.

U.S. Department of Health and Human Services, Administration for Children and Families, Administration on Children, Youth and Families, Children's Bureau: *Child maltreatment 2010*, 2011. Available from: <http://www.acf.hhs.gov/programs/cb/resource/child-maltreatment-2010>.

U.S. Department of Health and Human Services; Office of Population Affairs: *Title X family Planning Annual Report: 2012 National Summary*, 2013. https://www.hhs.gov/opa/title-x-family-planning/fp-annual-report/index.html.

U.S. Department of Health and Human Services, Health Resources and Services Administration, Maternal and Child Health Bureau: *Child Health USA*, Rockville, Maryland, 2014, U.S. Department of Health and Human Services, 2015. Online at http://mchb.hrsa.gov/chusa14/.

U.S. Department of Health and Human Services; Office of the Surgeon General: *The surgeon general's call to action to support breastfeeding*, Washington, DC, 2011, Author. <http://www.surgeongeneral.gov/library/calls/breastfeeding/index.htm>.

U.S. Department of Labor, Wage and Hour Division: *Break time for nursing mothers*, 2013. Available from: https://www.dol.gov/whd/nursingmothers/#Overview.

U.S. Department of Labor, Wage and Hour Division: *Family and medical leave act*, Final rule to amend the definition of spouse in the family and medical leave act regulations, revised February 2015. Available from: https://www.dol.gov/whd/fmla/spouse/.

Ventura SJ, Hamilton BE, Mathews TJ: *National and state patterns of teen births in the United States, 1940-2013*, National Vital Statistics Reports vol. 63, no. 4, Hyattsville, MD, 2014, National Center for Health Statistics. Available from: https://www.cdc.gov/nchs/data/nvsr/nvsr63/nvsr63_04.pdf.

White N, Lauritsen JL, Office of Justice Programs, Bureau of Justice Statistics: *Violent crime against youth, 1994-2010*, U.S. Department of Justice, 2012. Available from: https://www.bjs.gov/content/pub/pdf/vcay9410.pdf.

Widome R, Neumark-Sztainer D, Hannan PJ, et al.: Eating when there is not enough to eat: eating behaviors and perceptions of food among food-insecure youths, *Am J Public Health* 99:822–828, 2009.

Wolff T, Witkop CT, Miller T, et al.: Folic acid supplementation for the prevention of neural tube defects: an update of the evidence for the United States Preventive Services Task Force, *Ann Intern Med* 150:632–639, 2009.

Womenshealth.gov: *Breastfeeding*, n.d. Available from: <http://www.womenshealth.gov/breastfeeding/index.html>.

World Health Organization-Western Pacific Region: *Barriers to access to child healthcare*, n.d. Available from: www.wpro.who.int/publications.

World Health Organization: *Media centre. Youth violence facts*, 2016. Available from http://www.who.int/mediacentre/factsheets/fs356/en/.

Women's Health

Lori A. Glenn

OBJECTIVES

Upon completion of this chapter, the reader will be able to do the following:

1. Identify the major indicators of women's health.
2. Examine prominent health problems among women of all age groups (i.e., from adolescence to old age).
3. Identify barriers to adequate health care for women.
4. Discuss issues related to reproductive health.
5. Explain the influence of public policy on women's health.
6. Discuss issues and needs for increased research efforts focused on women's health.
7. Apply the nursing process to women's health concerns across all levels of prevention.

KEY TERMS

breast cancer
cesarean section
Civil Rights Act
cardiovascular disease
ectopic pregnancy

Family and Medical Leave Act
Hypertension
intimate partner violence
life expectancy
maternal mortality

multiple family configurations
osteoporosis
pelvic inflammatory disease
sexual harassment

To achieve "health for all" in the twenty-first century, health care services must be affordable and available to all. Although adequate health care for women is a key to realizing this goal, a significant number of women and their families face tremendous barriers to health care access. Additionally, knowledge deficits related to

health promotion and disease prevention activities prevent women of all educational and socioeconomic levels from assuming responsibility for their own health and well-being.

Beginning in the 1970s, the women's movement called for the reform of systems affecting women's health. Women were encouraged to become involved as consumers of health services and as establishers of health policy. More women entered health professions in which they were previously underrepresented, and those in traditionally female-dominated professions, such as nursing and teaching, became more assertive in their demands to gain recognition for their contributions to society. Health care for women has evolved from a focus on the pelvic area and breast to viewing the woman as a holistic being with specialized needs.

In "Preamble to a New Paradigm for Women's Health," Choi (1985) declared that collaboration and an interdisciplinary approach are necessary to meet the health care needs of women. She further stated, "[E]ssential to the development of health care for women are the concepts of health promotion, disease and accident prevention, education for self-care and responsibility, health risk identification and coordination for illness care when needed" (p. 14). To realize this paradigm, community-based health care focuses on health beyond the biophysical, disease-focused approach. Health from a social perspective considers the interaction of individual physiology along with work environment, living conditions, lifestyle choices, and health habits (Ruzek et al., 1997). Community health nurses must work with other health care professionals to formulate upstream strategies that modify the factors affecting women's health. Many *Healthy People 2020* objectives address health problems pertaining to women and include specific targets and strategies to improve the health of this aggregate. The *Healthy People 2020* boxes in this chapter present a small selection of these objectives. This chapter examines the health of women from adolescence to old age. It explores the major indicators of health, including specific health problems and the socioeconomic, sociocultural, and health policy issues surrounding women's health. The chapter also discusses identification of current and future research aimed at improving the health of women. An understanding of these points will enable community health nurses to appropriately apply this expertise in a community setting to help improve women's health.

MAJOR INDICATORS OF HEALTH

In the United States, data collected on major causes of death and illness appraise the health status of aggregates. These data are typically presented in terms of gender, age, or ethnicity and can help us interpret the levels of health in different groups. The primary indicators of health this chapter covers are life expectancy, mortality (i.e., death) rate, and morbidity (i.e., acute and chronic illness) rate.

♥ HEALTHY PEOPLE 2020

Selected Objectives for Women's Health

Objective	Baseline (Year)	Target (2010)	Final (Year)	Target (2020)
3-3: Reduce breast cancer death rate.	26.6 deaths per 100,000 (1999)	21.3 deaths per 100,000	22.9 deaths per 100,000 (2007)	20.6 deaths per 100,000
3-4: Reduce death rate from cervical cancer.	2.8 deaths per 100,000 (1999)	2.0 deaths per 100,000	2.4 deaths per 100,000 (2008)	2.2 deaths per 100,000
3-11b: Increase the proportion of women 21 years of age and older who have received a Papanicolaou smear test within the preceding 3 years.	79%* (1998)	90%	84.5%* (2008)	93%
3-13: Increase the proportion of women who have received breast cancer screening based on most recent guidelines in 2008.	67%[†] (1998)	70%	67% (2008)	81.1%
16-4: Reduce maternal deaths.	9.9 deaths per 100,000 live births (1998)	4.3 deaths per 100,000 live births	12.7 deaths per 100,000 live births (2007)	11.4 deaths per 100,000 live births
16-5a: Reduce maternal complications during labor and delivery.	31.2% (1998)	24%	31.1% (2007)	28%
16-6a: Increase the proportion of pregnant women who receive early and adequate prenatal care beginning in the first trimester.	83% (1998)	90%	70.8% (2007)	77.9%
16-15: Reduce the occurrence of neural tube defects (spina bifida and anencephaly).	60 cases per 100,000 live births (1996)	50 cases per 100,000 live births	60 cases per 100,000 live births (2007)	52 cases per 100,000 live births
25-1a: Reduce the proportion of females 15 to 24 years of age attending sexually transmitted disease clinics with *Chlamydia* infections.	5% (1997)	3%	7.4% (2008)	6.7%
25-6: Reduce the proportion of females 15 to 44 years of age who have required treatment for pelvic inflammatory disease.	8% (1995)	5%	4.2% (2006–2010)	3.8%

*Reflects a change in practice guidelines: Through 2008, women >18 years old were recommended for routine Pap smear screening, but guidelines changed the age to 21 years old in 2008.
[†]Reflects a change in practice guidelines. Prior to 2008, the measurement was mammograms within the past 2 years for women older than 40 years.
Data from U.S. Department of Health and Human Services: *Healthy People 2020*, ed 3, Washington, DC, 2010, Author; and National Center for Health Statistics: *Healthy People 2010* final review, 2012. http://www.cdc.gov/nchs/data/hpdata2010/hp2010_final_review.pdf Accessed 11-10, 17.

According to the Census Bureau (2017), there are an estimated 164 million women in the United States. Of these women, 11% are considered in fair to poor health and 12% have conditions that impair their daily functioning (Adams et al., 2011). Many factors that lead to death and illness among women are preventable or avoidable. If certain conditions receive early detection and treatment, a significant positive influence on longevity and the quality of life could ensue. Recognition of patterns demonstrated by these indicators can address problems preventively. This section presents an overview of these major indicators of health among women.

LIFE EXPECTANCY

Except in a few countries, such as Bangladesh, Malawi, Niger, Pakistan, Qatar, and Zimbabwe, women typically experience greater longevity than their male counterparts (World Health Organization [WHO], 2013). For example, women born in the 1970s in the United States have an average life expectancy of 74.7 years, or 7.6 years longer than men born in the same year.

Life expectancy for Americans is at an all-time high, but the discrepancy between males and females remains. Males born in 2014 have a life expectancy of 76 years, compared with 81 years for females. This suggests a trend toward narrowing the gap between male and female life expectancies. Ethnic/racial disparities in life expectancy unfortunately continued into the twenty-first century, as there is considerable variation among races. For example, black females gained an additional 7.1 years, from 69.4 years for those born in 1970 to 78 years for those born beginning in 2005. Although that is a significant gain, it falls behind the 81 years of life expectancy for white females born in 2014 and has not changed since 2005 (Hoyert and Xu, 2012).

Mortality Rate

Table 17.1 lists the six major causes of death among American women in 2009 by age group (Centers for Disease Control and Prevention [CDC], 2009, 2016). As age increases, the leading causes of death change. In the adolescent to early adulthood years, the leading cause is unintentional injuries (i.e., motor vehicle accidents, drug overdose). Changes since 2007 include (1) increased rate of suicide for 15- to 44-year olds, (2) increased proportion of deaths from chronic liver disease in 25- to 44-year-olds, and (3) stabilization or decrease in death from pregnancy complications in 20- to 34-year-olds. As middle age approaches, cancer becomes the number-one cause for women aged 35 to 85+ years, with the exception of the 75- to 84-year-olds who are more likely to die from heart disease.

◢ RESEARCH HIGHLIGHTS

Nurse Researchers Study the Inclusion of Women in Research

A group of nurse researchers (Crane et al., 2004) examined more than 1000 articles published in nursing journals between 1995 and 2001 to determine whether women had been included in research studies focusing on the leading causes of mortality. They found that 87% of the studies did include women participants. They also noted that there appeared to be a slight increase in inclusion of women from the earlier years to the later years.

TABLE 17.1 Six Leading Causes of Death Among American Women for All Races by Age Groups In 2009

Age Group (Years)	Cause of Death (in Rank Order)
15–19	Unintentional injury or accidents (43.9%)
	Suicide (9.1%)
	Homicide (8.1%)
	Cancer (8.1%)
	Heart disease (3.4%)
	Birth defects (3.1%)
20–24	Unintentional injury or accidents (36.8%)
	Suicide (9.1%)
	Homicide (8.1%)
	Cancer (7.8%)
	Heart disease (4.9%)
	Pregnancy complications (3.6%)
25–34	Unintentional injury or accidents (26.5%)
	Cancer (13.9%)
	Suicide (7.7%)
	Heart disease (7.6%)
	Homicide (5.6%)
	Pregnancy complications (3.0%)
35–44	Cancer (25.3%)
	Unintentional injuries (15.8%)
	Heart disease (11.9%)
	Suicide (5.5%)
	Stroke (3.1%)
	Chronic liver disease (3.0%)
45–54	Cancer (34.6%)
	Heart disease (14.4%)
	Unintentional injuries (9.0%)
	Stroke (3.8%)
	Chronic liver disease (3.6%)
	Chronic lower respiratory disease (3.3%)
55–64	Cancer (40.1%)
	Heart disease (26.6%)
	Chronic lower respiratory disease (5.7%)
	Stroke (3.8%)
	Diabetes mellitus (3.8%)
	Unintentional injuries (2.9%)
65–74	Cancer (36.5%)
	Heart disease (19.1%)
	Chronic obstructive pulmonary disease (8.9%)
	Stroke (4.7%)
	Diabetes mellitus (3.7%)
	Kidney disease (2.2%)
75–84	Heart disease (23.8%)
	Cancer (23.5%)
	Chronic obstructive pulmonary disease (8.0%)
	Stroke (7.0%)
	Alzheimer disease (4.6%)
	Diabetes mellitus (3.1%)
85+	Heart disease (31.1%)
	Cancer (10.5%)
	Stroke (8.0%)
	Alzheimer disease (8.0%)
	Chronic obstructive pulmonary disease (4.6%)
	Influenza and pneumonia (3.0%)

Data from Centers for Disease Control and Prevention: *Leading cause of death by age group, all females – United States, 2009.* http://www.cdc.gov/women/lcod/2009/index.htm.

Cardiovascular Disease

About one in four Americans has one or more forms of cardiovascular disease (CVD) (e.g., high blood pressure, coronary heart disease, stroke, congenital defects, or rheumatic heart disease). For women in the United States, CVD accounts for one out of every four deaths, making it the leading cause of death (CDC, 2016b). One in ten women under age 60 has some form of CVD; the ratio increases to one in three after age 65. Black women are more likely to die from CVD than are white women. In 2011, the CVD death rate among white women was 230.4 per 100,000, compared with 319.7 per 100,000 for black women. Black women are also more likely to die from stroke than white women (60.7 per 100,000 and 44 per 100,000, respectively) (American Heart Association [AHA], 2013).

CVD continues to be the number-one overall killer of women. One out of every 7.5 deaths is from CVD, whereas 1 out of every 30 deaths is from breast cancer. Since 1984, CVD caused more deaths among females than males. In 2011 51% of deaths from CVD were in women (AHA, 2013). The overall number of deaths due to CVD decreased dramatically from 424.2 per 100,000 in 1950 to 236 per 100,000 in 2010, with significant differences between white women (190.4 per 100,000) and black women (267.9 per 100,000). (CDC, 2016a)

Disparities have improved for women in relation to prevention, diagnosis, and management of heart disease through public awareness campaigns such as "Go Red for Women" and research focusing more on the unique aspects of women and heart disease (AHA, 2017). Despite an increased focus, 64% of women do not recognize that heart disease is their number-one cause of death. The number of cardiovascular deaths has decreased, but women were still more likely to die from a first myocardial infarction than men. In part, this phenomenon is due to the subtle or absence of symptoms of coronary artery disease (CDC, 2016d). Women have smaller arteries and higher rates of metabolic syndrome, diabetes, heart failure, and other comorbidities. They tend to be older at their first cardiovascular event, with more urgent and emergency presentations (Jacobs, 2003).

Rates of CVD among women can decline further when individuals become more aware of risk factors and accept responsibility for managing their own health and well-being (Kuehn et al., 1999). Concerned and motivated providers must encourage women to practice heart-healthy behaviors. In 2002, the American Heart Association launched the "Go Red" campaign for women and "The Heart Truth" program for health care providers, which were designed to educate both groups about the unique features of women and heart disease.

Cancer

Cancer is the second leading cause of death in the United States. One out of four deaths in the United States is due to cancer (Siegel et al., 2014). Cancer rates rose through the early 1990s for a number of reasons, including lifestyle choices (smoking, diet, sun exposure), increasing exposure to environmental carcinogens, and, probably most important, greater life expectancy. Because of improvements in early detection, screening, and treatment of the major cancers, incidence rates have leveled off and in some cases decreased. To illustrate, death rates from cancer among women have increased from 136 per 100,000 in 1960 to 167.3 per 100,000 in 2000 (CDC, 2004). Yet there was a decline in the cancer death rate from 2002 to 2004, about 2% per year, which was "large enough to overcome the impact of the growth and aging of the population" (ACS, 2013). In 2013, there were 277,319 deaths among women as a result of cancer.

According to the American Cancer Society (2017b) in 1987 lung cancer surpassed breast cancer as the leading cause of cancer deaths in women, and death rates from lung cancer increased sharply until about 1990. The percentage of cancer deaths due to lung cancer leveled off in 2005 to 26% and remained stable through 2013 at 25%. Breast cancer was the second most common cause, accounting for 14% of all cancer deaths. Colorectal cancer, the third most frequent cause of cancer deaths, accounts for 8% of such deaths.

Other female-specific cancers include ovarian cancer (fifth most common), uterine cancer (sixth most common), and cervical cancer. Cervical cancer, in particular, has received considerable attention of late because it has been determined that 90% of women with cervical cancer have evidence of cervical infection with human papillomavirus (HPV) (ACS, 2016a). In June 2006, the U.S. Food and Drug Administration (FDA) licensed Gardasil (Merck and Co, Inc.), the first vaccine to prevent HPV infection (CDC, 2015e). Through March 2013, 57 million doses have been given (CDC, 2017d). Gardasil has been shown to be highly effective in preventing the most common types of HPV infection and was approved for use in females between 9 and 26 years of age.

The good news is that healthy lifestyle changes and early detection and intervention have contributed to the decreases in mortality rates from some cancers. For example, the death rate for colorectal cancer has been dropping since the mid-1980s as a result of early detection and treatment (ACS, 2014). Lung cancer deaths are beginning to show a slight decline that parallels a lower incidence of smoking by women older than 18 years (ACS, 2017b).

Five-year survival rates vary according to the type of cancer and stage at diagnosis. For instance, the 5-year survival rate for all clients with lung cancer is 19%. For those with localized breast cancer, it is 91%, decreasing to 23% for those diagnosed with distant metastases. Of cancers related to the reproductive tract, ovarian cancer has the lowest survival rate, as only around 46% of women survive for 5 years (ACS, 2017c). The 5-year survival rate is 66% for women with colon cancer and 68% for those with rectal cancer; this rate improves significantly with early detection (ACS, 2014).

Early diagnosis and prompt treatment are major factors in surviving many types of cancer. Routine cervical cancer screening begins at age 21, at which time a Papanicolaou (Pap) smear should be done every 3 years. Colorectal cancer screenings include annual fecal occult blood tests along with sigmoidoscopy every 5 years or colonoscopy every 10 years (ACS, 2017c).

Certain health choices may reduce an individual's risk of cancer. Women reduce their risk for cancer by never smoking or by quitting if they already use tobacco products. Eating a nutritious, plant-focused, high-fiber diet along with adopting a physically active lifestyle and maintaining a healthy body weight protect against both heart disease and many cancers. Nutrition guidelines include avoiding salt-cured, smoked, nitrite-containing, and charred foods; high-fat foods; and excessive alcohol. Obesity has been associated with an increased risk for cancers of the colon and rectum, endometrium, and breast (ACS, 2016b). Finally, the practice of safe sex has been shown to reduce the spread of cancer associated with sexually transmitted diseases (STDs) such as HPV, hepatitis B and C, and HIV (ACS, 2016c; CDC, 2016b).

Community health nurses must encourage all females (i.e., from childhood to old age) to adopt these healthy lifestyle choices and pursue early cancer detection. Community health nurses play a major role in providing cancer control services that should be culturally sensitive and appropriate to the targeted aggregate. If providers and clients applied everything known about cancer prevention, approximately two thirds of cancer cases would not occur.

Diabetes

In 2014, the number of diabetics in the United States reached 29 million, 9.3% of the population. Of 86 million American adults over age 20, 37% are considered prediabetic, and 51% of those over age 60 are affected (CDC, 2014a). The CDC estimates that at the current rate, one third of adults will have diabetes by 2050 (CDC, 2016b).

Diabetes mellitus is a chronic disease that causes the premature death of many women and overall ranks sixth in mortality among that group, being highest after age 45. Diabetes is the fourth leading cause of death among several aggregates, including Native Americans, blacks, and Asians, and is fifth among Hispanics (National Center for Health Statistics, 2013). Women are more likely to be seriously affected by the complications of diabetes, including CVD, stroke, vision loss, and depression (USDHHS, 2017).

In addition to being a serious illness in itself, diabetes is a risk factor for the development of CVD; furthermore, it dramatically influences the severity and course of CVD. In death certificates from 2004 on which the cause of death was related to diabetes, 68% also listed CVD and 16% also listed stroke (CDC, 2009). When comparing men and women with diabetes, of those who suffer a myocardial infarction before age 65, women are more likely to die and suffer long-term health problems (Norhammar et al., 2009). The good news is that the number of women hospitalized for diabetes and its complications has dropped, indicating that better management with tighter control of blood glucose has decreased complications (CDC, 2014a). The community health nurse is an important resource for supporting the tight control of diabetes to prevent its complications. An upstream approach to this problem includes helping women maintain a desirable weight throughout life in an effort to avoid nutrition-related causes of death such as diabetes and CVD.

BOX 17.1   Centering Pregnancy: Model for Prenatal Care

Developed in 1993, the Centering Pregnancy model uses a group approach to prenatal care. The prenatal visit occurs with women of similar gestational ages and includes an assessment with the provider along with group learning, facilitated discussion, and support among women. The group dynamic contributes to health-promoting behaviors and to normalizing attitudes to pregnancy. Women report high satisfaction with the care and go on to have fewer preterm births and babies of optimal weight (Centering Health Care, 2013; Manant and Dodgson, 2011).

Maternal Mortality

According to the WHO (2012), 800 women die every day from complications of pregnancy and childbirth, which are the leading cause of disability and death among women worldwide between the ages of 14 and 49 years. Maternal mortality in developing countries is 240 per 100,000 live births, whereas it is 16 per 100,000 in developed countries. Forty percent of women experience complications during pregnancy, childbirth, and the postpartum period, 15% of which are life threatening. Reduction of maternal mortality is one of the *Healthy People 2020* objectives for the United States. See Box 17.1 for information on a group approach to prenatal care.

The United States ranks seventeenth in maternal mortality among all nations. Beginning in the 1950s, maternal mortality rates began to decline in the United States due to the use of blood transfusions, the availability of antimicrobial drugs, and the maintenance of fluid and electrolyte balance during serious complications of pregnancy and birth. The development of obstetrical training programs and obstetrical anesthesia programs was also important.

However, since 1987 the rate of maternal death has increased from 7.2 per 100,000 pregnancies to 17.3 in 2013 (CDC, 2016b). Some of this change may be due to updated methods for data collection. Before 2003, in the United States, maternal mortality was defined as the deaths of women while pregnant or within 42 days after termination of pregnancy. The U.S. Standard Certificate of Death and the tenth revision of WHO's *International Statistical Classification of Diseases and Related Health Problems* (ICD-10) revised this definition in 2003 to include late causes of maternal death, defined as occurring more than 42 days but less than 1 year after the end of the pregnancy (Hoyert and Xu, 2012; WHO, 2007). Although this change may explain the increase in the mid-2000s, the continued increase in the death rate is still without clear etiology. Researchers cite maternal obesity, older age, and chronic health conditions along with an increasing cesarean section rate as contributing factors (CDC, 2017; Kaiser Daily, 2009). In 2013 the leading cause of maternal death was CVD, followed by other medical conditions, infection/sepsis, cardiomyopathy, pulmonary embolism, and hypertensive disorders (CDC, 2017).

Beginning in the 1950s, maternal mortality rates began to decline in the United States due to the use of blood transfusions, the availability of antimicrobial drugs, and the maintenance of fluid and electrolyte balance during serious complications of pregnancy and birth. The development

TABLE 17.2 **Maternal Mortality Rate Per 100,000 Live Births—Selected Years**

Year	Total	Whites	Blacks	Other (Nonwhite)
1992	7.8	5.0	20.8	18.2
1999	13.2	9.5	32.2	14.5
2001	14.7	10.2	36.8	9.9
2003	16.8	11.7	43.5	18.9
2005	15.4	10.7	38.7	15.9

Data from Berg CJ, Callaghan WM, Syverson C, Henderson Z: Pregnancy-related mortality in the United States, 1998 to 2005, *Obstet Gynecol* 116(6):1302–1309, 2010.

of obstetrical training programs and obstetrical anesthesia programs was also important.

Racial discrepancy persists, however, in maternal mortality rates as in life expectancy. Table 17.2 illustrates how nonwhite women have a significantly higher incidence of death during pregnancy than white women. The gap in maternal mortality rates between black and white women has widened over the past several decades. Early in the twentieth century, black women were two times more likely to die of pregnancy-related complications than white women. Currently, black women are nearly four times more likely to die (CDC, 2017). Major risk factors for maternal death include lack of antepartum care and family planning services, inadequate health education, and poor nutrition. An additional risk factor, regardless of race, is advancing age. Women 40 years and older have more than three times the risk of dying from a pregnancy-related cause as women aged 30 to 39 years (National Center for Health Statistics, 2017). Intrinsic maternal factors, such as higher frequency of hypertension and greater likelihood of uterine hemorrhage, help explain this increase in the mortality rate among older mothers.

Death associated with legal surgical abortion is rare in the United States, with four cases reported in 2012 (Jatlaoui et al., 2016). Complications that result in death from legal abortion relate to the woman's age, the type of procedure, the gestational age of the fetus, and general health problems at the time of the abortion (Cates et al., 2004).

A medical, or induced, method of abortion using mifepristone (i.e., RU-486), an antiprogestin medication, together with prostaglandins has been used in the United States since September 2000. This method is as effective as surgical abortion and is considered a safe alternative to surgical abortion in pregnancies of less than 49 days (7 weeks). In 2013, 22% of the legal abortions in the United States employed this method. Curettage is still the most widely used abortion procedure.

Abortion is a controversial issue for providers and for the women in their care. Abortion rates have fallen significantly from 820,151 in 2005 to 664,435 in 2013, as has the rate of complications from this procedure. (Jatlaoui et al., 2016). Access to free contraception through the Affordable Care Act (ACA) and multiple long-acting methods have contributed to the decreased use of abortion. Nurses must continue to keep abreast of all available pregnancy prevention and termination options to provide the best counsel for women.

Ectopic pregnancy is the leading cause of maternal death in the first trimester. Since the 1980s, the incidence of ectopic pregnancy has decreased from 1.15 to 0.50 per 100,000 live births, the cause of death being hemorrhage in 67% of cases. Racial discrepancy is evident, with rates 6.8 times higher in African Americans. Rates are also 3.5 times higher in women older than 35 years than in those younger than 25 years. The rates are possibly higher because STDs are diagnosed more frequently in this older population and may cause damage and scarring of fallopian tubes, raising the risk of ectopic pregnancy (CDC, 2016b; Creanga et al., 2011).

The most significant risk for ectopic pregnancy is previous pelvic inflammatory disease (PID) or salpingitis. Early diagnosis and treatment greatly lower the mortality rate. Prevention interventions for women at risk for acquiring STDs are critical in reducing a woman's risk for an ectopic pregnancy. An important task of health care providers is to educate women and men about methods to reduce sexual health risk-taking behaviors. Additional risk factors for ectopic pregnancy include tubal pathology, previous ectopic pregnancy, tubal surgery, and the use of intrauterine contraceptive devices.

Morbidity Rate

Hospitalizations

The 2010 National Hospital Discharge Survey reported that more women than men are hospitalized each year in the United States (Hall et al., 2010). Pneumonia resulted in an average hospital stay of 5.0 days, which occurred most frequently among women aged 65 or older. Fractures accounted for an average 5.1 days, malignant neoplasms for an average 6.5 days, and diseases of the heart for an average 4.4 days. The primary reason for hospitalization was childbirth, followed by circulatory, digestive, and respiratory diseases, and finally injury or poisoning (DeFrances et al., 2008).

The prospective payment system for hospitalization resulted in a greater demand for skilled nursing services in the home. After community members have been hospitalized for any of several of these conditions, community health nurses may provide ongoing nursing care in the home by referral. Nurses practicing in home environments must be prepared to deliver "high-tech" and "high-touch" services. Chapter 33 discusses home health care in detail.

Chronic Conditions and Limitations

Women are more likely than men to be disabled by chronic conditions. Arthritis and rheumatism, hypertension, and impairment of the back or spine decrease women's activity level more often than they affect their male counterparts. In fact, twice as many women (24.3%) as men (11.5%) are limited in activity from arthritis and rheumatism. Women are more likely than men to have difficulty performing activities such as walking, bathing or showering, preparing meals, and doing housework (Arthritis Foundation, 2014; CDC, 2009b).

Functional limitations may require home health care that community health nurses supervise and deliver. Nurses plan and implement interventions on the basis of functional assessments.

Each care plan facilitates optimal resumption of the individual's independence in personal care activities.

Surgery

Women are more likely than men to have surgery. Hysterectomy is the second most frequently performed major surgical procedure among women of reproductive age after cesarean section. Approximately 600,000 hysterectomies are performed each year (CDC, 2015d). Hysterectomy rates for women in the South are slightly higher than those in the Northeast (6.3 and 4.9 per 1000 women, respectively). Overall, rates of hysterectomy decreased from 5.4 to 5.1 per 1000 in the years 2000 through 2004 (Whiteman et al., 2008).

According to the CDC (2016b), the most common reason for hysterectomy is uterine fibroids or leiomyoma, which contributes to more than one-third of all such surgeries, but considerably more in blacks (68%) than in whites (33%). White women are more often diagnosed with endometriosis and uterine prolapse, which are the second and third most common reasons for hysterectomy. Hysterectomy rates are the highest in women aged 40 to 44 years CDC, 2015c).

Optional procedures are becoming available to women. Myomectomy—removal of only the tumors with repair of the uterus—uterine artery ablation, and the use of a gonadotropin-releasing hormone to shrink the tumors can decrease the need for hysterectomy, but women may not know about these alternatives. Community health nurses function as advocates for women and can provide health education programs related to alternatives to hysterectomy, indications for hysterectomy and oophorectomy (i.e., removal of ovaries), and information regarding the type of surgical approach and the purpose of a second opinion. Second opinions and higher levels of education tend to lower the rate of hysterectomies (Finkel and Finkel, 1990).

Birth by **cesarean section** (C-section) is the most prevalent surgical procedure experienced by women in the United States and accounts for 32% of births. Several factors contribute to the high rates of C-section, including physician fear of malpractice suits, routine use of early induction of labor, and epidural anesthesia. The technology of fetal monitoring has been shown to increase the C-section rate without improving neonatal outcomes.

Mental Health

The most frequently occurring interruption in women's mental health relates to depression. Well-controlled epidemiological studies consistently demonstrate that women experience depression at two to three times the rate of men (American Psychological Association [APA], 2005). Symptoms of depression include depressed mood, apathy, anxiety, irritability, and thoughts of death and suicide (Evans et al., 1999). Unique to women are atypical symptoms including anxiety, increased appetite, weight gain, and somatic complaints along with increased rates of comorbid conditions. Women are more likely to attempt suicide but less likely to be successful (Urbanic, 2014). Women with socioeconomic barriers, such as lower income and lower educational levels, racial/ethnic discrimination, unemployment, poor

health, single parenthood, and high-stress jobs, are at greater risk for depression than women with higher educational levels or higher economic status. Other risk factors are childhood negligence and abuse, parental death, negligence, and alcoholism (Urbanic, 2009).

Nurses practicing in community health settings should be aware of the signs and symptoms of depression and should identify referral sources for professional help within the community. The community health nurse plays a vital role in identifying mothers who suffer from postpartum depression. The CDC (2008d) reports that up to 12% of women suffer postpartum depression that interferes with a woman's ability to care for herself, baby, and family. The nurse needs to also be aware of the impact a mother's depression may have on her child's development and family functioning. A woman experiencing depression displays a variety of symptoms, including depressed mood, weight changes, sleep disturbances, and fatigue, among others, which can be found in the *Diagnostic and Statistical Manual of Mental Disorders* (APA, 2013).

SOCIAL FACTORS AFFECTING WOMEN'S HEALTH

Health Care Access

In 2012, 18.2% of the U.S. population, or 48.2 million U.S. citizens, lacked health insurance coverage (NCHS, 2017). With the passing of the ACA in 2012, the number of uninsured citizens had dropped to 28.5 million by 2016 (NCHS, 2017). The ACA required all insurers to provide coverage for essential services to women, including preventive screenings (cervical and breast cancer), pregnancy care, breast-feeding support, and contraception (NCHS, 2017). Young adults (i.e., those between ages 16 and 24 years) previously made up approximately 50% of individuals without health insurance, but can now obtain coverage or stay on their parent's insurance until the age of 26. Women who choose not to enroll in the ACA are not likely to seek health care until they or a family member is in acute distress. Others may rely on home remedies, over-the-counter drugs, or folk healers for health care. Older women on fixed incomes may have difficulty meeting copayments required by Medicare and paying for prescription medications. Many senior citizens have paid hospitalization insurance premiums for policies that fail to meet the gap.

Education and Work

In the workplace, women traditionally predominated as secretaries, administrative assistants, registered nurses (RNs), teachers, cashiers, and retail sales people. However, in the 1980s, more women began to enter professions traditionally held by men (e.g., lawyers, physicians, and dentists), and in 2008, more than half (51%) of young professionals were women (U.S. Department of Labor, 2016). In 1970, 55.4% of all women aged 25 or older were high school graduates, compared with 81.6% in 1995 and 85% in 2003. Of this same age group in 2009, 35% had completed college, which was more than three times the 1970 rate of 8.1% (U.S. Census Bureau, 2012). A growing number of women have earned degrees in traditionally male-dominated professions. Table 17.3 reflects the changes occurring in percentages of women receiving degrees in medicine, dentistry, law, and theology.

Employment and Wages

In 2016, 57% of the workforce were women. In addition, more than half (64%) of women with young children (younger than 6 years) were working outside the home (U.S. Department of Labor, 2017). In 1950, only 12% of women were combining these roles (Chadwick and Heaton, 1992).

Several questions concerning women's health and well-being relate to employment issues. A review of female-dominated versus male-dominated jobs discloses inequalities in wage and salary scales; despite the diminishing gap between women's and men's incomes, there is still much room for improvement. Table 17.4 depicts median annual income by sex and ethnicity for both men and women (DeNavas-Walt et al., 2012). Disparities in income, based on sex and ethnicity, are clear.

Women heads of households and their children are the poorest aggregate in the United States. This phenomenon is labeled "the feminization of poverty." In 2014, the poverty rate for single female heads of household was 38.9%, compared with 8.2% for single male heads of households (National Women's Law Center [NWLC], 2017). Race is a factor in the poverty rate as follows:

- Asian American 28.9%
- Black 45.6%
- Hispanic 46.3%
- Foreign born 44.8%
- Native American 56.9 %
- White 32.0%

The nurse working with impoverished families should be aware of social services, child care programs, emergency services, and other resources for families in need. The community health nurse often needs to act as case manager and advocate for families with social service agencies and other public entities.

WORKING WOMEN AND HOME LIFE

Added to inequalities outside the home are inequalities within the home. A working woman is less likely to have a spouse or partner help with the home and children. Even when a spouse or partner is present, the burdens of housework and child care usually fall more heavily on the woman, regardless of ethnicity. Mothers generally spend more time than fathers preparing meals and training and disciplining their children. These multiple-role demands and conflicting expectations contribute to stress (American Academy of Pediatrics, 2003; Matthews and Power, 2002).

However, changes are occurring, as both younger and older men now report spending more time in family activities than middle-aged men. Black and Hispanic men tend to spend a little more time working at family tasks than white men. Books and articles encourage wives and husbands to make their needs known, encouraging greater communication between partners. Marriage enrichment programs, often offered through churches and synagogues, teach couples how to communicate more effectively with each other, fostering equality between partners.

Family Configuration and Marital Status

Women are members of **multiple family configurations** (e.g., nuclear families, extended family units, single-parent units, families of group marriages, blended family units, adoptive family units, nonlegal heterosexual unions, and lesbian family units). This diversity causes changes in women's roles within families. Whether or not they function in a traditional role, most women do whatever is necessary to maintain the integrity of their families. Early assessment of the strengths of family units by the community health nurse provides a database for positive nursing interventions established on upstream strategies to enhance each family's level of health and well-being.

Many women are delaying marriage, and an increasing number are not marrying. Overall, marriage rates have remained stable, perhaps because the increasing number of remarriages balances the declining rate of first marriages. When a relationship ends in divorce or separation, more women than men have the responsibility of providing for themselves and their children. Single mothers are most often the head of a single-parent family. Even in the face of changing lifestyles, divorce, and increased mobility, which leads to long-distance relationships, most Americans report that they remain connected to their extended families through parents, grandparents, siblings, aunts, and uncles.

One contemporary family configuration involves single women with one or more adopted children. Single-parent

TABLE 17.3 Percentages of Degrees Received by Women

Degree	1970	1980	1988	1996	2002	2007
Medicine (MD)	8.4	23.4	33.3	40.9	44.4	49.2
Dentistry (DDS or DMD)	0.9	13.3	26.7	35.8	38.5	44.5
Law (LLB or JD)	5.4	30.2	40.8	43.4	48.0	47.6
Theology (BD, MDiv, or MHL)	2.3	13.8	19.3	23.3	33.2	33.2

From U.S. Department of Education: *Digest of education statistics,* Washington, DC, 2008, Author.

TABLE 17.4 Median Annual Earnings by Type of Household in 7 Years Between 1969 and 2011

Household Type	1969	1979	1989	1999	2003	2007	2011
Married couple with children	41,453	47,793	50,613	56,827	62,405	72,785	74,130
Female householder with children	16,327	18,468	17,651	26,164	29,307	33,370	33,637
Male householder with children	33,749	36,619	34,646	41,830	41,959	49,839	49,567

From DeNavas-Walt C, Proctor D, Smith J: *Income, poverty, and health insurance coverage in the United States: 2011* (U.S. Census Bureau Current Population Reports), 2012. http://www.census.gov/prod/2008pubs/p60-243.pdf.

adoptions are legal, and a growing number of single women are becoming adoptive parents. An often-ignored family structure is one headed by a lesbian parent. Since the Supreme Court made gay marriage a right in 2015, same-sex couples have made progress in establishing families. Lesbians who become parents have needs similar to those of all mothers. Many cities have lesbian-gay parent groups that provide support, anticipatory guidance, and strategies for coping in society. However, lesbian women often neglect their own health. This self-neglect may be traced to hostile and rejecting attitudes of health care providers (Zeidenstein, 2004). However, the parents or guardians must remain healthy to ensure the child's well-being.

 ACTIVE LEARNING

Review county or state health department statistics for leading causes of death among women of varying ethnic or racial groups.

HEALTH PROMOTION STRATEGIES FOR WOMEN

A woman's ability to carry out her important roles can affect her entire family; therefore women should receive services that promote health and detect disease at an early stage. Early detection and improved treatments for disease allow women to return to work or remain working throughout the course of an illness. Although work is essential to the economic and social well-being of many women's families, the workplace itself creates physical and social stress. As more women enter the workforce and face many of the same risks and stressors as men do, it is not surprising that their formerly favorable mortality and morbidity rates have been declining.

Many women seek information that will allow them to be in control of their own health. Since the early 1970s, women have met in self-help groups to develop a better understanding of their own health needs. Some of the health behaviors that women learn in these groups are the importance of nutrition and exercise, health maintenance, pregnancy testing and contraceptive awareness; recognition of the early signs of vaginal infections and STDs; and awareness of the variations in female anatomy and physiology.

For women who desire to become more knowledgeable about their own health, books are available in bookstores, in public libraries, and among the holdings of traditional women's groups such as sororities and federated women's clubs. An excellent resource for women is the FDA Consumer (http://www.fda.gov/fdac/), the official consumer site of the FDA, which reports on studies that cover a variety of women's health issues such as mammography standards, menopause, treatment for STDs, eating disorders, infertility, cosmetic safety, silicone breast implants, and osteoporosis. Another resource is the U.S. Department of Health and Human Services' Office on Women's Health (www.WomensHealth.gov), which highlights positive health behaviors for women and girls. The community health nurse can use models such as Pender's Health Promotion Model in teaching health behaviors that lead to general health promotion among women. Pender notes that health-promoting behaviors are directed toward sustaining or increasing the level of well-being, self-actualization, and fulfillment of a given individual or group (Pender et al., 2006). However, because many models were developed for the middle class, they may not be useful to community health nurses working with low-income families.

Knowledge deficits related to body awareness prevail among all women, regardless of socioeconomic or educational level. For example, a woman may ask whether she will menstruate after a hysterectomy, whether she should perform a breast self-examination (BSE), or what she can do to prevent recurrent episodes of vaginitis. Nurses can play an instrumental role in helping women develop a greater sense of self-awareness. Furthermore, community health nurses can remove the mystery surrounding the woman's body and encourage clients to ask previously unmentionable questions.

Chronic Illness

Included among chronic diseases that may affect a woman during her life span are coronary vascular disease and metabolic syndrome, hypertension, diabetes, arthritis, osteoporosis, and cancer.

Coronary Vascular Disease and Metabolic Syndrome

Evidence suggests that CVD and metabolic syndrome in most women are preventable. CVD is caused by atherosclerosis, which results in buildup of plaque that in turn narrows arteries, decreasing blood flow to the heart muscle. Metabolic syndrome is a group of risk factors that have been linked to an increased risk of cardiovascular events. These factors are abdominal obesity (waist circumference more than 35 inches in women), dyslipidemia (elevated triglyceride and low high-density lipoprotein cholesterol values), insulin resistance, and elevated blood pressure. The underlying etiology of metabolic syndrome is related to the combination of inactivity, obesity, and genetics.

At-risk women have nonmodifiable risk factors such as increasing age, race, gender, or family history of CVD and diabetes. Where the greatest impact can be made is with the modifiable risk factors, which are as follows (AHA, 2013):

- Cigarette smoking
- Obesity
- Diet high in calories, total fats, cholesterol, refined carbohydrates, and sodium
- Glucose intolerance
- Elevated serum lipid values
- Sedentary lifestyle
- Personality type
- Hypertension
- Stress
- Alcohol use

Education by community nurses can assist women in identifying their risk of CVD and metabolic syndrome along with health behaviors that decrease modifiable risk factors. Also important are evidence-based recommendations for high-risk women with existing CVD, including aspirin therapy and omega-3 fatty acid supplementation (Mosca, 2007).

Hypertension

The latest report of the Joint National Committee on Prevention, Detection, Evaluation, and Treatment of High Blood Pressure defines **hypertension** as blood pressure of 140/90 mm Hg or greater diastolic. If the client is over the age of 60, the threshold is 150/90 (James et al., 2014). Essential hypertension is the most common type of chronic hypertensive disorder in women. Approximately one third of hypertension cases occur during pregnancy as gestational hypertension or preeclampsia. Essential hypertension is the most common type of chronic hypertensive disorder in women, accounting for 85% of such cases. It is also responsible for approximately one third of all hypertension cases during pregnancy. Hypertension is more common in women than in men and affects more blacks than whites. Hypertension usually starts with an asymptomatic phase; therefore every woman should be screened on an average of every 2 years beginning in her teenage years. Diagnosis is crucial to prevent or modify possible complications of this disease.

Diabetes

According to the CDC (2016b), 29 million people (9.3% of the population) have diabetes in the United States, and the number is growing every year. Furthermore, although an estimated 20.9 million have been diagnosed, some 8.1 million people are not aware they have the disease. In previous years, community health nurses have worked to educate women to assume responsibility in their management of diabetes mellitus. More recently, community health nurses have been actively involved in education and screening programs for groups at high risk. Included in these groups are individuals who have a family history of diabetes, those who are obese, and older adults. Nurses who design education programs need to be aware of the ethnic differences in the prevalence of diabetes. African American, Hispanic, American Indian, and Asian women are two to four times more likely to have diabetes than their non-Latino white counterparts (USHHS, 2011).

Pregnancy is potentially diabetogenic (Cunningham et al., 2010). Pregnancy may aggravate the condition, and clinical diabetes may appear in some women only during pregnancy. Consequently, screening for diabetes is routine in pregnancy. Annual screening for type 2 diabetes should occur beginning at age 45. Screening methods include the fasting blood glucose, hemoglobin A1C, or 2-hour oral glucose tolerance test (CDC, 2014a). The nurse is involved in explaining the purpose of the screening and how to prepare for the tests. In most public health settings, the nurse is responsible for explaining the results.

Arthritis

In 2009, 50 million people in the United States, nearly one in five adults, were afflicted with arthritis. The incidence of arthritis is higher in women than in men: approximately 25.9 million women have the condition, compared with 18.3 million men (CDC, 2010).

Osteoarthritis (OA) is the most common form of the disease. It is characterized by degeneration of the joints and is more common with increasing age and in women. OA of the knee is the leading cause of disability in the United States. Modifiable risk factors for OA include excess body mass, joint injury, occupation, and estrogen deficiency (CDC, 2017a).

Rheumatoid arthritis (RA) can affect anyone, but for every man affected, 2.5 women have the disease. Onset usually occurs between 30 and 50 years of age. RA often goes into remission in a pregnant woman, although symptoms tend to increase in intensity after the baby is born, and RA develops more often than expected the year after giving birth. Although women are two to three times more likely to have RA than men, men tend to be more severely affected when they do have it (Arthritis Foundation, 2014).

Arthritis is the leading cause of disability in the United States (CDC, 2017b). Nursing interventions focus on prevention of joint deformity and modification of lifestyle if necessary.

Osteoporosis

Osteoporosis is a major disorder affecting women, occurring in 25% to 50% of postmenopausal women. Although men may experience osteoporosis, it is four times more common among women. The National Osteoporosis Foundation (2014) estimates that of the 10 million Americans who have osteoporosis, 8 million are women and 2 million are men. An additional 34 million Americans have osteopenia. Half of all non-Hispanic white women in the United States will experience an osteoporosis-related fracture during their lifetimes. The most serious complication of osteoporosis is hip fracture, which is experienced by 280,000 Americans annually. Approximately 24% die within a year from complications of hip fracture.

Postmenopausal white women are at highest risk for osteoporosis. Loss of bone begins at an earlier age in women and proceeds twice as rapidly as in men. Guidelines issued by the National Osteoporosis Foundation recommend bone mineral density tests for selected postmenopausal women and the use of oral bisphosphonates as the first-line pharmacological treatment. In light of the results of the Women's Health Initiative Study showing that nonestrogen therapies fail or cause intolerable side effects, hormone replacement therapy is currently considered second-line therapy for the disease (Wei et al., 2003). Osteoporosis has no cure; therefore prevention is especially important early in life. Prevention involves an awareness of dietary practices such as maintaining a correct balance of calcium, vitamin D, and protein throughout life, in addition to regular weight-bearing, muscle-strengthening, and aerobic exercise.

Nurses in ambulatory health practices should encourage women to become more knowledgeable of the strategies to prevent osteoporosis. For women diagnosed with this condition, nurses can assist in various aspects of management (e.g., education regarding prescribed medication, follow-up care, avoidance of complications, and dietary modifications as needed).

Breast Cancer

The incidence of **breast cancer** has been rising since the 1950s. Currently, one out of every eight women will have breast cancer sometime in her life. The chance of dying from breast cancer is about 1 in 35. In 2013 230,815 women in the United States were diagnosed with breast cancer and 40,860 died from it (CDC, 2016b). Risk factors include aging, personal or family history (especially mother or sister) of breast cancer, early age at menarche, late age at menopause, never having children, and having a first child after age 30. Female gender and aging are the most significant risk factors for breast cancer (ACS, 2016b). An additional risk is a genetic mutation of tumor suppressor genes known as *BRCA1* and *BRCA2*. The lifetime risk for women with this mutation to be diagnosed with breast cancer is 60%, compared with 12% for the general population. Additional risks are for ovarian cancer, with a 40% lifetime risk for those who inherit the gene, compared with 1.4% for the general population (NCI, 2013a). Genetic testing is available, and the rights of those tested is protected legally, so insurers and employers cannot use this information to discriminate against those testing positive (Genetic Information Nondiscrimination Act, 2008; NCI, 2013a, 2013d).

In 2009 the United States Preventive Services Task Force published recommendations based on a review of scientific evidence that women should not have routine mammography screening between ages 40 and 49 years but should have biennial screenings between the ages 50 and 74 years. This was a major shift from the recommendation of annual screening mammograms for women older than 40 years. The researchers cited the reason for this recommended change as improvements in mammography screening films that led to more accurate diagnosing. They also cited the high cost and harmful psychological effect of screening on women related to unnecessary diagnostic testing resulting from the high number of false-positive results. Despite that recommendation, the American Cancer Society (2012) continues to recommend annual mammograms after age 40, whereas the National Cancer Institute (NCI) (2013c) recommends screening every 1 to 2 years, except in women at higher risk, who should begin before age 40. Key to mammogram screening is a woman's informed choice based on individual risk factors for development of breast cancer as well as the benefits (early detection and improved survival) and potential harms (false-positive results or missed cancer).

The current position of the U.S. Preventive Services Task Force is that there is insufficient evidence to recommend for or against the teaching of BSE (Thomas et al., 2002). The ACS (2016c) also no longer supports the routine use of self breast exam (SBE) or clinical breast examination (CBE) for screening because of this lack of evidence. Instead, women are encouraged to be familiar with the normal look and feel of their breasts and to report changes to a health care provider.

For women at low risk who are 40 years and older, the greatest potential to save lives from breast cancer is through early detection with mammography (ACS, 2016a). In addition to annual mammography and CBEs, breast cancer detection may involve ultrasound, MRI, positron emission tomography, and genetic testing for *BRCA1* and *BRCA2* (NCI, 2013a). Box 17.2 lists resources that provide information about breast cancer and early detection.

RESEARCH HIGHLIGHTS

Breast Cancer Study

A study of the data collected in the U.S. National Cancer Institute's Surveillance, Epidemiology, and End Results (SEER) program demonstrated an increase in the incidence of breast cancer with distant involvement in younger women. From 1976 to 2009 there was a 2.07% average compounded increase in this diagnosis in women 25 to 39 years old but not in older women. This increase was highest in Hispanic and African American women (Johnson, 2013).

The CDC looked at data from United States Cancer Statistics to determine whether race affected breast cancer outcomes. Black women had a lower incidence of breast cancer diagnosis than white women, yet cancers were diagnosed at more advanced stages and the death rate was 41% higher in the former group from 2005 through 2009 in the United States. Self-reports of mammogram frequency did not differ in the two groups. However, research shows that in black women, differences do exist in breast cancer screening, follow-up, and treatment after diagnosis, leading to greater mortality (Cronin et al., 2012).

Lung Cancer

Although breast cancer is the most common cancer among women after skin cancer, cancer of the lung and bronchus is responsible for more cancer deaths. In 2013, 219,709 women were diagnosed with lung cancer. Lung cancer is responsible for more deaths yearly in U.S. women than breast cancer. From 2005 to 2009, 39.6 of every 100,000 women died from lung cancer, compared with 21 per 100,000 from breast cancer (U.S. Cancer Statistics Working Group [USCSWG], 2016). In fact, lung cancer kills more women annually than breast, ovarian, and uterine cancers combined (ACS, 2016c). Between 1990 and 2003, there was a 60% increase in the number of new cases of lung cancer in American women, whereas the number of men diagnosed with lung cancer remained stable (Patel, 2005). The rise in the incidence of lung cancer in women is due primarily to an increase in their tobacco use: 85% to 90% of all clients who have lung cancer have a history of cigarette smoking. Yet lung cancer develops in only 20% of cigarette smokers, suggesting that the cause of lung cancer is multifactorial.

Widely accepted risk factors for lung cancer include exposure to environmental tobacco smoke, certain occupational exposures (especially asbestos), genetic predisposition, sex, gender, diet, chronic lung disease, and a history of tobacco-related cancer (Rivera and Stover, 2004). Studies have shown that the risks for development of lung cancer are different in women and men and that lung cancer appears to be a biologically different disease in women. Women smokers are more likely than men to have adenocarcinoma of the lung, and women who have never smoked are more likely to have lung cancer than men who have never smoked. These differences are due to hormonal, genetic, and metabolic differences between the sexes (Patel, 2005).

Although medical treatment may be similar for men and women, the symptom distress, quality of life, and demands of

BOX 17.2   Resource Materials for Breast Cancer

BCCCP (Breast and Cervical Cancer Control Program)
Federally funded free breast and cervical cancer screening through state departments of community health

American Cancer Society
Website
Breast Cancer: Early Detection (available from http://www.cancer.org/acs/groups/cid/documents/webcontent/003165-pdf.pdf)

Publications
Breast Cancer Awareness Information Packet
ABC's of Breast Health
The Older You Get, the More You Need a Mammogram (pamphlet)
Breast Health (card)
How to Check Your Breasts (pamphlet)
Let's Talk About Mammograms (pamphlet)
   For copies, call (800) ACS-2345. For more information, visit http://www.cancer.org/acs/groups/cid/documents/webcontent/003165-pdf.pdf.

National Cancer Institute
Website
General Information About Breast Cancer (available from http://www.cancer.gov/cancertopics/pdq/screening/breast/Patient/page2)

Publications and Videos
A Mammogram Once a Year . . . For a Lifetime (video)
Smart Advice for Women 40 and Over: Have a Mammogram (pamphlet)
Guidelines for Screening Mammography (pamphlet)
A Mammogram Could Save Your Life*
Take Care of Your Breasts
   For copies, call (800) 4-CANCER. For more information, visit http://www.cancer.gov/cancertopics/pdq/screening/breast/Patient/page2.

U.S. Department of Health and Human Services, and Health Care Financing Administration
Get a Mammogram: A Picture That Can Save Your Life (pamphlet)
Medicare Covers Mammograms (pamphlet)
   For copies and more information, call (800) 4-CANCER (breast cancer and mammograms) or (800) MEDICARE (Medicare coverage).

*Specifically designed for low-literacy audiences; some resources are available in Spanish and English.

illness experienced by women may be different from those in men, because the competing household, child care, and other role-related demands take a toll on many women (Sarna and McCorkle, 1996). Further, women with advanced lung cancer report more psychological symptoms than men (Hopwood and Stephens, 1995).

Lung cancer is often a fatal illness because it is diagnosed most commonly at an advanced stage; early detection is difficult, and treatment for advanced disease is not as effective. Women appear to have a slight survival advantage over men: the 5-year survival rate is 15.6% for women with lung cancer and 12.4% for men (Patel, 2005).

The primary factor in preventing lung cancer is for individuals either to never start smoking or to quit smoking. Nurses must work with other health care providers to reverse the morbidity and mortality rates related to this disease. The Agency for Healthcare Research and Quality has developed a useful guideline for health care professionals to assist women and their families in smoking cessation efforts plus summaries of more than 400 guidelines on a wide variety of topics, which can be found on their website (http://www.ahrq.gov).

Gynecological Cancers

About 20% of all malignant diseases in women occur in the genital tract. The incidence of invasive cervical cancer has declined dramatically as a result of regular Pap smears, which allow for identification of precancerous conditions. However, 4217 women died from the disease in 2013 (CDC, 2015c). Cervical cancer used to be the leading cause of cancer death, but the use of cytological screening has decreased the mortality rate. One major risk factor is infection with HPV, which is linked to nearly all cervical cancer cases. Other risk factors include coitus at an early age, multiple sexual partners, cigarette smoking, history of *Chlamydia* infection, long-term oral contraceptives, intrauterine device, multiple pregnancies, pregnancy at a young age, HIV, family history, and low socioeconomic status (ACS, 2016b). It is most commonly diagnosed in women between the ages of 30 and 50 years, because the cellular changes that lead to cancer are caused by chronic infection and inflammation. It is uncommon for women who undergo regular screening to be diagnosed with cancer.

Current guidelines recommend cervical cancer screening to begin at 21 years of age. Screening should then be performed every 3 years until age 65 using liquid-based Pap smear tests. After age 30, cotesting for HPV DNA (CDC, 2015b) is acceptable. Because HPV is a common virus affecting 80 million people, routine screening for HPV is not recommended in women younger than 30. HPV infection is responsible for the majority of these cancers: 90% anal, 70% vaginal and vulvar, 60% penile, and 70% throat (CDC, 2016a). Current recommendations are that girls and boys be vaccinated for HPV beginning at the age of 11 or 12 years. Between 2006 and 2016, 79 million doses of HPV vaccine had been administered without serious safety concerns (CDC, 2017d). Because of the ACA, vaccinations are covered by private insurers and through the Vaccines for Children Program for eligible children who would otherwise not have access (CDC, 2012).

According to the CDC (2017) and ACS (2017a), the incidence of endometrial cancer is highest among white women, but mortality is higher among black women, suggesting disparity in diagnosis and/or treatment. This cancer is commonly found in women during their sixth and seventh decades of life (i.e., 80% of women with this condition are postmenopausal). It is estimated that in 2017 61,380 women will be diagnosed with endometrial cancer and 10,920 will die. Factors related to its occurrence are obesity, low parity, diabetes mellitus, and conditions in which high circulating estrogen levels are not countered by adequate progesterone levels. The most common sign of endometrial cancer, occurring in 90% of women, is abnormal vaginal bleeding. Postmenopausal women experiencing vaginal bleeding should seek immediate gynecological evaluation.

Cancer of the ovary causes more deaths than any other pelvic malignancy, although the mortality rate has fallen 1.6% per year since 2001 (NCI, 2017). The lifetime risk of ovarian cancer is 1.38%. The incidence increases with age, peaking in women 75 to 79 years old at 56.7 per 100,000. Risk factors include increasing age, nulliparity, never having breast-fed, a history of breast cancer, postmenopausal use of hormone replacement therapy, obesity, a family history of breast and ovarian cancer, and testing positive for the *BRCA* mutation. Protective factors against ovarian cancer include use of oral contraceptives, having and breast-feeding children, tubal sterilization, hysterectomy, and prophylactic oophorectomy (NCI, 2017).

Ovarian cancer is a silent cancer. Early-stage detection is difficult; therefore it has usually reached an advanced stage when discovered. The health professional should be alert to ovarian enlargement on pelvic examination with suspicion that ovarian malignancy may be present, especially in a postmenopausal woman. The most common sign a woman experiences is abdominal enlargement. She may complain that her skirts and slacks are getting tighter in the waist. Any woman older than 40 years who experiences vague digestive complaints that persist and are not explained by another cause must have a thorough evaluation for ovarian cancer. According to the ACS (2017d), transvaginal ultrasound, MRI, or computed tomography scan along with a blood test for tumor marker CA-125 may assist in the diagnosis of ovarian cancer. These tests are not recommended for routine screening of all women, but are recommended for those with risk factors related to family history (strong family history of ovarian and breast cancer, positive for genetic mutations *BRCA1* and *BRCA2*).

Mental Disorders and Stress

Various circumstances and conditions influence the mental health of women. Women face stressful decisions about career and family, and many express anxieties about these decisions. A woman may feel pressured to make decisions regarding childbearing before she has fulfilled her career goals. Deciding to focus on a career may mean decreased authority and the suffering of stress in the workplace. More women are occupying middle-management positions, which are known for creating stress-related illnesses associated with high demands and little or no power. Women combining motherhood and a career have additional decisions, such as whether to work during pregnancy and choice of child care.

A woman's emotional state can be influenced by ovarian function from the onset of menstruation to the cessation of menstrual periods. Depression may be triggered or worsened by premenstrual hormonal changes. Women with a history of depression are also at increased risk for a recurrent episode of depression during the postpartum period, and they also are at risk for depression during the

perimenopausal transition (Blehar, 2003). Depression is more prevalent among women than among men. In all age groups from adolescents through the elderly, approximately two thirds of those affected with depression are women. According to Bhatia and Bhatia (1999), the higher prevalence of depression in women is most likely due to a combination of gender-related differences in cognitive styles, certain biological factors, and a higher incidence of psychosocial and economic stressors.

Mental disorders often go undiagnosed and untreated or undertreated despite the availability of effective treatments. Women may not recognize or correctly identify their symptoms, and even when they do, they may be reluctant to seek care because of stigma associated with mental illness (Blehar, 2003). Community health nurses are in a good position to assess women's moods in diverse aggregates. Being familiar with the symptoms of common mental disorders, nurses can identify these problems and can help women seek and maintain continuity of care.

Reproductive Health

Community health nurses provide a variety of services in the area of women's reproductive health from menarche through postmenopause. Nurses, in collaboration with other health care professionals, have identified a persistent group of preventable and correctable problems related to maternal-child health. *Healthy People 2020* (USDHHS, 2017) provides numerous recommendations for improving maternal and infant health, including reduction of cigarette smoking, reduction of alcohol and other drug use, optimal nutrition, improved socioeconomic opportunities (including education), and decreased environmental hazards.

For the *Healthy People 2020* initiative, some of the family planning objectives demonstrated progress. Adolescent pregnancy rates decreased until the year 2005, but a 5% increase occurred between 2005 and 2007 (CDC, 2009). Adolescent pregnancy (ages 15–19) rates have decreased since 1991, from 61.8 per 1000 to 26.5 per 1000 in 2013 (CDC, 2015a). The improvements have been attributed to reduced sexual activity, low-cost and long-acting contraceptives, and condom use. Health disparities remain an issue for Hispanic and black populations. With *Healthy People 2020* family planning objectives, the focus is on the positive that "all pregnancies should be intended." Examples of *Healthy People 2020* objectives related to family planning are shown in the *Healthy People 2020* box (National Center for Health Statistics, 2012).

Dysmenorrhea is another reproductive health problem affecting approximately 50% to 80% of the female population between ages 15 and 24 years (Nelson, 2004). At least 10% to 20% of women with dysmenorrhea are incapacitated for 1 to 3 days each month. Dysmenorrhea is the greatest single cause of absenteeism from school and work among young women and causes the loss of approximately 140 million working hours annually; therefore the economic influence of this condition is significant.

ETHICAL INSIGHTS

Working With Women's Health

Community health nurses working in the field of women's health will be exposed to ethical dilemmas during their careers. For this reason, nurses must have a working knowledge of the principles of health care ethics. The commonly accepted principles include the following:

- Respect for autonomy
- Beneficence
- Nonmaleficence
- Justice

Nursing care revolves around moral values such as compassion, empathy, honesty, trust, and respect. Most encounters will be nonproblematic. Occasionally, nurses may be exposed to clinical situations that challenge their values and beliefs. Clients and family members may, at times, also disagree with the nurse's professional advice/plan. It is important for the nurse to keep his or her personal philosophy, politics, religion, and moral values out of clinical work with individuals and families.

HEALTHY PEOPLE 2020

Selected Objectives for Family Planning

Objective	Baseline (Year)	Target (2010)	Final (Year)	Target 2020
9-1: Increase the proportion of pregnancies that are intended.	52% (2002)	70%	51% (2002)	56%
9-7: Reduce pregnancies among adolescent females (pregnancies per 1000 females 15–17 years of age).	63 (1996)	39	40.2 (2005)	36.2
9-11: Increase the proportion of women who have received formal instruction on birth control methods before turning 18 years of age.	70% (2002)	73%	70.5% (2006–2010)	77.6%
9-12: Reduce the proportion of married couples whose ability to conceive or maintain a pregnancy is impaired.	13% (1995)	10%	11% (2006–2008)	10.8%

Data from U.S. Department of Health and Human Services: *Healthy people 2020*, ed 3, Washington, DC, 2010, Author.

Examples of potential ethical dilemmas related to women's health care are emergency contraception, abortion, assisted reproductive technology, and end-of-life issues.

The average age of menopause in the United States is 51 years. *Menopause* is defined as the cessation of menses for at least 1 full year, but it is characterized by several years of symptoms as the hormonal shifts occur, called *perimenopause* (Schuiling and Likis, 2016). At this stage, women's health concerns become focused on the symptoms associated with this transition. The most common complaints are related to vasomotor changes causing hot flushes, increased heart rate, insomnia, and night sweats; urogenital atrophy causing incontinence; vaginal dryness and dyspareunia; and mood alterations, including irritability, depression, and anxiety (Schmidt, 2012). Community health nurses can play a key role in helping women find resources to deal with symptoms and develop an understanding of the normal processes associated with menopause. Also, women in menopause need guidance in promoting a healthy lifestyle because they have an increased risk for development of chronic conditions such as osteoporosis, coronary heart disease, hypertension, and type 2 diabetes.

Nutrition

One of the most important factors in a woman's reproductive health is her total life nutritional experience from infancy through childhood and adolescence. Obesity has become a major public health concern. The community health nurse is in an advantageous position to provide nutritional counseling. The U.S. Department of Agriculture updates the dietary recommendations every 5 years on the basis of current scientific information. In 2011, the "My Plate" approach to healthy eating was unveiled. This approach is intended to encourage persons to be mindful of the foods they eat in terms of both portion size and proportion to other foods. One-half of the plate should consist of fruits and vegetables, with one-quarter each for meats/proteins and grains, preferably whole grains. Recommendations also include eating less sodium and fewer sugary foods (U.S. Department of Agriculture, 2013).

Pregnancy may provide a motivational factor for developing an awareness of proper nutrition. During the nutritional assessment of a prenatal client, the community health nurse can take the opportunity to determine dietary habits and initiate a referral to the Special Supplemental Food Program for Women, Infants, and Children. This program provides food vouchers for pregnant or breastfeeding women, infants, and children who are at nutritional risk.

Good nutrition must include factors other than kinds and amounts of foods. Elements to consider include age, lifestyle, economic status, and culture. For example, when counseling a pregnant adolescent, the nurse can include the primary person responsible for meal preparation. The nurse should include the adolescent in the planning of her diet, asking her to identify foods that she likes from those recommended. The nurse should make the adolescent aware of the influence of her nutrition on fetal growth and development. This information must be balanced with the young woman's individual needs.

Sexually Transmitted Diseases

STDs are commonly found among U.S. women. Community health nurses and other health providers, including physicians, nurse practitioners (NPs), nurse midwives, and social workers, must be prepared to provide age-appropriate STD prevention, education, and counseling.

In 2016, the CDC reported STD rates were the highest ever, the most common was *Chlamydia trachomatis* (1,526,658 cases), followed by *Neisseria gonorrhea* (395,216 cases), gonorrhea (395,216), and syphilis (23,872). This was the largest number of *Chlamydia* cases ever reported. *Chlamydia* infection is diagnosed three times more in women than men, most likely because of the CDC's recommendation for routine screening of any sexually active woman of childbearing age to prevent infertility.

Gonorrhea is also diagnosed more often in women, but particularly in black women, who are diagnosed 15 times more often than white women. The Gonococcal Isolate Surveillance Project demonstrated that gonorrhea was becoming resistant to treatment with CDC-recommended fluoroquinolone drugs in 2007, prompting the CDC to revise treatment guidelines (CDC, 2017).

When rates of syphilis, another STD, dropped nearly 90% between 1990 and 2000, the CDC initiated the National Plan to Eliminate Syphilis. However, rates have increased yearly since 2001. Racial disparity in cases of syphilis has improved from 1999, when 29 times more blacks than whites were diagnosed, down to a rate that is now 7 times higher. The increase in syphilis began mostly among men, especially men having sex with men, and less in women (CDC, 2017b). In 2014–2015, there was a 19% increase in cases of syphilis.

Treatments of STDs are outlined in the CDC guidelines, which are updated regularly and available online (www.cdc.gov-/std/tg2015/default.htm). A vital role of the community health nurse is to follow up with the woman's sex partner(s) who require(s) evaluation and treatment. Partner notification and expedited treatment, along with avoidance of sexual activity until treatment/cure, are key to stopping the spread of STDs. In addition to medications, women and their partners need individualized counseling on reducing risky sexual behaviors.

Human Immunodeficiency Virus and Acquired Immunodeficiency Syndrome. Today, the HIV/AIDS epidemic represents a growing and persistent health threat to women in the United States, especially young women and women of color. In 2015, 19% of the 39,513 new HIV diagnoses in 2015 were women (CDC, 2017b). Among women diagnosed with HIV/AIDS, 61% are black, yet black women make up only 12% of the general U.S. population. The majority of infants born with HIV are black. For all ethnicities, primary transmission in men occurs through sexual contact with other men, whereas in women, the route is high-risk heterosexual contact. As of 2015, HIV/AIDS is no longer a top 10 cause of death globally, thanks to more available treatment and increased use of safe sex practices (WHO, 2017).

According to the CDC (2009), risk factors for and barriers to prevention of HIV/AIDS for women include the following:
- Young age at sexual initiation
- Lack of awareness regarding disease and condom use
- Sexual inequality in relationships
- Biological vulnerability to sexually transmitted infections
- Substance abuse
- Poverty; dropping out of school
- Stigma surrounding testing and treatment
- Working in the sex trade
- Participants in unprotected sex

In November 2008, the USDHHS released the updated Guidelines for the Use of Antiretroviral Agents in HIV-1 Infected Adults and Adolescents (USDHHS, 2013). Treatment guidelines continually evolve with new research and experience. The use of antiretroviral drugs has reduced the rate of death for HIV disease in women, which peaked in 1993–1994 at 6 per 100,000, down to 2.5 per 100,000 (CDC, 2009). It is imperative that the community health nurse working with this population stays abreast of the current trends for both counseling and treatment options. Community health nurses also must target at-risk populations and campaign for the use of safer sex practices and routine HIV testing for those at risk.

Other Issues in Women's Health

Unintentional Injury or Accidents and Intimate Partner Violence

Although unintentional injury affects women less commonly than men, several areas of concern still exist for women. For example, older women are at increased risk for accidents such as falls. Falls account for the majority of serious unintentional injuries and lead to 40% of all deaths from injury in people older than 75 years (Stevens, 2005). Factors that may be responsible for this major cause of injury among older adults are an unsteady gait, reduced vision, and a hazardous environment. Older women experience an increasing number of falls; therefore the nurse must identify the preventable factors. Whether working with older adults in the home or in institutional settings, nurses must be knowledgeable about hazards that may be corrected to decrease the incidence of falls.

Intimate partner violence (IPV), sometimes called domestic abuse, is the single largest cause of injury to women between the ages of 15 and 44 in the United States—more common than muggings, car accidents, and rapes combined. IPV is committed by a current or former boyfriend/girlfriend/spouse. In 2008, 552,000 females age 12 and over were victims of nonfatal, violent abuse.

Abuse in women is often explained as accidental injury. Approximately 6% of visits made by women to emergency departments are for injuries that result from physical battering by their husbands, former husbands, boyfriends, or lovers. Intimate partner violence includes physical, sexual, emotional, economic, and psychological abuse. A subset of intimate partner violence is dating violence, which occurs in a romantic relationship. Reports of teen dating abuse indicate that one in five teens reports some sort of abuse and one in four girls report being sexually coerced (CDC, 2013b).

Nurses employed in community health settings need to know how to make assessments, provide support, and make referrals to agencies dealing with intimate partner violence (see Boxes 17.3 through 17.5). Understanding the state laws related to reporting known or suspected intimate partner violence is important. The American Medical Association and American Nurses Association advocate that all women be assessed for IPV. Questions should be posed privately in nonjudgmental but specific terms (i.e., "Do you feel safe?" "Have you ever been hit, punched, slapped, or kicked?") with follow-up questions if the woman responds "yes" (Kovach, 2004). Many nurses are past or current victims of abuse; assessing abuse with clients can evoke painful emotions that the nurse may not be ready to confront. Chapter 27 contains additional information about intimate partner violence.

Disability

More women than men have disabilities resulting from acute conditions, but women experience fewer disabilities resulting

BOX 17.3 Intimate Partner Violence Strategies for Nurses

It is important not to revictimize the woman who admits to intimate partner violence. Avoid asking the woman "why" or talking negatively about the abuser. Sit down with her, give her time to talk, listen actively. Provide her with privacy and confidentiality as much as you can. Useful statements include:

"I believe what you are telling me."

"I am here for you."

"This will only get worse."

"You deserve better."

"I am afraid for your safety."

"You deserve to be treated with respect."

"It is a crime."

   This approach will empower the victim. Episodes of imminent danger must be reported to the police. An emergency plan should be formulated with the woman. Resources including phone numbers for hotlines and the local women's shelter should be provided in a format that is easy to conceal (such as on a business card).

Adapted from Perry SE, Hockenberry MJ, Lowermilk DL, Wilson D: *Maternal child nursing care*, Maryland Heights, MO, 2010, Mosby, p 62.

BOX 17.4 Signs of Intimate Partner Violence

- Overuse of health services
- Nonspecific, vague complaints
- Missed appointments
- Injuries without legitimate explanation
- Injuries not matching reported cause
- Untreated serious injuries
- Intimate partner describing the cause of injuries
- Intimate partner refusing to leave the woman's room

Adapted from Krieger CL: Intimate partner violence: a review for nurses, *Nurs Womens Health* 12(3):224–334, 2008.

BOX 17.5 Resources For Victims of Intimate Partner Violence

National Domestic Violence Hotline: 1-800-799-SAFE (7233) and http://www.thehotline.org

Dating Violence on Women's Health.gov: http://womenshealth.gov/violence-against-women/

National Coalition Against Domestic Violence: http://www.ncadv.org

Office on Violence Against Women: http://www.ovw.usdoj.gov

from chronic conditions because they report their symptoms earlier and receive necessary treatment. Women report proportionately more days of restricted activity than men.

   Disabling conditions limit the physical functional abilities of many women, but the health care delivery system has often overlooked the unique needs of this aggregate. In planning care for disabled women, community health nurses should focus attention on enabling women to strengthen their capabilities. In addition, nurses should be sensitive to barriers in the clinical setting that affect the access of disabled women to health care services. Chapter 21 discusses the needs of disabled people in greater detail.

MAJOR LEGISLATION AFFECTING WOMEN'S HEALTH

Several legislative acts have direct or indirect influence on the health of women. Many changes have been made in the past five decades that have the potential for improving the health and welfare of all women.

Public Health Service Act

The Public Health Service (PHS) Act, passed in 1944, provides for biomedical and health services research, information dissemination, resource development, technical assistance, and service delivery. In the area of women's health, the PHS Act supports activities related to general health issues, reproductive health, social and behavioral issues, and mental health. Aggregates of women targeted by the PHS Act include those disabled by specific diseases, victims of sexual abuse and intimate partner violence, recent immigrants, and occupational groups.

   Title X of the PHS Act is the Family Planning Public Service Act, which helped 5 million women obtain family planning services in 2008. Since 1970, federally subsidized family planning funds have been available to clinics and health departments throughout the country. These facilities provide access not only to contraception but also to routine preventive health services, education, and counseling. The program is an important part of the public effort to prevent low birth weight through addressing the relationship between lack of family planning and women at greatest risk for low-birth-weight infants (women who are adolescents, single, and/or low income) (Fowler et al., 2010).

Civil Rights Act

Title VII of the Civil Rights Act of 1964 prohibits discrimination based on sex, race, color, religion, or national origin in determining employment eligibility or termination, wages, and fringe benefits. The act has been amended to prohibit discrimination against pregnant women and conditions involving childbirth or pregnancy. This landmark legislation makes it unlawful for employers to refuse to hire, employ, or promote a woman because she is pregnant. In addition, employee benefit plans that continue health insurance, income maintenance during disability or illness, or any other income support program for disabled workers must include disabilities resulting from pregnancy, childbirth, and other related conditions. If employers allow disabled employees to assume lighter or medically restricted assignments, the same considerations must extend to pregnant women.

   Sexual harassment is unwelcome conduct of a sexual nature severe enough to create intimidating hostile work environment. Sexual harassment is a violation of the Civil Rights Act. Female and male workers may face unwelcome sexual advances or requests for sexual favors or other verbal or physical conduct of a sexual nature. Awareness of sexual harassment in the workplace has increased dramatically over the past decade, but sexual harassment has not been eliminated.

Social Security Act

The Social Security Act provides monthly retirement and disability benefits to workers and survivor benefits to families of workers covered by Social Security. Full retirement benefits are available after 10 years of covered employment, and workers can collect partial benefits beginning at age 62 and full benefits after age 67.

The Social Security Act permits a divorced person to receive benefits based on a former spouse's earning record when that spouse retires, becomes disabled, or dies if the marriage lasted at least 10 years. Since January 1985, a woman who has been divorced for at least 2 years can receive spousal benefits at age 62, if her former husband is eligible for benefits, regardless of whether he is actually receiving them.

Medicare and Medicaid also resulted from the Social Security Act. Medicare is the insurance plan that covers the majority of the health care expenses of older adults, including payments for hospital care, physicians, home health care, and other services and supplies after copayments and deductibles. Medicaid covers health care for indigent and eligible children and includes family planning, obstetrical care, and preventive cancer screening for women, such as mammography and Pap smears. Chapters 10 and 12 describe Medicare and Medicaid in detail, and they are further discussed later in this chapter.

Occupational Safety and Health Act

The Occupational Safety and Health Act, enacted in 1970, helps ensure safe and healthful working conditions for workers throughout the United States. Although there is a growing emphasis on the study of the health of women workers, gaps in knowledge exist. For example, little is known about women who work in cottage industries, as domestic workers, as prostitutes, in agriculture, and in the garment industry. In addition, the work of some women is classified as "women's work" and includes such things as housework, child care, caregiver of the sick, and farming (Misner, Beauchamp-Hewitt, and Fox-Levin, 1997). These women experience physical demands and hazards, yet government economic reports have not recognized them as workers. Investigations of factors that influence the health of these women workers are needed. Table 17.5 lists specific positions in which a large number of women are employed and the potential for health hazards within these positions. Community health nurses, occupational health nurses, and NPs need to be cognizant of environmental hazards wherever they find women at work. In taking a health history, the nurse should collect data regarding the client's occupational environment to assess the potential risk to emotional, general, and reproductive health. In addition, nurses must work individually and as an aggregate with their legislatures to maintain strong worker health and safety programs to protect the health of all women.

Family and Medical Leave Act

Enacted in 1993, the Family and Medical Leave Act (FMLA) allows an employee a minimum provision of 12 weeks unpaid leave each year for family and medical reasons such as personal illness; an ill child, parent, or spouse; and the birth or adoption of a child. In 2008, the FMLA was updated to include family providing care to members of the Armed Forces injured in the line of duty. This act guarantees the employee the same or an

TABLE 17.5	Hazardous Occupations in Which Women are Employed
Occupation	**Health Hazard**
Clerical workers	Organic solvents in stencil machines, correction fluids, and ozone from copying machines
Textile and apparel workers	Cotton dust, skin irritants, and chemicals
Hairdressers and beauticians	Hair, nail, and skin beauty preparations
Launderers and dry cleaners	Heat, heavy lifting, and chemicals
Electronics workers	Solvents and acids
Hospital and other health care workers	Infectious diseases, heavy lifting, radiation, skin disorders, and anesthetic gases
Firefighters	Exposure to hazardous materials and rescue environments
Laboratory workers	Biological agents; flammable, explosive, toxic, or carcinogenic substances; exposure to radiation; and bites from and allergic reactions to research animals
Construction workers	Exposure to hazardous materials, dangerous environments
Military personnel	Exposure to hostile persons, hazardous materials, harsh environments, and sexual assault

Data from Centers for Disease Control, National Institute for Occupational Safety and Health: *Workplace safety and health topics: Industries & occupations,* 2013. http://www.cdc.gov/niosh/topics/industries.html.

equivalent job with the same pay and benefits upon the employee's return to work. In addition, health benefits must continue throughout the leave. In 2011, 14 million people utilized FMLA. Of these 56% were women, 40% took less than 10 days, and those with a new child took an average of 22 days (National Partnership for Women & Families [NPF], 2012).

The FMLA is particularly important to female workers because they are more likely to use leave to care for seriously ill family members, whereas male workers more often use leave for personal illness. Employees who must be away from work for family or medical reasons lose income, with the most significant impact on those without job-protected leave. The FMLA is an important step toward equitable leave policies, but more change is needed.

⯑ ACTIVE LEARNING

1. Identify examples from everyday life that support or encourage violence against women (e.g., magazines, books, and television advertisements). Share findings with classmates.
2. Survey lay magazine advertisements and estimate the percentage of total pages that use a woman's image, including aging, menopause, overweight and obesity, and sexuality, to sell products. Share these with classmates.
3. Discuss the need for cancer screening with female relatives; refer to the ACS guidelines.
4. Discuss with female relatives the need for a heart-healthy nutritional plan based on AHA guidelines.
5. Identify resources for mammograms and Pap smears for low-income women.

HEALTH AND SOCIAL SERVICES TO PROMOTE THE HEALTH OF WOMEN

Major changes for women came with the signing of the ACA of 2010 (USDHHS, 2012). Particular to women are protections from being denied coverage by insurance companies and from being charged more for health care services because of gender. As of August 1, 2012, 47 million women gained access to preventive care without copays. Services include well-woman visits along with screening and counseling for gestational diabetes, HPV, STDs including HIV, contraception, and intimate partner violence. Also included were breastfeeding counseling, support, and supplies. The ACA mandated an expansion of Medicaid to include persons younger than 65 years with income below 133% of the federal poverty level. Medicaid is a health insurance program that was instituted in 1965 for the poor and is funded jointly by the federal and state governments but is administered by individual states. Medicaid is the largest source of funding for medical and health-related services for people with limited income, regardless of age eligibility. Medicaid is classified into five broad coverage groups: children, pregnant women, adults in families with dependent children, individuals with disabilities, and individuals 65 years or older.

Pregnant women who are eligible for Medicaid are at high risk for poor pregnancy outcome, including low birth weight. Ideally, a maternity care provider should examine women with high maternal risk immediately after conception. However, too often these women seek prenatal care late in pregnancy or arrive at the emergency department when delivery is imminent without having previously received prenatal care (Clinical Example 17.1). Barriers limit access to prenatal care for those most in need. Medicaid allows some access to care. Greater public awareness of facilities and maternity care providers who accept Medicaid are necessary.

Clinical Example 17.1

Anita Rogers, a 16-year-old unemployed single woman, arrived at the Family Services Health Center seeking initial prenatal care at 36 weeks of gestation. She stated that for a few days she noted some brown discharge from her vagina. She told the nurse she knew she should have begun prenatal care earlier, but when she called several health providers' offices, the receptionists told her they were not accepting patients with Medicaid insurance. She reported that the family did not have reliable transportation. Her father was unemployed, and her mother worked at a cafe as a waitress. Anita was sent to the hospital immediately for an ultrasound examination. The sonogram revealed twins, but one of them had died in utero. Anita was hospitalized and began to hemorrhage. She delivered a 3-lb infant.

Women's Health Services

Since the mid-1970s, women have sought health services beyond the conventional mode of care delivery. Women desire a participatory role in their health and have become more assertive. Health care facilities have recognized the importance of meeting women's health needs. A notable evolution has occurred in maternity care, in which the demands of women as consumers led to the emergence of freestanding and hospital-based birth centers and family- and sibling-attended births.

The National Women's Health Network has been a strong advocate for women's concerns and has provided testimony at congressional hearings dealing with women's issues. This organization is concerned with women's rights, environmental safety, reproductive rights, warnings about the effects of alcohol and drugs on the developing fetus, and safety in relation to medical devices and to drugs, especially those that may have teratogenic or carcinogenic effects. Examples of the organization's work include recall of the Dalkon Shield intrauterine device, identification of women who may have been exposed to diethylstilbestrol in utero, and promotion of well-woman health care.

Other Community Voluntary Services

Networking, the exchange of information among interconnected or cooperating individuals, has been one of the major movements during the past two decades. It is a means by which women seek to advance their careers, improve their lifestyles, and increase their income while helping other women become successful. Networking in business, professional support, politics and labor, arts, sports, and health is established throughout the United States enabling women to develop and become empowered to achieve mutual goals.

Many private voluntary organizations spend money, time, and energy in attempting to increase health awareness among its members and provide direct services to the public. Most urban areas have crisis hotline services in which women volunteer to provide counseling to battered women, battering parents, rape victims, those considering suicide, and those with multiple needs. One of the most effective, low-cost, voluntary efforts to assist abused women involves shelters and safe houses scattered throughout the United States. One of the goals of *Healthy People 2020* relates to this issue, as many women needing shelter are often denied emergency housing.

Women's organizations have a long history of voluntary involvement with the community. An increasing number have added activities to their agendas to improve pregnancy outcomes, prevent teen pregnancy, and support older women's rights. Organizations such as the Older Women's League, United Methodist Women, women's groups of other religious denominations, Urban League, sororities, Junior League, Young Women's Christian Association, and the National Association of Colored Women's Clubs, have made women's health a major item on their agendas.

? ACTIVE LEARNING

1. Visit with a women's group in the community (e.g., business, church, sorority, Parents Without Partners, Red Hat Society) to discuss members' health care needs and concerns. From these data, develop research questions.
2. Call a family planning clinic and determine the population served (i.e., eligibility), available services, and costs.

LEVELS OF PREVENTION AND WOMEN'S HEALTH

Primary Prevention

The focus of primary prevention is preventing disease from occurring. Women should recognize the risk of disease and target their health care behaviors accordingly. Types of primary prevention include never smoking, following a nutritious diet, practicing safe sex, avoiding drugs, limiting alcohol consumption, and staying physically active.

Consider Jackie, a 39-year-old woman with three first-order relatives diagnosed with breast and/or ovarian cancer. She is at risk for hereditary cancer and should seek genetic counseling and possibly testing. If genetic test results are positive, she should be given information on measures that could prevent cancer from occurring, a process that constitutes primary prevention. These measures include lifestyle choices (early childbearing/breast-feeding); prophylactic surgical procedures (oophorectomy/mastectomy); and medical treatment (contraceptive pills, tamoxifen). Vigilant screenings (pelvic ultrasound with Ca-125 measurement or breast MRI) to detect cancer early would be considered secondary prevention.

Secondary Prevention

The focus of secondary prevention is detecting the disease once it has begun but before it appears clinically. Examples of this level of prevention are routine screening for cervical cancer through Pap smears, for chlamydial infections through nucleic acid amplification tests on either urine or cervical specimens, and CBE and mammogram.

Tertiary Prevention

Tertiary prevention seeks to stop further complications after a disease has become clinically evident. For example, Sandra Smith, a 55-year-old Native American, has had diabetes mellitus for the past 3 years. She attended an urban clinic for monitoring of the diabetes. After the physician examined her, he suggested that she have her annual pelvic examination. She was overdue for one and agreed to be seen by the women's health care NP. Ms. Smith described symptoms of a yeast infection (e.g., increase in vaginal discharge and itching) to the nurse. Her examination and a wet mount examination confirmed the diagnosis of *Candida albicans* infection, a common problem among diabetic women. Sandra then learned about the nature of, predisposing factors for, and treatment of the infection.

CASE STUDY   Application of the Nursing Process

Pregnant Inmate in a Correctional Facility

John Lawrence, an educator at the state women's correctional center, contacted Donna Williams, a women's health care nurse practitioner and faculty member at the College of Nursing, and expressed concern for the health of an inmate, Lela Marvin. According to Mr. Lawrence, Lela, a 19-year-old pregnant primigravida, was being seen at the state-supported hospital for antepartal care; however, she was not permitted to attend perinatal education classes. He stated that other pregnant women in the facility could benefit from perinatal education. In fact, approximately 6.1% of female state prison inmates are pregnant when admitted to prison and could benefit from perinatal education (Snell, 1994).

Lawrence's call was followed by a call from Herman Martin, an RN who also expressed concern for the other women's needs for information regarding their personal hygiene. Although an RN, Mr. Martin was not knowledgeable of women's health because his primary clinical focus was emergency and trauma care. He indicated that many of the women were overweight, cared little about themselves, and lacked a general knowledge of how to maintain their health.

Assessment

After gaining clearance from the prison officials, Ms. Williams made an assessment of health care information needs and started offering classes for the inmates. The immediate need was for perinatal education for women in the last weeks of pregnancy. Lela said she wanted to learn about labor because she had heard only horror stories from other women. Ms. Williams noted that three other women were close to term and they also seemed eager to learn. She knew that students' readiness to learn was key to the course's success. Success of this course would be crucial to future course offerings.

The traditional perinatal education course was designed to promote healthy birth outcomes and an emotionally satisfying birth experience. These goals are also important to pregnant women in a correctional facility; however, perinatal education would have to be modified to meet this group's special needs. For example, information on newborn care is not appropriate because the infant born to an inmate is usually placed with the mother's family or in foster care.

Assessment of nonpregnant women provided opportunities for other health education classes. The next spring and each spring thereafter, junior nursing students under Ms. Williams's guidance were assigned to develop and carry out 1-hour weekly health education and awareness sessions at the correctional facility. Although each student expressed some initial anxiety about the experience, each evaluated it as being worthwhile.

Diagnosis

After assessment, the community health nurse developed community and aggregate diagnoses, which served as the basis for the care plan.

Individual

- Inadequate preparation for childbirth related to lack of resources in prison (Lela)
- Lack of family support related to separation secondary to incarceration (Lela)
- Potential for feelings of loss related to separation from infant after birth (Lela)

Family

- Lela's family visits were rare; therefore she looked for others to provide support during her pregnancy. Lela told Ms. Williams that her cellmate, Julieanna, offered to be her labor support person.
- Lack of knowledge of her role as a labor support person (Julieanna).

Community

- Lack of adequate health-seeking behaviors of women in the correctional facility (i.e., pregnant and nonpregnant women)
- Lack of programs to promote health and prevent diseases among women prisoners

Planning

After the nursing diagnosis was validated with the individual, family, or community, the plan of care was developed. Examples of long- and short-term goals follow.

CASE STUDY Application of the Nursing Process—cont'd

Pregnant Inmate in a Correctional Facility

Individual
Long-Term Goal
- Individual family members will have a positive birth experience (Lela).

Short-Term Goal
- Family members or friends will help Lela use relaxation techniques to cope with the discomforts of labor.

Family
Long-Term Goal
- The family members will be strengthened through their newly acquired knowledge and skills.

Short-Term Goal
- The family members will demonstrate increased ability to perform their role as labor support people.

Community
Long-Term Goal
- The health and well-being of incarcerated women (i.e., pregnant and nonpregnant) will improve.

Short-Term Goal
- Health education programs will be instituted for individuals, families, and aggregates in the correctional facility.

Intervention
The community health nurse worked with the individual, family, or community to achieve mutually established goals. Intervention was aimed at empowering individuals and groups to take responsibility for themselves and to form links with others to accomplish goals.

Individual
Providing a perinatal education program for Lela was Ms. Williams's first priority. In addition, counseling related to feelings of loss after birth might be appropriate. Referral to a counselor might be necessary, and Ms. Williams had to become familiar with available resources.

Family
Teaching the family the roles and responsibilities of a labor support person was an important intervention. In the correctional facility, interventions must ensure that Lela has a labor support person with whom to practice her relaxation techniques and to be available. In this case, Lela's cellmate, Julieanna, was willing to act in this role, and the nurse had to negotiate with prison officials to allow this arrangement.

Community
Specific interventions with a group of pregnant women in the correctional facility were based on the specific needs of the group. The community health nurse had to identify prison officials who were supportive of health education programs and request their input as to which women should be targeted for such programs. Then the nurse met with targeted women to assess their level of knowledge and skills regarding women's health. For example, the nurse surveyed what each woman perceived as learning needs (e.g., well-woman care, women's anatomy and physiology, self-care in health promotion, health protection, and disease prevention). Then the nurse tailored an intervention that was compatible with the community. Ms. Williams asked each nursing student to select a topic on the basis of the survey and to develop a teaching plan for presentation to female prisoners (i.e., pregnant and nonpregnant) at least once during the spring semester.

Evaluation
The community health nurse compared the actual and predicted outcomes to determine the efficacy of the plan of care and to make revisions.

Individual
For example, Lela learned necessary relaxation techniques that were useful to her in labor and helped make the birth experience positive. Follow-up of Lela's psychosocial concerns in postpartum was also important.

Family
Evaluation of this nontraditional family would include their level of satisfaction with their role in the birth experience. Evaluation would also include learning how this interaction between family members (i.e., Lela and Julieanna) prepared them for other situations.

Community
The aggregate evaluation focuses on the community. For example, in health education programs designed for pregnant and nonpregnant women in the correctional facility, it was important to do the following:
- Maintain attendance records.
- Seek feedback from women, the referring nurse-educator, and prison officials regarding changes in self-care behavior regarding health.
- Obtain student response to learning experience.
- Make changes in health education programs on the basis of evaluation.

Levels of Prevention
The following are examples of the three levels of prevention as applied to the individual, family, and community.

Primary
- Assessment and teaching perinatal education course to pregnant inmates
- Assessment and teaching health education classes to nonpregnant inmates
- Teaching the family the roles and responsibilities of a labor support person

Secondary
- Screening at the community level (correctional facility) of what is perceived as learning needs
- Educating the family and community of the signs of postpartum depression

Tertiary
- Educating HIV-positive pregnant inmates on the need for antiviral treatment and delivery by cesarean section
- Educating family members and foster parents about the need for neonatal follow-up with regard to HIV status
- Assessing available community resources for counseling and treatment of postpartum depression

ROLES OF THE COMMUNITY HEALTH NURSE

Direct Care

The community health nurse provides direct care in a variety of settings. Often, this care is considered the "hands-on" nursing care given to a client in the home or a clinic.

Educator

The nurse encounters many opportunities for teaching. To be successful with health education, the nurse must attempt to gain the client's trust and must be sensitive to any cultural issues present. The nurse must also be aware of the emotional and physical state of the client. If the client is anxious or in pain, teaching may be ineffective.

Counselor

The counseling role of the nurse occurs in almost every interaction in the area of women's health. Before counseling in the area of reproductive health is begun, it is essential for effective intervention that the nurse become aware of his or her value system, including how biases and beliefs about human sexual behavior affect the counseling role.

RESEARCH IN WOMEN'S HEALTH

Women have long been the major users of the health care system. Research involving women is beginning to provide information enabling prediction, explanation, or description of phenomena affecting health. In the past, medical treatment for women was based on findings of research performed with male subjects exclusively, even in conditions that caused more deaths in women. Since the federal mandate regarding women and research was instituted, research efforts to include women in studies have grown. If women are not included in a research project, a rationale must be given for their exclusion.

The National Institutes of Health established the Office of Research on Women's Health (ORWH) in 1990. Achievements include women in National Institutes of Health (NIH) research, increase research in women's health differences, prepare women's health researchers, and focus on interdisciplinary career and gender differences research. Nurse researchers are encouraged to test interventions and question rituals in nursing by conducting research. Following are some of the areas for exploration and research among women:

- Alcohol, tobacco, and other drug use
- Intimate partner violence
- Heart disease
- Health behaviors
- Genetic screening and breast cancer
- Bone and musculoskeletal disorders
- Cancer prevention, screening, diagnosis, and treatment
- Health education at various literacy levels
- Wellness throughout the life cycle
- Differences among women experiencing menopausal symptoms
- Dysmenorrhea
- Safe and effective contraception
- Promotion of breast-feeding
- Infertility
- Coping with chronic illness, such as systemic lupus erythematosus or arthritis
- Discomforts of pregnancy, including morning sickness
- Strengths of single, female heads of households
- Adolescent sexuality
- Multiple-role adaptation
- Menstrual cycle variations
- Control of obesity
- Substance abuse and its effect on pregnancy
- HIV infection and pregnancy
- Influence of diet on osteoporosis
- Effect of socialization on role
- Gender differences in pharmacology

The NIH supports research in women's health by the ORWH. Research done by the ORWH (2017) has strengthened knowledge about women's health, including:

- Certain medications affect women differently than men.
- Women have more difficulty in quitting smoking.
- HPV vaccines protect against most cervical cancers.
- HIV transmission between mother and baby can be prevented.
- Chronic pain disorders are more common in women.
- Deployed women are at greater risk of suicide.
- Heart disease and breast cancer can be prevented.
- The overall quality of life can be improved.

With the increased emphasis on community health, community health nurses can make significant contributions to the improvement of women's health through scholarly research, either as principal investigators or through data gathering. Furthermore, they can become consumers of research and develop nursing interventions based on sound research and recommendations.

▌ SUMMARY

Women's health care has multiple facets, with many areas for community health nursing intervention. Nurses are advocates and activists for women's health through their involvement in health policy making as a profession. Along with other multidisciplinary and consumer groups, professional nurses are in the forefront of making changes in the health care delivery system that will promote an overall quality and research-based health plan for women. Women are at the center of the health of the United States; therefore if better models are developed for improving the health of women, the health of the entire nation will benefit.

ⓔ EVOLVE WEBSITE

http://evolve.elsevier.com/Nies/community
- NCLEX Review Questions
- Case Studies

BIBLIOGRAPHY

Adams PF, Martinez ME, Vickerie JL: Summary health statistics for the US Population: National Health Interview Survey, 2010. National Center for Health Statistics, *Vital Health Stat* 10(251):1–117, 2011.

American Academy of Pediatrics: *Family pediatrics: report of the task force on the family*, 2003. Elk Grove Village, IL, 2005, The Author.

American Cancer Society: *About endometrial cancer*, Key Statistics, 2017a. The Author: Available at https://www.cancer.org/cancer/endometrial-cancer/about/key-statistics.html. Accessed March 09, 2017.

American Cancer Society: *American Cancer Society recommendations for early breast cancer detection in women without breast symptoms*, 2016a. The Author: https://www.cancer.org/cancer/breast-cancer/screening-tests-and-early-detection/american-cancer-society-recommendations-for-the-early-detection-of-breast-cancer.html. Accessed March 09, 2017.

American Cancer Society: *Cancer facts and figures 2017*, 2017b. The Author: https://www.cancer.org/content/dam/cancer-org/research/cancer-facts-and-statistics/annual-cancer-facts-and-figures/2017/cancer-facts-and-figures-2017.pdf. Accessed March 31, 2017. Accessed April 9, 2017.

American Cancer Society: *Colorectal facts & figures 2014-2016*, Atlanta, 2014. The Author: https://www.cancer.org/content/dam/cancer-org/research/cancer-facts-and-statistics/colorectal-cancer-facts-and-figures/colorectal-cancer-facts-and-figures-2014-2016.pdf. Accessed April 06, 2017.

American Cancer Society: *Guidelines for the early detection of cancer*, 2017c. The Author: https://www.cancer.org/healthy/find-cancer-early/cancer-screening-guidelines/american-cancer-society-guidelines-for-the-early-detection-of-cancer.html. Accessed March 30, 2017.

American Cancer Society: *Guidelines on nutrition and physical activity for cancer prevention*, 2016b. The Author: https://www.cancer.org/healthy/eat-healthy-get-active/acs-guidelines-nutrition-physical-activity-cancer-prevention.html. Accessed March 31, 2017.

American Cancer Society: *Tests for ovarian cancer*, 2017d. The Author: https://www.cancer.org/cancer/ovarian-cancer/detection-diagnosis-staging/how-diagnosed.html. Accessed March 30, 2017.

American Cancer Society: *What are the risk factors for cervical cancer?* 2016c. The Author: https://www.cancer.org/cancer/cervical-cancer/causes-risks-prevention/risk-factors.html. Accessed March 31, 2017.

American Heart Association: *Go red for women*, 2017a. https://www.goredforwomen.org. Accessed March 01, 2017.

American Heart Association: *High blood pressure and heart disease*, 2017b. The Author: https://www.goredforwomen.org/know-your-risk/factors-that-increase-your-risk-for-heart-disease/high-blood-pressure-heart-disease/. Accessed April 02, 2017.

American Heart Association: *Statistical fact sheet, 2013 update: Women and cardiovascular disease*, 2013. The Author: http://www.heart.org/idc/groups/heart-public/@wcm/@sop/@smd/documents/downloadable/ucm_319576.pdf. Accessed March 31, 2017.

American Heart Association: *Statistical fact sheet 2015 update: Women & cardiovascular diseases*, 2016. The Author: https://www.heart.org/idc/groups/heart-public/@wcm/@sop/@smd/documents/downloadable/ucm_472913.pdf. Accessed March 31, 2017.

American Psychological Association: *Diagnostic and statistical manual of mental disorders*, ed 5, Washington, DC, Author.

American Psychological Association: *Women and depression*, 2005. Available from: <http://www.apa.org.ppo/issues/pwomenanddepress.html>.

Arthritis Foundation: *Arthritis in Women*, 2014. The Author: <http://www.arthritis.org/conditions-treatments/disease-center/women/>.

Berg CJ, Callaghan WM, Syverson C: Pregnancy-related mortality in the United States, 1998 to 2005, *Obstet Gynecol* 116(6):1302–1309, 2010.

Bhatia SC, Bhatia SK: Depression in women: diagnostic and treatment considerations, *Am Fam Physician* 60(1):225, 1999.

Black MC, Basile KC, Breiding M, et al.: *The national intimate partner and sexual violence survey: 2010 summary report*, 2011. http://www.cdc.gov/violenceprevention/pdf/nisvs_report2010-a.pdf.

Blehar M: Public health context of women's mental health research, *Psychiat Clin North Am* 26:781–799, 2003.

Cates W, Ellertson C, Stewart F: Abortion. In Hatcher RA, Trussell J, Stewart F, editors: *Contraceptive technology*, ed 18, New York, 2004, Ardent Media.

Centering Health Care: *Centering pregnancy overview*, 2013. <http://www.centeringhealthcare.org/pages/centering-model/pregnancy-overview.php>.

Centers for Disease Control and Prevention: *Age-adjusted hospital discharge rates for diabetes as any-listed diagnosis per 1,000 diabetic population, by sex, United States, 1988-2009*, 2009. The Author: https://www.cdc.gov/diabetes/statistics/dmany/fig5.htm.

Centers for Disease Control and Prevention: *Arthritis types*, 2017a. The Author: <http://www.cdc.gov/arthritis/basics/types.htm>. Accessed February 28, 2017.

Centers for Disease Control and Prevention: *Birth Rates (Live Births) per 1,000 Females Aged 15–19 Years, by Race and Hispanic Ethnicity, Select Years*, 2015a. The Author: https://www.cdc.gov/teenpregnancy/about/alt-text/birth-rates-chart-2000-2011-text.htm. Accessed March 30, 2017.

Centers for Disease Control and Prevention: Cancer mortality surveillance United States, 1990-2000, *MMWR* 53(3):1–108, 2004.

Centers for Disease Control and Prevention: *Cervical cancer screening guidelines for average-risk women*, 2015b. The Author: <http://www.cdc.gov/cancer/cervical/pdf/guidelines.pdf>.

Centers for Disease Control and Prevention: *Cervical cancer statistics*, 2015c. Available from: <http://www.cdc.gov/cancer/cervical/statistics/#2>.

Centers for Disease Control and Prevention: *HIV among women, fast facts*, 2017b. The Author: https://www.cdc.gov/hiv/pdf/group/gender/women/cdc-hiv-women.pdf. Accessed April 7, 2017.

Centers for Disease Control and Prevention: *HPV-associated cancers*, 2016a. The Author: https://www.cdc.gov/cancer/hpv/statistics/index.htm. Accessed March 30, 2017.

Centers for Disease Control and Prevention: *National Diabetes Statistics Report: Estimates of Diabetes and Its Burden in the United States, 2014a*, Atlanta, GA, 2014, U.S. Department of Health and Human Services. The Author: https://www.cdc.gov/diabetes/pubs/statsreport14/national-diabetes-report-web.pdf.

Centers for Disease Control and Prevention: *Pregnancy related mortality in the United States*, 2016b. Available from: <http://www.cdc.gov/reproductivehealth/MaternalInfantHealth/Pregnancy-relatedMortality.htm>.

Centers for Disease Control and Prevention: *Key statistics from the National Survey of Family Growth*, 2015c. Available from: http://www.cdc.gov/nchs/nsfg/key_statistics/h.htm#hysterectomy.

Centers for Disease Control and Prevention: *Leading cause of death by age group, all females—United States, 2016*, 2016c. https://www.cdc.gov/women/lcod/2014/all-females/index.htm. Accessed February 28, 2017.

Centers for Disease Control and Prevention: *Prevalence of doctor-diagnosed arthritis and arthritis-attributable activity limitation United States, 2007–2009, Morbidity and Mortality Report*, 2010. https://www.cdc.gov/mmwr/preview/mmwrhtml/mm5939a1.htm.

Centers for Disease Control and Prevention: *Prevalence of Self-Reported Postpartum Depressive Symptoms in 17 states, 2004-2005*, 2008d. <http://www.cdc.gov/mmwr/preview/mmwrhtml/ss5610a1.htm>.

Centers for Disease Control and Prevention: Prevalence and most common causes of disability among adults—United States, 2005, *Morbid Mortal Wkly Rep* 58(16):421–426, 2009. Available from: <http://www.cdc.gov/mmwr/preview/mmwrhtml/mm5816a2.htm#tab1>.

Centers for Disease Control and Prevention: *STDs in Women & infants*, 2015d. https://www.cdc.gov/std/stats14/womenandinf.htm.

Centers for Disease Control and Prevention: *Syphilis strikes back*, 2017b. Available from: https://www.cdc.gov/std/sam/2017syphilis.htm.

Centers for Disease Control and Prevention: *Teen Dating Violence*, 2013b. Available from: <http://www.cdc.gov/violenceprevention/intimatepartnerviolence/teen_dating_violence.html>.

Centers for Disease Control and Prevention: *National Institute for Occupational Safety and Health: Workplace safety and health topics: Industries & occupations*, 2013c. Available from: <http://www.cdc.gov/niosh/topics/industries.html>.

Centers for Disease Control and Prevention: *Vaccine Safety: Frequently asked questions about HPV vaccine safety*, 2017d. The Author: https://www.cdc.gov/vaccinesafety/vaccines/hpv/hpv-safety-faqs.html#A7. Accessed April 07, 2017.

Centers for Disease Control and Prevention: *Vaccine safety: human papilloma virus*, 2015e. The Author: <http://www.cdc.gov/vaccinesafety/Vaccines/HPV/index.html>. Accessed April 07, 2017.

Centers for Disease Control and Prevention: *Women and heart disease fact sheet*, 2016d. The Author: https://www.cdc.gov/dhdsp/data_statistics/fact_sheets/fs_women_heart.htm. Accessed March 30, 2017.

Chadwick B, Heaton TB: *Statistical handbook on the American family*, Phoenix, AZ, 1992, Oryx Press.

Choi M: Preamble to a new paradigm for women's health, *Image* 17:14, 1985.

Crane PB, Letvak S, Lewallen, et al.: Inclusion of women in nursing research: 1995-2001, *Nurs Res* 53(4):237–242, 2004.

Creanga AA, Shapiro-Mendoza CK, Bish CL, et al.: Trends in ectopic pregnancy mortality in the United States: 1980-2007, *Obstet Gynecol* 117(4):837–843, 2011.

Cronin KA, Richardson LC, Henley SJ: Vital signs: Racial disparities in breast cancer severity—United States, 2005–2009, *Morbid Mortal Wkly Rep* 61(45):922–926, 2012. Also available from: <http://www.cdc.gov/mmwr/preview/mmwrhtml/mm6145a5.htm?s_cid=mm6145a5_w>.

Cunningham FG, et al.: *Williams' obstetrics*, ed 24, Norwalk, CT, 2010, Appleton and Lange.

DeFrances C, Lucas C, Buie V: 2006 National Hospital Discharge Survey, *Natl Health Statist Rep* 30(5):1–20, 2008.

DeNavas-Walt C, Proctor D, Smith J: *Income, poverty, and health insurance coverage in the United States: 2011, U.S. Census Bureau Current Population Reports*, 2012. Available from: <http://www.census.gov/prod/2008pubs/p60-243.pdf>.235.pdf>.

Elders J: Speech given at 2009 Public Health Practice Symposium: Public Health Leadership to Improve the Health of Young People, Ann Arbor, MI.

Evans DL, et al.: Depression in the medical setting: biopsychological interactions and treatment considerations, *J Clin Psychiatry* 60 (Suppl 4):4, 1999.

Finkel ML, Finkel DJ: The effect of a second opinion program on hysterectomy performance, *Med Care* 28:776, 1990.

Fowler CI, Gable J, Wang J: *Family planning annual report: 2009 National summary*, Research Triangle Park, NC, 2010, RTI International.

Genetic Information Nondiscrimination Act of 2008, 493 H.R., § 110 (2008).

Hall MJ, DeFrances CJ, Williams SN: National Hospital Discharge Survey: 2007 summary, *National Health Stat report*, 2010. https://www.cdc.gov/nchs/data/nhsr/nhsr029.pdf.

Holahan J, Buttgens M, Caroll C, et al.: *Kaiser Commission on Medicaid and the Uninsured: The cost and coverage implications of the ACA Medicaid expansion: National and state-by-state analysis*, 2012. Available from: <http://kaiserfamilyfoundation.files.wordpress.com/2013/01/8384.pdf>.

Hopwood P, Stephens RJ; Medical Research Council Lung Cancer Working Party: Symptoms at presentation for treatment in patients with lung cancer: implications for the evaluation of palliative treatment, *Br J Cancer* 71:633, 1995.

Hoyert DL, Xu JQ: Deaths: preliminary data for 2011. *National Vital Statistics Reports*, 61:6. Hyattsville, MD: National Center for Health Statistics, 2012.

Jacobs A: Coronary revascularization in women in 2003: sex revisited, *Circulation* 107:375–377, 2003.

James PA, Oparil S, Carter BL, et al.: Evidence-based guideline for the management of high blood pressure in adults report from the panel members appointed to the eighth joint national committee (JNC 8), *JAMA* 311(5):507–520, 2014. http://doi.org/10.1001/jama.2013.284427.

Jatlaoui TC, Ewing A, Mandel MG, et al.: Abortion surveillance — United States, 2013, *MMWR Surveill Summ* 65(SS-12):1–44, 2016. https://doi.org/10.15585/mmwr.ss6512a1.

Johnson RH, Chien FL, Bleyer A: Incidence of breast cancer with distant involvement among women in the United States, 1976 to 2009, *JAMA* 27(309):1229, 2013.

Kovach K: Trauma nursing: intimate partner violence, *RN* 67:38, 2004.

Krieger CL: Intimate partner violence: a review for nurses, *Nurs Womens Health* 12(3):224–334, 2008.

Kuehn J, McMahon P, Creekmore S: Stopping a silent killer. Preventing heart disease in women, *AWHONN Lifelines* 3(2):31–35, 1999.

Manant A, Dodgson JE: Centering pregnancy: an integrative literature review, *J Midwifery Women's Health* 56:94–102, 2011.

Matthews S, Power C: Socio-economic gradients in psychological distress: a focus on women, social roles and work-home characteristics, *Soc Sci Med* 54:799–810, 2002.

Misner S, Beauchamp Hewitt J, Fox Levin P: *Women and occupational health*, Ontario, Canada: Health Canada, 1997, Canada-USA Women's Health Forum.

Mosca CL: Evidence-based guidelines for cardiovascular disease prevention in women: 2007 update, *Circulation* 115:1481–1501, 2007.

National Cancer Institute: *BRCA1 and BRCA2: Cancer risk and genetic testing*, 2013a. Available from: <http://www.cancer.gov/cancertopics/factsheet/Risk/BRCA>.

National Cancer Institute: *HPV and cancer*, 2013b. Available from: <http://cancer.gov/cancertopics/factsheet/Risk/HPV>.

National Cancer Institute: *Mammograms*, 2013c. Available from: <http://www.cancer.gov/cancertopics/factsheet/detection/mammograms>.

National Cancer Institute: *Surveillance, Epidemiology, and End Results Program: SEER Stat fact sheets: Breast, surveillance epidemiology & end results*, 2013d. Available from: <http://seer.cancer.gov/statfacts/html/breast.html>.

National Cancer Institute: *Surveillance, Epidemiology, and End Results Program: SEER Stat fact sheets: Ovarian cancer*, 2017. Available from: <http://seer.cancer.gov/statfacts/html/ovary.html>.

National Center for Health Statistics: *Health insurance coverage*, 2017. The Author: https://www.cdc.gov/nchs/fastats/health-insurance.htm. Accessed March 30, 2017.

National Center for Health Statistics: *Healthy People 2010 Final Review*, 2012. The Author: <http://www.cdc.gov/nchs/data/hpdata2010/hp2010_final_review.pdf>.

National Institutes of Health: *Office of Research on Women's Health: Studying sex to strengthen science*. The Author: https://orwh.od.nih.gov/resources/pdf/ORWH-iGiant-Factsheet-Studying-Sex.pdf. Accessed April 8, 2017.

National Women's Law Center: *National snapshot: poverty among women & families*, 2014. The Author: <https://nwlc.org/resources/national-snapshot-poverty-among-women-families-2014/>. Accessed April 15, 2017.

National Partnership for Women & Families: *A look at the U.S. Department of Labor's 2012 family and medical leave act employee and worksite surveys*, 2013. The Author: <http://go.nationalpartnership.org/site/DocServer/DOL_FMLA_Survey_2012_Key_Findings.pdf?docID=11862.

National Osteoporosis Foundation: *What women need to know*, 2014. The Author: <http://www.nof.org/235>.

Nelson AL: Menstrual problems and common gynecologic concerns. In Hatcher RA, Trussell J, Stewart F, et al, editors: *Contraceptive technology*, ed 18, New York, 2004, Ardent Media.

Norhammar A, Stenestrand UJ, Lindbäck J: Women younger than 65 years with diabetes mellitus are a high-risk group after myocardial infarction: a report from the Swedish register of information and knowledge about Swedish heart intensive care admission (RIKS-HIA), *Heart* 94:1565–1570, 2009.

Patel JD: Lung cancer in women, *J Clin Oncol* 23(14):3212–3218, 2005.

Pender N, Murdaugh CL, Parsons MA: *Health promotion in nursing practice*, ed 4, Upper Saddle River, NJ, 2006, Prentice Hall.

Rivera MP, Stover DE: Gender and lung cancer, *Clinical Chest Med* 25(2):391–400, 2004.

Ruzek S, Olsen V, Clark A: *Social, biomedical, and feminist models of women's health. Women's health: complexities and differences*, Columbus, OH, 1997, Ohio State University Press.

Sarna L, McCorkle R: Burden of care and lung cancer, *Cancer Pract* 4:245, 1996.

Schuiling KD, Likis FE: *Women's gynecologic health*, Sudbury, MA, 2016, Jones and Bartlett.

Schulman KA, Berlin JA, Harless W: The effect of race and sex on physicians' recommendations for cardiac catheterization, *N Engl J Med* 340(8):618–626, 1999.

Schmidt P: The 2012 hormone therapy position statement of the North American Menopause Society, *Menopause* 19(3):265, 2012.

Siegel R, Ma J, Zou Z: Cancer statisitcs, 2014. CA, *Cancer J Clinicians* 64(1):9–29, 2014.

Snell T: *Survey of state prison inmates: 1991—women in prison*, U.S. Department of Justice, Bureau of Justice Statistics Special Report. Washington, DC, US GPO.

Stevens JA: Falls among older adults–risk factors and prevention strategies, *J Saf Res* 36(4):409–411, 2005.

Thibos M, Lavin-Loucks D, Martin M: *The feminization of poverty*, Dallas, TX, 2007, The J. McDonald Williams Institute and the YWCA.

Thomas B, et al.: Randomized trial of breast self-examination in Shanghai: final results, *J Natl Cancer Inst* 94:19, 2002.

Urbanic JC: Depressive disorders. In Urbanic JC, Groh CJ, editors: *Women's mental health: a clinical guide for primary care providers*, Philadelphia, 2009, Wolters Kluwer.

U.S. Cancer Statistics Working Group: *United States Cancer Statistics: 1999–2013 Incidence and Mortality Web-based Report*. Atlanta, GA, 2016, U.S. Department of Health and Human Services, Centers for Disease Control and Prevention and National Cancer Institute. Available at www.cdc.gov/uscs.

U.S. Cancer Statistics Working Group: *United States Cancer Statistics: 1999–2013 incidence and mortality web-based report*, 2017. Atlanta, GA, 2016, U.S. Department of Health and Human Services, Centers for Disease Control and Prevention and National Cancer Institute. Available at www.cdc.gov/uscs.

U.S. Census Bureau: *Educational Attainment in the United States 2009*, 2012. The Author: https://www.census.gov/prod/2012pubs/p20-566.pdf.

U.S. Department of Agriculture: *Choose my plate*, 2013. Available from: <http://www.choosemyplate.gov/weight management-calories.html>.

U.S. Department of Education: Digest of education statistics, Washington, DC, 2008, Author.

U.S. Department of Health & Human Services: Health Care: Improvements for Women, 2012. Available at <http://www.hhs.gov/healthcare/prevention/women/index.html>.

U.S. Department of Health and Human Services: *National diabetes statistics*, 2011. National Diabetes Clearinghouse. Available at <http://diabetes.niddk.nih.gov/dm/pubs/statistics/#fast>.

U.S. Department of Health and Human Services: *Panel on Antiretroviral Guidelines for Adults and Adolescents. Guidelines for the use of antiretroviral agents in HIV-1-infected adults and adolescents*, 2013. Department of Health and Human Services. Available at <http://aidsinfo.nih.gov/ContentFiles/Adultand AdolescentGL.pdf>.

U.S. Department of Health and Human Services: *Women's health: Diabetes*, 2017. The Author: https://www.womenshealth.gov/publications/our-publications/fact-sheet/diabetes.html. Accessed March 31, 2017.

U.S. Department of Labor: *Women in the labor force: a databook*, 2016. The Author: https://www.bls.gov/opub/reports/womens-databook/archive/women-in-the-labor-force-a-databook-2015.pdf. Accessed April 10, 2017.

Viens LJ, Henley SJ, Watson M, et al.: Human papillomavirus–associated cancers—United States, 2008–2012, *MMWR* 65(26):661–666, 2016.

Wei G, Jackson JL, Hatzigeorgiou C: Osteoporosis management in the new millennium, *Prim Care* 30(4):711–741, 2003.

Wenger NK: You've come a long way, baby: cardiovascular health and disease in women: problems and prospects, *Circulation* 109:558–560, 2004.

Whiteman MK, Hillis SD, Jamieson DJ, et al.: Inpatient hysterectomy surveillance in the United States, 2000–2004, *Am J Obstet Gynecol* 198(1):1–7, 2008.

World Health Organization: *International Statistical Classification of Diseases and Related Health Problems*, 10th revision, 2007. Available from: <http://apps.who.int/classifications/apps/icd/icd10online/>.

World Health Organization: *Maternal mortality (Fact Sheet No. 348)*, 2012. Available from: <http://www.who.int/mediacentre/factsheets/fs348/en/>.

World Health Organization: *Life expectancy by country*, 2013. Available from: <http://apps.who.int/gho/data/node.main.688>.

World Health Organization: *Top ten causes of death*, 2017. Accessed from: http://www.who.int/mediacentre/factsheets/fs310/en/.

Zeidenstein L: Health issues of lesbian and bisexual women. In Varney H, Kriebs J, Gegor C, editors: *Varney's Midwifery,* Sudbury, MA, 2004 Jones and Bartlett, pp 299–308.

Men's Health

Jené M. Hurlbut

OBJECTIVES

Upon completion of this chapter, the reader will be able to do the following:

1. Identify the major indicators of men's health status.
2. Describe physiological and psychosocial factors that have an impact on men's health status.
3. Discuss barriers to improving men's health.
4. Discuss factors that promote men's health.
5. Describe men's health needs.
6. Apply knowledge of men's health needs in planning gender-appropriate nursing care for men at the individual, family, and community levels.

KEY TERMS

Androgen
chronic condition
illness orientation

life expectancy
medical care

morbidity
mortality

It is common knowledge that women live longer than men and that health care use is greater among women than men. Death rates for men are higher than for women in terms of the major causes. Although the overall interest in health promotion and illness prevention has increased, men's health issues remain largely unaddressed (Baerolcher and Verma, 2008). Women's health has become a specialty practice with courses and programs available in many colleges of nursing. A specialty in men's health has not yet been established.

This chapter focuses on exploring the health needs of men and the implications for community health nursing. Specific areas that are discussed include the current health status of men; physiological and psychological theories that attempt to explain men's health; factors that impede men's health; factors that promote men's health; men's health needs; and planning gender-appropriate care for men at the individual, family, and community levels.

MEN'S HEALTH STATUS

Traditional indicators of health for all persons include rates of longevity, mortality, and morbidity. Reviewing these rates gives nursing students a better understanding of the community aggregate. Box 18.1 lists standardized terminology in the fields of demography and sociology.

Longevity and Mortality

Major gender differences in longevity and mortality rates reveal that men remain disadvantaged despite advances in technology. Although women are more likely to use health services and have higher morbidity rates, mortality rates for men remain higher. Gender differences are generally associated with both physiological and behavioral factors, which place men at greater risk of death. These behavioral factors, together with men's reluctance to seek preventive and health services, have marked implications for community health nursing.

Longevity

Rates of longevity are increasing for both men and women. People can now expect to live more than 20 years longer than their forefathers and foremothers lived at the turn of the nineteenth century. Infants born in the United States in 1996 can expect to live 77 years, whereas those born in 1900, when the death rate was highest, lived an average of 47.3 years. Life expectancy for both males and females has increased; however, since the 1970s this gender gap in longevity has decreased (Table 18.1). Between 2007 and 2008, men and women gained 0.2 year of longevity (Arias, 2012). This change in male longevity may be attributed to the advances in treatment of heart disease and cancer, which have been the major causes of death in U.S. males (Table 18.2).

Factors that influence the incongruencies between males and females are race or ethnic origin, socioeconomic status, and education. When reported by race, gender mortality rates show that less advantaged populations in the United States, especially

minorities, live significantly fewer years. African American males live 6 years less than white males (Arias, 2012). Hispanics have a life expectancy comparable with that of their white counterparts.

Mortality

The United States lags behind several other countries in premature mortality rates for males. In 2011 only six countries had premature mortality rates higher than that of the United States: Russian Federation, Mexico, Hungary, Estonia, Poland, and Slovak Republic (Organisation for Economic Co-operation and Development [OECD], 2011). In the United States, as in most industrialized countries, males lead females in mortality rates in each leading cause of death. Although males were the primary source of medical data before the 1970s, and most of the treatment advances have been developed from these data, gender-related disparity in death rates continues. Other factors also account for this mortality gender gap.

The gender disparity for disease-related deaths has narrowed. Heart disease remains the leading cause of death, but the ratio of death for heart disease decreased by 2.8 between 2005 and 2006. During this same period, the ratio of male deaths to female deaths increased by 1.4. Since the 1990s, cancer-related deaths in women have declined at a slower rate than those in men. Lifetime risk for lung cancer is estimated to be 9.8% among males and 3.8% among females (Lynch, 2008). The death rate for chronic lower respiratory tract disease among females has increased from 14.9 deaths per 100,000 population in 1980 to 37.1 in 2014, and among males from 49.9 in 1980 to 45.4 in 2014, indicating a 4.5 decrease (National Center for Health Statistics [NCHS], 2016). The rise in women may be associated with the increase in incidence of lower respiratory disease among the elderly (Lynch, 2008). Unintentional injury deaths for the whole population has increased 1.1 per 100,000 from 2013 to 2014 (NCHS, 2016). Males continue to be at risk for death due to unintentional injury with a rate of 54.7 compared with 27.3 for females per 100,000. Men are three to four times more likely to commit suicide. Males older than 85 years are 11 to 12 times more likely than females of the same age to commit suicide (NCHS, 2016).

Race and ethnic background also are factors to be considered in the evaluation of male mortality rates. Among males aged

---

BOX 18.1 Standardized Terminology

In the fields of demography and sociology, the following terms are standardized:

People of all ages: Males and females

Children younger than 18 years: Boys and girls

Adults 18 years of age or older: Men and women

Sex: The biological distinction between males and females

Gender: The attitudes and behavior of men and women that are shaped by socialization and have a potential to be changed

Role: The part one plays in society

Modified from Skelton R: Man's role in society and its effect on health, *Nursing* 26:953, 1988; and Verbrugge LM, Wingard DL: Sex differentials in health and mortality, *Women Health* 12:103, 1987.

TABLE 18.1 Life Expectancy at Birth According to Sex and Race, United States: 1900, 1950, 2000, 2005, 2007, and 2008

YR	ALL RACES			WHITE			BLACK		
	Both Sexes	Male	Female	Both Sexes	Male	Female	Both Sexes	Male	Female
1900	47.3	46.3	48.3	47.6	46.6	48.7	33.0	32.5	33.5
1950	68.2	65.6	71.1	69.1	66.5	72.2	60.8	59.1	62.9
2000	76.8	74.1	79.3	77.3	74.7	79.9	71.8	68.2	75.1
2005	77.4	74.9	79.9	77.9	75.4	80.4	72.8	69.3	76.1
2007	77.9	75.4	80.4	78.4	75.9	80.8	73.6	70.0	76.8
2008	78.1	75.6	80.6	78.5	76.1	80.9	74.0	70.6	77.2

Data from Arias E: *United States life tables, 2008* (National Vital Statistics Reports vol. 61, no. 3), Washington, DC, 2012, National Center for Health Statistics.

TABLE 18.2   Leading Causes of Death in Males, United States, 2014

	Percentage
All Males, All Ages	
Heart disease	24.5
Cancer	23.4
Unintentional injuries	6.4
Chronic lower respiratory diseases	5.2
Stroke	4.2
Diabetes	3.1
Suicide	2.5
Alzheimer disease	2.1
Influenza and pneumonia	2.0
Chronic liver disease	1.9
White Males, All Ages	
Heart disease	24.6
Cancer	23.6
Unintentional injuries	6.5
Chronic lower respiratory diseases	5.6
Stroke	4.0
Diabetes	2.9
Suicide	2.7
Alzheimer disease	2.3
Influenza and pneumonia	2.0
Chronic liver	1.9
Black Males, All Ages	
Heart disease	24.1
Cancer	22.2
Unintentional injuries	6.1
Stroke	4.9
Homicide	4.3
Diabetes	4.1
Chronic lower respiratory diseases	3.2
Kidney disease	2.6
Septicemia	1.9
Influenza and pneumonia	1.7
Asian or Pacific Islander Males, All Ages	
Cancer	26.4
Heart disease	23.0
Stroke	6.1
Unintentional injuries	5.3
Diabetes	3.9
Chronic lower respiratory diseases	3.4
Influenza and pneumonia	3.2
Suicide	2.6
Kidney disease	2.1
Alzheimer disease	1.6
Hispanic Males, All Ages	
Cancer	20.6
Heart disease	20.4
Unintentional injuries	9.7
Diabetes	4.5
Stroke	4.4
Chronic liver disease	4.2
Suicide	2.8
Chronic lower respiratory disease	2.6
Homicide	2.3
Influenza and pneumonia	2.1

From Centers for Disease Control and Prevention: Men's health: leading causes of death in males United States 2014, 2014. http://www.cdc.gov/men/lcod/.

15 to 24 years, African American males are more likely to die of vehicle accidents and seven times more likely to die of homicide (NCHS, 2016). Hispanic males fare somewhat better but are still more likely to die as a result of homicide than white males.

Morbidity

Despite the differences in mortality rates, men tend to perceive themselves to be in better health than women do (Brown and Bond, 2008). In the National Health Interview Survey (NHIS) of 2010, which asked people to rate their health status, men were more likely to rate their health as excellent or very good as opposed to fair or poor (Schiller et al., 2012). Morbidity rates, or rates of illness, are difficult to obtain and have been available usually only in Western industrialized countries. For example, in the United States, reports of analyses of morbidity rates by gender lag several years behind those of analyses of mortality rates by gender. Gender differences in morbidity rates reflect the latest available reports. The following are common indicators of morbidity rate:

- Incidence of acute illness
- Prevalence of chronic conditions
- Use of medical care

Although variations exist, women are more likely to be ill, whereas men are at greater risk for death. Box 18.2 lists several resources for morbidity data in the United States.

Chronic Conditions

A chronic condition is a condition that persists for at least 3 months or belongs to a group of conditions classified as chronic, regardless of time of onset, such as tuberculosis, neoplasm, and arthritis. In general, women have higher morbidity rates than men. Women are more likely than men to have a higher prevalence of chronic diseases that cause disability and limitation of activities but do not lead to death. However, men have higher morbidity and mortality rates for conditions that are the leading causes of death.

ACTIVE LEARNING

1. Examine the vital statistics in the community and compare the gender-specific differences in mortality rates.
2. During a 1-week period, determine the frequency of newspaper articles in the local major newspaper that identify the top 12 causes of death for men.
3. Review major nursing texts (e.g., medical-surgical); examine the tables of contents and the indexes for content on men's health versus women's health.

USE OF MEDICAL CARE

The use of medical care—the use of ambulatory care, hospital care, preventive care, or other health services—in the United States also illustrates different gender patterns.

Use of Ambulatory Care

Men seek ambulatory care less often than women. According to the 2010 NHIS (Schiller et al., 2012), the physician's office is the primary setting for ambulatory care for both men and women.

Responses to the survey indicated that men visited physician offices and clinics or health centers less often than women and emergency rooms more frequently. Additionally, 27% of men, compared with 14% women, had made no office visits to a health care provider in the past 12 months. Men were likely to visit a physician only if they experienced a specific health-related symptom (Brown and Bond, 2008). Injury-related visits to hospital emergency departments are higher for males than females. Males aged 18 to 24 years are twice as likely to visit hospital emergency departments for unintentional injuries as females in the same age range. Even though gender differences in ambulatory care utilization are lessening, males continue to delay medical treatment, so they are sicker when they do seek health care and therefore require more intensive medical care.

Use of Hospital Care

The literature indicates that hospitalization rates also vary by sex. In 2014, rates of hospital stays were lower for males than for females. Hospital stays increase for both men and women after 45 years of age; however, rates for men increase more rapidly. After 65 years of age, men's discharge rates continue to be higher than women's rates (NCHS, 2016).

Use of Preventive Care

Preventive examinations and appropriate health-protective behavior are necessary for health promotion and early diagnosis of health problems. Men do not engage in these health-protective behaviors at the same frequency as do females (Brown and Bond, 2008). Most men do not have routine checkups. National health surveys indicate that women overall are more likely than men to have visits to various health care providers (NCHS, 2016). Men are twice as likely to report no usual source of care, although eligibility for primary care in males exceeds that in females (Lynch, 2008).

Use of Other Health Services

Overall, the number of visits to health care provider offices and outpatient sites is lower for men aged 18 to 74 than for women in the same age span. Men tend to have fewer dental health care

visits (64.1) than do women (68.9) as a percentage of persons with a dental visit in the past year for 2014 (NCHS, 2016). In a research study conducted by Frisbee and colleagues (2010), findings supported the importance of oral hygiene as it relates to the overall health of the individual. Additionally, men have lower rates of use of colorectal testing and procedures (men, 56.7; women, 58.9, percentage of adults aged 50 to 75) (NCHS, 2016).

THEORIES THAT EXPLAIN MEN'S HEALTH

As discussed previously, a gender gap exists in health. The data reviewed raise many questions for community health nurses to explore regarding gender differences in health and illness. Although men have shorter life expectancies and higher rates of mortality for all leading causes of death, women have higher rates of morbidity, including rates of acute illness and chronic disease and use of medical and preventive care services. Verbrugge and Wingard (1987) asked why "females are sicker, but males die sooner." Several explanations exist for this paradox.

Nurses traditionally use developmental theories to explain individual behavior. Erickson's model was not gender specific; Levinson focused somewhat on male development. There remains a need for literature detailing the factors and combinations of factors that influence gender differences in the health and illness of populations.

The following explanations proposed by Waldron (1995d) and Verbrugge and Wingard (1987) attempt to account for gender differences in this important area:

- Biological factors, including genetics, effects of sex hormones, and physiological differences, which may be influenced by genetics, hormones, and environment
- Socialization
- Orientations toward illness and prevention
- Data collection of health behavior

Biological Factors

Several biological factors influence sex differences in mortality and morbidity rates, including genetics, effects of sex hormones, and physiological differences, which may be influenced by genetics, hormones, and environmental factors (Waldron, 1995a–d). The embryo is unisexual until the seventh week of gestation. **Androgen**, a hormone from the Y chromosome, coupled with the maternal androgen sources, results in the development of the male sex. More male births occur than female births. In 2008, 1048 male births occurred for every 1000 female births (Martin et al., 2010). However, during this period, infant mortality rates for males were 21% higher than for females, thus reducing this ratio (Mathews and MacDorman, 2012). Sex ratios at birth appear to be lower for births to American Indian and black fathers (Martin et al., 2010).

Whether sex ratios at birth are influenced by sex ratios at conception or sex differentials in mortality rates before birth is unknown. Current evidence suggests that more than two of every three prenatal deaths occur before clinical recognition of the pregnancy. Embryonic research shows excess male fetuses in early pregnancy and fewer males delivered at term. Males'

BOX 18.3 Four Dimensions of Stereotyped Male Gender-Role Behavior

- *No sissy stuff:* the need to be different from women
- *The big wheel:* the need to be superior to others
- *The sturdy oak:* the need to be independent and self-reliant
- *Give 'em hell:* the need to be more powerful than others, through violence if necessary

Modified from David DS, Brannon R: The male sex role: our culture's blueprint of manhood, and what it's done for us lately. In David DS, Brannon R, editors: *The forty-nine percent majority: the male sex role*, Reading, MA, 1976, Addison-Wesley.

---

experience of higher mortality rates for perinatal conditions is attributed to biological disadvantages such as males' greater risk of premature birth, higher rates of respiratory distress syndrome, and higher rates of infectious disease in infancy resulting from the influence of male hormones on the developing lungs, brain, and possibly the immune system of the male fetus (Heron et al., 2009). Sex chromosome–linked diseases, such as hemophilia and certain types of muscular dystrophy, are more common among males than females (Waldron, 1995b).

Biological advantages for females may also exist later in life because of the estrogen-related mechanism that protects against heart disease. Some evidence supports the hypothesis that men's higher testosterone levels contribute to their lower high-density lipoprotein cholesterol levels. Body fat distribution, specifically the tendency for men in Western countries to accumulate abdominal body fat versus the tendency for women to accumulate fat on the buttocks and thighs, may also contribute to sex differences in the development of metabolic syndrome (Kirby et al., 2006). Men's higher levels of stored iron also may contribute to risk for ischemic heart disease. Additional physiological gender differences are as follows (Tanne, 1997):

- During the process of aging, men's brain cells die faster than women's brain cells. This finding may explain why men are more often hospitalized for serious mental disease.
- Male immune systems are weaker than women's.

Socialization

A second theory for explaining sex differences in health is socialization, especially in the area of masculinity. Society emphasizes assertiveness, restricted emotional display, concern for power, and reckless behavior in males (Box 18.3). Pursuit of these attributes results in higher risks in work, leisure, and lifestyle. Internalization of these norms of masculinity reduces the likelihood of engaging in health promotion behaviors for fear these behaviors might be interpreted as a sign of weakness. Gender-role socialization may influence these differences. Peer pressure plays an important role in the adherence to masculine norms. Many men enculturate their sons to believe that risking personal injury demonstrates masculinity (Brown and Bond, 2008).

According to the National Institute for Occupational Safety and Health's NIOSH Workers Health Chartbook (2004), 53.4% of U.S. workers are males. Male workers account for 66.1% of the reported occupational injuries and for 92% of work-related fatalities. Men's higher exposure to carcinogens at the worksite is associated with high rates of mesothelioma and coal worker's pneumoconiosis. In the United States, men score higher than women on measures of hostility and lack of trust of others, which may place them at higher risk of ischemic heart disease. Although occupational hazards to women's health are being identified, evidence indicates that, unlike for men, employment outside the home has a positive effect for U.S. women.

Popular male leisure, sports, and play activities place men at high risk for injury. Males between the ages of 18 and 24 years are more likely than women to visit a hospital emergency department because of unintentional injuries, cuts, or piercings or intentional injury (NCHS, 2016). Statistics show that men drive faster than women, receive more traffic violations, and are less likely to wear seat belts, all of which contribute to a greater number of motor vehicle fatalities. Although prevalence of smoking is decreasing, 19.0% of males smoke (NCHS, 2016); 57.3% of men consume alcohol, and men are three times more likely than women to drink heavily. Additionally, males overall have a greater use of illegal substances and greater nonmedical use of psychotherapeutic drugs (NCHS, 2016).

Men are more likely to be involved in violent crimes, and violence is a typical precursor to homicide. Men are victims of homicide more often than women. For black males, the fifth leading cause of death is homicide. However, for white males, homicide is not one of the top 10 causes of death (NCHS, 2016).

Many barriers exist that prohibit positive changes in male health behavior, but female family members were seen as facilitators. Cheatham and colleagues (2008) reported that several studies show males to be more likely to change health behaviors when these changes are suggested and supported by female family members who the males thought were concerned about their well-being.

Orientation Toward Illness and Prevention

Illness orientation, or the ability to note symptoms and take appropriate action, also may differ between the sexes. Most diseases, injuries, and deaths prevalent among men are preventable. However, the stereotypical view of men as strong and invulnerable is incongruent with health promotion. Boys are socialized to ignore symptoms and "toughen up." Surveys done by the magazine *Men's Health* reveal that 9 million men have not seen a health care provider in 5 years. Men may be aware of being ill, but they make a conscious decision not to seek health care to avoid being labeled "sick." Brown and Bond (2008) suggest that men lack the somatic awareness and are less likely to interpret symptoms as indicators of illness. A desire to rationalize symptoms and denial of susceptibility to disease may contribute to the delay in treatment (Brown and Bond, 2008).

Health-protective behavior, or the ability to take action to prevent disease or injury, also may vary between the sexes. Perhaps as a result of the contraceptive developments of the 1970s, women are more likely to seek preventive examinations.

Routine reproductive health screening (e.g., the Papanicolaou smear test and breast examination) has been expanded to include some general screening, such as testing of blood pressure, urine, and blood for signs of chronic problems. Men do not have routine reproductive health checkups that include screening, which would detect other health problems at an early stage. Among respondents to the NHIS, more women than men reported contacting a dentist and a health care provider within the previous 6 months, and 22% of men were without a usual place of health care, compared with 13% of women (Schiller et al., 2012). Men reported spending more time in leisure activities and muscle-strengthening activities that met the federal physical activity guidelines. However, 41% of men were considered overweight, compared with 28% of women (Schiller et al., 2012).

Gender differences in preventive health behavior are a fertile ground for continued research. Meryn (2009) reported that 21% of research was devoted to men's health, compared with 53% for female health. He suggests that large-scale research in this area would add to the small evidence bases of health promotion behaviors among men. Specific national health objectives have only recently addressed the health care needs of this aggregate. Uniformly recognized preventive screening programs for males have only recently been developed. With the advent of managed care and initiatives for health care reform, men who are eligible for health care coverage will have access to these routine health screenings. For men coverage would be available for immunizations, colonoscopies, nutritional education, obesity screenings, cholesterol and blood pressure screenings, screenings for HIV, depression screenings, and tobacco counseling (Sommers and Wilson, 2012). However, whether men will take advantage of these programs is undetermined. Box 18.4 discusses matters related to men's reproductive health needs.

Reporting of Health Behavior

Data regarding health behaviors are collected from a variety of sources, such as interviews, surveys, questionnaires, and reports. Data from these sources may not be accurate because males are less likely than females to participate in such a data collection process. Men may be less willing to talk, may not recall health problems, and may lack a health vocabulary. Men may be more hesitant to talk about their illnesses. Not only do women participate more in the data collection process, but also they are often solicited in health surveys to report the health behavior of men. In this manner, women are proxies, and proxies have a tendency to underreport behavior. The accuracy of the data does increase with male participation, but men may not want to participate in the socialization of sickness and tend to make light of health problems. Males with an extreme conception of masculinity are less likely to admit their health problems and may conceal or suppress pain in an effort to appear strong (Naslindh-Ylispanger et al., 2008). Men are far less likely than women to seek counseling. Male socialization to suppress expressiveness may represent the explanation for gender differences in reporting health behaviors.

BOX 18.4 Men's Reproductive Health Needs

Reproductive health needs are beginning to be recognized as important to both men's health and women's health. Usually the term *reproductive health* is applied to women of childbearing age. Used here, the term applies to the health of reproductive organs, which develop in utero and with which a person is born, either male or female, regardless of whether he or she has sex or reproduces. Males may have reproductive health needs whether child or adult, straight or gay, or virgin or sexually experienced.

Many sexually transmitted diseases (STDs) are at epidemic proportions in the United States and are a major health hazard for many men and women. AIDS is twice as likely to occur in males as in females in the United States. In 2014, death due to HIV in males was 3.0 per 100,000, and for females it was 1.1 per 100,000 (NCHS, 2016). Less well known, perhaps, is that many STDs are considered intrinsically "sexist" because clinical evidence, more overt in men, is more likely to facilitate a correct diagnosis in men than in women. These STDs are easier to detect in men because men are more likely to be symptomatic; laboratory tests are more reliable in men; efficiency of transmission is greater from male to female; and men are more likely to seek care for STDs that are symptomatic. For example, the overall incidence rate for *Chlamydia* infection in 2015 for males was 305.2 per 100,000; for females, the rate was 645.5 per 100,000. The rate of gonorrhea was slightly higher among men (140.9 per 100,000 population) than among women (107.2 per 100,000 population). Syphilis was also more common in men than in women (13.7 per 100,000 males; 1.4 per 100,000 females) (Centers for Disease Control and Prevention, 2015).

Testicular cancer represents only 1% of cancers in males and is the most common cancer to affect young men between the ages of 15 and 35 years. Cancer of the prostate is a leading cause of death from cancer in men, was estimated to account for 19.0 deaths per 100,000 population in 2014, and remains twice as common in African American males as in white males (NCHS, 2016). The increase in the incidence of prostate cancer has been attributed to factors such as improved methods of detection and greater exposure to environmental carcinogens.

Mortality rates for all cancers remain high, especially in males older than 75 years. Men older than 85 years are twice as likely to die of cancer as those aged 75 to 84 years (NCHS, 2016).

Many occupational and environmental agents associated with adverse sexual and reproductive outcomes in men have been identified, including pesticides; anesthetic gases in the operating room and dental office; inorganic lead from smelters, paint, printing materials, carbon disulfide from vulcanization of rubber, inorganic mercury manufacturing, and dental work; and ionizing radiation from x-rays (Whorton, 1984). Nonchemical agents have also been identified as hazardous in men; for example, hyperthermia experienced by firefighters has been linked to male infertility.

Many pharmacological agents, including prescription, over-the-counter, and recreational drugs, have been found to affect the reproductive outcomes or sexual functioning of men. Examples are drugs from the following categories: antihypertensives, antipsychotics, antidepressants, hormones, sedatives, hypnotics, stimulants, chemotherapy agents used in cancer treatment, amphetamines, opiates, alcohol, marijuana, cocaine, barbiturates, and lysergic acid diethylamide (LSD). Erectile dysfunction has become a "socially acceptable" topic of discussion since many high-profile men, such as U.S. Senator Bob Dole, former National Football League coach Mike Ditka, and retired General Norman Schwarzkopf, have openly discussed their problem. Pharmaceutical companies market their products for treatment of this disorder via mass media. Controversy has arisen as to the use of public funding for these products.

A focus on homosexual men's health has come about largely through the advent of AIDS. Today, homosexuality encompasses not only the male but also the entire family. The community health nurse should develop nonjudgmental assessment skills that foster honest and open expression for all members of the community. Nurses may need specialized skills to work with these individuals.

Discussion of the Theories of Men's Health
Interpreting the Data

Community health nurses should be aware of gender disparity when collecting and interpreting data. To avoid bias, the community health nurse should consider the following issues:

Gender-specific interview techniques may be necessary to obtain the most accurate health history. Men respond better to direct questions than to open-ended questions.

How do data obtained by male nurses differ from those obtained by female nurses? Is there personal gender bias in data collection?

The accuracy of secondary sources of information is skewed toward the interpretation of the source. How do the data provided by women about male health behavior compare with the data collected from men regarding these same behaviors?

Men are not enculturated to be caregivers. They need assistance to learn how to provide support to a caregiver or to develop a caregiver role.

In response to the question why "females are sicker, but males die sooner," several reasons can be provided. Conditions that affect morbidity rates (e.g., arthritis and gout) do not significantly affect mortality rates. Conditions that affect mortality rates may not significantly affect day-to-day activity until the conditions are advanced. Men tend to delay seeking health care until their conditions are advanced. Although mortality rates are, in large part, the outcome of inherited or acquired risks, gender differences in illness and health promotion behaviors, as well as in the reporting of health behaviors, suggest that social and psychological factors also affect morbidity rates. Although males have higher prevalence and death rates for "killer" chronic diseases, injuries, and accidents, females have higher prevalence rates for a greater number of nonfatal chronic conditions.

Gender-Linked Behavior

The largest gender differences in mortality rates occur for causes of death associated with gender-linked behavior and suggest that gender-linked behavior, which is more prevalent and encouraged in men, correlates with the following major categories of death:

- *Tobacco use:* Lung cancer, bronchitis, emphysema, and asthma
- *Substance abuse:* Cirrhosis, accidents, and homicide
- *Poor preventive health habits and stress:* Heart disease
- *Lack of other emotional channels:* Cirrhosis, suicide, homicide, and accidents

Physical conditions can be seriously affected by social and environmental conditions, such as occupational hazards (e.g., carcinogens and stress), unemployment, and massive advertising campaigns that use gender and gender roles to sell alcohol and tobacco. These lifestyle factors are compounded by men's lack of willingness to seek preventive care such as screening and to seek health care when a symptom arises. To counter these types of factors, research is needed to determine gender-specific methods of data collection, education, and practice that are aimed at health promotion, illness prevention, and political processes for males.

RESEARCH HIGHLIGHTS

Health Education and Health Screening in a Sample of Older Men: A Descriptive Survey

Two nurse researchers (Dallas and Neville, 2012) conducted a study to describe the health education and health screening practices of older men living in an area of New Zealand and the perceived barriers to and benefits of healthy lifestyle choices. Data were collected using a self-reported instrument. The sample consisted of 59 men ranging in age from 65 to 91 years. The majority of the men in this sample (66%) reported no barriers to making a healthy lifestyle choice. However, of those men who did report barriers, the most common reason was lack of motivation (12%), followed by lack of knowledge related to availability of programs and screenings (8%). Reported external barriers included lack of programs, associated costs, and transportation challenges. The most common reported benefits of a healthy lifestyle choice were getting to be with other people (62%), having fun (56%), feeling healthier (54%), and feeling better about self (52%). The majority of the men reported their health as good (67%), and healthy lifestyle as always (43%) or frequently healthy (43%). Dallas and Neville (2012) contend that nurses can have a pivotal role in conducting future research endeavors aimed at understanding the health needs of older men that will ultimately improve their health outcomes.

Data from Dallas J, Neville S: Health education and health screening in a sample of older men: a descriptive survey. *Nurs Prax N Z* 28(1):6–16, 2012.

ACTIVE LEARNING

Survey the billboards in the community and determine the frequency of those that depict gender-linked behaviors of men that are associated with risk taking.

FACTORS THAT IMPEDE MEN'S HEALTH

Many factors function as barriers to men's health, including their risk-taking behaviors and infrequent use of the health care system. In addition, gaps in preventive health behavior and differences in illness and health orientations and reporting of health behavior all contribute to a diminished health status for men. Several other barriers have been proposed, including the patterns of medical care provided in the United States, access to care, and lack of health promotion.

Medical Care Patterns

Although the data that serve as a foundation for medical treatment were collected from males, the concept of a health care provider that specializes in men's health is a relatively new phenomenon. Many health professionals provide care for men with complex health needs in a wide variety of settings. A specialist to which a male could go to for care that "feels right" for him has not been developed. Little effort has been made to create a male-specific health care climate (Haines and Wender, 2006). Urologists, who may see men for genital abnormalities or diseases of the prostate, became the proxy "male health specialists." The medical specialty andrology, which originated in Europe to treat problems of fertility and sterility, is considered too narrow in focus to treat "the whole man." Without a primary care specialty that focuses specifically on men's needs and gender-role influences on health and lifestyle, the gender disparity will continue. Currently, male health concerns are addressed by specialists and generalists who have not received gender-specific training that would enable them to focus on men's health needs. In the current era of managed care and health care reform, men will still be left without gender-specific primary care providers who have training focused specifically on men's needs.

Access to Care
Mission Orientation

Historically, society's interest in men's health has focused on efforts necessary to maintain an effective workforce. Men are socialized to view health as a commodity or resource that enables the body to work. Mission-oriented health care is a priority for large industries and organized sports. Industries provide workers with preventive health care to maintain workplace productivity. Mission-oriented health care in the sports arena has given birth to the specialty of sports medicine. Insurance programs such as health maintenance organizations (HMOs) may provide more comprehensive health care to men. Perhaps the most complete care is currently offered by the military; however, marked deficiencies exist there in the lack of a focus on prevention and health promotion at the individual and aggregate levels and inattention to policy regarding environmental hazards.

Financial Considerations

Another barrier to health care for men is financial ability. A man may receive an annual physical examination if he belongs to an HMO or if he is an executive or an airline pilot, but many private insurance companies reimburse more fully for a diagnosed condition (e.g., for pathology) and less fully for preventive care. A man is more likely to be insured for acute or chronic illness conditions than for health education, counseling, or other types of preventive health care. Women have annual gynecological examinations that include screening for other conditions and allow a woman to express other physical or psychological needs; however, men have lacked entrance into the health care system for a physical examination on a routine basis. With the advent of managed care and societal interest in preventive health focus, gender differences in routine physical examinations for preventive reasons have narrowed. However, socialization has a marked influence on behavior, and current trends may prevail despite attitudinal changes in health care delivery. Men must become advocates for programs that meet their own health care needs (Porche, 2009).

Time Factors

Historically, medical care could be accessed between the hours of 9:00 AM and 5:00 PM Monday through Friday. Men were reluctant to take time from work for a medical visit, especially for reasons other than illness. Fear of loss of income or the stigmatization of being "weak," "ill," or "less of a man" inhibited medical care access for males. Men in the lower socioeconomic group may be too exhausted from working to access health care, especially preventive health care (Haines and Wender, 2006). Variety in the times and locations of care delivery clinics should improve male access.

> ### BOX 18.5 Precursors of Death
>
> The following precursors of death are frequently unaddressed by the present health care system:
> - Heart disease and stroke
> - Hypercholesterolemia
> - Hypertension
> - Diabetes mellitus
> - Obesity
> - Type A personality
> - Family history
> - Lack of exercise
> - Cigarette smoking
> - Cancer
> - Sunlight
> - Radiation
> - Occupational hazards
> - Water pollution
> - Air pollution
> - Dietary patterns
> - Alcohol
> - Heredity

More walk-in primary care clinics that provide evening and weekend appointments have appeared. These clinics may be housed in occupational settings, malls, and even grocery stores. Data must be collected regarding male utilization of these additional health care sites.

Lack of Health Promotion

Limiting the concept of health to being merely absence of disease eliminates health promotion. Using traditional mortality and morbidity rates as reflective of the state of "health" of a population represents only a biological basis of health. To provide the community health nurse with a clearer picture of male health, the presence of behavioral risk factors such as smoking, alcohol consumption, obesity, and sedentary lifestyle should be considered. When asked, men describe "healthy" people as those with proportional body weight and height who do not engage excessively in behaviors detrimental to health. Physical recovery after impairment, illness, or injury is also considered a factor in men's definition of "healthy." Disease prevention and health promotion are not often reflected in a man's perception of health. Addressing and limiting the precursors of death is a recent health care phenomenon (Box 18.5). Interventions by many disciplines are needed to prevent current health problems. Nursing can play a pivotal role in the contribution to practice and research in this area of concern.

The continued focus on disease cure in the present health care system reinforces men's perception of health. Coronary heart disease, cancer, and stroke are three conditions that account for two thirds of all deaths and require the greatest use of health care resources. The increase in life expectancy exhibits the effect these medical advances have had on mortality rates from these diseases. These advances have resulted in an increase in years of disability, which may account for the rise in suicide among men older than 65 years (NCHS, 2016). An increase in health care costs has also resulted.

ETHICAL INSIGHTS

Social Justice versus Market Justice Ethics

Community health nurses should be involved in political activities that develop health policies that will make a difference in the health of males and the entire population. Such activities are congruent with the philosophy of public health as "health for all" and a commitment to a social justice ethic of health care rather than a market justice ethic of health care. Examining men's health gives the community health nurse an opportunity to observe the market justice ethic of health care's influence on men's health in the United States and how this affects their traditional roles in the family and within the community. The community health nurse can play a vital role in contributing to a social justice ethic of health care, particularly in relation to promoting men's health. Nurses must focus on health promotion and prevention at the aggregate and population levels rather than on treatment and cure.

Financial resources are invested in traditional disease-curative care rather than health promotion action. An inordinate amount of funding is poured into the health care system each year, with only minimal amounts allotted to public health promotion, as discussed in earlier chapters. In 2014, total national health expenditures accounted for 17.5% of the gross domestic product (NCHS, 2016). Of every dollar spent on health care in 2014, more than half went to hospital care and physician services, which are in large part curative in focus. The current health care system is making limited advances in addressing the precursors of death. It is questionable whether medical care, or another medical specialty, is the answer to men's health needs when social, occupational, environmental, and lifestyle factors continue to place men at risk.

Healthy lifestyles are not a matter of free choice but rather a result of opportunities that are not always equally available to people. Although available, prevention and health promotion are not uniformly applied at the aggregate and population levels. Health policies shape these opportunities for a healthy lifestyle for individuals and aggregates. Policies related to environmental and occupational changes beyond an individual's control are required to significantly affect the health of the population (Meryn, 2009).

 ACTIVE LEARNING

Survey local businesses and industries in the community to determine what health promotion and prevention programs are available and used by men and women.

MEN'S HEALTH CARE NEEDS

Lynch (2008) delineated men's health care needs that draw from the biological and psychosocial causes of men's distinctive health situation, and these health care needs continue today. According to these writers, men need the following:

- Permission to have concerns about health and to talk openly to others about their concerns
- Support for the consideration of gender-role and lifestyle influences on their physical and mental health
- Attention from professionals regarding factors that may result in illness or influence a man's expression of illness, including such things as occupational factors, leisure patterns, and interpersonal relationships
- Information about how their bodies function, what is normal, what is abnormal, what action to take, and the contributions of proper nutrition and exercise
- Self-care instruction, including testicular and genital self-examination

- Physical examination and history taking that include sexual and reproductive health and illness throughout the lifespan
- Treatment for problems of couples, including interpersonal problems, infertility, family planning, sexual concerns, and sexually transmitted diseases (STDs)
- Help with fathering (i.e., being included as a parent in child care)
- Help with fathering as a single parent, in particular with a child of the opposite sex, in addressing the child's sexual development and concerns
- Recognition that feelings of confusion and uncertainty in a time of rapid social change are normal and that they may mark the onset of healthy adaptation to change
- Adjustment of the health care system to men's occupational constraints regarding time and location of health care sources
- Financial ways to obtain these goals

Additional health care needs of men are for primary prevention and for secondary and tertiary prevention at the individual, family, and community levels to address the precursors of death that influence males so greatly. Men are less likely than women to be consumers in the health care system; therefore alternative approaches must be developed that address their health needs. The most significant approaches in the future will be those that reach men in the community, schools, the workplace, and public settings. These approaches call for political processes that set policy, for health marketing techniques, and for advocacy (Meryn, 2009).

COMMUNITY HEALTH NURSING SERVICES FOR MEN

A male can be seen by a community health nurse in a well-baby clinic, by a school nurse, by an occupational health nurse, and by a community health nurse or home health nurse on a home visit for follow-up of a chronic disease. However, men are less likely than women to be seen by a community health nurse. Not only is maternal and child health a major focus of many health departments, but neither a medical nor a nursing specialty within a health department routinely exists to specifically address men's health. Preventive reproductive health care (e.g., family planning, prenatal care, and cancer screening) and associated general screening are not routinely available for men. The community health nurse's commitment to health for all requires an increased awareness of men's health issues in their social and cultural context as well as individual and group actions that will improve men's physical, psychological, and social well-being.

Meeting men's health care needs can be viewed in a traditional public fashion. By viewing the problem from a primary, secondary, and tertiary intervention method, the nurse can look at the problem in a holistic manner. Factors that promote men's health are in the community, including interest groups in men and men's health, men's growing interest in physical fitness and lifestyle, policy related to men's health, and health services for men.

Gaining Skills Necessary to Address Men's Health Needs

Assessment skills necessary to carry out screening activities with men to detect reproductive health needs may be lacking in nursing education. One community health nurse who worked in a rural health department felt unqualified to respond to male partners' requests for genital examinations when couples came to seek family planning services. This community health nurse requested to work for specified periods with a urologist and in an STD clinic in a large urban area to gain the necessary skills. On return to the rural health department, she felt comfortable with male patients and taught the skills she had learned to nurse colleagues. Cheatham and colleagues (2008) suggest that providers make efforts to establish a positive patient–provider relationship using nonjudgmental verbal and nonverbal communication techniques. The nurse should engage the male and the female significant other in a manner that is easily understood.

Primary Preventive Measures
Health Education

Health care professionals, including the community health nurse, find that health education is the cornerstone of prevention. Although criticized by some as too narrow, health education can be a means of empowerment that helps individuals make behavioral changes. Education about male health issues should begin early. At school, boys should learn the anatomical and physiological aspects of their bodies and the social aspects of taking responsibility for their health. Coeducational discussion classes that cover a variety of social and personal topics can be a venue to encourage boys to talk about their bodies and their feelings. Adolescent males are shown to lack the use of language in comparison with their female counterparts. This may lead to a less self-conscious attitude to health seeking when boys reach adulthood.

Access to health education should follow males into the workplace. Many employers have experienced benefits such as lower health care costs when their employees receive health education programs coupled with health screening. Government and private insurance incentives given to employers who provide such programs would provide further impetus. Men who are not in the workplace can access health education in other areas, such as shopping malls, barbershops, and local senior centers. Some health care professionals are concerned about such informal dispersion of health literature, citing possible issues with the literacy level of the population. Government benefits programs can function as a medium for health education by including it in their benefit mailings. More control over the readability and the information included can be exerted over this material. Educational material should be written in the context of male interests and should focus on making healthy living relevant to the male (Cheatham et al., 2008).

Interest Groups for Men and Men's Health

The consumer movement that occurred on behalf of women's health in the 1960s and early 1970s has no counterpart for advocation of men's health. However, a viable men's consumer movement is forming. The National Organization for Men Against Sexism is interested in redefining the male role, particularly those aspects of it that are detrimental to health and growth. The American Assembly for Men in Nursing sponsors annual meetings that address issues such as men's health, men's work environments, research on men's health, and networking and support among male nurses. Researchers are beginning to define and study men's health beyond men's occupational role (e.g., reproductive health). Marketing has changed to include male health promotion public service announcements. Peer-reviewed journals such as *International Journal of Men's Health* and *American Journal of Men's Health* are providing scholars with avenues to disseminate men's health concerns.

Men's Growing Interest in Physical Fitness and Lifestyle

Although cardiovascular diseases (CVDs) are a major health hazard for men, research on the validity and usefulness of preventive and treatment modalities is an issue of considerable debate (Harvard Men's Health Watch, 2009). Men's interest in altering behavior that places them at risk for cardiovascular and other major diseases is increasing, especially among older males (Shapiro and Yarborough-Hayes, 2008). For example, men's smoking behavior has changed dramatically. In 1965, more than 50% of males smoked compared with 21% in 2010. Today, 52.1% of men report engaging in aerobic activity three times a week or more, compared with 42.7% of females (Schiller et al., 2012).

However, those health behaviors that have shown the greatest change in a positive direction have been those most influenced by legislative action (e.g., seat belt use, use of smoke detectors, and drunk driving). Even with these legislative actions, males remain three times less likely to use seat belts as females of the same age. In the Southeast, use of seat belts in pickup trucks was 25%, compared with more than 75% in other vehicles. The states of Alabama, Florida, Georgia, Kentucky, Mississippi, North Carolina, South Carolina, and Tennessee have engaged in a campaign called "Buckle Up in Your Truck." The campaign's centerpiece is the use of targeted television and radio advertisements to encourage seat belt use. Intensive enforcement mobilizations in the form of Selective Traffic Enforcement Programs, like Click It or Ticket, have followed periods of pickup truck advertisements. According to Tison and Williams (2010), the Click It or Ticket program has been an important factor in the improved usage of seat belts across the nation. On the basis of data from this report, seat belt use has increased by 20 percentage points from 1991 through 2007.

Policy Related to Men's Health

Policies related to any group of people should include the opinions and perceptions of those directly affected. Policy related to men's health should include the male perception of health. Community health nurses can encourage and help males be advocates for policies regarding their health care. Male nurses can be extremely instrumental in this endeavor. Liaisons between male consumers and policy planners should be formed.

Secondary Preventive Measures
Health Services for Men

Fewer health care clinics are tailored to men's special needs than to women's special needs. The "well-man clinics" set up in the 1980s were designed to identify lifestyle risk factors, not to provide screening clinics like the women's clinics. Once they are identified, a method or resolution for these lifestyle risk factors is formulated. Although many well-man clinics exist in the United Kingdom, male use of these clinics is far below female use of women's clinics (Roberts and Gerber, 2003). Although not based on the medical model, the Men's Shed movement in Australia has provided men with the socialization needed to make positive health behavior changes. Male screening methods typically have been limited to detecting high blood cholesterol levels and cancers such as prostate cancer, skin cancer, and testicular lumps. The era of managed care and health care reform may not encourage the concept of gender-specific care, as men and women receive primary care from the same health services.

Screening Services for Men

The U.S. Preventive Services Task Force (2004) outlines the kinds of screening tests the population should receive. According to the Task Force, healthy men younger than 50 years should have the following evaluation schedule:

- Dental examination: Yearly
- Eye examination: Every 3 to 5 years
- Blood pressure check: Every 2 years
- Blood cholesterol check for men aged 53 years and older: Yearly
- Prostate examination: Every year after age 50; blacks every year after age 40
- Colorectal screening: Every 3 to 5 years
- Tobacco use and cessation information: Every year
- One-time screening for abdominal aortic aneurysm for any man 65 years old who has smoked

Community health nurses should be familiar with these recommended screening test frequencies and should take every opportunity to encourage men to have these screenings. Through the institution of male health care fairs and other organized screenings, nurses are able to work with other health care providers to ensure that such routine screenings are performed.

Tertiary Preventive Measures
Sex-Role and Lifestyle Rehabilitation

Traditional health services for males are available in both private and governmental arenas. The emphasis of these services is on diagnosis and treatment. The traditional male role may change dramatically from treatment modalities. Rehabilitation services for males must include counseling on lifestyle, role changes, and job retraining. Men must be given permission to express their emotions, such as fear and anxiety, over the resultant change (Cheatham et al., 2008).

Goal setting and possible methods for achievement must be acceptable to the man. For example, after a heart attack, a man may be told to stop smoking and begin an exercise program. For the plan to be successful, the male must be an active partner in its formation. (He may be able to exercise, for example, by walking to the nearest automotive shop to talk with friends rather than spending time on a stationary bicycle at a local gym.)

BOX 18.6 Door Openers: Ways to Address Men about Health Concerns

Strategies to address men about health concerns include the following:

Ask a man to talk about the last time he had a physical examination, what was done, why it was done, where it was done, and what the recommendations were.

Ask a man how he feels about his health insurance coverage. If he lacks health insurance, ask about the resources he used to obtain medical care for himself and for his family.

Ask a man about how he spends his leisure time, what he is doing to take care of himself, and what his usual physical activities are.

Observe a man for signs of stress such as moist palms, nail biting, posture (e.g., stooped with lack of eye contact), and nervous movements. If signs of stress are present, ask how he is coping with an identified health problem, family problem, or being unemployed.

Observe a man for difficulty clearing the airway (e.g., from smoking) and flushing of the face (e.g., from alcohol). Inquire as to habits of smoking and drinking and whether these habits have increased since the occurrence of the particular health or social problem.

Involve the man in decision making about health care to instill a sense of control over events.

Time taken away from work because of occupational injuries should be kept to a minimum. Males should be encouraged to return to work in an altered capacity rather than remaining away from work until injuries are completely healed. Occupational accommodation for the treatment regimen will help ensure compliance. Provision of medical care, supportive physical and occupational therapies, and "light-duty" jobs at the worksite help preserve the masculine persona. Box 18.6 lists some ways to address men about their health.

? ACTIVE LEARNING

1. Select a family that has a man in the household who is accessible. Select two "door openers" appropriate to initiate discussion of health concerns with this man. Devise a gender-appropriate nursing care plan that includes primary, secondary, and tertiary prevention for this man as an individual, for his family, and for his community.

2. Select a family that has a man in the household who is not readily accessible. Interview the female caregiver in the household and obtain information by proxy about the man's health. If possible, arrange to meet the man for lunch, at work, or after work and obtain information about his health. Compare the information obtained by proxy with that obtained from the client.

NEW CONCEPTS OF COMMUNITY CARE

Specific services for men within health departments continue to be lacking in the United States. With the exception of STD clinics and selected family planning service models, male health concerns remain unaddressed. Two male health visitors (the British term for public health nurses) from the National Health Service (NHS) started an innovative public health nursing program directed at men in Glasgow, Scotland. Health visitors Bill Deans and Bob Hoskins established a nurse-run well-man clinic with the help of the NHS and the Scottish Council for Health Education. During home visits with mothers and infants, Deans and Hoskins observed that fathers excused themselves and went to the local pub when they arrived.

Any intervention regarding men's health needs must include men as willing participants (Lynch, 2008). Noting the characteristics of the male population in their community (e.g., overweight, heavy smoking, drinking, and high unemployment), Deans and Hoskins decided to modify their practice to serve their clients' needs. One afternoon per week, the clinic, which is based on a nursing model rather than a medical model, offers health screening, health education, and primary prevention to men. Marketing is important, and men are referred from general practitioners' and specialists' practices and recruited through newspaper advertisements. Clients with clinical signs and symptoms are referred back to their physicians. Lifestyle counseling and education are offered in areas such as fat and fiber content in diet, smoking, alcohol use, and exercise.

Deans and Hoskins consider the clinic a way to extend the health visitor's role in the NHS's efforts in health education with an aim to "nip potential diseases in the bud." Deans and Hoskins are concerned that the NHS does not provide male services and are clear that "the unemployed chain-smoking husband needs as much care and health education from the health visitor as do his wife and baby" (Sadler, 1979, p. 18). The well-man clinic and well-woman clinic models can now be found in several communities throughout Great Britain and have been expanded to serve inmates in prison (Ballinger et al., 2009; Woodland and Hunt, 1994). After 10 years in existence, the well-man clinics in Great Britain are only sporadically used by males. Even when the services were expanded to the home, nurses found that men were purposely absent at the appointment time. Usage was highest with informal evening clinics directed by male nurses (Roberts and Gerber, 2003). An attempt to evaluate these nationally funded clinics was undertaken in 2003. It was suggested from the data that a collaborative approach to these interventions is a slow process and that adequate time should be provided before the evaluation (Reid et al., 2009).

In Australia, Men's Shed is a community-based health promotion initiative in men's health. Based on the social rather than medical model, the sheds promote well-being among older males by providing them with accepted and respected activities as well as a male-friendly space for socialization. Ballinger and colleagues (2009) found that participants in these activities reported an increase in recognition of the importance of health determinants and a sense of well-being.

Public health nurses working in the Benton County Health Department in Corvallis, Oregon, responded to the challenge of teen pregnancy in the 1970s by launching a community-wide effort that included developing a men's health clinic and marketing reproductive health services directly to teenage boys and men. An early effort established an advisory committee that included people from churches, schools, and health care facilities. A public health nurse health educator launched an extensive education program in the high school, which focused on decision-making processes and services available in the community. Later efforts involved the establishment of a clinic for men. Teenage boys were members of a consumer advisory committee established by the nurses that recommended the wording and format for advertisements about the clinic that ran in the high school newspaper. The advisory committee also recommended a flyer format that would be attractive to males. Specifically, they requested a card with information about the clinic and how to use condoms that would discreetly fit into their wallets and be available to share with peers.

The nurses have expanded their focus to create inclusive service environments in which teenage girls and boys and adult men and women will feel accepted and comfortable. Particular attention is given to the clinic decor and advertising, reading materials, and posters to transmit a message that includes offering health care for males and females. Clinic staff will see males or females at any time; however, a room in which staff members see men has decor geared toward men (e.g., no gynecological stirrups on the examining table) and pamphlets available for men on topics such as testicular cancer and chewing tobacco. Integrated services exist in the areas of family planning, STDs, and HIV counseling and testing.

CASE STUDY   Application of the Nursing Process

Gender-Appropriate Care for Men

Community health nurses are in an ideal position to address the health needs of men at individual, family, and community levels. The community health nurse may promote self-care in male members of the family, facilitate men's health by addressing needed changes at the family level, buttress women's roles as caregivers of the family's health, and bring about change that influences policies that affect men at the community level.

Planning gender-appropriate care for males is outlined in the following case study, which is an application of the nursing process at the individual, family, and aggregate levels initiated in a home visit, and applies the previous discussions about the levels of prevention, roles of the community health nurse, research, and men's health.

Application of the nursing process to aggregates is facilitated by the use of systems theory, in which the nurse identifies the system and subsystems involved. The nurse may use a deductive or an inductive approach. A deductive approach would involve carrying out a community assessment and identifying an area or areas, such as a program needed by the community. Planning,

implementation, and evaluation of the program would be carried out at the family or group level. An inductive approach would involve entering the community system through a person or client via a referral about a problem or concern. Assessment of the individual would be followed by identification of those groups to which the client belongs, such as family and community, and assessment of those groups.

Beth Lockwood, a community health nursing student at a health department, received a referral from the high school nurse to visit the Connors family to assess Richard Connors' mental health status. Richard was a 16-year-old sophomore whose academic work in school had declined rapidly after the premature death of his 46-year-old father. The father had died of a myocardial infarction, which he had while cleaning the garage with Richard one evening after school. Richard and the neighbors failed to revive Mr. Connors, and Richard carries feelings of guilt. Household members include Mrs. Connors, age 44 years, and Richard's sister Yvonne, age 12 years.

CASE STUDY Application of the Nursing Process—cont'd

Gender-Appropriate Care for Men

Assessment

The referral to assess the Connors family called for an inductive approach to assessment. Beth used a deductive approach later, when her experience with the Connors family piqued her concern about the status of men's health in her community. Beth assessed Richard, his mother, and his sister as household members of the family. However, she could not stop with the immediate family; she had to continue to identify the other groups within the community to which each individual family member belonged. Viewing the community as a system and focusing on systems and subsystems helped Beth organize the data she collected during assessment. Knowing that "the whole is greater than the sum of its parts," Beth prepared for her visit by reviewing adolescent theories of development and family theory. Beyond individual assessment, she noted factors related to the development of sex role–related behavior that may influence health. Examples of assessment areas include the following:

Family Configuration, Traditional or Nontraditional

- Sex role–related behavior of parents, including work patterns in and out of the home, division of household labor, and decision-making patterns
- Patterns of parenting: mothering, fathering, and substitute father figure(s)
- Ability of male children to disclose feelings to family members and others
- Degree of assertiveness in female children
- Ability of family members to give emotional and physical support during crises and noncrises
- Ability of family members to trade off role-related behavior during crises and noncrises
- Risk-taking health behaviors
- Processing of stress and grief
- Communal lifestyle patterns that place the individual or family at risk (e.g., lack of exercise, poor diet, smoking, and drinking)
- Family history of death and illness
- Health care–taking patterns of family members
- Preventive health behaviors
- Leisure activities

Assessment of other groups includes neighborhood and other peer groups, school environments, sports, and church and civic activities.

Diagnosis

Through induction, the nurse makes a diagnosis for each individual and each system component, including family and the community. The following are examples of diagnoses.

Individual

- Loss of interest or involvement in an activity related to conflicting stages of grief process secondary to premature death of father (Richard)
- Expressed dissatisfaction with parenting role related to feelings of helplessness and sadness secondary to premature death of husband (Mrs. Connors)
- Risk of interpersonal conflict resulting from prolonged, unrelieved family stress secondary to premature death of father (Yvonne)

Family

- Decreased ability to communicate related to family stress secondary to premature death of father
- Risk of family crisis related to disequilibrium

Community

- Inadequate systematic programs for linking families in crisis to community resources
- Inadequate systematic programs for populations at risk of premature death related to inadequate planning among community systems

Planning

Planning involves contracting and mutual goal setting and is an outcome of mutually derived assessment and diagnosis. A contract with the family alone is shortsighted and may provide little community benefit over time. The following are examples of other aggregates with which a contract may be established:

- The school subsystem that does not provide ongoing counseling but will meet periodically with family members to evaluate pupil progression
- The school subsystem that provides physical education in football, basketball, and baseball (i.e., nonaerobic, nonlifetime sports) but offers extramural aerobic, lifetime sports such as swimming, tennis, golf, and track after school hours
- The American Red Cross, which does not offer cardiovascular pulmonary resuscitation (CPR) courses on evenings or weekends but offers to consider doing so for a defined minimum-size community

Mutual goal setting requires collaboration regarding long- and short-term goals. Again, mutually defined needs and diagnoses are important to this process. Regardless of the diagnosis, each individual in the family and the subsystem must participate in development of a care plan. The following are examples of goals.

Individual
Long-Term Goal
- Individual family members will be able to trade off role-related behavior.

Short-Term Goal
- Individual family members will express feelings related to abandonment and loss.

Family
Long-Term Goal
- The family will exhibit an increased ability to handle crisis, as evidenced by ability to discuss roles and interdependencies.

Short-Term Goal
- The family will identify specific ways to recognize and use support services.

Community
Long-Term Goal
- Systematic programs, with ongoing program evaluation, will be established for populations at risk of premature death from coronary heart disease, as evidenced by local planning bodies.

Short-Term Goals
- Information is disseminated to individuals, families, groups, and planning bodies in the community about the incidence of coronary heart disease.
- Existing programs are identified that address coronary heart disease.
- Existing programs are coordinated to bridge gaps and avoid duplication of effort.

Intervention

The nurse, family, and other aggregates carry out interventions contracted during the planning phase to meet the mutually derived goals. Most important, the nurse empowers the family and community to develop the networks and linkages necessary to care for themselves.

Individual

Individual counseling regarding loss and grief may be beneficial to each family member, but options may need to be explored and referrals may need to be reevaluated for members of the rural family. Education regarding preventive measures that combat risk factors for heart disease include those aimed at individual family members and those that address areas such as diet, exercise, smoking, alcohol use, and stress management.

continued

Gender-Appropriate Care for Men

Family

Examples of interventions with the family include counseling, education, and referral aimed at family self-care promotion. For example, Beth's interventions with the Connors family depended on the family's ability to solve problems, investigate community resources, and create linkages between the family and resources. Periodic family conferences at school and more inclusive family therapy may enable the family to work through the death of Mr. Connors; this process results in the development of new roles and the communication necessary to maintain family equilibrium. Education regarding preventive measures to combat risk factors for heart disease may need discussion at the family and individual levels (e.g., diet, exercise, smoking, alcohol use, and stress management).

Community

The nurse must also carry out interventions with other aggregates. These may involve activities such as educating, facilitating program expansion, and tailoring programs to meet community needs. Intervention at the aggregate level calls for group and community work. The nurse carries out interventions at this level in several ways (e.g., by communicating community statistics from a community analysis, relating anecdotes from families served, or linking family experience to program needs by acting as an advocate and bringing family members to board meetings or hearings on community health issues).

Education regarding preventive measures to combat risk factors for heart disease also includes those interventions aimed at the community. A rationale for the development of lifetime aerobic sports is needed not only by Richard but also by school districts. Exploration of options with the school nurse and review of the school district health education curriculum would be beneficial. A community assessment of heart disease awareness, including determination of the availability of resources such as emergency response and CPR courses, is an aggregate intervention. Taking the outcome of the assessment in the form of statistics and the anonymous anecdotal story of the Connors family to planning bodies in the community is also intervention at the aggregate level. Creative programs other communities used (e.g., teaching CPR within the school system) should be investigated and proposed.

Evaluation

Evaluation is multidimensional and ongoing. Using a systems approach to evaluation, the nurse evaluates each component of the system, from individual family member to family and community, in terms of goal achievement. Evaluation consists of noting degrees of equilibrium established, extent of change, how the system handles change, whether the system is open or closed, and patterns of networking. Ongoing evaluation includes noting referrals and follow-up of the individual, the family, and other aggregates in resource use.

Individual

Use of resources such as support groups by the individual family member may be noted. These resources may include a teen support group, a women's support group, support groups for those experiencing the loss of a spouse or other family member, reentry programs for women at a local junior college or university, and Parents Without Partners.

Family

Evaluation of the Connors family would include follow-up of their use of support services specifically for the family, such as counseling options for the family as a unit. Evaluation would also focus on the family's ability to handle crises in the future.

Community

Aggregate evaluation would focus on the community. For example, to what extent do school programs encourage sports options that promote lifetime aerobic activities and prevent premature death from heart disease? Are programs systematically planned in the community for populations that are at risk of premature death from heart disease?

Levels of Prevention

Society's expectations of men and women are in transition. Application of levels of prevention by the community health nurse must take into account men's health status, men's socialization, men's use of health care services, men's primary needs for prevention and health promotion, and the role of women as caregivers in family health.

Primary

Men are more likely to engage in risk-taking behavior than women and are less likely to engage in preventive behaviors; therefore primary prevention must be marketed specifically to men. Examples of primary prevention for the Connors family are applied at the following individual, family, and community levels.

Individual

- Assessment, teaching, and referral related to diet and exercise behaviors

Family

- Assessment and teaching related to food selection and preparation at home and food selection at fast-food restaurants
- Teaching and role-modeling gender roles that allow male members of the family to use alternative expressions of emotion

Community

- Provision of CPR courses for members of the community; consultation with schools regarding need for aerobic activities in physical education and sports programs
- The nurse must pull men from the family, workplace, or other aggregates into involvement with family planning, education, antepartum and postpartum care, parenting, dental prophylaxis, and accident prevention. In addition, assessment of need for immunizations and classes (e.g., retirement preparation) is considered action aimed at primary prevention.

Secondary

Men have higher mortality, morbidity, and health care use rates for many of the leading causes of death, but they are second to women in overall use of health care services, including preventive physical examinations and screening; therefore early diagnosis and prompt intervention must also meet men's needs. Examples of secondary prevention regarding the Connors family include the following:

Individual

- Screen for risk factors related to CVD in the individual, such as how the individual handles stress.

Family

- Screen for risk factors related to CVD in the family, such as how the family processes stress.

Community

- Organize screening programs for the community, such as health fairs.
- The nurse must screen individuals and aggregates of men according to lifestyle risk factors, mortality rates at different age levels, morbidity rates, and occupational health risks.

Gender-Appropriate Care for Men

Tertiary

Activities that rehabilitate individuals and aggregates and restore them to their highest level of functioning are aimed at tertiary prevention. The nurse in the community is ideally situated to locate people in need of rehabilitation services. The nurse may provide evaluation and physical, mental, and social restoration services. Men in need of rehabilitation may have special needs because their disabilities influence them, their families, and ultimately their communities. Financial assistance and vocational counseling, training, and placement may be priorities for the well-being of the family. Socialization causes men to have difficulty admitting they need help. Community health nurses who teach men with chronic disease to rest at specified periods during the day or to continue with medical regimens or speech or occupational therapy are providing tertiary prevention. Working with couples as a unit is also important because caregiving patterns may shift as a result of chronic disease and disability. Encouraging

men to express their concerns about their health, families, and jobs and their frustration with themselves is important. The following are examples of tertiary prevention with the Connors family.

Individual

- Assist individual family members in dealing with grief from the loss of the father and husband.

Family

- Assist family in dealing with grief and assuming alternative roles.

Community

- Assist the community in dealing with loss of a fully functioning family by providing grief support services that include males or target males and females.

SUMMARY

As the information within this chapter shows, there is gender disparity in all areas of disease and all health entities. Health initiatives and programs are changing as more and more attention is given to the health care of men.

EVOLVE WEBSITE

http://evolve.elsevier.com/Nies/community

- NCLEX Review Questions
- Case Studies

BIBLIOGRAPHY

Arias E: *United States life tables*, 2008, (National Vital Statistics Reports vol. 61, no. 3) Washington, DC, National Center for Health Statistics. http://www.cdc.gov/nchs/fastats/lifexpec.htm.

Baerolcher MO, Verma S: *Men's health research: under researched and under appreciated. Medial Science Monitor* 14(Part 3), 2008.

Ballinger M, Talbot L, Verrinder G: More than a place to do woodwork: a case study of a community-based Men's Shed, *J Men's Health* 6(1):20–27, 2009.

Brown L, Bond M: An examination of influences on health protective behaviors among Australian men, *Int J Men's Health* 3(7):274–287, 2008.

Centers for Disease Control and Prevention: *Men's health: leading causes of death in males United States*, 2009. Available from <http://www.cdc.gov/men/lcod/>.

Centers for Disease Control and Prevention: *Sexually transmitted disease surveillance 2015*, Atlanta, 2012, U.S. Department of health and Human Services.

Cheatham C, Barksdale D, Rodgers S: Barriers to health care and health seeking behaviors faced by black men, *J Am Acad Nurse Pract* 20:555–562, 2008.

Frisbee S, Chambers C, Frisbee J: Associations between dental hygiene, cardiovascular disease risk factors and systemic inflammation in rural adults, *J Dental Hygiene* 84(4):177–184, 2010.

Haines C, Wender R: Men's health, *Prim Care* 33(1):xiii–xv, 2006.

Harvard Men's Health Watch, Volume 13:8, 2009.

Heron M, Hoyert DL, Murphy SL, et al.: *Deaths: final data for 2006*. (National Vital Statistics Reports vol. 57, no. 14) National Center for Vital Statistics: Washington, DC. https://www.ncbi.nlm.nih.gov/pubmed/19788058.

Kirby R, Kirby M, Aoroso P: Steps by which better overall health for men could be achieved, *BJU Int* 98(2):285–288, 2006. Also available from <www.bjui.org/ContentFullItem.aspx?id=81&SectionType=5>.

Lynch L: Men's Health, *Ir Med J* 101(1):5–6, 2008.

Martin JA, Hamilton BE, Sutton PD, et al.: *Births: final data for 2008* (National Vital Statistics Reports vol. 59 no. 1). National Center for Health Statistics: Hyattsville, MD.

Mathews TJ, MacDorman MF: *Infant mortality statistics from the 2008 period linked birth/infant death data set* (National Vital Statistics Reports vol. 60, no. 5). National Center for Health Statistics: Hyattsville, MD.

Meryn S: Global man and health, *J Men's Health* 6(1):2–3, 2009.

Naslindh-Ylispangar A, Sihvonen M, Kekki P: Health, utilization of health services, "core" information and reasons for non-participation: a triangulation study among non-respondents, *J Clin Nurs* 17:2972–2978, 2008.

National Center for Health Statistics: *Health, United States, 2015: with special feature on racial and ethnic health disparities*, Hyattsville, MD, 2016, Author.

National Institute for Occupational Safety and Health: *NIOSH workers health chartbook (NIOSH publ 2004–146)*, 2004. Available from <www.chc.gov/niosh/doc./chartbook>.

Organisation for Economic Co-operation and Development [OECD]: *Health at a glance*, 2011. Available from <http://www.oecd.org/health/health-systems/healthataglance2011.htm>.

Porche D: Men's health: building the science, *Am J Men's Health* 3(2):92, 2009.

Reid G, van Teijlingen E, Douglas F, et al.: The reality of partnership working when undertaking an evaluation of national well men's service, *J Men's Health* 1(6):36–49, 2009.

Roberts A, Gerber L: *Nursing perspective on public health programming in Nunavut, Iqaluit.* Department of Health and Social Services: Nunavut, Canada. <www.gov.nu.ca/health/Report%20on%20Nursing% 20Perspectives%20on%20Public%20Heatlh%20Programming%20in% 20Nunavut.pdf>.

Sadler C: DIY male maintenance, *Nurs Mirror* 160:16, 1979.

Schiller JS, Lucas JW, Ward BW, et al.: Summary health statistics for U.S. adults: National Health Interview Survey, 2010, *Vital Health Stat* 10(252):1–217, 2012.

Shapiro A, Yarborough-Hayes R: Retirement and older men's health, generations, *J Am Society on Aging* 32(1):49–53, 2008.

Skelton R: Man's role in society and its effect on health, *Nursing* 26:953, 1988.

Sommers B, Wilson L: *Fifty-four million additional Americans are receiving preventive services coverage without cost-sharing under the Affordable Care Act.* Available from: <http://aspe.hhs.gov/ health/reports/2012/PreventiveServices/ib.shtml>.

Tanne JH: Medicine's new motto: one sex does not fit all, *Am Health Women* 16(5):54–58, 1997.

Tison J, Williams A: *Analyzing the first years of the ticket or click it mobilizations (DOT HS 811 232),* 2010. Available from <www.nhtsa. gov/staticfiles/nti/pdf/811232.pdf>.

U.S. Preventive Services Task Force: *Men: stay healthy at 50+. Checklists for your health.* Available from: <http://www.ahrq. gov/patients-consumers/patient-involvement/healthy-men/men-over-50.html>.

Verbrugge LM, Wingard DL: Sex differentials in health and mortality, *Women's Health* 12:103, 1987.

Waldron I: Changing gender roles and gender differences in health behavior. In: Gochman DS, editor: *Handbook of health behavior research.* Plenum: New York, 1995a.

Waldron I: Contributions of changing gender differences in behavior and social roles to changing gender differences in mortality. In: Sabo D, Gordon DF, editors: *Men's health and illness: gender, power and the body.* Sage: Thousand Oaks, CA, 1995b.

Waldron I: Contributions of biological and behavioral factors in changing sex differences in ischaemic heart disease mortality. In: Lopez A, Caselli G, Valkonen T, editors: *Adult mortality in developed countries: from description to explanation.* Oxford University Press: New York, 1995c.

Waldron I: Factors determining the sex ratio at birth. In: *Sex differentials in infant and child mortality.* United Nations: New York, 1995d.

Whorton MD: Environmental and occupational reproductive hazards. In: Swanson J, Forrest K, editors: *Men's reproductive health.* Springer: New York.

Woodland A, Hunt C: Healthy convictions … well-man clinic for the inmates of Lindholme prison, *Nurs Times* 90:32, 1994.

Senior Health

*Mary Ellen Trail Ross**

OBJECTIVES

Upon completion of this chapter, the reader will be able to do the following:

1. Discuss the aging process.
2. Discuss the demographic characteristics of the elderly population.
3. Describe psychosocial issues related to aging.
4. Describe physiological changes due to aging.
5. Recognize *Healthy People 2020* wellness goals and objectives for older adults.
6. Describe health/illness concerns common to the elderly population.
7. Identify nursing actions that address the needs of older adults.
8. Identify resources available to older adults.

KEY TERMS

activities of daily living (ADLs)
advance directives
aging
alternative housing options
Alzheimer disease

anxiety disorder
cataract
crime
depression
do-not-resuscitate (DNR)

durable power of attorney for health care
elder abuse
falls
generalized anxiety disorder
glaucoma

*The author would like to acknowledge the contribution of Edith B. Summerlin, who co-wrote this chapter for the previous edition.

guardianship
instrumental activities of daily living
 (IADLs)
living will

macular degeneration
Medicaid
physician orders for life sustaining
 treatment (POLST)

Medicare
Social Security
suicide
traumatic brain injury (TBI)

In America, the number of individuals aged 65 years or older grew from 3 million in 1900 to 46 million in 2014 (Federal Interagency Forum on Aging-Related Statistics [FIFARS], 2016). Life expectancy is increasing; thus larger numbers of people are reaching 65 years and beyond. In view of the increasing number of seniors who potentially will remain living in the community, the role of the nurse becomes very important in helping these seniors continue to live independently and to increase their years of healthy life. For nurses to assist older adults, they must be familiar with the characteristics of seniors, their socioeconomic situations, their health behaviors, health status, health risks, and available community resources. This chapter discusses these issues and gives suggestions as to how nurses might address them.

CONCEPT OF AGING

Aging is a natural process that affects all living organisms. The concept of aging is most often defined chronologically. *Chronological age* refers to the number of years a person has lived. In the United States, an older adult is generally defined as one who is 65 years or older. However, it is important to remember that older adults cannot be grouped collectively as just one segment of the population. The older adult population is a heterogeneous group. The young-old (aged 65 to 74 years), the middle-old (aged 75 to 84 years), the old-old (aged 85 to 99 years), and the elite-old (more than 100 years old) are four distinct cohort groups (Touhy and Jett, 2012).

Functional age, on the other hand, refers to functioning and the ability to perform activities of daily living (ADLs), such as bathing and grooming, and instrumental activities of daily living (IADLs), such as cooking, shopping, and managing finances. This definition of aging is a better measure of age than chronological age. After all, most older adults are more concerned with their functional ability than their chronological age. Helping older adults remain independent and functional is a major focus of nursing care.

THEORIES OF AGING

Since early times, scientists have attempted to explain why humans age. There are many biological and psychosocial theories of aging. Biological theories answer questions such as "How do cells age?" and "What triggers the actual aging process?" (Miller, 2015). The biological theories can be subdivided into two main divisions: stochastic and nonstochastic. Stochastic theories explain aging as events that occur randomly and accumulate over time, whereas nonstochastic theories view aging as predetermined. Some of the popular biological theories are summarized in Box 19.1.

BOX 19.1   Biological Theories of Aging

Stochastic Theories
Error Theory
The error theory proposes that an accumulation of errors in protein synthesis occurs over time, resulting in impairment of cellular function. Defective cells are produced, which eventually interfere with biological function (Orgel, 1963).

Somatic Mutation Theory
Similar to the error theory, somatic mutation theory also suggests that when cells are exposed to x-ray irradiation or chemicals, alteration of DNA occurs, increasing the incidence of chromosomal abnormalities and decreasing cellular and organ function. The deleterious effects appear in later life (Morley, 1995).

Free Radical Theory
Free radicals are highly reactive molecules that possess an extra electric charge (free electron) that can damage protein membranes, enzymes, and DNA. The body produces antioxidants that scavenge the free radicals (Hayflick, 1996).

Cross-Linkage Theory
The cross-linkage theory posits that aging causes body chemicals (proteins, lipids, nucleic acid, and carbohydrates) to become cross-linked. The cross-linking causes abnormal metabolic activity and waste products to accumulate in the cells. The result is poor functioning of body tissues and structures (Hayflick, 1996).

Wear-and-Tear Theory
Cells and organs wear out after years of use. Proponents of the wear-and-tear theory view the human body as similar to a machine that eventually wears out because of decline in cellular function, death of cells, and mechanical injury and use (Hayflick, 1996).

Nonstochastic Theories
Programmed Theory
The programmed theory postulates that normal cells divide a specific number of times. The number of cell divisions is proportional to the lifespan of the species. Human cells double 40 to 60 times before the ability to replicate is lost and cellular death occurs (Hayflick, 1996).

Immunological Theory
According to immunological theory, alteration of the B and T cells causes a loss of a self-regulatory pattern between the body and the cells. Autoaggression occurs when cells normal to the body are misidentified as alien and are attacked by the body's immune system (Miller, 1996).

Neuroendocrine Control or Pacemaker Theory
Aging is described in neuroendocrine control theory or pacemaker theory as a programmed decline in the functioning of the nervous, endocrine, and immune systems. Cells lose their ability to reproduce, a process known as *replicative senescence* (De la Fuente, 2008).

The three classic psychosocial theories of aging are behavioristic and examine how humans experience late life. The disengagement theory, proposed by Cumming and Henry (1961), asserts that aging is inevitable, with mutual withdrawal or disengagement from society and decreased interaction between the aging person and others.

The activity theory posits that remaining active and involved is necessary to maintain life satisfaction (Havighurst et al, 1963). The continuity theory suggests that a person continues through life in a similar fashion as in previous years (Havighurst et al, 1968).

Concepts gleaned from the various theories are useful to nurses as they care for older adults. For example, knowledge that the immune system is affected by aging implies the need for nurses to be vigilant about preventing infections. Psychosocial theories of aging point out the uniqueness of older individuals as they age and make life adjustments. Knowledge of these theories may help nurses dispel common myths of aging.

DEMOGRAPHIC CHARACTERISTICS

Population

Americans are living longer than ever before, and it is expected that the older population will continue to grow. Currently, people who survive to age 65 years can expect to live an average of 19.3 more years. In 2014, the life expectancy of people who survive to age 85 years is 7 more years for women and 5.9 more years for men. Life expectancy varies by race, but the difference decreases with age. In 1900, people aged 65 years and older made up 4% of the population. In 2014, 46 million people aged 65 years and over lived in the United States, accounting for 15% of the total population. The oldest-old population (those 85 years and older) grew from just over 100,000 in 1900 to 6 million in 2014 (FIFARS, 2016). Lastly, in 2010, there were 53,364 centenarians in the United States (U.S. Census Bureau, 2012).

The baby boomers (individuals born between 1946 and 1964) started turning 65 years old in 2011, and the number of older adults will increase dramatically. By 2030, the number of Americans aged 65 years and older is expected to be more than twice as large as that of their counterparts in 2000, growing from 35 million to 74 million, and will represent nearly 21% of the total U.S. population. The greatest growth will occur in the population aged 85 years and older, whose numbers are projected to grow from 6 million in 2014 to nearly 20 million by 2060 (FIFARS, 2016).

Racial and Ethnic Composition

In addition to growing larger, the older population is becoming more diverse, as is the rest of the population in general. In 2014, non-Hispanic whites accounted for 78% of the U.S. older population. Blacks made up 9%, Asians made up 4%, and Hispanics (of any race) accounted for 8%. The older population will grow among all racial and ethnic groups; however, the older Hispanic population is projected to grow the fastest (FIFARS, 2016).

Geographic Location

The proportion of the population aged 65 years and over varies by state. In 2014, Florida had the highest proportion of people aged 65 years and over (19%). Maine, West Virginia, Vermont, Montana, Pennsylvania, Delaware, Hawaii, and Oregon also had high proportions, each more than 16% (FIFARS, 2016). More than half (54%) of persons 65 years or older lived in 10 states: California, Florida, Texas, New York, Pennsylvania, Ohio, Illinois, Michigan, North Carolina, and New Jersey (Administration on Aging, 2016).

Gender

Older women outnumber older men in the United States. In 2014, women accounted for 56% of the population 65 years and older and 66% of the population 85 years and older (FIFARS, 2016).

Marital Status

Older men are more likely than older women to be married. In 2015, about 74% of men aged 65 to 74 years were married, compared with 58% of women in the same age group. The proportion married was lower at older ages: 42% of women ages 75 to 84 and 17% of women 85 years and older were married in 2015. Widowhood is more common among older women than older men. Women aged 65 years and over were more likely than men of the same age to be widowed: 34% compared with 12%. Nearly 73% of women aged 85 years and over were widowed, compared with 34% of men. Relatively small proportions of older men (11%) and women (13%) were divorced in 2015, and a small proportion (5%) of the older population has never married (FIFARS, 2016).

Education

Educational attainment has increased among older adults. In 2015, 84% of older adults were high school graduates (compared with 24% in 1965). Eighty-nine percent of non-Hispanic whites age 65 and over had completed high school. The percentages of older Asians and blacks who had completed high school (74% and 75%, respectively) were not statistically different. In contrast, 54% of older Hispanics have completed high school. In 2015, 27% of older adults had a bachelor's degree or higher (compared with 5% in 1965). Older Asians had the highest proportion with a bachelor's degree or higher, at 34%, compared with 29% for non-Hispanic whites, 17% for blacks, and 12% for Hispanics. Older men had attained a bachelor's degree more often than older women (32% compared with 23%) (FIFARS, 2016).

Living Arrangements

As age increases and widowhood rates rise, the percentage of the population living alone increases accordingly. In 2015, 70% of older men lived with their spouse, whereas less than half (45%) of older women did. In contrast, older women were more likely than older men to live alone (36% vs. 20%). Older Hispanic (34%), black (30%), and Asian (26%) women were more likely than non-Hispanic white women (12%) to live with relatives other than a spouse. Older non-Hispanic white and black women were more likely than women of other races to live alone (37% of white and 43% of black women lived alone compared with 20% for Asian and 23% for Hispanic women). The percentage of older black men (30%) living alone was three times as high as the percentage of older Asian men (10%). Older Hispanic and black men were more likely (13% and 14%, respectively) than non-Hispanic white men (4%) to live with relatives other than a spouse (FIFARS, 2016).

Housing and Residential Services

Older adults typically prefer to "age in place," or live in their own homes for as long as possible. In 2013, 93% of the Medicare population aged 65 years and older resided in traditional community settings. Three percent of the Medicare population aged 65 years and over resided in community housing with at least one service available, such as meal preparation, housekeeping, laundry, and assistance with medication. Approximately 4% resided in long-term care facilities. The percentage of people residing in community housing with services and in long-term care facilities was higher for the older age groups. For example, among adults 85 years and older, 77% resided in traditional housing, whereas 8% resided in community housing with services and 15% resided in long-term care facilities (FIFARS, 2016). It is important to make services needed for independent living, such as meal preparation, medication assistance, and housekeeping, accessible to older adults who prefer this type of living arrangement.

Alternative Housing Options for Older Adults

The significant majority (93%) of adults aged 65 years and older reside in the traditional, single-family home; however, some choose to downsize to smaller housing, such as townhouses or condominiums, where maintenance needs are eliminated or minimized. The types of alternative housing options included retirement communities or apartments, continuing care retirement facilities, assisted-living facilities, and board and care homes. Services at these facilities include meal preparation, housekeeping, laundry, and medication administration. Approximately 4% of older adults reside in long-term care facilities that provide personal and/or skilled care 24 hours a day, 7 days a week. The percentage of people residing in community housing with services and in long-term care facilities is higher for individuals 85 years and older. These older adults generally have more functional limitations (FIFARS, 2016). It is important to note that many older adults who would like to change their current living arrangements find that organized senior housing is too expensive for middle-class and lower-middle-class citizens. On the other hand, these individuals often have too many assets to qualify for subsidized housing.

Although not considered a housing option, adult day care provides a safe and supportive environment during the day for adults who cannot or choose not to stay alone. This service is often needed for caregivers who work during regular hours or need respite. Socialization, recreational activities, medication supervision, and meals are provided on-site. Often transportation to and from the facility is provided.

Sources of Income

In 2014, the median household income of older adults was $36,895. Aggregate income for the population aged 65 years and over came largely from four sources: Social Security, earnings, pensions, and asset income. Social Security accounted for 49% of per capita family income. Among older Americans in the lowest fifth of the income distribution, Social Security accounted for 67% and earnings accounted for 13% of per capita family income, and public assistance accounted for 8%. For those in the highest fifth of the income distribution, Social Security accounted for 18% of per capita family income, pension income accounted for 26%, and earnings accounted for 40% (FIFARS, 2016).

With aging, a good percentage of income is spent on health care. Most older adults have Medicare, which provides health insurance for those who are 65 years or older, are disabled, or have end-stage renal disease. Medicare is funded, in part, by Social Security contributions from employers, employees, and the self-employed. Medicare Part A is a hospital insurance plan that covers acute care, short-term rehabilitative care, and some costs associated with hospice and home health care. For 2017, the Part A deductible for acute care was $1316 for the first 60 days of a hospital stay per benefit period. This amount increases for longer hospital stays. Medicare Part A will pay 100% of the first 20 days of a nursing home stay, with a $164.50 daily copay for days 21 to 100 of each benefit period and no coverage after that (U.S. Department of Health and Human Services [USDHHS]/Centers for Medicare and Medicaid Services [CMS], 2017).

Medicare Part B covers the costs for physician and nurse practitioner services; outpatient services, such as diagnostic procedures (e.g., laboratory and x-ray); qualified physical, speech, and occupational therapy; ambulance services; durable medical equipment; and some home health care services. Charges are paid by Medicare at a rate of 80% of what Medicare considers an "allowable charge." The client is responsible for the remaining 20% of the charge. In addition, the client is responsible for an annual Part B deductible ($183.00 in 2017) and a monthly premium of at least $134.00 (higher-income individuals pay more). This amount is generally deducted directly from the monthly Social Security check. Most Medicare enrollees have a supplemental insurance (Medigap) policy to pay for services not covered by Medicare. A Medicare Advantage Plan (sometimes called *Part C*) is another Medicare health plan choice. This plan is offered by private companies approved by Medicare. In addition to the Part B premium, there is usually a monthly premium for the Medicare Advantage Plan (USDHHS/CMS, 2017).

The newest component of Medicare is the prescription drug coverage (Part D). The prescription drug plan is designed to help lower prescription drug costs. The individual chooses the drug plan and pays a monthly premium, and most plans have an annual deductible. Most Medicare prescription drug plans have a coverage gap (also called the *donut hole*). This refers to a temporary limit on what the drug plan will cover. In 2017, once a member and his or her plan have spent $3700 on covered drugs (the combined amount plus the deductible), the member is in the coverage gap and will receive a 50% manufacture-paid discount on covered brand-name drugs (www.medicare.gov/part-d/costs/coverage-gap/part-d-coverage-gap.html) (USDHHS/CMS, 2017).

For older adults with low incomes, Medicaid may be available to offset the Medicare deductibles and copays and to provide additional health benefits. Each state establishes its own eligibility criteria within the broad guidelines established by the federal government. Medicaid generally covers more services than Medicare, including custodial care in nursing homes, without deductibles or copays. A very significant portion of Medicaid funds are used to offset the cost of long-term care for poor elders.

Poverty and Health Education

To determine who is considered poor, the U.S. Census Bureau compares family income (or an unrelated individual's income) with a set of poverty thresholds that vary by family size and composition and are updated annually for inflation. By 2014, the proportion of the older population (65 years and older) living in poverty had decreased dramatically to 10.1%, compared with 29% in 1966. Older women (12.1%) were more likely than older men (7%) to live in poverty. Older people who live alone have higher rates of poverty than those who are married. Race and ethnicity are also related to poverty among the older population. In 2014, older whites were less likely than older blacks, Hispanics, and Asians to be living in poverty (FIFARS, 2016).

Community nurses will be increasingly called upon to care for older adults of diverse backgrounds who have various living arrangements. Although educational attainment has increased among the elderly population, many older adults have less than a high school education; therefore nurses must be sensitive and creative when providing instruction and teaching. Nurses cannot assume that an older adult has had a formal education. In addition, instructions may need to be given at a slower pace. It may also be imperative to include family or significant others when providing instruction. Also, written information may be sent home for further reference.

On the other hand, increased educational levels of current and future elders also provide a challenge for the community health nurse. These elders are, and will be, more informed and will make greater demands for current and scientifically based information, thus requiring the nurse to be knowledgeable about the latest developments in health care.

Nurses Improving Care for Healthsystem Elders (NICHE) is a program developed by the Hartford Geriatric Institute in 1992 that assists hospitals and health care organizations improve the way in which care is provided to older adults. NICHE provides resources for nurses and other providers who care for older adults. The Geriatric Resource Nurse (GRN) model stems from this program. The GRN model guides nurses in addressing common concerns and complications related to aging using evidence-based practices (www.nicheprogram.org).

> **? ACTIVE LEARNING**
>
> Your 80-year-old client has become very frail and needs assistance with several activities of daily living. No family members are able or willing to take care of him full-time. The family has asked you for advice. What information would you share with them about alternative housing options?

PSYCHOSOCIAL ISSUES

In addition to adjusting to physiological changes related to aging and health concerns (discussed later in this chapter), older adults must cope with psychosocial and role changes such as retirement, relocation, widowhood, loss of family and friends, and possibly raising their grandchildren. Retirement may be a happy occasion when voluntary; however, the opposite may be true if it is involuntary. When older adults retire, they inevitably must cope with a change in social status and possibly income level; this may be especially difficult for people whose self-concept is related to job status. For retirees who are married, the spouse must also adjust to the changes related to retirement. Indeed, the adjustment may be more difficult for the spouse than the retiree as the retiree's leisure time will be increased. For elders who have no hobbies or interests, this extra leisure time may be a source of boredom. Nurses should encourage older retirees to pursue old hobbies and interests or establish new ones.

Relocation is another psychosocial issue that many older adults must manage. Often, relocation occurs as a result of health and functional impairment, lack of ability to maintain one's home, unsafe neighborhoods, and lack of assistance with ADLs or IADLs. The relocation may be prompted by the older adult's desire to be closer to family or medical care, or interest in moving to a new location or more supportive housing (as discussed in the section "Alternative Housing Options for Older Adults").

Widowhood is an event experienced by most older adults, especially elderly women. According to Miller (2015), common consequences of widowhood are loss of companionship and intimacy; loss of one's sexual partner; feelings of grief, loneliness, and emptiness; increased responsibilities and dependency on others; loss of income and less efficient financial management; and changes in relationships with children, married friends, and other family members. Widowhood may be especially traumatic for elders who have been married for many decades. In addition to the loss of a spouse, older adults must cope with loss of family members (sometimes their own children) and friends.

On the other hand, many older adults are faced with the responsibility of raising their grandchildren (Fig. 19.1). Substantial increases have occurred in the number of children under age 18 years living in households maintained by their grandparents, often without the presence of the grandchildren's parents

FIG. 19.1 A custodial grandmother doing homework with her grandson. (© 2013 Photos.com, a division of Getty Images. All rights reserved. Image # 86535689.)

(Clinical Example 19.1). Antecedents to children being raised by grandparents include neglect related to parental substance abuse, abandonment, emotional and physical abuse, parental death, mental and physical illness, incarceration, teen pregnancy, and grandparents assisting adult children who work or attend school. Although there may be rewards to raising grandchildren, such as satisfaction for keeping the family together, sense of purpose in life, and the opportunity to have a close relationship with one's grandchildren, this arrangement may contribute to both physical and psychological problems, such as stress, depression, and poorer health (Taylor et al, 2017; Trail Ross et al, 2015).

Clinical Example 19.1

Ms. Thomas, age 62, is divorced and has been raising her three grandchildren, ages 11 to 13, for the past 10 years. She was forced to retire from full-time teaching to assume this role. Her daughter, the children's mother, is bipolar and schizophrenic, and has tested positive for HIV. All of the grandchildren have medical problems and/or special needs, including asthma, attention-deficit hyperactivity disorder, and emotional/behavioral concerns. Ms. Thomas is very organized and keeps track of their many medications via a written schedule containing the name of each medication, dose, and time of administration. Ms. Thomas expressed increased stress, tension, and anxiety as a result of caregiving responsibilities and neglect of her own needs. She has hypertension, a "thyroid condition," asthma, gastroesophageal reflux disease, and allergies. She admits to occasionally forgetting to take her own medications because of her busy schedule. She rates her health as "fair" overall and "somewhat worse" in comparison with that of other people her age. She reports significantly less time for herself and leisure activities. Nonetheless, Ms. Thomas is determined to raise her grandchildren as well as possible. Despite her circumstances, she is very positive and optimistic that her grandchildren will grow up to be successful and respectable citizens.

Intimacy and Sexuality

Intimacy includes the need for close friendships and relationships, as well as spiritual connections and knowing that one matters in someone else's life (Syme, 2014). Expressing love and care, as well as exchanging intimate words and touch with another person, increases intimacy and expresses sexuality. Sexual expression tends to be consistent throughout life (Eliopoulas, 2018). Normal physiological changes of aging discussed in Table 19.1 may decrease older adults' frequency of sexual activity. For example, estrogen level in women decreases after menopause, which may lead to vaginal dryness and thinning and may make sexual intercourse uncomfortable. Effective treatments for vaginal dryness may range from over-the-counter moisturizers and lubricants to estrogen creams, tablets, and rings that are inserted vaginally. In men, testosterone levels decrease causing erections to be less firm and not last as long. Although erectile dysfunction (ED) is more common in older men, it is often due to underlying medical or emotional problems such as heart disease or diabetes, medication side effects, or anxiety. Some men who are impotent or have ED have taken advantage of the availability of medications like Viagra to remain sexually active.

Medical conditions, medications, chronic pain, and surgical procedures may also affect sexual performance and have a negative impact on sexual response, including a decrease in arousal and interest (HealthinAging.org, 2017).

The main reason many older adults experience a decrease in sexual activity is loss of a spouse or partner. The older adult may refuse to date or engage in a new relationship out of respect for their deceased spouse or because of fear of rejection. In addition, some individuals may believe sex is only appropriate in marriage, and sex with another person may create guilt and anxiety (Eliopoulas, 2018). On the other hand, with more "open attitudes toward sexuality, internet dating, and the availability of medications like Viagra, some older adults are remaining sexually active" (HealthinAging.org, 2017). It is important to note that older adults are particularly vulnerable to sexually transmitted diseases (STDs). Sexually active older adults who have sex with new or multiple partners may not consider using a condom, because pregnancy is no longer a risk. It is very important for older adults to practice safe sex. Methods might include knowing a partner's sexual background and sharing sexual histories, as well as getting tested—along with their partner—for HIV/AIDS and other STDs before having sex. Using a condom and water-based lubricant until test results are revealed is also advisable to decrease the risk of STDs (HealthinAging.org, 2017). If they do become symptomatic, older adults may be embarrassed to seek medical attention or may attribute the symptoms to normal aging (Clinical Example 19.2).

Clinical Example 19.2

It is very important that nurses educate their older adult clients/patients about normal physiological changes, safe sex practices, and STDs. An open approach to discussing sexuality will be very helpful to elders who are embarrassed about bringing these topics up.

"It is estimated that there are 2.4 million lesbian, gay, bisexual, or transgender (LGBT) adults over 50 living in the United States and that number is expected to double by 2030" (Choi and Meyer, 2016). LGBT individuals face societal stigma, isolation, stereotypes, and prejudices (Miller, 2015). These individuals are more likely to be single, particularly because legal marriages are fairly new, and are less likely to have children compared with heterosexual older adults. Thus they may have less support and fewer caregivers if assistance is needed. Gay and bisexual men have a higher risk of HIV and STDs. Nurses must recognize and address the health needs of these individuals by providing education and referral to appropriate community resources. In addition, the nurse should provide information about various community resources and make referrals to agencies that might be helpful.

PHYSIOLOGICAL CHANGES

Normal physiological changes occur in all body systems in response to aging. However, it is important to note that the rate and degree of these changes are highly individualized. These changes are influenced by genetic factors, diet, exercise, the environment, health status, stress, lifestyle choices, and many other elements. Table 19.1 depicts common physiological changes that occur with aging.

TABLE 19.1 Normal Physiological Changes Associated with Aging

Physiological Changes	Nursing Intervention(S) and Patient Instructions
Sensory Changes	
Vision	
Decreased visual acuity	Encourage use of corrective lenses as prescribed
Decreased visual accommodation	Use large print for teaching
Yellowing of lens	Encourage adequate lighting and night lights
	Avoid using shades of green, blue, and violet together
Hearing	
Decreased ability to hear (presbycusis)	Decrease extraneous sounds
Decreased ability to hear consonants with high-frequency sounds	Use concise sentences and speak slowly and distinctly in a low-pitched voice
	Encourage hearing examination and use of hearing aids, if needed
Taste	
Diminished taste sensation	Encourage well-balanced meals
Decreased saliva production	Advise to drink plenty of fluids
Decreased sensitivity to sweetness and saltiness	Observe for overconsumption of sweets and salt
	Give options for seasoning other than salt
Smell	
Decreased smell acuity	Advise to use other senses and other people to assist with monitoring the environment for safety (e.g., spoiled food and gas fumes)
Touch	
Decreased sensitivity to touch	Monitor for extreme temperature changes in the environment (e.g. water temperature); maintain adequate room temperature
Reduced capacity to sense pressure and pain	Ensure position changes frequently; monitor for pain
Nervous System	
Reduction in neurons and cerebral blood flow	Assess neurological status
	Ensure frequent position changes
Slower autonomic and voluntary reflexes	Assess for pain and unique responses to pain
Reduced capacity to sense pain and pressure	
Increase in amount of senile plaque and neurofibrillary tangles	
Cognitive Changes and Changes in Balance	
Slower reaction time	Allow adequate time for response, information processing, and performance of tasks
Slower learning time	Break instructions into small units
Memory: long-term memory better than short-term memory	Use shorter teaching sessions; use cues and gestures
Personality consistent with earlier years	Relate education to prior experience
Sleep	
Decrease in stages 3 and 4 sleep patterns	Assess quantity and quality of sleep
Increase in arousals during the night	Allow naps as needed
Slight reduction in total sleep time	Educate about effects of stimulants and caffeine
	Decrease interventions at night and avoid sleep medication use if possible
Cardiovascular System	
Decrease in tone and elasticity of aorta and great vessels	Pace activities and allow rest periods
Thicker and stiffer heart valves	Monitor for activity intolerance
Slowing down of heart's conduction system	Encourage use of ambulation aids when appropriate
Slower recovery of myocardial contractility and irritability	Encourage regular exercise program
Decreased cardiac reserve and output	Prevent or eliminate stressors
Decreased ability to increase heart rate when stress occurs	Monitor heart rate and blood pressure
Increased systolic blood pressure	
Respiratory System	
Reduced size of lungs, lung expansion, activity, and recoil	Encourage influenza and pneumococcal vaccinations
Increased rigidity of lungs and thoracic cage	Encourage regular exercise
Decreased cough response	Encourage adequate fluid intake
Decreased number of alveoli and gas exchange	Monitor oxygen administration

Continued

TABLE 19.1   **Normal Physiological Changes Associated with Aging—cont'd**

Physiological Changes	Nursing Intervention(S) and Patient Instructions
Musculoskeletal System	
Atrophy and decrease in muscle fibers	Prevent immobility
Decreased muscle mass and strength	Encourage regular exercise program
Reduced bone minerals and mass, causing porous and brittle bones	Teach safety precautions to prevent falls
Shortening of vertebra	Encourage adequate calcium and vitamin D intake
Gastrointestinal System	
Brittle teeth	Encourage dental health (i.e., brushing, flossing)
Decreased esophageal/colonic peristalsis	Encourage diet that is well balanced and has adequate protein and vitamins
Decreased stomach motility	Encourage adequate fluids and fiber intake
Decreased production of saliva, HCl, and digestive enzymes	Monitor diet for deficiencies
Decreased absorption of fat and vitamins B_1 and B_{12}	
Decrease in thirst response	
Renal System	
Decreased size of kidneys	Monitor drugs—smaller doses may be needed
Decreased number of nephrons	Observe for adverse responses to drugs
Reduced renal blood flow and tubular function	Monitor electrolytes and laboratory values
Decreased glomerular filtration rate	Prevent dehydration
Genitourinary System	
Weakening of bladder muscle, causing increased urinary frequency, urgency, and nocturia	Assess bladder function and assist with frequent toileting
Decreased bladder capacity	Encourage bladder training program, exercises, and medication when needed
Increased retention	Observe for signs of urinary tract infection
Increased nocturia	Ensure safety to bathroom at night
Reproductive System	
Women	
Atrophy of vulva and flattening of labia	Differentiate between changes due to normal aging and those due to disease or medications
Vaginal dryness and thinning	Advise about use of lubricants for comfort during intercourse
Atrophy of cervix, ovaries, and uterus	Recommend breast examinations and mammograms
Decreased amount and elasticity of breast tissue	
Men	
Atrophy of testes and decreased elasticity of scrotal skin	Differentiate between changes due to normal aging and those due to disease or medications
Prostatic enlargement	Recommend prostate examination
Erection takes longer to achieve and is not as firm	
Endocrine System	
Increased fibrosis and nodularity of thyroid gland	Recommend pneumococcal, influenza, and tetanus vaccinations
Shrinkage of pituitary gland	Monitor laboratory values and glucose
Decrease in adrenal gland secretion of glucocorticoid	Prevent infection
Decreased levels of aldosterone	Encourage good nutrition
Delayed insulin release	Observe for hypoglycemia or hyperglycemia
Reduced ability to metabolize glucose	
Decrease in testosterone, estrogen, and progesterone	
Immune System	
Shrinkage of thymus gland	Prevent infections and exposure to infectious diseases
Decreased production of thymic hormones	Encourage good hand washing
Decreased production of antibodies	Monitor laboratory values
Response to antigens diminishes	
Integumentary System	
Decreased skin elasticity	Encourage frequent position changes and inspect skin
Generalized thinning and dryness	Be careful of skin tears, bruising, and pressure ulcers
Atrophy of sweat glands and diminished sweating	Assess body and environmental temperatures to prevent hypothermia and hyperthermia
Altered thermoregulation	Ensure adequate clothing and comfortable room temperature
Variation in pigmentation (age spots)	

Adapted from Eliopoulos C: *Gerontological nursing,* ed 9, Philadelphia, 2018, Lippincott Williams & Wilkins.

WELLNESS AND HEALTH PROMOTION

Wellness is different from "good health." Wellness exists at one end of a continuum with illness at the other end. Health promotion programs focus on helping individuals maintain their wellness, prevent illness, and manage any chronic illnesses that they may have. Preventive health services are valuable in improving the health status of individuals to their maximum wellness potential.

Healthy People 2020

The USDHHS's program *Healthy People 2020* establishes national objectives for health promotion and disease prevention. A primary goal is to increase the quality and years of healthy life. Although people are living longer, many older adults have two or more chronic illnesses that interfere with their quality of life. *Healthy People 2020* has incorporated specific objectives related to older adults that are designed to promote healthy outcomes for this population.

 HEALTHY PEOPLE 2020

Summary of Objectives for Older Adults

Prevention

OA–1: Increase the proportion of older adults who use the Welcome to Medicare benefit.

OA–2: Increase the proportion of older adults who are up to date on a core set of clinical preventive services.

OA–3: (Developmental) Increase the proportion of older adults with one or more chronic health conditions who report confidence in managing their conditions.

OA–4: Increase the proportion of older adults who receive Diabetes Self-Management Benefits.

OA–5: Reduce the proportion of older adults who have moderate to severe functional limitations.

OA–6: Increase the proportion of older adults with reduced physical or cognitive function who engage in light, moderate, or vigorous leisure-time physical activities.

OA–7: Increase the proportion of the health care workforce with geriatric certification.

Long-Term Services and Supports

OA–8: (Developmental) Reduce the proportion of noninstitutionalized older adults with disabilities who have an unmet need for long-term services and supports.

OA–9: (Developmental) Reduce the proportion of unpaid caregivers of older adults who report an unmet need for caregiver support services.

OA–10: Reduce the rate of pressure ulcer–related hospitalizations among older adults.

OA–11: Reduce the rate of emergency department (ED) visits due to falls among older adults.

OA–12: Increase the number of States, the District of Columbia, and Tribes that collect and make publicly available information on the characteristics of victims, perpetrators, and cases of elder abuse, neglect, and exploitation.

From U.S. Department of Health and Human Services: *Healthy People 2020 summary of objectives: Older adults,* n.d. Retrieved from: http:// healthypeople.gov/2020/topicsobjectives2020/pdfs/OlderAdults.pdf.

BOX 19.2 Recommended Screenings and Examinations for Health Promotion and Disease Prevention in Older Adults

Examinations and Tests

For All Older Adults

Complete physical: Annually

Blood pressure: Annually; more frequently if hypertensive or at risk

Blood glucose: Annually; more frequently if diabetic or at risk

Serum cholesterol: Every 5 years; more frequently if at high risk

Fecal occult blood test: Annually

Sigmoidoscopy: Every 5 years
  OR
Colonoscopy: Every 10 years; more frequently if at high risk

Visual acuity and glaucoma screening: Annually

Dental examination: Annually for those with teeth with cleaning every 6 months; cleaning every 2 years for denture wearers

Hearing test: Every 2 to 5 years

For Women

Breast self-examination: Monthly

Clinical breast examination: Annually

Mammogram: Every 1 to 2 years if aged 40 years or older; check with health care provider if 74 years or older

Pelvic examination and Papanicolaou smear: Annually; may check with health care provider about discontinuation at 66+ years or after three consecutive negative Pap test results or >2 consecutive negative human papilloma virus (HPV) and Pap tests, no abnormal results in previous 10 years and not otherwise at risk, or have had a total hysterectomy

Digital rectal examination: Annually with pelvic examination

Bone density: Once after menopause and more frequently if at risk

For Men

Digital rectal examination and prostate examination: Annually

Prostate-specific antigen (PSA) blood test: Annually

Immunizations for All Older Adults

Tetanus, diphtheria, pertussis: Every 10 years

Influenza/flu vaccine: Annually

Pneumonia vaccine: Once after age 65 years; ask physician about booster every 5 years

Hepatitis A and B: For those at risk

Herpes zoster (shingles): One-time dose

Varicella: If evidence of lack of immunity and significant risk for exposure

Data from American Cancer Society: *Cancer facts & figures*, Atlanta, GA, 2013, Author; and Centers for Disease Control and Prevention: *Recommended adult immunization schedule, U.S., 2013,* 2013. https://www.cancer.org/content/dam/cancer-org/research/cancer-facts-and-statistics/annual-cancer-facts-and-figures/2017/cancer-facts-and-figures-2017.pdf, https://www.cdc.gov/vaccines/schedules/downloads/adult/adult-combined-schedule.pdf, and http://www.healthline.com/health/senior-health-tests#overview1

Recommended Health Care Screenings and Examinations

Many organizations, such as the American Cancer Society, the American Heart Association, the U.S. Preventive Services Task Force, and the Agency for Healthcare Research & Quality, have established guidelines for health promotion screenings and examinations. Box 19.2 depicts some of the more widely agreed-on

FIG. 19.2 Older adults participate in an exercise class. (© 2013 Photos.com, a division of Getty Images. All rights reserved. Image # 125557433.)

screenings and examinations for older adults. These recommendations are very useful to community nurses educating older adults about the benefits of screening and early detection of disease. Frequently, earlier detection of disease allows better treatment, lower health care costs, and the possibility of cure.

Physical Activity and Fitness

Physical activity is beneficial for the health of people of all ages (Fig. 19.2). Although there are various types of exercises, walking is one of the best forms of exercise, and it is free. Many older adults engage in walking, swimming, dancing, yoga, and tai chi for exercise. Regular exercise improves functional status, reduces blood pressure and serum cholesterol level, decreases insulin resistance, prevents obesity, strengthens bones, and reduces falls. Barriers to exercising that have been identified by older adults include lack of access to safe areas to exercise, pain, fatigue, and impairment in sensory function and mobility (Mauk, 2014).

Objective OA-6 of *Healthy People 2020* reads "increase the proportion of older adults with reduced physical or cognitive function who engage in light, moderate, or vigorous leisure-time physical activities" (USDHHS, Office of Disease Prevention and Health Promotion, 2018). Nurses may help older adults accomplish this goal by assessing their understanding of the beneficial effects of exercise and identifying barriers that prevent exercise. Nurses should also educate, encourage, and assist older adults with exercise. When applicable, antiinflammatory medications may be administered before physical activity to address accompanying pain.

Nutrition

The U.S. Department of Agriculture (USDA) and USDHHS provide authoritative advice on what constitutes a healthy diet. The USDA recommends using *MyPlate* as a means to consuming a healthy diet (U.S. Department of Agriculture, 2017). The plate picture helps an individual make smart choices from every food group, find balance between food and physical activity, get the most nutrition out of calories, and stay within caloric needs. Food groups emphasized are fruits, vegetables, grains, protein foods, dairy, and oils.

In *Healthy People 2020,* nutrition was identified as a priority area of health promotion for people of all ages. Similar to patterns among other age groups, poor nutrition in the elderly population is common. Obesity has been increasing in adults 65 years and older (FIFARS, 2016). Older adults require the same or higher levels of nutrients for optimal health outcomes, but poor diet quality is associated with cardiovascular disease, hypertension, type 2 diabetes, osteoporosis, and some types of cancer (World Health Organization [WHO], 2017). Also, an inappropriate diet is related to constipation, dental disease, physical inactivity, and depression. Normal physiological changes such as a diminished sense of smell may reduce the enjoyment of eating. Gastrointestinal changes can interfere with absorption of vitamin B_{12} and folic acid, leading to anemia. A diminished thirst sensation may lead to dehydration. Other factors that can affect the nutritional status of the elderly are income, functional status, taking multiple medications, social isolation, lack of transportation, and dependence on others for grocery shopping and cooking. The nutrition checklist presented in Table 19.2 lists warning signs of and risk factors for poor nutritional health described by the mnemonic DETERMINE. The nurse should use this tool to identify the elderly who need help with their dietary intake. The benefits of good nutrition are an important factor in helping maintain independence and quality of life.

> **? ACTIVE LEARNING**
>
> 1. Interview an elderly person you know to assess his or her physical activity level and nutritional status using the nutrition checklist and food pyramid. Review the results with the person and help him or her plan a nutritious menu for 1 day. What factors hindered or enhanced your interaction with the person?
> 2. Find the names, addresses, and phone numbers of local resources for someone interested in, for example, exercise programs for the elderly and smoking cessation programs.

COMMON HEALTH CONCERNS

Chronic Illness

About 80% of older adults have at least one chronic disease, and 68% have at least two chronic conditions, such as diabetes, arthritis, hypertension, and lung disease, that seriously compromise the quality of life of older adults (National Council on Aging, 2017). The prevalence of chronic diseases rises with age, and chronic illnesses are a major cause of disability and may cause limitations with ADLs and IADLs. The most common conditions are arthritis, hypertension, and diabetes. Chronic diseases are the leading causes of death among persons 65 years and older (Table 19.3).

Medication Use by Elders

The high prevalence of chronic diseases in the elderly population causes this group to use a large number of medications. In the United States, older adults are responsible for more than one third of total outpatient spending on prescription medications (National Institute on Drug Abuse, 2016). Older adults also consume many over-the-counter medications as well as "folk" or herbal remedies. The elderly population is vulnerable to the effects of drugs because of normal aging changes (see Table 19.1) and age-related differences in pharmacokinetics and

TABLE 19.2 Nutrition Checklist for Older Adults: Warning Signs of Poor Nutritional Health

Possible Problem	Question to Answer	Score For "Yes" Answer (Circle If "Yes")
Disease	Do you have an illness or condition that makes you change the kind and/or amount of food you eat?	2
Eating poorly	Do you eat fewer than two meals per day?	3
	Do you eat few fruits, vegetables, or milk products?	2
	Do you have three or more drinks of beer, liquor, or wine almost every day?	2
Tooth loss/mouth pain	Do you have tooth or mouth problems that make it hard for you to eat?	2
Economic hardship	Do you sometimes have trouble affording the food you need?	4
Reduced social contact	Do you eat alone most of the time?	1
Multiple medications	Do you take three or more prescribed or over-the-counter drugs a day?	1
Involuntary weight loss/gain	Have you lost or gained 10 pounds in the last 6 months without trying?	2
Needs assistance in self-care	Are you sometimes physically not able to shop, cook, or feed yourself?	1
Elder years >80 yr	Are you over 80 years old?	1
	TOTAL:	_____

Scoring:

0–2: Good! Recheck your nutritional score in 6 months.

3–5: You are at moderate nutritional risk. See what can be done to improve your eating habits and lifestyle. Your office on aging, senior nutrition program, senior citizens center, or health department can help. Recheck your nutritional score in 3 months.

6 or more: You are at high nutritional risk. Bring this checklist the next time you see your doctor, dietitian, or other qualified health or social service professional. Talk with them about any problems you may have. Ask for help to improve your nutritional health.

From The Nutrition Screening Initiative: *Determine your nutritional health*, n.d. http://www.rcaging.org/Portals/0/uploads/nutritional_health.pdf

pharmacodynamics. Polypharmacy may also make older adults vulnerable to drug interactions and dangerous adverse reactions.

RESEARCH HIGHLIGHTS

Beers Criteria for Adverse Drug Events

Shehab et al (2016) found that 34.5% of emergency department (ED) visits for adverse drug events occurred among older adults 65 or older. According to the Beers Criteria, medications that should always be avoided in older adults were associated with 1.8% of the ED visits, whereas medications that are potentially inappropriate in older adults were responsible for 3.4% of the ED visits for adverse drug events. Anticoagulants, diabetes agents, and opioids were the cause of 59.9% of older adult visits to the ED for adverse drug events. More efforts are needed among physicians and other health professionals to improve safety and prevent adverse drug events.

The "Beers Criteria" catalogs medications that cause adverse drug events in older adults because of the drugs' pharmacological properties and the physiological changes of aging. An updated version of the Beers Criteria for potentially inappropriate medications in older adults has been published by the American Geriatrics Society (AGS, 2015). A printable copy of the Beers Criteria pocket card is available at https://www.scribd.com/document/92092838/Printable-Beers-Pocket-Card

Nurses should closely monitor medication use in the home to ensure safety. An easy-to-use pill organizer may be helpful for older adults. In addition, such clients should be educated about potential adverse reactions as well as drug–drug and drug–food interactions. Pharmacists can be very helpful in answering questions about prescriptions and over-the-counter medications.

ADDITIONAL HEALTH CONCERNS

Sensory Impairment

Sensory disabilities increase with age and may seriously affect an older person's quality of life and ability to carry out routine daily activities. The National Health Interview Survey found that 7.3 million noninstitutionalized American adults 65 years and older reported significant vision loss. Vision loss refers to difficulty seeing, even when wearing glasses or contact lenses, as well as blindness (Centers for Disease Control and Prevention [CDC], 2015). This number will likely increase with the country's aging population. The four leading eye diseases affecting older individuals are age-related cataracts, macular degeneration, diabetic retinopathy, and glaucoma.

Cataracts

Cataracts are the leading cause, as well as the most reversible cause, of visual impairment in older adults. A **cataract** is

TABLE 19.3 Leading Causes of Death for Persons 65 Years of Age and Older

	White	Black	American Indian	Asian or Pacific Islander	Hispanic
1.	Heart disease	Heart disease	Heart disease	Heart disease	Heart disease
2.	Cancer	Cancer	Cancer	Cancer	Cancer
3.	Stroke	Stroke	Diabetes	Stroke	Stroke
4.	Chronic obstructive pulmonary disease (COPD)	Diabetes	Stroke	Diabetes	Diabetes
5.	Alzheimer disease	COPD	COPD	Pneumonia/influenza	COPD

From Gorina Y, Hoyert D, Lentzner H, Goulding M: *Trends in causes of death among older persons in the United States* (Aging Trends no. 6), 2006. www.cdc.gov/nchs/data/ahcd/agingtrends/06olderpersons.pdf.

a clouding of the normally clear lens of the eye. Risk factors that increase a person's chances of cataracts include increasing age, diabetes, excessive exposure to sunlight, smoking, obesity, hypertension, previous eye injury, inflammation, surgery, prolonged use of corticosteroids, and drinking excessive amounts of alcohol. Older adults should have annual eye examinations, which allow early detection of cataracts. The only effective treatment for a cataract is surgical removal of the clouded lens and replacement with a clear lens implant. Interventions that may be able to reduce risks are cessation of smoking, wearing of sunglasses, maintaining a healthy weight, choosing a healthy diet, and taking care of other coexisting health problems (Mayo Clinic Staff, 2016).

Macular Degeneration

There are two types of macular degeneration: dry and wet. Dry macular degeneration is more common and less severe. It causes blurred or reduced central vision due to thinning of the macula. It may affect one or both eyes (Mayo Clinic Staff, 2015a). With wet macular degeneration, symptoms appear suddenly and progress rapidly, and objects appear smaller or farther away than they really are (Mayo Clinic Staff, 2015b). Any changes in central vision and the ability to see colors and fine details indicate that the individual should be seen by an eye doctor. Treatment differs for the two conditions. Wet macular degeneration cannot be cured, but if treated early, it may slow down its progression. Dry macular degeneration usually progresses slowly, and many people with it can live relatively normal, productive lives. Nurses can recommend the following ways to cope with changing vision: use magnifiers, use alternative options for books, use brighter lights, join a support group, and make arrangements for traveling.

Glaucoma

Glaucoma is one of the leading causes of blindness in America. The condition causes damage to the optic nerve, often caused by an abnormally high pressure in the eye. The most common form of glaucoma, primary or chronic open-angle glaucoma, develops gradually without warning and progresses with few or no symptoms until the condition reaches an advanced stage. The drainage angle formed by the cornea and the iris remains open; however, the aqueous humor drains too slowly. This leads to fluid backup and a gradual buildup of pressure within the eye. Increased eye pressure continues to damage the optic nerve, and more and more peripheral vision is lost. Glaucoma cannot be cured, and its damage cannot be reversed, but treatment and regular eye examinations can prevent vision loss if the disease is found early, or can slow the disease or prevent further vision loss. Treatment consists of prescribed eyedrops or, if medications are ineffective, surgery (Mayo Clinic Staff, 2015c).

Nurses should educate clients about recommended vision screening. To determine the influence of visual impairment, the nurse should inquire about activity limitations associated with poor vision. Determining whether the client is using visual assistive devices such as glasses, contact lenses, magnifying lenses, or large-print books can be beneficial in recognizing the

degree of adaptation. The nurse should know about resources that help older adults with eye care and assistive devices. Organizations that provide information include the National Eye Institute, the American Foundation for the Blind, and Lighthouse International.

❓ ACTIVE LEARNING

Devise a nursing care plan for an elder with a visual disturbance (e.g., cataracts, glaucoma, or macular degeneration).

Hearing Loss

Hearing loss is one of the most common conditions affecting older adults. Approximately 15%, or 37.5 million American adults, report some degree of hearing loss. One in three adults 65 to 74 years of age and nearly half of adults 75 years old or older have difficulty hearing (NIHseniorhealth.gov, 2016a). There are two general categories of hearing loss: sensorineural hearing loss occurs when there is damage to the inner ear or the auditory nerve. This type of hearing loss is usually permanent. Presbycusis is the most common type of sensorineural hearing loss and is caused by gradual changes in the middle ear due to aging, loud noises, heredity, head injury, infection, illness, certain prescription drugs, and circulation problems. Conductive hearing loss occurs when sound waves cannot reach the inner ear. The cause may be ear wax buildup, fluid, or a punctured eardrum. Medical treatment or surgery can usually restore conductive hearing loss. A combination of both is known as *mixed hearing loss* (NIHseniorhealth.gov, 2016a).

Nurses should assess older adults for hearing impairment. The nurse should ask the individual whether he or she is having trouble hearing over the telephone, finds it hard to follow conversation when two or more people are talking, often asks people to repeat what they are saying, needs to turn up the volume of the radio or TV, or thinks that others are mumbling. If an individual is experiencing hearing problems, a qualified health professional such as an otolaryngologist or ear, nose, and throat specialist or an audiologist should be consulted. Box 19.3 contains tips for health care providers who work with older adults who have hearing difficulties.

BOX 19.3   Working With the Older Adult Who Has Hearing Difficulties

- Include the person with hearing loss in the conversation.
- Find a quiet place to talk to help reduce background noise, especially in restaurants and social gatherings.
- Stand in good lighting and use facial expressions or gestures to give clues.
- Face the person and talk clearly.
- Speak a little more loudly than normal, but do not shout.
- Speak at a reasonable speed; do not hide your mouth, eat, or chew gum.
- Repeat yourself if necessary, using different words.
- Try to make sure only one person talks at a time.
- Be patient. Stay positive and relaxed.
- Ask how you can help.

From National Institute on Aging: *Age page: hearing loss,* 2013. https://www.nia.nih.gov/health/hearing-loss-common-problem-older-adults

Dental Concerns

Age brings a host of dental problems that are often neglected because of inadequate dental care, limited mobility and transportation, poor nutrition, the myth that it is natural for older adults to become edentulous, and lack of finances and reimbursement. With proper care it is possible to retain one's natural teeth if one adheres to good dental hygiene and has regular dental checkups. Common dental problems of the elderly are dry mouth, receding gums, tooth cavities, hypersensitivity of the teeth, and tooth discoloration. Full or partial dentures may be needed to replace missing or badly damaged teeth. Regular dental visits for cleaning and dental evaluation are essential prevention strategies. The National Institute on Aging (2016) Age Page "Taking Care of Your Teeth and Mouth" may be very useful in educating patients on proper dental and mouth care.

Incontinence

Aging does not cause incontinence; however, this condition is common among the elderly population. About 50% of women and 25% of men 65 years or older who are noninstitutionalized suffer from urinary incontinence (CDC, 2014). Urinary incontinence can occur for many reasons. Urinary tract infections, vaginal infection or irritation, constipation, and certain medicines can cause short-term bladder control problems. Weak bladder muscles, overactive bladder muscles, blockage from an enlarged prostate, and damage to nerves that control the bladder may cause longer-lasting incontinence. However, in most cases, urinary incontinence can be treated or controlled, if not cured.

The choice of treatment depends on the type of bladder control problem. Types of urinary incontinence are stress incontinence, urge incontinence, and overflow incontinence or functional incontinence. One of the treatments that health care providers may suggest is Kegel exercises.

Approximately 8% of older adults have moderate, severe, or very severe bowel leakage (CDC, 2014). Loss of control of the bowels, or fecal incontinence, leads to leakage of stool from the large intestine. Medical evaluation to determine the cause should be recommended. Treatment varies, depending on the cause.

ELDER SAFETY AND SECURITY NEEDS

Each year, many elderly are injured in and around their homes. Older people are often targets for robbery, purse snatching, pickpocketing, car theft, and home repair scams. There are safety measures that the individual can take to avoid crime and to stay safe.

Falls

The risk of falling rises with age. **Falls** are the number one cause of fractures, hospital admissions for trauma, loss of independence, and injury deaths. Each year, 2.8 million older adults are treated in emergency departments because of falls. Over 800,000 patients a year are hospitalized because of a fall injury, most often because of a broken hip or head injury deaths (CDC, 2016a). Many of the physiological changes that normally occur with aging, as well as a variety of chronic illnesses, can affect balance and make falls more likely. Medications such as blood pressure pills, heart medicines, diuretics, and tranquilizers may increase the risk of falling. Osteoporosis, a disease that causes a gradual loss of bone tissue or bone density, makes bones more susceptible to breaking. There is a link between osteoporosis and broken bones from falls. A person who falls and sustains a fracture may become afraid of falling again and thus will limit his or her activities. Seniors living independently before a fall may be institutionalized for as long as a year after a fracture. Loss of footing and loss of traction are factors that can lead to a fall. Uneven surfaces such as sidewalks, curbs, and floor elevations; wet or slippery ground; and climbing up on household items not intended for climbing can result in loss of footing or loss of traction. In addition, drinking alcoholic beverages increases the risk of falling, because alcohol slows reflexes and response time and may cause dizziness, sleepiness, lightheadedness, and poor balance.

Steps can be taken to reduce the chance of falls. Simple exercises that strengthen leg muscles and exercises that can improve balance are recommended (Box 19.4). Seniors can also improve their environment in order to reduce their risk of falling by checking floor surfaces and curb heights; identifying weather-related problems before venturing outside; wearing supportive, low-heeled shoes; making sure that rooms are well lit; and ensuring that safety equipment is installed in bathrooms and stairwells. Another factor older adults should consider is having a cellular phone with them at all times to call for help directly. Telephone systems providing personal emergency response services may be available on a subscription basis, thus allowing seniors to be monitored; if such a service receives no answer to the call, help can be sent.

Traumatic Brain Injury

Traumatic brain injury (TBI) is a major cause of death and disability and contributes to about 30% of all injury deaths in the

---

BOX 19.4 Improving Balance

Focus on the Following Areas

Perform muscle-strengthening exercises.

Obtain maximum vision correction.

When using bifocal or trifocal glasses, practice looking straight ahead and lowering the head.

Practice balance exercises daily.

Balance Exercises

While holding onto a stable item like a chair or counter, practice standing on one leg at a time for a minute. Gradually increase time, try balancing with eyes closed, and try balancing without holding onto anything.

Practice standing on toes, then rock back to balance on heels. Hold each position for count of 10.

Hold onto a stable item with both hands, then make a big circle to the left with hips. Repeat to the right. Do not move the shoulders or feet. Repeat five times.

Modified from National Institutes of Health Osteoporosis and Related Bone Diseases, National Resource Center: *Preventing falls and related fractures*, 2015. //www.niams.nih.gov/Health_Info/Bone/Osteoporosis/Fracture/prevent_falls.asp.

United States (Taylor et al, 2017). TBI is a result of a bump, blow, or jolt to the head or a penetrating head injury, often after a fall, that disrupts the normal function of the brain (CDC, 2016b).

TBI symptoms may be mild, moderate, or severe. Mild symptoms include headache, confusion, lightheadedness, dizziness, blurred vision or tired eyes, ringing in the ears, bad taste in the mouth, fatigue or lethargy, and a change in sleep patterns or thinking. Moderate or severe TBI may cause the same symptoms as mild TBI plus a headache that gets worse or does not go away; repeated vomiting or nausea; convulsions or seizures; an inability to awaken from sleep; dilation of one or both pupils of the eyes; slurred speech; weakness or numbness in the extremities; loss of coordination; and increased confusion, restlessness, or agitation (CDC, 2016b). Medical attention should be sought for monitoring and treatment of symptoms. Referral for rehabilitation may be required for persons with disabilities resulting from TBI.

Driver Safety

One of the quality-of-life factors that is important to most seniors is the ability to drive. Many older adults depend on driving in order to maintain independence and personal mobility. Seniors overwhelmingly prefer to drive as their means of transportation, with being a passenger their second preferred option. The number of elderly drivers will be increasing with the extension of life expectancy.

Age alone should not be the determining factor of whether or not a senior can drive safely. Driving skills vary from one elderly person to another. Age-related declines in vision, hearing, and other abilities, as well as certain medical conditions and medications, can affect driving skills (NIHseniorhealth.gov, 2015). Most older drivers monitor their own driving ability and gradually limit or stop driving, whereas others risk personal injury rather than give up their driver's license. Motor vehicle crashes increase with age, especially after age 75 (NIHseniorhealth.gov, 2015). The nurse should be alert to signs of driving impairment in older clients and should offer practical advice so that the driver may either continue to drive safely or be encouraged to find alternative transportation (Box 19.5). The nurse can discuss issues with the senior driver, family, or friends such as drifting out of a lane, becoming confused when entering or exiting a highway, getting lost in familiar places, stopping inappropriately, failing to yield the right of way, and speeding or driving too slowly.

Some interventions that older adults could implement are limiting their driving to daylight hours and good weather conditions, planning their trips to avoid rush hour, not listening to the radio, and avoiding talking with passengers while driving. The driver should also be encouraged to find other methods of transportation, such as family and friends, public transportation, taxis, and other private transportation options available in the community.

When the question of driving safely becomes personal, elderly drivers might become very defensive. Therefore it is important that elderly persons, if at all possible, be involved in the decision-making process of evaluating their ability and deciding what should be done. However, if the individual is greatly impaired and therefore is dangerous to self or others,

BOX 19.5 Warning Signs That Indicate a Person Should Begin to Limit or Stop Driving

- Physical challenges or limitations
    1. Increasing vision and hearing difficulties
    2. Physical limitations or difficulties including moving foot between pedals, difficulty turning head
- Cognitive problems
    3. Decreasing confidence while driving
    4. Getting lost in familiar places
    5. Becoming easily distracted or confused while driving
    6. Failing to recognize dangerous situations
- Diminishing driving skills
    7. Improper use of turn signals
    8. Difficulty making turns or maintaining correct lane of traffic
    9. Difficulty judging distance between vehicles in traffic
    10. Poor parking abilities
- Potentially hazardous driving
    11. Driving too slowly or too fast for road conditions,
    12. Failing to stop at traffic lights or stop signs,
    13. Frequent "close calls,"
    14. Damage (scrapes or dents) to vehicle or surroundings
    15. Warnings or tickets for moving violations
    16. Multiple accidents

Adapted from https://www.aarp.org/auto/driver-safety/info-2013/warning-signs-unsafe-driving.html?intcmp=AE-ATO-ADS-ASSESS-ROW1-SPOT3

it may be necessary to involve the family, family physician, or department of motor vehicles in determining whether to suspend or revoke an older person's license. In addition, it may be necessary to take the keys, disable the car, or move it to a location beyond the individual's control to protect the senior and others from injury or accidents.

Residential Fire-Related Injuries

Older adults and people with limited physical and cognitive abilities are at a higher risk of death from fire. In 2014, older adults accounted for 38% of all fire deaths and 14% of fire injuries. With the increasing number of older adults, there is likely to be an increase in fire deaths and injuries (U.S. Fire Administration, 2017).

This risk of fire-related injuries may be attributed to reduced sensory abilities such as smell, touch, vision, and hearing; diminished mental faculties; slower reaction time; increased disabilities; and economic and social concerns that may prevent necessary home improvements that could reduce fire risk. The predominant causes of fires that result in injuries to older adults are cooking, open flames, smoking, and heating (U.S. Fire Administration, 2017). Nurses making home visits can assess their elderly client's home for fire risk and teach fire safety, including the importance of home smoke detectors and fire extinguishers. In many communities, the fire department installs free smoke detectors for older adults. In addition to the U.S. Fire Administration's public information campaign, A Fire Safety Campaign for People 50-Plus, organizations such as the National Fire Protection Association and the American Burn Association have active fire prevention and education programs for older adults.

Cold and Heat Stress

Cold Stress Disorders

Hypothermia is the most serious of the cold stress–related disorders and is the one elderly individuals might experience in the home because of failure of the heating systems or lack of financial resources to pay for sufficient heat. Factors that contribute to the development of hypothermia are age, health, nutrition, exhaustion, exposure and duration of exposure, wind, temperature, wetness, and medications that may decrease heat production, increase heat loss, or interfere with thermostability. Signs of hypothermia are confusion or sleepiness; slowed, slurred speech; weak pulse; a lot of shivering; and poor control over body movements (National Institute on Aging [NIA], 2017b).

Initial management is to prevent further loss of heat. Rewarming of the core temperature at a safe, slow rate is important in order to avoid lethal side effects. The reason for rewarming the core first is to prevent vasodilation that would put the individual into ventricular fibrillation (NIA, 2017b). Measures that can be taken are (1) remove the individual from the cold area as soon as possible; (2) add more clothing, especially to the head (e.g., use a hat or scarf); (3) provide a warm sweetened drink (no coffee or tea); and (4) apply mild heat to the head, neck, chest, and groin areas using hot water bottles or warm moist towels. Emergency care is imperative, and hospitalization may be needed, depending on the stage of hypothermia.

Heat Stress Disorders

The heat stress disorders are heatstroke, heat syncope, heat exhaustion, and heat cramps. As the environment becomes warmer, all methods of heat elimination become less effective, especially for older adults, who may have altered thermoregulation, diminished sweating, and decreased thirst sensation. These conditions should be taken seriously, and they require immediate attention; heatstroke is life threatening. Heat cramps are painful spasms of muscles of the arms, legs, or abdomen that occur during or after work. Signs and symptoms of heat exhaustion are fatigue, nausea, headache, and giddiness. The skin is clammy and moist, and the complexion may be pale or flushed. The individual may faint on standing, with a rapid, thready pulse and low blood pressure. Signs and symptoms of heatstroke include hot, dry skin that is usually red, mottled, or cyanotic; confusion, loss of consciousness, or convulsions might occur (NIA, 2017a). All of these heat stress disorders may occur in the home without fans or air conditioning, or from being in the sun for prolonged periods, either in recreation or working in extremely hot temperatures and high humidity. In all instances, the individual should be moved to a cooler environment and encouraged to lie down and rest. With heatstroke, immediate and rapid cooling with chilled water or by wrapping in a wet sheet, as well as being moved to a cooler area, should be done while immediate emergency care is being sought (NIA, 2017a).

Elder Abuse

Elder abuse is a serious problem throughout the United States. It is important to remember that abuse is not only a health concern but also a legal problem. States have laws defining abuse and identifying who is required to report abuse to the local Adult Protective Services. *Abuse* is generally defined as the willful infliction of pain, injury, or debilitating mental anguish; unreasonable confinement; or deprivation by a caretaker of services that are necessary to maintain mental and physical health. The categories of abuse are domestic, institutional, and from self-neglect. Domestic abuse is abuse that occurs in the home. Institutional abuse is abuse that occurs in a nursing home or other residential care facility. Self-neglect is defined as abuse that occurs when a person living alone threatens his or her own health or safety.

There are four common types of elder abuse: physical abuse, psychological/emotional abuse, financial or material exploitation, and neglect. Physical abuse involves slapping, pushing, pinching, and beating or use of physical restraint that results in broken bones, sprains, dislocations, bruises, black eyes, cuts, and rope marks, or sexual assault. Psychological or emotional abuse includes humiliation, intimidation, threats, and destruction of belongings (e.g., glasses). Financial or material exploitation refers to the improper or illegal use of the resources of an older person without consent (e.g., use of automated teller machine card). The most common type of abuse is neglect, which may be self-imposed or caused by another person. Signs of neglect include dehydration, malnutrition, untreated health problems, bedsores, unclean or inappropriate clothing, and weight loss.

Approximately 1 in 10 Americans 60 years of age or older have experienced some form of elder abuse. It is estimated that 5 million older adults are abused each year; however, only 1 in 14 cases of abuse are reported (National Council on Aging, 2017). This problem will steadily increase as more and more elderly are living longer and remaining in their homes. Abuse of the elderly is underreported for a number of reasons, including denial, fear of retaliation and further abuse, no other place to go, love of the abuser and not wanting him or her arrested, dependence on an abuser, shame and embarrassment that a loved one could act in an abusive manner, and lack of physical and/or cognitive ability to report the abuse. In addition, elder abuse may be missed by professionals working with older adults because of lack of training on detecting abuse.

Diagnosis is very difficult because many of the signs and symptoms may truly be the result of normal physiological aging. Ways to tell the difference include conflicting stories about how physical injuries were obtained, "physician shopping," clusters of signs and symptoms, increasing depression of the elder, new poverty, poor personal care, malnutrition, unresponsiveness, hostility, anxiety, confusion, new health problems, improper medication, dehydration, and longing for death.

The abuser is frequently the spouse, adult child, sibling, friend, or caregiver. The family member profile of an abuser is an individual who is middle-aged or older, a daughter or son of the elder, someone with low self-esteem and impaired impulse control. Caregiver behavior to look for includes aggression, defensive or increasingly resentful attitude toward the elder, blaming of the victim for an injury, and treating the elder like a child. Alternatively, the caregiver may show new affluence while withholding food or medication from the elder. Factors that lead to abuse are a lack of knowledge about normal aging, caregiver exhaustion, anger and frustration with the elder, financial problems, and drug and alcohol use by the caregiver. The elders who are most vulnerable are women who are widows or single and more than 75 years of age; those dependent on a caregiver for their shelter and food; and individuals who are frail, ill, incontinent, or mentally disabled.

Prevention activities include professional training of health care personnel, public education about elder abuse and its seriousness, and use of reliable assessment tools for the detection of abuse. The Elder Assessment Instrument developed by Fulmer is one accessible assessment for reviewing signs, symptoms, and subjective complaints of elder abuse, neglect, exploitation, and abandonment and is appropriate in all clinical settings (see http://consultgerirn.org/ for access to the tool). Nurses should report suspected abuse to the local Adult Protective Services through their state's hotline. Suggestions the community health nurse can give to the elder are to stay sociable, maintain friendships, and participate in senior citizen activities; have pension and Social Security checks deposited directly into bank accounts and obtain a durable power of attorney when no longer able to manage property and assets; consider coguardians so more than one person knows the elder's situation and can act on the elder's behalf; ask for help if needed; keep records, property, and a will in order; and plan ahead for possible disability. Community health nurses also should advise elders to avoid leaving cash, jewelry, and other valuables lying around visible; refuse to sign a document unless someone the elder trusts reviews it first; and resist letting anyone isolate them from others. Educational resources from the National Center on Elder Abuse (ncea.acl.gov/) may be useful.

Crime

Older adults are less likely to be victims of crime than teenagers and young adults; however, the older person who becomes a victim of a crime is more likely to be seriously hurt than someone who is younger. Crime against the elderly occurs in the form of robbery, purse snatching, pocket picking, car theft, and various scams (e.g. home repair, credit card fraud) (NIA, 2013).

The key to crime prevention for the senior is to be careful and alert to what is going on in the environment and to the types of crimes to which elders are vulnerable. The elderly person can take measures to lessen the risk of experiencing crime. In the home, safety measures include making sure that door and window locks are strong. Bars on doors and windows need to be installed with caution because they may increase the risk of harm in the event that public officials need to access the home during a fire or to assist the elderly person who may be ill or injured from a fall. The use of a safe deposit box should be recommended to store a list and pictures of expensive belongings and other important documents, such as a copy of the individual's will. Installation of a monitored alarm system with its accompanying outdoor security sign would also help deter criminals. Caution should always be used before answering the door.

Measures that elderly people should observe when out in the community are to stay away from unsafe places, to keep car doors locked and windows up at all times, and to park in well-lit areas. Inside pockets of clothing should be used for valuables such as a wallet, money, and credit cards. A purse should be carried close to the body and kept closed. In addition, the elderly person should be advised not to resist a thief, but to hand over immediately what the person is requesting.

Fraud is the crime that is frequently mentioned in the media as happening to elders. Older people are vulnerable to con games, insurance scams, home repair scams, and telephone scams. Types of Internet fraud include auction fraud, nondelivery of products ordered, securities fraud, credit card fraud, identity theft, bogus business opportunities, and unnecessary professional services. One strategy that can be recommended to seniors to prevent fraud from happening to them is to hang up the phone on telephone salespeople. The elder should request caller identification for the telephone; if no number or individual is identified, the elder may choose not to answer the call. No personal or financial information should be given over the phone unless the elder made the phone call. When in doubt about an inquiry or opportunity, the elder should be encouraged to say "no." The elder should check the references of anyone seeking to do home repairs and should be sure to obtain, in writing, the details of the work to be completed as well as the cost. A job should never be paid for in advance.

Identity theft is on the increase, and elderly individuals are particularly vulnerable. To avoid this problem, Social Security and monthly pension checks should be deposited directly into a bank account. Any information that is sent to the home with credit card offers, personal information, and so forth should be shredded so that the information cannot be used illegally. The elder should check bank statements and credit card account statements carefully for any discrepancies and report them immediately to the respective business. Caution should be used in using the Internet to buy products or pay bills because of websites without security (NIA, 2013).

> **?** **ACTIVE LEARNING**
>
> 1. Speak with police officers in a local community about elder abuse and crimes against elders. Identify community strengths and weaknesses. Discuss needs and solutions.
> 2. The family of your elderly client is considering taking his car keys from him. They asked you how to decide whether their loved one should stop driving. How would you respond?

PSYCHOSOCIAL DISORDERS

Psychosocial disorders account for a significant number of suicides, especially among older men. Depression is often likely to lead to suicide. The rate of Alzheimer disease increases with age. Alcohol and drug abuse are less common in older individuals but are still a concern. Depression and abuse of drugs and alcohol can coexist with one or more anxiety disorders. These conditions are discussed in the following sections.

Anxiety Disorders

Anxiety is a normal human emotion that everyone experiences at one time or another. For elderly individuals, normal age-related worries experienced are financial concerns, health problems, and reduced social interactions due to loss of friends through death and relocation, but these do not mean that the individual has an anxiety disorder. Anxiety disorders cause people to have feelings of intense fear and distress that prevent one from doing everyday tasks. Up to 15% of older adults are affected by anxiety disorders in a given year. (National Alliance on Mental Illness [NAMI], 2017). Anxiety disorders often occur with other mental or physical illnesses, including alcohol or substance abuse, depression, heart disease, diabetes, and other medical problems. The three most common types of anxiety disorders are generalized anxiety disorder, social phobia, and panic disorder (NIHseniorhealth.gov, 2016b).

Generalized anxiety disorder is characterized by excessive, exaggerated anxiety and worry about everyday events and is accompanied by physiological problems, including headaches, muscle tension, and nausea, (NAMI, 2017). The worry is often unrealistic or out of proportion to the real situation, because anxiety dominates the individual's thinking to such a point that it interferes with daily activities. Social phobia involves overwhelming worry and self-consciousness about everyday social activities. Worry centers on fear of being judged by others or fear of behaving in a way that might cause embarrassment. Panic disorder involves sudden, unexplainable attacks of terror and fear of impending doom or loss of control (NIHseniorhealth.gov, 2016b).

Anxiety disorders cannot be prevented. Some things that can be suggested to control or lessen symptoms are good diet, adequate sleep, regular exercise, reduced consumption of caffeine, and checking over-the-counter medicines or herbal remedies for any chemicals that can increase anxiety symptoms. Effective treatment for anxiety disorders includes a combination of counseling or psychotherapy, medications, and relaxation techniques (NAMI, 2017). The nurse can help elders realize that what they are experiencing does not need to interfere with their lives if they seek medical help.

Depression

Depression is a condition that interferes with daily life such as ability to work, sleep, concentrate, eat, and enjoy life (National Institute of Mental Illness[NIMH], 2016). It is a common problem among older adults, but it is not a normal part of aging. It may be overlooked as older adults experience death of loved ones, retirement, stressful life events, or health problems. The risk of depression in the elderly increases with other illnesses and when ability to function becomes limited. Estimates of major depression in older people living in the community range from less than 1% to about 5% but rises to 13.5% in those who require home health care and to 11.5% in hospitalized elders (CDC, 2017) Depression may last for days, weeks, months, or even years without treatment. It is a serious condition that increases the risk of death in the elderly population and may even lead to suicide. People with depression may experience several or all of the following symptoms: persistent (2 weeks or longer) sad, anxious, or "empty" mood; loss of interest or pleasure in hobbies or activities; feelings of hopelessness; pessimism; decreased energy; fatigue; difficulty concentrating or remembering; difficulty sleeping or oversleeping; appetite and/or unintended weight changes; thoughts of death or suicide; irritability; aches or pain; headaches; or digestive problems (NIMH, 2016). If any

BOX 19.6 Geriatric Depression Scale–Short Form

Choose the best answer for how you have felt over the past week:
1. Are you basically satisfied with your life? YES / **NO**
2. Have you dropped many of your activities and interests? **YES** / NO
3. Do you feel that your life is empty? **YES** / NO
4. Do you often get bored? **YES** / NO
5. Are you in good spirits most of the time? YES / **NO**
6. Are you afraid that something bad is going to happen to you? **YES** / NO
7. Do you feel happy most of the time? YES / **NO**
8. Do you often feel helpless? **YES** / NO
9. Do you prefer to stay at home, rather than going out and doing new things? **YES** / NO
10. Do you feel you have more problems with memory than most? **YES** / NO
11. Do you think it is wonderful to be alive now? YES / **NO**
12. Do you feel pretty worthless the way you are now? **YES** / NO
13. Do you feel full of energy? YES / **NO**
14. Do you feel that your situation is hopeless? **YES** / NO
15. Do you think that most people are better off than you are? **YES** / NO

Answers in **bold** indicate depression. Score 1 point for each bolded answer.
A score >5 points is suggestive of depression and should warrant a follow-up comprehensive assessment.
A score ≥10 points is almost always indicative of depression.

From Yesavage JA, Sheikh JI: Geriatric Depression Scale (GDS): recent evidence and development of a shorter version, *Clin Gerontol* 5(1/2):165–173, 1986; Yesavage JA: Geriatric Depression Scale, *Psychopharmacol Bull* 24(4):709–711, 1988; and Yesavage JA, et al.: Development and validation of a geriatric depression screening scale: a preliminary report, *J Psychiatr Res* 17(1):37–49, 1982–1983. Also available at <http://consultgerirn.org/uploads/File/trythis/try_this_4.pdf>.

of these symptoms exist, the client should be referred to his or her health care provider for diagnosis and treatment. Treatment consists of medication alone or medication with psychotherapy. How long depression lasts depends a great deal on identifying the condition and seeking treatment early. Depression is often undiagnosed or underdiagnosed. Delay in treatment in the elderly can be very dangerous.

Thus the community health nurse can play an important part in recognizing individuals who may be experiencing depression and who need to be referred for medical diagnosis and supervision. Short assessment tools such as the Geriatric Depression Scale–Short Form (Box 19.6) may be used to assess for this problem and assist the nurse in recognizing those at risk.

Substance Abuse

Data from the 2014 National Survey on Drug Use & Health sponsored by the Substance Abuse and Mental Health Services Administration (SAMHSA, 2015) revealed that 8.4% of the noninstitutionalized population 65 years and older currently smoke. According to the National Council on Alcoholism and Drug Dependence, Inc. [NCADD] (2015), 2.5 million older adults have alcohol or drug problems. Between 2013 and 2014, 14.9% of older adults had "binged" in the past month. A *binge drinker* is defined as a person who drinks five or more drinks on the same occasion on at least 1 day in the past 30 days.

Nearly 17 million prescriptions for tranquilizers are prescribed for older adults each year. Benzodiazepines are the most commonly misused and abused prescription medications

BOX 19.7   Cage Alcohol Screening Instrument

The CAGE screening test is short and simple to administer. Two or more positive answers are correlated with alcohol dependence in 90% of cases.

This screening instrument may not pick up problems in those who are fearful of negative consequences of disclosure, such as those looking for accommodation, people who are fearful of child protection agency staff, and those with mental health problems.

A short questionnaire about your alcohol use:

C: Have you ever thought you should **CUT DOWN** on your drinking?

A: Have you ever felt **ANNOYED** by others' criticism of your drinking?

G: Have you ever felt **GUILTY** about your drinking?

E: Do you have a morning **EYE OPENER**?

From National Institute on Alcohol Abuse and Alcoholism: *Assessing alcohol problems: a guide for clinicians and researchers,* ed 2 (NIH Pub. No. 03–3745), 2003. http://pubs.niaaa.nih.gov/publications/arh28-2/78-79.htm.

(NCADD, 2015). Opioid use is also increasing, and older adults are not immune to the opioid abuse crisis. Indeed, the Medicare population has among the highest and most rapidly growing prevalence of opioid use disorder (Lembke and Chen, 2016).

Many older adults with substance abuse problems are continuing a pattern of behavior or addiction that began earlier in life. Substance abuse that begins in later life may be due to losses associated with aging such as loss of family and friends, a job, retirement, failing health, or relocation. The warning signs of abuse are less obvious in older adults (NCADD, 2015). For example, many older adults are retired and drink alone at home so they are less likely to be noticed or get into trouble. Also, many of the diseases caused by substance misuse (e.g., hypertension, stroke, dementia, or ulcers) are common disorders in later life, so health care providers and family members may not recognize substance abuse as an underlying cause.

As a result of normal physiological changes discussed earlier in this chapter, older adults generally experience increased sensitivity and decreased tolerance to alcohol and drugs. Because of loss of body mass, reduced absorption rate in the gastrointestinal system, slower kidney function, and slower metabolism, drugs and alcohol remain in the body longer and at higher concentrations, thus prolonging and increasing their effects. The problem is compounded when alcohol and illicit drugs interact with prescribed or over-the-counter medications. This situation may be dangerous because the medications may have a stronger or weaker effect on the body.

Careful screening for such problems must include a thorough review of factors that may be directly affecting substance use and abuse. Several instruments have been utilized with the elderly population, including the CAGE, the Short Michigan Alcohol Screening Test—Geriatric Version (SMAST-G), and the Alcohol Use Disorders Identification Test (AUDIT). The CAGE is an easy-to-use, four-question interview (Box 19.7). The SMAST-G (10 questions) and AUDIT (10 items) are screening instruments that provide a more detailed description of alcohol use. All three of these instruments rely on client self-report.

If substance abuse is identified, the nurse should provide education about the increased health risks. Referral to addiction support groups, counseling or behavioral therapists, or addiction rehabilitation may be useful. Alcoholics Anonymous is a community peer self-help group that may be very beneficial; however, elderly individuals may believe that they do not fit into the group or may have differing concerns from those of younger members. In addition, they may have age-related mobility or hearing problems that prevent participation in peer self-help groups.

Suicide

Suicide, the act of intentionally taking one's own life, is a serious health concern that may be underreported among older adults. Omitted are "silent suicides," for example, deaths from medical noncompliance or overdoses, self-starvation or dehydration, and "accidents." The suicide rate is highest among men aged 75 and over (38.8 per 100,000), especially among white males (CDC, 2016c). Elderly individuals have a high success rate for suicide because they use firearms, hanging, and drowning. "Double suicides" involving spouses or partners occur frequently among the aged.

Elder suicide is associated with depression, chronic illness, physical impairment and medical conditions that significantly limit functioning or life expectancy, unrelieved pain, financial stress, loss and grief, social isolation, and alcoholism. Warning signs to watch for in the elderly are loss of interest in things or activities that are usually found enjoyable; social isolation; self-care neglect ; not following medical regimens (e.g., going off diets, not taking prescriptions); experiencing or expecting a significant personal loss (e.g., spouse or friend); feeling hopeless or worthless; putting affairs in order; giving things away; making changes in a will; and stockpiling medications or obtaining other lethal means of committing suicide. The most significant warning sign is any expression of intent. Risk factors that should also be considered in determining whether an elder might be at risk are previous suicide attempts, history of mental disorders, alcohol and substance abuse, family history of suicide, and local epidemics of suicide.

Prevention activities include dispelling any myths that exist relating to suicide. Myths that need to be discussed and debunked are that those who kill themselves must be crazy, asking someone about suicide can lead to suicide, and if someone is determined to kill himself or herself, no one can stop that person. Other prevention concepts are to promote awareness, develop broad-based support, reduce stigma associated with aging and being a consumer of mental health, urge use of psychiatric and mental health resources and suicide prevention services, develop community-based suicide prevention programs if none exist, reduce access to lethal means of self-harm, promote participation in education programs related to recognition of at-risk behaviors, and, lastly, promote and support research. The National Suicide Prevention Lifeline is available 24 hours/day, 7 days/week. 1-800-273-TALK (8255) and www.suicidepreventionlifeline.org.

Alzheimer Disease

Alzheimer disease (AD) is a slowly progressive brain disorder that begins with mild memory loss and progresses through stages to total incapacitation and eventually death. It is the sixth leading cause of death in the United States and the fifth leading cause of death among those 65 or older. An estimated 5.5 million

BOX 19.8 The Mini-Cog

Administration

1. Instruct the patient to listen carefully to and remember three unrelated words and then to repeat the words. The same three words may be repeated to the patient up to three tries to register all three words.
2. Instruct the patient to draw the face of a clock, either on a blank sheet of paper or on a sheet with the clock circle already drawn on the page. After the patient puts the numbers on the clock face, ask him or her to draw the hands of the clock to read a specific time. The time 11:10 has demonstrated increased sensitivity.
3. Ask the patient to repeat the three previously stated words.

Scoring (out of total of 5 points)

Give 1 point for each recalled word after the clock drawing test (CDT) distractor. Recall is scored 0–3.

The CDT distractor is scored 2 if normal and 0 if abnormal.

(Note: The CDT is considered normal if all numbers are present in the correct sequence and position and the hands readably display the requested time. Length of hands is not considered in the score.)

Interpretation of Results

0–2: Positive screen for dementia
3–5: Negative screen for dementia

From Borson S, et al.: The Mini-Cog: a cognitive "vital signs" measure for dementia screening in multi-lingual elderly, *Int J Geriatr Psychiatry* 15(11):1021–1027, 2000; Borson S, et al.: Improving identification of cognitive impairment in primary care, *Int J Geriatr Psychiatry* 21(4):349–355, 2006; and Lessig M, et al.: Time that tells: critical clock-drawing errors for dementia screening, *Int Psychogeriatr* 20(3):459–470, 2008. Copyright S. Borson. All rights reserved. Reprinted with permission.

Americans, mostly older adults, are living with AD (Alzheimer's Association, 2017a). The number of new cases of AD and other dementias is expected to increase as people are living longer. Diagnosing whether an individual has AD is very difficult, because the disease mimics conditions such as depression and other types of dementia. Usually, a tentative diagnosis is reached after all other conditions have been ruled out. The only sure way to diagnose AD is by autopsy, although cerebrospinal fluid analysis and magnetic resonance imaging are being investigated for their diagnostic accuracy. There is no cure, and limited treatment options are available.

A number of screening tools to assess for cognitive impairment have been developed. The clock drawing test (CDT) has become one of the most widely used cognitive screening instruments in clinical and research settings. It has been found to be an effective and easy-to-administer tool to screen for dementia. The CDT has also been incorporated into other widely used cognitive screening instruments such as the Mini Cog (Box 19.8). In addition to the CDT, the Mini Cog assesses for a three-item recall. The Mini-Mental State Examination is another tool used to assess for cognitive impairment. These tools may be accessed from www.consultgerirn.org.

Research is ongoing for development of a diagnostic test that could improve recognition of the disease in early stages, resulting in better management using available drugs and therapies. The U.S. Food and Drug Administration has approved five different drugs for treatment of AD. Aricept (donepezil), Exelon (rivastigmine), and Razadyne (galantamine) are cholinesterase inhibitors and are used to treat mild to moderate stages of the disease.

Namenda (memantine) is used for moderate to severe cases, and there is a new medication known as *Namzaric*, made from a combination of Aricept and Namenda (Alzheimer's Association, 2017c). These drugs appear to slow down memory loss, confusion, and problems with thinking and reasoning, but they do not stop the progression of the disease. Research regarding etiology, risk factors, diagnosis, treatment, and care issues continues.

The behavioral and physical changes due to AD create many challenges for caregivers, family, and friends. Some of the behavioral symptoms are agitation, aggression, wandering, and sleep disturbances. For the individual living alone, inadequate self-care, social isolation, falls, unattended wandering, and injuries occur in addition to problems such as fires from leaving the stove on and having the electricity turned off because bills have not been paid. Communication with a person with AD requires patience, understanding, and good listening skills. The Alzheimer's Association (2017b) provides useful communication strategies for the early, middle, or late stage of AD.

Management strategies for caring for the individual with AD include appropriate use of available treatment options, effective management of coexisting conditions, coordination of care among health care professionals and lay caregivers, participation in activities and adult day care programs, and taking part in support groups and support service such as counseling. Caregivers should contact the Alzheimer's Association for their many publications, experts, and local chapter programs. Medical supervision of the physical condition and medications (if clinically indicated) is essential. In addition, AD centers throughout the country offer diagnosis and treatment; provide information about the disease, services, and resources; and give volunteers an opportunity to participate in drug trials and other research projects. A number of resources are available for respite for the caregiver, support groups for both client and family, and day care facilities for the client. For the patient with AD who wanders, the local police should be informed of the potential problem, current pictures of the individual should be available, and safety measures such as installing locks and bells on doors should be taken.

ACTIVE LEARNING

You are asked to lead a 1-hour discussion (see following topic list) for a group of 10 seniors at a senior citizens' center. What would be your goal? What physiological aspects would you include? What psychosocial aspects would you consider?

- Issues related to urine control
- Fall prevention
- Prevention of influenza and pneumonia
- Medications and aging
- Normal aging changes

SPIRITUALITY

As people age and face life's challenges, such as loss of loved ones, declining physical health, and a realization that life's end may be near, spirituality may become more important (Ebersole and Touhy, 2016). Spirituality involves "finding core meaning in life, responding to meaning, and being in relationship with God/Other" (Manning, 2013). Spirituality is a broader concept than religion, encompassing a person's values or beliefs, search for meaning, relationships with a higher power, nature, and other people. It includes religion, which is defined as a social institution that unites people in a faith in God, a higher power, and in common rituals and worshipful acts (Ebersole and Touhy, 2016). More than 90% of older adults in the United States consider themselves religious or spiritual (Kaplan and Berkman, 2016).

RESEARCH HIGHLIGHTS

Spirituality and Depression

In a 2-year prospective study of 1992 depressed and 5740 nondepressed older adults (mean age 68.12), Ronneberg et al (2016) found that religiosity both protected against and helped individuals recover from depression. The older adults who were depressed at the beginning of the study were more likely to be depression-free at follow-up if they had been engaging in frequent private prayer. Those who were depression-free at the beginning of the study were more likely to remain depression-free at the end of the study if they attended religious services frequently.

Addressing the spiritual needs and concerns of a client is part of providing holistic nursing care. If nurses are comfortable with their own spirituality, they will be more attentive to the spiritual needs of their clients. Visible cues, such as the wearing of a religious article or the presence of religious symbols (e.g., Bible, Koran, rosary beads, prayer or inspirational books) can provide useful insights and a means to open discussion about spiritual needs (Eliopoulos, 2018). Furthermore, use of open-ended questions to begin dialogue about spiritual concerns and use of established spiritual assessments such as the FICA Spiritual History Tool (available at www.consultgerirn.org) are helpful. The FICA, which stands for faith, importance/influence, community, and address, provides nurses with a quick and simple means to conduct a spiritual assessment.

Nursing interventions that may be helpful in addressing spiritual needs include the nurse's presence, active listening, caring touch, reminiscence, prayer, hope, conveying a nonjudgmental attitude, facilitation of religious practices, and referral to spiritual care experts (Eliopoulos, 2018).

END-OF-LIFE ISSUES

Advance Directives

Decision making at the end of life is complex. Older adults often experience multiple chronic illnesses, some life threatening; therefore it is especially imperative that this population have advance directives. An older person who is approaching death may not be able to make end-of-life decisions. For such a person, confusion as to how to provide appropriate care may develop.

The Patient Self-Determination Act is a federal law enacted in 1990 that requires health care facilities that receive Medicare and Medicaid funds to ask patients on admission whether they possess an **advance directive** (Miller, 2015). There are three types of advance directives: the living will, do-not-resuscitate order, and durable power of attorney for health care. A **living will** is a legal document that allows individuals to specify what type of medical treatment they would or would not want if they became incapacitated or had an irreversible terminal illness. Living wills

can direct physicians to withhold life-sustaining procedures and can assist family members in making decisions when they are unable to consult a comatose or medically incompetent relative. An individual must be competent to initiate a living will, and he or she can revoke or change it at any time (Miller, 2015).

A **do-not-resuscitate (DNR)** order alerts medical personnel that the individual does not wish to have cardiopulmonary resuscitation in the event the person stops breathing and has no heartbeat. Individuals should place their requests on advance directive forms and inform their physicians. Afterward, a DNR order is written in the medical chart by the physician.

The **physician orders for life sustaining treatment (POLST)** paradigm is a nationally recognized program that promotes discussions about end-of-life care between patients and their health care professionals. The POLST paradigm is intended to support the medically-related wishes of patients who are frail or seriously ill and expected to die within a year. It specifically focuses on decisions made when patients are transitioning between facilities or for patients who live outside of a facilities. It differs from the DNR in that POLST forms are a physician's orders in a standardized format which communicates the patient's treatment wishes to emergency personnel. For more information on this program, see http://polst.org/.

A **durable power of attorney for health care** allows a competent individual to designate a health care proxy or surrogate to make decisions about medical care if the person becomes incapacitated. When an individual has no advance directive, is incompetent, or is unable to handle his or her affairs adequately, a guardian may be appointed by the court to direct the individual's medical treatment, housing, personal needs, finances, and property. Because the guardian manages all the individual's affairs and assumes legal rights, a **guardianship** is generally considered a last resort (Miller, 2015).

Advance directives not only make a person's wishes known but may also decrease the stress of decision making experienced by family members at the end of a loved one's life. State-specific advance directives can be ordered from the national organization Caring Connections or downloaded from its website (http://www.caringinfo.org/i4a/pages/index.cfm?pageid=1).

ETHICAL INSIGHTS

Making End-of-Life Decisions

Al Smith is 76 years old, lives alone, and suffered a massive stroke in his home. He was found by his older brother, Joe, who had come to visit him. Joe immediately called 911, and Al was rushed to a nearby hospital. Joe informed the health care providers at the hospital that he wanted everything done for his brother.

Complications from the stroke included irregular breathing, paralysis on one side of the body, aphasia, severe confusion, and problems with vision. Because of subsequent worsening of his breathing and nonresponsiveness, Al was started on ventilation therapy.

Joe called to inform their sister, Rose, who lives out of town, about the incident and condition of their brother. Rose was very upset with Joe for allowing Al to be connected to a ventilator. She claimed that Al would not have wanted this.

Questions
- What should Al Smith have done to make his wishes known?
- What discussion should his siblings have had to prevent disagreement?
- What are the ethical principles involved in this case?
- What are the legal implications?

The Nurse's Role in End-of-Life Issues

The nurse is encouraged to discuss and educate clients about end-of-life issues. These issues include advance directives and prefuneral considerations when death is imminent. When a client enters a health care facility with an advance directive, nurses should ensure that it is current and reflects the client's wishes. The nurse should inform other members of the health care team and make sure that the document is visible and accessible in the client's chart. The nurse should also encourage clients to discuss their wishes regarding the decisions in these documents with their families. Clients should provide copies of advance directives such as living wills to their family members in case of emergency. Furthermore, clients should discuss their living wills with their physicians so that the documents are made part of their medical records. A copy of advance directives should also be kept in the individual's automobile.

? ACTIVE LEARNING

Your elderly client has a terminal illness. You note that she does not have an advance directive. What issues surrounding this topic would you discuss with her?

CASE STUDY   Application of the Nursing Process

75-Year-Old Widow

Mrs. Darren, a 75-year-old widow, was referred to the community health nurse by her physician, who did not believe she could care for herself sufficiently. Her diagnoses were hypertension, mild congestive heart failure, arthritis, and occasional confusion after transient ischemic attacks.

During the initial home visit, the nurse observed that Mrs. Darren lived in a run-down house in an inner-city neighborhood. The roof leaked, and the house had no functioning heat unit. Mrs. Darren told the nurse that she did not have children and her only relative was a sister who lived with her family in another state. She was used to the neighborhood and knew her neighbors, but she was frightened of the teenagers who lingered when she took the bus to the supermarket .

Mrs. Darren received Supplemental Security Income, Medicare, Medicaid, and food stamps. She ate mostly bread and butter and drank coffee, but she enjoyed fried chicken and oranges after going to the supermarket. Constipation was sometimes a problem, and she took a laxative every night. She said she did not always remember whether she took her medication and held out a small bottle containing an assortment of pills of different colors, shapes, and sizes.

Assessment

With Mrs. Darren as the system, or central planning focus, the nurse identified her strengths and weaknesses and looked for actual or potential connections to her family and community . Considering aging theories, the nurse believed Mrs. Darren was undergoing disengagement from her physical and social circumstances and decided that this process might be reversed if her health could be maintained and her links to the community strengthened. On a practical level, the nurse also checked with Mrs. Darren's physician regarding the prescriptions and identified the assortment of pills by taking them to the pharmacist who filled them.

The nurse used a problem-solving approach to data gathering and identified Mrs. Darren's assets as the following:
- Being basically able to care for herself
  - Receiving medical treatment
  - Receiving income from various sources
  - Being accustomed to the neighborhood and knowing her neighbors

Her liabilities were more extensive:
- Inadequate nutrition
- Confusion with medications and improper use of laxatives
- Condition of the house, which was not supportive of health
- Threat of violence in neighborhood
- Physical impairment resulting from age and illness
- No children or other family living nearby
- Probable progression of confusion
- Possibility of a health episode at home while unattended

Diagnoses

Diagnoses and related short- and long-term goals address Mrs. Darren's situation. The nurse wrote plans at the three levels of prevention for the diagnoses and included suggestions for intervention with families.

Individual
- Inadequate nutrition, which was related to difficulty or inability to procure food
- Risk for exploitation due to possibility of theft, or fraud, aging, and progression of disease

Family
Potential for social isolation related to unanticipated loss of interaction with only relative who lives a distance away and Mrs. Darren's declining health.

Community
- Lack of knowledge regarding community resources for nutritional services and financial assistance
- Lack of support programs for medication consistency related to unrecognized need

Planning
Individual
Long-Term Goals
- Mrs. Darren will maintain a nutritionally adequate diet through self-care and use of community programs as evidenced by a steady weight and normal results on tests for nutritional status.
- in her medication regimen related to forgetfulness and mild confusion.
- Mrs. Darren will continue to take medications as ordered, as evidenced by stabilization of disease processes and intermittent demonstration to a nurse.
- Mrs. Darren will explore sheltered housing for older adults and continue contact neighborhood friends.

Short-Term Goals
- Mrs. Darren will improve her diet to include a recommended daily allowance of nutrients, including fiber and fluids, as evidenced by diet recall, and she will report regular bowel habits without use of laxatives.
- Mrs. Darren will utilize memory aids for a consistent medication regimen.
- Mrs. Darren will identify medications and know when to take them, as evidenced by demonstration to a nurse.
- Mrs. Darren will improve her home to allow healthy habitation, avoid victimization, expand her social network, and maintain health care appointments.

Family
Long-Term Goal
- Mrs. Darren will maintain family contact by mail, telephone, or possible visits.

continued

CASE STUDY   Application of the Nursing Process—cont'd

75-Year-Old Widow

Short-Term Goal

- Family members' addresses are included in Mrs. Darren's record to facilitate emergency contact.

Community

Long-Term Goals

- Promote publicity campaign to advertise nutritional services for older adults in the community.
- Support community pharmacists in the campaign to increase public awareness of the need to take medications as prescribed.
- Identify and support programs that will assist with provision of prescribed medications for people who have difficulty obtaining prescriptions because of a lack of insurance, money, transportation, or other problems.
- Have community groups work together to maximize use of resources.

Short-Term Goal

- Identify existing programs for older adults in the community.

Intervention
Individual

When the nurse discussed the nursing diagnoses and plans with Mrs. Darren, Mrs. Darren agreed with the short-term goals, but she was not sure that she wanted to leave her home for other housing and agreed to try to meet other people through community activities. During the the next few visits, the nurse explained basic nutritional principles and helped make a shopping list and menus for 1 week. Together, they developed a plan to assist with medication scheduling.

The nurse encouraged Mrs. Darren to talk about her earlier life. She had been widowed soon after her marriage, and she had never remarried. She lived in the neighborhood where she grew up, although it had deteriorated over the years. She had worked as a secretary until her retirement; there was no pension plan.

Family

Because Mrs. Darren's family did not live close by, the nurse worked to increase Mrs. Darren's social contacts by introducing her to a group that met frequently and offered several activities she might enjoy. If she were unexpectedly absent, the group would check on her. A neighbor invited her to a senior center, where she became involved in a domino-playing group.

Community

Referrals initiated by the nurse resulted in a greatly improved living situation. A home health aide from the same program came for half a day each week to assist with shopping and cleaning. A local Area Agency on Aging fixed her roof, and a church-sponsored group painted the house and cleaned the yard. A small heater was purchased from the Salvation Army store, and application was made to the utility company for help with bills during the winter months.

Evaluation
Individual

With the nurse as intermediary for and coordinator of community services, Mrs. Darren easily accepted help with the problems related to security. When her home improvements were completed, Mrs. Darren was able to maintain herself more comfortably with the help of the weekly visit from the home health aide.

Family

In the absence of family support, the establishment of an orderly routine, and safer financial arrangements increased Mrs. Darren's feelings of belonging and self-esteem. The nurse reduced her home visits but maintained contact with Mrs. Darren during her visits to the health clinic for blood pressure checks and preventive health care.

Community

Discussion with the home health aide informed the nurse of proposed funding cuts to the city's Supportive Services to the Elderly program, which would result in reduced services. The nurse spoke to the president of the district branch of the professional nurses' association. The association assisted the nurse in working with other local agencies for older adults to establish a publicity campaign against funding cuts through writing letters, speaking at public hearings on the city budget, and speaking at city council meetings. Although funds were reduced, the cuts were less severe than they would have been without the campaign, and most services were able to continue

Levels of Prevention
Primary Prevention

Goal: Promote good nutrition.

Individual

- Instruct about nutritional needs.
- Plan a shopping list and menus incorporating a prescribed diet for health problems.

Primary Prevention

Goal: Promote safety and prevention of injury.

Individual

- Provide immunizations as appropriate.
- Provide community services for assistance to maintain property and prevent deterioration.
- Encourage a network of friends and family members.

Family

- Provide services of community health nurse or case manager.
- Provide counseling.
- Provide respite care.

Community

- Provide community education programs for older adults.
- Be aware of potential hazards for older adult residents and provide intervention as needed.

Secondary Prevention

Goal: Assess and treat nutrition-related disorders.

Individual

- Provide referral for assessment of possible nutrition-related disorders.
- Provide hospitalization or prescribed nutritional supplements for illness resulting from inadequate nutrition.

Family

- Provide referral for nutritional assessment and counseling.

Community

- Encourage emergency food supplies.

Secondary Prevention

Goal: Diagnose and treat medication-related injuries.

CASE STUDY Application of the Nursing Process—cont'd

75-Year-Old Widow

Individual
- Provide referral for apparent overmedication or undermedication symptoms.
- Diagnose and treat drug or food reactions.

Family
- Reassess the client's understanding of medications.

Community
- Provide a 24-hour poison hotline.
- Provide an emergency department with 24-hour response.
- Provide medical services.

Tertiary Prevention

Goal: Maintain improved nutrition.

Individual
- Encourage use of community services.

Family
- Encourage exchange of family recipes.
- Encourage attendance at home economics classes.

Community
- Provide campaigns for nutritional awareness and healthy eating.
- Encourage healthy snacks in food machines.
- Encourage use of funding of community food services for emergencies.
- Encourage use of services providing access to food (e.g., food banks, Meals on Wheels, and food stamps).
- Encourage use of transportation to grocery stores or nutrition services.

Tertiary Prevention

Goal: Be consistent with prescribed medications and prevent medication error.

Individual
- When medications are dispensed, provide written and oral instructions at the level of understanding and in the language of the client.
- Have the client repeat instructions to the health care provider.

Family
- Have the client repeat instructions to family members.

Community
- Provide a community education program about understanding medications.

SUMMARY

Increasing life expectancy, coupled with the aging of the baby boomer generation, will cause a dramatic rise in the number of older adults. In addition to successful aging, older adults desire to function independently for as long as possible. This chapter has described aging, demographic characteristics, normal aging changes, health promotion and illness prevention interventions, common health and psychosocial concerns, end-of-life issues, and various resources that may assist older adults. Community health nurses should be aware of and address these issues and concerns so that they may help elders have a better quality of life.

EVOLVE WEBSITE

http://evolve.elsevier.com/Nies/community
- NCLEX Review Questions
- Case Studies

BIBLIOGRAPHY

Administration on Aging: *A profile of older Americans*, Washington, DC, 2016, U.S. Department of Health & Human Services. https://www.giaging.org/documents/A_Profile_of_Older_Americans__2016.pdf.

Alzheimer's Association: *2017 Alzheimer's disease facts and figures*, 2017a. www.alz.org/facts/.

Alzheimer's Association: *Communication and Alzheimer's*, 2017b. www.alz.org/care/dementia-communication-tips.asp#early.

Alzheimer's Association: *Medications for memory loss*, 2017c. www.alz.org/alzheimers_disease_standard_prescriptions.asp.

American Geriatrics Society: *AGS updated Beers criteria for potentially inappropriate medication use in older adults*, 2015. https://guideline.gov/summaries/summary/49933/American-Geriatrics-Society-2015-updated-Beers-Criteria-for-potentially-inappropriate-medication-use-in-older-adults.

Centers for Disease Control and Prevention: *Prevalence of incontinence among older Americans*, National Center for Health Statistics, 2014. http://www.cdc.gov/nchs/data/series/sr_03/sr03_036.pdf.

Centers for Disease Control and Prevention: *National health interview survey (NHIS)*, National Center for Health Statistics, 2015. www.cdc.gov/nchs/nhis.htm.

Centers for Disease Control and Prevention: *Web-based injury statistics query and reporting system (WISQARS)*, National Center for Injury Prevention and Control, 2016a.

Centers for Disease Control and Prevention: *Basic information about traumatic brain injury and concussion*, National Center for Injury Prevention and Control, 2016b. https://www.cdc.gov/traumaticbraininjury/basics.html.

Centers for Disease Control and Prevention: *Increase in suicide in the U.S., 1999-2014*, National Center for Health Statistics, 2016c. https://www.cdc.gov/nchs/products/databriefs/db241.htm.

Centers for Disease Control and Prevention: *Depression is not a normal part of growing older*, National Center for Chronic Disease Prevention and Health Promotion, 2017. https://www.cdc.gov/aging/mentalhealth/depression.htm.

Choi SK, Meyer IH: *LGBT aging: a review of research findings, needs, and policy implications*, Los Angeles, 2016, The Williams Institute. https://williamsinstitute.law.ucla.edu/research/lgbt-older-adults-highlighting-isolation-discrimination.

Cumming E, Henry W: *Growing old*, New York, Basic Books.

De la Fuente M: Role of neuroimmunomodulation in aging, *Neuroimmunomodulation* 15:213, 2008.

Ebersole P, Touhy T: Self-actualization, spirituality, & transcendence. In *Ebersole & Hess' Toward healthy aging: human needs & nursing response*, ed 9, St. Louis, 2016, Elsevier, pp 508.

Eliopoulos C: *Gerontological nursing*, ed 9, Philadelphia, 2018, Wolters Kluwer.

Federal Interagency Forum on Aging-Related Statistics: *Older Americans*, Washington, DC, 2016, Author. http://www.air.org/project/federal-interagency-forum-aging-related-statistics.

Havighurst RL, Neugarten BL, Tobin SS: Disengagement and patterns of aging. In Neugarten BL, editor: *Middle age and aging*, Chicago, 1968, University of Chicago Press.

Havighurst RL, Neugarten BL, Tobin SS: Disengagement, personality, and life satisfaction in the later years. In Hansen PF, editor: *Age with a future*, Copenhagen, 1963, Munksgaard.

Hayflick L: *How and why we age*, New York, 1996, Ballantine Books.

HealthinAging.org: *Sexual health*, 2017. http://www.healthinaging.org/aging-and-health-a-to-z/topic:sexual-health/.

Kaplan DB, Berkman BJ: *Religion and spirituality in the elderly*, 2016. https://www.merckmanuals.com/home/older-people%E2%80%99s-health-issues/social-issues-affecting-older-people/religion-and-spirituality-in-older-people.

Lembke A, Chen J: Use of opioid agonist therapy for medicare patients in 2013, *JAMA Psychiatry* 73(9):990–992, 2016.

Manning LK: Navigating hardships in old age: exploring the relationship between spirituality and resilience in later life, *Qual Health Res* 23(40):568–575, 2013.

Mauk K: *Gerontological nursing competencies for care*, ed 3, Boston, 2014, Jones and Bartlett.

Mayo Clinic Staff: *Cataracts*, 2016. www.mayoclinic.org/diseases-conditions/cataracts/symptoms-causes/dxc-20215129.

Mayo Clinic Staff: *Dry macular degeneration*, 2015a. http://www.mayoclinic.org/diseases-conditions/dry-macular-degeneration/home/ovc-20164874.

Mayo Clinic Staff: *Glaucoma*, 2015c. http://www.mayoclinic.org/diseases-conditions/glaucoma/basics/definition/con-20024042.

Mayo Clinic Staff: *Wet macular degeneration*, 2015b. http://www.mayoclinic.org/diseases-conditions/wet-macular-degeneration/home/ovc-20164274.

Mental Health America: *Preventing suicide in older adults*, 2017. www.mentalhealthamerica.net/preventing-suicide-older-adults.

Miller CA: *Nursing for wellness in older adults: theory and practice*, ed 7, Philadelphia, 2015, Wolters Kluwer.

Miller RA: The aging immune system: primer and prospectus, *Science* 273:70, 1996.

Morley A: The somatic mutation theory of aging, *Mutat Res* 338(1–6):19–23, 1995.

National Alliance on Mental Illness: *Anxiety disorders*, 2017. https://www.nami.org/Learn-More/Mental-Health-Conditions/Anxiety-Disorders.

National Council on Aging: *Chronic disease management*, 2017. https://www.ncoa.org/healthy-aging/chronic-disease/.

National Council on Aging: *Elder abuse facts*, 2017. https://www.ncoa.org/public-policy-action/elder-justice/elder-abuse-facts/#intraPageNav1.

National Council on Alcoholism and Drug Dependence, Inc: *Alcohol, drug dependence and seniors*, 2015. https://www.ncadd.org/about-addiction/seniors/alcohol-drug-dependence-and-seniors.

National Institute of Mental Illness [NIMH]: *Older adults and depression*, 2016. https://www.nimh.nih.gov/health/publications/older-adults-and-depression/qf-16-7697_153371.pdf.

National Institute on Aging: *Age page: crime and older people*, 2013. https://www.nia.nih.gov/print/health/publication/crime-and-older-people.

National Institute on Aging: *Age page: hyperthermia: too hot for your health*, 2017a. https://www.nia.nih.gov/health/publication/hyperthermia.

National Institute on Aging: *Age page: hypothermia: a cold weather hazard*, 2017b. https://www.nia.nih.gov/newsroom/2017/02/hypothermia-cold-weather-hazard.

National Institute on Aging: *Age page: taking care of your teeth and mouth*, 2016. https://www.nia.nih.gov/health/publication/taking-care-your-teeth-and-mouth.

National Institute on Drug Abuse: *Misuse of prescription drugs*, 2016. https://www.drugabuse.gov/publications/research-reports/prescription-drugs/trends-in-prescription-drug-abuse/-adults.

NIHseniorhealth.gov: *What is hearing loss?* 2016a. https://nihseniorhealth.gov/hearingloss/hearinglossdefined/01.html.

NIHseniorhealth.gov: *Anxiety disorders*, 2016b. https://nihseniorhealth.gov/anxietydisorders/aboutanxietydisorders/01.html.

NIHseniorhealth.gov: *How aging affects driving*, 2015. http://nihseniorhealth.gov/olderdrivers/howagingaffectsdriving/01.html.

Nurses Improving Care for Healthsystem Elders [NICHE]: *Our story*, 2017. www.nicheprogram.org.

Nutrition Screening Initiative: *Determine your nutritional health*, Washington, DC, Author.

Orgel LE: The maintenance of the accuracy of protein synthesis and its relevance to aging, *Proc Natl Acad Sci* 49:517–521, 1963.

Ronneberg CR, Miller EA, Dugan E, et al.: The protective effects of religiosity on depression: a 2-year prospective study, *Gerontologist* 56(3):421–431, 2016.

Shehab N, Lovegroe M, Geller A, et al.: U.S. Emergency department visits for outpatient adverse drug events, 2013-2014, *JAMA* 316(20):2115–2125, 2016.

Substance Abuse and Mental Health Services Administration: *Results from the 2014 National Survey on Drug Use & Health: summary of national findings*, Rockville, MD, 2015, Center for Behavioral Statistics & Quality.

Syme M: The evolving concept of older adult sexual behavior and its benefits, *Generations* 38(1):35–41, 2014.

Taylor CA, Bell JM, Breiding MJ, et al.: Traumatic brain injury–related emergency department visits, hospitalizations, and deaths — United States, 2007 and 2013, *MMWR Surveill Summ* 66(No. SS-9):1–16, 2017. https://doi.org/10.15585/mmwr.ss6609a1.

Taylor MF, Marquis R, Coall DA, et al.: The physical health dilemmas facing custodial grandparent caregivers: policy considerations, *Cogent Medicine* 4(1), 2017.

Touhy T, Jett K: *Ebersole & Hess' toward healthy aging: human needs & nursing response*, St. Louis, Elsevier.

Trail Ross ME, Kang DK, Cron S: Psychological profile, salivary cortisol, C-reactive protein, and perceived health of grandmothers with childrearing responsibility, *J Family Issues* 36(14):1904–1927, 2015.

U.S. Census Bureau: *Centenarians: 2010 census special reports (C2010SR-03)*, Washington, DC, 2012, U.S. Government Printing Office.

U.S. Department of Agriculture: *What is my plate?* 2017. www.choosemyplate.gov/MyPlate.

U.S. Department of Health and Human Services/Centers for Medicare and Medicaid Services (USDHHS/CMS): *Medicare and you*, 2017. www.Medicare.gov.

U.S. Department of Health and Human Services, Office of Disease Prevention & Health Promotion: *Healthy people 2020: leading health indicators*, Washington, DC, n.d., Author. https://www.healthypeople.gov/2020/Leading-Health-Indicators

U.S. Department of Health and Human Services, Office of Disease Prevention & Health Promotion: *Healthy people 2020: older adults*, Washington, DC, 2018, Author. https://www.healthypeople.gov/2020/topics-objectives/topic/older-adults

U.S. Fire Administration: *Fire in the United States 2005-2014*, ed 18, 2017. https://www.usfa.fema.gov/downloads/pdf/publications/fius18th.pdf.

World Health Organization: *Diet, nutrition and the prevention of chronic diseases*, Report of the joint WHO/FAO expert consultation, 2017. http://www.who.int/dietphysicalactivity/publications/trs916/summary/en/.

20

Family Health

Beverly Cook Siegrist and Tonya Bragg-Underwood

Family is not an important thing, it's everything.

Michael J. Fox

OUTLINE

OBJECTIVES

Upon completion of this chapter, the reader will be able to do the following:

1. Give a definition of *family.*
2. Identify characteristics of the family that have implications for community health nursing practice.
3. Describe strategies for moving from intervention at the individual level to intervention at the family level.
4. Describe strategies for moving from intervention at the family level to intervention at the aggregate level.
5. Discuss a model of care for families.
6. Apply the steps of the nursing process to individuals within the family, the family as a whole, and the family's aggregate.

KEY TERMS

Cohabitation
ecological framework
ecomap
expressive functioning
external structure
family

family health assessment
family health tree
family interviewing
general systems theory
genogram
instrumental functioning

internal structure
nuclear family
sandwich generation
social network framework
transactional model

To understand changing American families, many sociologists suggest that one needs to only view television and movies. Stereotypical television families have allowed American families to identify with developmental landmarks and to understand changing family demographics and structure. Whether one's view of families is parallel with *All in the Family, Family Ties,* or *Modern Family,* television shows illustrate that definitions of American families are unique, diverse, and ever changing.

TABLE 20.1	A Comparison of Families by Type in the United States 2003–2007	
	2003	**2007**
Married-Couple Households	50,130,111 (68%)	49,932,000 (69%)
Father-Only Households	4,425,000 (6%)	5,076,000 (7%)
Mother-Only Households	21,138,000 (31%)	22,282,000 (32%)
Children in Care of Grandparents	3,194,000 (4%)	3,457,000 (5%)
Children Living with Cohabiting Domestic Partners	4,186,000 (6%)	4,343,000 (6%)
Children Living with Neither Parent	4,126,000 (6%)	4,343,000 (6%)
Children Living in Married-Couple Immigrant Families	10,935,000	12,774,000
Children Living in Single-Parent Immigrant Families	2,944,000	3,680,000
Children Living in Single-Parent Immigrant Families (U.S.-born children)	17,967,000	18,602,000

From Annie E. Casey Foundation: *National kids county key indicators,* 2009. http:www.kidscount.org.

Legal definitions of family have tended not to keep current with modern representations of American families because the definitions have more to do with statistics. For example, the U.S. Census Bureau (2014) definition of family has remained basically unchanged since 1930:

> *A family includes a householder and one or more people living in the same household who are related to the householder by birth, marriage, or adoption…*

Although these definitions are important, is enough direction provided to health care providers who work with many families in many situations? In reality, modern families may be much more complex than families defined by statute or on television because of chronic health issues and the changing societal forces that are affecting the family in ways never before imagined by health care professionals. Table 20.1 provides a summary of the changes in family type by year.

A diverse American family, 2017.

CHALLENGES FACING U.S. FAMILIES

The dynamic forces affecting families are not new, but when combined result in new challenges to families and family nurses. For example, it is well documented that the increase in the number of aging Americans is expected to present new challenges to families and society. "The older population—persons 65 years or older—numbered 46.2 million in 2014. They represented 14.5% of the U.S. population, about one in every seven Americans. By 2060, there will be about 98 million older persons, more than twice their number in 2014. People 65+ represented 14.5% of the population in the year 2014 but are expected to grow to be 21.7% of the population by 2040" (U.S. Dept. of Health and Human Services [DHHS], 2016) . The oldest subgroup in this population is the "oldest-old," or those over 85 years of age, with the greatest increase in the 90- to 94-year-old age group (Werner, 2010). It should be noted that the older population comprises 23.1% of the total disease burden worldwide (World Health Organization [WHO], 2010). The largest U.S. disease increases in the over-60 age group are noted in the 2010 census as dementia (113%) and diabetes (79%) (Prince et al., 2013). Prince et al. (2013) also list the most burdensome (in cost and resources) diseases in this same population as ischemic heart disease, stroke, chronic obstructive pulmonary disease, and diabetes. When combined with the declining economy, the increasing population of aging persons has resulted in challenging living arrangements, draining economic resources, and growing numbers of families without sufficient health care coverage. Increasing numbers of elderly have created a **sandwich generation** or sandwich family structure, in which adults care for elderly parent(s) either in their homes or by providing financial support (Parker and Patten, 2013). Added to this financial burden is the number of adults also providing financial support to adult children. According to a report from the Pew Research Center (PRC) (2013), "47% of adults in their 40s and 50s have a parent aged 65 or older, are raising a young child, or financially supporting a grown child. And about one-in-seven middle-aged adults (15%) is providing financial support to both an aging parent and a child." The primary caregiver of the sandwich family also requires attention by health care providers. The increased stressors of caregiving, financial concerns, and related family and marital conflicts has resulted in reports of depression of between 20% and 50% for the caregiver, indicating a potential area of concern for health care providers (University of Michigan, 2016).

The financial burden of the cost of health care is a major challenge for families. The Patient Protection and Affordable Care Act (ACA), when implemented in 2010, made sweeping changes resulting in large numbers of families receiving health insurance either through expanded Medicaid programs or the availability of insurance markets offering lower insurance rates (Cantor et al., 2012). One popular change allowed families to insure dependent adult children up to the age of 26 on the family policy. Table 20.2 lists the changes implemented by the ACA by year.

One study found that the number of young adults (aged 19 to 25 years) who received health insurance increased by 2.5 million (Sommers and Schwartz as cited in Cantor et al., 2012). For

TABLE 20.2   ACA Provision Timeline, 2010–2015

Year	Provision
2010	• Dependents up to age 26 covered by parents • Patient-Centered Outcomes Research Institute (PCORI) created • Expansion of 340B drug discount • Health plans provide certain preventive services without cost sharing • Consumer protections take effect (no preexisting condition exclusions for children, lifetime limits, or rescinding coverage)
2011	• Prescription drug discounts • Free preventive care for senior citizens • Increased access to services at home and in the community
2012	• Incentives for physicians to form Medicare Accountable Care Organizations • Medicare Advantage plan payment reductions and bonuses • Annual fees imposed on pharmaceutical manufacturers • Medicare value-based purchasing program established • Medicare hospital readmissions penalties
2013	• Medicare bundled payment pilot program established • Temporary Medicaid payment increase for primary care • Medical device tax takes effect • Reduction in Medicare and Medicaid • Disproportionate Share Hospital payments • Medicaid expansion • Individual mandate takes effect • Essential health benefits package created • First individual exchange open enrollment period closes with approximately 8 million signed up • Additional consumer protections (no pre-existing condition exclusions, no annual limits)
2015	• Physician payment based on value, not volume • Delayed employer mandate takes effect

Data from Reisman M: The Affordable Care Act, five years later: policies, progress, and politics, *Pharm Ther* 40(9):575–600, 2015.

non–income-eligible families purchasing insurance through the health markets, the benefits included limits on cost, including out-of-pocket maximums (Abramowitz and O'Hara, 2014). Health care researchers are currently evaluating the possible impact of loss of health care insurance should current lawmakers repeal the ACA without new legislation. Eighty-one percent of those losing health care coverage will be in working families; 40% will be young adults; and 50% will be non-Hispanic white families. Family nurses must beware of the impact of not only the burden of the cost of health care but the impact of the loss of health care coverage (UI, 2016).

Globalization has also affected the family. In many areas manufacturing has replaced agriculture as primary employmentLoss of jobs results in financial decline, personal bankruptcies, and downward social mobility. All of these forces impact individual and family health.

The families described in Clinical Examples 20.1 through 20.4 depict broad contemporary definitions of family and are the kinds of families carried in caseloads by undergraduate community health nursing students. Assessments made by students during home, office, and hospital visits with these families triggered interventions that linked the families to resources provided by the community and, in turn, led to questions about health needs of groups of families or larger aggregates living in the same communities.

Clinical Example 20.1

Rebecca Martin is a 72-year-old widow of 10 years who lives in a rural town in Tennessee. She resides in the home that she and her husband purchased before his death. Her primary source of income is her deceased husband's Social Security benefits, and she also receives a small income from providing child care for infants at her church. Medicare benefits are her only source of payment for health care. Her only child, a daughter from whom she has been estranged for many years, recently died. The daughter was a never-married, single mother of an 8-year-old, medically fragile child with asthma. As the only surviving relative, Rebecca has become the custodial parent for her granddaughter.

Clinical Example 20.2

Joe Hudson is a 74-year-old alcoholic who is being treated at an outpatient department in a large medical center. He lives in a hotel room in downtown Salt Lake City, Utah. He has one living relative, a 76-year-old brother. Mr. Hudson states, "I had a falling out with my brother 20 years ago. I never hear from him. I reckon he's still in Boston, if he's alive at all." Mr. Hudson frequently falls out of bed, dislodging the telephone that the desk clerk has placed precariously close to the bed, which signals the desk clerk that something is amiss. The clerk then goes to Mr. Hudson's room and puts him back in bed. Mr. Hudson's source of income is a check sent to him the first day of each month by a minister who lives in a town 75 miles away. The desk clerk cashes Mr. Hudson's check and helps him pay his bill from the hotel, which provides congregate dining facilities.

Clinical Example 20.3

Lyn Nguyen is a refugee from Vietnam who moved with her family to San Francisco 3 months ago. Mrs. Nguyen is a single parent; Mr. Chan died in an automobile accident shortly after arriving in the United States. Mrs. Nguyen has two children, an 11-year-old son and a 5-year-old daughter. The family resides in a one-room efficiency apartment in the Tenderloin district in downtown San Francisco.

Clinical Example 20.4

Jaime Gutierrez, a 72-year-old Mexican American man, lives with his 36-year-old son, Roberto; his 34-year-old daughter-in-law, Patricia; and his three grandchildren, who are 14, 13, and 12 years of age. Mr. Gutierrez was in good health until he fell from a tree while helping his son make roof repairs on the house in 1995. He suffered a concussion, right hemothorax, and fracture of vertebrae T11 and T12. Confined to bed, he is receiving home health care. He requires intermittent catheterization but feels uncomfortable when the nurse suggests that his daughter-in-law is willing to carry out this procedure for him. Therefore Roberto quit work to provide this personal care to his father. Consequently, the family of six lives on Mr. Gutierrez's retirement income, which consists of $239 from Social Security and $244 from a pension plan per month. Roberto would like to improve his job skills while at home. He has finished the fourth grade and has failed the Graduate Equivalency Degree (GED) examination twice. Patricia also would like to return to school and pursue job training. Although agreeable to Patricia's interests, Roberto is hesitant to support active steps taken by Patricia to initiate her plan.

Working with families has never been more complex or rewarding than now. Nurses understand the actual and potential impact that families have in changing the health status of individual family members, communities, and society as a whole. Additionally, families have challenging health care needs that are not usually addressed by the health care system. Instead, the health care system most frequently addresses the individual. This holds true for nursing interventions within the health care system. This chapter helps the nurse understand and address complex issues that affect family health and suggests methods to improve family health.

UNDERSTANDING FAMILY NURSING

Family nursing is not a new concept and has been taught in schools of nursing since Nightingale's "district nursing" concept (Cook, 1913) and Lillian Wald's (1904) principles on how to nurse families in the home.

The family is composed of many subsystems and, in turn, is tied to many formal and informal systems outside it. The family is embedded in social systems that have an influence on health (e.g., education, employment, and housing). The International Family Nursing Association provides family characteristics that explain "why family nursing?" (2015):

Families have inherent competencies, strengths, and unique interactional processes that influence family health beliefs, goals, and actions. All families have the capacity for transforming their quality of life and family health. All verbal & non-verbal family communication is meaningful. All families possess a cultural heritage that is integral to family health and family life.

(p. 1)

These competencies explain the importance of including families as a population of interest for nurses. Many disciplines are interested in the study of families; interdisciplinary perspectives and strategies are necessary to understand the influence of the family on health and the influence of the broader social system on the family. This chapter addresses how community health nurses (CHNs) work with families within communities to bring about healthy conditions for families at the family, social, and policy levels. It focuses on the following five areas:

- The changing family
- Approaches to meeting the health needs of families
- The family theory approach to meeting the health needs of families
- Extending family health interventions to larger aggregates and social action
- An example of the nursing process applied to a family

THE CHANGING FAMILY

Definition of Family

Many definitions of **family** exist, such as the traditional definition from U.S. Census Bureau experiences. Definitions of family vary by professional discipline and the type of family described. For example, psychologists may define family in terms of personal development and intrapersonal dynamics; the sociologist has used a classic definition of family in terms of a "social unit interacting with the larger society." Other professionals have classically defined family in terms of kinship, marriage, and choice: "a family is characterized by people together because of birth, marriage, adoption, or choice" (Allen et al., 2000, p. 7). Friedman et al. (2003) incorporate the idea of many nontraditional definitions: "a family is two or more persons who are joined together by bonds of sharing and emotional closeness and who identify themselves as being part of the family" (p. 10). Again, this definition supports the idea of letting the family define their composition and relationships (Wright and Leahey, 2012).

Wright and Leahey (2012) state "the family is who they say they are" (p. 70). Current advocacy groups find these definitions even too narrow. The Human Rights Campaign (2017) urges that health professions acknowledge all types of families, even too narrow. The Human Rights Campaign (2014) urges that health professions acknowledge all types of families, including gay, lesbian, and even grandparents as heads of family by using this definition:

"Family" means any person(s) who plays a significant role in an individual's life. This may include a person(s) not legally related to the individual. Members of "family" include spouses, domestic partners, and both different-sex and same-sex significant others. "Family" includes a minor patient's parents, regardless of the gender of either parent . . . without limitation as encompassing legal parents, foster parents, same-sex parent, step-parents, those serving in loco parentis, and other persons operating in caretaker roles.
(Human Rights Campaign, 2017, Inclusive definition of family)

In the past, the dominant American definition focused on the intact **nuclear family**. African American families focus on a wide network of kin and community. The "nuclear" family does not exist for Italian families. To them, family means a strong, tightly knit, three- or four-generational group that includes godparents and old friends. Some families of early- (e.g., first- or second-) generation Chinese Americans go beyond this and include in their definition of family multigenerational family members and ancestors (Li et al., 2009).

The CHN interacts with communities made up of many types of families. When faced with great diversity in the community, the CHN must formulate a personal definition of family and must be aware of the changing definition of family held by other disciplines,

U.S. teen birth rate has fallen dramatically over time

Births per 1,000 females ages 15-19, 1940-2014

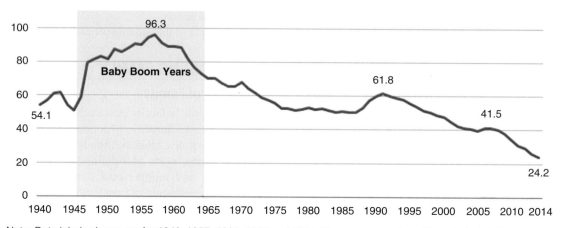

Note: Data labels shown are for 1940, 1957, 1991, 2007 and 2014. Teens younger than 15 not included. These data only account for live births and do not include miscarriages, stillbirths or abortions.

FIG. 20.1 U.S. teen birth rate has fallen. (From CDC National Center for Health Statistics: Births and natality, 2016. https://www.cdc.gov/nchs/fastats/births.htm.)

professionals, and family groups. The CHN who interacts with Mr. Hudson, the alcoholic described in Clinical Example 20.2 who lives in a hotel, must have a broad conceptualization of the family. That is, the group of people that the patient defines as significant for his or her well-being" (2005, p. 2).

Regardless of the accepted definition of family, what is evident is the importance of the family unit to society. The family fulfills two important purposes. The first is to meet the needs of society, and the second is to meet the needs of individual family members (Friedman et al., 2003). The family meets the needs of society through procreation and socialization of family members. "The basic unit (family) so strongly influences the development of an individual that it may determine the success or failure of that person's life" (Friedman et al., 2003, p. 4). The family is the "buffer" between individuals and society. The family meets individual needs through provision of basic needs (food, shelter, clothing, affection). The family supports spouses or partners by meeting affective, sexual, and socioeconomic needs. For children, the family is the "first teacher," instructing the children in societal rules and providing values needed for growth and development.

Characteristics of the Changing Family

The characteristics of the U.S. family continue to change. The PRC (Krogstad, 2014) found that 16.1% of the total U.S. population in 2012 lived in families composed of at least two adult generations or a grandparent and one other adult. PRC reported in 2014 a report that describes "5 Facts About the Modern American Family":

- Americans are putting off life's big milestones. The median age for first marriage is 29 for men and 27 for women compared with 2013 when more than one-in-four of people ages 18 to 32 years were married.
- Today, an American woman is expected to have 1.9 children. This is below what is considered 'replacement rate' of 2.1 children per woman.
- Three million (37% of lesbian, gay, bisexual and transgender [LGBT]) will have a child at some point in their life.

- Families are more blended today and constructed differently. Nearly 44% of young people ages 18 to 29 years have a step-sibling. More babies are born to unmarried women than ever before (5% in 1960).
- Intermarriage among people of different races is increasingly common. In 1980 there were only 7% of people who married a spouse of another race, and in 2010 this had doubled. (Krogstad, 2014, p.1)

The rate of **cohabitation**, which is defined as "a living arrangement in which an unmarried couple live together in a long-term relationship that resembles a marriage," has also increased over time (U.S. Census Bureau, 2008, 2011). The U.S. Census Bureau (2010) reported a 15% increase in the number of cohabitating families with significant changes in the family structure. The household more likely included at least an adult parent of one of the individuals, and it was more likely that one half of the couple was unemployed. This was a significant change from 2007 findings, in which both individuals were employed in more than half of the couples. It is hypothesized that this change is due to the economy (Pew Research Center, 2010). The nurse should be aware of the potential need for additional support and intervention with such families.

The birth rate among teenagers is the lowest it has been in four decades. During the years 1980 to 2006, the birth rate for unmarried women 15 to 17 years of age increased from 21 to 41.9 per 1000 in the United States, before dropping back 23% in 2012, resulting in a rate of 31.3 births per 1000 teens (Guttmacher Institute, 2016). The Annie E. Casey Foundation (2016) reports that the incidence of single teen parenting continues to rise in all ethnic groups. Single parenting is associated with greater risks because of reduced social, emotional, and financial resources, which affect the general well-being of children and families. In 2012, 34% of all U.S. children lived in single-parent homes. Single parenting is a key indicator of risk for well-being in children (Annie E. Casey Foundation, 2013). Fig. 20.1 provides an overview of the declining birth rate by age of mother.

The proportion of children younger than 18 years who are living with their grandparents has increased since 2007 (American Association for Marriage and Family Therapy [AAMFT], 2016). In 2007, grandparent-headed families accounted for 5% of all families; in 2016 census data document that 2.4 million grandparents are raising 4.5 million children (AAMFT, 2016). The American Academy of Child & Adolescent Psychiatry (2016) suggests that parenting by grandparents may be "due to serious societal issues and problems including increasing numbers of single parent families, the high rate of divorce, teenage pregnancies, AIDS, incarcerations of parents, substance abuse by parents, death or disability of parents, parental abuse and neglect" (p. 3).

The gay or lesbian family is made up of a cohabiting couple of the same sex who have a sexual relationship. The 2010 U.S. Census reports 594,000 same-sex couple households, 84% of which include children. A 2016 Gallup poll found that approximately 3% of adults in the United States are in same-sex married relationships and another 5% report same-sex cohabitation. This translate to 2 million U.S. adults in LBG relationships (Gallup, 2016). All of the described population groups have the potential to be considered families at risk for health problems and may require additional CHN interventions.

APPROACHES TO MEETING THE HEALTH NEEDS OF FAMILIES

Community health nursing has long viewed the family as an important unit of health care, with awareness that the individual can be best understood within the social context of the family. Observing and inquiring about family interaction enables the nurse in the community to assess the influence of family members on one another. However, direct intervention at the family rather than the individual client level is a new frontier for many nursing students, most of whom have experience in acute care settings before the community setting. A family model, largely a community health nursing or psychiatric–mental health intervention model, also includes the areas of birthing and parent–child interventions, adult day care, chronic illness, and home care. Nursing assessment and intervention must not stop with the immediate social context of the family; it must also consider the broader social context of the community and society. Friedman and colleagues (2003, pp. 5–6) suggest reasons why it is important for nurses to work with families:

The family is a critical resource: The importance of the family in providing care for its members has already been established. In this caregiver role, the family can also improve individual members' health through health promotion and wellness activities.

In a family unit any dysfunction (illness, injury, separation) that affects one or more family members will affect the members and unit as a whole: Also referred to as the *ripple effect,* changes in one member cause changes in the entire family unit. The nurse must assess each individual and the family unit.

Case finding is another reason to work with families: As the nurse assesses an individual and family, he or she may identify a health problem that necessitates identifying risks for the entire family.

Improving nursing care: The nurse can provide better and more holistic care by understanding the family and its members.

Moving from Individual to Family

The rationale of Friedman and colleagues (2003) for the importance of moving to family nursing is still relevant. Community health and home care nurses have traditionally focused on the family as the unit of service. With health care system changes throughout the United States, many CHNs continue to focus their practices on individuals residing in the home. As a result of the current era of cost containment, constraints on the CHN and on nurses working within hospitals and in other settings will increase. For example, reimbursement, which is almost entirely calculated for services rendered to the individual, is a major constraint against moving toward planning care for the family as a unit. However, current methods of reimbursing hospitals depend on keeping patients at home, so all nurses must consider the importance of not only the entire health care team but also the patient's family unit in meeting health and rehabilitation goals. Moving from individual to family nursing becomes more important than ever. Various creative approaches to meeting the health needs of families are needed, also reflecting interventions appropriate to the needs of the population as a whole.

Family Interviewing

Approaches to the care of families are needed and must be creative, flexible, and transferable from one setting to another. CHNs are generalists who bring previous preparation in communication concepts and interviewing to the family arena. Wright and Leahey (2012) proposed the realm of **family interviewing** rather than family therapy as an appropriate model. In this model, the CHN uses general systems and communication concepts to conceptualize the health needs of families and a family assessment model to assess families' responses to "normative" events such as birth and retirement or to "paranormative" events such as chronic illness and divorce. Intervention is straightforward, as in helping parents educate prepubescent teenage family members about sex by providing appropriate educational materials, or consists of making a referral to another health professional if the level of intervention is beyond the preparation of the nurse. For the purposes of this text, the model is extended to include intervention at the level of the larger aggregate. For example, the index of suspicion based on the health needs of a particular family would prompt the CHN to assess the need for similar information and the resources for intervention with other families in the community, schools, churches, or other institutions. Family interviewing requires thinking "interactionally," not only in terms of the family system, but also in terms of larger social systems.

Wright and Leahey (2005, 2012) identify the following critical components of the family interview: manners, therapeutic conservation and questions, family genogram (and ecomap when indicated), and commendations. Family theorists and practitioners suggest that, with experience, the nurse can accomplish the family interview in 15 minutes (Bell, 2012; Martinez et al., 2007; Wright and Leahey, 2012).

Manners. Manners are common social behaviors that set the tone for the interview and begin the development of a therapeutic relationship. Wright and Leahey (2012) believe that erosion of these social skills prevents the family nurse from collecting essential data. Many nurses argue that too much formality establishes artificial barriers to communication; however, studies have shown that the essentials of a therapeutic relationship begin with manners. The nurse introduces himself or herself by name and title, always addresses the client (and family members) by name and title (i.e., Mr., Mrs., or Ms., unless otherwise directed by client), keeps appointments, explains the reason for the interview or visit, and brings a positive attitude. Other behaviors (manners) that invite rapport include being honest with the client and checking attitude (the nurse's) before each client encounter.

Therapeutic Conversations. The second key element in the interview is the therapeutic conversation. This type of conversation is focused and planned and engages the family. The nurse must listen and must remember that even one sentence has the potential to heal or help a family member. The nurse encourages questions, engages the family in the interview and assessment process, and commends the family when strengths are identified. Every encounter, whether brief or extended, has "healing potential." Therapeutic conversation may initiate further discussion that brings the family together on issues (Wright and Leahey, 2012). Bell (2016) suggests that therapeutic conversations are "contextually sensitive to language, culture, setting, time available, and theoretical orientation" (p. 442) and are practiced and intentional.

Genogram and Ecomap. The genogram and ecomap constitute the third element and are described in detail later in this chapter. These tools provide essential information on family structure and together are an efficient way to gather information such as family composition, background, and basic health status in a way that engages the family in the interview process.

Therapeutic Questions. Therapeutic questions are key questions that the nurse uses to facilitate the interview. The questions are specific for the context or family situation but have the following basic themes (Wright and Leahey, 2012): family expectations of the interview or home visit; challenges, concerns, and problems encountered by the family at the time of the interview; and sharing of information (e.g., who will relate the family history or information).

Commending Family or Individual Strengths. The fifth element of the family interview is commending the family or individual strengths. Wright and Leahey (2012) suggest identifying at least two strength areas and, during each family interview, sharing them with the family or individual. Sharing strengths reinforces immediate and long-term positive relationships between the nurse and family. Interviews that identify and build on family strengths tend to progress to more open and trusting relationships and often allow the family to reframe problems, thereby increasing problem solving and healing (Wright and Leahey, 2012).

Issues in Family Interviewing. Creative family interviewing requires interviewing families in many types of settings. The prediction of decreased hospitalization, supplemented by a wide variety of health care settings ranging from acute to ambulatory to community centers, calls for flexible, transferable approaches.

Clinical settings for family interviewing are reviewed by Wright and Leahey (2012) and include inpatient and outpatient ambulatory care and clinical settings in maternity, pediatrics, medicine, surgery, critical care, and mental health. According to Wright and Leahey, CHNs have many opportunities besides the traditional home visit to engage the family in a family interview. CHNs are employed in ambulatory care centers, occupational health and school sites, housing complexes, day care programs, residential treatment and substance abuse programs, and other official and nonofficial agencies. At each of these sites, CHNs meet families and can assess and intervene at the family and community levels.

The family interview assists the nurse in identifying family health risks because the family experiences similar risk factors (i.e., physiological, behavioral, and environmental). Studies have documented the familial predisposition to the three major diseases resulting in morbidity and mortality in the United States: cardiac disease, cancer, and diabetes. Family health practices also influence lifestyle habits among family members. Recognizing the importance of a family health history related to individual and public health, the U.S. Surgeon General initiated the National Family History Initiative in 2003 with a goal to educate individuals about inherited predispositions to disease (McNeill et al., 2008). This website has proved to be successful in engaging American families in learning about their family history and familial and genetic health risk for family members. The project was renamed "My Family Health Portrait Tool" and has been redesigned to be more user friendly for individuals (USDHHS, 2017). Another example would be a Hispanic American family in which a family member has diabetes; the nurse could implement a family health promotion plan based on the needs of the individual within an at-risk family. The family plan for diabetes prevention is based on the nurse's understanding that the National Institutes of Health (NIH) reports that this group has the second highest rate of diabetes among a nonwhite ethnic group in the United States (Spanakis and Golden, 2013) (Table 20.3).

Involving family members in newborn assessments can aid the CHN in determining the family's adjustment to the newborn and parenthood. The nurse can do this in the home, clinic, or other health care center. Family members should be involved during the first contact or visit, and, if they do not attend, a

TABLE 20.3 Age-Adjusted Prevalence of Diabetes Mellitus in the United States by Race/Ethnicity in Adults >20 Years of Age

Race/Ethnic Group	Age-Adjusted Prevalence
Non-Hispanic whites	7.1
Asian Americans	8.4
Hispanic Americans overall	11.8
Non-Hispanic Blacks	12.6
Alaskan Natives	5.5
Native Americans	33

From Spanakis E, Golden SH: Race/ethnic differences in diabetes and diabetes complications. *Curr Diab Rep* 13(6), 2013, https://doi.org/10.1007/s11892-013-0421-9.

telephone call explaining the nurse's interest in them should take place (Wright and Leahey, 2012).

Children and parents in these families need a chance to express their concerns; the family interview is important and may provide the nurse with necessary information needed to care for these families.

Intervention in Cases of Chronic Illness

The Centers for Disease Control and Prevention (CDC) (2017) reports that as many as 90% of families are dealing with chronic illness in a family member. Chronic disease is responsible for 7 to 10 deaths, and the care of chronic disease uses 86% of the nation's health care costs (CDC, 2017). For the family with a member who has a chronic illness, it is important to the individual's and family's adjustment, as well as to the patient's symptom management, that the family is prepared to be emotionally and physically supportive. The CHN can intervene to assist the family coping with related stressors. Also significant is the fact that a resource such as third-party reimbursement forces most families to learn to manage the chronic problems with limited or infrequent intervention from health professionals. The CHN working with families coping with chronic illness in a child, adult, or older adult is aided by the family interview. As Glaser and Strauss (1975) stated, chronic illness injects change into various areas of family life:

> Sex and intimacy can be affected. Everyday mood and interpersonal relations can be affected. Visiting friends and engaging in other leisure time activities can be affected. Conflicts can be engendered by increased expenses stemming from unemployment and the medical treatment . . . [D]ifferent illnesses may have different kinds of impact on such areas of family life, just as they probably will call for different kinds of helpful agents.
>
> (p. 67)

Changes in family patterns, fears, emotional responses, and expectations of individual family members can be assessed in the family interview. Special needs of the primary caretaker (i.e., often the spouse, daughter, or daughter-in-law) can be assessed. The CHN making family visits to older adults and the terminally ill is able to assess intergenerational conflict and stress and positively influence family interaction (Wright and Leahey, 2012).

Moving from Family to Community

The health of families can affect the health of society as a whole, in both positive and negative ways. The health of a community is measured by the well-being of its people and families. Circumstances such as low-birth-weight infants, lack of health insurance, homelessness, violence, poverty, and low employment rates provide a description of families and nations. CHNs provide family nursing to improve individual and family health; however, the potential result may be improving the health of society. The care of entire populations is the major focus, as stated by Freeman (1963) in her classic work, *Public Health Nursing Practice*:

> The selection of those to be served . . . must rest on the comparative impact on community health rather than solely on the needs of the individual or family being served . . . The public health nurse cannot elect to care for a small number of people intensely while ignoring the needs of many others. She must be concerned with the population as a whole, with those in her caseload, with the need of a particular family as compared to the needs of others in the community.
>
> (p. 35)

The challenge to the CHN is to provide care to communities and populations and not to focus only on the levels of the individual and the family. The CHN, who traditionally carries a caseload of families, extends his or her practice to the community. To do so, an aggregate, community, and population focus must serve as a backdrop to the entire practice.

For example, families must be viewed as components of communities. The CHN must know the community. As stated in previous chapters, a thorough community assessment is necessary to practice in the community. By way of review, the nurse must remember that communities must be compared not only in terms of different health needs but also in terms of different resources to effect interventions that influence policies and redistribute resources to ensure that community and family health needs are met.

CHNs must then compare city data with county data and then county data with state data and national data. In addition, they may need to compare local census tract data and areas of a city or county with other areas of the city or county. For example, community health nursing students in San Antonio, Texas, who were planning home visits to families of pregnant adolescents attending a special high school compared local, state, and national statistics on infant mortality rates as part of a community assessment. They found higher rates of infant mortality in San Antonio in census tracts on the south side of the city, in which the population was predominantly Mexican American. They also found this population to be younger, to have a higher rate of functional illiteracy among adults, to be less educated, to be more likely to drop out of high school, to have higher fertility rates, to have higher birth rates among adolescents, and to be more likely to be unemployed. They found that specific health needs varied among census tracts. Common major health needs of this subpopulation were identified from the community assessment, which helped the students plan care for these families. For example, their goals were broadened from carrying out interventions at the individual level to interventions at the family and community levels. In addition to targeting good perinatal outcomes for the individual teenage parent, nursing students planned to include assessments of functional literacy at the individual and family levels and arranged for group sessions in clinic waiting rooms that offered information about and referral of individuals and family members to alternative resources to enable teenage parents to complete school, take classes in English as a second language, and use resources for family planning and employment at the community level.

In addition to the cross-comparison of communities, the CHN cross-compares the needs of the families within the communities and sets priorities. The nurse in the community finds that specific health needs vary among families. The nurse must account for time spent with families and choose those families on the basis of their needs in comparison with the needs of others in the community.

 HEALTHY PEOPLE 2020

Access to Health Care

In relation to improving family health, all of the leading health indicators listed as priorities in *Healthy People 2020* can serve as a guide for family nursing interventions. Access to quality health care affects every aspect of family nursing because it affects prevention of disease and disability, quality of life, preventable death, and overall life expectancy. The objectives for measurement of this goal include the following:

- Increase the proportion of persons with health insurance.
- Increase the proportion of insured persons with coverage for clinical preventive services.
- Increase the proportion of persons with a usual primary care provider.
- Increase the proportion of persons who have a specific ongoing care.

This chapter has discussed the disparities that exist among families and populations with regard to health care access. The community nurse should use political skills, advocacy, and education to influence policy that will result in increased access to health care. The nurse can educate families about available resources and help communities develop resources to improve health care access.

Data from U.S. Department of Health and Human Services: *Healthy People 2020: objectives*. https://www.healthypeople.gov/2020/topics-objectives/topic/Access-to-Health-Services/objectives. Accessed February 12, 2018.

Delegation of Scarce Resources

Although the CHN serves the community or population as a whole, fiscal constraints hold the nurse accountable for the best delegation of scarce resources. Time spent on home visits has traditionally allowed the CHN to assess the environmental, social, and biological determinants of health status among the population and the resources available to them. Fiscal accountability, nevertheless, means setting priorities. In 1985, Anderson and colleagues listed the factors that influence public health nursing practice, especially home visits, as "the need to justify personnel costs in a time of fiscal constraint, the increasing number of medically indigent who turn to local public health services for primary care, and the change in reimbursement mechanisms by the federal government and some states" (p. 146). These observations still hold true. In 2009, more than 46 million Americans, including 9 million children, lacked health insurance (Robert Wood Johnson Foundation, 2009). In 2010 the number of uninsured rose to 49.9 million, or 16.3% of the U.S. population; however, in 2011 there was a drop to 48.6 million (U.S. Census Bureau, 2013). This drop is attributed to the increase in the number of young adults ages 19 to 26 who could for the first time remain on their parent's primary insurance following graduation from college. The Children's Health Insurance Program (CHIP) of 1997 has greatly increased access to health care for many low-income children. When the CHIP program was initiated, there were 10 million children in the United States and 14% were uninsured; in 2008, 7.4 million children were enrolled in state CHIP plans (Centers for Medicare and Medicaid Services, 2015). The majority of these children lived in families with working, low-income parents. On February 4, 2009, President Obama signed the Children's Health Insurance Program Reauthorization Act, which renewed and expanded coverage of CHIP from 7 million children to 11 million children. The Affordable Care Act of 2010 keeps the CHIP program in place until 2019 (Medicaid.gov, n.d.).

ACTIVE LEARNING

Define the term *family* with a group of three colleagues. Compare definitions and list similarities and differences. Develop a list of criteria for being a member of a family.

APPROACHES TO FAMILY HEALTH

Many schools of thought regarding the approaches to meeting family health needs exist among community health, community mental health, and public health nursing professionals. Dreher (1982) wrote that the traditional basis for community health nursing intervention has a focus that has long endorsed psychological and social-psychological theories to explain variations in health and patterns of health care, such as those set forth by Erikson (1963), Maslow (1970), and Duvall (1977). Dreher (1982) stated that what is needed are "more encompassing theories which explain the relationship between society and health [and] the policies which will be most effective in assuring health and health care" (p. 508). To help bridge this gap, four frameworks for meeting family health needs are presented here: family theory, systems theory, structural-functional conceptual framework, and developmental theory.

Family Theory

Many reasons exist for why the CHN should work with families. Friedman (1998) listed the following six reasons:

- Any "dysfunction" (e.g., separation, disease, or injury) that affects one or more family members probably affects other family members and the family as a whole (Clinical Example 20.5).
- The wellness of the family is highly dependent on the role of the family in every aspect of health care, from prevention to rehabilitation.
- The level of wellness of the whole family can be raised through care that reduces lifestyle and environmental risks by emphasizing "health promotion, 'self-care,' health education, and family counseling" (p. 5).
- Commonalities in risk factors and diseases shared by family members can lead to case finding within the family.
- A clear understanding of the functioning of the individual can be gained only when the individual is assessed within the larger context of the family.
- The family as a vital support system to the individual member needs to be incorporated into treatment plans.

Nurses have relied heavily on the social and behavioral sciences for approaches to working with families. These approaches include psychoanalytical, anthropological, systems or cybernetic, structural-functional, developmental, and interactional frameworks (for reviews, see Friedman et al., 2003, and Wright and Leahey, 2012). The use of a framework for assessing a family helps the nurse understand the health potential for the family. Three conceptual frameworks (systems, structural-functional, and developmental), often used by nurses in providing health care to families, are described here. These models help the nurse empower the family in the process of family health promotion.

Clinical Example 20.5

Ten-year-old Jean Wilkie was referred by her teacher to the school nurse. She was withdrawn, had no school friends, and was dropping behind in her schoolwork. The school nurse talked to Jean in her office. Jean said that she had no friends because the other girls stayed overnight with one another "all the time" and that she did not want to bring her friends home because her father "drank all the time." The school nurse decided that Jean's problems needed assessment within the context of the family and arranged to visit the family at home. The father refused to participate in the family interview, but Jean's mother, her 13-year-old brother Peter, and Jean expressed concerns that the father had changed jobs several times in the past year, was frequently absent from work, and had been in two recent car accidents while "drinking." The school nurse was able to verify the family context as the basis of Jean's "problems," continue her family assessment, and plan for intervention at the family level. In addition, she was prompted to assess the community's preventive efforts directed toward drinking and the ability to provide ongoing care for families of alcoholics.

Systems Theory

The systems approach has been used in such diverse areas as education, computer science, engineering, and communication. General systems theory (Minuchin, 2002; von Bertalanffy, 1968, 1972, 1974) has been applied to the study of families. General systems theory is a way to explain how the family as a unit interacts with larger units outside the family and with smaller units inside the family (Friedman et al., 2003). The family may be affected by any disrupting force acting on a system outside the family (i.e., suprasystem) or on a system within the family (i.e., subsystem). Parke (2002) stated that there are three subsystems of the family that are most important: parent–child subsystem, marital subsystem, and sibling–sibling subsystem. Dunst and Trivette (2009) reviewed 20 years of systems theory and its importance to early childhood interventions, adding that systems theory provides direction for understanding how health care providers can expand family capacity by changing parenting and therefore changing child behaviors. Table 20.4 presents definitions of the major terms used in the systems approach.

The past two decades have resulted in what many sociologists identify as imposing community subsystems with actual or potential negative influence on the family system. These include communities where violence has become the norm, dangers related to community-acquired diseases—both manmade and natural, disasters, biohazards, and so on. These subsystems have the potential to complicate the care planned by the CHN and require interventions from several subsystems interacting with the family system and community. It is important that the CHN understand systems theory as a tool for both assessing families and communities and identifying resources and support services for families.

Characteristics of Healthy Families

Otto (1973) and Pratt (1976) characterized healthy families as "energized families" and provided descriptions of healthy families to guide the assessment of strengths and coping. DeFrain (1999) and Montalvo (2004) helped identify healthy families. These writers suggest the following traits of a healthy family:

- Members interact with one another; they communicate and listen repeatedly in many contexts.
- Healthy families can establish priorities. Members understand that family needs are priority.
- Healthy families affirm, support, and respect each other.
- The members engage in flexible role relationships, share power, respond to change, support the growth and autonomy of others, and engage in decision making that affects them.
- The family teaches family and societal values and beliefs and shares a religious core.
- Healthy families foster responsibility and value service to others.
- Healthy families have a sense of play and humor and share leisure time.
- Healthy families have the ability to cope with stress and crisis and to grow as a result of positive coping. They know when to seek help from professionals.

Structural-Functional Conceptual Framework

With the structural-functional conceptual framework approach, the family is viewed according to its structure, or the parts of the system, and according to its functions, or how the family fulfills its roles.

Structural

Wright and Leahey (2005, 2012) stated that three aspects of family structure can be examined (internal structure, external structure, and context). Internal structure of the family refers to the following five categories:

- Family composition, the family members, and changes in family constellation
- Gender
- Rank order, or positions of family members by age and sex
- Subsystem, or labeling of the subgroups or dyads (e.g., spouse, parental, and interest) through which the family carries out its functions
- Boundary, or who participates in the family system and how he or she participates (e.g., a single-parent mother who does not allow her 17-year-old son to have his girlfriend spend the night in their home)

TABLE 20.4 Major Definitions From Systems Theory

Term	Definition
System	"A goal-directed unit made up of interdependent, interacting parts which endure over a period of time" (Friedman, 1992, p. 115). A family system is not concrete. It is made up of suprasystems and subsystems and must be viewed in a hierarchy of systems. The system under study at any given time is called the focal, or target, system. In this chapter, the family system is the focal system.
Suprasystem	The larger system of which the family is a part, such as the larger environment or the community (e.g., churches, schools, clubs, businesses, neighborhood organizations, and gangs).
Subsystem	Smaller unit within the family, such as the relationship between spouses, parent and child, sibling and sibling, or extended family.
Hierarchy of systems	The levels of units within the system and its environment, which, in their totality, make up the universe. Higher-level units are composed of lower-level units (e.g., the biosphere is made up of communities, which are made up of families). Families are made up of family subsystems, and, in turn, family subsystems are made up of individuals, who are made up of organs, which are made of cells, which are made of atoms.
Boundary	An imaginary definitive line that forms a circle around each system and delineates the system from its environment. Auger (1976) conceptualized the boundary of a system as a "filter" that permits the constant exchange of elements, information, or energy between the system and its environments. "The more porous the filter, the greater the degree of interaction possible between the system and its environment" (p. 24). Families with rigid boundaries may lack information necessary and resources pertinent to maintaining family health or wellness.
Open system	A system that interacts with its surrounding environment and gives outputs and receives inputs necessary to survival. An exchange of energy occurs. All living systems are open systems. However, if a boundary is too permeable, the system may be too open to input of new ideas from the outside and may be unable to make decisions on its own (Wright and Leahey, 1994).
Closed system	A system that theoretically does not interact with the environment. This is a self-sufficient system; no energy exchange occurs. Although no system has been found that exists in a totally closed state, if a family's boundaries are impermeable (i.e., less open as a system), needed input or interaction cannot occur. An example is a refugee family from Vietnam living in San Francisco; they may remain a closed family for some time because of their differences in culture and language.
Input	Information, matter, or energy that the open system receives from its environment that is necessary for survival.
Output	Information, matter, or energy dispensed into the environment as a result of receiving and processing the input.
Flow and transformation	The system's use of input may occur in two forms. Some input may be used in its original state, and some input may have to be transformed before it is used. Both original and transformed input must be processed and flow through the system before being released as output (Friedman, 1992).
Feedback	"The process by which a system monitors the internal and environmental responses to its behavior (i.e., output) and accommodates or adjusts itself" (Friedman, 1992, p. 117). The system controls and modifies inputs and outputs by "receiving and responding to the return of its own output" (Friedman, 1992, p. 117). Internally, the system adjusts by making changes in its subsystems. Externally, the system adjusts by making boundary changes.
Equilibrium	A state of balance or steady state that results from self-regulation or adaptation. As with the concept of a system as a mobile in the wind, balance is dynamic and, with change, is always reestablishing itself.
Differentiation	The tendency for a system to actively grow and "advance to a higher order of complexity and organization" (Friedman, 1992, p. 117). Energy inputs into the system make this growth possible.
Energy	Energy is needed to meet a system's demands. Open systems require more input through porous boundaries to meet the high energy levels necessary to maintain high levels of activity.

External structure refers to the extended family and larger systems (Wright and Leahey, 2005). It consists of the following two categories:

- Extended family, including family of origin and family of procreation
- Larger systems, such as work, health, and welfare

Context refers to the background or situation relevant to an event or personality in which the family system is nested (Wright and Leahey, 2005, 2012). It comprises the following five categories:

- Ethnicity
- Race
- Social class
- Religion
- Environment

Functional

Wright and Leahey (2005, 2012) also dichotomized family functional assessment, or how family members behave toward one another, into two categories: instrumental functioning and expressive functioning. **Instrumental functioning** refers to routine activities of daily living (e.g., elimination, sleeping, eating, giving insulin injections) (Box 20.1). This area takes on important meaning for the family when one member of the family becomes ill or disabled, is unable to carry out daily functions, and must rely on other members of the family for assistance (Clinical Example 20.6). For example, an older adult may need assistance getting into the bathtub, or a child may need to have medications measured and administered.

The second type of family functional assessment is **expressive functioning**, or affective or emotional aspects. This aspect has the following nine categories:

- *Emotional communication*: Is the family able to express a range of emotions, including happiness, sadness, and anger?
- *Verbal communication* focuses on the meaning of words. Do messages have clear meanings rather than distorted meanings? Wright and Leahey (2005, 2012) gave the example of

BOX 20.1 Summary of Family Functional Assessment

Instrumental functioning (i.e., activities of daily living)
Expressive functioning
    Emotional communication
    Verbal communication
    Nonverbal communication
    Circular communication
    Problem solving
    Roles
    Influence
    Beliefs
    Alliances and coalitions

Data from Wright LM, Leahey M: *Nurses and families: a guide to family assessment and intervention,* ed 2, Philadelphia, 1994, FA Davis.

BOX 20.2 Family Life Cycle

1. Leaving home
2. Beginning family through marriage or commitment as a couple relationship
3. Parenting the first child
4. Living with adolescent(s)
5. Launching family (youngest child leaves home)
6. Middle-aged family (remaining marital dyad to retirement)
7. Aging family (from retirement to death of both spouses)

Adapted from Duvall EM, Miller BC: *Marriage and family development,* ed 6, New York, 1985, Harper and Row; and Carter B, McGoldrick M: *The expanded family life cycle: individual, family, and social perspectives,* Boston, 2005, Pearson Allyn & Bacon.

masked criticism when a father states to his child, "Children who cry when they get needles are babies."

- *Nonverbal communication,* which includes sounds, gestures, eye contact, touch, or inaction. An example is a husband remaining silent and staring out the window while his wife is talking to him.
- *Circular communication* is commonly observed between dyads in families. A common example is the blaming, nagging wife and the guilty, withdrawn husband.
- *Problem solving* refers to how the family solves problems. Who identifies problems? Someone inside or outside the family? What kinds of problems are solved? What patterns are used to solve and evaluate tried solutions?
- *Roles* refers to established patterns of behavior for family members (Wright and Leahey, 2000, 2012). Roles may be developed, delegated, negotiated, and renegotiated within the family. It takes other family members to keep a person in a particular role. Formal roles, with which the larger community agrees, may come into conflict with roles set by family members and influenced by religious, cultural, and other belief systems.
- *Influence* refers to methods used to affect the behavior of another. Instrumental influence is the use of reinforcement via objects or privileges (e.g., money or use of technology tools). Psychological influence is the influence of behavior through the use of communication or feelings. Corporeal control is the use of body contact (e.g., hugging and spanking).
- *Beliefs* refer to assumptions, ideas, and opinions that are held by family members and the family as a whole. Beliefs shape the way families react to chronic or life-threatening illness. For example, if a family of a person with colon cancer believes in alternative treatments, then acupuncture may be a viable option.
- *Alliances and coalitions* are important within the family. What dyads or triads appear to occur repeatedly in the family? Who starts arguments between dyads? Who stops arguments or fighting between dyads? Is there evidence of mother and father against child? When does this change to parent and child against the other parent? The balance and intensity of relationships between subsystems within the family are important. Questions may be asked regarding the permeability of the boundary. Does it cross generations?

Clinical Example 20.6

When Edna Smith, a 64-year-old client with severe arthritis, received a diagnosis of diabetes, her longtime friend, Frank Gardens, a widower of several years, moved in with her and assumed a caregiver role. The community health nurse assessed the dietary habits of Mr. Gardens and Mrs. Smith and found that Mr. Gardens did the shopping and the cooking because Mrs. Smith's mobility was severely restricted by her arthritis. Mr. Gardens did the cooking; therefore he purchased canned fruits and vegetables rather than fresh or frozen. Mr. Gardens perceived cooking, which was a new role for him, as demanding. After several visits, he disclosed to the nurse that his resistance to preparing fresh or frozen fruits and vegetables came from "the time it takes to clean the darn things, cook 'em, store 'em, and clean up the fridge when they go bad on ya." He stated unequivocally that it was stressful caring for Mrs. Smith and that he wanted to do it, but it was "much easier" to just "open a can" and "heat it in a pan" than to take the time and energy that preparation of fresh or frozen foods would require. The shift in roles that is often required of couples when a chronic illness is diagnosed in one can have an influence on the health of the family. Lubkin and Larsen (2013) provide additional reading about how couples manage with chronic illness.

Developmental Theory

Nurses are familiar with developmental states of individuals from prenatal through adult. Duvall, a noted sociologist, is the forerunner of a focus on family development (Duvall and Miller, 1985). In her classic work, she identified stages that normal families traverse from marriage to death (Box 20.2).

To assess the family, the CHN must comprehend these phases and the struggles that families experience while going through them. Wright and Leahey (2005, 2012) called attention to the need to distinguish between "family development" and "family life cycle." They stated that the former is the individual, unique path that a family goes through, whereas the latter is the typical path many families go through.

The developmental categories listed in Box 20.3 outline the six stages of the middle-class North American family life cycle (Carter and McGoldrick, 1988; Wright and Leahey, 2005) and the tasks necessary for the family's resolution of each stage. Nurses may use the stages to delineate family strengths and weaknesses.

RESEARCH HIGHLIGHTS

Work Hours and Perceived Time Barriers to Healthful Eating Among Young Adults

Young adults, though identified as underinsured and having limited access to primary care, are also identified as a group knowledgeable about the benefits of healthy eating. This age group (20 to 31 years) has been confirmed in numerous national surveys as not regularly engaging in healthy eating habits, especially eating fewer than the recommended daily servings of fruits and vegetables and consuming a diet high in fast foods. Earlier studies among college students identified the following barriers: cost, stress, lack of knowledge related to food preparation, peer influence, and lack of time to balance busy lives.

A population study survey involved responses from 2287 individuals who were originally among a population of 4776 high school juniors and seniors participating in a program called Project EAT-III (Eating and Activity in Teens and Young Adults), a program that looked at dietary intake, weight control, and weight control behaviors during 1998 and 1999. Ten years later, the original participants were mailed letters asking them to participate in a new questionnaire, to which 1030 men and 1257 women agreed. Information was collected on time-related beliefs and behaviors about healthful eating, their fast-food intake, fruit and vegetable intake, work hours, and sociodemographics.

This group reported time-related beliefs such as being too rushed to eat breakfast, eating on the run, and no time to eat healthy. They reported eating fast food weekly. Working at least 40 hours per week was associated with an increase in time-related poor eating habits for men but not for women. Recommendations included workplace programs—free fruit and vegetables for break, flex time, and other interventions.

Data from Escoto KH, et al: Work hours and perceived time barriers to healthful eating among young adults. *Am J Health Behav* 36(3):786–789, 2012.

ASSESSMENT TOOLS

There are many tools for the CHN to use in assessing the family (Butler, 2008; Friedman et al., 2003; Wright and Leahey, 2005, 2012). Reviewed here are the genogram, family health tree, and ecomap. The nurse can use these tools for assessment with families in every health care setting. They help increase the nurse's awareness of the family within the community and help guide the nurse and the family in the assessment and planning phases of care.

Genogram

The **genogram** is a tool that helps the nurse outline the family's structure. It is a way to diagram the family. Generally, three generations of family members are included in a family tree, with symbols (Fig. 20.2) denoting genealogy. Children are pictured from left to right, beginning with the oldest child.

The CHN may use the genogram during an early family interview, starting with a blank sheet of paper and drawing a circle or a square for the person initially interviewed. The nurse tells the family that he or she will ask several background questions to gain a general picture of the family. The nurse may draw circles around family members living in separate households.

For example, as depicted in the Case Study at the end of the chapter, family order across generations can be illustrated and specific personal characteristics can be noted in the drawing (Fig. 20.3). Mr. and Mrs. Garcia do not speak English, a factor that will be of importance to the nurse as he or she plans nursing interventions. At times, the usefulness of the genogram is

BOX 20.3   Stages and Tasks of Middle-Class North American Family Life Cycle

I. Launching: single young adult leaves home
   A. Coming to terms with the family of origin
   B. Development of intimate relationships with peers
   C. Establishment of self: career and finances
II. Marriage: joining of families
   A. Formation of identity as a couple
   B. Inclusion of spouse in realignment of relationships with extended families
   C. Parenthood: making decisions
III. Families with young children
   A. Integration of children into family unit
   B. Adjustment of tasks: child rearing, financial, and household
   C. Accommodation of new parenting and grandparenting roles
IV. Families with adolescents
   A. Development of increasing autonomy for adolescents
   B. Midlife reexamination of marital and career issues
   C. Initial shift toward concern for the older generation
V. Families as launching centers
   A. Establishment of independent identities for parents and grown children
   B. Renegotiation of marital relationship
   C. Readjustment of relationships to include in-laws and grandchildren
   D. Dealing with disabilities and death of older generation
VI. Aging families
   A. Maintenance of couple and individual functioning while adapting to the aging process
   B. Support role of middle generation
   C. Support and autonomy of older generation
   D. Preparation for own death and dealing with the loss of spouse and/or siblings and other peers

Data from Wright LM, Leahey M: *Nurses and families: a guide to family assessment and intervention,* ed 2, Philadelphia, 1994, FA Davis.

limited by how freely the family member relates significant information such as divorces and remarriages and family health concerns. Other families may be sensitive to the sharing of such information, particularly when it is shown to recur with each generation. For example, a family history of alcohol or substance abuse or depression may be a sensitive issue. For other families, the development of the genogram is an excellent opening to the discussion of family history or hereditary health problems, or highlights the need for health education and promotion.

Family Health Tree

The **family health tree** is another tool that is helpful to the CHN. Based on the genogram, the family health tree provides a mechanism for recording the family's medical and health histories (Butler, 2008; Friedman 2003, 1992; USDHHS, 2010, 2017). The nurse should note the following information on the family health tree:

- Causes of death of deceased family members
- Genetically linked diseases, including heart disease, cancer, diabetes, hypertension, sickle cell anemia, allergies, asthma, and mental retardation
- Environmental and occupational diseases
- Psychosocial problems, such as mental illness and obesity
- Infectious diseases

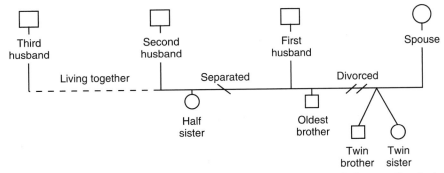

FIG. 20.2 Commonly used genogram symbols. (Redrawn from Genopro Software: *Symbols used in genograms, 2016.* www.genopro.com.)

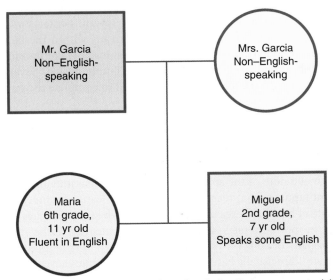

FIG. 20.3 Sample genogram of the Garcia family (see case study).

- Familial risk factors from health problems
- Risk factors associated with the family's methods of illness prevention, such as having periodic physical examinations, Papanicolaou smears, and immunizations
- Lifestyle-related risk factors (elicited by asking what family members do to "handle stress" and "keep in shape")

The family health tree can be used in planning positive familial influences on risk factors such as diet, exercise, coping with stress, and the pressure to have a physical examination. The USDHHS (2017), under the direction of U.S. Surgeon General Richard Carmona, launched the Family History Initiative. Included in this

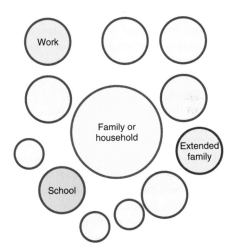

FIG. 20.4 Ecomap. (Redrawn from Hartman A: Diagrammatic assessment of family relationships, *Soc Casework* 59:496, 1978.)

initiative is an online interactive tool, My Family Health Portrait, to help families learn about their risk for disease (www.hhs.gov/familyhistory). Included are questions to ask family members about common diseases, questions that suggest health promotion activities, and goals as established in *Healthy People 2020*. When completed, the "family tree" can be printed. This tool could be incorporated into the family assessment and utilized by the nurse to plan family interventions to improve health.

Ecomap

The **ecomap** (Fig. 20.4) is another classic tool that is used to depict a family's linkages to their suprasystems (Hartman, 1979; Wright and Leahey 2000, 2005, 2012). As originally stated by Hartman (1979),

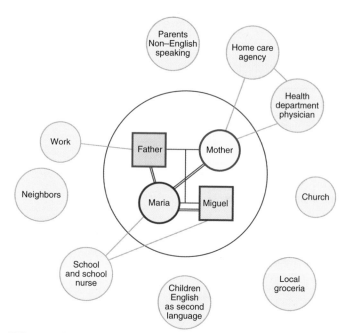

FIG. 20.5 Sample ecomap of the Garcia family (see Case Study).

The ecomap portrays an overview of the family in their situation; it depicts the important nurturant or conflict-laden connections between the family and the world. It demonstrates the flow of resources, or the lacks and deprivations. This mapping procedure highlights the nature of the interfaces and points to conflicts to be mediated, bridges to be built, and resources to be sought and mobilized.

(p. 467)

As with the genogram, the nurse can fill out the ecomap during an early family interview, noting people, institutions, and agencies significant to the family. The nurse can employ symbols used in attachment diagrams (see Fig. 20.2) to denote the nature of the ties that exist. For example, in Fig. 20.5, the sample ecomap of the Garcia family suggests that few contacts occur between the family and the suprasystems. The community health nursing student was able to use the ecomap to discuss with the Garcia family the types of resources available in the community and the types of relationships they wanted to establish with them.

 ACTIVE LEARNING

Complete a personal genogram. What are the high-risk factors in the family history? Current risk factors? Categorize current risk factors into physical, interpersonal, and environmental. Identify needed health education and determine who needs the education. Identify sources of appropriate screening in the community for the identified risk factors.

Complete a personal ecomap. Is the family an "open" or "closed" family system? What resources do families currently use for mental, physical, emotional, social, and community health? What referrals are needed?

FAMILY HEALTH ASSESSMENT

Many agencies in the community have developed guidelines for assessment of the family that help practitioners identify the health status of individual members of the family and

aspects of family composition, function, and process. Often included in family health assessment guidelines is information about the environment, or community context, and information about the family. A **family health assessment** form can be used as a guide to help the nurse with both collection of data and organization of the data collected from families over time.

The nurse can obtain information for the family health assessment through interviews with one or more family members individually, or with interviews of subsystems within the family (e.g., mother–child, parent–parent, and sibling–sibling dyads. The nurse can also obtain information through observing the environment in which the family lives, including housing, the neighborhood, and the larger community.

Family assessment tools are used with many health disciplines and are useful to assess a range of dimensions of the family, such as marital satisfaction, parental coping abilities, and family dysfunction.

The family health assessment addresses family characteristics, including structure and process and family environment (i.e., residence, neighborhood, and community). Not all dimensions of the family health assessment will be appropriate for every family; therefore the nurse should modify content of the assessment guidelines and adapt it as necessary to fit the individual family. The guidelines are a means to record pertinent information about the family that will assist the nurse in working with them. The nurse should gather information in the assessment spontaneously over several contacts with the family and various members and dyads within the family. It should also include multiple forays into the community, neighborhood, and home in which the family resides. Several contacts with the family will be required to complete the family health assessment.

Social and Structural Constraints

In addition to the tools just reviewed, an important aspect of family assessment and planning for intervention is the need to make note of the social and structural constraints that prevent families from receiving needed health care or achieving a state of health. These constraints explain why some families differ in mortality rates, ability to achieve "integrity" rather than "despair," or ability to "self-actualize." Social and structural constraints are usually based on social and economic causes, which affect a wide range of conditions (e.g., literacy, education, and employment) associated with major health indicators (i.e., mortality and morbidity rates). Families frequently served by the CHN are disadvantaged in that they lack the financial resources to purchase health care. However, constraints to obtaining needed health and social services are well documented and may come from characteristics of health and social services rather than individual family limitations. The nurse can note these constraints on the ecomap because they influence each family's ability to interact with a specific agency. For example, in addition to noting the strength of the relationship between family and agency or institution, the nurse should note those constraints that prevent use of the resource. Constraints include hours of service, transportation, availability of interpreters, and criteria

FAMILY HEALTH ASSESSMENT: THE GARCIA FAMILY

The school nurse, Jana, works with multiple city schools, including this inner-city school, which has a low-income, ethnically diverse population.

Jana assesses the community as she drives to the Garcias' home, noting the availability of resources such as the local groceria.

Local churches are a community resource, offering socialization and spiritual support for immigrant families such as the Garcia family.

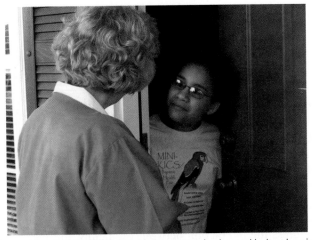

Jana arrives at the Garcias' home. Maria answers the door and invites Jana in.

Jana completes the family assessment of the Garcia family with the help of Maria as interpreter for Mrs. Garcia. Mrs. Garcia listens intently as Jana asks questions about the family's health needs.

Jana reviews the plan of care and confirms the family's commitment to the plan of care they developed with her.

for receiving services (e.g., age, sex, and income barriers). Specific examples are the different guidelines posed by each state for Medicaid and by each community for home-delivered meals to the homebound.

Helping families understand constraints and linking them to accessible resources is necessary, but intervention at the family level is not sufficient. The common basic human needs of families in a community add up, and the CHN must tally structural constraints faced repeatedly by families and compare them with those faced by families in other communities. The nurse can then plan and implement interventions at the aggregate level. The following section is an overview of how CHNs can extend intervention at the family level to larger aggregates and social action.

 ACTIVE LEARNING

Identify family types or situations (e.g., families of different cultures, gay or lesbian families, or never-married-mother families) that elicit "discomfort" in working situations. Identify ways to overcome barriers in working with these types of families.

EXTENDING FAMILY HEALTH INTERVENTION TO LARGER AGGREGATES AND SOCIAL ACTION

Institutional Context of Family Therapists

Many theories exist to help bridge the gap between the application of nursing and family theory to the family and broader social action on behalf of communities of families. Most family theorists view the family as a system that interfaces with outside suprasystems or institutions only when a problem is to be addressed, such as in the school or a courtroom. The following three approaches go beyond the family as a system to address the interaction between the family and the larger social system:

- Ecological framework
- Network therapy
- Transactional model

Ecological Framework

The ecological framework is a blend of systems and developmental theory that focuses on the interaction and interdependence of humans (families) as biological and social beings with the environment. Using this framework the CHN would assess the family as a system within the context of its environment. Bronfenbrenner (2005) identified four basic systems that make up our ecological environment. The microsystem is our immediate environment that supports our development—the family, school, church, etc. The environment interacts with "age, health, sex, [and] genetic predispositions." The mesosystem recognizes the links between two or more microsystems and the individual. The exosystem includes those settings or institutions that may not directly come in contact with an individual but still influence development in less direct ways, such as government agencies, what is happening in the world, and the media. Lastly, there is the chronosystem, or the future development. This takes into account the notion of time.

What happens to the individual and family over time depending on events, and so on (Smith and Harmon, 2011)?

This approach explains the results of health care specialization and fragmentation of care based on Western concepts of time and space. It focuses on providing a more complex and flexible structure. For example, Kogan and colleagues (2004) investigated parent–health care provider discussions of family and community health risks during well-child examinations. Additionally, they studied the gaps between the issues discussed by the practitioner and the information the parent desired. On the basis of the results of the National Survey of Early Childhood Health, health topics for discussion were identified, including family financial difficulties, the presence of a support partner, parent's emotional support, alcohol and/or drug use in the home, cigarette smoking in the home, the parent's physical health, and community violence. Cigarette smoking was discussed nearly 80% of the time, and alcohol and drug use was discussed 45% of the time; however, community violence was discussed less than 10% of the time, and financial needs 12%. The results indicate the need for better communication and education between health care providers and clients.

Social Network Framework

The social network framework (Christakis and Fowler, 2011) is based on earlier network therapy work involving all the connections and ties within a group. In network theory, an identified family member feels marginalized and seeks to replace the family network with others from the wider system to provide more support, hoping to enhance his or her role or functioning in the family. The concept of social network in this instance is related to social support. "Social network refers to a weblike structure comprising one's relationships and social support focuses on the nature of the interactions taking place within social relationships" (Friedman et al., 2003, p. 462). A family's social network includes friends, community groups, church, and agencies. Social network also can be explained as the structure of relationships, and social support as the function of relationships. Examples of network therapy are drawn from community mental health. In the social network framework, a *group* is defined as a collection of individuals with a common attribute. A social network is composed of connected groups. A network has structure (also called *typology*); contagion that flows across connections (e.g., money, violence, fashion, organs, obesity, etc.); connection, who is connected to whom (e.g., family, friends, colleagues); and homophily, or the tendency we have to be with those who are similar to ourselves. To some extent individuals and families control the density of our connectedness, our centrality to the group, and how we are viewed by others. This model has been used to explain health-related issues, such as the spread of sexually transmitted diseases and the obesity epidemic in the United States. It has also been used to understand the issue of hyperconnectivity and technology. The PRC (2014) states that the average adult Facebook user has 338 friends; younger Facebook users, aged 18 to 29, tend to have about 500 friends in their network.

Perhaps then, using the research on social marketing, the CHN needs to become familiar with the use of social networks and other technology to ensure individuals and families have accurate health information. Rsearchers have found that individuals with the following demographics are more likely to seek medical answers online: women, younger, white, income of $75,000 or more, and a college degree. Fifty-nine percent of Americans looked online for health information in 2012 (Parker and Patten, 2013), and the majority began with a search engine, such as Google, Bing, or Yahoo, instead of a website that a CHN might identify as a reliable source such as the NIH or the CDC. Nearly one half of this group was seeking a diagnosis; these individuals are called *online diagnosers*. Thirty-eight percent of this group believed that they could take care of the problem at home and did not seek the advice of a health professional (Parker and Patten, 2013). This presents new issues for the CHN, such as teaching families how to evaluate appropriate online sites.

Transactional Model

In the **transactional model**, the term *transaction* refers to a system that focuses on family processes. The family as an institution, along with other institutions (e.g., religious, educational, recreational, or governmental), is culturally anchored (i.e., each holds a distinct set of beliefs and values about the nature of the world and human existence). An awareness of culture (e.g., beliefs and values) as it is expressed in each system is important (i.e., as it is expressed in mainstream U.S. values versus the value patterns of the family).

VanderValk and colleagues (2007) used a transactional model to explore the relationship between parental marital distress and adolescent emotional adjustment. In a 6-year prospective study of 531 parent–adolescent dyads, they found such a relationship, especially for late adolescent and young adult girls and less so for males. The findings suggest that "girls' greater sensitivity to interpersonal problems may be reciprocal and that the parental marriage is still associated with adjustment for girls in late adolescence and early adulthood" (p. 130).

Models of Care for Communities of Families

Models exist to guide the CHN in providing care to communities of families in special need of services that improve access, equality between consumer and provider, and sensitivity to human need. There is generally an increase in the number and type of models that emerge as traditional public and private models of health care decline due to shrinking funding and resources. Many of the programs develop as the result of community efforts or partnerships with existing health care providers. The following are examples of such models.

The Kentucky Partnership for Farm Family Health and Safety

The Kentucky Partnership is a community coalition, originally funded by the W. K. Kellogg Foundation, involving farm families, universities, and various community-based organizations.

The coalition was originally established to improve the health of farm families in rural Kentucky. Farming is identified as one of the most dangerous occupations in the United States, and few resources have been developed to support the unique needs of farm families. The Partnership identified farm women as the primary "health officers" for farm families. The farm women were provided with opportunities to develop skills in leadership, conflict resolution, and team building. Nurse educators and nursing students provided health education and assisted the farm women in developing a self-sustaining structure to support their efforts to improve family health. Cardiopulmonary resuscitation and first aid classes, the development of unique emergency medical subsystems, and other activities helped improve the health of the farm families. The local members reported an increase in personal knowledge, self-esteem, and personal satisfaction through the Partnership efforts. The Kentucky Partnership for Farm Family Health and Safety continues to affect the health of farm families in south-central Kentucky. The efforts are supported through the help of the South Central Kentucky Area Health Education Center at Western Kentucky University. The coalition has been replicated in three states (Texas, Louisiana, and Florida) and continues to connect universities and farm families in research efforts. Outcome assessment research was conducted to evaluate the impact of the coalition efforts on farm family health (Palermo and Ehlers, 2001; Siegrist and Jones, 2005). This organization continues as a positive force improving the health of farm families. In 2017, they provided an annual Farm Safety Day Camp for area children and screening and education for farm families on such topics as preventing work-related accidents, tractor safety, and chronic disease management and prevention. The Farm Safety Day Camp is funded in part by the *Progressive Farmer* magazine and is duplicated in five other states. Since 1995 the day camps have educated more than 100,000 children (Progressive Farmer, 2017).

The Health Access Nurturing Development Services Program

The Health Access Nurturing Development Services (HANDS) program is a voluntary home visitation program for any new parent targeting at-risk families that include first-time parents. Implemented through interdisciplinary teams consisting of social workers, nurses, and parent resource persons, the program serves first-time pregnant mothers and their families. HANDS was originally funded through tobacco settlement monies allocated through the state legislature to the Kentucky Cabinet for Health and Family Services. The program services are provided through district health departments and currently are available throughout the Commonwealth of Kentucky. Counseling, education, and support services are provided until the child reaches 2 years of age. On the basis of a systems approach, home visits are made for the purpose of screening, assessment, referrals, care coordination, case management, and policy advocacy. The program implements the "Growing Great Kids" and evidence-based curriculum (http://www.greatkidsinc.org/ggk-curriculum.html) based on building family strengths through parenting, child safety, and connecting families with many resources. Initially the program focused on teen and first-time mothers,

TABLE 20.5   Health Access Nurturing Development Services (Hands) Program: Outcomes and Potential Related Medical Cost Savings

Outcome	Estimated Cost Per Case*	Hands Impact	Estimated Annual Cost Savings
Preterm birth	$49,000	32% reduction	$16,900,000
Emergency department use	$420	50% reduction	$5,700,000
Child abuse	$10,400	n/a	$685,940
Child neglect	$1,900	33% reduction	$90,900
Infant mortality	N/A	70% reduction	N/A

*The original calculations used estimated costs per case drawn from the Children's Safety Network. The estimated cost per case for child abuse and child neglect are hospitalization costs only and do not consider costs associated with child protective services or other expenditures. Source: Kentucky Cabinet and Family Services and Department for Public Health: *Home visiting: a healthy return on investment—a presentation for the Prichard committee*, 2011; table reprinted from The Pew Center on the States: *Home visiting issue brief, Kentucky: joining HANDS for a comprehensive system of care*, 2012, page 8. Retrieved from http://www.pewtrusts.org/~/media/legacy/uploadedfiles/pcs_assets/2012/02012home20kentucky20briefwebpdf.pdf © 2012. The Pew Charitable Trusts.

but data collected have revealed that at-risk mothers include individuals with previous children but poor support and parenting skills.

Programs such as HANDS require time in order to show outcomes. Ten years after the inception of the program the Kentucky Cabinet for Health and Family Services documented the positive impact of HANDS services, which can be seen in decreases in the number of preterm births, emergency department uses, rates of child abuse and neglect, and infant mortality rates in Kentucky as well as a cost savings to the Kentucky Medicaid program (Pew Center on the States, 2012) (Table 20.5). Currently, services have been expanded in eight counties targeting mothers identified as at risk or diagnosed with depression or other mental illness. Home visitors have been taught to use Home Cognitive Behavior Therapy to integrate into the HANDS curriculum for these families (Kentucky Cabinet for Health and Family Services, 2017; Pew Center on the States, 2012; USDHHS, 2014).

These alternative health programs are strategies to change the structural barriers that prevent low-income families' access to care. Professional role functions changed as nurses, rather than physicians, provided health care. Active self-care was promoted, and health and medical knowledge was shared. Assistance by family and social networks was encouraged. Both of these programs address aspects of the health needs of populations at risk, but they do not address the social determinants of disease. Neither program addresses the health-damaging conditions that poor people face, such as poor housing, malnutrition, and environmental hazards at the workplace and in the community. Although these programs represent steps in the right direction, changes in access to medical and health services are not enough. Social changes also are necessary.

APPLYING THE NURSING PROCESS

Home Visit

The case study presents the application of the nursing process to a family on a home visit. The example notes the use of

the home visit to identify health needs of the family within the community and programs planned to meet those needs, which ultimately will benefit a population of families in the future.

The home visit is a crucial experience for the nursing student and family (Friedman et al., 2003). Important factors that may influence the home visit include the family's background experience with the health care system, the agency in which the nursing student is working, the family's experience with previous nursing students who have visited the family, and the student's background. For example, nursing student characteristics may vary; students bring differing levels of knowledge of medical and nursing practice, self, and the community.

The nursing student brings previous learning about families, family-related theory, the growth and development of members of different ages within a family, disease processes, and access to the health care system. Curricula within schools of nursing vary; therefore some students will also bring preparation in all specialties—medical-surgical nursing, childbearing, parent–child nursing, and psychiatric and mental health nursing—to the experience. Others may be taking basic clinical courses, such as pediatrics and psychiatric–mental health nursing, concurrently with community health. Thus the need for review of appropriate theory, health education, and standard assessment tools for individuals and families will vary.

The nursing student's knowledge of self, previous life experiences, and values also are important in planning for home visits. Nursing students must recognize their strengths and weaknesses in preparation for entering a new community and working with families. Additional preparation by all nursing students is necessary before the first home visit, depending on the content of the referral. The student should gather referral information, review assessment forms, and intervention tools (e.g., screening materials, supplies) before going to the home. Flexibility is important in working with families, because the nursing student will not know the family's priority needs until the home visit.

CASE STUDY Application of the Nursing Process

Student Absenteeism

Jana Parks is a community health nurse employed by the district health department. She is a school health nurse, providing services for six schools in a moderately sized community. After receiving a referral from school officials related to a student's absenteeism, Jana plans to assess the student and family. (See the photo novella in this chapter for photos that depict this case study.)

Assessment

Jana knows that the school is located in the inner city where 75% of the children come from families with a median family income at or below the federal poverty level. English is the second language for approximately 25% of the students, and 5% are not fluent in spoken or written English. Each year, more than 20% of the student body moves into or out of the school district.

She reviews the school records for the student, Maria Garcia, and learns that this is the first year of enrollment for the sixth grader and her second-grade brother, Miguel. Maria's family moved to the area 6 months ago from the Dominican Republic. School records note that the girl is adequately fluent in spoken English but that the parents do not speak English. The student's father works part-time at a local furniture manufacturer. There has been a noticeable decline in grades over the previous quarter, there have been no disciplinary actions, and teacher comments are positive regarding the student's classroom performance. The health record indicates that she is up to date with required immunizations; no chronic illnesses are noted on the school physical examination record. Jana notes that Maria's brother does not have the same school absence pattern.

Jana contacts the family and identifies her role as the school health nurse. She explains the need for a meeting with the student and family to discuss concerns about Maria's school attendance. A time is scheduled when both parents and the student are available. She confirms the home address and directions.

Jana notes that the house is in need of paint and some windows have been replaced with cardboard; however, the yard is free of clutter and there are containers of blooming plants on the small porch. Maria Garcia opens the door, and Jana enters a small, dimly lit room. As the student makes introductions, Mr. Garcia stands and greets Jana with a nod and handshake while Mrs. Garcia remains recumbent on the sofa but raises her hand in greeting. Mrs. Garcia's appearance surprises Jana, as she appears much older than Mr. Garcia. Her skin is pale, her eyes are sunken, and she appears frail, with a distended abdomen and generalized muscle wasting.

Jana is aware that the exchange of social conversation is important in establishing a relationship with Hispanic clients. She mentions the beautiful picture in the room and learns that a family member painted it as a wedding gift for the Garcias. Jana learns that the family has no other relatives in the community and moved to the city through the work of a refugee assistance organization. In this interview, Jana plans to collect information related to individual, family, and/or community functioning.

Throughout the conversation, Jana has noted that both Maria and Mr. Garcia appear tense; Mrs. Garcia is quiet and rarely speaks or smiles. Maria has translated throughout the conversation, although Jana senses that the parents may have limited understanding of spoken English. To lessen anxiety, Jana begins the interview by saying, "I am here because the school and I are concerned about Maria's absences. I want to learn why Maria misses school and to see if there are ways that the school can help."

Through the interview process, Jana learns that Maria likes school and has made friends there. She observes that Miguel stays close to Maria and frequently hides his face into her shoulder when Jana speaks to him. She also notes that Mr. and Mrs. Garcia rarely look at each other, and Mr. Garcia chooses a seat on the opposite side of the room. The family rents the home, and the father has been able to supplement his part-time income by working as a day laborer for a lawn service. The family was beginning to establish connections at a local church and with neighbors when Mrs. Garcia was diagnosed with an abdominal tumor that has required numerous operations over the past 3 months.

She is still receiving home care visits for a surgical wound that has not healed. Although Medicaid has covered most physician and hospital expenses, the family has experienced out-of-pocket expenses for noncovered medications. These problems have contributed to family financial stress. Mr. Garcia has to drive his wife to medical appointments; as a result, he is in danger of losing his job. Maria also attends these appointments to serve as the interpreter, resulting in her frequent school absences.

In addition, Jana learns that Maria has assumed responsibility for the household cooking, cleaning, and laundry since her mother's illness. Mr. Garcia shops at a small neighborhood groceria. Jana determines that with food stamps the family has adequate resources to purchase food, although Maria admits that she is still learning to cook. The family eats the evening meal together, frequently rice and beans. Maria and Miguel are eligible for subsidized breakfast and lunch at school. Maria believes that it is her responsibility to help Miguel complete his homework, get to bed on time, and attend school regularly. Mr. Garcia disciplines both children. Jana asks questions regarding family health practices and learns that they see a provider at the health department only when ill or for school requirements and do not seek dental care. She observes a number of medication bottles on a table near the sofa.

Diagnosis
Individual

- Risk for excessive stress related to time-consuming activities, insufficient finances, and insufficient recreation (Mr. Garcia and Maria)
- Risk for personal injury related to improperly stored medications (Miguel)
- Ineffective health promotion related to language and cultural differences and lack of routine dental hygiene (Mr. and Mrs. Garcia, Maria, and Miguel)

Family

Risk for poor parenting and family crisis related to change in Mrs. Garcia's ability to function, financial burden of treatments for ill family member, and disruption of family routines, mother's illness, and mother's prolonged illness

Community

Inadequate systematic programs for linking Hispanic families to community resources

Planning

A plan of care is developed to meet the needs of the individuals, family, and community. Planning involves mutual goal setting between the nurse and family; mutual setting of objectives to meet goals, prioritizing or setting short- and long-term goals with the family, contracting or establishing the division of labor between nurse and family that will meet the objectives, and evaluating the process and outcome.

Individual
Long-Term Goals

- Mr. Garcia will recognize appropriate roles and responsibilities for Maria. He will identify and use resources to allow her to resume suitable educational, social, and family duties.
- Mr. Garcia will identify and use community resources to assist with transportation needs and medication costs.
- Jana noted a long-term need to discuss dental care.
- Mr. and Mrs. Garcia will improve their English comprehension and speaking skills.

Short-Term Goals

- Relieve Maria of interpreting at medical appointments by identifying alternative interpretive resources.
- Store medications in a secure location.

continued

CASE STUDY Application of the Nursing Process—cont'd
Student Absenteeism

Family
Long-Term Goal
- The family will be able to find and use appropriate services for physical and social support.

Short-Term Goal
- The family will learn to appropriately express their feelings related to the mother's illness, social isolation, role strain, and/or fear.

Community
Long-Term Goal
- The community will establish programs to support immigrant family needs for transportation, interpretation, and enculturation to the American medical system.

Short-Term Goal
- Mr. Garcia will identify existing programs available to support Hispanic immigrants.

Intervention
- Jana recognizes that many interventions must be carried out at the individual, family, and community levels.

Individual
- Education regarding safe medication storage.
- Referral to the Refugee Assistance Society or local churches for interpretive assistance.

Family
Direct nursing interventions aimed at family functioning include the following levels:
- *Cognitive:* New information is provided to the family that promotes problem solving. An example is referring the Garcias to the community free clinic for medical and dental care.
- *Affective:* Families are encouraged to express their feelings, which may be blocking their efforts at problem solving. An example would be Jana's planned validation of Mr. Garcia's concerns regarding finances and the threat of losing employment.
- *Behavioral:* Tasks are negotiated to be carried out either during the family interview or as homework between visits. An example is Mr. Garcia's planned call to the Refugee Assistance Society.

Community
Jana recognizes that her referral of Mr. Garcia to the Refugee Assistance Society to obtain support through existing programs is also an intervention at the community level. She engages in ongoing parafamily work to identify how the community can be mobilized to provide physical, mental, and social support to immigrant families. Does anyone at the community free clinic speak Spanish? Are interpreters available at health care facilities? Where do most immigrant families receive health care and social support? Are classes on English as a second language free of charge for Hispanic families? Are job skill training programs available for Mr. Garcia? Questions such as these bring up many areas of assessment that Jana will need to make with the Garcia family and the community in the future.

Evaluation
Individual/Family
Jana helps the Garcias obtain a small lockable box in which to store medications. Mr. Garcia establishes contact with a local church, which provides a volunteer interpreter and driver for medical visits and twice-weekly delivery of meals. Mr. Garcia takes Maria and Miguel to the free clinic, where dental sealants are applied to their molars. The social worker at the community's free clinic meets with Mr. Garcia to offer him assistance in obtaining low-cost medications. Through this conversation, Jana identifies his reluctance to ask for financial assistance. He states that he should provide for his family and that Maria should not have to assume the role of mother for Miguel. However, he does not see any other options at this time. She identifies that Mr. Garcia may be in need of ongoing support and suggests that he talk with a counselor about his concerns. Mr. Garcia refuses to see a counselor but agrees that he will talk to the pastor of his church. Maria and Miguel meet with the school counselor as needed to discuss feelings related to their mother's illness and the resulting family strain.

Community
Jana identified that many community resources are available to immigrant families; however, information about them is limited and not readily accessible. She contacts the director of the Refugee Assistance Society, and together they initiate a community coalition to address this issue.

Levels of Prevention
Society's expectations of the family are in transition. Application of the levels of prevention to families by the community nurse must take into account the changing family configuration; the financial, emotional, and physical burdens often compounded in the single-parent family; and the lack of resources, such as nonexistent or inadequate health insurance.

Primary Prevention
This chapter has established the importance of the family to individuals and society. Primary prevention with families becomes an essential element of any comprehensive family health plan. From the family perspective, health education must address actual and potential challenges to health, such as immunizations of all family members, educating about resources to support the family financially and emotionally, encouraging exercise and activity, and empowering the family to build on strengths. An example is using the family genogram to teach the family about predisposition to diseases and helping the family develop a health prevention plan.

Secondary Prevention
The focus of secondary prevention for the family includes ensuring that the family has continued access to health care and resources for individual and family health problems. The changing economy in the United States has "closed the door" to regular health providers for some families. The challenge to the nurse is helping the family locate and access continued care and teaching the family to move through the system of government assistance, which may be new and unacceptable for the family. The nurse must be politically active in lobbying legislators for continued resources to support families.

Tertiary Prevention
Tertiary prevention for family includes assuring that the needed resources are available to support long-term care of each family member. An example of a community-based organization established and funded solely by volunteers is the Kelly Autism Program (KAP). KAP is "designed to provide services to adolescents and young adults diagnosed along the Autism Spectrum Continuum, as well as their families, while serving as a training opportunity for future professionals in a variety of disciplines. KAP has programs for middle school, high school and post-secondary participants including higher education, vocational training, and job support" (Western Kentucky University, 2016, p. 1). It includes a comprehensive screening program and one-on-one support for young adults with autism capable of living and studying on a university campus.

Developed by Mary Kovar, RN, MSN, and Barbara Minix, RN, MSN.

SUMMARY

This chapter highlights the CHN's work with families and identifies the major family-related health care needs that the health care system has not adequately addressed. The nature of the family is changing and challenging traditional definitions and configurations. Approaches to meeting the health needs of families must go beyond that of the traditional health care system, which addresses the individual as the unit of care. Strategies are given in this chapter for expanding notions of care from the individual to the family and from the family to the community. To guide intervention with families, nurses have traditionally relied on common theoretical frameworks from the disciplines of psychology and social psychology. These frameworks often target individuals; frameworks are needed that go beyond the individual to the family and community and that address social and policy changes needed to alter the social, economic, and environmental conditions under which families must function.

This chapter provides tools for assessing the family and the family within the community and gives examples of the extension of family health intervention to larger aggregates, which involves social action to overcome constraints to accessing health services. Nonnursing and community health nursing models of care provided for communities of families are presented and critiqued. The nursing process is applied in a case study at individual, family, and community levels on a home visit. Examples of interventions by the CHN at individual, family, and community levels are presented.

Families remain the core of society, with diversity as the constant for families in the United States. Family nursing must be understood and practiced by CHNs. An understanding of family theory provides a mechanism for assessing and intervening with families to improve their level of wellness and increase the health of the community as a whole.

ⓔ EVOLVE WEBSITE

http://evolve.elsevier.com/Nies/community

- NCLEX Review Questions
- Case Studies

BIBLIOGRAPHY

Abramowitz J, O'Hara B: The financial burden of medical spending, *Med Care Res Rev* 72(2):187–199, 2014. http://doi.org/10.1177/1077558714563173.

Allen DR, Fine MA, Demo HD: An overview of family diversity: controversies, questions, and values. In Demo DH, Allen KR, Fine MA, editors: *Handbook of family diversity,* New York, 2000, Oxford Press.

American Academy of Child & Adolescent Psychiatry: *Grandparents raising grandchildren,* 2016. Available from: <https://www.aacap.org/AACAP/Families_and_Youth/Facts_for_Families/FFF-Guide/Grandparents-Raising-Grandchildren-077.aspx>.

American Association for Marriage and Family Therapy: *Grandparents raising grandchildren,* 2016. Available from: https://www.aamft.org/imis15/AAMFT/Content/Consumer_Updates/Grandparents_Raising_Grandchildren.aspx.

Anderson MP, O'Grady RS, Anderson IL: Public health nursing in primary care: impact on home visits, *Public Health Nurs*(2):145, 1985.

Annie E. Casey Foundation: *Kids Count Faststats data book online,* 2016. Available from: <http://www.aecf.org/resources/the-2016-kids-count-data-book/>.

Auger JR: Behavioral systems and nursing, *AJN* 77(11):1856–1857, 1976.

Beard M: Home nursing, *Public Health Nurs Q* 7:44–51, 1999.

Bell J: The central importance of therapeutic conversations in nursing: Can talking be Healing? *J Family Nurs* 22(4):439–448, 2016. http://doi.org/10:1177/107480716680837.

Bell JM: Making ideas "stick": the 15-minute family interview, *J Fam Nurs* 18:171, 2012.

Bronfenbrenner U: *Making human beings human: bioecological perspectives on human development,* Thousand Oaks, CA, 2005, Sage Publications.

Butler JF: The family diagram and genogram: comparisons and contrast, *Am J Family Therapy* 36:169–180, 2008.

Cantor J, Monheit AC, Delia D: Early impact of the Affordable Care Act on health insurance coverage of young adults, *Health Serv J* 47(5):1773–1790, 2012. http://doi.org/10.1111/j.1475-6773.2012.01458.x.

Carter E, McGoldrick M: *The changing family life cycle: a framework for family therapy,* ed 2, New York, 1998, Gardner Press.

Centers for Disease Control and Prevention: *Faststats: Teen births,* 2017. http://www.cdc.gov/nchs/fastats/teen-births.htm.

CDC: National Center for Health Statistics (NCHC): *Births and natality,* 2016. Available from: https://www.cdc.gov/nchs/fastats/births.htm.

CDC: *Chronic disease prevention and health promotion,* 2017. Available from: https://www.cdc.gov/chronicdisease/.

Centers for Medicare and Medicaid Services: *The children's health insurance program,* 2015. Available from: <https://www.cms.gov/Outreach-and-Education/American-Indian-Alaska-Native/AIAN/CHIP-Grantees/Overview.html>.

Christakis NA, Fowler JA: *Connected: The surprising power of our social networks and how they shape our lives,* Boston, 2009, Little, Brown & Company.

Cody WK: Nursing frameworks to guide practice and research with families, *Nurs Sci Q* 13(4):277–284, 2000.

Cook E: *The life of Florence Nightingale,* vol. 2, London, 1913, Macmillan.

DeFrain J: Strong families, *Family Matters* 53:6–13, 1999.

Dreher MC: The conflict of conservatism in public health nursing education, *Nurs Outlook* 30:504, 1982.

Dolgin JL: The Constitution as family arbiter: a moral in the mess? *Columbia Law Rev* 102:337–407, 2002.

Dunst CJ, Trivette CM: Capacity-building family-systems intervention practices, *J Fam Soc Work* 12(2):119–143, 2009.

Duvall EM: *Marriage and family relationships,* ed 5, Philadelphia, 1977, JB Lippincott.

Duvall EM, Miller BC: *Marriage and family development,* ed 6, New York, 1985, Harper and Row.

Erikson E: *Childhood and society,* ed 2, New York, 1963, WW Norton.

Escoto KH, Laska MN, Larson N, et al.: Work hours and perceived time barriers to healthful eating among young adults, *Am J Health Behav* 36(3):786–789, 2012.

Freeman R: *Public health nursing practice,* ed 3, Philadelphia, 1963, WB Saunders.

Friedman MM: *Family nursing: theory and assessment*, ed 3, East Norwalk, CT, 1998, Appleton-Lange.

Friedman MM, Bowden VB, Jones EG: *Family nursing: research, theory and practice*, ed 2, Upper Saddle River, NJ, 1992, Prentice Hall.

Friedman MM, Bowden VB, Jones EG: *Family nursing: research, theory and practice*, ed 3, Upper Saddle River, NJ, 2003, Prentice Hall.

Gallup Poll: *An estimated 780,000 Americans in same-sex marriages*, 2016. Available from: http://www.gallup.com/poll/182837/estimated-780-000-americans-sex-marriages.aspx.

Glaser B, Strauss AL: *Chronic illness and the quality of life*, St. Louis, 1975, Mosby.

Guttmacher Institute: *U.S. teen pregnancy, birth and abortion rates reach the lowest level In almost four decades*, 2016. Available from: https://www.guttmacher.org/news-release/2016/us-teen-pregnancy-birth-and-abortion-rates-reach-lowest-levels-almost-four-de.

Hartman A: *Finding families: an ecological approach to family assessment in adoption*, Beverly Hills, CA, 1979, Sage.

Human Rights Campaign: *Inclusive definition of family*, 2017. Available from: <http://www.hrc.org/hei/lgbtq-inclusive-definitions-of-family>.

International Family Nursing Association (IFNA): *Position statement on generalist competencies for family nursing practice*, 2015. Available from: http://internationalfamilynursing.org/resources-for-family-nursing/family-nursing-links/family-nursing-conferences/.

Kaakinen JR, Gedaly-Duff V, Hanson SM: *Family health care nursing: theory, practice and research*, ed 4, Philadelphia, PA, 2009, FA Davis.

Krogstad JM: *PEW: 5 facts about modern American family*, 2014. Available from: http://www.pewresearch.org/fact-tank/2014/04/30/5-facts-about-the-modern-american-family/.

Kentucky Cabinet for Health and Family Services: *HANDS program*, 2017. Available from: <http://chfs.ky.gov/dph/mch/ecd/hands.htm>.

Kogan MD, Schuster MA, Yu SM, et al.: Routine assessment of family and community health risks: parent views and what they receive, *Pediatrics* 113:1934–1943, 2004.

Li L, Lin C, Cao H: Intergenerational and urban-rural health habits in Chinese families, *Am J Health Behav* 33(2):172–180, 2009.

Lubkin IM, Larsen PD: *Chronic illness: Impact & intervention*, ed 8, Burlington, MA, 2013, Jones & Bartlett.

Martinez AM, D'Arois D, Rennick JE: Does the 15-minute or less family interview influence family nursing practice? *J Fam Nurs* 31(2):157–178, 2007.

Maslow A: *Motivation and personality*, ed 2, New York, 1970, Harper and Row.

McNeill JA, Cook J, Mahon M, et al.: Family history: value-added information in assessing cardiac health, *AAOHN* 56(7):297–305, 2008.

Medicaid.gov: *Children's health insurance program reauthorization Act*, n.d. Available from: <https://www.medicaid.gov/chip/chip-program-information.html>.

Minuchin P: Looking toward horizon: present and future in study of family systems. In McHale JP, Grolnick WS, editors: *Psychological study of families*, Mahwah, NJ, 2002, Lawrence Erlbaum.

Montalvo B: Useful coincidences and family strengths, *Contemp Fam Ther* 26(2):117–119, 2004.

National League for Nursing: *A curriculum guide for schools of nursing*, New York, 1937, Author.

National Institute of Health: *Better diabetes care for systems change: Cultural competency tips*, 2017. Available from: <http://diversityrx.org/resources/better-diabetes-care-improving-cultural-competency>.

Office of Disease Prevention and Health Promotion: *Healthy People. gov*, 2017. Available from: https://www.healthypeople.gov/2020/topics-objectives/topic/Access-to-Health-Services/objectives.

Otto H: A framework for assessing family strengths. In Reinhard A, Quinn M, editors: *Family-centered community health nursing*, St. Louis, 1973, Mosby.

Palermo T, Ehlers J: *Coalitions: building partnerships to promote agricultural health and safety*, Washington, DC, 2001, National Institutes for Occupational Health and Safety.

Parke RP: Family & peer systems, *Psychol Bull* 128(4):596–601, 2002.

Parker K, Patten E: *The sandwich generation: Rising financial burden for middle-aged Americans (Pew Research Social & Demographic Trends)*, 2013. Available from: <http://www.pewsocialtrends.org/2013/01/30/the-sandwich-generation/>.

Pew Center on the States: *Home Visiting Issue Brief, Kentucky: Joining HANDS for a comprehensive system of care*, 2012. Available from: <http://www.pewtrusts.org/en/research-and-analysis/reports/0001/01/01/joining-hands-for-a-comprehensive-system-of-care>.

Pew Research Center: *Social & demographic trends: The return of the multi-generational family household*, 2010. Available from: <http://www.pewsocialtrends.org/2010/03/18/the-return-of-the-multi-generational-family-household/>.

Pew Research Center: *Health online*, 2013. Available from: <http://www.pewinternet.org/2013/01/15/health-online-2013/>.

Pew Research Center: *Facttank news in the numbers: 6 new facts about Facebook (2014)*. Available from: http://www.pewresearch.org/fact-tank/2014/02/03/6-new-facts-about-facebook/.

Pequegnat W, Bray JH: Families and HIV/AIDS: Introduction to the special section, *J Fam Psychol* 11(1):3–10, 1997.

Pratt LV: *Family structure and effective health behavior: The energized family*, Boston, 1976, Houghton Mifflin.

Prince M, Prina M, Guerchet M: *World Alzheimer Report 2013: Journey of caring:an analysis of long-term care for dementia*, London, 2013, Alzheimer's Disease International.

Progressive Farmer: *Progressive Farmer safety days*, 2017. Available from: http://dtnpf-igital.com/article/Progressive+Agriculture+Safety+Days%C2%AE/2688460/375735/article.html.

Reisman M: The affordable care act, five years later: policies, progress, and politics, *Pharm Ther* 40(9):575–600, 2015.

Robert Wood Johnson Foundation: *Let's cover the uninsured*, NI. Available from: <http://covertheuninsured.org/>.

Rothausen TJ: 'Family' in organizational research: A review and comparison of definitions and measures, *J Org Behav* 20:817–836, 1999.

Siegrist B, Jones S: Nursing education beyond classroom walls: Service learning through collaboration with community partners. In *Exploring the scholarship of teaching*, Bowling Green, KY, 2005, Faculty Center for Excellence in Teaching, p 87. https://web.tcc.edu/faculty/facultyacademy/newfaculty/documents/sotl_0complete.pdf#page=91.

Spanakis E, Golden SH: Race/ethnic differences in diabetes and diabetes complications, *Curr Diab Rep* 13(6), 2013. http://doi.org/10.1007/s11892-013-0421-9CDC.

Smith SR, Harmon RR: *Exploring family theories*, New York, 2011, Oxford University Press.

Stack CB: *All our kin*, New York, 1996, Basic Books.

University of Michigan: *Depression in the sandwich generation*, 2016. Available from: http://www.depressiontoolkit.org/news/depression_in_the_sandwich_generation.asp.

U.S. Census Bureau: *Statistical definition of family unchanged since 1930*, 2014. Available from: https://www.census.gov/newsroom/blogs/random-samplings/2015/01/statistical-definition-of-family-unchanged-since-1930.html.

U.S. Department of Health and Human Services (DHHS): *Administration for Community Living: Aging statistics*, 2016. Available from: https://aoa.acl.gov/Aging_Statistics/Index.aspx.

U.S. DHHS: *My family health portrait: A tool of the surgeon general*, 2017. Available from: https://familyhistory.hhs.gov/FHH/html/index.html#.

U.S. DHHS: *Implementing HANDS program: Home visit effectiveness*, 2014. Available from: https://homvee.acf.hhs.gov/Implementation/3/Health-Access-Nurturing-Development-Services–HANDS–Program-Implementation/37.

U.S. Census Bureau: *Population profile of the nation: dynamic version*, Washington, DC, 2005, Author.

U.S. Census Bureau: *Income, poverty and health insurance: coverage in the US in 2007*, 2008. Available from: <www.census/prod/2008/pub/p60>.

U.S. Census Bureau: *2010 American community survey*, Washington, DC, 2011, Author. http://www.census.gov/prod/2011pubs/acsbr10-03.pdf>.

U.S. Census Bureau: *2013 Families and living arrangements*. Available from: <https://www.census.gov/topics/families/families-and-households.html>.

U.S. Department of Health and Human Services: New family history tool promotes prevention, *Nations Health* 34(10):33, 2005.

U.S. Department of Health and Human Services: *My family health portrait: A tool from the US Surgeon General*, 2017. Available from: <https://familyhistory.hhs.gov/fhh-web/home.action>.

U.S. Department of Health and Human Services: *Administration on Aging: A profile of older Americans*, 2012. Available from: <http://aoa.gov/AoARoot/Aging_Statistics/Profile/index.aspx>.

Werner CA: *The older population: 2010*. U.S. Census Bureau, 2010. Retrieved from: https://www.census.gov/prod/cen2010/briefs/c2010br-09.pdf.

World Health Organization (WHO): *2010 The World Health Report: Health systems financing: The path to universal coverage*, Geneva, 2012, World Health Organization.

VanderValk I, de Goede M, Spruijt E, et al.: A longitudinal study on transactional relations between parental marital distress and adolescent emotional adjustment, *Adolescence* 42(165):116–136, 2007.

von Bertalanffy L: *General systems theory: foundations, development, applications*, New York, 1968, George Braziller.

von Bertalanffy L: The history and status of general systems theory. In Klir G, editor: *Trends in general systems theory*, New York, 1972, Wiley.

von Bertalanffy L: General systems theory and psychiatry. In Arieti S, editor: *American handbook of psychiatry*, New York, 1974, Basic Books.

Wald L: The family as a unit of care: a historical review, *Public Health Nurs* 3:427–428, 515–519, 1904.

Western Kentucky University: *Kelly Autism Program*, 2014. http://www.wku.edu/kellyautismprogram/index.php.

Wright LM, Leahey M: *Nurses and families: a guide to family assessment and intervention*, Philadelphia, 1994, FA Davis.

Wright LM, Leahey M: *Nurses and families: a guide to family assessment and intervention*, ed 4, Philadelphia, 2000, FA Davis.

Wright LM, Leahey M: *Nurses and families: a guide to family assessment and intervention*, ed 5, Philadelphia, 2005, FA Davis.

Wright LM, Leahey M: *Nurses and family: a guide to family assessment and intervention*, ed 6, Philadelphia, 2012, FA Davis.

21

Populations Affected by Disabilities

*Allison P. Edwards, Lisa W. Thomas, and
Meredith Troutman-Jordan*

OUTLINE

OBJECTIVES

*Upon completion of this chapter, the reader will be able to do the
following:*

1. Differentiate among the definitions, models, and social
   constructs of disability.
2. Describe historical attitudes and perspectives surrounding
   disability that have contributed to treatment of people with
   disabilities.
3. Summarize the prevalence of various disabilities.
4. Outline federal legislation that supports the rights of people
   with disabilities.

5. Identify the unique living experiences of disabled persons
   and their families.
6. Provide evidence-based interventions to promote function
   and health management for persons with disabilities and/or
   chronic illnesses.
7. Identify ethical issues related to the care of people with
   disabilities.

KEY TERMS

activity limitation
activities of daily living (ADL)
Americans with Disabilities Act
child(ren) with disabilities (CWD)
developmental disability
disability
fatal four

functional activities
handicap
impairment
independent living
Individuals with Disabilities
   Education Act (IDEA)
instrumental activities of daily living
   (IADL)

intellectual and developmental
   disabilities (IDD)
Patient Self-Determination Act
   (PSDA) of 1990
people/person with disabilities
   (PWD)

quality of life
Rehabilitation Act of 1973
reasonable accommodations

Social Security Disability Insurance (SSDI)
Supplemental Security Income (SSI)

Ticket to Work and Work Incentives Act (TWWIIA)

SELF-ASSESSMENT: PERCEPTION OF DISABILITY

Picture what it's like to be born with a disability. Envision yourself unable to use your arms or legs or being confined to a wheelchair and dependent on the assistance of others. Imagine not being able to view anything above chair height. Consider having to prepare yourself for the day with the use of only one arm, from a wheelchair. What might seem like a simple task, like dressing or grooming, may take hours of preparation and assistance for an individual with a physical or cognitive disability. To further complicate the situation, imagine that the person with a disability has a significant health concern such as high blood pressure or diabetes that requires close monitoring or medications.

Now consider individuals who were healthy since birth but became disabled by a disease or accident. How do they adapt to living in their old environment with new physical challenges? How would their employment be affected? Will financial resources and personal and emotional support systems be available?

Finally, think about living in a family affected by disability. Consider the impact of a child with a disability on parental activities, family roles, and siblings. Imagine dilemmas encountered by parents faced with the possibility of having a child with a disability who may not survive without extensive surgeries and, even then, a good and productive quality of life is not guaranteed. These are examples of some of the many different situations experienced by persons with disabilities (PWD).

This chapter discusses general information about the various types of disabling conditions encountered in the community. It summarizes some of the more commonly occurring comorbidities and presents basic information on public policy and legislation that affect PWD. Last, it suggests some interventions that may be used by public health nurses to help care for this vulnerable population.

DEFINITIONS AND MODELS FOR DISABILITY

Disability is an umbrella term describing impairments, activity limitations, and participation restrictions. The Americans with Disabilities Act of 1990 and the Rehabilitation Act of 1973 define having a disability by how it limits carrying out a major life activity, such as the ability to breathe, walk, see, hear, speak, work, care for oneself, perform manual tasks, and learn. The International Classification of Functioning, Disability and Health (ICF) (World Health Organization [WHO], 2016a) proposes the scope of disability encompasses impairments, activity limitations,

and participation restrictions. These definitions frame the evolution of policy as it pertains to disabilities and are often used to facilitate eligibility determination for federal or state financial assistance.

Disability affects people irrespective of class, culture, race, and economic level. Depending on the term's definition, disability affects nearly one out of every five Americans. Disability increases with age, often influencing a person's ability to maintain self-care, which is essential to remaining in one's preferred living environment. A physical disability may be readily apparent, as with someone confined to a wheelchair or an individual who is visually impaired, or it may be less obvious, such as an individual's intellectual, sensory, or neurologic deficit.

People who are born with a disability describe their experience somewhat differently from those who acquire a disability. For example, people with a sensory disability, a physical disability, or an intellectual disability from birth adapt to the world as they know it. Compare this situation with that of a 20-year-old who becomes blind, deaf, or paralyzed because of an accident. In this case, adaptation is likely necessary and lengthy, and the loss may never be fully grieved. If an 80-year-old becomes blind because of diabetes-induced retinopathy, the loss of sight was chronic, progressive, and predictable. There will be loss and grief, but the blindness occurs as part of the aging process. Thus, rather than viewing PWD as "all the same," nurses must be able to see each person as unique, with different goals, knowledge, and experiences.

Physical disabilities, sensory disabilities, intellectual disabilities, serious emotional disturbances, learning disabilities, significant chemical and environmental sensitivities, and health problems such as asthma or diabetes are examples of disabilities that may substantially limit at least one major life activity. Current nomenclature categorizes disabilities in different ways. Developmental disabilities encompass those conditions that are manifested by limitation before the legal age of adulthood, which is 18. This includes issues that limit or present challenges to the performance of activities of daily living (ADLs). Developmental disabilities encompass those lifelong conditions that are chronic in nature and may incorporate either or both intellectual and physical disabilities. Developmental disabilities are often the result of maternal illness or infection, genetic disorders, or trauma. Examples include fetal alcohol syndrome, spina bifida (SB), Down syndrome (DS), or cerebral palsy (CP), among others.

Disabilities are often categorized according to their onset. They may be conditions from birth, such as DS or CP; conditions diagnosed during early childhood, such as autism spectrum disorder (ASD) or attention-deficit disorder/attention-deficit hyperactivity disorder (ADD/ADHD); conditions acquired as a result of an injury, such as spinal cord injury or traumatic brain

TABLE 21.1	Terminology for Impairment, Disability, and Handicap		
Characteristic	**Impairment**	**Disability**	**Handicap**
Definition	Physical deviation from normal structure, function, physical organization, or development	May be objective and measurable	Not objective or measurable; is an experience related to the responses of others
Measurability	Objective and measurable	May be objective and measurable	Not objective or measurable; is an experience related to the responses of others
Illustrations	Spina bifida, spinal cord injury, amputation, and detached retina	Cannot walk unassisted; uses crutches and/or a manual or power wheelchair; blindness	Reflects physical and psychological characteristics of the person, culture, and specific circumstances
Level of analysis	Micro level (e.g., body organ)	Individual level (e.g., person)	Macro level (e.g., societal)

injury (TBI); conditions that are progressive with age, such as cognitive decline/dementia and Alzheimer disease; or conditions associated with chronic illness, such as multiple sclerosis or diabetic neuropathy or retinopathy.

In comparison to the term *disability*, an impairment is a problem in body function or structure; an activity limitation is a difficulty encountered by an individual in executing a task or action (WHO, 2016a. A disability resulting from an impairment involves a restriction or an inability to perform an activity in a normal manner or within the normal range resulting from a loss or abnormality of psychological, physiological, or anatomical structure or function. A handicap is a disadvantage resulting from an impairment or a disability that prevents fulfillment of an expected role; it refers to an obstacle imposed on people by some constraint in the environment (Dunn and Andrews, 2015). A handicap is not a characteristic of a person, but rather a description of the relationship between the person and the environment. In other words, impairment affects a human organ on a micro level, whereas disability affects a person on an individual level; a handicap results when a person with an impairment cannot fulfill a normal life role in society on a macro level of analysis (University of Iowa, 2016). Table 21.1 compares and contrasts these definitions related to disability.

Measurement of Disability

Healthy People 2020, the Affordable Care Act (ACA), and the U.S. Department of Health and Human Services (HHS) helped establish a framework for accurately surveying the extent of disabilities among the U.S. population. *Healthy People 2020* urged inclusion of standard questions pertaining to surveillance of disabilities, and the ACA advanced this objective by mandating that data collection include race or ethnicity, sex, primary language, and disability status. In 2011, HHS established standard questions required for all public health surveys. They determined or assumed a disability if the respondent replied positively to any of these:
- Deafness or difficulty hearing
- Blindness or difficulty seeing
- Difficulty concentrating, remembering, or making decisions due to physical, mental, or emotional issues among those 5 years and older
- Difficulty walking, climbing stairs, dressing, or bathing among those 5 years and older

- Difficulty doing errands independently, such as grocery shopping or going to a doctor's appointment, secondary to a physical, mental, or emotional condition among those 15 years and older

The U.S. Census Bureau administers the Survey of Income and Program Participation (SIPP), which examines the confluence of income, employment, health insurance, and government transfer programs. The SIPP is a longitudinal survey that is administered over a 4-year period among the same respondents. It contains a broad but extensive set of disability questions that inquire about limitations in functional activities (e.g., seeing, hearing, speaking, walking, using stairs, lifting, and carrying items), activities of daily living (ADLs) (e.g., getting around inside the home, bathing, dressing, eating, or toileting), and instrumental activities of daily living (IADLs) (e.g., going outside the home, shopping, light house cleaning, preparing meals). The SIPP also gathers data on whether an individual has used an adaptive mobility device (e.g., wheelchair, cane, and walker); has been diagnosed with a mental or emotional disability; or has an impairment that produces on-the-job limitations or the inability to perform housework, or that involves the disability status of children (Brault, 2008). The complement to the SIPP is the American Community Survey (ACS), which asks respondents to assess disabilities from a more narrow perspective, such as whether they have a disability limitation that affects a certain function or activity, including sensory perception, physical activities, mental or emotional state, self-care, ability to leave home, or employment options (U.S. Census Bureau, 2010).

National Agenda for Disability Model

The Committee on a National Agenda for the Prevention of Disabilities (NAPD) conceptualized a model for disability (Fig. 21.1). The NAPD model complements the concepts defined in the WHO/ICF model, in that disability is noted by the NAPD to be any condition of the body or mind (impairment) that makes it more difficult for the person with the condition to do certain activities (activity limitation) and interact with the world around them; this will in turn influence quality of life (CDC, 2015). The NAPD model provides an alternative framework for viewing four related and distinct stages in the disabling process. Pathology at the cellular and tissue levels may produce impairment in structure or function at the organ

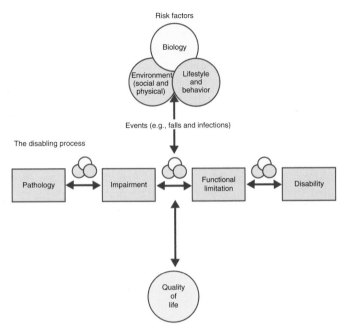

FIG. 21.1 Model of disability. (Reprinted with permission from Pope AM, Tarlov AR, editors: *Disability in America: toward a national agenda for prevention*, Washington, DC, 1991, National Academy Press. Copyright 1991 by the National Academy of Sciences. Courtesy National Academy Press, Washington, DC.)

level. An individual with an impairment may experience a functional limitation, which restricts their ability to perform an action within the normal range. The functional limitation may result in a disability when certain socially defined activities and roles cannot be performed. Although the model appears to indicate unidirectional progression from pathology to impairment, to functional limitation, to disability, stepwise or linear progression may not occur. Disability prevention efforts can limit or reduce many of the risk factors or stages in the disabling process.

Disability: A Social Construct

Disability is a complex phenomenon, reflecting the interaction between features of a person's body and features of the society in which the person lives (WHO, 2016b). Diverse approaches to defining and measuring disability have led to considerable variation in disability rates. Much of the complexity in defining disability stems from its socially constructed nature. Because disability is conceptualized as the inability to perform important life functions, it becomes a product of interaction between health status and the demands of one's physical and social environment. Thus, using a wheelchair is disabling in a workplace with steps and narrow doorways, but much less so in one with ramps and wide passageways. An individual with a less visible disability, such as deafness, may not be conscious of the disability until immersed in a social situation with others who cannot communicate via sign language. The interactive relationship between a person and the demands of the environment characterizes disability across many conceptual definitions or models (Costa-Black et al., 2013). Similarly, culture, education, and the social organization can shape how all individuals perceive disability.

🔬 RESEARCH HIGHLIGHTS
The Social Meaning of Disability

Grue (2016) provided a historical perspective on the social meaning of disability. She wrote that medicine continues to exercise great influence on the social meaning of disability, as well as the social valuation of various illnesses and impairments. Moreover, Grue maintained that people with long-term physical, mental, intellectual, or sensory impairments may be hindered from full and effective participation in society on an equal basis with others. Disability today, according to Grue, is a label that signifies social marginalization. She concluded with two key points: it is possible for a person to be disabled without recognizing himself as such, and it is possible for one to be disabled without being recognized as such by others.

❓ ACTIVE LEARNING

Ask an experienced nurse about their encounters with people with disabilities. Listen to their language and perceptions of disability. Compare these with the perspectives reflected in the social construct model for disability.

A HISTORICAL CONTEXT FOR DISABILITY

Current models and definitions for disability cannot be understood apart from their historical-sociopolitical context. As cultures have changed, and with them images of beauty and value, *exceptional* people have experienced a wide range of treatment. They have sometimes been viewed as mascots and fascinating freaks. In other cases, people with disabilities have been isolated, ridiculed, and discriminated against or, worse, marked for extermination.

Early Attitudes Toward People With Disabilities

Since the beginning of recorded history, people with disabilities have been set apart from others and viewed as different or unusual. Early Greek and Roman cultures emphasized bodily and intellectual perfection, and babies who were sick, weak, or born with obvious disabilities were commonly killed or left to die (Barnes, 1996). In biblical times, people with disabilities were often viewed as unclean and/or sinful, though Jewish culture prohibited infanticide on the basis of belief in the sanctity of life. Jesus facilitated an expansion of Christian acceptance of individuals with disabilities. Many of the Bible's accounts of miracles performed by Jesus involved him listening, accepting, embracing, and healing those shunned by society.

In early European history, people with disabilities sometimes served as entertainers, circus performers, and sideshow exhibitions. Historically, appearing disabled has often been a matter of risking censure or hostility. The hostility was often linked to the suspicion of malingering or an attempt to profit from the sympathy of others.

Attitudes Toward People With Disabilities: Eighteenth Through Twentieth Centuries

In the absence of a scientific model for understanding and treating disability, people saw disability as an irreparable condition caused by supernatural agency (Longmore, 1987). People with disabilities were viewed as sick and helpless. They were expected to participate in whatever treatment was deemed necessary to cure or produce a reasonable level of social or vocational performance. During the nineteenth century, the Industrial Revolution stimulated a societal need for better education. People who were unable to achieve the equivalent of a contemporary third-grade education (e.g., those with intellectual disability) were labeled "feebleminded" (Pfeiffer, 1993). Soon, the label was applied to people with vision, hearing, speech, and mobility impairments. Schools for people who were deaf and blind were established in the early 1800s. Although these early efforts demonstrated that people with disabilities could be educated and integrated into society, institutionalization and segregation of people with disabilities were the norm.

Disability in the Twentieth Century

Special-interest groups for PWD began to develop in the twentieth century. The first federal vocational rehabilitation legislation, passed in the early 1920s, focused on limitations in the amount or type of work that people with disabilities could perform (Longmore, 1987). In the early 1900s, social Darwinism and the eugenics movement conducted involuntary sterilization of many people with intellectual disabilities (Pfeiffer, 1993). The eugenics philosophy was first advanced by Francis Galton, a relative of Charles Darwin. The root of the word *eugenics* relates to "good birth" or "well born." This movement was characterized by selective genetic breeding meant to advance desirable hereditary traits to improve a culture's intellect. The eugenics philosophy was adopted in the United States in the 1920s to 1930s and advanced by biologist Charles Davenport (Norrgard, 2008). The focus of the U.S. movement was to inhibit individuals with any malady or disability from procreation. Ultimately, legislation was enacted in over 28 states that mandated forced sterilization of individuals who were "mentally handicapped."

The atrocities of Adolf Hitler's decrees, which ordered euthanasia of mentally ill and disabled individuals, helped reverse these civil rights abuses. Hitler empowered physicians to grant "mercy killings" of all individuals deemed incurable. Initially, in the *good death* program at least 5000 mentally and physically disabled children, from newborn to age 17 years, were killed by starvation or lethal overdoses. Soon extermination was extended to adults with mental or physical disabilities who lived in institutional settings, resulting in the deaths of over 70,000 adults with disabilities. After widespread public and private protest led by the German clergy, Hitler cancelled the adult euthanasia program in late 1941.

Killing resumed in August 1942, however, and continued until the last days of World War II, although in a more concealed manner. Ultimately, an estimated 200,000 people were exterminated through Hitler's euthanasia program because they were regarded as "unworthy of life" (Eskay, 2012). Disguised as humanitarian, the basis of the decree was to eliminate genetically defective individuals from the Aryan race. Propaganda films perpetuated a utilitarian philosophy that the costs of care for mentally ill and disabled individuals did not benefit the greater good.

Particularly ironic is that the president and U.S. commander-in-chief during wartime, Franklin Delano Roosevelt (FDR), disabled by polio, administered the nation's highest office from a wheelchair. Interestingly, FDR was rarely photographed in his wheelchair. He utilized various adaptive devices to simulate his ability to stand alone or move to a speaking podium (Hamiwka et al., 2009). Contemporary disability activists often view his disguise of his disabilities as promoting an image of individuals with disabilities as weak and infirm, contradicting efforts of integration in later years.

Contemporary Conceptualizations of People With Disabilities

Soon after the conclusion of WWII, in 1950 a group of parents opposed to the concept of institutionalization for their disabled children formed the Association for Retarded Children (now called The Arc). This group began to advocate strongly for children with intellectual disabilities. Today, the Arc is the "world's largest community-based organization of and for people with intellectual and developmental disabilities" (The Arc, 2013).

The concept of **independent living** began with the deinstitutionalization movement in the 1960s and 1970s, when parents' groups and professionals improved institutional care and established community-based independent living centers for PWD. This corresponded with the Rehabilitation Act of 1973, which promoted disabled individuals' efforts to form community based, nonresidential programs and find resources within their geographic area. Although some PWD moved into a limited number of community settings, most remained in institutional settings.

PWD are seldom portrayed in the modern media as having a full range of personality types and unique abilities. When a television or movie role portrays people with disabilities as fully functioning, integral members of society, this is often viewed by the public as unusual or unexpected.

Global Perspective on Culture and Disability

Individuals from other parts of the globe may have varying perspectives and experiences of disability. For example, in Nigerian society, children with disability have been perceived as cursed by God for gross disobedience, having ancestral violations of societal norms, or being witches and wizards, among the range of common societal misperceptions, leading to poor treatment from others (Eskay et al., 2012). Similarly, in Chinese culture, Confucian ideology, which otherwise views all people as deserving respect and kindness, also recognizes a social hierarchy in which those with disabilities were regarded as having the lowest status (Campbell and Uren, 2011). Traditional Chinese culture focuses on the cause of disability because, culturally, there is assumed to be a link between disability and previous wrongdoing. In those areas, someone with a disability is believed to bring shame and guilt to the family (Chiang and Hadadian, 2010).

Likewise, thematic assumptions derived from qualitative research on disability in South India include the notion that increased biomedical knowledge imparted via health education programs will reduce the incidence of disability because people will learn to take preventive measures and will decrease suffering caused by disability (Staples, 2012). A common belief is that many conditions are caused or made worse by a failure to access biomedical resources or by carelessness. This implies that many disabled people, and especially those from rural, uneducated, and economically poor backgrounds, do not obtain suitable treatment for their conditions (Staples, 2012).

PREVALENCE OF DISABILITY

Worldwide, over 1 billion people, or 15% of the population, has some form of a disability, with between 110 and 190 million people experiencing significant functional disabilities (WHO, 2016a). In the United States, prevalence estimates range from 12% to 20% of the U.S. population, with approximately 18.7% of those aged 5 years and older having a long-term condition or disability (U.S. Census Bureau, 2012). Of those with a disability, 12.6% have a disability considered severe (Brault, 2012).

Among those 15 years and older, wheelchairs are utilized by 3.6 million individuals in the United States, accounting for 1.5% of this population (Brault, 2012). An additional 4.8% of the disabled population utilizes a mobility aid such as a cane, crutches, orthotics, and/or a walker. About 9.2 million people reported hearing, visual, and speech disabilities.

Collectively, more than 15 million people (about 6.3%) experienced a mental disability as defined by one or more of the following: a learning disability, intellectual disability, cognitive disability (dementia), other mental/emotional condition, and/or difficulty managing money/bills. An emotional disability, experienced by nearly 8.4 million people, consisted of one or more of the following: depression and/or anxiety, interpersonal challenges, concentration difficulties, and/or difficulty coping with stress (Brault, 2012). Fig. 21.2 from the U.S. Census Bureau's ACS illustrates disability prevalence as of 2014 by age and type. Note the proportion of sensory deficits—hearing and vision—that constitutes a disability prevalence.

Disability Prevalence by Age, Race, and Sex

U.S. Census Bureau SIPP data indicate prevalence differences by race and sex (Brault, 2012). Blacks (22.2%) had a higher rate of disability than Asians (14.5%) and Hispanics (17.8%), although the higher rate was not statistically different from that of non-Hispanic whites (17.6%). Females had a higher disability rate (19.8%) than males (17.4%) in all racial groups. In a Medicaid expenditure study, Caucasian females represented the largest percentage of physically disabled older (60–80 years) adults (Shireman et al., 2013). Higher disability rates in females can be explained by proportionally larger groups of older women than of older men.

As acquired age-related conditions occur during the lifespan, disability prevalence and disability severity levels rise with aging. In the United States, there is a shifting demographic of individuals living beyond the age of 65. Individuals with disabilities of all types are part of that demographic. In 2005, roughly half (49.8%) of people aged 65 years and older had a disability, with 36.6% of people 65 years and older having disabilities considered severe (Brault, 2012). The highest incidence of disability (70.5%) occurred in people 80 years and older; of these, 55.8% had a severe disability and 30.2% needed personal assistance. Approximately 1.3 million of the 40.4 million people age 65 and older were living in nursing facilities in 2010 (Brault, 2012). As of 2005, people residing in nursing facilities had a disability prevalence of 97.3% (Brault, 2008). Notably, the need for assistance with one or more ADLs or IADLs increases as severity of disability increases. As a result, more than 16 million people require personal care services in their homes (Brault, 2012).

Prevalence of Disability in Children

More than 8% of U.S. children under the age of 15 have some kind of disability, and about half of them were classified as having severe disabilities (Brault, 2012). Children with special health care needs require a broad range of comprehensive health services, including prescription medications (86%), specialty medical care (47.5%), vision care (35.3%), mental health care (27.6%), specialized

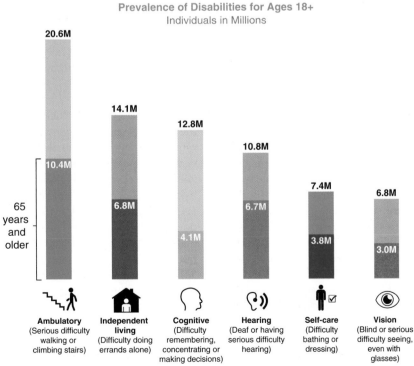

Prevalence of Disabilities for Ages 18+
Individuals in Millions

FIG. 21.2 Prevalence of disabilities for individuals ages 18 and over. (From U.S. Census Bureau: *American community survey: population: question on disability,* 2014. Available from https://www.census.gov/library/visualizations/2016/comm/cb16-ff12_disabilities.html.)

therapies (21.53%), and medical equipment (11.3%) (Child and Adolescent Health Measurement Initiative, 2012). Among children with special health care needs, almost 32% had ongoing emotional, behavioral, or developmental conditions requiring treatment, and almost 60% reported difficulty with one or more emotional or behavioral factors—feeling anxious, depression, acting out, fighting, bullying or arguing, and making and keeping friends (Child and Adolescent Health Measurement Initiative, 2012).

🏠 COMMUNITY FOCUS

Zika Virus

In January 2016, the Centers for Disease Control and Prevention issued an advisory for pregnant women to avoid travel where cases of the Zika virus were identified. The Zika virus is transmitted by the *Aedes agypti* mosquito, sex, mother to fetus, and possibly blood transfusion. Zika has been determined to cause a cadre of birth defects, including microcephaly, abnormal brain development, damage to the eye, loss of muscle tone, and joint-related issues including clubfoot. The epidemic has created a population that will require additional support mechanisms, including the possibility of long-term care, parental support services, and medical interventions related to the disabilities. The Centers for Disease Control and Prevention has published a number of references and resources to support parents in the acquisition of services, support, and care.

Centers for Disease Control and Prevention. Zika virus. Available at https://www.cdc.gov/zika/index.html. Accessed February 8, 2018.

Intellectual and developmental disability (IDD) is defined as limitations in intellect measured by intelligence quotient (IQ) ranging from mild (IQ 50–70), moderate (IQ 35–49), severe (IQ 20–34), to profound (IQ <20). Etiology includes genetic disorders and syndromes and TBI (Maenner et al., 2016). Two recent U.S. national surveys examined the prevalence of common developmental disabilities. Among the findings, the prevalence rates of intellectual disability were about 12.2%. Some of the most commonly reported developmental disabilities and IDDs are described here.

Autism Spectrum Disorder

ASD is a developmental disability that affects social, emotional, and behavioral skills. ASD is comprehensive term for a set of similar developmental disabilities, including autistic disorder, pervasive developmental disorder, and Asperger syndrome. It has been estimated that about 1 in 88 children (or slightly more than 1.1%) have autism (CDC, 2013). Alarmingly, between 2000 and 2010, autism's prevalence increased 119%, with estimates at 1 in 68 births (CDC, 2014). Autism has no known etiology, but more frequently occurs among older parents. It is about 4.5 times more common among boys than girls and co-occurs with chromosomal abnormalities such as Down syndrome and fragile X syndrome. Early identification of autism is important for effective implementation of interventions and improvement of outcomes.

📋 RESEARCH HIGHLIGHTS

Prevalence of Autism Spectrum Disorder

A large survey was conducted through the Early Autism and Developmental Disabilities Monitoring Network in 2016. Among the findings were a prevalence estimate for 4-year-olds at 13.4 per 1000 (20.3 male and 6.1 female). This illustrated a 30% lower prevalence than 8-year-olds, but prevalence with ASD and cognitive deficits was 20% higher among the 4-year-old age group. Additionally, female and white non-Hispanic children were more likely to be evaluated at an earlier age, 36 months, than male and non-Hispanic black children. Most importantly, 93% of 4-year-olds and 87% of 8-year-olds had a documented record of developmental issues before age 3. Emphasis on early diagnosis is therefore imperative to improved outcomes.

From Christensen DL, et al.: Prevalence and characteristics of autism spectrum disorder among 4-year-old children in the autism and developmental disabilities monitoring network. *J Dev Behav Pediatr* 37(1):1–8, 2016.

Down Syndrome

DS is a chromosomal disorder occurring in 1 in 700 people. Six thousand children are born with this alteration in genetic makeup each year (CDC, 2017). There are three types of DS: trisomy 21 (95%), translocation in chromosomal pairing (4%), and mosaics (1%–2%) (CDC, 2017). Children born with DS have distinctive physical characteristics as a result of changes on chromosome 21. Assessments of these children typically reveal proportionally shorter necks, small hands, almond-shaped eyes, small ears, a short stature, poor muscle tone, and "loose" joints. Of note, approximately half of children with DS present with serious cardiac anomalies, creating inadequate pulmonary and cardiovascular circulation (see the Case Study at the end of the chapter).

Cerebral Palsy

CP is a disorder of motor movement and posture due to complications occurring during the development of the brain during the prenatal or perinatal period. Prevalence of CP of children 2 to 17 years old is estimated at 2.75/1000 children (Maenner et al., 2016). Etiologies of CP include hypoxiischemic injury, congenital abnormalities from brain malformation or genetic disorders, prematurity, infections, and intracranial hemorrhage. CP can be classified by type of motor disorder (spasticity, dyskinesia, ataxia, or mixed), distribution of the motor disorder (hemiplegia, diplegia, quadriplegia), or the severity of the mobility impairment. Sensory deficits are typically present with CP, such as hearing issues and strabismus or other visual acuity–related issues.

Spina Bifida

SB occurs when there is failure of the neural tube to close during the twenty-eighth day of gestation. SB is associated with deficits in motor, sensory, and physical differences that may be largely prevented with proper folic acid intake during gestation. Children born with SB also experience higher rates of epilepsy and hydrocephalus. Adequate folic acid supplementation is important for prevention of neural tube development. In the United States, mandatory fortification was instituted in 1998, to include wheat flour and maize. Estimates of mandatory folic acid fortification in 58 countries in 2015 resulted in a prevention rate of 13.2% for spina bifida (Arth et al., 2016). Many developing countries experience a high prevalence of spina bifida, cleft lip/palate, hydrocephalus, and anencephaly secondary to subpar nutritional standards—for example, cereals and flour in these areas may not be fortified with folic acid.

Morbidity and Mortality of PWD

Epidemiological data could offer insight not only into disparities in care involving lack of access, income, advocacy, and quality of care historically present but also primary intervention priorities.

Unfortunately, standardized data are not captured comprehensively in many health visits or from national surveys, even those that aim to illuminate the extent of the data gap in both disability surveillance and morbidity and mortality reporting. In part, the variances in definitions for disability complicate the collection of measurable and generalizable data. The most relevant estimate to date, collected from Medicaid data, has estimated that individuals with IDD experience premature mortality of approximately 20 years earlier than the general population (Lauer and McCallion, 2015). This was illustrated in a study examining health services data of individuals with CP. Among the findings were that increased CP severity was associated with more frequent hospital admissions, predominantly associated with respiratory illnesses (Meehan et al., 2016).

Extensive surveillance and research are warranted to determine the extent of the etiology as a consequence of the underlying disability, as opposed to the definitive disparities and inequalities that are known to occur in this vulnerable population. In the following section, fairly frequently occurring comorbidities that increase the overall risk of mortality of those with selected conditions within the disabled population will be outlined.

Epilepsy

Among those with developmental disabilities, epilepsy is prevalent as a comorbidity. Epilepsy is a significant contributor to other risk factors such as the inability to feed or care for oneself, poor communication ability, and lower IQ. Prevalence of epilepsy varies by diagnosis. For example, a meta-analysis of studies concluded that the overall prevalence of epilepsy was 22.2% in those with CP (Robertson et al., 2015). Estimates from a 2017 meta-analysis of epilepsy within the intellectual and CP (motor disability) population revealed a significantly higher rate, at 70% for this combination of comorbidities(van Timmeren et al., 2017). Autism is also correlated with a higher prevalence of epilepsy, among other comorbidities, including schizophrenia, cranial anomalies, inflammatory bowel disease, sleep disorders, and muscular dystrophy (Kohane et al., 2012). Other risk factors within this population that are also associated with a higher mortality include the inability to feed or care for oneself, poor communication ability, inability to ambulate, and lower IQ (van Timmeren et al., 2017). Finally, prevalence of epilepsy increases with age in individuals diagnosed with DS (Robertson et al., 2015).

Obesity, Diabetes, and Cardiovascular Disease

Individuals with IDD are more vulnerable to obesity and type 2 diabetes than the general population due to medications that alter their appetite, genetic disorders, limited mobility, limited opportunities for physical activity, and poorly controlled eating habits (Grondhuis et al., 2014). It is estimated that individuals with CP, dependent on their caregivers for nutritional support, are also at an increased risk for nutritional deficits. Studies have suggested that the diagnosis of ASD is complicated by the correlation of physical activity decreasing with age and neighborhood or physical environments that are not conducive to physical activity (Jones et al. 2017). The prevalence of obesity among children ages 10 to 17 years old analyzed from a nationally representative sample with autism was significantly higher, at 23.1%, than in children without autism, at 14.1% (Must et al., 2017). Although incidence of cardiovascular disease may be

similar to that of the general population, among individuals with intellectual disabilities, a 3-year prospective study indicated that predictive factors included abdominal obesity, use of atypical antipsychotics, and a history of heart failure, resulting in a 32% mortality in the cohort (de Winter et al., 2016).

Fatal Four

The term **fatal four** refers to four common medical conditions that could result in complications and fatality more frequently for the IDD population and other PWD. Nurses and primary care providers should be knowledgeable about the fatal four, which includes (1) constipation/bowel obstruction, (2) aspiration/gastroesophageal reflux disease (GERD), (3) dehydration, and (4) seizures, as complications related to these conditions could result in death if not assessed, diagnosed, and treated swiftly (Smith and Escude, 2015). The etiology of the fatal four includes polypharmacy, improper positioning, obesity, and dysphagia. Individuals with intellectual disabilities and/or motor disabilities are also predisposed to a variety of dental issues, including dental erosions as a consequence of GERD, dental caries, sialorrhea (drooling) due to inadequate swallowing, bruxism (grinding of teeth), malocclusion, and enamel defects (Jan and Jan, 2016).

DISABILITY AND PUBLIC POLICY

Early American public policy viewed people with disabilities as "deserving poor" who required governmental protection and provision and had little capacity for self-support or independence (Rubin and Millard, 1991). Contemporary disability policy minimizes this disadvantaged view and maximizes opportunities for people with disabilities to live productively in their communities. Public policy on disability includes civil rights protections, skill enhancement programs, and income and in-kind assistance programs (e.g., Social Security Disability Insurance [SSDI] and Medicare).

Legislation Affecting People With Disabilities

Consistent with historical and social changes and the recognition of barriers and discrimination, key federal legislation has been enacted that supports the rights of people with disabilities. This section describes a few of the most significant acts and their impact.

The Individuals With Disabilities Education Act

The **Individuals with Disabilities Education Act (IDEA)** (PL 94-142) ensures a free and appropriate public education to children with disabilities that is based on their needs, in the *least restrictive setting* from preschool through secondary education. Addressing special education needs requires appropriate evaluation and transition services. Parents, the student, and professionals are to join together to develop an individualized education plan (IEP) that includes measurable educational goals and related services specific for the child. The National Association of School Nurses (NASN, 2013) asserts that the registered professional school nurse is an essential member of the team participating in the identification and evaluation of students who may be eligible for services. Within the legally required process, the school nurse's responsibilities could include:

- Assisting in identification of special educational or health-related service needs

- Working collaboratively with child/parent/guardian/health care provider assessing functional and physical health status
- Developing individualized health care plans and emergency care plans
- Making recommendations to the team of any health-related accommodations or services required
- Assisting the team in developing an IEP or accommodation plan that provides for required health needs and enables the student to participate in their educational program
- Assisting with identification and removal of health-related barriers to learning
- Providing in-service training for teachers and staff regarding the individual health needs of the child
- Providing and/or supervising unlicensed assistive personnel or direct service providers for provision of specialized health care services in the school setting
- Evaluating the effectiveness and revising as necessary the IEP health-related components (Gibbons et al., 2013).

It is the school nurse's responsibility to understand the law and to refer students who may be eligible for the services as outlined in the law. The nurse will also participate on school teams that determine eligibility for services (NASN, 2013).

The Americans With Disabilities Act of 1990 and ADA Amendments Act of 2008

The Americans with Disabilities Act (ADA) (PL 101-336) became law in July 1990. This landmark civil rights–styled legislation prohibits discrimination against people with disabilities by guaranteeing equal opportunities for people with disabilities in relation to employment, transportation, public accommodations, public services, and telecommunications (U.S. Department of Justice, 2009). It provides protection to people with disabilities similar to those provided to any person on the basis of race, color, sex, national origin, age, and religion. The U.S. Equal Employment Opportunity Commission is charged with enforcement of the employment provisions.

The ADA refers to a "qualified individual" with a disability as a person with a physical or mental impairment that substantially limits one or more major life activities or bodily functions, a person with a record of such an impairment, or a person who is regarded as having such an impairment. The ADA prohibits discrimination against people who have a known association or relationship with an individual with a disability. A qualified individual with a disability must meet legitimate skill, experience, education, or other requirements of an employment position. The person must be able to perform the essential job functions, such as those contained within a job description, with or without reasonable accommodation(s). Reasonable accommodations should make it easier to be successful in job duties and may either involve altering the duties or the tasks of the job performed. Qualifying organizations must provide reasonable accommodations unless they can demonstrate that the accommodation will cause significant difficulty or expense, producing an undue hardship.

Ticket to Work and Work Incentives Improvement Act

Historically, national public policy has defined disability as the inability to work. Typically, people with disabilities could qualify only for such benefits as health care, income assistance programs,

and personal care attendant services if they chose not to work. To address employment and benefit issues for persons with disabilities, in December 1999, the Ticket to Work and Work Incentives Improvement Act (TWWIIA) was signed into law. The TWWIIA reduced the disincentives to work for PWD by increasing access to vocational services and provided new methods for retaining health insurance after they returned to work. In 2008, the Ticket to Work program experienced a significant overhaul when new regulations were produced that dramatically revised the payment structure available to employment networks. This provided a higher cap to accommodate earnings when beneficiaries make progress in their employment plans but before they reach the level of earnings that would terminate their benefits (U.S. Department of Education [USDE], 2008). The Ticket to Work revision is intended to improve program effectiveness in order to maximize the economic self-sufficiency of beneficiaries.

? ACTIVE LEARNING

- Can a client who uses a wheelchair obtain mammography for breast cancer screening, or is the lack of adaptive equipment a barrier to participation? What can you discover online about the availability and cost of accessible transportation to the screening site? Can a woman get onto an examination table for collection of a Papanicolaou smear specimen? Office staff and equipment *should* accommodate people's limitations. Think about the office where you receive health care or the imaging laboratories in the area where you live. Can they accommodate someone in a wheelchair?
- In a primary care office, a woman presents with symptoms of a urinary tract infection. She has experienced decreased mobility due to past lower extremity amputation and is morbidly obese, so is unable to sit down on a standard toilet and hold a cup, both of which are required to collect a urine sample. How can the nurse make modifications to the environment to assist the client and collect the sample?

Public Assistance Programs

Public assistance programs include cash assistance (monetary payments, like Social Security), food stamps, and subsidized housing. In 2010, 59% of people with a severe disability received public assistance, compared with 8.8% of people with a nonsevere disability, whereas only 2.6% of people with no disability received public assistance (Brault, 2012).

Supplemental Security Income and Social Security Disability Insurance

The Social Security Administration (2017) defines disability as the "inability to engage in any substantial gainful activity because of a medically determinable physical or mental impairment(s) that is expected to result in death, or that has lasted or is expected to last for a continuous period of not less than 12 months." Most people who receive disability benefits qualify on the basis of their personal inability to work because of a disability; however, exceptions include people who are blind or have low vision, benefits for widows or widowers who are disabled, and benefits for children who are disabled. Table 21.2 provides a comparison of Supplemental Security Income (SSI) and Social Security Disability Insurance (SSDI) programs. Information about SSI and SSDI can also be accessed online (www.ssa.gov/disability/) or be obtained at a Social Security office.

TABLE 21.2 Comparison of SSI and SSDI

Supplemental Security Income (SSI)	Social Security Disability Insurance (SSDI)
Funded through general tax revenues	Funded through disability trust fund monies (Social Security taxes paid by workers, employers, and self-employed workers)
To qualify for SSI, the person with disabilities (PWD) must have limited income and resources	To qualify for SSDI, the PWD must be "insured" through Federal Insurance Contributions Act (FICA) earnings of self, parents, and/or spouse
SSI disability benefits are payable to adults and children who are disabled or blind and are eligible	SSDI disability benefits are payable to workers or widow(er)s who are disabled or adults who have been disabled since childhood and are eligible
SSI recipients receive Medicaid health benefits	SSDI recipients receive Medicare health benefits
Some states may elect to pay a state supplement to some PWD in SSI programs	PWD in SSDI programs are never provided with state supplements

THE EXPERIENCE OF DISABILITY

Persons with disabilities are commonly thought to constitute the largest minority group in the United States. Of note, most people whose lives do not end abruptly will experience disability in their later years. Regardless of the specific condition, many experiences are common in the lived experience of disability. However, the personal meaning of disability differs significantly with the time frame and the duration of the event or disease process. Those who have a temporary disability, such as a sprained ankle, have a very different experience from someone with chronic illness or permanent disability. Although the former may experience the frustrations of mobility associated with the use of a wheelchair or crutches, this condition is temporary and the full impact of the disability is not experienced. With a temporary disability, ADLs are adjusted as needed and additional or long-term resources are generally not necessary.

In contrast, those who have a permanent disability from an accident or from a disease process, such as limb loss or stroke, must learn to incorporate the modifications required for living into their daily routines and identities. People who become disabled from the progressive decline of a chronic illness, such as multiple sclerosis, may be reluctant to use assistive devices. They might believe that accepting such a device would mean accepting the label of being disabled. Unfortunately, many falls could be prevented by the use of walkers or canes that were declined because the people did not want to appear disabled. In many progressive diseases, a benchmark event forces the person to accept their disability—for example, a driving accident caused by failing eyesight or a change in mental capacity, or a leg amputation from diabetic complications. The person can no longer plan daily activities and expect to accomplish them independently. Because the incidence of chronic illness and disability increases with longevity, often elderly persons experience increasingly disabling changes in their daily lives.

In many cases, a disability can result in a downward spiral. For example, when people with disabling symptoms are unable to return to work, they may lose their jobs and their benefits and exhaust personal resources, which could result in the loss of their home. They may apply for state and federal disability benefits, feeling fully qualified, but are warned there is a waiting period and to expect to be initially rejected. Nurses should engage active listening to better understand a client's situation. Finally, nurses play a role in helping clients connect with comprehensive social services by maintaining knowledge of available resources.

Sexual Health, Education, and the Potential for Abuse

PWD are no different from the general population in their desire for social inclusion and intimacy. Many parents or caregivers are not comfortable addressing what is integral to the quality of life and well-being of PWD, and conservative standards may label sexual activity, marriage, or child bearing as unorthodox or difficult to condone. Health care professionals often consider sexual behavior as less acceptable, somehow unsafe, or inappropriate for PWD, assuming they are asexual, and consequently eliminate sexual assessment and conversation from client education (Shandra and Chowdhury, 2012). The exclusion of PWD from a discussion about sexual health has been highlighted in recent research (Groce et al., 2013). Studies support that a lack of sexual health knowledge can lead to sexually transmitted diseases or pregnancy (Jahoda and Pownall, 2014).

Various obstacles may interfere with the sexual health of PWD, including the societal views noted, functional or physical limitations, difficulty conceptualizing abstract concepts, and personal boundaries/privacy issues. As advocates of PWD, community health nurses should establish a rapport and initiate therapeutic conversations about healthy sexual relationships and facilitate the identification of the health-related consequences of sexual behaviors, while also assessing for potentially abusive situations.

Violence and abuse in the disabled community are more prevalent than among other populations, as there may be a lack of inhibition as well, predisposing some individuals to perpetrate the sexual abuse (Euser et al., 2016; Normand and Sallafranque-St-Louis, 2016). Explanations for the IDD population, in particular, being at a greater risk for sexual abuse include the potential desire for social inclusion, powerlessness, or naiveté. The psychological impact of sexual abuse can result in posttraumatic stress disorder and have long-lasting negative effects (Shabalala and Jasson, 2001). In one population-based study, children with IDD represented 25.9% of the maltreatment allegations, with 29% of those allegations validated (Maclean et al., 2017).

The Family of a Child With a Disability

Challenges and stressors encountered by parents with a child with a disability (CWD) are definitively different, and more numerous. Caregiver burden in terms of quality of life, employment disruption, and financial impact has been frequently documented. Uncertainty in the future of the child and worry about who will care for the child if the child outlives the parent are common themes of parents of CWD (Redquest et al., 2015).

In the past, research concerning children with disabilities has emphasized pathology, personal deficits, and impaired family functioning (Cuskelly, 2009). More recently, efforts have examined more positive and creative aspects of the family experience, including coping behaviors. Humor and exercise have been cited as the most frequent and effective coping mechanisms utilized by parents of CWD (Redquest et al., 2015). A qualitative exploration of coping among parents of children with intellectual disabilities yielded positive themes of coping, including increased sense of personal strength and confidence, changed priorities, greater appreciation of life, pleasure in the child's accomplishments, increased faith/spirituality, more meaningful relationships, and a positive effect on the community at large (Beighton and Wills, 2016). Public health nurses can facilitate positive coping mechanisms by accentuating these same themes with parents.

Parents of a child with a disability grieve the loss of the idealized or expected child over time and redefine their image of and expectations for the child, and also themselves as individuals/parents/marital partners/members of a culture and society. Whether or not a parent anticipated a child's disability, the birth of any child with a disability is a shock, and denial, the first stage of grief, may be the behavior witnessed by health care professionals and others close to the family. In some cases, the child will be rejected, more commonly by one parent.

Sibling responses to a brother/sister who is disabled may be influenced by such factors as the age of the sibling, their reservoir of coping strategies, strength of other peer relationships, perception of the parent's burden in caring for the CWD, desire of a sibling to protect parents from their concerns about the CWD, and the impact of the CWD on family plans and social activities. The following comments of a mother with two children, the younger one with serious disabilities, illustrate these points (Dwight, 2001):

> *My first son, Timmy . . . had taught my husband, Phil, and me many things . . . But I don't think I came face to face with the true meaning of motherhood until Aidan entered our lives. As I pored over the books and talked with these other parents, I found the factual side of Down syndrome fairly easy to piece together . . . Of course, there was nothing in those reference books that could fully explain the other side of the story—the ups and downs of raising a child with Down syndrome in our society . In many ways, our lives have been transformed. We have found loving support from people who used to be strangers. We look at the world differently . . . We have an appreciation for a slower pace . . . And we have a newfound understanding of the preciousness of all people.*

Families quickly learn that neither governmental support nor private health plans offer adequate community-based or in-home assistance for disabled family members. Literature findings describe the associations between low income and children with special needs, associations that might go both ways. In other words, children with a disability are often born into low-income families (Rauch and Lanphear, 2012); however, families who care for a child with a disability often find themselves sliding toward financial insufficiency (Stabile and Allin, 2012). Furthermore, the extent of financial and other resources available, which can determine the possibility of compensatory strategies (such as home modifications), often is the key factor in determining whether effective adaptation can be achieved (Palmer, 2016). Being denied or delayed access to needed health services can negatively affect the health and well-being of any person.

Parents will likely experience some degree of caregiver role strain, which can affect relationships. For example, one study reported an 85% divorce rate among parents of autistic children (Freedman et al., 2012). In contrast, another study did not yield any difference in marriage termination or separation than the general population among parents of children with IDD (Tossebro and Wendelborg, 2017). Among adolescents with CP, predictors of lower quality of life were found to be pain, psychological problems, and the presence of parenting stress (Rapp et al., 2017). Another study evaluated caregiver burdens' effect on quality of life for parents of children with neurodevelopmental conditions and determined that an indirect relationship of care burden to the parent's quality of life exists, but is not related to the child's quality of life (Carona et al., 2014).

🏠 COMMUNITY FOCUS
Bullying of Children With Disabilities

Experiences of school-age children may range from teasing to *bullying,* which is defined as unwanted, aggressive behavior among school-age children, involving a real or perceived power imbalance that is repeated or has the potential to be repeated over time (stopbullying.gov, 2013). Bullying is a very serious problem for children, regardless of disability status. Although a commonly encountered phenomenon in many situations, children with physical, developmental, intellectual, emotional, and sensory disabilities are more likely to be bullied than their peers (stopbullying.gov, 2013).

Children with special health needs may be at greater risk of being bullied or abused. Emerging research validates the magnitude of the problem, indicating that children with ASD are more than three times as likely as other children to be bullied and left out by peers (Twyman et al., 2010). Along with children who have medical conditions that affect their appearance (such as CP and SB), children with seizure disorders and learning disorders are also more likely to be bullied by peers (Hamiwka et al., 2009; Twyman et al., 2010). For the child coping with a disability, the threat of bullying is an added challenge, as bullying often contributes to depression, anxiety, health complaints, and decreased academic achievement.

For individuals with disabilities, bullying may be considered "disability harassment," a behavior that is prohibited under the Rehabilitation Act of 1973 and The Americans with Disabilities Act. Intimidation or abusive behavior toward a child that is based on disability and creates a hostile environment by interfering with or denying the child's participation in or receipt of benefits, services, or opportunities in an institution's program constitutes disability harassment (USDE, 2000). If such an event occurs, there are actions parents of children with disabilities can take to support the bullied child. This involves communicating through the proper channels within the school system. A number of resources, such as "Stopybullying.gov," provide information on how to address the problem of bullying, including strategies for bullying prevention, identification of risk factors for victimization, and resources for help.

⚗ RESEARCH HIGHLIGHTS
Body Image After Amputation

A study conducted by a team led by Freysteinson et al. (2017) described body image and self-esteem experiences that occurred when individuals viewed themselves in the mirror for the first time after the loss of a limb. Previously explored in burn patients, after mastectomy, and in the elderly, this study adds a description of the mirror trajectory of experience among amputees.

A qualitative design was employed to explore this concept with focus groups. Researchers then utilized hermeneutic phenomenology, the study of

Body Image After Amputation

the words and meaning ascribed to them, in dwelling with the content of the discussions and shared the concepts emerging from the experience.

The mirror experience had three key moments: decision, seeing, and consent. There were four key themes: mirror shock, mirror anguish, recognizing self, and acceptance of a new normal. Participants in focus groups also shared ways that staff members could better facilitate the introduction of a mirror after an amputation, such as using it as a small tool to check skin integrity and to correct gait and balance in the larger view. As this is a little-known phenomenon, further research on educational aspects, such as preparation of patients, families, and interprofessional staff members to better support the experience, is needed. Support of a family member or friend is suggested during this experience, but as nurses develop trust and intimacy with their patients, they could be a facilitator of the discussion of what to expect.

ACTIVE LEARNING

Ask your friends, neighbors, or family if they know someone with a serious disability. Discover and inquire about what challenges or concerns are most important to the PWD.

HEALTH PROMOTION AND DISEASE PREVENTION FOR PWD

Worldwide, health care problems frequently are unrecognized and untreated, particularly among those with IDD who may not be able to communicate their symptoms and/or are unable to share in decision making. Despite the higher prevalence of chronic conditions that can significantly compromise physical function, such as arthritis, asthma, cardiovascular disease, diabetes, high blood pressure, high cholesterol, and stroke among individuals with disabilities, improvements in primary preventative care and surveillance are slow to occur (Reichard and Stolzle, 2011). Clients with disabilities may exhibit behavioral problems that discourage health care providers from caring for them, or they may resist others' attempts to care for them because of their discomfort or unfamiliarity with the health care setting or equipment. There may be difficulties in obtaining a client history and in determining the nature and cause of a problem. This might easily be alleviated with teaching health care providers about health care problems that accompany a specific disability (May and Kennedy, 2010).

For example, it is widely acknowledged that socioeconomic disadvantages account for a significant proportion of variation in health status. Specifically, women with disabilities often experience disparities in primary care services, particularly in women's health issues. Because osteoporosis develops at higher rates in women with decreased mobility, recommendations include screening at earlier and more frequent intervals, special gynecological examination techniques, and "thoughtful well-coordinated" care from primary care providers (Wilkinson and Cerreto, 2008). Similarly, women with cognitive limitations and functional disabilities have been noted as less likely to receive a Pap smear within the past 3 years or a mammogram within the past 2 years. Primary care assessments for this population should also include immunizations and preventive screenings, such as those for breast, colon, and testicular cancer in males (Reichard et al., 2011). Further, health promotion questions that assess diet, exercise, alcohol, drug use, smoking, and sexual health should be routine in primary care visits for disabled individuals (Bakker-van Gijssel et al., 2017).

Strategies for the Public Health Nurse Caring for People With Disabilities

Nurses have the responsibility of caring for the needs of varying populations. Regardless of whether the nurse chooses to work in a setting that specializes in health care services for people affected by disabilities, disability is a common experience that all practicing nurses will encounter in their professional career. This will require the professional nurse to be familiar with effective strategies for communicating and caring for individuals with a variety of disabilities. The scope of responsibility in caring for individuals with disabilities includes procuring the knowledge related to health conditions that may result from or lead to the disability, as well as being aware of the resources available and legal implications that affect the PWD.

Health care professionals are taught to assess and provide interventions that promote health, and they usually assume they know what people with disabilities need. Regardless of the provider's professional experience or familiarity with disability, clients may question a provider's ability to understand their experience. Moreover, literature supports that nurses and physicians who have not had experience caring for individuals with disabilities lack confidence and exhibit attitudes that are not conducive to caring for this vulnerable population (Bu et al., 2016).

Nurses must work with the interprofessional care team to form alliances with the client and family and reduce or eliminate barriers. People affected by disabilities may have some common health care needs or utilize similar resources, but other issues will be unique to each individual situation. The public health nurse's perspective on disability will influence the nursing role and the level of care provided to PWD and their families. Delivery of passionate, person-centered care is essential and includes concepts of care, compassion, competence, communication, courage, and commitment and ensures patients' values are a component of clinical decisions (Brown et al., 2016). The Association of Rehabilitation Nurses has proposed a competency model for nursing that can be a guide for public health nursing care of clients with disabilities in the current dynamic health care environment (Fig. 21.3).

Nursing care must incorporate the true essence of advocacy, where it is defined as representing the needs of the client or patient. The nurse's role should be to discern the needs and resources of the client and his or her family. Only then may the nurse act effectively as a resource themselves, working to provide information, make connections, and manage accommodations. The acronym developed that spells ADVOCATE (Table 21.3) can help remind and guide the nurse of essential principles that are integral to the care of PWD. The table provides specific strategies to ensure the nurse practices effective care, communication etiquette, and advocacy in his or her care of PWD.

Nursing Interventions

Public health nurses should partner with clients and families affected by disabilities to address barriers that negatively affect quality of life, a measure of satisfaction that reaches across physical, psychological, social, and environmental domains. Nurses cannot remedy health concerns without attending to interacting systems, such as

**ARN Competency Model for
Professional Rehabilitation Nursing**

FIG. 21.3 Rehabilitation nursing professional role competency model. (Reprinted with permission from the Association of Rehabilitation Nursing.)

knowledge and educational background, personal and family belief systems, religious/spiritual beliefs and supports, finances, social networks, physical resources, and cultural influences. Health promotion interventions for the community health nurse should include:

- Provision of age-related health screenings
- Early surveillance of diseases based on knowledge of common comorbidities
- Maintenance of proper weight: counseling on appropriate nutrition and social inclusion through enhanced physical activity
- Identification of caregivers and support systems
- Identification of access to care issues: transportation, financial, and environmental barriers
- Safety of the physical environment: assistive technology (such as health monitoring devices and alarms, voice-activated technology, and mobility devices) and potential for abuse
- Knowledge of resources

Differentiating Illness From Disability

Nurses who work in community settings must be able to differentiate between the person who has an illness and becomes disabled secondary to the illness and the person who has a disability but may not need care. Rather than assuming a need for intervention, the nurse should ask whether the client wants assistance, ask the client/family to describe the goal(s), and ask how and in what way(s) the nurse can help. PWD often confront *medicalization* issues when others view

them in the *sick role* rather than as people first. Nurses should listen to understand, collaborating with the person/family to make plans and goals that meet the identified needs and that draw on strengths and improve weaknesses. Collaboration empowers and affirms the worth and knowledge of the person/family with a disability. Collaboration promotes self-determination and allows choices that foster personal values and preferences.

📋 NURSING CARE GUIDELINES

Assistive Technology and Creative Solutions

A diagnosis of autism or ASD presents a myriad of issues for the provision of health care to this population. Unfamiliar individuals, places, or loud noises can hyperstimulate individuals with ASD. Primary care sites, including health care facilities or physicians' offices, may produce anxiety for someone with ASD. Telemedicine offers an ideal avenue for providing treatment in a convenient manner. Telemedicine involves the use of remote access to a primary care physician. Equipment necessary for accessing the primary care provider may include a video conference camera and a telephonic stethoscope, digital camera, and otoscope for a nurse-assisted visit (Langkamp et al., 2015). Telemedicine is utilized predominantly to improve access to care for individuals living in rural or underserved geographic areas; however, use in the IDD/developmental disability population could produce positive results if counseling may be more realistically delivered via conference call.

TABLE 21.3 Nurse Strategies for Care, Communication, and Advocacy

Advocate	Don't assume the client has a physical or cognitive deficit until you have validated it.
	Be knowledgeable and educate yourself about community resources and those pertaining to various disabilities
	Know the client's payer sources or other financial resources, as it may determine the level of assistance they obtain
	Be knowledgeable of risk for injury and abuse
	Practice forensic nursing, as clients may not be able to articulate their issues
Deficits	Determine sensory, visual, and hearing deficits
	Allocate additional time for care
	Eliminate physical environmental barriers
	Select the client's optimal time of day for education and ADLs
Vocation	Encourage vocation or "avocation," including recreational therapy that encourages social interaction (i.e., intramural teams, physical activity, hippotherapy, art classes)
	Assess employment history, interests, and employment obtainment
Outcomes	Observe for polypharmacy: side effects/ interactions
	Observe patterns of multiple hospitalizations and etiology
	Adopt the client's perspective as to what works best with no bias; cultural preferences may be a factor
	Be knowledgeable about evidence-based treatment options specific to the disability or disease
	Establish bowel and bladder routine and adequate hydration: observe for signs and symptoms of urinary tract infection (UTI) or constipation
	Encourage weight-bearing exercises, T.E.D. hose, observe potential for postural hypotension with immobile clients
Communicate	Listen and learn from client, family, and caregiver
	Always say "Hello," "Good morning," and "Good afternoon," regardless of the client's ability to respond
	Directly speak with or to the client unless there are deficits that make it not feasible (communication, cognitive, hearing)
	At wheelchair level, by client's name, not their disability
	Reduce background noises or distractions during discussions
	Rephrase rather than repeat information if something is not understood
	Collaborate with interprofessionals for care outcomes, issues, facilitators, and barriers to care
	Professional boundaries if necessary
Assess	Determine what deficits the client deems a challenge or an issue
	Skin integrity of the immobilized and incontinent client
	Self-care ability: ADLs, feeding, bathing, and time of day where energy is optimal
	Necessary accommodations to environment (ramp, access), with communication (Braille, sign language) or adaptive devices that are used or needed; wheelchair, hearing aids, long-handled combs or shoe horns, hand braces for toothbrushes or utensils, drinking cups with weighted bases, Velcro, voice-activated technology
	Home environment, care providers, social networks
	Primary transportation preferences or use
Transition	Provide resources, information, and support when there is a change in level of care, care providers, school, or role responsibility within the family unit
Empower	Encourage learning, memory, coping skills, independence
	Reinforce abilities and success in ADLs, mobility, employment

© Allison Edwards.

"Knowledgeable Client" and "Knowledgeable Nurse"

Regardless of the cause of disability, the nurse must see beyond the disabling impairment, carefully assessing each affected person's perceptions of the disability experience. A person who lives with a disability commonly becomes an expert at knowing what works best for his or her body. This case differs significantly from the person with a new disabling illness or injury, or the parent of a child with a newly diagnosed disability, who needs information and time to adapt to their new change in circumstance. The Intersystem Model (Artinian et al., 2011) refers to the first-described person as the "Knowledgeable Client." In this case, a client has been living with disability for an extended time and has become sensitive to the needs of his or her body. The nurse should ask the client what works best for him or her and what goals the client is pursuing. The client wants the nurse to listen to his or her concerns and may benefit from a referral to health-related resources. However, if the nurse attempts to tell the Knowledgeable Client what to do without seeking input, the client may become angry and seek help elsewhere.

The clients in the second situation need the services of the "Knowledgeable Nurse" (Artinian et al., 2011). The client with a newly diagnosed condition can benefit from the nurse's information about the disability and the available community and governmental resources. It is important to note that if the nurse is unable to help a newly diagnosed client learn how to manage the disability and accept himself or herself as disabled, the nurse may compromise the client's adaptation and future client/nurse interactions.

Active collaboration between the client and nurse is required to develop a plan of care that both will find acceptable. Health care for PWD must incorporate remedies that address issues surrounding access to health care and the resolution of environmental and social barriers that prevent their full participation in society. Encouraging recreational time and physical activity provides a positive stimulus for PWD and multiple psychosocial and physiological benefits—for example, hippotherapy, a therapeutic method of horseback riding, shows evidence that it enhances motor strategies, which can improve functional task performance by enhancing reaction time among individuals with intellectual disabilities. Not only does the activity of horseback riding provide a rich social environment with the interaction between the PWD and the animal as well as other equestrians, but it also has demonstrated improvement in balance and strength in individuals with IDD, which could have a profound impact on their quality of life (Giagazoglou et al., 2012).

ETHICAL ISSUES FOR PEOPLE AFFECTED BY DISABILITIES

PWD and their families are concerned about the same contemporary ethical and legal issues that concern all people. However, some of the associated issues carry particular interest for PWD and their families, including questions and problems surrounding definitions of respect for human beings, beneficence (do good), and nonmaleficence (do no harm), as well as the rights of PWD. The Patient Self-Determination Act (PSDA) of 1990 is one example. This law mandated that health decisions are communicated and protected and that patients, upon admission to a health care facility, are asked if they have a durable power of attorney or an advance directive. Families, guardians, or individuals are reluctant to address end-of-life decisions when health is good, so when conditions decline, bioethical principles must be balanced and applied, sometimes by a team or committee.

Determining the appropriate care for infants, children, and adults with disabilities is a complex issue for families to consider. Associated issues include choosing between abortion and continuing the pregnancy when prenatal screening suggests the presence of impairments and health problems. In 2009, parents filed a $14 million malpractice suit when prenatal testing failed to correctly diagnose Down syndrome. They stated that an accurate test result would have led them to end the pregnancy (Green, 2009). Health care professionals may convey negative attitudes about life with a disability, so it is vital that accurate and balanced information be provided. The Prenatally and Postnatally Diagnosed Awareness Act of 2008 (PL 110-374) uses federal resources to produce and distribute information about prenatally and postnatally diagnosed conditions (Dresser, 2009).

Clients' spiritual perspectives play an important role in decision making when there is a change in health status or a life-threatening illness. People who establish hope and meaning in their lives may choose to positively reframe the difficulties associated with functional limitations that others may find intolerable. Holistic caregiving requires the nurse to assess and promote spiritual health along with physical and psychological well-being.

Differences in quality of life and justice perspectives intersect with concerns about the control of health care costs. Advances in neonatology are responsible for increasing numbers of very-low-birth-weight babies, who are at high risk for cognitive disorders and other serious health problems (Reichman et al., 2008). Many parents of CWD desire or incur (costly) life-sustaining treatment. In contrast, some people who are either newly disabled or nondisabled may see future life as a disabled person so burdensome that they may refuse extraordinary medical treatments and/or actively seek to end their lives (Hahn and Belt, 2004).

For health care professionals to understand the end-of-life desires of the disabled population, more research is needed. Focus groups can yield beneficial information; however, feasibility is challenging. Participants may struggle to understand abstract concepts such as death; furthermore, physical environment supports and consulting for recruitment and consent among this vulnerable population are difficult (Savage et al., 2015). End-of-life decision making for children with severe developmental disabilities must involve a determination of whether the caregiver or parent will continue care necessary to sustain life, such as maintenance of a ventilator or artificial nutrition via gastrostomy tube, or cease support. In a meta-analysis of end-of-life decisions among the severe IDD population aged 0 to 18, parents felt physician information regarding their child's situation was insufficient and that to speak with other parents who had faced similar dilemmas would be most helpful (Zaall-Schuller et al., 2016). Shared final decision making was favored 40% of the time, whereas independent decisions without the physician were favored 41% of the time. A key influence was perceived suffering evidenced by visible facial expressions and eye movement and declining quality of life (Zaall-Schuller et al., 2016).

Genetic technology, such as prenatal cell-free DNA screening for chromosomal abnormalities, may lead to elective abortions but also offer hope for the prevention and cure of diseases. A recent study reported the elective termination rate at 67% for singleton and 60% for twins after prenatal testing resulting in aneuploidy, an abnormal number of chromosomes (Dobson et al., 2016). At the other end of the life continuum, advocacy groups, such as Not Dead Yet, have taken a strong stance against physician-assisted suicide, fearing it will lead to the early or forced death of PWD. Disability rights proponents recognize that the devaluation of PWD may promote their unnecessary and untimely deaths (Ne'eman, 2009). The case of Terri Schiavo, described in the Ethical Insights box, illustrates some of these issues.

ETHICAL INSIGHTS

When Is Life Worth Continuing?

The world watched while Terri Schiavo's situation unfolded amid numerous legal and legislative challenges surrounding whether her feeding tube should be discontinued, and conflict developed between her parents and her husband/guardian, Michael. Disability rights groups and right-to-life advocates kept vigil for weeks outside the nursing home where Terri resided. Terri, at age 34, experienced an anoxic event that led to brain damage. Although previous court decisions have clearly established a person's right to discontinuation of treatment, including the provision of food and fluids, there was no documentation or advance directive indicating Terri's wishes. Terri's parents offered to assume guardianship of their daughter, believing her to be both responsive to her environment and desiring life in her current condition. Michael fought to have her feeding tube removed, stating that in previous discussions Terri had said that, in a similar situation, she would not want to continue living. Medical discussions focused on the extent of her "vegetative state" and capacity to respond to her environment. Seven years later, amid numerous court challenges and Michael's obtaining a reported million-dollar-plus malpractice settlement designated for his wife's care, the court ordered that Terri's feeding tube and all hydration be stopped as requested by her husband. She died several days later.

What are the relevant issues when families are in conflict about what medical treatment the person with a severe disability would want in the absence of written advanced directives? What values and ethical principles should be considered? As health care professionals, evaluate this case in terms of the principles of utilitarianism and beneficence or nonmaleficence.

Blake is in his early 20s. His parents reported that they were told many times throughout Blake's life about what he "can't do" or "won't do." But they chose to focus on what he "can do" and even "could do" in the future. Blake was named a two-time captain of the varsity football team, Prom King, and Texas Citizen of the Year. At 20 years old, Blake became the first business owner in Texas with Down syndrome when he opened a snow cone stand, *Blake's Snow Shack*. Blake's business has achieved local, national, and international acclaim. (Courtesy of Blake's Snow Shack. www.blakessnowshack.com.)

Rosa is a Hispanic female with intellectual disabilities. She is her own guardian and lives with her sister and attends a day habilitation program.

Sam is an African American in his mid-30s. Sam has autism (ASD). He is nonverbal but follows directions and performs all ADLs independently.

Max, age 60, is a Caucasian male, born with intellectual disabilities. He has lived in a variety of settings since the age of 12, including a specialized residential school, residential-vocation facility, long-term care, and currently a group home. He feeds and dresses himself, but personal care activities are assisted.

Catalina is a 32-year-old Hispanic female who was born with cerebral palsy. She has some upper extremity mobility, and needs assistance eating and with ADLs. She has discernible language skills, although limited to monosyllabic words.

Anthony is a 30-year-old African American who was born with Down syndrome and severe cardiac anomalies and lived his first 4 years at a children's hospital. Now, Anthony is healthy and involved in his day habilitation program.

CASE STUDY   Application of the Nursing Process
A Child With Down Syndrome

Ginger Johnson was 37 years old when she conceived her third pregnancy. Per her doctor's recommendation, Ginger underwent genetic screening tests, which revealed that the fetus was positive for Down syndrome. A very intense and emotional time followed as Ginger and her family planned to welcome the new baby they recognized would likely have physical and developmental challenges. During the pregnancy, Ginger developed gestational diabetes, and baby Jack was born 6 weeks premature by emergency caesarean section.

Assessment

Jack had feeding difficulties due to low muscle tone requiring oral motor therapy every 3 hours at birth followed by once-weekly therapy until age 2. He could not tolerate any dairy or gluten products from birth. His low muscular tone also required physical and occupational therapy one to three times per week. He had hip dysplasia that required various adaptive measures, and his feet, ankles, and lower calves required orthotic braces. Unlike over 50% of children with Down syndrome, Jack had no cardiac anomalies.

Jack had strabismus from birth, which required eye patching and glasses for far-sighted vision at approximately 18 months. He also had bilateral eustachian tubes and underwent an adenoidectomy at age 3. Jack was plagued with chronic diarrhea for his first 6 years, which resolved with elimination of intestinal bacteria and use of digestive enzymes.

His growth chart illustrated no growth from ages 2 to 3, and he was diagnosed with a pituitary deficiency. Human growth hormone treatment was initiated at age 3 and will continue through puberty. Jack was also diagnosed with attention-deficit hyperactivity disorder (ADHD) but did not respond well to stimulant medications at age 5; therefore a second-line medication was prescribed.

As Jack's immune system improved, he experienced fewer illnesses, with the exception of contracting pneumonia at age 7. He was hospitalized for 10 days of which 3 days were in the intensive care unit (ICU). Jack was diagnosed as borderline diabetic, and his physician recommended a Paleo diet to help normalize glucose. Jack began puberty at 10½ and was diagnosed with scoliosis at age 11. Jack attends a public elementary school that has a special program for children with IDDs, where he has had the same teacher for the last 4 years. But he will be transitioning to middle school this year and be introduced to a new teacher.

Jack's family lives in a middle-class area of a small city and consists of his mother Ginger, father Sam, and sisters Jill (15) and Jessica (17). Ginger is a stay-at-home mother, and Sam is an accountant for an insurance company. Health insurance is provided by Sam's company, but the deductible and copayments have risen dramatically in the last few years. With Jessica starting college next year, money is tight and expected to become more difficult.

Jack participates weekly in hippotherapy and maintains the horse stalls as part of his activities. His only sibling, a sister, will leave for college in a few months.

Jack, age 12, Caucasian male, was born with Down syndrome. Jack uses variety of interprofessional medical services that have yielded success in the day-to-day management of Jack's health issues.

Jack has struggled with an immune-based response, alopecia.

■ SUMMARY

Community health nurses must recognize that there are a variety of personal and societal perspectives on disability with accompanying moral or ethical issues. They should practice holistic nursing care that incorporates mind, body, and spiritual care considerations into health care practice. To this end, nurses can do the following:

- Become familiar with a variety of ethical frameworks for decision making and adopt a strategy to analyze ethical problems related to health care for people with disabilities.

- Help clients and families access information needed to make informed decisions that reflect their interests and priorities.
- Help educate the public on health care issues within the nurse's scope of practice and knowledge and skill level.
- Participate in the development of institutional policies and procedures for ethical and legal issues related to disability.
- Take a position on an ethical issue with political implications.
- Work to influence governmental policies and laws related to disability.

ⓔ EVOLVE WEBSITE

http://evolve.elsevier.com/Nies/community
- NCLEX Review Questions
- Case Studies

BIBLIOGRAPHY

Arc: *The first 50 years*, 2013. Available from: www.thearc.org/NetCommunity/Page.aspx?pid=269.

Arth A, Kancherla V, Pachon H, et al.: A 2015 global update on folic acid-preventable spina bifida and anencephaly, *Birth Defects Res Part A, Clin Mol Teratol* 106(7):520–529, 2016. https://doi.org/10.1002/bdra.23529. [doi].

Artinian BM, West K, Conger M, editors: *The Artinian Intersystem Model: integration theory and practice for the professional nurse*, ed 2, New York, 2011, Springer Publishing Company.

Barnes C: Theories of disability and the origins of the oppression of disabled people in Western society. In Barton L, editor: *Disability and society: emerging issues and insights*, New York, 1996, Longman.

Bakker-van Gijssel EJ, Lucassen PL, Olde Hartman TC, et al.: Health assessment instruments for people with intellectual disabilities-A systematic review, *Res Develop Disabil* 64:12–24, 2017. https://doi.org/S0891-4222(17)30070-7. [pii].

Beighton C, Wills J: Are parents identifying positive aspects to parenting their child with an intellectual disability or are they just coping? A qualitative exploration, *J Intellect Disabil*, 2016. 174462951665607; 174462951665607.

Brault M: *Americans with disabilities: 2005*, 2008. Available at https://www.census.gov/prod/2008pubs/p70-117.pdf.

Brault M: *Americans with disabilities: 2010*, 2012. Available at https://www.census.gov/prod/2012pubs/p70-131.pdf.

Brown M, Chouliara Z, MacArthur J, et al.: The perspectives of stakeholders of intellectual disability liaison nurses: a model of compassionate, person-centred care, *J Clin Nurs* 25(7-8):972–982, 2016. https://doi.org/10.1111/jocn.13142. [doi].

Bu P, Veloski JJ, Ankam NS, et al.: Effects of a brief curricular intervention on medical students' attitudes toward people with disabilities in healthcare settings, *Am J Phys Med Rehabil* 95(12):939–945, 2016. https://doi.org/10.1097/PHM.0000000000000535. [doi].

Campbell A, Uren A: 'The invisibles'... : Disability in China in the 11st Century, *Intl J of Special Ed* 26(1):12–24, 2011.

Carona C, Silva N, Cresp C, et al.: Caregiving burden and parent-child quality of life outcomes in neurodevelopmental conditions: the mediating role of behavioral disengagement, *J Clin Psychol Med Settings* 21(4):320–328, 2014. https://doi.org/10.1007/s10880-014-9412-5. [doi].

Centers for Disease Control and Prevention: *Autism (ASD) spectrum disorders: data and statistics*, 2014. Available from: http://www.cdc.gov/ncbddd/autism/data.html.

Centers for Disease Control and Prevention: *Disability and health: disability overview*, 2015. Available from: https://www.cdc.gov/ncbddd/disabilityandhealth/disability.html.

Centers for Disease Control and Prevention: *Disability and health: related conditions*, 2016. Available from: https://www.cdc.gov/ncbddd/disabilityandhealth/relatedconditions.html.

Centers for Disease Control and Prevention: *Facts about down syndrome*, 2017. Available from: https://www.cdc.gov/ncbddd/birthdefects/DownSyndrome.html.

Center for Health Care Strategies: *Inc: Structuring new service delivery models for individuals with intellectual and developmental disabilities*, 2013.

Chiang LH, Hadadian A: Raising children with disabilities in China: the need for early interventions, *Int J Special Educ* 25(2):113–118, 2010.

Child and Adolescent Health Measurement Initiative: *2009/10 National Survey of Children with Special Health Care Needs*, Available from: http://www.childhealthdata.org/browse/survey/.

Christensen DL, Bilder DA, Zahorodny W, et al.: Prevalence and characteristics of autism spectrum disorder among 4-year-old children in the autism and developmental disabilities monitoring network, *J Dev Behav Pediatr* 37(1):1–8, 2016. https://doi.org/10.1097/DBP.0000000000000235. [doi].

Costa-Black K, Feuerstein M, Loisel P: Work disability models: past and present. In Loisel P, Anema J, editors: *Handbook of work disability: prevention and management*, New York, 2013, Springer, pp 71–93.

Cuskelly M: Challenging the myths and redressing the missteps in family research, *J Policy Practice Int Disabil* 6(2):86–88, 2009.

de Winter CF, van den Berge AP, Schoufour JD, et al.: A 3-year follow-up study on cardiovascular disease and mortality in older people with intellectual disabilities, *Res Dev Disabil* 53–54:115–126, 2016. https://doi.org/10.1016/j.ridd.2016.01.020. [doi].

Dobson LJ, Reiff ES, Little SE, et al.: Patient choice and clinical outsomces following positive noninvasive prenatal screening for aneuploidy with cell-free DNA, *Prenat Diagn* 36(5):456–462, 2016.

Dresser R: Prenatal testing and disability: a truce in the culture wars? *Hastings Cent Rep* 39(3):7–8, 2009.

Dunn D, Andrews E: *There is a difference between having a handicap and a disability, in the publich interest newsletter*, American Psychological Association, 2015. Retrieved December 10, 2016 from: http://www.apa.org/pi/about/newsletter/2015/11/handicap-disabilities.aspx.

Dwight V: Aidan's gift. In Klein SD, Schive K, editors: *You will dream new dreams: inspiring personal stories by parents of children with disabilities*, New York, 2001, Kensington, pp 31–37.

Eskay M, Onu VC, Igbo JN: Disability within the African culture, *US-China Rev* B4:473–484, 2012.

Euser S, Alink LR, Tharner A, et al.: The prevalence of child sexual abuse in out-of-home care: increased risk for children with a mild intellectual disability, *J Appl Res Intellect Disabil* 29(1):83–92, 2016, https://doi.org/10.1111/jar.12160. [doi].

Freedman BH, Kalb LG, Zablotsky B: Relationship status among parents of children with autism spectrum disorders: a population-based study, *J Autism Dev Disord* 42:539–548, 2012. https://doi.org/10.1007/s10803-011-1269-y.

Freysteinson W, Thomas L, Sebastian-Deutsch A, et al.: A study of the amputee experience of viewing self in the mirror, *Rehabil Nursing J* 42(1):22–32, 2017. https://doi.org/10.1002/mj.256.

Giagazoglou P, Arabatzi F, Dipla K, et al.: Effect of a hippotherapy intervention program on static balance and strength in adolescents with intellectual disabilities, *Res Dev Disabil* 33(6):2265–2270, 2012. https://doi.org/10.1016/j.ridd.2012.07.004. [doi].

Gibbons LJ, Lehr K, Selekman J: Federal laws protecting children and youth with disabilities in the schools. In: (ed: Selekman J.) *School nursing: a comprehensive text*, ed 2, Philadelphia, PA, F.A. Davis & Company, pp 257–283.

Green A: Prenatal testing goes to court OregonLive.Com/The OregonianJune 14, 2009. Available from: www.oregonlive.com/news/oregonian/index.ssf?/base/news/1244872511325030.xml&;coll=7&thispage=3

Groce NE, Rohleder P, Eide AH, et al.: HIV issues and people with disabilities: a review and agenda for research, *Soc Sci Med (1982)* 77:31–40, 2013. https://doi.org/10.1016/j.socscimed.2012.10.024. [doi].

Grondhuis SN, Grondhuis SN, Aman MG: Overweight and obesity in youth with developmental disabilities: a call to action, *J Intellec Disabil Res* 58(9):787–799, 2014.

Grue J: The social meaning of disability: a reflection on categorisation, stigma and identity, *Sociol Health Illness* 38(5):557–564, 2016.

Hahn H, Belt TL: Disability identity and attitudes toward cure in a sample of disabled activists, *J Health Soc Behav* 45:453–464, 2004.

Hamiwka LD, Yu CG, Hamiwka LA, et al.: Are children with epilepsy at greater risk for bullying than their peers? *Epilepsy & Behav* 15:500–505, 2009.

Health Media Lab: Franklin Delano Roosevelt (1933–1945), the dying president, Available from: www.healthmedialab.com/html/president/roosevelt.html.

Healthy People.gov: *Healthy People 2020: immunization and infectious diseases*, Available from: http://healthypeople.gov/2020/topicsobjectives2020/objectiveslist.aspx?topicId=23.

Jahoda A, Pownall J: Sexual understanding, sources of information and social networks; the reports of young people with intellectual disabilities and their non-disabled peers, *J Intellect Disabil Res* 58(5):430–441, 2014. https://doi.org/10.1111/jir.12040. [doi].

Jan BM, Jan MM: Dental health of children with cerebral palsy, *Neurosciences (Riyadh, Saudi Arabia)* 21(4):314–318, 2016. https://doi.org/10.17712/nsj.2016.4.20150729. [doi].

Jones RA, Downing K, Rinehart NJ, et al.: Physical activity, sedentary behavior and their correlates in children with autism spectrum disorder: a systematic review, *PloS One* 12(2):e0172482, 2017. https://doi.org/10.1371/journal.pone.0172482. [doi].

Kohane IS, McMurry A, Weber G, et al.: The comorbidity burden of children and young adults with autism spectrum disorders, *PloS One* 7(4):e33224, 2012. https://doi.org/10.1371/journal.pone.0033224. [doi].

Langkamp DL, McManus MD, Blakemore SD: Telemedicine for children with developmental disabilities: a more effective clinical process than office-based care, *Telemed J e-Health* 21(2):110–114, 2015. https://doi.org/10.1089/tmj.2013.0379. [doi].

Lauer E, McCallion P: Mortality of people with intellectual and developmental disabilities from select US state disability service systems and medical claims data, *J Appl Res Intellect Disabil* 28(5):394–405, 2015. https://doi.org/10.1111/jar.12191. [doi].

Longmore PK: Uncovering the hidden history of people with disabilities, *Rev Am Hist* 15(3):355–364, 1987.

Maclean MJ, Sims S, Bower C, et al.: Maltreatment risk among children with disabilities, *Pediatrics*, 2017. https://doi.org/e20161817 [pii].

Maenner MJ, Blumberg SJ, Kogan MD, et al.: Prevalence of cerebral palsy and intellectual disability among children identified in two U.S. national surveys, 2011–2013, *Ann Epidemiol* 26(3):222–226, 2016. https://doi.org.ezproxyhost.library.tmc.edu/10.1016/j.annepidem.2016.01.001.

May M, Kennedy C: Health and problem behavior among people with intellectual disabilities, *Behav Anal Pract* 3(2):4–12, 2010.

Megargee GP, editor: *Euthanasia program*, The United States Holocaust Memorial Museum Encyclopedia of Camps and Ghettos (vol. 1). Available from: www.ushmm.org/wlc/article.php?lang=en&;ModuleId=10005200.

Meehan E, Reid SM, Williams K, et al.: Hospital admissions in children with cerebral palsy: a data linkage study, *Dev Med Child Neurol*, 2016. https://doi.org/10.1111/dmcn.13350. [doi].

Must A, Eliasziw M, Phillips SM, et al.: The effect of age on the prevalence of obesity among US youth with autism spectrum disorder, *Child Obes* 13(1):25–35, 2017. https://doi.org/10.1089/chi.2016.0079. [doi].

National Association of School Nurses (NASN): *Section 504 and individuals with disabilities education improvement act—the role of the school nurse*, Available from: http://www.nasn.org/PolicyAdvocacy/PositionPapersandReports/NASNPositionStatementsFullView/tabid/462/ArticleId/491/Section-504-and-Individuals-with-Disabilities-Education-Improvement-Act-The-Role-of-the-School-Nurse.

Ne'eman A: *Health care reform and the disability community, The Huffington Post*, 2009. Available from: www.huffingtonpost.com/ari-neeman/health-care-reform-and-th_b_206492.html.

Normand CL, Sallafranque-St-Louis F: Cybervictimization of young people with an intellectual or developmental disability: risks specific to sexual solicitation, *J Appl Res Intellect Disabil* 29(2):99–110, 2016. https://doi.org/10.1111/jar.12163. [doi].

Norrgard K: Human subjects and diagnostic genetic testing, *Nat Educ* 1(1):82–86, 2008.

Palmer S: Family adaptation and intervention, Budd MA, Hough S, Wegener ST, Stiers W, editors: *Practical psychology in medical rehabilitation*415–422, 2016.

Pfeiffer D: Overview of the disability movement: history, legislative record, and political implications, *Policy Stud J* 21(4):724–734, 1993.

Pope AM, Tarlov AR: *Disability in america: toward a national agenda for prevention*, Washington, DC, 1991, National Academy Press.

Rapp M, Eisemann N, Arnaud C, et al.: Predictors of parent-reported quality of life of adolescents with cerebral palsy: a longitudinal study, *Res Dev Disabil* 62:259–270, 2017. https://doi.org/S0891-4222(16)30271-2 [pii].

Rauch S, Lanphear B: Prevention of disability in children: elevating the role of environment, *Child Disabil* 22(1):193–217, 2012.

Redquest BK, Reinders N, Bryden PJ, et al.: Raising a child with special needs: The perspective of caregivers, *Clin Nurse Spec* 29(3):E8–15, 2015. https://doi.org/10.1097/NUR.0000000000000122. [doi].

Reichard A, Stolzle H: Diabetes among adults with cognitive limitations compared to individuals with no cognitive disabilities, *Intellect Dev Disabil* 49(3):141, 2011.

Reichard A, Stolzle H, Fox MH: Health disparities among adults with physical disabilities or cognitive limitations compared to individuals with no disabilities in the United States, *Disabil Health J* 4(2):59–67, 2011. https://doi.org.ezproxyhost.library.tmc.edu/10.1016/j.dhjo.2010.05.003.

Reichman NE, Corman H, Noonan K: Impact of child disability on the family, *Matern Child Health J* 12(6):679–683, 2008. Also available from: www.medscape.com/viewarticle/581577_2.

Robertson J, Hatton C, Emerson E, et al.: Prevalence of epilepsy among people with intellectual disabilities: a systematic review, *Seizure* 29:46–62, 2015. https://doi.org/10.1016/j.seizure.2015.03.016. [doi].

Rubin SE, Millard RP: Ethical principles and American public policy on disability, *J Rehabil*, 1991. Available from: http://findarticles.com/p/articles/mi_m0825/is_n1_v57/ai_10684712/?tag=content;col1.

Savage TA, Moro TT, Boyden JY, et al.: Implementation challenges in end-of-life research with adults with intellectual and developmental disabilities, *Appl Nurs Res* 28(2):202–205, 2015. https://doi.org/10.1016/j.apnr.2014.10.002. [doi].

Shabalala N, Jasson A: PTSD symptoms in intellectually disabled victims of sexual assault, *South African J Psychol* 41(4):424–436, 2011. https://doi.org/10.1177/008124631104100403.

Shandra C, Chowdhury Afra R: The first sexual experience among adolescent girls with and without disabilities, *J Youth Adolesc* 41:515–532, 2012. https://doi.org/10.1007/x10964-011-9668-0.

Shireman TI, Reichard A, Hunt SL: Learning your ABDs: variation in health care utilization across Kansas Medicaid disability groups, *Disabil Health J* 6(3):220–226, 2013. https://doi.org/10.1016/j.dhjo.2013.02.001. [doi].

Smith MA, Escude C: *Intellectual and Developmental Disabilities: The fatal four. The Clinical Advisor, CME*, 2015. http://www.clinicaladvisor.com/cmece-features/cme-ce-credit-intellectual-and-developmental-disabilities/article/395169/4/.

Social Security Administration: A Summary guide to employment supports for persons with disabilities under the Social Security Disability Insurance (SSDI) and Supplemental Security Income (SSI) programs. Available. 2017 Retrieved from: https://www.ssa.gov/redbook/documents/TheRedBook2017.pdf

Stabile M, Allin S: The economic costs of childhood disability, *The Nature of Children* 1:65–96, 2012.

Staples J: Culture and carelessness: constituting disability in South India, *Med Anthropol Q* 26(4):557–574, 2012.

Stopbullying.gov. *Bullying definition*. Available from: http://www.stopbullying.gov/what-is-bullying/definition/index.html.

Ticket to Work and Work Incentives Advisory Panel: *Annual report to the President, Congress, and the Commissioner of SSA, Year Eight*, Available from: www.ssa.gov/work/panel/panel_documents/FORMAT%20-%20Final%20Report–;121707.pdf.

Tossebro J, Wendelborg C: Marriage, separation and beyond: a longitudinal study of families of children with intellectual and developmental disabilities in a Norwegian context, *J Appl Res Intellect Disabil* 30(1):121–132, 2017. https://doi.org/10.1111/jar.12225. [doi].

Twyman KA, Saylor CF, Saia D, et al.: Bullying and ostracism experiences in children with special health care needs, *J Dev Behav Pediat* 31:1–8, 2010.

University of Iowa: *Impairment, disability, or handicap?*, 2016. Retrieved December 10, 2016 from: http://www.continuetolearn.uiowa.edu/nas1/07c187/Module%201/module_1_p3.html.

U.S. Census Bureau: *How common are specific disabilities?*, 2014. Retrieved from: https://www.disabled-world.com/disability/statistics/census-stats.php.

U.S. Census Bureau: *American community survey: population: question on disability*, Available from: http://www.census.gov/acs/www/Downloads/QbyQfact/disability.pdf.

U.S. Census Bureau: *Survey of income and program participation*, Available from: http://www.census.gov/prod/2012pubs/p70-131.pdf.

U.S. Census Bureau: *Housing and Household Economic Statistics Division. Definition of disability varies by survey*, Available from: http://www.census.gov/hhes/www/disability/disab_defn.html#CPS.2010.

U.S. Census Bureau: *Newsroom. Nearly 1 in 5 people have a disability in the U.S., Census Bureau reports*, Available from: http://www.census.gov/newsroom/releases/archives/miscellaneous/cb12-134.html.

U.S. Department of Education: *Prohibited disability harassment: reminder of responsibilities under Section 504 of the Rehabilitation Act of 1973 and Title II of the Americans with Disabilities Act*, Available from: www.ed.gov/about/offices/list/ocr/docs/disabharassltr.html.

U.S. Department of Education: *Family educational rights and privacy; final rule*, Available from: http://www2.ed.gov/legislation/FedRegister/finrule/2008-4/120908a.html.

U.S. Department of Justice: *Civil Rights Division. ADA home page*, 2009. Available from: www.ada.gov/.

van Timmeren EA, van der Schans CP, van der Putten AA, et al.: Physical health issues in adults with severe or profound intellectual and motor disabilities: a systematic review of cross-sectional studies, *J Intellect Disabil Res* 61(1):30–49, 2017 https://doi.org/10.1111/jir.12296. [doi].

Wilkinson JE, Cerreto MC: Primary care for women with intellectual disabilities, *J Am Board Fam Med* 21:215–222, 2008.

World Health Organization: *International Classification of Functioning, Disability and Health (ICF)*, 2016a. http://apps.who.int/classifications/icd10/browse/2016/en.

World Health Organization (WHO): *Disability and health*, 2016b. Available from: http://www.who.int/mediacentre/factsheets/fs352/en/index.html.

Zaall-Schuller IH, Willems DL, Ewals FV, et al.: How parents and physicians experience end-of-life decision-making for children with profound intellectual and multiple disabilities, *Res Dev Disabil* 59:283–293, 2016.

Veterans' Health

Bridgette Crotwell Pullis, Angelic Denise Chaison, Alison C. Sweeney,
Joanna Lamkin, Robert Pullis, Sarah G. Candler,
Rex Marsau, Tina Doyle-Hines, and Rola El-Serag

OUTLINE

OBJECTIVES

Upon completion of this chapter, the reader will be able to do the following:

1. Explain basic terms and the culture associated with U.S. military service personnel.
2. Describe elements of the Veterans Health Administration, including benefits, eligibility, costs of care, and outreach programs.
3. Explain some of the commonly occurring health issues encountered among veterans of different wars and conflicts.
4. Describe risk factors and manifestations for frequently encountered health risks among veterans.
5. Identify assessment strategies to improve the health of veterans.
6. Describe nursing interventions to improve the health of the veteran.

KEY TERMS

active duty
Agent Orange
burn pit
CHAMPVA
military sexual trauma (MST)
National Guard

Polytrauma
posttraumatic stress disorder (PTSD)
Reserves
service-connected disability
substance use disorder (SUD)
traumatic brain injury (TBI)

TRICARE
Veteran
Veterans Health Administration
  (VHA)

We might speak of an individual as a "World War II veteran," "a Vietnam vet," or a "veteran of the Persian Gulf war" to denote service in a specific conflict or place, but a veteran is not necessarily a person who fought in war or who served in wartime. Put simply, the definition of a veteran is a person who has served in the military. As we'll see, this experience can impart a distinctive culture and value system, and it is also associated with certain health risks. Thus, the veteran aggregate can present in the health care system with unique health problems or issues associated with their experiences.

Public health nurses and others providing care in the community must be aware of the needs, histories, and experiences of this particular population. This chapter describes some of the more common health threats and issues among veterans. Also included is an overview of some of the services provided by the Veterans Health Administration (VHA), as well as an assessment of methods and strategies to help veterans manage reintegration with civilian life.

OVERVIEW OF THE AMERICAN UNIFORMED SERVICES

People join the uniformed services for many reasons: to serve their country, to learn job skills, to have the opportunity to pursue a higher education, for a sense of pride and belonging, for financial stability, for a chance to travel, or to carry on a family tradition. The U.S. Army is the largest branch of the military, making up 39% of all military personnel. Other branches of service include the Air Force, the Navy, the Marine Corps, and the Coast Guard. Table 22.1 lists the appropriate designations for persons in each branch of the uniformed services.

Veteran Status

Legally, a veteran is an individual who has served in the active military, naval, or air service and who was discharged or released under conditions other than dishonorable. Any individual who completed service for any branch of armed forces is a veteran as long as they were not dishonorably discharged. This legal status is important to understanding a patient's eligibility for veteran benefits from the U.S. government. Note that people who have served in the United States Public Health Service and some persons employed by the National Oceanic and Atmospheric Administration are also veterans. There were 18.8 million veterans in the United States in 2015 (U.S. Department of Veterans Affairs [VA], 2016). Table 22.2 enumerates the size of the veteran population living today from various armed conflicts. Women are the fastest-growing segment of the veteran population, with one fifth of veterans being female (Fig. 22.1).

As discussed in Chapter 13, culture is the set of shared attitudes, values, goals, and practices characterizing a group of people. Military culture is one of structure and uniformity; it is governed by rules and standards. Though each branch of the military has a different mission, common core values and norms direct the behavior of all military members. These values include leadership, teamwork, loyalty, hierarchy, obedience, and discipline. Common norms among military personnel are a strong sense of service, a hierarchal class system, solutions-focused actions, unique dialogue and expressions, and a reluctance to show weakness. These norms affect how veterans seek care and how they manage their health. For example, veterans

TABLE 22.1 Branches of the Uniformed Services	
Branch	**Service Member**
Army	Soldier
Air Force	Airman
Navy	Sailor
Marine Corps	Marine
Coast Guard	Guardian

TABLE 22.2 Summary of Status of Veterans of Past Wars Involving U.S. Service Members				
War	**Number of U.S. Service Members**	**Estimated Deaths**	**Estimated Wounded**	**Estimated Living Veterans**
World War II (1941–1945)	16,112,566	405,399 (291,557 in battle)	670,846	1,711,000
Korean War (1950–1953)	5,720,000	54,246 (36,574 in theater)	103,284	2,275,000
Vietnam War (1964–1975)	8,744,000 (estimated 3,403,000 deployed)	90,220 (58,220 in theater)	153,303 number of service members	7,391,000
Desert Shield/Desert Storm (1990–1991)	2,322,000 (694,550 deployed)	1,948 (383 in theater)	467	2,244,583 (2009 estimate; may include veterans who served in Iraq and Afghanistan)
The Global War on Terror (2000 to present) (e.g., actions in Afghanistan, Iraq and Syria)	2.9 million (2016 estimate)	6,855	52,351	2.9 million (2016 estimate)

FIG. 22.1 During the All Female Honor Flight, veterans from World War II, the Korean War, the Vietnam War, and the post-9/11 era visit the Women in Military Service Memorial at Arlington National Cemetery, which honors them. (Robert Turtil/ US Department of Veterans Affairs)

may avoid getting needed care due to the stigma of appearing weak or out of fear of letting their colleagues down. They may not trust their information to be kept confidential, or they may fear that seeking treatment will jeopardize future promotions. They may also be concerned that seeking treatment will cause financial hardship, or they may have negative attitudes regarding providers.

ETHICAL INSIGHTS

Sexual Orientation in the Armed Forces

Prior to 1993 homosexuals were prohibited from serving in the military and were dishonorably discharged if their sexual orientation was discovered. Don't Ask Don't Tell (DADT) was an administrative regulation established by President Clinton that allowed LGB individuals to serve in the military, but required them to hide their sexual orientation. Between 1993 and 2010 more than 13,000 military members were discharged for being gay. DADT was declared unconstitutional in 2010 and repealed in 2011. Despite this change, LGB service members may face challenges to seeking health care due to concerns over:

- Threats to career advancement
- Internalized stigma and shame
- A loss of benefits after a dishonorable discharge

Active Duty, National Guard, and Reserves

The military is composed of both active duty, or full-time personnel, and members of the National Guard and Reserves. The service member is typically assigned to a group or unit, which is stationed either domestically or overseas. Overseas deployments generally last between 6 and 15 months; when on deployment, individuals may have periods of working nearly 24 hours every day, 7 days a week. Further, military personnel may be separated from their family for long periods, even when not deployed, due to long training cycles.

Personnel serving in the National Guard or Reserves are considered part-time employees. The key difference among them is that the Reserves report to the federal government, whereas the National Guard is administered by each state (e.g., the Pennsylvania National Guard is called into action by the governor of Pennsylvania). These individuals serve no more than 39 days a year, unless called into action. Usually, their service consists of monthly drills and two-week annual trainings. Reservists may be called very suddenly to active duty (full-time) for deployments, requiring that they leave their family, regular job, and community for a time.

Military Rank

The military is a hierarchal organization consisting of enlisted personnel, who perform tasks according to their specific job, training and skills, and commissioned officers, who plan missions and direct the enlisted personnel. Each person in the uniformed service is assigned a rank (or *rate* in the Navy) indicating his or her position in the hierarchy:

- Enlisted Personnel (E-1 through E-9)—includes noncommissioned officers and petty officers
- Warrant Officers (W-1 through W-5)—highly specialized experts
- Commissioned Officers (0-1 through 0-10)—highest ranks, similar to managers/leaders of a company

Enlisted personnel comprise over 80% of the military workforce. Officers outrank the enlisted personnel and are referred to as "sir" or "ma'am." One can be promoted in rank based on knowledge, time in service, work performance, skills, and vacancies.

The Veterans Health Administration

Most veterans receive all or part of their health care through the Veterans Health Administration (VHA) under the U.S.

Department of Veterans Affairs (VA). In order to understand the ways that veterans interact with the VHA, it is important to begin with an understanding of the VA itself. As a federal program, the overarching rules about the functions of the VA are determined at a national level. However, the implementation of those rules and guidelines is variable according to the leadership at regional and hospital levels.

Framework of the VA

The Department of Veterans Affairs has three subdivisions: the VHA, the Veterans Benefits Administration (VBA), and the National Cemetery Administration. The VHA provides all types of health care in every setting, including inpatient, outpatient, and long-term care. The VBA is an administrative arm responsible for unemployment and pension payments, home loans, vocational training, and educational benefits. In total the VA has 377,000 employees working at 144 hospitals, 1055 outpatient clinics, 300 vet centers, 11 stand-alone residential and extended care facilities, and 56 regional offices—as well as 240 national, state, or tribal cemeteries (VA, 2016).

Eligibility and Enrollment

Veterans—and sometimes their survivors and dependents—are eligible for VA benefits when they fulfill two requirements related to service and separation. 1) Service: they must have served in active duty for 24 consecutive months or for a full period of call (Reserves and Guard). There are some exceptions to the length of service minimum, the most important being when a person is discharged for disability incurred or aggravated in the line of duty. 2) Separation: they must have been separated under any condition other than dishonorable (Scott 2012).

Reservists and members of the National Guard can qualify for some veteran benefits depending on the length of time they were on active duty; for example, if a Guard or Reserve member is activated and serves in Afghanistan for a period of 14 months, then he or she meets eligibility requirements because the member has completed a full period of call—even though it is shorter than 24 consecutive months. However, the "active duty" requirement can prove difficult for these groups to meet. If while in the Guard or Reserves an individual is never activated for federal active duty military service, that person does not meet the active duty requirement for the definition of a veteran for VA benefits (Scott, 2012). Crucially, members of the National Guard and Reserves can face the same health issues and challenges as their active duty counterparts without being eligible for full veteran benefits. Relatedly, individuals who have been dishonorably discharged may experience the same health risks as the veteran cohort, though they are ineligible for VA benefits.

In order to receive care through the VHA, a veteran must enroll in the benefits program. It is important to understand that not all veterans who are eligible for benefits can enroll. The VA determines which veterans are able to enroll by stratifying them according to eight *priority groups* (Table 22.3), depending on urgency and need. Based on current VA funds, veterans in priority groups 1 through 7 are able to enroll in and receive care from the VHA.

TABLE 22.3 VA Enrollment Priority Groups

Priority Group	Qualifications
Priority Group 1	SC ≥50% or unemployable as a result of SC conditions
Priority Group 2	SC 30%–40%
Priority Group 3	POWs, recipients of Purple Heart, Medal of Honor, disability discharge, 10%–20%, "disabling SC disability, disabled by treatment orf vocational rehabilitation"
Priority Group 4	Receiving aid and attendance or housebound benefits from VA, or catastrophically disabled
Priority Group 5	Non-SC or noncompensable SC rated 0% disabled with income < income limits, receiving VA pension benefits, eligible for Medicaid programs
Priority Group 6	Compensable 0% SC veterans, exposed to ionizing radiation, Vietnam, Persian Gulf, Camp Lejune, combat veterans 1998–2003 enrolled within 5 years of discharge
Priority Group 7	Gross household income < income limits, who agree to pay copays
Priority Group 8	Income > income limits, who agree to pay copays

SC, Service connected; *POWs,* prisoners of war; *VA,* Veterans Affairs.

One's priority group does not, however, determine which services a veteran can utilize. Instead, all veterans who enroll in care receive the same services and benefits (with the exception of dental coverage). Once a veteran is enrolled, he or she remains enrolled and maintains access to VA benefits, regardless of whether his or her priority group changes (VA, 2017a).

An individual's priority group is determined in a large part by the extent to which he or she suffers a disability related to military service. A service-connected disability is a disease or injury that was incurred as a result of or during the veteran's active duty, or one that was aggravated by military service. A percentage associated with service-connectedness measures the degree of disability that the veteran faces as a result of that diagnosis. For example, one veteran may be 20% service-connected for tinnitus because he gets debilitating migraines and has associated hearing loss as a result; another veteran is 0% service-connected for the same diagnosis (tinnitus) because it does not cause him any disability. These determinations are made by a third party at the regional VA offices, not by the patients' regular providers (VA, 2017b).

Notice that VA funding prohibits Priority Group 8 from enrolling in VHA services at this time. This group has no service-connected disabilities and has a higher annual income than the VA income limits.

Cost of Care

Many veterans do not realize that their care at their VA hospitals and clinics is not a type of health insurance. Instead, it is a benefit that they receive in compensation for their duty and service to the country. The difference between health insurance and VA health benefits is twofold. First, veterans do not have to "pay into" their VA benefits the way one would pay premiums for a health insurance plan. Second, the "coverage" received in the form of VA benefits is not transferable to other non-VA providers, except through formal contracts deemed appropriate by the VA and its providers.

Once veterans are enrolled, the cost of care is relatively straightforward. At the time of publication, primary care copays are $15 per visit, and outpatient specialist copays are $50 per visit (VA, 2017c). Some services are free for all veterans: care for service-connected conditions, registry exams for exposures (such as chemical exposures), compensation and pension exams, counseling/care for military sexual trauma, research, readjustment and mental health services, smoking and weight loss classes, health fairs, combat-related care post-1998, laboratory tests, electrocardiographs, and hospice (VA, 2017c).

Medications are also affordable through the VHA, and the cost is a predictable and standardized set of copays. Additionally, veterans have an annual cap (currently $700) on the amount of money they must spend on their medications (VA, 2017c).

 COMMUNITY FOCUS

The Role of Private Insurance

When they enroll, veterans are required to divulge any other health coverage they have—personally or through a spouse. The VA always bills an individual's private insurance for medical care, supplies, and prescriptions provided for nonservice-connected conditions. Any monies collected from a veteran's private insurance offset his or her copayments, and furthermore, the veteran is not responsible for any balance the private insurance does not cover.

Patient-Centered Community Care and Veterans Choice Program

There are some services that the VHA may not be able to provide—either at all or in a timely manner. For these circumstances, there are programs that coordinate transfer of that care on a VA contractual basis. *Patient-Centered Community Care (PC3)* is one program for veterans needing certain primary care or inpatient-related care, particularly for female veterans after delivery and requiring limited newborn care. PC3 also covers some skilled home health care and home infusion therapy.

The *Veterans Choice Program* outsources veteran care when they cannot receive needed services at the VHA in a timely manner (within 30 days of the date clinically indicated by the veteran's VHA provider) or within reasonable distance (within 40 miles of the veteran's home). The care that is received in the community is only paid for by VA benefits if that care was approved by the veteran's VHA physician.

 COMMUNITY FOCUS

Rural Outreach for the Veteran Population

Veterans are an underserved population—with 4,638,100 veterans across the nation living in rural areas far removed from the nearest VHA or comprehensive medical center. Over 70% of rural veterans are over the age of 55 and are more likely than their urban counterparts to have at least one disabling condition. Though the VHA is seeking outreach to these veterans through community-based outpatient clinics (CBOCs), this mission is hampered by a lack of primary care providers. The Veterans' Choice Act, allowing veterans unable to secure an appointment for care at a VHA within 30 days to receive care from a community provider, will increase the number of veterans seen by providers in the community. Most veterans are covered by private insurance, Medicare, Medicaid, or Tricare and do not receive care in the VHA system (Heisler et al., 2013).

CHAMPVA and TRICARE

The Civilian Health and Medical Program of the Department of Veterans Affairs (CHAMPVA) is a program in which the costs of *some* health care services for eligible civilian beneficiaries are covered by the VA. According to Benefits.gov (2017), to be eligible for CHAMPVA benefits and services, individuals must be in *one* of these categories:

- The spouse or child of a veteran who has been rated permanently and totally disabled for a service-connected disability by a VA regional office **OR**
- The surviving spouse or child of a veteran who died from a VA-rated service-connected disability **OR**
- The surviving spouse or child of a veteran who was at the time of death rated permanently and totally disabled from a service-connected disability **OR**
- The surviving spouse or child of a military member who died in the line of duty, not due to misconduct (in most of these cases, these family members are eligible for TRICARE, not CHAMPVA)

Application for CHAMPVA is made through the VHA (Benefits.gov, 2017). It is important to recognize that CHAMPVA and TRICARE are not the same. TRICARE is sponsored by the Department of Defense (DoD) and provides health care for active duty military personnel, their families, and their survivors. In contrast, CHAMPVA is sponsored by the VA, and eligibility for TRICARE disqualifies one for CHAMPVA.

VETERAN HEALTH RISKS

There are several health risks or threats that occur among military personnel, regardless of where or when they served. Many have experienced life-altering trauma, such as dismemberment, loss of hearing or sight, burns, or neurological conditions such as traumatic brain injuries (TBIs). In addition, mental and emotional health risks are equally important: veterans have faced many and varied stressors, such as threats to their life, loss of friends, inner conflict regarding their role in combat, survivor's guilt, and separation from family. Some may even find the quest for peace and reintegration to be harder than fighting in a war. Included in this section are common health risks for the veteran aggregate.

Traumatic Brain Injury

A traumatic brain injury (TBI) is a disruption of brain function caused by an external mechanical force, including blunt force trauma, penetration by a foreign object, acceleration or deceleration movements, and pressure waves from explosive blasts (Johnson et al., 2013). TBIs are categorized as mild (abbreviated mTBI), moderate, and severe (Table 22.4). The mTBI is the most common, and is synonymous with the term *concussion*.

Technological advancements, such as Kevlar body armor and helmets, have greatly reduced penetrating injuries and the mortality rates from bullets and shrapnel; however, this higher survival rate has worked to increase the incidence of TBIs among veterans of combat in Iraq and Afghanistan. In addition, protective helmets do not prevent injury from pressure waves caused by blasts from improvised explosive devices (IEDs), a type of bomb favored by insurgents (Okie, 2005). Over 370,000 service members were diagnosed with TBI from 2000 to 2017 (DoD Worldwide Numbers for TBI, n.d.).

Symptoms of mTBIs can include headaches, tinnitus, sleep disorders, irritability, memory problems, mood and anxiety disorders, suicidality, chronic pain, and dizziness or balance problems (Johnson et al., 2013). Because these symptoms are often comorbid, mTBI can be difficult to identify, and beginning in 2007, all veterans who seek care at a VHA facility are screened for TBI.

Noise

Many veterans have been exposed to various levels and types of noise. This can include sound from gunfire, machinery, explosives, rockets, and heavy weapons. Others have been exposed to loud engines from tanks, large machinery, and aircraft. This exposure can lead to hearing loss and tinnitus, the top two most prevalent disabilities of all compensation recipients in 2016, affecting over 2.5 million veterans (VA, 2016a).

TABLE 22.4	**Severity Rating for Traumatic Brain Injury**			
Severity	GCS	AOC	LOC	PTA
Mild	13–15	≤24 hr	0–30 min	≤24 hr
Moderate	9–12	>24 hr	>30 min to <24 hr	>24 hr to <7 days
Severe	3–8	>24 hr	≥24 hr	≥7 days

GCS, Glasgow Coma Score; *LOC,* loss of consciousness; *AOC,* alteration of consciousness; *PTA,* posttraumatic amnesia.
From U.S. Department of Veterans Affairs Office of Public Health and Environmental Hazards (13A), Force Health Protection (DoD), and the VA-DoD Deployment Health Working Group: Mild traumatic brain injury – concussion: pocket guide for clinicians, October 2010. Available at https://www.publichealth.va.gov/docs/exposures/TBI-pocketcard.pdf.

Radiation

Some veterans are particularly at risk from diseases caused by ionizing radiation exposure. This exposure was of particular concern among those who participated in nuclear weapons testing or who served near Hiroshima and Nagasaki after the bombings—later known as *atomic veterans.* Complications of prolonged or intense exposure to even low levels of radiation can lead to many types of cancer. It is also associated with other diseases such as thyroid and parathyroid disease, cataracts, and nervous system disorders.

Cold Injuries

The major cold injuries veterans suffer include frostbite, nonfreezing cold tissue damage, immersion foot (formerly called *trench foot*), and hypothermia (Fig. 22.2). Cold injuries may result in long-term health problems, including the following signs and symptoms (at the site of exposure):
- Changes in muscle, skin, nails, ligaments, and bones
- Skin cancer in frostbite scars
- Neurological injury with symptoms such as bouts of pain in the extremities, hot or cold tingling sensations, and numbness
- Vascular injury with Raynaud phenomenon with symptoms such as extremities becoming painful and white or discolored when cold

Amputations

Modern body armor has increased the survival rate among troops who experience an explosive ordnance in combat, and medical advances further increase the likelihood that a soldier will survive the loss of a limb (Fig. 22.3). Around 1650 men and women have lost hands, arms, legs, or feet since combat began in Afghanistan and Iraq in 2001 (Fischer, 2015). The majority of the 11,879 amputation surgeries performed in 2016, however, were not combat related. Rather, the main etiology was diabetes and peripheral vascular

FIG. 22.2 Veterans may suffer from injuries related to their exposure to cold temperatures during their time of service. (Air Force photo by Senior Airman Curt Beach.)

FIG. 22.3 Jack Farley, a retired federal judge and peer amputee visitor at Walter Reed Army Medical Center, talks with Marine Lance Cpl. Josh Bleill, who lost both legs in Iraq when the Humvee in which he was riding struck a bomb. (Fred W. Baker III/U.S. Department of Defense)

disease, with a 78% incidence of diabetes in veterans undergoing surgery in 2016. Besides the obvious physical impairment affecting activities of daily living (ADLs), body image issues from limb amputations or disfigurement may create multiple social and employment barriers (Johnson et al., 2013).

Occupational Hazard Exposures

A veteran's particular service branch, time period of service, and activities in which the individual was engaged may have contributed to exposure to a number of other potentially harmful toxins or substances. These include exposure to asbestos, lead, industrial solvents, and other harmful chemicals. Symptoms and subsequent problems or complications might develop years later and be very hard to determine.

Posttraumatic Stress Disorder

Although the terminology is relatively new, for centuries people have observed psychological disturbances among soldiers returning from war. Amid the devastation of the First World War (1914–1918), British medical personnel noticed a series of symptoms among troops at the front lines, including anxiety attacks, hallucinations, nightmares, irritability, sleeplessness, and cardiovascular and gastrointestinal disorders. Some psychiatrists of the day theorized that these symptoms were caused by exploding artillery shells inflicting damage to the brain and dubbed the condition "*shell shock*." Others argued it was psychological in origin, the result of witnessing killing, torture, and other horrors of war, a position confirmed by the success of psychotherapeutic treatments. Among psychiatrists and military officers, there were several different names for the condition throughout the conflicts of the twentieth

TABLE 22.5 Names for Trauma-Related Conditions in History	
Time Period	**Nomenclature**
Seventeenth century through the American Civil War	Nostalgia
Mid-to-late nineteenth century	Soldier's heart
	Irritable heart
	Da Costa syndrome
	Railway spine
World War I	Shell shock
World War II	Battle fatigue
Korean War	Gross stress reaction
Vietnam War	Combat stress reaction (CSR)
DSM-III (1980)	Posttraumatic stress disorder

century (Table 22.5) until the publication of DSM-III in 1980, which codified the diagnosis as **posttraumatic stress disorder (PTSD)**.

Put simply, PTSD is a mental illness that develops in some individuals who have experienced a shocking, frightening, or dangerous event (NIMH, 2017), and although PTSD is of special concern to the veteran cohort, it is important to recognize that the condition is not unique to the experience of warfare. For example, PTSD can develop among those involved in car accidents, natural disaster survivors, and victims of rape or incest. Factors that contribute to an individual developing PTSD include getting injured or seeing another person injured, viewing a dead body, feeling helpless, having little or no social support after a traumatic event, dealing with extra stress after the event (e.g., loss of a loved one, pain and injury), or having a history of mental illness or substance abuse (NIMH, 2017).

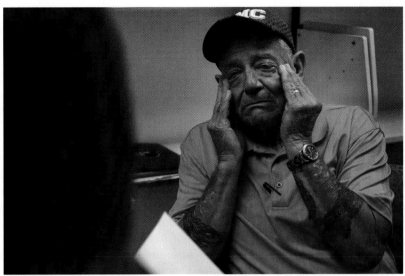

FIG. 22.4 Jim Alderman, a Vietnam veteran, receives treatment for PTSD at a VA medical center. (EJ Hersom/U.S. Department of Defense)

NURSING CARE GUIDELINES

Prevalence of PTSD

The nurse should note that not everyone exposed to dangerous events develops symptoms of PTSD; however, combat veterans are at a higher risk for the disorder. Among the general population, an estimated 8% of men and 20% of women who experience a traumatic event will develop PTSD, whereas 36% of men and 18% of women in war zones develop the disorder (Kulka, 1990).

The VA indicates that in 2011, more than 476,000 veterans received treatment at VHA facilities for primary or secondary diagnosis of PTSD (Fig. 22.4). In addition, it is estimated that PTSD will affect between 11% and 20% of veterans who served in Operations Iraqi Freedom and Enduring Freedom in a given year (VA, 2016b).

Diagnosis

Typically, PTSD symptoms begin within 3 months of the traumatic incident, but they may begin years afterward. To be diagnosed with PTSD, an individual must have experienced a "stressor criterion," which means that the person has been exposed to an event that is considered traumatic (Friedman, 2016). In addition, an adult must experience all of these symptoms for at least a month:

- At least one re-experiencing symptom (e.g., flashbacks, bad dreams, frightening thoughts)
- At least one avoidance symptom (e.g., staying away from places, events, or objects that are reminders of the experience; avoiding thoughts or feelings related to the event)
- At least two arousal and reactivity symptoms (e.g., being easily startled, feeling tense or on edge, difficulty sleeping, angry outbursts)
- At least two cognition and mood symptoms (e.g., trouble remembering key features of the event, negative thoughts about oneself or the world, distorted feelings of guilt or blame, loss of interest in enjoyable activities) (NIMH, 2017)

In general, a diagnosis of PTSD has been found to be associated with chronic pain, hypertension, coronary artery disease, thyroid disorder, insomnia, back pain, swollen joints, dizziness, chronic fatigue, difficulty concentrating, high blood pressure, and heart palpitations. Women with PTSD have more than twice the number of clinic visits over a year as do women without a lifetime history of PTSD (Gill et al., 2009).

Military Sexual Trauma

Sexual assault and sexual harassment during military service are associated with myriad deleterious health consequences among the veteran population. The VA defines **military sexual trauma (MST)** as a broad continuum of traumatic experiences that are sexual in nature. As such, MST may be a physical assault of a sexual nature, battery of a sexual nature, or sexual harassment that occurred while the veteran was serving on active duty. The VA further specifies that "sexual harassment" refers to "repeated, unsolicited verbal or physical contact of a sexual nature which is threatening in character" (Counseling and Treatment for Sexual Trauma, 2006).

Based on data from a nationally representative survey, it is estimated that 7.6% of all veterans have experienced MST. MST is more common among women veterans, with 32.4% reporting MST compared with 4.6% of their male counterparts (Klingensmith et al., 2014). Box 22.1 lists common sociodemographic characteristics of MST victims. It is estimated that in one of seven women who report MST, the trauma was perpetrated by an intimate partner (Mercado et al., 2015).

A number of health conditions are more prevalent among women with a history of sexual trauma, including sexually transmitted infections, diabetes, obesity, arthritis, irritable bowel syndrome, hypertension, and eating disorders (Schnurr and Jankowski, 1999). MST is also associated with the development of significant mental health consequences and related functional impairment. In a nationally representative sample of veterans, individuals who have a history of MST are also more

BOX 22.1   **Risk Factors and Characteristics of Veterans Experiencing MST**

- Female
- Younger (18–29 years of age)
- Racial ethnic minority
- Unemployed
- Single/divorced
- Enlisted
- Navy veteran

Klingensmith K, et al.: Military sexual trauma in US veterans, *J Clin Psychiatry*, 2014, doi:10.4088/jcp.14m09244

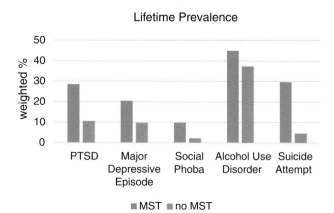

FIG. 22.5 Association between MST and mental health threats. (Data from Klingensmith K, et al.: Military sexual trauma in US veterans, *J Clin Psychiatry* 75(10):1133–1139, 2014, doi:10.4088/jcp.14m09244.)

likely to have lifetime and current mental health conditions (Fig. 22.5). Higher rates of eating disorders—especially among male veterans—have also been documented among veterans who screen positive for MST (Blais et al., 2017). Insomnia is also a prevalent condition among veterans and is more common and more severe among veterans who report a history of MST (Jenkins et al., 2015). MST is also independently associated with poorer cognitive functioning and quality of life as well as increased somatic symptoms (Klingensmith et al., 2014).

Among veterans seeking treatment for PTSD, sexual trauma has been associated with more severe PTSD than any other type of trauma, including combat trauma (Goldstein et al., 2017). Similar trends are found on the impact of MST on mental health among veterans returning from Afghanistan and Iraq. Veterans deployed to Iraq or Afghanistan who screen positive for MST when seeking services with the VHA were more likely to be diagnosed with PTSD, depressive disorders, and substance use disorders (Gilmore, Brignone, et al., 2016).

Polytraumatic Injuries

The term **polytrauma** refers to two or more injuries sustained in the same incident, affecting multiple body parts or organ systems, and resulting in various kinds of impairments and functional disabilities. Polytrauma is often the result of a blast-related event, and frequently includes TBI. For example, a soldier who has lost a limb, suffered a TBI, and lost his eyesight

from a rocket-propelled grenade attack is said to have a polytraumatic injury. Like other types of combat health risks, incidence of polytrauma is on the rise because of IED attacks and because soldiers now survive events that would have killed them in the past (Geiling et al., 2012). Care for veterans with these injuries is especially complicated because of the presence of several overlapping physical and cognitive impairments affecting their ability to perform ADLs.

Chronic Pain

Combat operations impart physical stress on the bodies of soldiers. They work long hours, carry heavy packs, and wear heavy armor, increasing the burden on the musculoskeletal system. According to a 2009 study, 29% of Operation Enduring Freedom (OEF) and Operation Iraqi Freedom (OIF) veterans report chronic widespread pain (Helmer et al., 2009). Pain is not limited to load-carrying service members in the infantry, however: one study of U.S. Marines found that lower back pain was even more prevalent among troops in trade occupations such as construction and law enforcement than among their counterparts in the infantry (MacGregor et al., 2012). In 2015, more veterans received treatment for service-connected musculoskeletal disorders than for any other body system (Table 22.6).

Chronic pain is often comorbid with TBI and PTSD, and for some individuals, muscle tension associated with PTSD can exacerbate pain. Furthermore, constant pain can serve as a reminder of traumatic events (Johnson et al., 2013). As mirrored by the opioid epidemic in the general population, the increased use of long-term opioid therapy for the management of chronic pain has been matched by an increase in opioid-related morbidity, mortality, and substance use disorders among veterans (VA, DoD, 2017).

Substance Use Disorders

Substance use disorders (SUDs) involve a pattern of use of alcohol, tobacco, and illegal and prescription drugs that results in marked distress and/or impairment (American Psychiatric Association [APA], 2013). Although problems with alcohol or other drugs affect veterans at about the same rates as the general population, there is a strong relationship between SUD and PTSD: more than 2 of 10 veterans with PTSD also have SUD (VA, 2017d). SUDs are also associated with other substantial negative correlates such as depression and anxiety, medical problems and disabilities, and increased rates of suicidal ideation and attempts (Teeters et al., 2017).

Binge drinking and cigarette smoking are the most prevalent types of substance use problems among male and female veterans, affecting about 11% of the veteran population, with disorders more common among males younger than 25 years of age. That this younger, male demographic associated with higher rates of SUDs in the general civilian population makes up a greater proportion of the military population could explain an increased risk of certain SUDs relative to civilians. About 4.8% of male veterans have drug use disorders, double the rate of their female counterparts (Teeters et al., 2017).

TABLE 22.6	Number of SC Disabilities of All Compensation Recipients FY 2011 to FY 2015					
Body system	2011	2012	2013	2014	2015	% Chg. FY 2014 to 2015
Musculoskeletal	4,721,091	5,189,302	5,780,195	6,397,255	7,117,586	11%
Auditory	1,679,146	1,883,919	2,116,528	2,352,609	2,613,285	11%
Skin	1,407,126	1,542,739	1,726,884	1,910,027	2,111,444	11%
Neurological	1,183,512	1,345,832	1,557,654	1,788,151	2,058,164	15%
Mental	878,417	986,904	1,110,050	1,230,063	1,368,427	11%
Cardiovascular	675,434	786,826	834,775	878,381	919,068	5%
Respiratory	582,933	644,675	719,770	798,353	889,002	11%
Digestive	732,523	719,598	772,021	825,345	884,368	7%
Genitourinary	464,634	515,282	570,093	627,252	684,965	9%
Endocrine	396,121	422,786	447,399	469,910	488,942	4%
The Eye	187,440	200,546	216,955	233,430	252,069	8%
Gynecological	72,512	77,882	85,043	92,164	101,008	10%
Dental/ Oral	58,705	64,724	72,588	80,526	89,713	11%
Hemic/ Lymphatic	39,147	42,770	46,517	50,677	55,075	9%
Infection/ Immune/Nutrition	47,756	48,318	48,928	49,495	50,275	2%
Total	**13,126,497**	**14,472,103**	**16,105,400**	**17,783,638**	**19,683,391**	**11%**

From U.S. Department of Veteran's Affairs, Veterans Benefits Administration: Annual Benefits Report, Fiscal Year 2015. Available at https://www.benefits.va.gov/REPORTS/abr/ABR-Compensation-FY15-05092016.pdf.

RESEARCH HIGHLIGHTS

Smoking Habits Among Veterans

Veterans are significantly more likely than nonveterans to be current smokers (28% vs. 20%). Although almost three fourths of veterans report that they want to quit, most don't take advantage of tobacco cessation advice or counseling. A recent study at a large VHA setting by Fore and colleagues (2014) underscored the importance of nurses being prepared to promote smoking cessation interventions. The nurses at the facility received training on behavioral and pharmaceutical interventions that focused on evidence-based protocols to promote smoking cessation. The nurses were encouraged to provide patients with educational videos and materials as well as access to helplines and follow-up phone calls for those who wanted to stop smoking. The nurses who received the education were significantly more likely to recognize the importance of delivering smoking cessation interventions and to report confidence in their counseling efforts. The researchers concluded that nurse-delivered tobacco cessation interventions have widespread potential to increase quit rates among veterans.

Fore AM et al.: Nurses' delivery of the Tobacco Tactics intervention at a Veterans Affairs Medical Center, *J Clin Nurs* 23:2162–2169, 2014.

Veteran Suicide

An August 2016 report by the VA provided the first comprehensive assessment of differences in rates of suicide among veteran and the U.S. civilian populations. This report confirmed that veterans as a cohort are at an increased risk for suicide. Increased suicide rates were particularly evident among female veterans and veterans who did not use VHA services. Of significance, among male veterans, suicide rates were highest in the 18 to 29 and 75 and older age groups, whereas suicide rates for females were highest in the 18 to 29 age group. The report highlighted additional key findings, including:

- An average of 20 veterans died by suicide each day
- Veterans accounted for 18% of all deaths by suicide among U.S. adults, although veterans only account for 8.5% of the U.S. population

- Risk for suicide was 21% higher among veterans compared with U.S. civilian adults after adjusting for differences in age and gender
- Approximately 67% of all veteran suicides resulted from firearm injuries
- Approximately 65% of all veterans who died by suicide were age 50 or older
- Risk for suicide was 18% higher among male veterans and 2.4% higher among female veterans when compared with U.S. civilian adult males and females, respectively, after adjusting for differences in age

Risk factors for suicide among veterans identified in the literature include non-Hispanic white race/ethnicity, male (Logan et al., 2015), sexual minority status (Blosnich et al., 2014), preenlisted and/or current mental health conditions (Ramsawh et al., 2014), history of self-directed violence (Lemaire and Graham, 2011), substance use (LeardMann et al., 2013), poor physical health and functioning (Magruder et al., 2012), intimate partner conflict (Alexander et al., 2014), lack of social support (Monteith et al., 2015), and sexual trauma (Lutwak and Dill, 2013). Veterans with any of these risk factors need to be closely screened and referred for follow-up services. Additional information on the VA's efforts to prevent suicide is described later in the chapter.

COMMUNITY FOCUS

Suicidality Following PTSD and MST

Perhaps the most crucial sequelae for both PTSD and MST is suicidality. Veterans who experienced MST are two to four times more likely to report suicidal ideation, suicide plans, and suicide attempts (Bryan et al., 2015; Monteith et al., 2016a). Suicide risk is more strongly associated with MST among male veterans compared to female veterans (Bryan et al., 2015; Monteith et al., 2016b).

Health Risks Common to Cohorts

Beyond the basic health threats, there are several health risks or problems commonly encountered for specific cohorts based on their theater, time of service, or experiences.

WWII Veterans

World War II veterans were exposed to high levels of noise. Veterans were exposed to radiation at Hiroshima and Nagasaki. WWII veterans who were in the Battle of the Bulge, fought in December 1944 through January 1945, were exposed to extreme cold and may have sustained cold injuries. Some volunteers were exposed to mustard gas experiments, in which the DoD evaluated equipment for their protection against mustard gas attacks. About 4000 soldiers were subjected to severe, full-body exposures during testing.

In addition to these, WWII veterans suffer from PTSD, at the time called *battle fatigue* or *combat stress reaction.* Despite efforts to screen soldiers for mental health as well as treatments offered on the lines, about 500,000 patients received disability pensions for neuropsychiatric disorders in 1947 (Pols and Oak, 2007).

Korean War Veterans

The Korean War, sometimes referred to as the *Korean conflict,* lasted from 1950 to 1953, with more than 5.7 million Americans serving during this time and ending in more than 54,000 American fatalities. The Korean War is often called "the forgotten war" because it received so little attention compared with WWII.

Health concerns for Korean War veterans center around three main categories: extreme cold injuries, noise, and occupational hazards. Korean War veterans who served in the Chosin Reservoir Campaign during October through December of 1950, in particular, could have been exposed to temperatures of −50°F. Indeed, there were more casualties from cold than from battle during this campaign (NVF, 2017).

Vietnam Veterans

Approximately 8,744,000 U.S. troops served during the Vietnam War (about 2.6 million in the theater), with 58,220 deaths, and 1611 missing in action. Actually serving "in country" is dramatically associated with increased health problems, as research indicates that veterans who were stationed in Vietnam during the war have worse health status than those who were elsewhere during the same time period. Those who served in the war theater self-report poor health status. Further, they experience significantly higher rates of other health conditions, including cancer, stroke, hypertension, and lung conditions (Brooks et al., 2008).

In addition to the common health risks of noise and occupational hazards mentioned earlier, Vietnam veterans suffer health disorders related to exposure to Agent Orange—an herbicide used to kill the vegetation that provided cover for the enemy. The VA (2017e) presumes certain cancers and other conditions to be caused by Agent Orange exposure. Because of this presumptive nature, the VA awards disability compensation for the following conditions to anyone who served in the Republic of Vietnam from 1962 to 1975:

- AL amyloidosis
- Chronic B-cell leukemia
- Chloracne
- Diabetes mellitus type 2
- Hodgkin disease
- Ischemic heart disease
- Multiple myeloma
- Non-Hodgkin lymphoma
- Parkinson disease
- Peripheral neuropathy
- Porphyria cutanea tarda
- Prostate cancer
- Respiratory cancers
- Soft tissue sarcomas
- Lou Gehrig disease, or AML
- Spina bifida among children of exposed service members

Besides the physical health risks associated with serving in Vietnam, the veterans of this war contended with the effects of the political and social environment of the day. Antiwar sentiment increased in the United States from the mid-1960s to the end of the war, both among those who found the war pointless and unjust, and those who blamed the troops for the lack of a victory. When they returned home, many veterans did not speak of their experiences out of fear of criticism. Wishing to distance themselves from the war, many Vietnam veterans never received treatment for the mental impacts of their time in combat.

Gulf War and the Global War on Terror

The Gulf War, codenamed Operation Desert Shield and Operation Desert Storm, took place from 1990 to 1991 in Kuwait, Iraq, and the Saudi Arabian border. The Global War on Terror (GWOT) refers to the series of campaigns launched primarily in Iraq and Afghanistan after the September 11, 2001, attacks in the United States. Veterans of this broad series of missions includes those involved in Operation Freedom's Sentinel (OFS, Afghanistan), Operation Inherent Resolve (OIR, Iraq and Syria), Operation New Dawn (OND, Iraq), Operation Iraqi Freedom (OIF, Iraq), and Operation Enduring Freedom (OEF, Afghanistan). Veterans who served in Iraq and Afghanistan have many potential health risks to consider. About 900,000 Gulf War veterans and 1 million veterans of the GWOT have received benefits from the VHA (VA, 2016a). In desert conditions, they were exposed to a number of health threats, including:

- Sand, dust, and particulate matter, which can cause respiratory disorders
- **Burn pits**, open pits where waste was burned during deployment (Fig. 22.6). Toxic smoke can damage the respiratory, gastrointestinal, reproductive, peripheral nervous, and cardiovascular systems, as well as the skin and eyes (VA, OPH, WRIISC, 2013).
- Shrapnel from IEDs, bombs, mines, and shells
- TBIs from blast injuries
- Heat stroke or heat exhaustion
- Chemical exposures such as mustard agents, which can irritate the airways and cause cancer, and sarin, a nerve agent
- Chromium, which can cause cancer

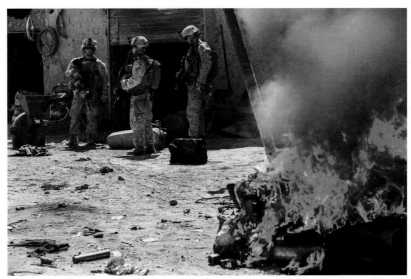

FIG. 22.6 Marines burn materials used to make IEDs in Afghanistan, 2014. (U.S. Department of Defense)

In addition to these threats, veterans serving in Iraq or Afghanistan may have been exposed to a number of infectious diseases. Among them are malaria, brucellosis, *Campylobacter jejuni, Coxciella burnetii* (Q fever), tuberculosis, salmonella, *Shigella, Visceral leishmanisis*, rabies, and West Nile Virus. Furthermore, many servicemen were given mefloquine (Lariam) to prevent malaria. Long-term use of this medication can cause serious neurological or psychiatric side effects (VA, 2015).

Chronic Multisymptom Illness. Approximately 250,000 veterans of the 1991 Gulf War (about 25% to 32%) returned home with multiple varied, unexplained symptoms, including fatigue, dizziness, headaches, cognitive dysfunction, musculoskeletal pain, respiratory problems, rashes, and diarrhea. Popular media of the time referred to the disorder as *Gulf War Syndrome* or *Gulf War Illness*, although today the VHA refers to this cluster of symptoms as *chronic multisymptom illness (CMI)*.

In the years immediately following the conflict, various causes for CMI were suggested, including chemical weapons exposures, depleted uranium, sarin gas, smoke from burning oil wells, vaccinations, and PTSD, many of which have been ruled out. Studies since then have narrowed in on two consistent risk factors: exposures to pesticides and pyridostigmine bromide, given to U.S. troops as a prophylactic against nerve gas agents (White et al., 2016). The VA presumes certain illnesses to be related to service in southwestern Asia:

- Chronic fatigue syndrome
- Fibromyalgia
- Gastrointestinal illnesses (irritable bowel syndrome, for example)
- Undiagnosed illnesses with symptoms that may include but are not limited to abnormal weight loss, fatigue, cardiovascular disease, muscle and joint pain, headache, menstrual disorders, neurological and psychological problems, skin conditions, respiratory disorders, and sleep disturbances (VA, 2017f)

Homelessness Among Veterans

Though most veterans successfully transition into civilian life, there are many who struggle, eventually becoming homeless. Though exact numbers are hard to come by, the U.S. Department of Housing and Urban Development estimates that there are 39,471 veterans homeless on any given night. The majority of homeless veterans are single males between the ages of 31 and 50 (Fig. 22.7). The numbers of young veterans who are homeless is increasing, with approximately 12,700 veterans of OEF/OIF/OND being homeless in 2010 (Clinical Example 22.1). Only 9% of homeless veterans are females. Most homeless veterans live in urban areas and have mental health and/or substance abuse disorders. Approximately 45% of all homeless veterans are African American or Hispanic (National Coalition for Homeless Veterans, 2017).

Clinical Example 22.1

Bobby Jackson, 24, ducked into the Pontiac Health Department to get out of the January wind and settled in to one of the hard plastic chairs in the waiting room for a nap. Because everyone is required to leave the overnight shelter by 7 AM each morning, he has a long 14 hours to fill until the shelter opens for the night. Since his discharge from the army, Bobby hasn't been able to find work, other than odd jobs shoveling walkways for strangers or washing windshields for stopped cars. Typically he spends any money he makes on a bottle or a fix—anything to calm his nerves and stop the flashbacks.

Amy Butler, RN, has worked at the Health Department for 6 months. She has noticed the young African American man asleep in the waiting room several times recently, and she knows that the army boots and flak jacket he usually wears are not warm enough for the Michigan winters. Today, she observed him twitching and trembling while he slept. Although a colleague suggested, "Ignore him, he's just a street person," Amy approached him after he awoke to offer the services of the Health Department.

When asked by Amy, Bobby explained that he had served in Operation Iraqi Freedom. Although Bobby was very polite, like many combat veterans, he seemed reluctant to seek assistance. As with every vet she cares for, Amy looked him in the eye and thanked him for his service. Then she reminded him that he is entitled to health care and other benefits through the VA. She

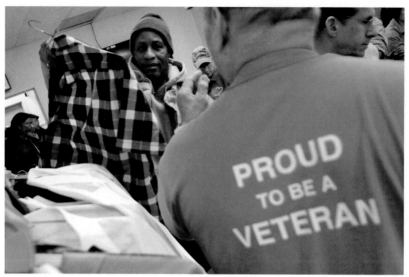

FIG. 22.7 Volunteers distribute clothing at an event for homeless veterans.

also gave him contact information for the VHA clinic a few miles away, the local Veterans Center, so he can connect with other vets, and a flyer from the Michigan Veterans Trust Fund, which provides for temporary basic living needs of veterans. Then she pointed out the Alano Club across the street, where recovering alcoholics would be available to help Bobby with his substance abuse problem. Finally, she made an appointment for Bobby to be evaluated by the Health Department's nurse practitioner for possible elevated blood pressure and frostbite.

Before he left, Bobby promised to follow up with the VA and report back to the Health Department within 1 week.

Created by Kathleen Walsh Spencer, DNP, MA, ACNS-BC.

Nearly half of homeless veterans served during the Vietnam era, and two-thirds served our country for at least 3 years; one third were stationed in a war zone. Approximately 89% of homeless veterans have an honorable discharge. About 1.4 million veterans are considered at risk of homelessness due to poverty, lack of support networks, and overcrowded or substandard housing (National Coalition for Homeless Veterans, 2017).

Veterans become homeless due to a number of factors. In addition to the complex set of factors influencing all homelessness—a shortage of affordable housing, lack of a livable income, and access to health care—a large number of displaced and at-risk veterans live with lingering effects of PTSD and substance abuse, which are compounded by a lack of family and social support networks. Additionally, military occupations and training are not always transferable to the civilian workforce, placing some veterans at a disadvantage when competing for employment.

Incarceration also significantly increases the risk of a veteran becoming homeless; even a brief incarceration will increase the likelihood of homelessness. About one half of veterans participating in VA homeless assistance programs are also involved in the criminal justice system. Homelessness and criminal justice system involvement can be a vicious cycle, with the impact of one problem increasing the risk of the other. Many behaviors associated with homelessness such as trespassing, loitering, and petty theft are criminalized. Incarceration, in turn, often leads to barriers to obtaining housing and reintegrating into society. Though the incarceration rate for veterans is lower than that of civilians, 181,500 veterans were incarcerated in 2012. A greater percentage of veterans (64%) were incarcerated for violent offenses compared with nonveterans (48%).

Female Veterans and Homelessness

Men and women veterans, two groups within the homeless veteran subpopulation, have health problems similar to those of nonveteran individuals experiencing homelessness. However, women veterans who experience homelessness have problems specific to their military service experience and their roles as child caregivers. A brief sketch of these problems follows. Women veterans are three to four times more likely to be homeless than their nonveteran counterparts in virtually all age groups (Gamache et al., 2003). The U.S. Government Accountability Office (2011) reported a study in which minor children accompanied 33% of homeless women veterans, almost two thirds of the women were between the ages of 40 and 59 years, and more than one third had disabilities. Additional research has demonstrated that being unemployed, disabled, or unmarried strongly predicts homelessness among women veterans (Washington et al., 2010).

Pavao and colleagues (2013) found that 39.7% of the women veterans in the VHA experience MST. The U.S. Government Accountability Office (2011) also documented that 60% of the housing programs serving homeless women veterans did not accommodate children and that women reported concerns about their safety in the housing facilities with regard to incidents of sexual harassment or assault. The report recommended that services for women veterans address privacy, safety, and gender-specific concerns, including accommodations for minor children.

VETERANS HEALTH ASSESSMENT

Veterans, especially those who access care at the VHA hospitals and clinics, tend to be older, sicker, and require more complex care than nonveterans. Veterans have more diagnosed conditions such as PTSD, diabetes, hearing loss, cancer, hypertension, heart disease, and chronic conditions such as chronic obstructive pulmonary disease (COPD). Veterans are 13 times more likely to have PTSD than nonveterans. The rate of PTSD is higher among veterans who are 35 and under. These young veterans also have higher rates of TBI, amputations, blindness, and severe burns than do older veterans. Veterans of the wars in Iraq and Afghanistan are more likely to have health conditions linked to their military service than do other veterans (Watkins et al., 2011). As most veterans will access care in the community, all health care professionals must appropriately assess veterans, be aware of their unique needs, and develop skills to meet those needs.

It is important to ask if the person has ever served in the military, rather than asking if the person is a veteran (American Academy of Nursing, 2017). This is because many prior military service members—especially younger veterans—do not self-identify as "veterans," as they see the term as referring to "the old guys." Others may feel that if they were not deployed to a combat zone that they are not veterans. Asking if they have served in the military will allow them to tell you how they identify.

A veteran's health may be related to their theater of deployment, injuries related to combat, possible MST, and PTSD, yet over half of community providers do not ask their patients about prior military service. Training in health risks such as PTSD, CMI, MST, and TBI is an essential element of quality veteran care (Miltner et al., 2013). Box 22.2 contains assessment questions to ask the patient with prior military service.

As mentioned, PTSD is a risk factor for many veterans due to their exposure to life-threatening situations, seeing their friends killed or injured, training accidents, sexual trauma, or exposure to natural disasters. Many veterans with PTSD do not seek mental health services but present in the primary care setting, where their symptoms may go unrecognized. Traumatic stress is associated with increased health complaints, increased health services utilization, and higher morbidity and mortality (Schnurr and Jankowski, 1999). It is crucial for primary care providers to recognize signs and symptoms suggestive of a trauma history (e.g., PTSD or MST). These may include substance abuse, hostility and mistrust of the medical community, noncompliance, and frequent missed or canceled appointments. Patients who present with multiple health complaints and diagnoses, particularly those who do not respond to treatment, should alert the provider to the underlying possibility of MST or PTSD.

All veterans seeking care at the VHA are screened for MST. Models to identify women at risk for MST suggest that lower sociocultural and organizational power (young age, low education, single, lower rank, short time in service and duty unit) are predictors of administratively reported sexual assault in the military, but not self-reported MST (Street et al., 2016). Due to stigma and shame, many veterans will not volunteer information regarding sexual trauma exposure. When screening for history of MST, it is best to avoid words that are emotionally or politically loaded (e.g., "rape") or words that are poorly defined (e.g., "sexual harassment"). Nonjudgmental, descriptive general questions are recommended (National Center for Posttraumatic Stress Disorder, 2004) (see Box 22.2).

BOX 22.2 Assessment Questions

General Questions

- In what branch of the military did you serve?
- Where did you serve?
- Did you serve in combat?
- What was your job in the military?
- Did you sustain any injuries related to your military service?
- What were you exposed to: chemical (pollution, solvents, etc.), biological (infectious disease), or physical (radiation, heat, vibration, etc.)?
  - What precautions were taken (avoidance, personal protective equipment [PPE], treatment, etc.)?
  - How were you exposed (inhaled, on skin, swallowed, etc.)?
  - How concerned are you about the exposure?
  - Where were you were exposed?
  - When were you exposed?
  - Who else may have been affected?

Posttraumatic Stress

- Have you ever experienced a traumatic or stressful event that caused you to believe your life or the lives of those around you were in danger?
- Are you experiencing trauma-related thoughts or feelings?
- Are you having nightmares, vivid memories, or flashbacks of the event?
- Are you feeling anxious, jittery?
- Are you experiencing a sense of panic that something bad is about to happen?
- Are you having difficulty sleeping or concentrating?

Military Sexual Trauma

- During military service did you receive uninvited or unwanted sexual attention, such as touching, pressure for sexual favors, or sexual remarks?
- Did anyone ever use force or threat of force to have sexual contact with you against your will?
- Did you report the incidents to your command and/or military or civilian authorities?

Blast Concussions/Traumatic Brain Injury

- During your service, did you experience:
  - Heavy artillery fire, vehicular, or aircraft accidents
  - Explosions (improvised explosive devices, rocket-propelled grenades, land mines, grenades) or fragment or bullet wounds above the shoulders
- Did you have any of these symptoms immediately afterward:
  - Loss of consciousness or being knocked out
  - Being dazed or seeing stars
  - Not remembering the event
  - Diagnosis of concussion or head injury

INTERVENTIONS FOR VETERAN HEALTH PROBLEMS

Nurses who encounter veterans in community-based care situations, as well as those who work with veterans on a routine basis, need to be knowledgeable about the health problems and threats common among this population. This section describes a few resources and interventions that may be helpful during these instances.

Management of PTSD

Friedman (2016) described the most effective treatment strategies for those experiencing PTSD. He noted that the most successful interventions include cognitive-behavioral therapy and medication (e.g., selective serotonin reuptake inhibitors such as sertraline [Zoloft] and paroxetine [Paxil]). Other trauma-focused psychotherapies are evidence based and highly recommended for PTSD. Here treatment focuses on the memory of the traumatic event or its meaning.

To ensure that veterans receive high-quality mental health care, the VA has increased access to evidence-based psychotherapies. Research has shown that participation in psychotherapy protocols for diagnoses such as PTSD has been shown to decrease suicidal ideation for veterans (Cox et al., 2016). There are variations of trauma-focused therapies. These include 1) prolonged exposure therapy (where the individual is repeatedly questioned by the therapist about the trauma to encourage control of the thoughts and feelings to reduce fear of the memories); 2) cognitive processing therapy, which involves talking with the therapist about the negative thoughts and beliefs and development of strategies to manage the recollection of the trauma in a way that is less upsetting; and 3) eye movement desensitization and reprocessing, which involves identification of the negative thoughts, emotions, and feelings while focusing on specific sounds or movements, helping the brain work through the traumatic memories (National Center for PTSD/VA, 2017a).

The VA supports a number of programs, strategies, and experts to help veterans identify, assess, and treat PTSD. Each VHA center has PTSD specialists who provide therapy, and there are almost 200 PTSD treatment programs in the country (see the PTSD program locator at https://www.va.gov/directory/guide/PTSD.asp). These programs offer education, evaluation, and treatment, including mental health assessment, medications, one-on-one therapy, family therapy, and group therapy. Specialized Intensive PTSD Programs provide care in inpatient or resident settings (National Center for PTSD/VA, 2017b).

Home-based telemedicine is another intervention strategy that is currently being employed and investigated to increase access to PTSD treatment (Gilmore, Davis, et al., 2016). This is an option that may be used in situations in which the veteran is located in a remote area or when travel is particularly difficult (e.g., when the person is bedbound or cannot leave the home).

Suicide Prevention Measures

Recognizing that even one veteran suicide is one too many, the VA has worked diligently to develop and improve suicide prevention programs to help all veterans at risk for suicide, whether or not the veteran is enrolled in the VHA system. These efforts include developing better screening and assessment processes to identify veterans at risk for suicide, developing partnerships with organizations and agencies in the public and private sector to assist veterans with psychosocial concerns, and increasing access to timely and high-quality mental health services for mental health concerns such as PTSD, substance use, depression, and suicidal ideation (Pheister et al., 2014; VA, 2016c).

In February 2007, the VA created a suicide prevention coordinator (SPC) position at every VHA center. The SPC's primary role is to help veterans access timely mental health care, particularly in times of crises, and to assist health care treatment teams with managing the care of suicidal veterans. SPCs are able to "flag" veterans' charts to prompt treatment providers to assess for suicide when appropriate. Utilizing findings from suicide research in military and veteran populations, VHA medical record templates were updated to include suicide risk factors that providers should determine when doing suicide risk assessments.

Suicide prevention coordinators also maintain weekly contact with the veteran and ensure that the veteran's treatment team works with him or her to develop a suicide prevention safety plan that helps the veteran cope with suicidal ideation. The safety plan is tailored to each patient and identifies crisis warning signs, internal coping resources, places the patient can go in order to maintain his or her safety, people to call with whom the veteran has close relationships, professional resources and contact information, and a plan for means restriction. Components of the safety plan can be found on the VA's website: https://www.mentalhealth.va.gov/docs/VA_Safety_Planning_manual.pdf.

A well-known suicide prevention effort is the establishment of the National Veterans Crisis Line in 2007 to provide veterans with immediate access to mental health crisis intervention and support 24 hours a day/7 days a week. Veterans may call the national suicide prevention hotline number (1-800-273-TALK), or text 838255, or use the chat service via VeteransCrisisLine.net. Hotline responders who are trained in suicide prevention and crisis intervention assist callers by initiating dispatch of emergency services to callers in imminent suicidal crisis and referring veterans to VA suicide prevention coordinators to ensure that veterans are connected to local mental health care.

Interventions for Mental Health Issues and Substance Abuse

The VA also expanded veteran access to timely and high-quality mental health treatment and assistance with substance use problems.

Part of increasing access has involved increased numbers of VHA CBOCs available in rural areas to provide needed mental health services, including telemental health services, available both at CBOCs and directly into the veteran's home. Free mobile phone apps have also been developed to facilitate veteran engagement in mental health treatment by providing them with tools and coaching to manage emotional and behavioral concerns.

The VA has created veteran peer support specialist positions within mental health programs. Peer support specialists are veterans who have been trained to provide recovery-oriented support and outreach that encourages other veterans to utilize VHA health services, particularly mental health, to assist with their recovery. Peer support specialists often share personal stories of recovery from mental health and substance use disorders using VHA resources with the purpose of helping other veterans connect to the VHA system and feel more comfortable seeking assistance.

Recognizing the mental health problems faced by female veterans and increasing numbers of female veterans accessing the VHA system, the VA has bolstered mental health services for this population. Designated women's health providers have been trained and established at 100% of VHA centers and 90%

of CBOCs to ensure that women veterans can receive a variety of health care services from providers who are trained specifically on women's health issues. The VA has also created a Women Veterans Call Center to contact women and inform them about eligible services.

In addition to seeking help at VHA facilities, veterans who served on active military duty in any combat theater or area of hostility are eligible to receive services at vet centers, which are community-based counseling centers that provide professional readjustment counseling to veterans and active duty service members. Vet center services typically include social services; psychotherapy (individual, group, and family); outreach and networking; benefits counseling; and referrals for follow-up at federal, state, and local community agencies to assist veterans with basic needs such as shelter, financial assistance, etc. There are currently 300 community-based vet centers and 80 mobile vet centers across the United States.

The VA recognizes the association between many mental health issues and substance abuse. Indeed, substance use and abuse may be the underlying problem or a way to manage the problem. Overuse or misuse of alcohol, tobacco, or drugs (both street drugs and prescription medications) can harm health, cause mood problems, destroy relationships, and result in financial problems. Effective treatment for both mental health threats, including PTSD, depression, and relationship issues, often necessitates addressing substance abuse problems. In addition to individual and group therapy focusing on treatment of substance abuse, medications are available to treat alcohol dependence or tobacco use. Medications may also be used to treat addiction to opioids; in severe cases, management may be inpatient (VA, 2015).

Finally, the VA proactively engages in education and outreach efforts that connect veterans and their families with the resources they need. Efforts often focus on increasing awareness of VA suicide prevention efforts, reducing stigma about seeking mental health treatment, and strengthening and expanding community resources available to veterans by training community providers to provide culturally competent care. The VA *Make the Connection* campaign, in particular, has been effective in highlighting veterans' true stories of mental health recovery, reducing stigma and negative perceptions about mental health care, and connecting veterans and family members with local mental health resources (accessible at https://maketheconnection.net).

Management of TBI

Nurses may be involved with community-based or long-term management of TBI. Even mild TBI can result in postconcussion symptoms, including headache, dizziness, nausea/vomiting, trouble concentrating, memory issues, irritability, tinnitus, and sensitivity to noise and light. If symptoms of TBI persist, referral to a specialist (e.g., neurologist or rehabilitative therapist) may be necessary (VA, 2010).

Management of moderate to severe TBI will initially be implemented in an acute care setting. Depending on the severity and response, treatment will often be moved to a long-term care facility before the veteran goes home. With moderate to severe TBI, the individual will require treatment from a multidisciplinary team. Patient care coordination among the various providers (e.g., physical, occupational, or speech therapists) is essential, and the nurse may act as the case manager. The nurse may be called upon to assist, identify, and intervene with physical, cognitive, and emotional sequelae and help administer and evaluate the individualized treatment plan. Finally, nurses are often responsible for educating the patient and their family about available rehabilitative interventions, strategies, and options (VA, 2010).

Caring for Patients With Amputations

Veterans who undergo amputations will experience a number of specific health issues and threats. The VHA (2002) described how clinicians, including nurses, should be involved in management of the physical and emotional issues related to the amputation. Specific areas that were mentioned in this report are the need for assistance during rehabilitation and long-term care, pain management, and prevention of secondary complications. Further, when the patient is physically ready for prosthetics, the nurse may be involved in prosthetic fitting and training, as well as vocational rehabilitation.

To help meet the needs, the Amputation System of Care (ASoC) was implemented by the VHA in 2007 to improve access to rehabilitation techniques and prosthetic technology for service members. The ASoC works to ensure that the veterans will have the expertise they require by incorporating the best practices in rehabilitation therapies and prosthetic technology. Using regional VHA settings, goals of the ASoC include providing state-of-the-art, holistic, interdisciplinary care; optimizing each individual's activity and participation in social roles; employing wellness and preventive strategies to minimize secondary condition, impairments, and activity limitations; and developing treatment interventions through research and outcome assessment (VA, 2015b).

Interventions for Health Problems Associated With Environmental Exposures

As explained, active duty service members are at risk for exposure to environmental toxins or agents from several sources. Interventions and resources for several of these are described here.

Chemicals

Threats to the health of veterans include exposure to a number of different chemicals, as discussed earlier. Of particular concern are Agent Orange and other herbicides. In addition is potential exposure to pesticides, industrial solvents, and polychlorinated biphenyl, which were commonly used as coolants and in insulation.

As mentioned, Agent Orange is associated with a number of significant health problems. The VA provides health care, disability compensation, and other benefits to eligible veterans and sometimes their dependents and survivors. The VA (2008) maintains a comprehensive program for health providers to educate them about health effects of exposure to Agent Orange and other pesticides. The "Agent Orange Newsletter" is a resource for health providers and exposed veterans to learn more about the health issues and the VA's programs (see https://www.publichealth.va.gov/exposures/publications/agent-orange/agent-orange-summer-2017/index.asp). Nurses working with veterans, particularly those from the Vietnam era, should be well versed in the effects and resources related to Agent Orange exposure.

Cold Injuries

The major cold injuries suffered by veterans include frostbite, immersion foot (trench foot), and hypothermia. The risks are dependent on temperature, wind, and moisture in combination with the duration of exposure and the amount of protection. Damage from cold exposure can include changes in muscle, skin, nails, ligaments, and bones; skin cancer in frostbite scars; or neurological or vascular injuries in the involved extremities (VA, 2017g). Those with potential health problems associated with cold injuries from military service may be eligible for disability compensation and are encouraged to contact their environmental health coordinator (https://www.publichealth.va.gov/exposures/coordinators.asp).

Radiation

Exposure to radiation among service members could have come from several situations. Some individuals from these groups might have been affected: those stationed in Japan during the Fukushima nuclear accident; the "atomic veterans" (described earlier as those involved in nuclear weapons testing and the occupation of Hiroshima and Nagasaki); nuclear weapons technicians; those exposed to pieces of depleted uranium after an explosion; Coast Guard veterans who worked at Long Range Navigation stations from 1942 to 2010; naval veterans stationed at McMurdo Station in Antarctica from 1964 to 1973; and service members (e.g., divers, submariners, and some pilots) who were given radium irradiation treatment between 1940 and the mid-1960s to prevent ear damage from pressure changes (VA, 2015c). Veterans from any of these groups are urged to discuss the potential radiation exposure to their health care provider or to contact their local VA environmental health coordinator (see https://www.publichealth.va.gov/exposures/coordinators.asp).

The VA reports that some diseases may be related to exposure to radiation during military service. These include many different cancers (e.g., bile duct, bone, brain, breast, colon, esophagus, gall bladder, liver, and lung, among others), as well as leukemia, lymphomas, and multiple myeloma. Other potentially related health problems include nonmalignant thyroid disease, parathyroid adenoma, subcapsular cataracts, and tumors of the brain and central nervous system (VA, 2015c). Health care providers, including nurses, should be aware of the resources available to address problems caused by exposure to radiation. For example, "atomic veterans" have special eligibility to enroll in VA health care (priority level 6). In addition, they are eligible to participate in the Ionizing Radiation Registry Examination Program, which coordinates care for affected veterans (VA, 2015c). Veterans should be informed of service benefits and be referred to the nearest VHA for comprehensive management and other benefits.

Air Pollutants

Exposure to a variety of air pollutants has been commonplace for veterans. Of particular concern are health threats from the burn pits that were employed to dispose of waste at military sites in Iraq and Afghanistan. Health effects associated with the smoke from burn pits include irritation of the skin and eyes as well as harm to the respiratory and cardiovascular systems and other internal organs. The health threats are dependent on the type of waste being burned, length of exposure, and wind direction. High levels of dust and other pollutants also posed a threat to respiratory health (VA, 2017h).

Veterans of OEF/OIF, Operation Desert Shield, or Operation Desert Storm may be eligible for care and compensation. The Airborne Hazards and Open Burn Pit Registry allows veterans to document exposure and report health concerns. Findings from data analysis indicate that burn pit exposure has resulted in COPD, chronic bronchitis, or emphysema as well as asthma in a significant number of cases (VA, 2015d). Additionally, exposure to dust storms increase the likelihood of asthma, COPD, and chronic bronchitis. Hypertension was the most common cardiovascular condition associated with both burn pit and dust storm exposure. Health providers caring for veterans from these conflicts should be aware of the potential health problems and refer accordingly.

Addressing Homelessness

Addressing veteran homelessness must include initiatives to decrease incarceration, such as jail diversion programs, and efforts to help veterans obtain identification, housing, and substance abuse treatment.

Another successful initiative to divert veterans from jail is veterans' court. These courts allow veterans to avoid jail if they agree to and successfully complete a prescribed program of rehabilitation and counseling. Veterans treatment courts have been demonstrated to be an important diversion from the cycle of incarceration and homelessness. Veterans who participate in VA services have experienced a 30% increase in stable housing in the year after court admission and an 88% reduction in arrests (VA, 2012). By implementing veterans treatment courts, justice system officials, the VA, and community organizations are able to attack the cycle between homelessness and incarceration, giving these veterans a much better chance for success. The majority of these courts were established between 2011 and 2012.

Due to efforts from the VA, local and state governments, community organizations, and law enforcement, there has been dramatic progress in ending veteran homelessness. Between 2015 and 2016 veteran homelessness declined by 17%, with an overall decrease of 47% between 2010 and 2016. A housing-first orientation increases the likelihood of a veteran being successful in treatment for drug abuse, mental health disorders, and other health conditions and gaining employment. The housing-first orientation means that a veteran is housed or rehoused as quickly as possible, regardless of their state of sobriety or poor credit or financial situation or criminal history. Once housed the veteran is linked to resources to meet his or her mental and physical needs (National Coalition for Homeless Veterans, 2017).

Transition from Military to Civilian Life

Military service can be rewarding, positive, and life changing; however, it is sometimes difficult, demanding, and dangerous. Whether one served for a short period or retired after a long career, returning to civilian life will most often present challenges (Box 22.3). Approximately 72% of all veterans report having a smooth readjustment to civilian life, but approximately 44% of GWOT veterans report difficulty with readjustment (Morin, 2011).

Veterans' attitudes, experiences, and demographic characteristics can have a significant impact on their transition and readjustment to civilian life (Fig. 22.8). Veterans who participate in preseparation seminars, transition assistance programs, and job fairs are more likely to have easier and more successful transitions than those who do not take advantage of these resources. Military commanders require all service members to attend transition briefings to prepare these personnel for separation; however, it is imperative that veterans begin planning for civilian life 1 year, or earlier, before separation from the military.

Veterans who were commissioned officers tend to have a more positive experience transitioning, as these veterans have experienced a more focused career; they also tend to be planners and understand the importance of preparation and order. As leaders they are thorough and follow through with the "mission" of transitioning, in the same way as they would carry out their active duty job and mission.

Veterans who were noncommissioned are typically high school graduates who often held nonleadership positions. They are more likely to experience a negative transition, as they may lack the guidance, experience, and knowledge needed to prepare for separating from the military. These members tend to be younger and have not experienced a career in the military. Their separation may be based on administrative action, military downsizing, or their decision to not reenlist. Another factor that

---

BOX 22.3 Voices of Veterans Upon Their Return Home

"Home—the place many think is the safe haven to find relief from the stress of war—may initially be a letdown. When a loved one asks, 'What was it like?' and you look into eyes that have not seen what yours have, you suddenly realize that home is farther away than you ever imagined."

—From Down Range: From Iraq and Back, by Cantrell and Dean, 2005.

"I went with my wife to a new church. I sat down in the pew. All of a sudden, I was in a different church in Germany—in the middle of the war—and there were lots of bombs going off. The roof of the church was blown off and there was a woman singing."

—World War II veteran

"When in uniform, you follow orders, no matter how you feel. When given a command, you use whatever force is necessary. Then you come back to civilian life and those things land you in jail."

—Vietnam veteran

"I will only speak to another combat Marine about my experiences in the desert. No one else can understand what it means to be a Marine or what it means to be a combat Marine."

—Gulf War veteran

"After returning home, I find that I get frustrated easily with others. People here at home get upset so quickly over the little things—long lines at the grocery store, busy traffic. Don't they know that these are small things and we all need to be simply grateful that we live in a free country?"

—Afghanistan veteran

"Three weeks ago I was driving Humvees and kicking down doors, and now after three weeks of demobilization, signing papers and getting medical checkups, I am suddenly back on the streets at home, but I can't yet make myself understand it or believe it."

—Iraq veteran

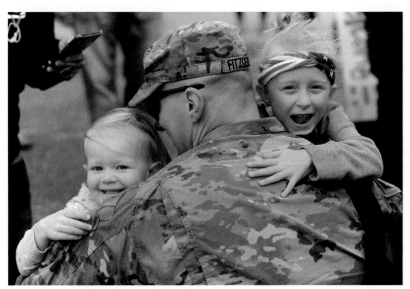

FIG. 22.8 An Army National Guardsman returns home to his family after a 10-month deployment. (South Dakota National Guard photo by Staff Sgt. Heather Trobee)

makes transitioning difficult for them may be a lack of career planning. Some veterans can transition to a civilian job similar or identical to their military job; however, this is not true for all service members. Veterans continue to have difficulty translating their job experience, qualifications, and training to the civilian job market.

COMMUNITY FOCUS

Veteran Employment

Every year thousands of veterans transition to the civilian sector to start a new life and career. With a challenging economic environment, much attention is focused helping veterans transition into civilian careers. The unemployment rate for veterans was 4.3% in April 2017—only slightly higher than the total national unemployment rate of 4%. Veterans with a service-connected disability had an unemployment rate of 4.8%. Whether veteran or civilian, younger people had higher rates of unemployment than older persons. The unemployment rate for female veterans was 5% in April 2017 (U.S. Bureau of Labor Statistics, 2017).

Enlisted service members and veterans can face unique challenges in gaining civilian credentials for military occupations because much of their education and training are attained primarily through their military service, as opposed to the traditional approaches to civilian career preparation. The military invests extensively in formal training for its enlisted personnel, complemented by extensive on-the-job training and hands-on experience. Military training is state of the art and, early in their careers, service members have direct experiences that are unprecedented in the civilian sector. However, the eligibility requirements for civilian credentials seldom recognize military training and experience as a means of qualification (The American Legion, 2017). It is important that future employers recognize, accept, and value the experiences, education, and training of this vital population.

An estimated 200,000 women will transition from the military during the next several years. Women veterans are younger than male veterans, with about 84% of female veterans being working age. Despite the experience and skills gained during their military service, nearly 2 in 10 female veterans aged 17 to 40 live in poverty, with about 10% of all female veterans being in poverty. A key to understanding the high poverty rate among female veterans is the perception among female veterans that their military training and experience are not relevant or helpful in transitioning to civilian jobs. Women veterans are also the fastest-growing segment of the homeless veteran population. Women veterans are two to four times more likely to be homeless than are nonveteran women. Unemployment is the biggest risk factor for homelessness among women veterans, with a lack of child care being the greatest barrier for employment. MST and PTSD are other barriers to employment for women veterans. Access to affordable housing can be a barrier for women with children; 60% of programs that serve women veterans do not house children, and the remaining programs have restrictions on the ages and numbers of children housed (Easter Seals, 2015).

Veterans who experienced emotional or physical trauma while serving are at a greater risk of having difficulty readjusting to civilian life (Morin, 2011). Having an emotionally distressing experience while in the military reduces the chances that a veteran will have a relatively easy transition by 26% compared with a veteran who did not have an emotionally distressing experience while on active duty. Similarly, suffering a serious injury while serving reduces the probability of an easy transition—from 77% to 58% (Morin, 2011).

It is important to understand that distress during the initial weeks of reintegration is expected and should not be medicalized. Most veterans can function well within a few weeks of returning home. If, after several months, veterans are not reintegrating well, they may be experiencing a mental health disorder and professional help should be sought.

Veterans who have families may be more likely to have a difficult time reintegrating to life after the military. Approximately 43% of service members have children. It is important that the veteran realize the changed dynamics of the family, their role within that dynamic, and how to transition into the family with as little disruption as possible. When a family member is absent due to military service, the family dynamic changes to redistribute the roles of the absent member.

Multiple deployments are common in today's military, complicating readjustment to home life. Multiple deployments are a common cause of family stress attachment problems and increase the rate for divorce among military families. The average deployment durations vary by branch of service. Military personnel often rate home life as the most stressful component of military service. Fig. 22.9 illustrates some of the sources of stress for military personnel and the impact of deployment on family life.

Predeployment is the period of training and equipping before deployment (30 to 90 days). Deployment is the period of a combat or humanitarian mission anywhere in the world (3 to 18 months). Redeployment is the return from operations to home base (30 days).

Family members need time to readjust to the veteran being home, transitioning to a new career and/or dealing with physical or mental health disorders. Veterans and their families will need time to transition into a new routine and to rebuild relationships. This could take months, as routines and responsibilities may change. The veteran and their family should seek relationship, parenting, and family counseling or classes as appropriate. In 2009 military children sought outpatient mental health care approximately 2000 times.

When moving to a new base or post, the military offers assistance to active duty military personnel and their families to adjust to the new environment. However, this support is not available when the veteran separates from the military. The veteran and their family will have to navigate the challenges of reintegrating and joining a new community without the assistance of the military. The VA has extensive initiatives to assist service members with the reintegration process. Counseling services and a host of resources are available (see https://www.benefits.va.gov/TAP/index.asp).

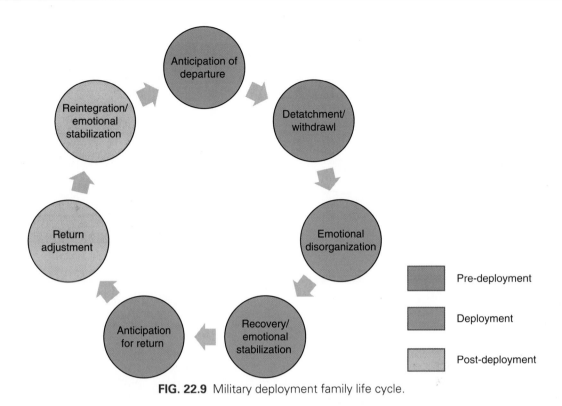

FIG. 22.9 Military deployment family life cycle.

CASE STUDY Application of the Nursing Process

A Community Intervention: Give a Vet a Smile

One of the many problems faced by homeless veterans is access to health care, and access to dental care is particularly challenging. It is difficult to obtain health care when one does not have an address or identification, and most homeless veterans have neither. The result is they go without needed health care, which leads to harmful physical and psychological consequences. Further, even if they are able to obtain health care, homeless veterans usually have no place to store medication or even personal items such as a toothbrush. Compounding the problem, many homeless veterans have mental illness, substance abuse disorders, and chronic health conditions such as diabetes and hypertension.

The U.S. Veterans' Initiative (U.S. Vets) is the largest nonprofit organization in the nation that serves homeless and at-risk veterans. U.S. Vets provides transitional housing, job training, mental health services, permanent housing to disabled veterans, and crisis care to homeless veterans. The goal of U.S. Vets is to return veterans to independent living in a home of their own.

While overseeing a community health nursing clinical group with the veterans housed at U.S. Vets-Houston and other homeless veterans served through the drop-in center, it was observed that many veterans were reporting dental pain. The community health students and faculty saw several who had facial swelling and fever from dental infections or missing or decaying teeth. Many veterans also spoke of difficulty finding employment due to the impact of poor health and oral hygiene.

As the nursing students worked with the veterans, it become clear they had no access to dental care and therefore had neglected their oral health for years. Most sources for dental care and services are based on income and require that the patient or insurance make payment. But many of the veterans served by U.S. Vets had very little money and no income, putting even low-cost dental care out of reach. Lack of transportation was another barrier to care faced by this population, as most homeless veterans do not have cars or transportation to clinic appointments.

Following a comprehensive assessment of the situation and validation of the needs, community-based faculty from UTHealth School of Dentistry at Houston were approached and told of the plight of these veterans. Many veterans are among the faculty, staff, and students of both the School of Dentistry and the School of Nursing, and there was considerable excitement about serving their fellow veterans. After a number of planning meetings, faculty from the nursing and dental schools developed a collaborative intervention called "Give a Vet a Smile" to provide free dental care for homeless veterans.

For the program, the faculty, students, and residents of UTHealth School of Dentistry provided dental care such as cleaning, x-rays, extractions, and other emergent care. Nursing students publicized the event at several community agencies that serve homeless veterans and completed health histories on those who chose to participate. Nursing students also solicited donations from local businesses to provide a light breakfast for the volunteers on Give a Vet a Smile Day, plus lunch for the volunteers and patients. Many veterans do not have Medicare or Medicaid and were not enrolled for care at the local VHA, so a source for medications was needed. A local pharmacist agreed to donate medications for the veterans so that they could get their prescriptions for antibiotics and pain medication filled free of charge. The veterans were given cards to remind them of the date for their appointments.

Transportation to and from the School of Dentistry was set up for the day of the event, and the veterans arrived early in the morning. Each was assessed by the dental staff for needed care, and plans of care were developed. As the process unfolded, the veterans received their requisite procedures and were scheduled for appointments for follow-up if needed.

Though the first year of Give a Vet a Smile was implemented with no donor funds—just in-kind donations such as food and dental supplies—39 veterans received dental care worth more than $18,000. The program is now in its third year, and community support is building. In year two a local private foundation donated $2000, and in year three, a local bank donated $5000 to finance the cost of the event and to provide follow-up care such as root canals, dentures, and other complex procedures. In the third year of the event, 70 veterans received care worth more than $36,000, with several veterans receiving follow-up care.

continued

A Community Intervention: Give a Vet a Smile

It is gratifying for the participating professionals and volunteers to see veterans who have been helped by "Give a Vet a Smile." One veteran now has dentures and is enjoying being able to eat again. Another veteran received care that might have been lifesaving, as he had a dental infection so severe that he required several extractions and long-term antibiotics. Finally, enhanced, directed outreach to the homeless veteran community has resulted in a more trusting relationship with the veterans—encouraging and enabling them to access needed services.

Planning is under way for year four of Give a Vet a Smile.

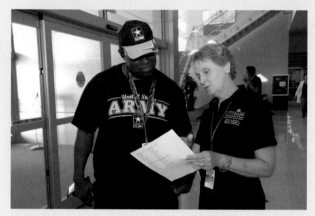

Initial intake and screening by UTHealth faculty

Welcome banner.

Initial health assessment by nursing students

Check in for veterans

An Army Veteran and US Vets employee receives care.
Initial oral assessment by a hygienist

CASE STUDY **Application of the Nursing Process—cont'd**

A Community Intervention: Give a Vet a Smile

Health assessment and vital signs by nursing students

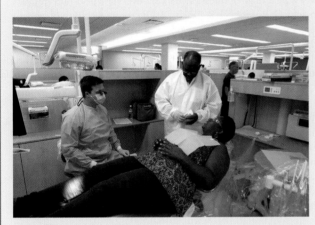

Many of the dental professionals caring for the veterans are veterans as well. They are delighted to care for other vets.

Post care instructions

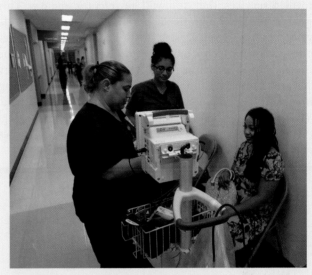

A veteran nursing student - a US Marine, welcomes fellow veterans to the event.

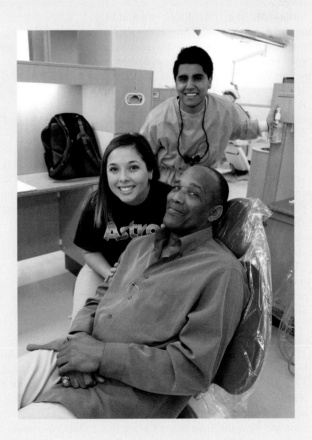

◼ SUMMARY

The Census Bureau (2017) reports that there are almost 20 million veterans in the United States. Furthermore, there are around 2 million men and women currently serving in the uniformed services; they, too, will be veterans one day. This very large and very significant population requires a wide range of health care services. Many of these services are specific to health problems and threats directly related to the veterans' roles or activities while in the military, but many of the problems are simply those commonly found among their nonservice member contemporaries. For example, WWII veterans will have problems associated with aging, and women veterans may have health concerns and issues because they are female.

Nurses working in community settings will encounter veterans in many different situations. During the assessment process, we are encouraged to include a question to elicit information on veteran status, as it may be important either with respect to underlying health problems or as a potential source for additional resources.

This chapter has presented basic information on some of the health issues and threats that commonly occur among those who have served in the military. It has also provided an overview of the veterans health system and described resources that are available for those who have served and those with service-connected health problems. All nurses should learn more about these problems and resources and be prepared to provide appropriate and specific care to meet the health needs of members of this vital population.

ⓔ EVOLVE WEBSITE

http://evolve.elsevier.com/Nies/community
- NCLEX Review Questions
- Case Studies

BIBLIOGRAPHY

Alexander CL, Reger MA, Smolenski DJ, et al.: Comparing U.S. Army suicide cases to a control sample: initial data and methodological lessons, *Mil Med* 179(10):1062–1066, 2014.

American Academy of Nursing (AAN): *Have you ever served in the military? A service for America's veterans by the American Academy of Nursing*, 2017. http://www.haveyoueverserved.com/.

American Psychiatric Association: *Diagnostic and statistical manual of mental disorders (DSM-5®)*, Washington, DC, 2013, American Psychiatric Publishing.

Benefits.gov: *Health Care Benefits for Dependents (CHAMPVA)*, 2017. https://www.benefits.gov/benefits/benefit-details/318.

Blais RK, Brignone E, Maguen S, et al.: Military sexual trauma is associated with post-deployment eating disorders among Afghanistan and Iraq veterans, *Int J Eating Disord*, 2017. http://doi.org/10.1002/eat.22705.

Blosnich JR, Mays VM, Cochran SD: Suicidality among veterans: implications of sexual minority status, *Am J Public Health* 104(Suppl 4):S535–S537, 2014.

Brooks MS, Laditka SB, Laditka JN: Evidence of greater health care needs among older veterans of the Vietnam War, *Mil Med* 173(8):715–720, 2008.

Bryan CJ, Bryan AO, Clemans TA: The association of military and premilitary sexual trauma with risk for suicide ideation, plans, and attempts, *Psychiatry Res* 227(2–3):246–252, 2015. http://doi.org/10.1016/j.psychres.2015.01.030.

Counseling and Treatment for Sexual Trauma: § 38 U.S. Code Sec. 1720D violence as a form of MST: an initial investigation, *Psycholog Serv* 12(4):348–356, 2006. http://doi.org/10.1037/ser0000056.

Cox KS, Mouilso ER, Venners MR, et al.: Reducing suicidal ideation through evidence-based treatment for posttraumatic stress disorder, *J Psychiatr Res* 80:59–63, 2016.

Defense and Veterans Brain Injury Center. (n.d.): DoD Worldwide Numbers for TBI. (n.d.). Retrieved 11 27, 2017. from: http://dvbic.dcoe.mil/dod-worldwide-numbers-tbi.

Easter Seals: *Call to action: support communti efforts to iprove athe trnasiion to civilial Lf for women veterans*, 2015. Retrived from: http://www.easterseals.com/shared-components/document-library/study-on-female-veteran.pdf.

Fischer H: *A Guide to U.S. military casualty statistics: operation freedom's sentinel, operation inherent resolve, operation new dawn, operation Iraqi freedom, and operation enduring freedom*, Congressional Research Service, 2015. Available at: https://fas.org/sgp/crs/natsec/RS22452.pdf.

Friedman MJ: *PTSD history and overview*, 2016. Retrieved from: https://www.ptsd.va.gov/professional/PTSD-overview/ptsd-overview.asp.

Gamache G, Rosenheck R, Tessler R: Overrepresentation of women veterans among homeless women, *Am J Public Health* 93(7):1132–1136, 2003.

Geiling J, Rosen JM, Edwards RD: Medical costs of war in 2035: long-term care challenges for veterans of Iraq and Afghanistan, *Mil Med* 177(11):1235–1244, 2012.

Gill JM, Szanton S, Taylor TJ, et al.: Medical conditions and symptoms associated with posttraumatic stress disorder in low-income urban women, *J Women's Health* 18(2):261–267, 2009. https://doi.org/10.1089/jwh.2008.0914.

Gilmore AK, Brignone E, Painter JM, et al.: Military sexual trauma and co-occurring posttraumatic stress disorder, depressive disorders, and substance use disorders among returning afghanistan and iraq veterans, *Women's Health Issues* 26(5):546–554, 2016. http://doi.org/10.1016/j.whi.2016.07.001.

Gilmore AK, Davis MT, Grubaugh A, et al.: "Do you expect me to receive PTSD care in a setting where most of the other patients remind me of the perpetrator?": home-based telemedicine to address barriers to care unique to military sexual trauma and veterans affairs hospitals, *Contemp Clin Trials* 48:59–64, 2016. http://doi.org/10.1016/j.cct.2016.03.004.

Goldstein LA, Dinh J, Donalson R, et al.: Impact of military trauma exposures on posttraumatic stress and depression in female veterans, *Psychiatry Res* 249:281–285, 2017. http://doi.org/10.1016/j.psychres.2017.01.009.

Heisler EJ, Panangala SV, Bagalman E: Health care for rural veterans: the example of federally qualified health centers, 2013, Congressional Research Service. Available at: https://www.aachc.org/wp-content/uploads/2014/04/Health-Care-for-Rural-Veterans-The-Example-of-Federally-Qualified-Health-Centers.pdf. Accessed 3 November 2017.

Helmer D, Chandler HK, Quigley KS, et al.: Chronic widespread pain, mental health, and physical role function in OEF/OIF veterans, *Pain Med* 10(7):1174–1182, 2009. Retrieved 11 28, 2017, from: https://ncbi.nlm.nih.gov/pubmed/19818029.

Jakob JM, Lamp K, Rauch SA, et al.: The Impact of trauma type or number of traumatic events on PTSD diagnosis and symptom severity in treatment seeking veterans, *J Nerv Ment Dis* 205(2):83–86, 2017. http://doi.org/10.1097.

Jenkins MM, Colvonen PJ, Norman SB, et al.: Prevalence and mental health correlates of insomnia in first-encounter veterans with and without military sexual trauma, *Sleep* 38(10):1547–1554, 2015. http://doi.org/10.5665/sleep.5044.

Johnson BS, Boudiab LD, Freundl M, et al.: Enhancing veteran-centered care: a guide for nurses in non-VA settings, *Am J Nurs* 113(7):24–39, 2013; quiz 54, 40. http://doi.org/10.1097/01.NAJ.0000431913.50226.83.

Kimerling R, Pavao J, Greene L, et al.: Access to mental health care among women veterans, *Med Care* 53, 2015. http://doi.org/10.1097/mlr.0000000000000272.

Klingensmith K, Tsai J, Mota N, et al.: Military sexual trauma in US veterans, *J Clin Psychiat* 75(10):1133–1139, 2014. http://doi.org/10.4088/jcp.14m09244.

Kulka RA: *Trauma and the Vietnam War generation: report of findings from the National Vietnam Veterans Readjustment Study*, New York, 1990, Brunner/Mazel Publishers.

Lemaire CM: Graham DP: factors associated with suicidal ideation in OEF/OIF veterans, *J Affect Disord* 130:231–238, 2011.

LeardMann CA, Powell TM, Smith TC, et al.: Risk factors associated with suicide in current and former U.S. military personnel, *J Am Med Assoc* 310(5):496–506, 2013.

Logan JE, Skopp NA, Reger MA, et al.: Precipitating circumstances of suicide among active duty U.S. Army personnel versus U.S. civilians, 2005-2010, *Suicide Life Threat Behav* 45(1):65–77, 2015.

Lutwak N, Dill C: Military sexual trauma increases risk of post-traumatic stress disorder and depression thereby amplifying the possibility of suicidal ideation and cardiovascular disease, *Mil Med* 178(4):359–361, 2013.

MacGregor AJ, Dougherty AL, Mayo JA, et al.: Occupational correlates of low back pain among US Marines following combat deployment, *Mil Med* 177:845–849, 2012.

Magruder KM, Yeager D, Brawman- Mintzer O: The role of pain, functioning, and mental health in suicidality among Veterans Affairs primary care patients, *Am J Public Health* 102(Suppl 1):S118–S124, 2012.

Mercado R, Foynes MM, Carpenter SL, et al.: Sexual intimate partner violence as a form of MST: an initial investigation, *Psychol Serv* 12(4):348–356, 2015. http://doi.org/10.1037/ser0000056.

Miltner RS, Selleck CS, Moore RL, et al.: Equipping the nursing workforce to care for the unique needs of veterans and their families, *In Nurse Leader* 11(5):45–48, 2013. ISSN 1541-4612. https://doi.org/10.1016/j.mnl.2013.05.013.

Monteith LL, Pease JL, Forster JE, et al.: Values as moderators of the association between interpersonal-psychological constructs and suicidal ideation among veterans, *Arch Suicide Res* 19(4):422–434, 2015.

Monteith LL, Bahraini NH, Matarazzo BB, et al.: Perceptions of institutional betrayal predict suicidal self-directed violence among veterans exposed to military sexual trauma, *J Clin Psychol* 72(7):743–755, 2016a. http://doi.org/10.1002/jclp.22292.

Monteith LL, Bahraini NH, Matarazzo BB, et al.: The influence of gender on suicidal ideation following military sexual trauma among veterans in the veterans health administration, *Psychiat Res* 244:257–265, 2016b. http://doi.org/10.1016/j.psychres.2016.07.036.

Monteith LL, Bahraini NH, Menefee DS: Perceived burdensomeness, thwarted belongingness, and fearlessness about death: associations with suicidal ideation among female veterans exposed to military sexual trauma, *J Clin Psychol*, 2017. http://doi.org/10.1002/jclp.22462.

Morin R: *The difficult transition from military to civilian life*, Washington, DC, 2011, Pew Research Center, December.

National Center for Posttraumatic Stress Disorder: *Iraq war clinician guide*, ed 2, Department of Veterans Affairs, 2004.

National Center for PTSD/U.S. Department of Veterans Affairs: *understanding PTSD and PTSD Treatment*, 2017a. Retrieved from: https://www.ptsd.va.gov/public/understanding_ptsd/booklet.pdf.

National Center for PTSD/ U.S. Department of Veterans Affairs: *PTSD: National Center for PTSD: PTSD Treatment Programs in the U.S. Department of Veterans Affairs*, 2017b. Retrieved from: https://www.ptsd.va.gov/public/treatment/therapy-med/va-ptsd-treatment-programs.asp.

National Coalition for Homeless Veterans: *Background and statistics*, 2017. Retrieved from: http://nchv.org/index.php/news/media/background_and_statistics/.

National Institute of Mental Health (NIMH): *Post-traumatic stress disorder*, 2017. Retrieved from: https://www.nimh.nih.gov/health/topics/post-traumatic-stress-disorder-ptsd/index.shtml.

National Veterans Foundation (NVF): *Who are Korean War Veterans? What Risks did these veterans face in addition to the enemy?* 2017. https://nvf.org/korean-war-veterans-risks/.

Okie S: Traumatic brain injury in the war zone, *New Eng J Med* 352(20):2043–2047, 2005. Retrieved November 27, 2017, from: http://nejm.org/doi/full/10.1056/nejmp058102.

Pavao J, Turchik JA, Hyun JK, et al.: Military sexual trauma among homeless veterans, *J Gen Int Med* 28(Suppl 2):536–541, 2013. http://doi.org/10.1007/s11606-013-2341-4.

Pols H, Oak S: WAR & Military Mental Health: The US Psychiatric response in the 20th century, *Am J Public Health* 97(12):2132–2142, 2007. http://doi.org/10.2105/AJPH.2006.090910.

Pheister M, Kangas G, Thompson C, et al.: Suicide prevention and postvention resources: what psychiatry residencies can learn from the veteran's administration experience, *Acad Psychiat* 38:600–604, 2014.

Ramsawh HJ, Fullerton CS, Heberman Mash HB, et al.: Risk for suicidal behaviors associated with PTSD, depression, and their comorbidity in the U.S. Army, *J Affect Disord* 161:116–122, 2014.

Schnurr PP, Jankowski MK: Physical health and post-traumatic stress disorder: review and synthesis, *Semin Clin Neuropsychiatry* 4:295–304, 1999.

Scott C: Who is a veteran?" – basic eligibility requirements for veterans' benefits, *Congressional Research Service*, 2012. Available at: http://www.ncdsv.org/images/CRS_WhoIsAVeteran-BasicEligibilityForVeterans'Benefits_1-23-2012.pdf.

Street AE, Rosellini AJ, Ursano RJ, et al.: Developing a risk model to target high-risk preventive interventions for sexual assault victimization among female U.S. army soldiers, *Clin Psychol Sci* 4(6):939–956, 2016. http://doi.org/10.1177/2167702616639532.

Teeters JB, Lancaster CL, Brown DG, et al.: Substance use disorders in military veterans: prevalence and treatment challenges, *Subst Abuse and Rehabil* 8:69–77, 2017. http://doi.org/10.2147/SAR.S116720.

The American Legion. The State of Credentialing of Service Members and Veterans Challenges, Successes, and Opportunities 2017. Retrieved from: https://www.legion.org/sites/legion.org/files/legion/publications/25VEE0517%20The%20State%20of%20Credentialing_0.pdf

Turchik JA, Rafie S, Rosen CS, et al.: Preferences for gender-targeted health information, *Am J Men's Health* 8(3):240–248, 2014. http://doi.org/10.1177/1557988313508304.

U.S. Census Bureau: *Veterans/United States*. Retrieved from: https://census.gov/search-results.html?q=veterans&search.x=0&search.y=0&search=submit&page=1&stateGeo=none&searchtype=web&cssp=SERP, 2017.

U.S. Department of Veterans Affairs (VA): *Traumatic amputation and prosthetics: independent study course*, 2002. Retrieved from: https://www.publichealth.va.gov/docs/vhi/traumatic_amputation.pdf.

U.S. Department of Veterans Affairs (VA): *Veterans and radiation: independent study course*, 2004. Retrieved from: https://www.publichealth.va.gov/docs/vhi/radiation.pdf.

U.S. Department of Veterans Affairs (VA): *Vietnam veterans and agent orange: independent study course*, 2008. Retrieved from: https://www.publichealth.va.gov/docs/vhi/VHIagentorange_text508.pdf.

U.S Department of Veterans Affairs (VA): *Mild traumatic brain injury – concussion: Pocket guide for clinicians*, 2010. Retrieved from: https://www.publichealth.va.gov/docs/exposures/TBI-pocketcard.pdf#.

U.S. Department of Veterans Affairs (VA): *Vets in crisis get a chance, not a cell*, 2012. Retrieved from: https://www.va.gov/health/News-Features/20120216a.asp.

U.S. Department of Veterans Affairs (VA): *Iraq war exposures*, 2015a. https://www.publichealth.va.gov/exposures/wars-operations/iraq-war.asp.

U.S. Department of Veterans Affairs (VA): *Rehabilitation and prosthetic services: Amputation System of Care (ASoC)*, 2015b. Retrieved from: https://www.prosthetics.va.gov/PROSTHETICS/asoc/index.asp.

U.S. Department of Veterans Affairs (VA): *Exposure to radiation during Military Service*, 2015c. Retrieved from: https://www.publichealth.va.gov/exposures/radiation/sources/index.asp.

U.S. Department of Veterans Affairs (VA): *Report on data from the Airborne Hazards and Open Burn Pit (AH&OBP) Registry*, 2015d. Retrieved from: https://www.publichealth.va.gov/docs/exposures/va-ahobp-registry-data-report-june2015.pdf.

U.S. Department of Veterans Affairs: *Veterans Benefits Administration: annual benefits report, Fiscal Year 2015*, 2016a. Available at: https://www.benefits.va.gov/REPORTS/abr/ABR-Compensation-FY15-05092016.pdf.

U.S. Department of Veterans Affairs: *PTSD: Basics*, 2016b. Retrieved from: https://www.ptsd.va.gov/public/PTSD-overview/basics/how-common-is-ptsd.asp.

U.S. Department of Veterans Affairs Office of Suicide Prevention: VA Suicide Prevention Program, *Facts about veteran suicide*, 2016c. Retrieved on 4/19/17 from: https://www.va.gov/opa/publications/factsheets/Suicide_Prevention_FactSheet_New_VA_Stats_070616_1400.pdf.

U.S. Department of Veteran's Affairs (VA): *Health Benefits: Priority groups*, 2017a. Retrieved from: https://www.va.gov/HEALTHBENEFITS/resources/priority_groups.asp.

U.S. Department of Veteran's Affairs (VA): *Health benefits: compensation*, 2017b. Retrieved from: https://www.benefits.va.gov/COMPENSATION/.

U.S. Department of Veteran's Affairs (VA): *Health benefits*, 2017c. Retrieved from: https://www.va.gov/healthbenefits/cost/copay_rates.asp.

U.S. Department of Veteran's Affairs (VA): *PTSD: National Center for PTSD*, 2017d. https://www.ptsd.va.gov/public/problems/ptsd_substance_abuse_veterans.asp.

U.S. Department of Veteran's Affairs (VA): *Veteran's Diseases associated with agent orange*, 2017e. https://www.publichealth.va.gov/exposures/agentorange/conditions/.

U.S. Department of Veteran's Affairs (VA): *Gulf war veterans' medically unexplained illnesses*, 2017f. https://www.publichealth.va.gov/exposures/gulfwar/medically-unexplained-illness.asp.

U.S. Department of Veteran's Affairs (VA): *Cold injuries*, 2017g. Retrieved from: https://www.publichealth.va.gov/exposures/cold-injuries/index.asp.

U.S. Department of Veteran's Affairs (VA): *Military exposures: burn pits*, 2017h. Retrieved from: https://www.publichealth.va.gov/exposures/burnpits/index.asp.

U.S. Department of Veteran's Affairs (VA), Department of Defense (DoD), The Opioid Therapy for Chronic Pain Work Group: *VA/DoD clinical practice guideline for opioid therapy for chronic pain*, 2017. Available at: https://www.healthquality.va.gov/guidelines/Pain/cot/VADoDOTCPG022717.pdf.

U.S. Department of Veteran's Affairs (VA), Office of Public Health (OPH), War Related Illness & Injury Study Center (WRIISC): *Burn Pits (Trash and Human Waste Exposures)*, 2013. https://www.warrelatedillness.va.gov/education/factsheets/burn-pits.pdf.

U.S. Government Accountability Office: *Homeless women veterans: actions needed to ensure safe and appropriate housing (Report to Congressional Requesters No. GAO-12-182)*, Washington, DC, 2011, Author. Also available from: <http://www.gao.gov/assets/590/587334.pdf>.

Washington DL, Yano E, McGuire J: Risk factors for homelessness among women veterans, *J Health Care Poor Underserved* 21(1):81–91, 2010.

Watkins KE, Smith B, Paddock SM, Mannle TE, Woodroffe A, Solomon J, et al.: *Veterans Health Administration mental health program evaluation: Capstone report*, 2011. Retrieved on 4/22/17 from: http://altarum.org/sites/default/files/uploaded-publication-files/Final%20Capstone%20Technical%20Report%20TR956_compiled.pdf.

White RF, Steele L, O'Callaghan JP, et al.: Recent research on Gulf War illness and other health problems in veterans of the 1991 Gulf War: Effects of toxicant exposures during deployment, *In Cortex* 74:449–475, 2016. ISSN 0010-9452. https://doi.org/10.1016/j.cortex.2015.08.022.

Zinzow HM, Britt TW, Pury CL, et al.: Barriers and facilitators of mental health treatment-seeking in U.S. active duty soldiers with sexual assault histories, *J Trauma Stress* 28(4):289–297, 2015, http://doi.org/10.1002/jts.22026.

Zogas A: *U.S. Military veterans' difficult transitions back to civilian life and the VA's response*, Watson Instituted; International & Public Affairs; Brown University, 2017. http://watson.brown.edu/costsofwar/files/cow/imce/papers/2017/Zogas_Veterans%27%20Transitions_CoW_2.1.17.pdf.

23

Homeless Populations

*Meredith Troutman-Jordan**

OBJECTIVES

Upon completion of this chapter, the reader will be able to do the following:

1. Discuss conceptual and legal approaches used to define *homelessness.*
2. Describe strategies used to estimate the prevalence of homelessness in the United States.
3. Identify demographic characteristics of the homeless population and its subpopulations.
4. Analyze three factors that contribute to homelessness.
5. Identify major health problems among various homeless aggregates.
6. Analyze the health status of populations who are homeless using the World Health Organization (WHO) definition of health.
7. Describe the federal health centers that provide health care services to homeless populations.
8. Plan community health nursing services based on knowledge of the social determinants of health and health status in this population.

KEY TERMS

Annual Homeless Assessment Report
chronically homeless
continuum of care
European Federation of Organisations Working with the Homeless

Federally Qualified Health Centers
FQHC Look-A-Likes
market justice

point-in-time (PIT) count
social justice
U.S. Conference of Mayors

The purpose of this chapter is to describe the scope of the homeless problem. The chapter presents definitions, prevalence, and demographic characteristics of homelessness, and it describes the health status of selected aggregates of the homeless population. The chapter includes a discussion of the relationship between the factors that contribute to homelessness and the social determinants of health and of the implications of this relationship for community health nursing practice.

---

* The author would like to acknowledge the contribution of Nellie S. Droes and Diane C. Hatton, who wrote this chapter for the previous edition.

DEFINITIONS, PREVALENCE, AND DEMOGRAPHIC CHARACTERISTICS OF HOMELESSNESS

Definitions of Homelessness

Defining "homeless" and "homelessness" is not only complex but contested. Although a generally accepted agreement on the meaning of these terms is lacking, definitions are important in determining who should be counted, described, planned for, and assisted (HUD.Gov, 2017; Perl et al., 2015; Shumsky, 2012).

An exploration of the national and international homeless literature for the past decade reveals two approaches to defining homelessness: conceptual and legal. A brief overview of the conceptual approach used in Europe and Canada is presented next, followed by a discussion of the legal approach used in the United States.

Conceptual Approaches to Defining Homelessness

In 2005, the European Federation of Organisations Working with the Homeless (FEANTSA) launched the *European Typology of Homelessness and Housing Exclusion* (ETHOS) (European Federation of National Associations Working with the Homeless, 2017). In developing ETHOS, members of the European Observatory on the Homeless, the research arm of FEANTSA, used "home" as a basis for developing a definition of homelessness. From the ETHOS perspective, home was conceptualized as having three domains: *physical, social,* and *legal.* The *physical domain* meant having an adequate dwelling for which a person/family has exclusive possession; the *social domain* meant being able to maintain privacy and enjoy relations; the *legal domain* meant having exclusive possession, security of occupation, and legal title to occupation (Edgar, 2009). Building on the three domains of home, the European researchers designated four broad types of living situations to classify homeless people: *rooflessness, houselessness, insecure housing,* and *inadequate housing.* Each of these four categories is subdivided into more specific living situations to provide classifications useful for different purposes, such as determining the extent of homelessness, developing policies, and evaluating interventions (European Federation of National Associations Working with the Homeless, 2017).

In 2012, building on ETHOS, the Canadian Homelessness Research Network provided a conceptual definition of homelessness that has four major categories: *unsheltered, emergency sheltered, provisionally accommodated,* and *at risk of homelessness.* Similar to ETHOS, the Canadian definition is divided into more specific living situations, thereby providing more details to facilitate its use by different groups, such as governmental agents, service providers, and researchers. In contrast to ETHOS, the Canadian Research Network's definition includes a category that indicates an at-risk population (Canadian Homelessness Research Network, 2012).

For a more complete understanding of these two conceptual approaches to defining homelessness, the reader is encouraged to visit the websites of the respective organizations. Setting the browser to search for FEANTSA and then searching within the site for ETHOS should provide access to the complete typology. To locate the Canadian definition, one should access the Research Hub website and search for "homeless definition."

Legal Approaches to Defining Homelessness

In contrast to these previously discussed European and Canadian definitions of homelessness, which were developed by researchers, the U.S. definition has been determined by federal governmental legislative and administrative actions. These federal actions provide the statutory and regulatory basis for local homeless service providers, including program direction, funding resources, and eligibility criteria. Responsibility for implementing and managing the many federal homeless initiatives is assigned to seven different departments within the executive branch of the federal government: the departments of (1) Housing and Urban Development (HUD), (2) Education (ED), (3) Health and Human Resources (HHS), (4) Veterans Affairs (VA), (5) Homeland Security (DHS), (6) Justice (DOJ), and (7) Labor (DOL) (Perl et al., 2015).

Both HUD and ED administer homeless programs that hold considerable significance for community health nursing: HUD's Homeless Assistance Grants (U.S. Department of Housing and Urban Development HUD Exchange, 2017) and the ED's Education for Homeless Children and Youth (U.S. Department of Education, 2016). A brief overview of these two programs and their definitions of homelessness follow.

HUD's Definitions of Homelessness. The *U.S. Code,* Title 42, Chapter 119 (U.S. House of Representatives, Office of the Law Revision Center, 2017), which is named "Homeless Assistance," contains two subchapters that provide homeless definitions. These are Subchapter I: General Provisions and Subchapter VI: Education and Training. The definitions in Subchapter I were broadened by the McKinney-Vento Homeless Assistance (MVHA) Act as Amended by the Homeless Emergency Assistance and Rapid Transition to Housing (HEARTH) Act of 2009 (U.S. Department of Housing and Urban Development; Office of Community Planning and Development [USHUD, OCPD], 2017). Subsequent to the enactment of the HEARTH Act, the HUD issued regulations that summarized the statutory definitions in four descriptive categories, as follows (USHUD, OCPD, 2011):

Category 1. *Literally Homeless:* Individuals and families who lack a fixed, regular, and adequate nighttime residence and includes a subset for an individual who resided in an emergency shelter or a place not meant for human habitation and who is exiting an institution where he or she temporarily resided;

Category 2. *Imminent Risk of Homelessness:* Individuals and families who will imminently lose their primary nighttime residence;

Category 3. *Homeless Under Other Federal Statutes:* Unaccompanied youth and families with children and youth who are defined as homeless under other federal statutes who do not otherwise qualify as homeless under this definition; and

Category 4. *Fleeing/Attempting to Flee Domestic Violence (DV):* Individuals and families who are fleeing, or are attempting to flee, domestic violence, dating violence, sexual assault, stalking, or other dangerous or life-threatening conditions that relate to violence against the individual or a family member.

ED's Definition of Homeless Student. The ED administers the law known as the McKinney-Vento Homeless Education Assistance Improvements Act of 2001, which is located in Subchapter VI of the *U.S. Code.* One of the intents of this law is to direct state and local educational agencies to take action to ensure that each child and each homeless youth has equal access to the same free, appropriate public education, including a public preschool education, as provided to other children and youths. The definitions, located in Part B, Section 11434a, are broader than the HUD definitions listed previously. These definitions include children and youth who are (NHCHC, 2017):

- Sharing the housing of other persons (frequently referred to as *doubling up*)
- Abandoned in hospitals
- Awaiting foster care placement

U.S. Department of Health and Human Services Definition of Homelessness. The U.S. Department of Health and Human Services (HHS) also has definitions of who is considered homeless. The Runaway and Homeless Youth (RHY) Program is located in the Administration for Children & Families, Family and Youth Service Bureau, which are agencies within the HHS. The RHY program operates under legislation that has definitions for who is eligible for services; as defined in the statute, *runaway youth* is "a person under 18 years of age who absents himself or herself from home or place of legal residence without the permission of his or her family" and *homeless youth* is "a person under 18 years of age who is in need of services and without a place of shelter where he or she receives supervision and care" (USDHHS, Administration for Children & Families, Family and Youth Service Bureau, 2014).

In addition to these two definitions of youth, HHS uses a different definition in determining who is eligible for services provided through the Health Care for the Homeless (HCH) Program (see the later section "Health and Homeless Populations").

The next section presents information related to the number of people in the total U.S. homeless population and also in smaller subpopulations. HUD and ED are the two primary federal agencies with responsibility for reporting U.S. homeless prevalence estimates. The departments use their own, but differing, definitions in their enumeration efforts.

Prevalence of Homelessness

Determining prevalence of homelessness requires not only definitions of who is counted but also how data are collected. Given the characteristics of the population and subpopulations of homeless people, obtaining accurate counts is difficult. Efforts to enumerate the homeless have evolved over the past three decades. Earlier efforts included the U.S. Census Bureau's collections of national data on the homeless population in Census 1990 (U.S. Department of Housing and Urban Development Office of Policy Development and Research, 2010) and Census 2000 (U.S. Department of Commerce, 2009). A brief sketch of more recent approaches to counting the homeless—those conducted by HUD and ED—follows.

HUD's Efforts to Count the Homeless

Two strategies used by HUD to strengthen the nation's efforts to reduce homelessness, including improvement in collecting prevalence data, are the **continuum of care** (CoC) concept and the Homeless Information Management System (HMIS). A brief overview of these two strategies follows.

HUD requires homeless service providers in each local community to collaborate and submit just one CoC application to HUD for funding, rather than allowing multiple providers to submit individual applications. If successful in obtaining funding, these CoC providers are then responsible for providing to persons in the local area who are experiencing homelessness a range of housing and related services, including emergency and preventive responses (USHUD, 2015).

 HEALTHY PEOPLE 2020

Objectives for Social Determinants of Health

Economic Stability

SHOH-1: Proportion of children aged 0 to 17 years living with at least one parent employed year round full time.

SDOH-3: Proportion of persons living in poverty.

Education

SDOH -2: Proportion of high school completers who were enrolled in college the October immediately after completing high school.

From U.S. Department of Health and Human Services: *Healthy People 2020: social determinants of health,* 2010. https://www.healthypeople.gov/2020/topics-objectives/topic/social-determinants-of-health Accessed September 15, 2017.

The CoC providers are also responsible for implementing and managing the HMIS at the local level. The HMIS is a computerized database designed to facilitate collection of client-level data used to plan for service needs of homeless populations.

As a requirement of HUD funding, all groups of CoC providers conduct a **point-in-time (PIT) count** of *sheltered* homeless people on a single night in late January of *every year* and submit these data to HUD via HMIS (USHUD, 2015). In addition to the annual PIT count of sheltered homeless people, HUD requires that *every 2 years*, on odd years, the PIT count include both *sheltered and unsheltered* homeless people. Although not required, some CoC providers include unsheltered homeless people in their PIT counts on both even and odd years.

Since 2007, HUD has used the data submitted by local CoC providers via the HMIS to prepare an **Annual Homeless Assessment Report** (AHAR) that is delivered to Congress. The populations and subpopulations HUD used in the AHAR reflect the legislative and administrative definitions outlined previously. In addition to total population prevalence, the AHAR includes subpopulations—individuals, families, the chronically homeless, and veterans. Homeless children and youth enrolled in public schools are not included in HUD's HMIS. Responsibility for reporting information about this important subpopulation lies with the ED. "Unaccompanied youth"—children and youth who are homeless and on their own—that is, not living with their families, are often excluded from estimates of the homeless population (Childtrends.org, 2015).

ED's Efforts to Count the Homeless

One of the main differences between the HUD and ED approaches to counting homeless people is based on definitions of who is considered homeless. As previously described, the ED

TABLE 23.1 Pit Estimates of Homeless People January 2015–2016

Population	Sheltered and Unsheltered Single Night, January 2016	Change	Previous Year of Estimates
Households			
Individuals[1]	355,212	–3%	2015
Families with children	194,716	–6%	2015
Total	549,928	–3%	2015
Subpopulations[2]			
Veterans	39,471	–17%	2016
Chronically homeless	77,486	–7%	2015

[1]Person who is not part of a family; single adults, unaccompanied youth, or in multiple-adult or multiple-child households.

[2]Categories are not mutually exclusive; it is possible for a chronically homeless person to be a veteran.

Data from U.S. Department of Housing and Urban Development: *The 2015 point-in-time estimates of homelessness,* 2016. https://www.hudexchange.info/resource/5178/2016-ahar-part-1-pit-estimates-of-homelessness/.

uses a broad definition of homelessness that includes youth and families that are living with other households, or "doubled up." Consequently, the ED provides services to homeless children and youth who are not included in HUD's programmatic services. Children and youth whom the ED defines as homeless receive services through the Education for Homeless Children and Youth (EHCY) program.

To meet ECHY requirements the ED collects data on program performance from all state education agencies and local education agencies (LEAs). The number of homeless students enrolled in LEAs during each school year is part of the annual performance report. In addition, the ED collects information on students' nighttime residence at the time they were determined eligible for EHCY services. This information is included in the Consolidated State Performance Record, which the ED issues on an annual basis (National Center for Homeless Education, 2016).

Homeless Prevalence Estimates

These two federal departments, HUD and ED, issue summary reports of the sizes of homeless populations and subpopulations. Both departments provide annual estimates. HUD provides a PIT count as well; the results of the January 2015 count are summarized in Table 23.1.

The prevalence estimates outlined in Table 23.1 provide a "snapshot" of the homeless population taken on one night in January 2015 as reported in Part I of the 2016 AHAR. HUD also uses a different lens—the annual estimate—to produce another picture of the homeless population. In contrast to the one-night view, HUD's annual estimate is a count of the total number of people who used either shelters or transitional housing during the course of a year. As of this writing, the most recently available annual estimates are for fiscal year 2015–2016; this information follows.

Annual National Estimate of Homeless Persons' Use of Shelters and Transitional Housing 2015–2016

HUD reported the following numbers of people in the total population and in subpopulations who used shelters or transitional housing between October 1, 2015, and September 30, 2016 (USHUD, OCPD, 2016):

- 549,928 people in the total homeless population, a decrease of 2.6% since 2015
- 355,212 *individuals,* accounting for 65% of the homeless population, with a decline by less than 1% between 2015 and 2016
- 194,716 *people in families with children,* a decrease of 5% between 2015 and 2016
- 39,471 *veterans,* a decrease of 17% between 2015 and 2016 alone

The population and subpopulations HUD included in the 2016 annual estimate of shelter use are based on the legislatively and administratively derived definitions outlined previously. The ED, using a broader definition of homeless families than HUD, provides information on the population of children and youth enrolled in public schools.

ED's Annual National Estimate of Homeless Students for 2015–2016 School Year

According to the ED (National Center for Homeless Education, 2016):

- 1,263,323 *homeless students* were enrolled during the 2014–2015 school year (SY), an increase of 3.4% over the 3-year period 2012–2013 to 2014–2015.

The *nighttime residences* of homeless students for the 2014–2015 data collection period were:

- 181,386 in shelters or transitional housing awaiting foster care
- 958,495 doubled up
- 39,421 unsheltered
- 82,159 in hotels/motels

The following subpopulations of homeless students received services during SY 2014–2015:

- 95,032 *unaccompanied youths,* a 21% increase since SY 2012–2013
- 17,748 *migratory children/youths,* a 9% increase since SY 2012–2013
- 216,477 *children with disabilities,* a 13% increase since SY 2012–2013
- 181,949 *limited-English-proficient students,* a 4% increase since SY 2012–2013

The subpopulations listed here are not mutually exclusive; homeless students may be counted in one or more subpopulations.

U.S. Conference of Mayors' Hunger and Homelessness Survey 2012

In addition to the previously outlined national counts based on data generated by HUD and ED, the U.S. Conference of Mayors provides an urban-local perspective on homelessness. Information on homeless populations in the cities whose mayors are members of the **U.S. Conference of Mayors** Taskforce on Hunger and Homelessness is reported each year. According to the 2016 report, between September 1, 2015, and August 31,

2016, homelessness has been declining across the nation for several years—a 12.9% decrease from 2009 to 2016, including a 2.6% decrease from 2015 to 2016. Two thirds (65%) of cities providing data followed the long-term trend, reporting decreases from 2009 to 2016, and two-thirds (62%) also reported decreases from 2015 to 2016. The number of people in families reported to be experiencing homelessness in the United States decreased 18.5% from 2009 to 2016. From 2015 to 2016, homelessness among people in families decreased 5.6% nationally. The authors of the report recommend caution in interpreting the information, however, because they note that the cities reporting data are not a representative sample of cities and hence the report is not a national report (U.S. Conference of Mayors, 2016).

A Caveat

This section presented a sketch of HUD's and ED's approaches to enumerating homeless populations and the latest available national prevalence estimates. Also included were pertinent prevalence rates in cities represented in the annual U.S. Conference of Mayors report. Although structure and processes for enumerating the homeless are important and have improved, Kozol (1988, p. 10) cautioned a quarter-century ago:

> We would be wise to avoid the numbers game. Any search for the "right number" carries the assumption that we may at last arrive at an acceptable number. There is no acceptable number. Whether the number is "1 million or 4 million," there are too many homeless people in America.

Demographic Characteristics

This section reports selected demographic characteristics of the sheltered homeless population and subpopulations. The data CoC providers reported to Congress, from between 2014 and 2015, provided the demographic characteristics of the following subpopulations: all homeless people, individuals, families with children, and veterans.

All Homeless People

Among all sheltered homeless adults in 2015, there was an estimated 1.48 million people ; 62.1% were men and 37.9% women. The sheltered homeless population is younger than the general population. More than one fifth of people experiencing sheltered homelessness (22.3%) were children under age 18, and 11% percent were youth between the ages of 18 and 24. About one third of sheltered homeless individuals (33.8%) were ages 31 to 50, the most numerous age group among all people experiencing sheltered homelessness. Although 17.9% of all people in the United States were age 62 or older, this population comprised only 4.2% of people experiencing sheltered homelessness (U.S. HUD, 2016). Minorities accounted for 61.9% of the total sheltered population. African Americans represented more than 41%, though they comprised only 13% of all people in the United States (U.S. HUD, 2016). Adults with disabilities were over three

times more likely to be experiencing sheltered homelessness than adults without disabilities (1 in 86 adults with disabilities, compared with 1 in 313 adults without disabilities) (U.S. HUD, 2016).

Individuals

"Individual" as used by HUD refers to a person "who is not part of a family during his/her episode of homelessness. They are homeless as single adults, unaccompanied youth, or in multiple-adult or multiple-child households." Among this group, 70.4% were men and 29.6% women; each gender constitutes about half the general U.S. population. Nearly half of individuals (42.5%) were between 31 and 50 years of age; just over one-quarter (25.4%) were 51 to 61 years old; 23.6% were ages 18 to 30; 6.3% were age 62 or older; and 2.2% were under age 18. Minorities accounted for 46.3% of sheltered individuals; African Americans (37.2%) were overrepresented in comparison with the racial composition of the general population. Disability rates of sheltered individuals were higher than those of the general population, 44.8%, about 2.3 times the national rate for individuals (USHUD, OCPD, 2016).

Families

A family is composed of at least one adult and one child. On a single night in January 2015 206,286 people experienced homelessness as part of a family with children (USHUD, OCPD, 2016). Among all adults experiencing sheltered homelessness, men considerably outnumbered women (62.1% of adults versus 37.9%). Adults in homeless families are younger than adults in poor families; 1 in 220 adults in the United States who were between the ages of 18 and 30 and in families with children used a shelter program at some point during the year 2015. This proportion is more than three times larger than the proportion of adults over age 30 in families with children (U.S. HUD, OCPD, 2016). Minorities (77.6%) remain overrepresented in sheltered homeless families in comparison with the general population (46.6%). African Americans made up 50.1% of the sheltered homeless population. The 15.8% of Hispanic/Latino sheltered families was slightly higher than the rate of Hispanic/Latino families in the general population (15.6%). The homeless family disability rate, 20.7%, is 2.4 times higher than that in all U.S. families (8.5%) (USHUD, OCPD, 2016).

Veterans

Men accounted for 90.2% of the sheltered homeless veteran population, which is less than the 92.8% in the entire U.S. veteran population. Among sheltered homeless veterans, 9.1% were between 18 and 30 years old, 39.1% were 31 to 50 years old, 42.3% were between 51 and 61 years old, and 9.5% were 62 or older. This pattern differs from that of the entire veteran population, more than half of which were 62 years or older. Minority sheltered veterans were overrepresented in comparison with the total veteran population. Of sheltered veterans, African Americans accounted for 35.5%, compared with 11.0% of all veterans. Although Hispanic/Latino veterans are 3% of the entire veteran population, they accounted for 6.3% of sheltered veterans.

Minorities were also more likely to be in poverty and to have a disability than the general veteran population (USHUD, OCPD, 2012). Men and women veterans, two groups within the homeless veteran subpopulation, have health problems similar to those of nonveteran individuals experiencing homelessness. However, women veterans who experience homelessness have problems specific to their military service experience and their roles as child caregivers.

> **? ACTIVE LEARNING**
>
> Compare the information contained in the most recent U.S. Department of Housing and Urban Development *Annual Homeless Assessment Report* (AHAR) to Congress with the information contained in the previous 3 years. What has changed?

FACTORS THAT CONTRIBUTE TO HOMELESSNESS

In the larger society, three broad factors singly and interactively contribute to homelessness. They are (1) shortage of affordable housing, (2) insufficient income to meet basic needs, and (3) inadequate and scarce support services.

Shortage of Affordable Housing

Housing is considered affordable if it costs a renter or owner no more than 30% of his or her income (HUD, 2017). In cooperation with state and local governments and nonprofit housing organizations, HUD operates programs that provide financial housing assistance to low-income families. This assistance may be provided as (1) direct payment to apartment owners, who in turn lower rents for low-income tenants; (2) access to apartments located in public housing facilities; or (3) housing choice vouchers, which may be used by low-income persons to "pay" all or part of the rent. Option 3's arrangements continue to be more commonly known as *Section 8 housing* (Center on Budget and Policy Priorities, 2015). Although these programs are intended to alleviate housing problems for low-income renters, the demand for these assisted housing programs has far exceeded the supply.

Factors contributing to the shortages include market forces that inhibit the private housing sector's production of affordable rental housing, decreases in the federal government's spending on assisted housing for low-income families, and the increasing inequality of incomes among groups within the larger population. The national housing market has now regained enough momentum to provide an engine of growth for the U.S. economy; however, lingering pressures on homeownership, the eroding affordability of rental housing, and the growing concentration of poverty continue to hamper the housing recovery (Joint Center for Housing Studies [JCHS], 2016). The foreclosure crisis that began in 2007 exacerbated the obstacles that people with low incomes face in obtaining affordable housing. As noted by HUD, the rates of worst-case housing need—a renter whose income is 50% of the area median income and who paid more than half of his or her income for rent—decreased between 2011 and 2013 but persist at high levels across demographic groups, household types,

and regions (JCHS, 2016; National Alliance to End Homelessness, 2013; National Low Income Housing Coalition, 2013; USHUD, Office of Policy Development and Research [OPDR], 2015).

Income Insufficiency

More than 10 years ago, Burt (2007) documented that insufficient incomes and lack of employment prevented people from leaving homelessness. A 2015 U.S. Census Bureau American FactFinder Report reveals that in 2015, the median household income was $53,889 The proportion of people in poverty and poverty rates in 2015 (11.3%) did not differ statistically from those over the previous 5 years (less than 1 percentage point). The poverty rate in 2015 among children younger than 18 years was 21.7% (U.S. Census Bureau, 2015). Moreover, in 2013 among the poor, 19.9 million people lived in families with an income below one half of their poverty threshold, representing 6.3% of all people and 43.8% of those in poverty (the U.S. Census Bureau's weighted average poverty threshold for a family of four in 2013 was $24,028; DeNavas-Walt and Proctor, 2014).

A consequence of the shortage of affordable housing and insufficient income is that an increasing number of low-income people end up paying much more than they can afford for rent. Since 2009, the number of renters who pay more than half of their income for rent has increased dramatically (USHUD, OPDR, 2015).

With the lack of affordable housing in combination with insufficient income, people have to spend much of their income on rent, leaving them without adequate resources for other necessities, such as food, clothing, and health care. This situation substantially increases their risk for homelessness (Kaiser Commission on Medicaid and the Uninsured, 2012).

Inadequacy and Scarcity of Supportive Services

Some people experiencing homelessness have individual characteristics that, in interaction with the structural conditions of shortage of affordable housing and insufficient income, perpetuate their homeless condition. Supportive services for these people are deficient in quality and quantity. Some people need services to work and earn money. They are able to function in the workforce, whereas others need services to maintain their housing status. Included in this latter group are people whose serious chronic mental health and/or substance abuse problems preclude their functioning in the workforce and whose behaviors frequently interfere with their ability to obtain housing stability. People in this group need income assistance and comprehensive and accessible behavioral and physical health care.

What these two groups have in common is the need for affordable health care—that is, care that reflects health in its broadest sense as outlined by the World Health Organization (WHO, 2017), a state of complete physical, mental, and social well-being, and not merely the absence of disease or infirmity (WHO, 2017). "In 2013, 21.6 percent of people in households with an annual household income less than $25,000 had no health insurance coverage, compared with 18.7 percent of people in households with income ranging from $25,000 to $49,999, and 13.1 percent of people in households with income ranging from $50,000 to $74,999" (Smith and Medalia, 2014, p. 6).

Homelessness and Causation

This section has addressed three broad factors—shortage of affordable housing, insufficient income, and scarcity of supportive services—as societal conditions that contribute to homelessness rather than cause homelessness. Within both popular literature and scholarly literature, these factors are frequently referred to as "causes" of homelessness. However, one can assert that evidence is insufficient to infer causation. Closer analysis of the claim that people are homeless because they choose to be reveals that persons as active agents do make decisions that result in homelessness. However, these decisions are made in highly contextualized conditions—frequently, in the midst of mental illness or addiction to alcohol and/or other substances (National Law Center on Homelessness and Poverty, 2015). Whether or not these addictive conditions permit free choice entails philosophical issues that are beyond the scope of this chapter.

HEALTH AND HOMELESS POPULATIONS

As discussed in Chapter 1, the WHO has defined health from a broad perspective. This classic definition, which purports that health is "a state of complete physical, mental, and social well-being and not merely the absence of disease or infirmity" (WHO, 2017), is particularly useful when considering the health status of the homeless. For these individuals, a continual interaction exists among these three dimensions (physical, mental, and social) that has enormous consequences for health. The boundaries of these dimensions overlap; therefore it is difficult, if not impossible, to address health among the homeless without a concomitant analysis of physical, mental, and social dimensions.

The definitions of homelessness, prevalence rates, and demographic characteristics previously outlined were based for the most part on activities of two federal agencies: HUD and ED. To provide a background for exploring health and homeless populations, this section presents a sketch of three aspects of the HHS, the federal agency with designated responsibility for provision of primary health care services to underserved populations. The three aspects of HHS's homeless services are (1) federal health centers, (2) the Health Care for the Homeless (HCH) program, and (3) the definition of the homeless individual used by the HCH program.

Federal Health Centers

Two types of federal health care centers provide services to generally underserved populations (low income): **Federally Qualified Health Centers** (FQHCs) and **FQHC Look-A-Likes** (FQHCLAs). Although both types of centers are located administratively within the HHS's Health Resources and Service Administration (HRSA), Bureau of Primary Health Care (BPHC), and both serve underserved populations, their sources of funding differ. FQHCs receive federal grants to fund services to underserved populations, whereas FQHCLAs do not. Both types of health centers may receive reimbursement under Medicare and Medicaid (USDHHS, HRSA, BPHC, n.d.).

Health Care for the Homeless

Some FQHCs receive additional federal funding to provide primary health care and substance abuse services to homeless populations through the HCH program. In addition to the homeless population, there are two other categories of special populations that federal health centers may serve: migrant seasonal farmworkers and their families and/or residents of public housing.

The definition used by health centers funded by HHS, as cited by the National Health Care for the Homeless Council (2017), follows:

A homeless individual is defined in section 330(h) (4) (A) as "an individual who lacks housing (without regard to whether the individual is a member of a family), including an individual whose primary residence during the night is a supervised public or private facility (e.g., shelters) that provides temporary living accommodations, and an individual who is a resident in transitional housing." A homeless person is an individual without permanent housing who may live on the streets; stay in a shelter, mission, single room occupancy facilities, abandoned building or vehicle; or in any other unstable or non-permanent situation. [Section 330 of the Public Health Service Act (42 U.S.C., 254b)]

An individual may be considered to be homeless if that person is "doubled up," a term that refers to a situation in which individuals are unable to maintain their housing situation and are forced to stay with a series of friends and/or extended family members. In addition, previously homeless individuals who are to be released from a prison or a hospital may be considered homeless if they do not have a stable housing situation to which they can return. Recognition of the instability of an individual's living arrangements is critical to the definition of homelessness.

The HHS definition of a homeless individual differs from the HUD and ED definitions. The differences are based on the specific legislative and administrative actions that authorize each agency's services. Both ED and HHS operate with broader definitions of homeless individuals than HUD. Using WHO's definition of health and HHS's definition of homeless individuals provides a perspective from which to view the health status of homeless populations.

HEALTH STATUS OF THE HOMELESS POPULATION

This section is organized according to the most prominent subpopulations within the larger homeless population: adults, women, families, youth, veterans, and persons experiencing chronic homelessness.

Adults

An exploration of the literature over the past two decades related to the health of the homeless population reveals that morbidity rates in the adult homeless population are higher than those occurring in comparable groups in the general population. Acute physical health problems occurring at higher rates in adults in the homeless population include respiratory infections and trauma. Chronic disorders experienced at higher rates than in the general population include hypertension, musculoskeletal disorder, gastrointestinal problems, respiratory problems (asthma, chronic bronchitis, emphysema), neurological disorders including seizures, and poor dentition. Serious mental illnesses and minor emotional problems also occur more frequently in the homeless population than in the general population. High rates of alcohol and drug use exacerbate the existing acute and chronic physical and mental health problems (National Coalition for the Homeless, 2014; National Policy and Advocacy Council on Homelessness, 2014). The excessive morbidity rates are associated with mortality rates that are also higher than those in the general population (Baggett et al., 2015; Fazel et al., 2014; Henwood et al., 2015).

Lebrun-Harris and associates (2013) published a study that provides a national perspective on the self-reported health status of adult homeless patients in comparison with that of non-homeless federal health center patients. The researchers analyzed data collected in 2009 by the BPHC for the Health Center Patient Survey. Trained interviewers elicited respondents' housing status by asking patients whether they currently had a place to live, such as a house, apartment, or room. If they answered "yes" they were classified as non-homeless. Those patients who indicated they lived in an emergency or transitional shelter or hotel/motel room were categorized as homeless. In addition to housing status, interviewers elicited information regarding sociodemographic characteristics, medical conditions, access to care, and utilization of services.

On the basis of their analysis, Lebrun-Harris and associates (2013) reported that more males were homeless (57%) than were housed (37%). Unmarried patients made up 93% of the homeless group compared with 70% in the housed group. In the group of homeless patients, 6% were employed, in contrast to 37% of the housed group. More patients in the homeless group (84%) were 100% below the federal poverty level, in contrast to 50% of the housed group. Seventy-two percent of patients in the homeless group had experienced at least two homeless episodes versus 7.6% in the housed group.

A larger proportion of homeless patients reported substance use problems than their housed counterparts. Problems included higher rates of smoking, binge drinking, risk of alcohol and drug dependence, ever having injected drugs, and receiving treatment for alcohol or drug use in the past year. Larger percentages of homeless patients (52%) than of housed patients (36%) judged their health status as fair/poor. A higher proportion of patients in the homeless group (26%) than in the housed group (10%) reported that sometimes or often they did not get enough to eat—the definition of food insufficiency.

A larger proportion of individuals in the homeless group reported mental health problems in comparison with the housed individuals. The mental problems included psychological distress in the past month, lifetime anxiety, and receipt of mental health treatment in the past year. A higher proportion of homeless patients than housed patients reported needing medical care and using hospital emergency departments as their usual sources of care.

Summarizing the results of the study, Lebrun-Harris and associates (2013) stated that a larger proportion of homeless patients reported worse health status and more chronic physical disease, mental health problems, and substance use problems than nonhomeless patients. This conclusion substantiates results of previous research on the health status of a large segment of the homeless population—adults. Within the homeless population that the Lebrun-Harris group's work addresses, there are subpopulations that, although they share similar mortality and morbidly problems, also have characteristics and circumstances that render a different health status.

Women

As noted earlier in this chapter, national data suggest that nearly 38% of sheltered individuals are women (USHUD, OCPD, 2016). Women constituted nearly 30% of the 2938 homeless persons sampled in the National Survey of Homeless Assistance Providers and Clients. Of these women, nearly 55% were accompanied by at least one minor child and the remaining 45% were living as unaccompanied adults; one third of the women reported experiences indicative of long-term homelessness (Zlotnick et al., 2012).

Homeless women have higher rates of pregnancy, including unintended pregnancy, than their housed counterparts, and researchers have demonstrated that the severity of homelessness increases the likelihood of preterm births and low-birth-weight infants (Begun, 2015). The majority of chronically homeless adults are male, though anywhere between 22,000 and 28,000 females experience chronic homelessness and its associated risks on any given day (Edens et al., 2011). Women with substance use disorders are a growing group in the United States and are increasingly represented among the chronically homeless, though few gender differences in rates of alcohol and drug problems have been reported over time (Edens et al., 2011). Research has revealed that many homeless women have extraordinary histories involving substance use, criminal activity, serious mental health concerns, marital dissolution, escape from domestic violence, housing accidents, limited employment options or job loss, and poor physical health that prevented gainful employment (Moxley et al., 2012). Vijayaraghavan et al. (2011) reported that between 30% and 90% of homeless women have experienced high rates of intimate partner violence. Moreover, homeless young women have been found to have high rates of childhood sexual abuse, dependency and delinquency systems involvement, and psychiatric hospitalization (Warf et al., 2013). Advocates for the homeless continue to argue that the immediate cause of homelessness among women is typically violence and that the vast majority has experienced violence at some point in their lives. Sexual assaults are associated with worse physical and mental health outcomes, including use/abuse of alcohol and other drugs (WHO, 2013), and, as may be expected, women living in unsheltered locations on the street have higher risk for victimization than women living in shelters.

Young (homeless) women involved in survival sex (participating in sexual acts in exchange for money, food, lodging, clothing, or drugs) are motivated primarily by desperation to meet basic needs, including a place to stay, food, and money, and one third mentioned that peers commonly were influential in decisions to engage in survival sex. Others were influenced by coercion (10%) or pursuit of drugs (10%) (Warf et. al, 2013)

Families

The health status of adults and women, the two subpopulations discussed in the previous sections, is also relevant to the health status of families experiencing homelessness. The histories of chronic physical and mental health conditions, substance abuse, victimization, and low education and job training of adults are also risk factors for compromised caregiver–child relations. Because women are often the single or major caregivers in homeless families, their compromised physical, mental, and social health status is of even more concern.

Reviews of published literature about children in families experiencing homelessness show that research-based studies indicate these children have physical health problems, including asthma, iron-deficiency anemia, and obesity; mental health problems, including behavior problems; and developmental delays at rates higher than those reported for children in the general population. These reviews also note that such problems interact and adversely affect homeless children's educational achievement on standardized tests covering reading, language usage, and/or mathematics. Missing days of school due to family mobility, homeless children are more likely than other children to repeat grades. Homeless children may lack resources for clothing and school supplies and access to facilities for maintenance of personal hygiene. Moreover, they are at risk for high rates of alcohol and drug use, depression, risky sexual behaviors, and victimization (Lim et al., 2015; Saddichha et al., 2014).

Youth

This section sketches the health problems occurring within the subpopulation of homeless youth. It includes those individuals federally defined as unaccompanied, runaway, and homeless youth.

As indicated by several substantial reports and reviews of studies, youth from all sectors of society engage in health-risking behaviors that result in serious health problems (Eaton et al., 2012). These problems include unintended pregnancy, sexually transmitted disease (STDs, including HIV/AIDS), alcohol and drug abuse, depression, and suicide. One and a half to 2 million youth per year are homeless or have run away from home; homeless youth are highly likely to experience early sexual debut, have multiple sex partners, engage in unprotected sexual intercourse, and use alcohol or other drugs before sex, resulting in a high risk of acquiring HIV (Centers for Disease Control and Prevention [CDC], 2015; Warf et al., 2013).

Homeless youth experience STDs, physical and sexual abuse, skin disorders, anemia, drug and alcohol abuse, and unintentional injuries at higher rates than their counterparts in the general population. Depression; suicidal ideation; and disorders of behavior, personality, or thought also occur at higher rates among homeless youths. Family disruption, school failures, prostitution or "survival sex," and involvement with the legal system indicate that homeless youths' social health is severely compromised (Edidin et al., 2012; Kennedy et al., 2012; Nyamathi et al., 2012; Tucker et al., 2012a; Warf et al., 2013).

Homeless youth who are pregnant; engage in prostitution; or identify themselves as gay, lesbian, bisexual, transgender, or questioning (LGBTQ) experience more health problems than other homeless youth. "Compared to their housed counterparts, homeless youth become pregnant at exceptionally high rates" (Begun, 2015, p. 444). Pregnant homeless youth have more severe mental health problems and use alcohol and drugs more than nonpregnant homeless peers. In addition to increased pregnancy rates, homeless young women who engage in survival sex are also significantly more likely to attempt suicide (Warf et al., 2013). Not surprisingly, they have higher rates of birth complications and newborns who are more likely to be born preterm, at low birth weights, and with health problems due to prenatal nutritional deficits (Begun, 2015).

Both female and male homeless youth make up a large percentage of all youth involved in prostitution. Many become involved because they need money to meet subsistence needs (survival sex). They are more likely to have serious mental health problems and to be actively suicidal. Alcohol and drug use, HIV infection, suicide attempts, criminal arrests, and victimization (robbery, assault) occur at higher rates among this group than among homeless youth not engaged in prostitution. Those involved in prostitution are more likely to report histories of physical and sexual abuse (Begun, 2015; National Sexual Violence Resource Center, 2017).

Rates of attempted suicide are higher among gay homeless youth. A large majority of males involved in survival sex identify themselves as gay or bisexual. Many of these young people are on the streets because of the effects of homophobia and prejudice (National Runaway Safeline, 2017).

Between 11% and 37% of youth aging out of foster care experience homelessness after they transition (National Alliance to End Homelessness and Mitchell, 2014). Homeless youth who have a history of foster care are at increased risk of psychiatric disorders. They are more likely to report psychiatric disorders than homeless youth without a history of foster placement (Thompson and Hasin, 2012).

Youth in the general population are at risk, those who are homeless are at even higher risk, and the special subpopulations of youth—including those who are LGBTQ-identified, those who are pregnant, those who are practicing survival sex, and those who have a history of foster care—are particularly vulnerable. Health for many of these groups is severely jeopardized.

Chronically Homeless

As noted previously, many homeless individuals experience both mental and substance use disorders. These are the individuals included in the HUD definition of the **chronically homeless**. More specifically, they are unaccompanied adults who are homeless for extended or numerous periods and have one or more disabling conditions, which are very often severe mental and substance use disorders (Collins et al., 2012; SAMHSA, 2016). This subpopulation is also at increased risk for the health problems outlined in previous sections on the health status of subpopulations of adults and women.

As of 2015, approximately two thirds (or 54,815) of the chronically homeless were unsheltered—sleeping on the street or in places not meant for human habitation (USHUD, OCPD, 2015). Homeless service providers, concerned about the high mortality risk among the "street" homeless population, constructed the Vulnerability Index (Hwang et al., 1998), a screening tool for identifying and prioritizing the need for housing. Those at high risk for death are individuals who have been homeless for 6 months or more with one or more of the following features (Community Solutions, 2017; Pedersen, 2016):

- More than three hospitalizations or emergency room visits in a year
- More than three emergency room visits in the previous 3 months
- 60 years or older
- Cirrhosis of the liver
- End-stage renal disease
- History of frostbite, immersion foot, or hypothermia
- HIV/AIDS
- Co-occurring psychiatric, substance abuse, and chronic medical conditions
- Suicide
- Drug or alcohol abuse

❓ ACTIVE LEARNING

1. Analyze at least three or four factors that contribute to homelessness in the United States.
2. Discuss common health problems found among homeless adults, families, women, and youth.
3. Identify two special subgroups of the homeless and describe their health problems.
4. Describe social determinants of health. What is their significance for community health nursing practice with homeless individuals and families?

COMMUNITY PUBLIC HEALTH NURSING: CARE OF HOMELESS POPULATIONS

An examination of the reports of the health status of persons experiencing homelessness reveals that physical and mental health problems predominate. Stated differently, the studies reflect a biological-psychological basis—social health is rarely addressed. Although many of the studies noted that homelessness, as a form of extreme poverty, contributed to poor health and poor health in turn was a risk for homelessness, the interventions focused on resolving the physical and mental health problem rather than ameliorating the conditions that contributed to homelessness. This section discusses concepts that suggest directions for community/public health nursing care of the homeless population that is broader in scope than the biological-psychological approach.

Framework for Community/Public Health Nursing Care for Homeless Populations

This section presents a framework for developing approaches to providing community/public health nursing care of homeless populations. The framework has four elements: models of justice, thinking upstream, social determinants of health (SDH), and the Public Health Intervention Wheel (Minnesota Department of Health, 2001) that supports upstream interventions for homeless populations.

Models of Justice

Beauchamp (1979) distinguished between the two types of justice (i.e., market justice and social justice) that influence public health policy in the United States. Market justice, which has been the dominant model, purports that people are entitled to valued ends (i.e., status, income, and happiness) according to their own individual efforts. Moreover, this model stresses individual responsibility, minimal collective action, and freedom from collective obligations other than respect for another person's fundamental rights. In contrast, under a social justice model, all people are equally entitled to key ends (i.e., access to health care and minimum standards of income). Consequently, all members of society must accept collective burdens to provide a fair distribution of these ends. Moreover, social justice is a foundational aspect of public health (Krieger and Birn, 1998) and nursing (Kagan et al., 2014). Others have noted the limits of the market approach; citing the many problems inherent in the current health care system, they call for a social justice approach to health care (Rhodes et al., 2012).

Thinking Upstream

McKinlay's (1979) work of more than 30 years ago (see Chapter 3) suggests conceptualizing homelessness as the river and the homeless as the people in the river. Building on McKinlay's "river" metaphor, McKinlay and Marceau (2000) hold that government and private efforts to address homeless health care problems largely focus on "pulling the bodies out of the river of homelessness." Such downstream interventions, aimed at treating or alleviating health care problems such as physical disease and mental illnesses, are worthy and needed. However, these interventions, when used alone, are far less adequate in alleviating homeless people's social health problems. To improve the social health of the homeless, it is necessary to go upstream and focus on the primary contributors to homelessness itself (i.e., lack of affordable housing, inadequate income, and insufficient services). An upstream approach to homelessness is provided by the concept of *social determinants of health.*

Social Determinants of Health

In 2008 the World Health Organization Commission on Social Determinants of Health published its final report, *Closing the Gap in a Generation: Health Equity through Action on the Social Determinants of Health.* As defined by WHO, "The social determinants of health are the circumstances in which people are born, grow up, live, work and age, and the systems put in place to deal with illness. These circumstances are in turn shaped by a wider set of forces: economics, social policies, and politics" (WHO, 2017).

Building on WHO's extensive work, the United States included in *Healthy People 2020* a new overarching goal to "create social and physical environments that promote good health for all" (HealthyPeople.gov, 2017) and a new topic area, the SDH (USDHHS, 2013).

Five broad dimension of SDH are defined within *Healthy People 2020* as follows: (1) economic stability, (2) education, (3) social and community context, (4) health and health care, and (5) neighborhood and built environment. Each of these dimensions includes key issues that identify more specific factors (HealthyPeople.gov,

TABLE 23.2 Social Determinants of Health And Factors Contributing to Homelessness	
Healthy People 2020 Social Determinant of Health Dimensions and Key Issues	**Factor(s) Contributing to Homelessness**
Economic Stability	
Poverty	Income insufficiency
Employment status	Income insufficiency
Access to employment	Income insufficiency
Housing stability (e.g., homelessness foreclosure)	Shortage of affordable housing
Health and Health Care	
Access to health services—including clinical and preventive care	Inadequacy and scarcity of supportive services
Access to primary care—including community-based health promotion and wellness programs	Inadequacy and scarcity of supportive services

Adapted from U.S. Department of Health and Human Services: *Healthy People 2020: determinants of health,* 2012. http://www.healthypeople.gov/2020/about/DOHAbout.aspx.

2017). Two of the dimensions, economic stability and health and health care, hold significant relevance for homelessness in that the key issues are those defined as contributing to homelessness. Table 23.2 lists the key issues that *Healthy People 2020* identifies as underlying economic stability, health and health care, and the associated factors contributing to homelessness.

SDH, as noted by the CDC (2010, p. 1), are the "complex, integrated and overlapping social structures and economic systems that include the social and physical environments, and health services." These determinants are shaped by the levels of income, power, and resources at global, national, and local levels. They are also often influenced not only through personal choices but through policy choices as well. As defined, the SDH call for an upstream approach to deal with the "causes of the cause"—those factors embedded in the social fabric of communities at all levels. However, as cautioned by governmental entities and individual writers, both upstream and downstream approaches are needed (CDC, 2010; Koh et al., 2011; Martins and Burbank, 2011; USDHHS, 2012, 2013). Interventions are needed upstream at community or systems levels and downstream at the individual or family levels.

Public Health Intervention Wheel

Developed more than 10 years ago, the Public Health Intervention Wheel provides guidance in identifying the types of interventions and the most appropriate level for providing public health nursing care to homeless populations (Minnesota Department of Health Division of Community Health Services, 2001). The 17 interventions are graphically displayed and defined in Chapter 1. One of the major strengths of the Intervention Wheel is that it directs practice at individual and family levels, a downstream approach, as well as at the community or systems level, an upstream approach.

Although nurses may use all interventions at all three levels, community/public health nurses, working downstream with individuals, families, or groups use surveillance, disease and other health event investigation, outreach, screening, case finding referral and follow-up, case management, delegated functions, health teaching, counseling, and consultation. In contrast, community/public health nurses working more upstream at the system level employ collaboration, coalition building, community organizing, advocacy, social marketing, and policy development and enforcement.

❓ ACTIVE LEARNING

Discuss at least two community health nursing interventions and locate them on the Public Health Intervention Wheel.

SUMMARY

This chapter provides an overview of homelessness from a national perspective. Definitions of homeless, prevalence estimates and demographic characteristics of subpopulations (adults, families with children, veterans, and the chronically homeless) are presented. Factors contributing to homelessness (lack of affordable housing, insufficient income, and lack of supportive services) are compared with the social determinants of health. Health status of homeless subpopulations, as reported in the literature, is outlined and noted to be focused mainly on physical health, reflecting a downstream focus. A framework for community/public health nursing care of the homeless population based on social justice, upstream thinking, SDH, and the Public Health Intervention Wheel and supporting both upstream and downstream interventions is outlined. The interventions identified reflected macro-upstream factors and more micro-downstream conditions of individuals and families experiencing homelessness.

ⓔ EVOLVE WEBSITE

http://evolve.elsevier.com/Nies/community
- NCLEX Review Questions
- Case Studies

BIBLIOGRAPHY

Anderson DG: Homeless women's perceptions about their families of origin, *West J Nurs Res* 18(1):29–42, 1996.

Austin EL, Andersen R, Gelberg L: Ethnic differences in the correlates of mental distress among homeless women, *Womens Health Issues* 18(1):26–34, 2008.

Baggett TP, Change Y, Singer D, et al.: Tobacco-, alcohol-, and drug-attributable deaths and their contribution to mortality disparities in a cohort of homeless adults in Boston, *Am J Public Health* 105(6):1189–1197, 2015.

Bassuk EL, Buckner JC, Weinreb LF: Homelessness in female-headed families: childhood and adult risk and protective factors, *Am J Public Health* 87(2):241–248, 1997.

Bassuk EL, Melnick S, Browne A: Responding to the needs of low-income and homeless women who are survivors of family violence, *J Am Med Womens Assoc* 53(2):57–64, 1998.

Bassuk EL, Weinreb LF, Buckner JC: The characteristics and needs of sheltered homeless and low-income housed mothers, *JAMA* 276(8):640–646, 1996.

Beauchamp DE: Public health as social justice. In Jaco EG, editor: *Patients, physcians, and illness,* ed 3, New York, 1979, Free Press.

Begun S: The paradox of homeless youth pregnacyL A review of challenges and opportunities, *Soc Work Health Care* 54(5):444–460, 2015.

Bowman D, Dukes C, Moore J: *Summary of the state of research on the relationship between homelessness and academic achievement among school-aged children and youth.* Available from: <http://center.serve.org/nche/downloads/nche_research_pub.pdf>.

Budetti PP: Market justice and US health care, *JAMA* 299(1):92–94, 2008.

Burt MR: *Understanding homeless youth: numbers, characteristics, multisystem involvement and intervention options* (testimony submitted to Subcommittee on Income Security and Family Support, U.S. House Committee on Ways and Means), 2007. Available from: <http://www.urban.org/UploadedPDF/901087_Burt_Homeless.pdf>.

Busen NH, Engebretson JC: Facilitating risk reduction among homeless and street-involved youth, *J Am Acad Nurse Pract* 20(11): 567–575, 2008.

Canadian Homelessness Research Network, The Homeless Hub: *Canadian definition of homelessness,* 2012. Available from: <http://homelesshub.ca/homelessdefinition>.

Caton CL, Dominguez B, Schanzer B: Risk factors for long-term homelessness: findings from a longitudinal study of first-time homeless single adults, *Am J Public Health* 95(10):1753–1759, 2005.

Caton CL, Wilkins C, Anderson JA: *People who experience long-term homelessness: characteristics and interventions,* Washington, DC, March 1-2, 2007, Presented The National Symposium on Homelessness Research. Available from: <http://aspe.hhs.gov/hsp/homelessness/symposium07/caton/report.pdf>.

Centers for Disease Control and Prevention: *Strategy summaries for PS13-1308,* 2015. Available from: https://www.cdc.gov/healthyyouth/fundedpartners/1308/strategies/index.htm.

Center on Budget and Policy Priorities: *Policy basics: federal rental assistance,* 2015. Available from: <http://www.cbpp.org/cms/index.cfm?fa=view&id=3890>.

Centers for Disease Control and Prevention: *Establishing a holistic framework to reduce inequities in HIV, viral hepatitis, STDs, and tuberculosis in the United States.* Available from: <http://www.cdc.gov/socialdeterminants/docs/SDH-White-Paper-2010.pdf>.

Childtrends.org: *Databank indicator: homeless children and youth,* 2015. Available from: http://www.childtrends.org/indicators/homeless-children-and-youth/.

Collins S, Malone D, Clifasefi S, et al.: Individuals with alcohol problems: within-subjects analyses of 2-year alcohol trajectories, *Am J Public Health,* 2012. Available from: http://scholar.google.com/scholar_url?url=http://www.academia.edu/download/41481572/ProjectBased_20HF_20for_20Chronically_20Homeless_20Indiv_20with_20Alcohol_20Problems.collins_20et_20al.pdf&hl=en&sa=X&scisig=AAGBfm3RgAu1u63adFuGWMg5I7ttg_FLVA&nossl=1&oi=scholarr.

Community Solutions: *Vulnerability index: prioritizing the street homeless population by mortality risk,* 2017. Available from: 100khomes.org/sites/default/files/About%20the%20Vulnerability%20Index.pdf.

DeNavas-Walt C, Proctor B: *Income and poverty in the United States: 2013,* 2014. Available from: <https://www.census.gov/prod/www/population.html>.

DeNavas-Walt C, Proctor BD, Smith JC: *Income, poverty, and health insurance coverage in the United States: 2011* (Current Population Reports, P60–243), Washington, DC, 2012, U.S. Census Bureau. Also available from: <http://vuwne.census.gov/prod/2012pubs/p60-243.pdf>.

Eaton DK, Kann L, Kinchen S: Youth risk behavior surveillance—United States, 2011, *MMWR Surveillance Summaries* 61(4):1–162, 2012.

Edens E, Mares A, Rosenheck R: Chronically homeless women report high rates of substance use problems equivalent to chronically homeless men, *Women's Health Issues* 21(5):383–389, 2011.

Edgar W: *European review of statistics on homelessness.* Available from: <http://eohw.horus.be/files/freshstart/European%20Statistics%20Reports/2009%20European%20Review%20of%20Statistics/chapter2_EN.pdf>.

Edidin JP, Ganim Z, Hunter SJ: The mental and physical health of homeless youth: a literature review, *Child Psychiatry Hum Dev* 43(3):354–375, 2012.

European Federation of National Associations Working with the Homeless: *ETHOS typology on homelessness and housing exclusion,* 2017. Available from: http://www.feantsa.org/en/toolkit/2005/04/01/ethos-typology-on-homelessness-and-housing-exclusion?bcParent=27.

Fazel S, Geddes J, Kushel M: The health of homeless people in high-income countries: descriptive epidemiology, health consequences, and clinical and policy recommendations, *Lancet* 384(9953):1529–1540, 2014.

Fernandes AL: *Runaway and homeless youth: demographics, programs and emerging issues (No. RL33785),* Washington, DC, 2007, Congressional Research Services.

Gamache G, Rosenheck R, Tessler R: Overrepresentation of women veterans among homeless women, *Am J Public Health* 93(7): 1132–1136, 2003.

Grace PJ, Willis DG: Nursing responsibilities and social justice: an analysis in support of disciplinary goals, *Nursing Outlook* 60(4):198–207, 2012.

HealthyPeople. gov: *Social determinants of health,* 2017. Available from: https://www.healthypeople.gov/2020/topics-objectives/topic/social-determinants-of-health.

Henwood BF, Byrne T, Scriber B: Examining mortality among formerly homeless adults enrolled in housing first: an observational study, *BMC Public Health* 15:1209, 2015. http://doi.org/10.1186/s12889-015-2552-1.

HUD.GOV: *Homeless assistance,* 2017. Accessible at https://portal.hud.gov/hudportal/HUD?src=/program_offices/comm_planning/homeless.

Huntington N, Buckner JC, Bassuk EL: Adaptation in homeless children: an empirical examination using cluster analysis, *Am Behavioral Scientist* 51(6):737–755, 2008. 10.1177/0002764207311985.

Hwang S, Lebow J, Bierer M, et al.: Risk factors for death in homeless adults in Boston, *Arch Intern Med* 158:1454–1460, 1998.

Joint Center for Housing Studies of Harvard University: *State of nation's housing,* 2016. Available from: <http://www.jchs.harvard.edu/sites/jchs.harvard.edu/files/son2012.pdf>.

Kagan P, Smith M, Chinn P: *Philosophies and practices of emancipatory nursing: social justice as praxis,* New York, 2014, Routledge.

Kaiser Commission on Medicaid and the Uninsured: *The uninsured and the difference health insurance makes.* Available from: <http://www.kff.org/uninsured/1420.cfm>.

Kanis R, Mccannon J, Craig C: An end to chronic homelessness: an introduction to the 100,000 homes campaign, *J Health Care Poor Underserved* 23(1):321–326, 2012.

Kennedy DP, Tucker JS, Green Jr HD: Unprotected sex of homeless youth: results from a multilevel dyadic analysis of individual, social network, and relationship factors, *AIDS Behav* 16(7):2015–2032, 2012.

Kilmer RP, Cook JR, Crusto C: Understanding the ecology and development of children and families experiencing homelessness: implications for practice, supportive services, and policy, *Am J Orthopsychiatry* 82(3):389–401, 2012.

Koh HK, Piotrowski JJ, Kumanyika S: Healthy people: a 2020 vision for the social determinants approach, *Health Educ Behav* 38(6):551–557, 2011.

Kozol J: *Rachel and her children: homeless families in America*, New York, 1988, Crown.

Krieger N, Birn AE: A vision of social justice as the foundation of public health: commemorating 150 years of the spirit of 1848, *Am J Public Health* 88(11):1603–1606, 1998.

Larimer ME, Malone DK, Garner MD: Health care and public service use and costs before and after provision of housing for chronically homeless persons with severe alcohol problems, *JAMA* 301(13):1349–1357, 2009.

Lawrence RS, Gootman JA, Sim LJ: *Adolescent health services: missing opportunities*, Washington, DC, 2009, National Academies Press.

Lebrun-Harris LA, Baggett TP, Jenkins DM: Health status and health care experiences among homeless patients in federally supported health centers: findings from the 2009 patient survey, *Health Serv Res* 48(3):992–1017, 2013. 10.1111/1475-6773.12009.

Lim C, Rice E, Rhoades H: Depressive symptoms and their association with adverse environmental factors and substance use in runaway and homeless youths, *J Adolesc Res* 26(3):403–417, 2015.

Martins D, Cocozza Burbank PM: Critical interactionism: an upstream-downstream approach to health care reform, *Adv Nurs Sci* 34(4):315–329, 2011. 10.1097/ANS.0b013e3182356c19.

McCoy-Roth M, Mackintosh BB, Murphey D: When the bough breaks: the effects of homelessness on young children, 2012. Available from: <http://www.caction.org/CAN-Research/Reports/2012/Child_Trends-2012_02_16_ECH_Homelessness.pdf>.

McKinlay JB: A case for refocusing upstream; the political economy of illness. In Jaco EG, editor: *Patients, physicians, and illness*, ed 3, New York, 1979, Free Press.

McKinlay JB, Marceau LD: To boldly go…, *Am J Public Health* 90(1):25–33, 2000.

Metraux S, Eng N, Bainbridge J: The impact of shelter use and housing placement on mortality hazard for unaccompanied adults and adults in family households entering New York City shelters: 1990-2002, *J Urban Health* 88(6):1091–1104, 2011.

Minnesota Department of Health Division of Community Health Services: *Public health interventions: applications for public health nursing practice*. Available from: <http://www.health.state.mn.us/divs/cfh/ophp/resources/docs/phinterventions_manual2001.pdf>.

Molino A: Characteristics of help-seeking street youth and non-street youth. Available from: <http://aspe.hhs.gov/hsp/homelessness/symposium07/molino/index.htm;>.

Moxley D, Washington O, Calligan H: Narrative insight into risk, vulnerability, and resilience among older homeless African American women, *The Arts in Psychotherapy* 39(5):471–478, 2012.

Murphy J, Tobin K: Homelessness comes to school, CA, Corwin, 2011, Thousand Oaks.

National Alliance to End Homelessness: *The state of homelessness in America*, 2013. Available from: <http://www.endhomelessness.org/library/entry/the-state-of-homelessness-2013>.

National Alliance to End Homelessness & Mindy Mitchell: *HUD report explores options for youth aging out of foster care*, 2014. Available from: http://www.endhomelessness.org/blog/entry/hud-report-explores-options-for-youth-aging-out-of-foster-care#.WMhoTfI-jGl.

National Center for Homeless Education: *Education for homeless children and youths program: data collection summary school year 2010-11.* Available from: <http://center.serve.org/nche/downloads/data_comp_0909-1011.pdf>.

National Center on Family Homelessness: *America's youngest outcasts*, 2010. Available from: <http://www.homelesschildrenamerica.org/media/NCFH_AmericaOutcast2010_web.pdf>.

National Health Care for the Homeless Council: *Frequently asked questions about health care for the homeless*. Available from: <http://bphc.hrsa.gov/technicalassistance/taresources/hchfaqupdated.pdf>.

National Health Care for the Homeless Council: *What is the official definition of homelessness?*, 2017. Available from: https://www.nhchc.org/faq/official-definition-homelessness/.

National Center for Homeless Education: *Federal data summary: school years 2012-2013 to 2014-2015: education for homeless children and youth*, 2016. Available at https://nche.ed.gov/ibt/sc_data.php.

National Coalition for the Homeless: *Homelessness in America*, 2014. Available at http://nationalhomeless.org/about-homelessness/.

National Law Center on Homelessness and Poverty: *Homelessness in American: overview of data and causes*, 2015. Available from: https://www.nlchp.org/documents/Homeless_Stats_Fact_Sheet.

National Low Income Housing Coalition: America's affordable housing shortage, and how to end it, *Housing Spotlight* 3(2):1–6, 2013. Also available from <http://nlihc.org/sites/default/files/HS_3-1.pdf>.

National Low Income Housing Coalition: *Out of reach 2016. How much do you need to earn to afford a modest apartment in your state?* Available from: <http://nlihc.org/oor>http://nlihc.org/sites/default/files/oor/2013_OOR.pdf>.

National Policy and Advocacy Council on Homelessness: *Homelessness risk factors*, 2014. Available from: http://www.npach.org/homelessness-risk-factors.html.

National Runaway Safeline: *Runaway statistics: third party statistics*, 2017. Available from: https://www.1800runaway.org/runaway-statistics/third-party-statistics/#LGBTQ.

National Sexual Violence Resource Center: *Housing, homelessness, and sexual violence statistics*, 2017. Available from: www.nsvrc.org/sites/default/files/NSAC11.../NSAC11_Handout_With_Statistics.pdfmwww.nsvrc.org/sites/default/files/NSAC11.../NSAC11_Handout_With_Statistics.pdf.

Nyamathi A, Hudson A, Greengold B: Characteristics of homeless youth who use cocaine and methamphetamine, *Am J Addictions* 21(3):243–249, 2012.

Nyamathi A, Leake B, Gelberg L: Sheltered versus nonsheltered homeless women differences in health, behavior, victimization, and utilization of care, *J Gen Intern Med* 15(8):565–572, 2000.

Obradovic J, Long JD, Cutulia A: Academic achievement of homeless and highly mobile children in an urban school district: longitudinal evidence on risk, growth, and resilience, *Dev Psychopathol* 21:493–518, 2009.

Park JM, Fertig AR, Allison PD: Physical and mental health, cognitive development, and health care use by housing status of low-income young children in 20 American cities: a prospective cohort study, *Am J Public Health* 101(Suppl 1):S255–S261, 2011.

Pauly BM, MacKinnon K, Varcoe C: Revisiting "Who gets care?": health equity as an arena for nursing action, *Adv Nurs Sci* 32(2):118–127, 2009.

Pedersen T: Homeless youth in San Francisco face high risk of death, *Psych Central*, 2016. Available from: https://psychcentral.com/news/2016/04/18/homeless-youth-in-san-francisco-face-high-risk-of-death/101921.html.

Perl L, Bagalman E, Fernandes-Alcantara A, et al.: *Homelessness: targeted federal programs and recent legislation (CRS Report for Congress No. 7–5700)*, 2015. Available from: <http://www.fas.org/sgp/crs/misc/RL30442.pdf>.

Minnesota Department of Health: *Public Health Nursing Section: Public Health Interventions–Applications for Public Health Nursing Practice*, St. Paul, 2001, Minnesota Dept. of Health. Available from: http://www.health.state.mn.us/divs/opi/cd/phn/wheel.html.

Rayburn RL, Pals H, Wright JD: Death, drugs, and disaster: mortality among New Orleans' homeless, *Care Manag J* 13(1):8–18, 2012.

Rew L, Grady M, Whittaker TA: Interaction of duration of homelessness and gender on adolescent sexual health indicators, *J Nurs Scholarsh* 40(2):109–115, 2008.

Rew L, Rochlen AB, Murphey C: Health educators' perceptions of a sexual health intervention for homeless adolescents, *Patient Educ Couns* 72(1):71–77, 2008.

Rhodes R, Battin M, Silvers A: *Medicine and social justice: essays on the distribution of health care*, Oxford, 2012, Oxford University Press.

Saddichha S, Linden L, Krausz M: Physical and mental health issues among homeless youth in British Columbia, Canada: Are they different from older homeless adults? *J Can Acad Child Adolesc Psychiatry* 23(3):200–206, 2014.

Sadowski LS, Kee RA, VanderWeele TJ: Effect of a housing and case management program on emergency department visits and hospitalizations among chronically ill homeless adults: a randomized trial, *JAMA* 301(17):1771–1778, 2009.

SAMHSA: *Homelessness and housing*, 2016. Available at: https://www.samhsa.gov/homelessness-housing.

Shumsky NL: *Homelessness: a documentary and reference guide*. Santa Barbara, CA, 2012, Greenwood.

Smith J, Medalia C: *Health insurance coverage in the United States: 2013*, 2014. Available from: *https://www.census.gov/content/dam/Census/library/publications/2014/.../p60-250.pdf*.

Tevendale HD, Lightfoot M, Slocum SL: Individual and environmental protective factors for risky sexual behavior among homeless youth: an exploration of gender differences, *AIDS & Behavior* 13(1):154–164, 2009.

Thompson RG, Hasin D: Psychiatric disorders and treatment among newly homeless young adults with histories of foster care, *Psychiatric Services* 63(9):906–912, 2012.

Toro P, Dworsky A, Fowler P: *Homeless youth in the United States: recent research findings and intervention approaches*, Washington, DC, March 1-2, 2007, Presented by The National Symposium on Homelessness Research. Available from: <http://aspe.hhs.gov/hsp/homelessness/symposium07/Toro/report.pdf>.

Tucker JS, Hu J, Golinelli D: Social network and individual correlates of sexual risk behavior among homeless young men who have sex with men, *J Adoles Health* 51(4):386–392, 2012a.

Tucker JS, Ryan GW, Golinelli D: Substance use and other risk factors for unprotected sex: results from an event-based study of homeless youth, *AIDS & Behavior* 16(6):1699–1707, 2012b.

U.S. Census Bureau: *American fact finder*, 2015. Available from: https://factfinder.census.gov/faces/tableservices/jsf/pages/productview.xhtml?pid=ACS_15_5YR_DP03&prodType=table.

U.S. Conference of Mayors: *Hunger and homelessness survey: a status report on hunger and homelessness in America's cities*, 2016. Available from: <https://usmayors.org/pressreleases/uploads/.../1213-hh-survey.pdf>.

U.S. Department of Commerce: *History: 2000 census of population and housing*, Washington, DC, 2009, US Government Printing Office.

U.S. Department of Education: *Education for homeless children and youths grants for state and local activities*, 2016. Available from: <https://www2.ed.gov/programs/homeless/index.html>.

U.S. Department of Health and Human Services: *Healthy people 2020: determinants of health*. Available from: <http://www.healthypeople.gov/2020/about/DOHAbout.aspx>.

U.S. Department of Health and Human Services: *Healthy people 2020: social determinants of health*. Available from: <http://www.healthypeople.gov/2020/topicsobjectives2020/overview.aspx?topicId=39>.

U.S. Department of Health and Human Services; Administration for Children & Families; Family and Youth Service Bureau: *Runaway and homeless youth program authorizing legislation*, 2014. Available from: <http://www.acf.hhs.gov/programs/fysb/resource/rhy-act>.

U.S. Department of Health and Human Services, Health Resources and Services Administration, Bureau of Primary Health Care: *Health center program terminology tip sheet*, n.d. Available from: <http://bphc.hrsa.gov/technicalassistance/healthcenterterminologysheet.pdf>.

U.S. Department of Housing and Urban Development: *Affordable housing*, 2015. Available from: https://portal.hud.gov/hudportal/HUD?src=/program_offices/comm_planning/affordablehousing/.

U.S. Department of Housing and Urban Development: *The 2015 annual homeless assessment report (AHAR) to Congress*, 2016. Available from: https://www.hudexchange.info/resource/5162/2015-ahar-part-2-estimates-of-homelessness/.

U.S. Department of Housing and Urban Development: *The point-in-timecount methodology guide*, 2015. Available from: <https://www.hudexchange.info/resource/4036/point-in-time-count-methodology-guide/>.

U.S. Department of Housing and Urban Development; Office of Community Planning and Development: *Continuum of care 101*. Available from: <https://www.onecpd.info/resources/documents/coc101.pdf>.

U.S. Department of Housing and Urban Development; Office of Community Planning and Development: *Preview of 2015 worst case housing needs*, 2017. Available from: https://www.huduser.gov/portal/publications/Preview-2015-Worst-Case-Housing-Needs.html.

U.S. Department of Housing and Urban Development; Office of Community Planning and Development: *McKinney-Vento homeless assistance act as amended by S.896 HEARTH Act of 2009*, 2017. Available from: <http://portal.hud.gov/hudportal/documents/huddoc?id=HAAA_HEARTH.pdf>.

U.S. Department of Housing and Urban Development Office of Community Planning and Development: *The 2015 annual homeless assessment report (AHAR) to congress: Part 1: point-in-time estimates of homelessness*, 2015. Available at: https://www.hudexchange.info/resources/documents/2015-AHAR-Part-1.pdf.

U.S. Department of Housing and Urban Development; Office of Community Planning and Development: Homeless emergency assistance and rapid transition to housing: defining "homeless", *Federal Register* 76(233):75994–70619, 2011. Also available from: <http://www.gpo.gov/fdsys/pkg/FR-2011-12-05/pdf/2011-30942.pdf>.

U.S. Department of Housing and Urban Development; Office of Community Planning and Development: *The 2015 annual homeless assessment report: Part 2-Estimates of homelessness in the U.S*, 2016. Available from: <https://www.hudexchange.info/resource/5162/2015-ahar-part-2-estimates-of-homelessness/>. <https://www.hudexchange.info/resources/.../2016-AHAR-Part-1.pdf>.

U.S. Department of Housing and Urban Development; Office of Policy Development and Research: *Worst case housing needs: 2015 report to Congress*, 2015. Available from: https://www.huduser.gov/portal/publications/affhsg/wc_HsgNeeds15.html.

U.S. Department of Housing and Urban Development Office of Policy Development and Research: Evidence matters: *transforming knowledge into housing and community development policy*, 2012. Available from: https://www.huduser.gov/portal/periodicals/em/summer12/highlight2.html.

U.S. Department of Housing and Urban Development: *Continuum of care program*, 2017. Available from: https://portal.hud.gov/hudportal/HUD?src=/hudprograms/continuumofcare.

U.S. Department of Housing and Urban Development HUD Exchange: *Homelessness assistance*, 2017. Available from: https://www.hudexchange.info/homelessness-assistance/.

U.S. Government Accountability Office: *Homeless women veterans: actions needed to ensure safe and appropriate housing (Report to Congressional Requesters No. GAO-12-182)*, Washington, DC, 2011, Author. Also available from: <http://www.gao.gov/assets/590/587334.pdf>.

U.S. House of Representatives: *Office of the Law Revision Center: U.S. Code*, 2017. Available from: <http://uscode.house.gov/view.xhtml?-path=/prelim@title42/chapter119/subchapter1&edition=prelim>.

Vijayaraghavan M, Tochterman A, Hsu E, et al.: Health, access to health care, and health care use among homeless women with a history of intimate partner violence, *J Community Health* 37(5):1032–1039, 2011.

Warf C, Clark L, Desai M, et al.: Coming of age on the streets: survival sex among homeless young women in Hollywood, *J Adoles* 36(6):1205–1213, 2013.

Washington DL, Yano E, McGuire J: Risk factors for homelessness among women veterans, *J Health Care Poor Underserved* 21(1):81–91, 2010.

Weinstein LC, LaNoue M, Collins E: Health care integration for formerly homeless people with serious mental illness, *J Dual Diagn* 9(1):72–77, 2013. https://doi.org/10.1080/15504263.2012.750089.

Wenzel SL, Leake BD, Gelberg L: Health of homeless women with recent experience of rape, *J Gen Intern Med* 15(4):265–268, 2000.

Wiersma P, Epperson S, Terp S: Episodic illness, chronic disease, and health care use among homeless persons in metropolitan Atlanta, Georgia, 2007, *Southern Med J* 103(1):18–24, 2010.

World Health Organization: *Social determinants of health: key concepts*, n.d. Available from: <http://www.who.int/social_determinants/thecommission/finalreport/key_concepts/en/>.

World Health Organization; Commission on Social Determinants of Health: *Closing the gap in a generation: health equity through action on the social determinants of health, final report*. Available from: <http://www.who.int/social_determinants/thecommission/finalreport/en/index.html>.

World Health Organization: *Progress on the implementation of the Rio Political Declaration*. Available from: <http://www.who.int/social_determinants/en/>.

World Health Organization: *Global and regional estimates of violence against women: prevalence and health effects of intimate partner violence and non-partner sexual violence*, Italy, 2013, World Health Organization.

World Health Organiztation: *Constition of WHO: principles*, 2017. Available at http://www.who.int/about/mission/en/.

World Health Organization: *Social determinants of health: key concepts*, 2017. Available at http://www.who.int/social_determinants/thecommission/finalreport/key_concepts/en/.

Zlotnick C, Tam T, Zerger S: Common needs but divergent interventions for U.S. homeless and foster care children: results from a systematic review, *Health Soc Care Community* 20(5):449–476, 2012. Available from: <https://doi.org/10.1111/j.1365-2524.2011.01053.x>.

24

Rural and Migrant Health

Patricia L. Thomas and Lori Wightman

OUTLINE

OBJECTIVES

Upon completion of this chapter, the reader will be able to do the following:

1. Compare and contrast characteristics of rural and urban communities.
2. Describe features of the health care system and population characteristics common to rural aggregates.
3. Discuss the impact of structural and personal barriers on the health of rural aggregates.
4. Identify factors that place farmers and migrant workers at risk for illness and accidents.
5. Discuss the importance of the informal care network to rural health and social services.
6. Describe the characteristics of rural community health nursing practice.
7. Apply an upstream perspective to health promotion and illness prevention for rural and migrant populations.

KEY TERMS

disparities
frontier
metropolitan

migrant
pesticide
rural

seasonal
urban

RURAL UNITED STATES

There are many different versions of rural America, in that each rural area is somewhat unique but shares certain features with other rural regions. Geographic, demographic, environmental, economic, and social factors all influence health, access to health care, and quality of health care. When aggregated, these characteristics may be contrasted with those of urban populations. In this section, we present a "snapshot" of rural population and health characteristics that contribute to challenging health disparities for many of the people living in the most rural areas of America.

Although the urban growth rate has been steadily climbing since 1890, with numbers of urban dwellers surpassing those in rural areas around 1920, the number of rural residents is the highest in the country's history (U.S. Department of Agriculture [USDA], 2016). In 2010–2015 population loss in nonmetro areas occurred in the United States as a whole. In 2014 nonmetro populations stabilized after 4 years of decline, likely related to improved rural employment growth (USDA, 2016). Opportunities for population growth and economic expansion vary widely from one nonmetro county to the next, and new regional patterns of growth and decline have emerged in recent years. Current census estimates are that 15% of the nation's elderly and more than 50% of the nation's poor live in rural areas (USDA ERS, 2013).

Rural residents have long been thought to be family farmers and ranchers, but today, rural America is a diverse and important marketplace to marketers of consumer products, and demographers and economists consider trends in farm and farm-related employment much more broadly. They characterize agriculture as a "food and fiber system" that encompasses all aspects of agriculture, from core materials sectors (farm, food processing, textiles, and other manufacturing) to wholesale and retail trade and the food service sector (USDA, National Institute of Food and Agriculture, 2017). Despite the shrinking number of family farms and full-time farmers, agriculture continues to be an important part of the rural and U.S. economy, with agriculture-related employment representing 5% of the gross domestic product (GDP) and farms representing 1% of the GDP.

Poverty, a key health determinant, continues to be greater in rural America than in urban areas. Whereas the nonmetropolitan population had a poverty rate of 16%, the metropolitan poverty rate was 14% in 2013, and child poverty rates were 23% nonmetropolitan and 19% metropolitan (U.S. Department of Agriculture, ERS, Poverty Overview, 2017). This overall gap may not seem large, but when the degree of rurality or the poverty rate for particular subpopulations (e.g., minorities, children under 18 years of age, or the elderly) are examined, the gap increases greatly. For example, the poverty rate for non-Hispanic blacks in nonmetropolitan areas in 2012 was 41%, compared with a rate of 25% for the same group in metropolitan areas (U.S. Census Bureau, 2013). See Box 24.1 for the 2017 U.S. Department of Health and Human Services' Poverty Guidelines.

Not only is the economic base shifting but the age composition is as well. For the first time in decades, 2010–2014 showed a decline in nonmetropolitan populations, stabilizing in 2015. Younger people are leaving rural areas for jobs in urban centers, so that those who remain behind are increasingly older and isolated and have diminished access to health care. Recent demographic changes in rural areas identify the 18% of rural areas are 65 and older and 2% are 85 and older (Rural Health Information Hub, Rural Aging, 2016). Three trends—aging in place, outmigration of young adults, and immigration of older persons from metro areas—present challenges to already stressed communities that must provide adequate health care, housing, transportation, and other human services (Rural Health Information Hub, Rural Aging, 2016).

The rural population is also becoming more ethnically diverse. Generations ago, many families began farming when

BOX 24.1 The 2017 U.S. Department of Health and Human Services Poverty Guidelines

In concept, the U.S. Department of Health and Human Services (DHHS) determines the poverty guidelines by estimating the minimum income level needed by a family or individual to just meet the basic needs of food, shelter, clothing, and other essential goods and services. Official poverty guidelines adjusted for family size and composition are set by DHHS for use by all federal agencies to determine financial eligibility for certain federal programs (e.g., Medicaid). Some programs (e.g., State Children's Health Insurance Program) also use multiples of the guidelines to determine eligibility of participants. For example, participants may be eligible for programs if they are classified as being at or near poverty, with poverty being defined as 100%, and near poverty as 125% or 150%, of the poverty level. Poverty guidelines are adjusted periodically by DHHS to reflect price changes and are published in the *Federal Register*. The 2017 guidelines reflect just the size of the "family unit" rather than the family composition. The poverty level for a family unit of one in the contiguous 48 states, for example, was $12,060; it was $24,600 for a family unit of four, and $41,320 for a family unit of eight. Each household's cash income (including pretax income and cash welfare assistance, but excluding in-kind welfare assistance, such as food stamps and Medicare) is compared with the poverty line for the household.

From U.S. Department of Health and Human Services: *The 2017 HHS poverty guidelines: one version of the [U.S.] federal poverty measure,* 2017. https://www.federalregister.gov/documents/2017/01/31/2017-02076/annual-update-of-the-hhs-poverty-guidelines.

they came to the United States as European immigrants. In the 1990s, new immigrants began buying and operating their own small family farms, and others found employment in rural agriculture and manufacturing. Today, more than one half of rural Hispanics live outside the Southwest, and "high-growth Hispanic counties" are mostly in the South and Midwest (U.S. Census Bureau, 2011).

Policies and programs developed to close the health disparities gap must take a population health view of the special circumstances of rural life. Although 75% of U.S. counties are classified as rural, they contain only 20% of the U.S. population. Members of rural populations also are more likely to be older, to be less educated, to live in poverty, to lack health insurance, and to experience a lack of available health care providers and access to health care (Farrigan and Parker, 2012). Only 10% of U.S. physicians practice in rural counties, and the ratio of physicians in rural population size is 36 per 100,000 people, compared with nearly double that number in urban settings (American Academy of Family Practitioners [AAFP], 2014).

Rural residents more often assess their health as fair or poor and have more disability days associated with acute conditions than their urban counterparts. Rural people also tend to have more problems related to negative health behaviors (e.g., untreated mental illness; obesity; and alcohol, tobacco, and drug use) that contribute to excess deaths and chronic disease and disability rates. The literature suggests, for example, that the highest death rates for children and young adults are in the most rural counties. Residents of rural areas are nearly twice as likely to die from unintentional injuries, including motor vehicle accidents, than urban residents (National Rural Health Association [NRHA], n.d.).

Noting a prominent and persistent pattern of risky health behaviors in rural dwellers, McClelland et al. (2010) suggests that "rural culture" may itself be a key determinant of health in rural communities and that these behaviors vary along the rural–urban continuum and within rural populations by geographical areas. These behaviors, including unintentional injury, smoking, and suicide, are discussed in more detail in the section titled "Composition: Health Disparities Related to Persons."

Defining Rural Populations

Multiple definitions of rural populations have been formulated to describe the characteristics of areas with low population density. Previous definitions have simply included either those towns with a population of less than 2500 or towns located in open country as rural. This definition has often been further differentiated into the subcategories farm and rural nonfarm. A second classification of interest used the term *rural* for populations with fewer than 45 persons per square mile and the term frontier for geographical areas with fewer than 6 persons per square mile (Rural Assistance Center, n.d.). Many counties of the Great Plains, Intermountain West, and Alaska are designated as frontier.

The rural–urban continuum distinguishes counties by population and adjacency to metropolitan areas. Residences can range from small towns to large metropolitan areas. Statistical reporting has been in use since 1990 with the term *metropolitan statistical areas (MSAs)* used to differentiate nonmetropolitan and metropolitan areas. In June 2003, the Office of Management and Budget (OMB) released a new classification scheme to better reflect trends in population distribution across the nation (OMB, 2016). The MSA designation has been replaced by county-level *core-based statistical areas (CBSAs)* to simplify the multilevel designations. Within CBSAs, *metropolitan areas* are those counties that contain at least one urbanized area of 50,000 or more people. A micropolitan area contains a cluster of 10,000 to 50,000 persons. Counties that are neither metropolitan nor micropolitan are called "outside CBSAs," also known as *noncare areas* (U.S. Census, 2013).

Describing Rural Health and Populations

Rural populations differ in complex geographical, social, and economic ways. Although older, poorer, and less educated people are usually overrepresented in rural areas, this finding may not apply to all rural areas or to everyone in a particular rural area.

The health profiles discussed here are shared by rural areas in general and may be contrasted with overall patterns of health, health habits, and health care in urban settings. However, the reader should note that it is difficult to interpret differences between urban health and rural health. First, statistically significant differences between urban and rural health indicators may seem small when data are aggregated to "rural areas" in general. The differences tend to become larger when data are available for particular rural areas (e.g., certain counties), particular rural subgroups (e.g., minorities), or specific characteristics (e.g., percentage of uninsured children). Second, heterogeneity of race, age, economic status, regional distribution, and cultural groupings makes health data for rural populations useful only as estimates of individual health. For example, in 2011, about 15.9% of the U.S. population had an income below the poverty level, an increase from 15.3% in 2010. The number of people in poverty rose from 46.2 million to 48.5 million during the same time, representing the fourth consecutive increase in the poverty rate (Bishaw, 2012). The family poverty rate in 2011 was 11.8% (representing 9.5 million), not statistically different from the 2010 estimates (U.S. Census Bureau, 2012).

Infant mortality, a major health status indicator, varies greatly by geographical area, even within rural areas, and dramatizes the importance of both contextual and compositional data. The infant mortality rate plateaued between 2005 and 2010 and then declined from 6.86 deaths per 1000 live births to 6.14 between 2005 and 2010. The largest decline was for non-Hispanic black women (from 13.63 to 11.46), followed by non-Hispanic whites (5.76 to 5.18) and Hispanic women (from 5.62 to 5.25). During 2000 and 2005, the non-Hispanic black infant mortality rates were 2.4 times the non-Hispanic white rates, but the difference narrowed in 2010 with a non-Hispanic black rate 2.2 times that of non-Hispanic whites (Mathews and MacDorman, 2010).

The rate of infant deaths in 2009 for black Americans is 2.3 times that for whites and Hispanics per 1000 births. In both the South and West, rural counties experienced the highest rates (24% and 30% higher, respectively, than fringe areas of large metro areas) (Office of Minority Health, 2013). Overall, the infant mortality rate declined 10% between 1995 and 2004 (7.57); however, the rate has not declined much since 2000 (6.89). From 1995 until 2004, small declines were observed for all races and ethnic groups. Significant decreases were noted for infants of Central and South American (16%), Puerto Rican (12%), Asian or Pacific Islander (11%), non-Hispanic white (10%), Mexican (9%), and non-Hispanic black (7%) mothers (Centers for Disease Control and Prevention [CDC], 2011).

Mortality rates for white infants in rural areas adjacent to population centers with fewer than 2500 people varied from a high of 9.85 per 1000 in the South to 6.46 per 1000 in the West. Although infant mortality rates have changed since 1993, infant mortality data provide insight into the heterogeneity of rural populations and show why national or even regional data may or may not reflect the status quo for a particular county or local population.

One might also consider the health disparities that exist among rural racial and ethnic minorities. Although limited because the phenomenon has only recently been studied, research findings support the conclusion that rural racial and ethnic minorities—Native Americans, Alaska Natives, Hispanics/Latinos, and African Americans—concentrated in the South and West are more disadvantaged relative not only to rural majority members but also to urban racial and ethnic minorities. The disparities include employment, income, education, health insurance, mortality, morbidity, and access to health care (*Healthy People 2020* Disparities, 2010).

Because population numbers are small, national rural data, limited as they are, can only suggest the health needs of a particular area, racial or ethnic mix, or age distribution, for example. Program planners still need to determine whether certain health or health care delivery problems apply to their specific service area. Useful data sources include state-, county-, and census tract–level data on health and demographics available from state and federal government agencies, such as those cited in the References at the end of this chapter. In planning for health-related programs, nurses can also gather community-level data from health care providers, local records, focus groups, and older residents who know the area's history.

RURAL HEALTH

 ### Minority Health and *Healthy People 2020*

Healthy People 2020 represents the health promotion and disease prevention agenda for the nation (U.S. Department of Health and Human Services [USDHHS], Office of Disease Prevention and Health Promotion, n.d.) Additionally, *Healthy People 2020* is the United States' contribution to the World Health Organization "Health for All" program. The framework for *Healthy People 2020,* developed through public consensus, builds on the national health program established since the 1980s. It has the broad goals of increasing quality of life and years of life, eliminating disparities in health among different population groups, and improving access to preventive health services (see Fig. 1.1 in Chapter 1).

Healthy People 2020 is an evidence-based, 10-year plan with the goal to "attain high-quality, longer lives free of preventable disease, disability, injury, and premature death." Achieving this goal will accomplish health equity, elimination of disparities, and improvement of the health of all groups through social and physical environments to promote quality of life, healthy development, and healthy behaviors across all life stages (Bolin and Bellamy, n.d.). The challenges are great, but public health professionals and planners in every state have a plan patterned on *Healthy People 2020* goals to direct their efforts.

RURAL HEALTH DISPARITIES: CONTEXT AND COMPOSITION

To improve understanding of the health of populations and health disparities, there is a growing emphasis on the distinction between context, which is defined by the characteristics of places of residence, and composition, which is the collective health effects that result from a concentration of persons with certain characteristics. Most public health problems include elements of both context and composition, though they may be predominantly one or the other. The Centers for Disease Control is the primary public health organization in the United States and, working with its partners, focuses on factors leading to health disparities among racial, ethnic, geographic, and socioeconomic barriers (CDC Health Disparities & Inequalities Report, 2013). The 2013 CDC Health Disparities & Inequalities Report, published in the CDC *Morbidity and Mortality Weekly Report,* highlighted disparities across diseases, behavioral risk factors, exposures, social determinants of care, and health care access by sex, race and ethnicity, income, education, disability status, and other social characteristics (CDC Health Disparities & Inequalities Report, 2015).

It is noteworthy that rural health, particularly for children, identified mental, behavioral, and developmental disorders begin early in childhood affecting lifelong health and well-being. People in rural areas report more health-related disparities, including less access to health resources, poorer health, and more health risk behaviors, than counterparts in urban areas (Robinson et al., 2017).

Health issues in rural areas are contextual when they derive from characteristics of place. Characteristics of place include not only natural features of geography and environment but also the political, social, and economic institutions that build and support communities within a given geographical area. For example, limited economic opportunities, low wages, or agricultural accidents might be considered to have contextual effects on the health of populations. Problems in rural areas are compositional when they derive from individual characteristics of groups of people residing in rural settings. Examples of compositional sources of health disparities include such characteristics as age, education, income, ethnicity, and health behaviors.

Consideration of both context and composition enables us to take a more deliberate and refined approach to study, plan programs for, and deliver health care services to rural populations. Although the overall health of rural Americans is worse than that of urban Americans, the relationship between rurality and health is not necessarily linear. Many differences exist among rural areas in both the nature and extent of health problems. Furthermore, some rural populations share more in common with people in urban core areas than with people in other rural areas. Effective planning depends on understanding and documenting needs that take into account context, composition, and their interaction. The next section presents data for problems of both contextual and compositional sources of health disparities in rural America.

Context: Health Disparities Related to Place

Regardless of their diverse demographic and geographical attributes, rural groups share certain health patterns, difficulties, and delays in obtaining health care (see Ethical Insights box). Many of the contextual issues that contribute to rural health disparities are described in the introduction to the chapter ("Rural United States"). Many rural regions that are already sparsely populated are losing residents, a process that often triggers a downward spiral. People leave and services are lost; the local drugstore closes; the tax base will not support an ambulance service, so most seriously ill persons must be transported long distances to get health care; jobs become scarce and younger people leave the area. Retirees may be attracted to the lower costs, but they need public health and other services that must be provided by counties without the tax base to support them. Racial and ethnic minorities are migrating to rural areas to find employment opportunities. Structural, financial, and personal barriers to accessing health care services exist in all environments, but rural residents are unique in how they experience structural barriers.

Access to Care

Rural health leaders have identified 10 priorities for health care in rural America, with access to and affordability of care topping the list. Because most people in rural America are self-employed or part of small businesses, insurance tied to employment will not serve them (Bailey, 2009). Ziller et al. (2012), using data from the 2002–2007 Medical Expenditure Panel Survey to examine uninsured rural and urban residents and the factors associated with access to care, found the rural uninsured more likely to have a usual source of care than their urban counterparts. Controlling for demographic and health characteristics, the access and use differences between the uninsured and insured in rural areas are smaller than those observed in urban areas, suggesting that providers in rural areas may impose fewer barriers on the uninsured who seek care.

ETHICAL INSIGHTS

Racial and Ethnic Disparities in Health Care

Because public health is a societal approach to protecting and promoting health that usually acts through social rather than individual means (Sorrell, 2012), many of the most pressing ethical dilemmas are considered in public domains. Perhaps no more important ethical challenge facing our public today revolves around the just distribution of health care resources. With the enactment of the Patient Protection and Affordability Act, ethical concerns persist related to access to care, the underserved, and coverage (Sorrell, 2012).

For example, among 47 million rural adults in 2015, nearly 16% were uninsured and in poverty (Holder et al., 2016). The uninsured distribution by race in 2015 was 11% of blacks, 7.5% of Asians, and 6.7% of non-Hispanic whites. Hispanics had the highest uninsured rate at 16% (Barnett and Vornovitsky, 2016). These data may help explain why minorities are more likely to seek care, use less prenatal care, and make fewer visits to physicians.

Differences in care resulting from patient or care process-level variables (e.g., patient attitudes, preferences or expectations, provider bias, stereotyping, or uncertainty) are problems of professional ethics. Disparities in care resulting from system-level variables, such as financing, accessibility, and geographical location, are problems of justice (Institute of Medicine [IOM], 2003; Rural Health Information Hub, 2014). Subsequently, solutions for justice issues in disparities in care require public discourse aimed at solving system-level problems.

From an ethical perspective, the theory of justice as fairness was formulated to specify terms of social cooperation that are "fair" and ensure that people of equal basic liberties have equal opportunity (Daniels et al., 1999). The Civil Rights Act of 1964 specifically bars discrimination in health care for all entities that receive federal funds, and both the American Nurses Association (ANA) and American Medical Association codes of ethics endorse the principle of justice. However, despite overall agreement that justice is an important practice concept, difficulty arises in implementing changes in the health system to address disparities in care.

Solutions to disparities in care have been suggested by the IOM (2003) and include the following policy, health system, and patient education and empowerment interventions:

Policy Interventions

1. Medical care financing should discourage fragmentation of health care into separate tiers of providers who adhere to different standards of care and serve separate racial and ethnic minority segments of society. Government programs that require enrollment in managed care should be prepared to pay plans at rates comparable to those paid to plans for privately insured patients.
2. Strengthen the stability of patient–provider relationships in publicly funded health plans and create policy to create consistency, limit patient loads for providers, and provide reasonable time allowances for initial and follow-up visits.
3. Increase the proportion of underrepresented U.S. racial and ethnic minorities among health professionals.
4. Apply the same managed care protections to publicly funded health maintenance organization (HMO) enrollees that apply to private HMO enrollees.
5. Provide greater resources to the U.S. Department of Health and Human Services Office for Civil Rights to enforce civil rights laws.

Health Systems Interventions

1. Promote the consistency and equity of care through evidence-based guidelines. These guidelines should be published to allow public and professional scrutiny.
2. Construct payment systems to enhance available services to minority patients, and limit provider incentives that may promote disparities.
3. Enhance patient–provider communication and trust by providing financial incentives for practices that reduce barriers.
4. Support the use of interpretation services where community need exists.
5. Institute programs that use community health workers among medically underserved and racial and ethnic minority populations.
6. Support greater use of multidisciplinary treatment and preventive care teams to improve and streamline care for racial and ethnic minority patients.

Patient Education and Empowerment Interventions

1. Implement patient education programs to increase patients' knowledge of how to access care and participate in treatment decisions.

With the enactment of the Patient Protection and Affordability Act, improvements have been made related to care access and Medicaid expansion; however, issues persist related to equity.

Primary Care. Rural areas have fewer primary care physicians than urban areas, fueling concerns about inadequate access and gaps in U.S. health care equity in many rural areas. Several improvements have been made since the inception of the Affordable Care Act (ACA) in 2010 through training grants, reimbursement modifications, expanded scope of practice for nurse practitioners (NPs) in select states, and Medicaid expansion. Despite these efforts, the disparities for access to and availability of primary care providers still exist.

About 20% of the U.S. population lives in rural areas, yet only 10% of the nation's physicians practice in a rural area. This is a contributing factor for the higher death rates, disabilities, and chronic conditions rural populations experience compared with urban populations. "Of the 2,050 rural U.S. counties, 77% are designated as health professional shortage areas (HPSAs). Notably, nearly 30% of rural primary care practitioners are at or nearing retirement age, and those under 40 account for 20% of the current rural workforce. Existing shortages coupled with replacement requirements for retirees escalate concerns regarding equitable care for rural populations. As a result of the ACA, an additional 5 million rural Americans (16%) will have health insurance coverage by 2019, so when combined with demands of an aging population, an already burdened rural health care delivery system will be stretched further. Recommendations for scholarships, loan repayment, focused recruitment for rural practitioners, and medical residencies in rural health are being considered. Today, nonphysician primary care practitioners (NPs and physician assistants) make up nearly half (46%) the providers in rural federally qualified health centers (National Conference of State Legislatures, 2017). In a joint statement, the NRHA and the American Academy of Family Physicians said medicine has become specialized, centralized, and urban and challenged educators to be responsive to the needs of rural underserved communities (AAFP, 2013).

Availability of providers and health care facilities in rural areas is an important determinant of the quality of the health care delivery system and the likelihood of positive health outcomes for rural residents (Bailey, 2009). Gordon (2014) identified that 44% of rural areas in the United States have a shortage of primary care practitioners. A good example of the lack of specialists is the lack of mental health services available for rural dwellers of any age. The incidence of mental illness in rural areas is the same as that of urban areas, but there is far less access to mental health services in rural areas. Additionally, primary care doctors, nurses, and physician assistants, rather than mental health specialists, provide most of the mental health care in rural regions (Bailey, 2009; Hanrahan and Hartley, 2008). A recent survey found that 41% of rural Medicare beneficiaries saw a physician assistant or NP for all (17%) or some (24%) of their primary care in 2012 (National Conference of State Legislatures, 2017).

General Health Services. A study by the National Academy of Medicine (NAM), formerly called the Institute of Medicine (IOM), reported rural medical access problems in these areas, with some hospital and pharmacy closures, greater distances to travel for physician services, and limited (if any) choice of providers (IOM, 2005). Lack of local access to primary care and health care facilities forces rural residents to either go without or travel long distances—often over rural roads in dangerous weather conditions—to access needed care. Access to health care may become a particularly challenging and expensive proposition for the elderly who do not drive and depend on limited public transportation. Geography, health care costs, and lack of available services also are contextual problems that keep many rural adults and children from obtaining needed primary, secondary, and tertiary preventive services.

Health Insurance. With economic decline and rising costs of health care, health insurance—or, more importantly, the lack of health insurance—for Americans has become a major issue for the health of the nation. An estimated 45.7 million people were without health insurance in 2010 (U.S. Census Bureau, 2011).

As with poverty and unemployment data, insurance coverage varied with race and ethnicity coverage in 2007, as did age and residence (rural or urban). For example, 10.4% of non-Hispanic whites, 19.5% of blacks, and 16.8% of Asians were uninsured for all or part of 2007; young adults were more likely to lack health insurance than older persons; and 18% of poor or near-poor children lacked coverage (U.S. Census Bureau, 2012). Lack of insurance coverage was greatest in the South (14.2%) and West regions (12%) in 2007, and in general, rural residents were more likely than urban residents to lack insurance (20% versus 17%) (IOM, 2005). In 2015 about 18% of the persons living in rural counties were at the poverty level, with 14% of rural children living in poverty (USDA, 2016). See Resource Tool 23C for a map of the United States detailing estimations of populations in poverty.

The impact of health insurance and decision making related to health care practices since the Patient Protection and Affordability Act of 2010 have not been published. What is known is that the number of uninsured patients nationwide has decreased to 13% from a high of 18% in 2013 (Levy, 2015), and in some rural areas, Medicaid expansion has been beneficial. However, nearly two thirds of uninsured people in rural areas live in states that did not expand Medicaid coverage (Newkirk, 2014). Additionally, the linkage of provider influence on health promotion and health literacy cannot be assumed. Although early research points to a strong relationship among health insurance status, chronic illnesses, and poverty the Patient Protection and Affordability Act does not provide equity in coverage in rural areas comparable to urban counterparts (Newkirk, 2014). Rural people are often employed in industries characterized by seasonal work, economic uncertainty and decline, high unemployment risk, and occupational accidents and death (e.g., agriculture, mining, forestry, and fisheries). Rural industries are often small and offer low wages, thereby contributing to the growing number of uninsured rural families. Farm families also tend to be two-parent households, so they are less likely to qualify for Medicaid, even with incomes below the federal poverty level. Unlike the uninsured population nationally, individuals in rural areas face challenges in accessing care related to transportation and workforce shortages in providers (Newkirk, 2014).

Health insurance has been identified as one of the 10 leading health indicators because it is generally a reliable predictor of overall health status (Bailey, 2009; Center on Budget and Policy Priorities, 2012). Public health professionals and health planners are most concerned with the impact of increasing numbers of uninsured children. In 2010, the overall percentage of children who were uninsured was 9.4%, which works out to 7 million (DeNavas-Walt et al., 2012). The uninsured rate of children has declined, in large part because of state programs, between 2009 and 2011; however, rural children are still uninsured at a slightly higher rate (7.7%) than the national average (7.5%) and their urban counterparts (7.4%) (Alker et al., 2012). In the absence of health insurance, poverty becomes an even more powerful predictor of poor health for all age groups and particularly for children.

In 1997, the State Children's Health Insurance Program was enacted to improve health insurance coverage of children less than 19 years of age in poor and near-poor families (see the "Legislation and Programs Affecting Rural Public Health" section in this chapter). In the years following passage of this program, the overall percentage of children who were uninsured fell and the number of uninsured children declined. The number of uninsured children declined to 5.5 million in 2011, from 6.4 million in 2009, and the percentage of children with insurance increased to 93% in 2011 (Alker et al., 2012). Health insurance coverage of children as well as adults varies from state to state and is influenced by employment patterns, the percentage of children in the population, state Medicaid policies, poverty levels, and racial and ethnic composition.

Composition: Health Disparities Related to Persons

To review, health problems in rural areas are compositional when they result from a concentration of persons with certain

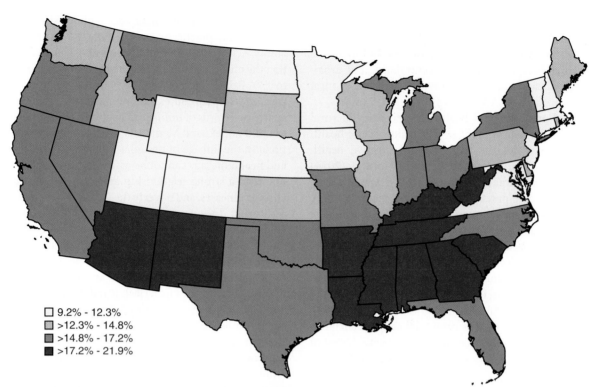

FIG. 24.1 Percentage of total population in poverty, 2015. (From U.S. Census Bureau: *Small area income and poverty estimates. 2014 All ages in poverty.* https://www.census.gov/did/www/saipe/data/interactive/saipe.html?s_appName=saipe&map_yearSelector=2014&map_geoSelector=aa_ss.)

characteristics. Examples of compositional sources of health disparities include such characteristics as income, health behaviors, education, occupation, gender, and ethnicity. In the *Rural Healthy People 2020* survey, 80% of respondents listed access to health care as the top rural health priority (Bolin and Bellamy, n.d.). Additional priorities listed by respondents as leading health problems are largely compositional but may also have a contextual dimension. For example, problems such as obesity, chronic pulmonary disease, and higher levels of infant mortality have a strong compositional component because their variation is related to the health behaviors and the educational, socioeconomic, racial, and ethnic characteristics of the rural groups. The variation may also be contextual, because the groups have fewer educational opportunities, have low-wage jobs, lack insurance, or have genetic propensities for certain health problems.

Income and Poverty

Income, education, and type of employment help determine socioeconomic status, and in the aggregate, rural dwellers have lower educational levels, higher unemployment rates, higher poverty rates, and lower income levels than urban aggregates (National Advisory Committee on Rural Health and Human Services, 2013). The poverty rate is one of the most important indicators of the health and well-being of all Americans, regardless of where they live (see Ethical Insights box).

The U.S. Department of Agriculture's ERS tracks economic trends and demographic characteristics of rural dwellers to help develop policies and services. In the most recent report, the ERS reported continued unemployment declines, falling close to levels last seen before the Great Recession. Employment and

populations in rural areas have also stabilized. The population of rural counties was 46.2 million representing 14% of the U.S. population. The rural population declined 0.3% between 2010 and 2014, before leveling out in 2015. Rural employment rose 1.3% between 2013 and 2015, with seasonally adjusted rural employment rising another 0.5% in mid-2016. Poverty rates in 2015 marked the greatest decline since the Great Recession as unemployment continued to fall. Poverty rates rose in both rural and urban areas until 2013 and 2011, respectively. Poverty rates declined in 2014 and 2015 by 0.9% in rural areas and 0.8% in urban areas, still above pre-recession levels (USDA, ERS, 2016).

In 2015, the U.S. Census Bureau identified nonmetro poverty rates at 17.2%, whereas the metro poverty rate was nearly 3% lower. Historically, poverty rates for rural people have been higher than those for urban dwellers (Fig. 24.1 and Table 24.1). As noted earlier in this section, however, data averaged across all rural counties in the United States do not give planners and providers much information about their own counties, or even regions. The following discussion gives examples of available data that can be used to make an analysis of local and regional conditions and characteristics.

Regional Differences. Consistent with the idea that there are many rural Americas in rural America, rural poverty varies by rural region. For example, there are 353 counties with persistent poverty rates in the United States (persistent poverty is defined as being in poverty over the last 30 years), comprising 11% of all U.S. counties. Of these, 301 are in nonmetropolitan areas. Persistent poverty is highest in the South (22%), followed by the West (16.2%), and then the Northeast and Midwest (13%). The higher persistent poverty rate in the South is particularly important, because an estimated 43% of the nonmetro population lived in this

TABLE 24.1	Percentage of Population in Poverty by State (2015)					
	ALL PEOPLE IN POVERTY (2015)			**CHILDREN AGES 0–17 IN POVERTY (2015)**		
		90% CONFIDENCE INTERVAL OF ESTIMATE			**90% CONFIDENCE INTERVAL OF ESTIMATE**	
NAME	**PERCENT**	**LOWER BOUND**	**UPPER BOUND**	**PERCENT**	**LOWER BOUND**	**UPPER BOUND**
Alabama	18.5	18.2	18.8	26.5	25.8	27.2
Alaska	10.4	9.9	10.9	14.5	13.5	15.5
Arizona	17.4	17.1	17.7	24.7	23.9	25.5
Arkansas	18.7	18.3	19.1	26.4	25.5	27.3
California	15.4	15.3	15.5	21.2	20.9	21.5
Colorado	11.5	11.2	11.8	14.8	14.2	15.4
Connecticut	10.6	10.3	10.9	14.6	13.8	15.4
Delaware	12.6	12	13.2	19.1	17.9	20.3
District of Columbia	17.7	16.8	18.6	28.3	25.4	31.2
Florida	15.8	15.6	16	23.4	22.9	23.9
Georgia	17.2	16.9	17.5	24.7	24.1	25.3
Hawaii	10.7	10.3	11.1	14.5	13.5	15.5
Idaho	14.7	14.1	15.3	17.7	16.8	18.6
Illinois	13.6	13.4	13.8	19.1	18.6	19.6
Indiana	14.4	14.1	14.7	20.4	19.7	21.1
Iowa	12.1	11.8	12.4	14.9	14.2	15.6
Kansas	12.9	12.5	13.3	16.9	16.1	17.7
Kentucky	18.3	17.9	18.7	25.3	24.5	26.1
Louisiana	19.5	19.1	19.9	28.1	27.3	28.9
Maine	13.2	12.7	13.7	17.5	16.5	18.5
Maryland	9.9	9.6	10.2	13.9	13.2	14.6
Massachusetts	11.5	11.2	11.8	14.9	14.3	15.5
Michigan	15.7	15.5	15.9	22.2	21.6	22.8
Minnesota	10.2	10	10.4	13.1	12.5	13.7
Mississippi	22.1	21.6	22.6	31.5	30.5	32.5
Missouri	14.8	14.5	15.1	20.4	19.7	21.1
Montana	14.4	13.9	14.9	18.8	17.7	19.9
National	14.7	14.6	14.8	20.7	20.5	20.9
Nebraska	12.2	11.8	12.6	15.9	15	16.8
Nevada	14.9	14.5	15.3	21.6	20.7	22.5
New Hampshire	8.4	7.9	8.9	11	10.1	11.9
New Jersey	10.8	10.6	11	15.5	14.9	16.1
New Mexico	19.8	19.3	20.3	27.2	26.2	28.2
New York	15.5	15.3	15.7	22.3	21.8	22.8
North Carolina	16.4	16.2	16.6	23.4	22.8	24
North Dakota	10.7	10.2	11.2	12.1	11.1	13.1
Ohio	14.8	14.6	15	21.2	20.6	21.8
Oklahoma	16	15.7	16.3	22	21.3	22.7
Oregon	15.2	14.8	15.6	19.8	18.9	20.7
Pennsylvania	13.1	12.9	13.3	19.1	18.6	19.6
Rhode Island	14.1	13.5	14.7	20.6	19.5	21.7
South Carolina	16.8	16.4	17.2	24.4	23.6	25.2
South Dakota	13.5	12.9	14.1	17.7	16.6	18.8
Tennessee	16.7	16.4	17	24.1	23.4	24.8
Texas	15.9	15.7	16.1	22.9	22.5	23.3
Utah	11.2	10.8	11.6	12.8	12.1	13.5
Vermont	10.4	9.9	10.9	13.7	12.5	14.9
Virginia	11.2	11	11.4	15	14.5	15.5
Washington	12.2	11.9	12.5	15.7	15.1	16.3
West Virginia	18	17.5	18.5	24.7	23.6	25.8
Wisconsin	12.1	11.9	12.3	16.5	15.9	17.1
Wyoming	10.6	9.9	11.3	13	11.8	14.2

Data from U.S. Census Bureau: *Small area income and poverty estimates.* Table modified from U.S. Department of Agriculture, Economic Research Service: *County-level data sets: Poverty,* 2015. http://www.ers.usda.gov/data-products/county-level-data-sets/poverty.aspx?reportPath=/State_Fact_Sheets/PovertyReport.

region in 2010 (USDA, ERS, 2014). Poverty is also highest in the most rural areas and in completely rural counties (i.e., not adjacent to any metropolitan counties), the poverty rate is 35% with 26% residing in persistent poverty counties (USDA, ERS, 2014).

Racial and Ethnic Minorities. When poverty rates among rural dwellers are analyzed by race, ethnicity, age, and family structure, the statistics on poverty are even more dramatic than residence or region. Racial and ethnic minorities (mainly nonwhite Hispanics, blacks, and Native Americans) constitute 22% of the rural population, according to the 2010 Census (USDA, ERS, 2012f). This segment of the rural population grew 30% from 1990 to 2000, largely due to the dramatic increase in non-white Hispanics (up 70.4%) (IOM, 2005). In 2012, according to the ERS, poverty rates among rural and racial minorities were two to three times higher (67%) than poverty rates for rural whites (13%) (USDA, ERS, 2012c).

Family Composition. Families with two or more adults are less likely to be poor, whether in rural or urban areas, because they are more likely to have multiple sources of income. Families with more than one adult have lower out-of-pocket child care costs and are less likely to have to limit their working hours. More than 75% of rural families are headed by a married couple, and these constitute only 7% of families living in poverty. On the other hand, people living in female-headed families have higher poverty rates (40%) than single male–headed families (21.2%) in rural areas. The ERS attributes the high rate of poverty for female-headed families to "lower labor force participation rates, shorter average work weeks, and lower earnings" (USDA, ERS, 2011).

Children. Children are particularly vulnerable to outcomes of poverty, and they are among the poorest citizens in rural America, constituting 2.8 million, or 27.4%, of the overall population of rural poor in 2010 (Farrigan and Parker, 2012). The heaviest concentrations of child poverty are in the South and West. Understanding how poverty is distributed in rural populations is important for planning and delivering programs that ameliorate the impact of poverty, such as food stamps, school lunch programs, school health nursing interventions, and health insurance coverage (Farrigan and Parker, 2012).

When race and ethnicity are taken into account, the poverty profile of children worsens dramatically. Racial and ethnic minorities fare far worse than the general rural population of children from birth to18 years of age. When family composition is also taken into account, we find that almost half of non-Hispanic black children, 34% of Native American children, and 18% of rural children who live in a female-headed household are poor (Farrigan and Parker, 2012).

Health Risk, Injury, and Death

Health behaviors vary along the rural–urban continuum and within rural populations by geographical area. For example, researchers have noted that adults in nonmetropolitan areas use seat belts less often and are less likely to use preventive screening (although the latter trend is confounded by access problems). Elliot et al. (2008) compared the prevalence of unlicensed teenaged drivers and that of licensed drivers and found that the former were more likely to be black or Hispanic and to live in rural areas. Rural teens are equally likely as or more likely than both suburban and urban teens to report being victims of violent behavior, to engage in suicide behaviors, and to use drugs (Johnson et al., 2008). Rural residents in the Southern states are more likely to be obese, to smoke more heavily if they do smoke, to use smokeless tobacco, and to engage in sedentary lifestyles. In the rural West, rates of smoking, seat belt use, and obesity are lower and those of alcohol and smokeless tobacco use are higher. For example, 19% of adolescents living in the most rural counties are smokers, compared with 11% in large metropolitan counties (National Rural Health Association, n.d.).

Other risk factors include alcohol use (higher in rural areas and highest among persons living in the most rural areas and more commonly among men than women), obesity (higher in rural areas, most particularly rural areas of the South), and physical inactivity during leisure time, which varies by level of urbanization (National Rural Health Association, 2014).

Intentional injuries, against the self or another, are most often the result of firearms usage. In rural counties, nonfatal firearm injuries occur most often at home, whereas in urban counties such injuries occur most often in the streets. Furthermore, numerous studies have noted that firearm suicide in rural counties is an important public health concern. Nationally, suicide is the eleventh leading cause of death, but in rural America, it is the second leading cause of death. The rate of suicide in some rural areas is 800% higher than the national average. Nationally, 14 people in 100,000 died by suicide between the years 1901 and 2009, the latest year for which data are available from the CDC (CDC, Injury Center, 2013). There was also variation by race and ethnicity. Decreased access to mental health services for treatment of depression may contribute to these higher rates. Among suicide victims, racial and ethnic disparities exist. Suicide rates among American Indian/Alaskan Natives ages 15 to 34 years are 2.2 times higher than the national average for that age group, and Hispanic female high school students in grades 9 through 12 reported more suicide attempts (14.0%) than non-Hispanic white (7.7%) or non-Hispanic black (9.9%) students (CDC, 2008). The suicide rate for non-Hispanic white men 65 years of age and over is higher than that rate for other groups. In 2004, the suicide rate for older non-Hispanic white men was about two to three times the rate for older men in other race or ethnicity groups and nearly eight times the rate for older non-Hispanic white women (CDC, 2007).

Unintentional injuries are the leading cause of death in the United States for both sexes, for all races and ethnicities, and for all age groups from ages 1 to 44 years. Overall, unintentional injuries occur most often as the result of driving a vehicle (automobile, all-terrain vehicle, bicycle). In the latest available reports, unintentional injuries continue to be higher in rural areas of the United States. The mortality rate for unintentional injuries reported in the *Urban and Rural Health Chartbook* was 54.1 per 100,000 rural residents, which is twice the rate for large metropolitan counties (CDC, 2007). Unintentional injuries are highest among males and in rural counties with the lowest population densities (Castillo and Alexander, 2004).

According to the CDC's National Center for Health Statistics, unintentional injury was ranked fifth in the leading causes of death in 2009. This category of death includes "transport accidents," including motor vehicle accidents, and "nontransport accidents," which include falls, firearm accidents, drowning, fire-related deaths, and accidental poisoning. Males aged 15 to 24 years are the most likely victims of unintentional injuries. In four of the least populated states, the percentage of deaths from unintentional injuries was much higher than the national average: 7.7% in Idaho, 8.0% in Montana, 9.1% in Wyoming, and 14.3% in Alaska. Overall, deaths from unintentional injuries were approximately 80% to 85% higher for females and males in the most rural counties than for those in suburban areas of metropolitan counties in 1996 to 1998, and highest of all in the West (Castillo and Alexander, 2004). Driving at high speeds, driving long distances, driving in winter conditions, not using seat belts, and consuming alcohol have been cited as contributing to higher levels of injury deaths and disability for rural residents in the West. Lack of ready access to counseling, emergency medical services, and rehabilitation are also thought to be contributing factors to these high levels.

Vulnerable Groups

Demographic and personal characteristics, such as age, education, gender, race, ethnicity, language, and culture, round out the examples of factors that affect health and that may block access to existing services. Age is an important consideration in the planning of health care services for rural communities. As noted in previous sections, many retirees are moving into rural areas, and many younger people are moving out. Because the incomes of many elderly may be lower, the tax base of counties and municipalities may be inadequate to cover the disproportionate share of the health care services used by the elderly (age 65 years and over) (Bailey, 2009).

The population of the elderly is expected to double by 2050. Elderly women tend to live at or near the poverty level and to achieve poverty status twice as often as men (Cawthorne, 2010; USDA, ERS, 2012c). Along with educational attainment, this is a critical indicator of well-being for the elderly and the young. The elderly poor tend to be isolated and to lack access to support services, health care, prescription drugs, adequate nutrition, and transportation.

The number of children in rural areas increased by 2% from 2008 to 2009 and another 0.9 percentage points from 2009 to 2010. More than 2.8 million children in nonmetro areas were in poverty in 2010 (USDA, ERS, 2012c). In addition to population growth, racial and ethnic diversity has increased. Today, the proportion of Hispanic children is the fastest-growing component of the rural population, regardless of region. The population of black children has remained steady, and the majority of rural black children are still concentrated in the South. Native American children constitute only 3% of the total nonmetropolitan population, although in areas of the country (mainly West and Central) with high concentrations of Native Americans, this percentage is, of course, much higher. Evidence suggests that fetal, infant, and maternal mortality rates are slightly higher in nonmetropolitan than metropolitan areas and that prenatal care in the later pregnancy stages is problematic. Nonmetropolitan children, like nonmetropolitan adults, are more likely to live in poverty, and proportionately fewer rural children were covered by health insurance (Kandel, 2005; USDA, ERS, 2012c).

Education and Employment

Research on the socioeconomic determinants of health has revealed a strong positive correlation between health and length of schooling (Cutler and Lleras-Muney, 2006; USDA, ERS, 2012d). Demographics of a minority group often influence and result from social and economic factors. Age and education are indicators for employment. For the aged and for ethnic and racial minorities, a pattern of lower educational attainment and unfavorable economic circumstances emerges with increasing rurality (Fig. 24.2). Although the education picture is changing, many women now in their 70s and 80s grew up before public education was mandatory. Families could not afford to send them to school, or they were simply expected to learn to read and write, seek employment, and marry. Education, with its links to economic and health variables, is still a serious problem for rural America (Fig. 24.3). Low education and employment levels characterize all rural minority groups except Asians. Children living in precarious economic conditions have additional challenges to doing well in school and remaining in school through high school graduation. In 2010, 70% of rural dwellers held high school diplomas or Graduate Equivalency Diplomas (GEDs), compared with 77% in 2000 (USDA, 2012a). The college completion rate of rural students was almost half (17%) that of urban students (30%). There are also large gaps in educational completion by region, race, and ethnicity, with the Western and Midwestern rural students exceeding the high school completion rates of students in the rural South (USDA, 2012a). Generally, rural students perform better than students in cities and town, but not as well as suburban students, on the National Assessment of Educational Progress (NAEP). Students in rural districts had higher graduation rates than in cities and towns. Nationally, during the 2008–2009 school year (the latest year for which these data are available), the averaged freshman graduation rate for the 47 states and the District of Columbia was 77% and rural rates were 80%. City rates were 68%, towns 79%, and suburban rates were highest at 81% (National Center for Education Statistics, n.d.) Educational attainment is a challenge in rural America, and skill requirements for rural employment continue to rise. Lack of education is correlated with persistent poverty, and poverty is a predictor of poor health.

Furthermore, counties that have a low-wage economy have difficulty providing the infrastructure needed to provide education, public health, and health care services for low-wage families. They also have difficulty attracting new employers who might contribute to the economic development of a rural area but need a more highly educated workforce.

Occupational Health Risks

In the United States, approximately 4693 workers died from work-related illnesses and injuries in 2011 (Bureau of Labor Statistics, 2012a). Fatal occupational injuries declined 23.1% from 1992 to 2002. The overall fatal work injury rate for the United States in 2011 was 3.5 fatal injuries per 100,000 full-time equivalent workers, down slightly from the final rate of 3.6 reported for 2010. The published fatal injury rate for 2011 equals the lowest rate reported by the program since the conversion to hours-based rates in 2006. Tractors contributed to 12% of the

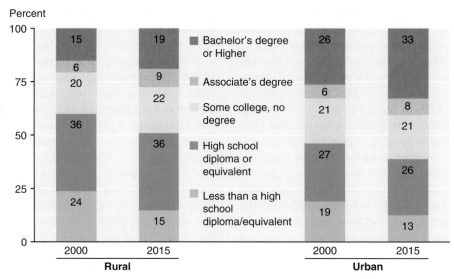

Note: Educational attainment for adults ages 25 and older; urban/rural status is determined by 2015 metropolitan area definitions from the Office of Management and Budget.

FIG. 24.2 Educational attainment rates for rural adults. (From U.S. Department of Agriculture, Economic Research Service: *Employment & education: high school completion rates (adults 25 and older)*, 2016. http://www.ers.usda.gov/topics/rural-economy-population/employment-education/rural-education.aspx.)

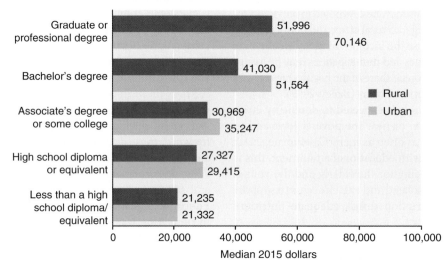

Note: Median earnings in 2015 dollars for all earners age 25 and older; urban/rural status is determined by 2015 metropolitan area definitions from the Office of Management and Budget.

FIG. 24.3 Rural and urban earnings by educational level. (From Marré A. From USDA Rural Education: *Rural education,* 2017. https://www.ers.usda.gov/topics/rural-economy-population/employment-education/rural-education/.)

deaths (Bureau of Labor Statistics, 2012b). Occupational injuries, fatalities, and illnesses play a significant role in rural health, because rates of disabling injuries and injury-related mortality are dramatically higher in the rural population. Industries with the highest death rate were mining, agriculture, forestry, and fishing, followed by construction, transportation, and public utilities. The majority of job-related deaths due to workplace injuries were in the following categories: transportation-related motor vehicle accidents, machinery-related events, homicides, falls, electrocution, and chemical and thermal injuries.

Agriculture ranks among the most hazardous industries. Farmers are at very high risk for injury, and often family members who live on the land work together. In 2012, there were 955,000 people aged 20 and younger working on farms. In 2012, there were 1,854,000 full-time workers in production agriculture. Annually there are 1.4 to 2.1 million adult hired crop workers in the United States.

Fatalities on farms were 20.2 per 100,000 workers in 2012, with tractor overturns the leading cause of death. On average, 113 youth less than 20 years of age die annually from farm-related injuries (1995–2002), with 34% being 16–19 years old. The leading cause of fatal injuries to youth involved machinery (23%), with motor vehicles (19%) and drownings (16%) following (National Institute for Occupational Safety and Health [NIOSH], 2014).

Occupational death and disability can also be attributed to nonfatal injuries and occupational diseases, such as cancer, asbestosis, silicosis, and anthracosis, associated with both organic and inorganic exposures (CDC, NIOSH Program Portfolio, 2012). Work-related injuries, deaths, and illness data must be interpreted with caution. Although surveillance of occupational injuries, illnesses, and fatalities has improved through the collaboration of the states and NIOSH, data still come from many sources, and underreporting continues to be problematic.

Perceptions of Health
Gender, Race, and Ethnicity

Both rural men and rural women are less likely than metropolitan residents to report their health as good or excellent. Rural areas, particularly in the rural South, have higher incidents of heart disease and cancer. Higher prevalence of chronic disease is consistent with the composition of rural populations, which tend to be older, poorer, and less educated (Artnak et al., 2011). Rural men and women also smoke or use smokeless tobacco more. In the aggregate, they exercise fewer preventive behaviors, have less contact with physicians, and often have less access to care than people with similar problems in urban areas (NRHA, 2014). Rural men and youths are also more likely to die or become disabled from unintentional injuries due to risky behavior or work-related causes and are more likely to commit suicide than women or urban men and youths.

Although rural populations overall are at lower risk for most cancers, certain rural subpopulations are at greater risk. For example, Appalachia has a much higher rate than the national figure. The CDC (2017) reported rural Americans are more likely to die from preventable disease, including heart disease (25,000), cancer (19,000), unintentional injury (12,000), chronic lower respiratory disease (11,000), and stroke (4000). The percentages of deaths that were potentially preventable were higher in rural areas than in urban areas. Residents in low-income areas and the uninsured, particularly African Americans, tend to have more late-stage cancer diagnoses; and rural residents in general may have less access to quality health care, including both medical care and screening and prevention programs. A particularly serious problem for minorities and the elderly is the lack of cancer screening, including screening for breast and cervical cancer for women and prostate cancer for men. Preventive care is especially important for African American men, for whom the prostate cancer rate is higher than for any other racial or ethnic group.

From 1987 to 2005 the age-adjusted percentage of women more than 40 years of age who had had a mammogram improved from 29% to 70% according to the CDC's National Center for Health Statistics (CDC, 2009b). The percentages were lower for all racial and ethnic minorities: 55% for Asian American, 65% for African American, and 58% for Hispanic American women. Use of mammography was the lowest among the poor, most particularly in the 40- to 49-year age bracket (47.4%), and among the least educated (CDC, 2009b). Health objectives for 2010 called for at least 80% of American women aged 40 years and older to have received a mammogram and clinical breast examination in the previous 2 years (National Advisory Committee on Rural Health and Human Services, 2013). Similarly, women who are poor, elderly, and less educated are less likely to receive Papanicolaou (Pap) smear tests. In racial and ethnic groups, the percentages of women who get Pap tests are lower for Hispanics, American Indians, and Alaska Natives. The lowest percentage is found in Asian women.

The percentage of Hispanics and Latinos in the U.S. population was about equal to that of African Americans (13% vs. 16% during the year 2011), and the former will soon become the largest minority group in the United States (U.S. Census Bureau, 2010). They are already the predominant minority in the West. Hispanics have diverse cultures, histories, and socioeconomic and health status. The largest Hispanic subgroups are of Mexican, Cuban, and Puerto Rican descent, although Mexican is the largest by far (accounting for 58% of the Hispanic population living in the United States). In nonmetropolitan areas, the population of Hispanics has doubled, and almost half of all Hispanics in rural areas are living outside the traditional areas of settlement in the Southwestern states. As emphasized previously, this growing segment of the population continues to be overrepresented among the rural poor. In 2010, the U.S. Census Bureau reported that 27% of Hispanics live below the federal poverty level, compared with 13% of the white non-Hispanic population. Elderly Hispanics were also 2.5 times more likely to live below the poverty line than white non-Hispanics. Hispanics are most likely to report barriers to obtaining needed health care and are least likely to have a usual source of care; for those blacks and Hispanics reporting a usual source of care, the source is most likely to be hospital based (U.S. Census Bureau, 2010).

SPECIFIC RURAL AGGREGATES
Agricultural Workers
Health Disparities

An example of health disparities among agricultural workers is the group of farm workers that support fruit and vegetable production. In general, migrant and seasonal farmworkers (MSFWs) may have the poorest health of any aggregate in the United States and the least access to affordable health care. Eighty-five percent of MSFWs are Hispanic, Latino, or African American. The rest are largely white seasonal workers who follow the harvests to drive combines or haul crops from the fields to storage, market, or seaports. These populations, estimated as between 3 and 5 million people each year, are vulnerable to a host of health problems and diseases that center on occupational and environmental hazards and other health correlates (USDA, 2013c, 2013d).

Accidents and Injuries

Working in highly variable environmental conditions (e.g., temperature extremes, a wide variety of work tasks, and unpredictable circumstances) is associated with an increased frequency of accidents and fatalities. Farm-related activities are extremely heterogeneous and vary significantly with the season, types of crops produced, and types of machinery used. Farmers are located in geographically isolated areas and often work alone. This constellation of factors puts farmers and their families at increased risk for accidental injury and delayed access to emergency or trauma care.

In 2012, the rate of fatal injuries per 100,000 full-time equivalents employed in the agricultural sector was 21.2 compared with manufacturing (2.1), retail trade (1.9), transportation (13.3), and governmental employees (2.0) (Bureau of Labor Statistics, 2012a). According to the CDC's NIOSH Program (2012), agricultural machinery is the most common cause of fatalities and nonfatal injuries of U.S. agricultural workers, including on-farm fatalities among youth (<20 years). Tractor-related accidents, especially rollovers, are the most frequent causes of farm accidents, accounting for more than one fourth of farm fatalities. The actual causes of death and serious injury are associated with rollovers of equipment that lacks rollover protective structures and seat belts (CDC, NIOSH Program, 2012). With such statistics, it is easy to see why accident prevention programs for farm children and families have focused heavily on tractor safety awareness.

Acute and Chronic Illnesses

Several types of farming activities are associated with more occurrences than expected of acute and chronic respiratory conditions. Individuals with long-term exposure to grain dusts, such as grain elevator workers and dairy workers, have diminished respiratory function and increased frequency of respiratory symptoms (National Center for Farmworker Health [NCFH], 2013). Occupational asthma and more exotic fungal or toxic gas–related conditions also occur in higher frequency in agricultural than nonagricultural populations. Community health nurses, who are familiar with local farming practices in rural areas, often make links between farm work and respiratory symptoms. In such situations, the role of the nurse is to refer patients to appropriate health care providers and to provide support and education for affected people and their families.

Exposure to pesticides, herbicides, and other chemicals is also a major concern for farmers and their families. From an occupational perspective, farming is unusual because the home and the worksite are the same. Exposure risks to children and spouses may be heightened when farmers wear contaminated clothing and boots into the home. Homes are often located in close proximity to fields and animal containment facilities, which are treated with a variety of chemicals.

Nurses in rural emergency rooms or other ambulatory care settings may be the first providers to encounter farmers and others with acute **pesticide** poisoning. During discussions with farmers, ranchers, or other high-risk groups (e.g., nursery workers and tree planters), community health nurses may note a pattern of headaches and nausea that occurs during planting or spraying seasons. In such an instance, the nurse can serve as an important resource by obtaining a careful history of signs and symptoms, the temporal nature of symptom occurrence,

and the types of pesticides and personal protection used (e.g., respirators and protective clothing). When evidence suggests pesticide-related illness, appropriate referral and follow-up are imperative to ensure the safety of the affected person and the family.

Signs and symptoms of acute pesticide poisoning are fairly clear, and most health providers in rural communities would recognize them. Common symptoms include headache, dizziness, diaphoresis, nausea, and vomiting. If left untreated, those affected may experience a progression of symptoms, including dyspnea, bronchospasm, and muscle twitching. Deaths are relatively uncommon, but they do occur.

Several demographic, environmental, economic, and social factors might put rural residents at higher risk of death from these public health conditions. Residents of rural areas in the United States tend to be older and sicker than their urban counterparts. They have higher rates of cigarette smoking, high blood pressure, and obesity. Rural residents report less leisure-time physical activity and lower seat belt use than their urban counterparts. They also have higher rates of poverty, have less access to health care, and are less likely to have health insurance (CDC, 2017).

Migrant and Seasonal Farmworkers

Although the discussion of agricultural issues has focused primarily on farmers and farm families, it is important to understand the role of **migrant** (i.e., migrate to find work) and **seasonal** (i.e., reside permanently in one place and work locally when farm labor is needed) farmworkers in U.S. agricultural production and the health risks to this population. Older references to farmworkers often referred to three "migrant streams," in which workers entered the country through Mexico and migrated north. The current reality is that migrant workers enter the country through a variety of access points and follow any route necessary to obtain work. Seasonal workers reside in agricultural areas permanently and take various farm jobs during harvesting times. For example, a seasonal worker may be employed in restaurant work during the winter and may spend the summer months picking apples or working in a local apple shed or cannery (USDA, ERS, 2013). MSFWs comprise a vulnerable population in regard to health risks because they have a low-income and migratory status. In many rural areas, community health nurses form the central link between farmworkers and health services. Through standing or mobile clinic sites, nurses have established a leadership role in the provision of episodic and preventive services for workers and their families. Lacking access to many types of preventive services, farmworkers often visit a migrant clinic with any number of health problems, including severe dental problems, unresolved communicable diseases, and untreated injuries. In addition to the direct provision of care, nurses in many communities have served as important advocates on behalf of farmworkers and have worked to ensure health care access for those traveling through their areas.

Cultural, linguistic, economic, and mobility barriers all contribute to the nature and magnitude of health problems observed in farmworkers. Cultural and linguistic barriers are the most overt because many of the communities where farmworkers work consider them outsiders. In many settings, migrant workers live isolated from the agricultural communities they serve. Although some workers travel in extended family groups and have the support that comes with being together, other workers leave their families at home. Often the latter are male workers who work and live together. A common misconception among U.S. health care providers is that these farmworkers are from Mexico and that Spanish is their primary language. Farmworkers originate from many communities in Mexico, the Caribbean, and Central and South America, and they may speak the language of their home country, English, or several languages.

Enumeration of Migrant and Seasonal Farmworkers

To increase access to primary and preventative care for MSFW populations, information is needed on the numbers and distribution of farmworkers at the national, state, and local levels. Because MSFWs move frequently for work, census estimates generally provide a poor assessment of this population's needs for health care services. Additionally, the legislation that created the Migrant Health Program (MHP) (Section 330g of the Public Health Service Act), under the direction of the Bureau of Primary Health Care (BPHC) (2000) and the Health Resources and Services Administration (HRSA), requires that priorities be established according to where the greatest need exists. Hence the MHP has supported the ongoing and comprehensive assessment of the numbers of MSFWs and published the Migrant and Seasonal Farmworker Enumeration Profile Study (Bureau of Health Professions, 2016).

Health Needs and Opportunities for Preventive Care

Similarities in exposure and work practices make some of the farmworkers' health needs similar to those of farmers and their families. Generally, these health needs reflect the increased rates of accidents and injuries, dermatological conditions, and pulmonary problems observed in the two populations. However, there are additional challenges in both the identification and the treatment of farmworkers with health problems. One of the biggest problems that nurses face in designing health programs is understanding the full magnitude of these health problems. Many farmworkers who become ill eventually return to their countries of origin to obtain treatment and to be with family. This phenomenon makes it difficult to get complete, reliable numbers about disease rates. A variety of public health indicators are likely to undercount farmworkers as a group, ranging from tumor registries to workers' compensation injuries (NCFH, 2013). In addition, farmworkers may be less likely to seek treatment for health problems that do not require emergency treatment or surgery.

Studies of farmworkers' health status have provided data indicating that they are less likely to receive preventive care from any health source. Preventive needs include dental care, vision screening and treatment, and gynecological and breast examinations. Many farmworkers, because they move from community to community, are often unaware of clinical and social services they could receive and that are available at reduced or no cost to low-income families.

⊘ ACTIVE LEARNING

1. University libraries commonly subscribe to newspapers published within the state. Visit the library and select three to four small town or rural county newspapers. Read them for information about health care activities and concerns related to the health of the individuals, families, and community.
   - Report findings to the class about rural health concerns and activities.
   - Identify one priority problem that could be researched in the community and has relevance to rural community health nursing practice.
2. Choose one of the major causes of morbidity and mortality in migrant populations.
   - On the basis of risk factor and natural history, specify interventions for primary, secondary, and tertiary prevention of this problem.
   - Identify which of these interventions are examples of upstream thinking.
3. Locate a telephone book, a community resource directory, or a resource website from a rural community.
   - List and evaluate the resources that are available for prevention, assessment, intervention, and follow-up care for the major cause of mortality and morbidity identified in Learning Activity 2.
   - Would it be necessary to go outside the rural town or county for any of the needed resources? Which ones? Where might they be located?

RURAL HEALTH CARE DELIVERY SYSTEM

Health Care Provider Shortages

In a National Advisory Committee on Rural Health and Human Services brief (2013) the authors indicate that the quality and functionality of a health care delivery system depend on the availability of medical personnel and infrastructure to provide needed services. Rural communities generally have fewer physicians, nurses, specialists, and other health care workforce, and the small population size and scale make the loss or shortage of a single health provider likely to have far-reaching impacts.

The health care labor shortage in the United States has been widely documented and is expected to last for the foreseeable future. The increase in population—aging and growing racial and ethnic diversity—is partially responsible for the health care labor shortage. As the health care workforce ages, the U.S. population is expected to rise by 18% by 2030, and the population over the age of 65 is expected to increase three times that rate (USDA, State Fact Sheets: United States, 2011). In addition to the shortage of health professionals, maldistribution is another prevalent obstacle rural Americans face in accessing timely and appropriate primary health care services (Rural Information Center Health Service, 2014). Workforce shortages are especially serious in remote frontier communities, many of which are located in the Western region of the United States.

Nursing is by far the largest health care profession in the United States, with more than 2.6 million registered nurses (RNs) practicing in hospitals and other settings nationwide. Despite their large numbers, many more qualified nurses must be prepared in programs offered by community colleges and 4-year institutions to meet the nation's growing demand for health care and to replace a large wave of nurses nearing retirement. By 2020, the Bureau of Labor Statistics projects that more than 1.2 million additional RNs will be needed to work in acute care hospitals, long-term care facilities, community health centers, nursing schools, and other areas. Although approximately

25% of the U.S. population lives in nonmetropolitan counties, only 18% of RNs practice there (American Association of Colleges of Nursing, 2012). See "Primary Care."

Clearly the growing nursing shortage will affect all of America. This is both a supply shortage and a demand shortage. Declining school enrollments, retirement of current nurses, and the increased need for care of an aging population make the situation especially critical (Sigma Theta Tau International, n.d.). A survey by the American Organization of Nurse Executives found that it takes significantly longer to fill vacancies in small hospitals, usually located in rural areas, than in larger urban facilities (Thrall, 2007). Rural nurses earn less than their urban counterparts, compounding recruitment difficulties. Nurses with baccalaureate and master's degrees, other than master's degree–prepared NPs, are compensated less for this additional education (Thrall, 2007).

A solution proposed for the shortage of health care providers is for rural communities to "grow their own." A rural community, a group of small communities, or a county could support local students attending college and recruit students currently attending professional schools. The students would make a commitment to work in the community in return for monetary support for their educations (Thrall, 2007). Tuition reimbursement and access to distance learning programs can assist practicing nurses. Continuing education and baccalaureate and master's degrees are available through e-mail, Internet-based courses, interactive video classes, and by-mail videos. Some programs are provided exclusively via the Internet. Nebraska's rural communities are enthusiastic about the University of Nebraska College of Nursing Internet courses. The program is helping them grow their own nurses. Research shows that nurses educated in rural communities are more apt to stay and work there than those who move away to attend school (Thrall, 2007).

Once new graduates are hired into health care positions in rural communities, it is imperative that they are assisted in their transition to practice. An opportunity exists to transform nurses' professional development and to improve health care quality and affordability through nurse residency programs. These programs need to go beyond basic orientation and provide a clinical preceptorship focused not just on delivering competent care, but also in how to develop and grow in the nursing profession. A survey of new nurses found many challenges: a lack of confidence, difficulty with work relationships, frustrations relating to the work environment, lack of time and guidance for developing organizational and priority-setting abilities, and overall high levels of stress. These factors likely contribute to the high turnover rate among new nurses, estimated at between 35% and 60% within the first year (Kosman, 2011).

Telemedicine

In light of provider storages and recruitment difficulties with the physician, nurse, and other health care worker shortages, coupled with the difficulty in recruiting them to rural areas, alternatives to improve access must be identified. Telemedicine is an alternative that is expanding across the country. Telemedicine is viewed as a cost-effective alternative to the more traditional face-to-face way of providing medical care (Medicaid.gov, 2013).

The American Telemedicine Association largely views telemedicine and telehealth to be interchangeable terms, encompassing a wide definition of remote health care, although telehealth may not always involve clinical care. Yet regardless of how you refer to it, what is now indisputable is how telemedicine greatly improves the quality, equity, and affordability of health care throughout the world.

Distinctions can be made between telehealth and telemedicine. *Telehealth* includes technologies such as telephones, facsimile machines, electronic mail systems, and remote patient monitoring devices for the collection and transmission of patient data for monitoring and interpretation. Conversely, telemedicine seeks to improve a patient's health by permitting two-way, real-time, interactive communication between the patient and the physician or practitioner at the distant site and is centered on efficiency, effectiveness, and safety. This electronic communication means the use of interactive telecommunications equipment that includes, at a minimum, audio and video equipment. This definition is modeled on Medicare's definition of telehealth services (Medicaid.gov, 2013).

Recent projects geared toward extending telemedicine services to rural areas include the Frontier Health Projects support of new models of health care. Although several states in the Midwest and West have taken advantage of telemedicine in rural areas, the patchwork approach in legislation has contributed to varying degrees of implementation and financial support for its implementation (Braum, 2013).

Managed Care in the Rural Environment

Managed care has recently changed health care delivery in the United States. In rural areas, health care delivery networks with managed care elements are being developed. Potential benefits and risks of managed care for rural areas have been identified, with recognition of the difficulty rural providers in solo or small group practices face in delivering cost-effective, complex health care. Possible benefits to managed care include lowering primary care costs, improving the quality of care, and stabilizing the local rural health care system. Risks are also apparent, including probable high startup and administrative costs and the volatile effect of large, urban-based, for-profit, managed care companies (Allender et al., 2010).

Outside of Medicaid, managed care has yet to become a major presence in much of rural America because small disperse populations, few visits per individual, and large numbers of elderly on Medicare with low-level reimbursements do not make the aggregate financially attractive to a managed care organization (MCO). In fact, despite the existence of federally qualified health centers that provide care to underserved populations through Medicare or Medicaid or on sliding fee scales, few rural people were enrolled in sponsored health plans (Allender et al., 2010). Providers in rural markets face severe financial constraints as health maintenance organizations (HMOs) increasingly cope with smaller numbers of enrollees and continue to reduce provider reimbursement (IOM, 2005).

Patient-centered medical homes (PCMHs) and patient-centered medical neighborhoods play a vital role in delivering care to rural communities. The medical home model holds promise as a way to improve health care in America by transforming how primary care is organized and delivered. Building on the work of a large and growing community, the Agency for Healthcare Research and Quality defines a medical home not simply as a place but as a model of the organization of primary care that delivers the core functions of primary health care. The medical home encompasses five functions and attributes: comprehensive care, patient centered, coordinated care, accessible services, and quality and safety.

We conceptualize the medical neighborhood as a PCMH and the constellation of other clinicians providing health care services to patients within it, along with community and social service organizations and state and local public health agencies. Defined in this way, the PCMH and the surrounding medical neighborhood can focus on meeting the needs of the individual patient, but also incorporate aspects of population health and overall community health needs in its objectives.

COMMUNITY-BASED CARE

In the mid-1990s, the phrase *community-based care* became a popular term for the myriad of services provided outside the walls of an institution. Health care services are no longer provided exclusively in the hospital setting. Community-based care includes services that are provided where individuals live, work, or go to school. Examples of community-based services are home health and hospice care, occupational health programs, community mental health programs, ambulatory care services, school health programs, faith-based care, and elder services such as adult day care. The concept also includes community participation in decisions about health care services, a focus on all three levels of prevention, and an understanding that the hospital is no longer the exclusive health care provider.

Home Health and Hospice Care

Rural populations are disproportionately older than their urban counterparts, and this disparity will only increase as baby boomers continue to age. The elderly growth rates in nonmetropolitan areas are expected to triple from 6% in 2000–2010 to 18% in 2010–2020. Aside from being older, rural residents have higher rates of age-adjusted mortality, disability, and chronic illness than their urban counterparts. As the elderly comprise a larger percentage of the rural population, access to high-quality end-of-life care in rural areas will become increasingly important.

Home health and hospice programs vary in structure. A national study on Medicare hospice use found that only one third of rural counties have a hospice based within the county, but nearly two thirds of urban counties do (Vernig et al., 2004). Urban hospices are more likely to be freestanding, whereas rural hospices tend to be hospital based. Larger communities may support a hospital-based home care agency with hospice service, a freestanding full-service agency, or both. In sparsely populated rural locations, home health and hospice services may be contracted from a larger regional agency, with a local nurse hired to provide services.

Vernig and associates (2004) found that the more remote the rural environment, the less likely hospice services were used.

Nurse case management and development of local resources, using the county extension services as a bridge for outreach services, can improve home care for patients needing hospice care and provide support for their families. A partnership between the public health nurse and county extension service could provide support and information groups and caregiving classes for the important informal provider network.

Given the more fragile financial margins and lower patient volume in rural areas, rural hospice providers face different challenges from their urban counterparts, and one-size-fits-all policy reform may have negative consequences for rural hospice providers. Despite data indicating that hospice provider density in rural areas is comparable to and even higher than in urban areas, rural and frontier Medicare decedents continue to utilize hospice at lower rates than their urban peers (National Advisory Committee on Rural Health and Human Services, 2013). Chapter 33 discusses home health and hospice in greater detail.

Faith Communities and Parish Nursing

Rural residents are perceived as having strong traditional values. At the heart of these values is a strong sense of community, family life, and religious faith. Since the conceptualization of parish nursing in the early 1980s, RNs have developed and expanded the role. The Canadian Association for Parish Nursing Ministry defines the role of the parish nurse as to promote the integration of faith and health in a variety of ways that reflect the context of the faith community. Specific examples include health advocacy, health counseling, health education, and resource referral. The Westberg Institute develops and supports faith community or parish nurses. They define the role as licensed, registered nurses who practice holistic health for self, individuals, and the community using nursing knowledge combined with spiritual care. They function in paid and unpaid positions as members of the pastoral team in a variety of religious faiths, cultures, and countries. The focus of their work is on the intentional care of the spirit, assisting the members of the faith community to maintain and/or regain wholeness in body, mind, and spirit.

In a comparison of experiences of rural and urban faith-based programs, rural nurses are more likely to be involved in case management and coordination of services than their urban counterparts (Molanari et al., 2011). In urban settings, contact with parishioners is primarily at the church, whereas contacts in rural settings are most often in the home, on the phone, or in other community-based settings. Collaboration between faith communities and other organizations can help extend limited rural community health resources. Such partnerships have been promoted by federal and state governments to enhance the public health efforts (Zahner and Corrado, 2004). Chapter 33 provides an in-depth discussion of parish nursing.

In 1997, the ANA designated parish nursing a specialty practice. At the same time, the Health Ministries Association, a membership organization for parish nurses and others in health ministry, developed the "Scope and Standards of Parish Nursing Practice." Revised in 2004, these standards are now called "Faith Community Nursing: Scope and Standards of Practice" (Patterson, 2010).

Informal Care Systems

Limited availability of and accessibility to formal health care resources in rural areas, combined with the self-reliance and self-help traits of rural residents, have resulted in the development of strong informal care and social support networks in rural communities. Rural residents are more apt to entrust care to established informal networks than to new formal care systems. Examining perceptions of rural health and social systems, Thorngren (2003) found that rural residents agreed that experiences inherent in rural life both contribute to and ameliorate health-related concerns attributed to higher levels of family and community involvement, problem-solving abilities, and connections to the land, which may be a factor in the formation and use of informal systems.

Informal care systems or networks include people who have assumed the role of caregiver on the basis of their individual qualities, life situations, or social roles. These informal care providers are often referred to as *lay caregivers*. Family caregivers play an important role in patient-centered health care. Lay caregivers are individuals who are not licensed health professionals, but often care for patients after a hospital stay. Those designated caregivers are usually friends or members of a patient's family (Miller, 2015). People who participate in these networks may provide direct help, advice, or information.

Informal caregivers often find themselves in stressful circumstances (Sanford et al., 2004). Rural residents who are in need of assistance are usually elderly, have chronic illness, have few resources, and must travel long distances for health care. Rasheed and Rasheed (2003) suggest that by 2050, 21% of all Americans will be members of a minority group. Disparities already exist in the physical and mental health status, service availability, service access, and socioeconomic status for minorities. Americans in rural communities and in the black community rely heavily on community-based informal care systems. Van Exel, de Graaf, and Brouwer (2008) studied caregiver attitudes toward respite care and found that those who could potentially benefit were reluctant to seek it for various reasons. This finding has enormous implications for nursing practice. Because informal health care is an important, cost-effective component of health care systems, different forms of respite care have been implemented to support caregivers. Not only do many patients have a preference for receiving care from someone familiar in their home environment; in many cases such care will help them avoid placement in a long-term care facility. Nurses have a role in discussing the potential benefits of support for both the family and the care recipient.

Rural Public Health Departments

There are more than 2800 local health departments in the United States, yet less than 5% serve populations of fewer than 50,000 people (Weisbecker, 2010). The purpose of *Healthy People 2010* objective 24-11 was to increase the proportion of state and local public health departments (LHDs) that meet national performance standards for public health services. In *Healthy People 2020*, the health disparities in rural health have been highlighted and specific areas of focus for rural health have been established (*Healthy People 2020*, Disparities, 2013).

Uniquely positioned within rural communities, LHDs are a potential catalyst for addressing the long-standing challenges associated with urban–rural health disparities. While focused on improving the health of populations, LHDs provide a wide array of services focused on assessing health status, mobilizing action to address health-related issues, and ensuring the delivery of important health services in the community. The ability of rural health departments to develop and cultivate partnerships is important for the integration of public health within the larger health care delivery system.

Nonetheless, rural LHDs remain subject to the same persistent challenges facing the larger health care delivery system in rural communities. Limited by budget, staffing, and capacity constraints, both the number and type of public health services provided in rural health departments often differs markedly from what is observed among urban LHD counterparts. These differences ultimately limit the ability of rural health departments to respond to national public health and health care policy initiatives. Even so, some examples point to important advances in meeting the health needs of rural communities (Hale, 2015).

Rural Mental Health Care

The economic crisis that affected much of the rural population in the 1980s contributed to mental health problems. Natural disasters, such as drought and flood, and economic downturns in the late 1990s have contributed to continuing chronic stress. Those affected are most apt to work in the traditional ranching, farming, mining, forestry, and fishing industries. Although mental health disorders widely affect rural and urban residents throughout the lifespan, factors such as poverty, race, age, and rural dwelling lower the prospect of accessing mental health services. Clearly, large sections of at-risk rural populations are without mental health care (Bailey, 2009).

Three key factors have been identified as contributing to mental illness in rural areas. First, there is a lack of specialized mental health providers in rural areas. The most recent figures show that 75% of rural counties with populations between 2500 and 20,000 do not have a psychiatrist and that 95% do not have a child psychiatrist. Next, because of the lack of qualified mental health care providers, rural residents often receive services from primary care providers. Many rural primary care providers are ill equipped to provide mental health services, and there are limited NP and physician assistant resources to support the mental health care that is needed. Both specialized mental health care and primary health care providers are confronted with barriers related to rural practice. These include a more diverse practice, fewer opportunities for ongoing education, and fewer professionals to consult than their colleagues in urban practice. Lastly, rural residents often do not seek mental health services because of perceived stigma and because they do not always recognize a need for mental health services (Bailey, 2009).

Emergency Services

Access to emergency medical services (EMS) has been identified as one of the most significant health care issues for rural residents (Bailey, 2009; Bryant, 2009). EMS include prehospital care, hospital- or health center–based emergency care, and trauma systems.

Rural residents depend on EMS because of their high risk for unintentional injury. Low population density has been shown to be a strong predictor of higher injury-related morbidity and mortality rates in rural areas (Peek-Asa et al., 2004). In medically underserved areas, EMS systems play an increasingly important role in decreasing the morbidity and mortality of individuals needing emergency care. Getting patients from the place of injury to the trauma center within the "golden hour" is frequently not possible in rural areas because of barriers imposed by distance, terrain, climatic conditions, and communication methods. Some rural facilities are more than 1 hour away by air from the nearest trauma center or tertiary care hospital (Hsia and Shen, 2011). For those rural residents, the death rate remains twice that of urban residents.

Challenges faced by rural EMS systems include a shortage of volunteers, a lower level of training than among urban providers, training curricula that often do not reflect rural hazards (e.g., farm equipment trauma), lack of guidance from physicians, and lack of physician training about and orientation to the EMS system (Bryant, 2009). Low population density; large, isolated, or inaccessible areas; severe weather; poor roads; and lower density of telephones or other communication methods also contribute to difficult public access for emergency care. These problems make the challenges of developing EMS in rural areas substantial (Branas et al., 2005).

Emergency Preparedness in Rural Communities

Emergency preparedness refers to actions that should be performed before an emergency, such as planning and coordination meetings, procedure writing, team training, emergency drills and exercises, and positioning of emergency equipment. Emergency response is generally described as the tactical planning and practical activities designed to protect life and property immediately after some type of event. Some of the key elements of an emergency response program include evacuation planning and assembly; escalation protocols; damage assessment and reporting; hazmat response and spill control; medical response; salvage and reclamation; and specialty issues such as fire brigades, first aid, high angle or confined space rescue, etc. (Blanchard, 2008). Rural areas are not exempt from disasters. Challenges of emergency preparation and management are different for rural communities from those for urban ones. Bryant (2009) categorized these challenges into four major themes: resource limitation, separation and remoteness, low population density, and communication.

Resources needed in a disaster include human capital, financial capital, and social capital. Due to the increase in urbanization, the decline in the rural overall population, and the rise in rural population age, the human and financial resources available to prepare and respond to disasters are limited. Social capital becomes the focus to meet the challenges of rural communities. Building relationships among emergency agencies, community organizations, and local businesses is essential to secure human and financial resources. Rural areas also depend on networks of volunteers (e.g., first responders).

The remoteness of rural areas results in longer response times. Population density may affect funding of rural communities'

emergency preparedness. State and federal programs often consider population size and density in many funding decisions, so densely populated areas receive the most attention for mitigation and recovery activities (Bryant, 2009). Finally, communication education about emergency preparation is more expensive in rural areas. This higher cost leads to reduced outreach before disasters and throughout the event. Warning systems are often absent or neglected in remote areas, placing the burden on the individual to access emergency information.

> ### ❓ ACTIVE LEARNING
>
> Select a rural community health nurse (i.e., public health or home care) and conduct an interview in person or by telephone if distance prohibits a face-to-face meeting.
> - Identify what the nurse sees as the pros and cons of rural nursing.
> - If negative aspects of rural nursing are identified, discuss how the nurse deals with them.
> - Ask the nurse to discuss the three highest-priority efforts related to his or her rural practice.

Upstream Interventions

Upstream and prevention-oriented approaches have several implications for nurses in rural practice. Descriptions of three strategies for upstream interventions follow: attack community-based problems at their roots, emphasize the "doing" aspects of health, and maximize the use of informal networks.

Attacking Community-Based Problems at Their Roots

Upstream approaches to community health problems direct the nurse toward an understanding of the precursors of poor health within populations of interest. Individual nurses can be effective forces in uncovering and enhancing community awareness of health-endangering situations. Environmental health issues in rural communities, such as pesticide exposure and health hazards from point-source factory emissions, are more effectively assessed and remedied on a community level than on a case-by-case basis. Nurses' involvement in helping people understand health problems in a larger context can be the genesis of change. Nurses and other community members can take social action on behalf of those affected. For example, by heightening awareness of sulfur dioxin levels from a local refinery and the relationship of those emission levels to respiratory problems in vulnerable populations, nurses can help citizens gain an understanding of the collective rather than individual burden of the refinery on their community's health.

Emphasizing the "Doing" Aspects of Health

There are consistent differences between the ways rural and nonrural residents perceive health. The primary one may be the relative importance of "work" and "being able to work" in self-reported definitions of health (Weinert and Long, 1987). Rural attitudes generally emphasize the "doing" aspects of health in functioning and performing the activities fundamentally important in their daily lives. The high value placed on "being able to do" can give astute nurses intervention opportunities for both families and communities. Examples of nursing intervention strategies that capitalize on this attitude include accident prevention programs for children, exercise and nutrition programs for seniors, and participation of local industries in risk reduction programs for workers. Active involvement of the target population in all phases of program planning and implementation is key to the success of these programs.

Maximizing the Use of Informal Networks

Recognizing and using informal networks in the community is essential to the "doing" concept of prevention programs. The name used, such as empowerment model or community action model, is less important than soliciting the involvement of informal networks and local leaders in planning health interventions. As most people who have been involved in community empowerment programs will attest, accomplishing the involvement of these important entities is not easy or straightforward. Turf issues and collateral agendas can obstruct rather than facilitate change. However, failure to elicit community involvement in population-based health interventions will have unfavorable consequences. Frequently, superimposed change tends to fit poorly with the community it is intended to serve. Rural change strategies will be short-lived unless community members understand them and invest in their own well-being.

LEGISLATION AND PROGRAMS AFFECTING RURAL PUBLIC HEALTH

Programs That Augment Health Care Facilities and Services

Several programs are particularly important for meeting the public health needs of rural people. One is the Community Health Centers (CHC) program administered by the United States Public Health Service. The CHC program benefits underserved areas and populations by providing primary health care and, in some cases, supplemental secondary and tertiary health care, such as hospital care, long-term home health care, and rehabilitation. Rural health clinics (RHCs) are designed to improve access to primary care. As an incentive to rural communities to apply for RHCs, Medicare and Medicaid are reimbursed at a higher rate than usual at such centers.

The Migrant Health Clinic (MHC) program and the MHP also come under the Division of Community and Migrant Health and HRSA. The MHC program provides comprehensive nursing and medical care and support services to MSFWs and their families. The centers provide culturally sensitive care to a racially and culturally diverse farm labor force from many countries in Latin America and the Caribbean. Bilingual, bicultural health personnel, including lay outreach workers, use culturally appropriate protocols to provide primary care, preventive health care, transportation, dental care, pharmaceuticals, and environmental health services. The MHCs must provide the same services as the CHC and may also offer supplemental services, such as environmental health services, infectious disease and parasite control, and accident prevention programs.

Medicare's Rural Hospital Flexibility (RHF) grant program replaces earlier demonstration programs. According to information provided by the Office of Rural Health Policy (ORHP), the RHF program "allows small hospitals the flexibility to reconfigure operations and be licensed as Critical Access Hospitals (CAHs)" (HRSA, Medicare Rural Hospital Flexibility Grant, n.d.). The program also provides cost-based reimbursement for inpatient Medicare and outpatient services. Grants are also awarded for planning, implementing, and establishing networks of care and improving EMS.

Primary care cooperative agreements facilitate the development of primary care services and attract primary care providers to rural health professional shortage areas (HPSA). Special legislation for HPSAs has also created programs to provide acute care facilities and services. The Rural Transition Grants Program, administered by Health Care Financing Administration (HCFA), helps small rural communities with nonprofit hospitals adjust to changes in clinical practice patterns and in-hospital use, shifts from hospital- to community-based care, and changes in emergency care delivery patterns.

RURAL COMMUNITY HEALTH NURSING

Perhaps a more accurate title than rural community health nursing would be "community health nursing along the rural continuum." Nonmetropolitan areas would be at one end of the continuum, with metropolitan areas at the other end.

Practice in a rural area may require working as the only nurse at a health department in a remote Western Great Plains frontier county with a population of 6000, at a full-service health department in a town of 50,000 people, or at a large health department in a rural area next to an urban population. A practice in a rural area adjacent to a large metropolitan area often appears to have more in common with the urban end of the continuum in terms of agency size, distances, and resources. For the purposes of this discussion, the practice setting is at the more "rural" end of the continuum.

The following definition illustrates the broad-based, generalist focus of the modern rural community health nurse. It includes the important geographical and cultural environment in which community health practice is implemented and helps define appropriate nursing interventions.

Rural nursing is the practice of professional nursing within the physical and sociocultural context of sparsely populated communities. It involves the continual interaction of the rural environment, the nurse, and his or her practice. Rural nursing includes the diagnosis and treatment of a diversified population of people of all ages and a variety of human responses to actual (or potential) occupational hazards or to actual (or potential) health problems existent in maternity, pediatric, medical/surgical, and emergency nursing in a given rural area (Bigbee, 1993; Lee and Winters, 2004; Rosenthal, 2005; Williams et al., 2012).

Characteristics of Rural Nursing

The uniqueness of rural nursing practice has been in question. Some believe that nursing care for rural clients is the same as for other individuals and that health problems and patient care needs are similar, regardless of the setting. Others argue that rural practice should be designated as a specialty or subspecialty area because of factors such as isolation, scarce resources, and the need for a wide range of practice skills that must be adapted to social and economic structures. Whether generalist or specialist, nurses being prepared for rural practice must be equipped with other community health assessment skills (Kulbok et al., 2012).

Molanari et al. (2011) identified several positive aspects of rural nursing in the ability to provide holistic care, to know everyone well, and to develop close relationships with the community and coworkers where they enjoyed rural lifestyle as reasons to practice rural nursing. Autonomy, professional status, and being valued by the agency and community have been reported components of positive job satisfaction. Of those components identified as negative, agencies and professional organizations are most actively addressing professional isolation. The use of distance education technologies is one way to address the isolation many rural nurses experience. University degree programs and continuing education courses are readily available online or through full-motion interactive television. Using these technologies, rural nurses are able to update their skills and network with other nurses without having to leave their home communities.

Scharff (1998) considered the distinctive nature of the rural nurse's practice. She found that the rural nurse is a generalist and remarked that "generalist" is not synonymous with "boring." Interviews with rural nurses show that they feel an "intensity of purpose" that makes rural nursing distinctive. Nurses living and practicing in the same place have a strong sense of integration and continuity between practice and community:

> The newcomer practices nursing in a rural setting, unlike the more experienced nurse, who practices rural nursing. Somewhere between these extremes lies the transitional period of events and conditions through which each nurse passes at her or his own pace. It is within this time zone that nurses experience rural reality and move toward becoming professionals who understand that having gone rural, they are not less than they were, but rather, they are more than they expected to be. Some may be conscious of the transition, and others may not, but in the end, a few will say, "I am a rural nurse."
>
> *(Scharff, 1998, p. 38)*

Rural community health nursing is rewarding and challenging. Services can include maternal and child health, elder health, school health, mental health, and occupational health. The nurse practicing with the autonomy common in rural practice brings knowledge and competence in other clinical specialties. The work requires a discriminating, solid practitioner who can perform general nursing at a skill level beyond that of the outdated "mile wide and inch deep" general nursing. The rural nurse must be an "expert generalist."

Rural Health Research

The HRSA provides access to and support for research through the Research Centers Program. The Research Centers Program is the only federal research program entirely dedicated to producing policy-relevant research on health care and population health in rural areas. Each research center has its own identity

(although it may be part of a larger organization), website, and core staff that include a disciplinary mix of health services research, epidemiology, public health, geography, medicine, and mental health. Over the 4-year award cycle, each research center develops a portfolio of several research projects per year in conjunction with input from the Federal Office of Rural Health Policy and other experts.

To strengthen the dissemination of research results, the Rural Health Research Gateway was launched in early 2006. The gateway is a "one-stop shop" for the research centers, providing easy access to projects funded by ORHP and summaries of research in progress. The gateway's research alerts provide e-mail updates when new publications become available.

The Community-Based Division (CBD) grant programs provide funding to increase access to care in rural communities and to address their unique health care challenges. Most of the CBD's programs require community organizations to share resources and expertise using evidence-based models of care in networks of two or more health care services providers.

Universities across the country have created centers for rural health research. North Dakota State University has The Center for Rural Health, which undertakes research initiatives to support rural and tribal communities by identifying and describing health disparities; examining issues related to health care service delivery and systems, health workforce, and population health; and supporting the development of research expertise. The University of Minnesota has the Rural Health Research Center. The research center has been producing focused, top-quality research for two decades now. The Rural Health Research Center was first established with funding from the Federal Office of Rural Health Policy in 1992. Their projects address key forces that are shaping quality of care and quality improvement in rural areas. For example:

- Employing quality measurement and public reporting as tools to upgrade quality of care
- Using technology and health professional staffing in innovative ways to improve quality of care and patient safety
- Devising financial incentives that can help improve care in rural hospitals and clinics

Capacity of Rural Public Health to Manage Improvements in Health

Healthy People 2020 (HealthyPeople.gov, 2013) outlines health-related objectives for Americans and forms the rationale for efforts to intervene in disease trends to improve health where disparities have been identified. Determining the status of health indicators, such as rates of morbidity, mortality from common diseases or injury, and, perhaps most important, access to health care services, allows for priorities to be determined for which improvements in health are needed. Importantly, *Healthy People 2020* objectives and intervention strategies have been analyzed for rural–urban disparities that may exist along geographic, demographic, and cultural dimensions to provide a more specific picture of potential research priorities concerning improvements in health. The *Healthy People 2020* box presents data from a survey of 44 national and state rural health experts that identify percentages of respondents who indicated giving priority status for various health issues.

HEALTHY PEOPLE 2020

Rural Health Priorities

Rural Priorities (Identified By 25% or More)	Percentage (%) of Respondents (N = 44)
Access to health care (includes one of the following):	73
Access to emergency medical services	32
Access to health workforce	29
Access to health services (general)	29
Access to health insurance	26
Access to primary care	24
Mental health	49
Oral health	41
Educational and community-based programs	29
Diabetes	26
Injury and violence prevention	26
Nutrition and overweight	21
Public health infrastructure	21
Tobacco	21
Maternal, infant, and child health	18
Occupational safety and health	18
Cancer	15
Environmental health	15
Heart disease and stroke	15

Data from Gamm LD, Hutchison L, Dabney RJ, Dorsey AM, editors: *Rural Health People 2010: A companion document to Healthy People 2010* (vols 1–3). College Station, TX, 2003, The Texas A&M University System Health Science Center, School of Rural Public Health, Southwest Rural Health Research Center.

Research questions directed toward improving health may be suggested for any of the *Healthy People 2020* objectives, but may have the greatest potential to address salient rural trends if they relate to issues of access to care, mental health, oral health, educational and community-based programs, diabetes, or injury and violence prevention. Additionally, investigators may want to consider how these established rural priorities may be consistent or different within specific populations of concern. Because availability of surveillance data are often limited as researchers concern themselves with increasingly smaller populations (e.g., from state to county), efforts to gather additional primary data may be needed to set research priorities for improvements to health.

Information Technology in Rural Communities

As the distribution of technology expands across rural populations, more research is needed to examine the impacts of readily accessible information on both rural citizens and the health care delivery system. Rural patients are able to access specialty services such as radiological or dermatological examinations through telemedicine, and rural people are increasingly taking advantage of the World Wide Web to access information to make health decisions. The federal government has tied health care reimbursement to compliance with requirements of hospitals and physician practices to implement an electronic health record. Federal efforts directed toward disaster and terrorism preparedness have strengthened rural technological

infrastructure so that communication pathways remain open during times of need. Just as patients access health care services from isolation, rural citizens are accessing health education through distance programs both for continuing education for entry-level and advanced degree programs in various health sciences. The need to address new research questions has grown alongside rapid expansion of information technology (IT), and questions abound relating to the application and evaluation of technology for improving systems of care and care outcomes (see the Research Highlights box).

Telehealth (or telemonitoring) is the use of telecommunications and IT to provide access to health assessments, diagnosis, intervention, consultation, supervision, and information across distance. Telehealth includes technologies such as interactive video (e.g., teleconsultation, teleradiology), patient monitoring (e.g., home monitoring, electronic intensive care unit [ICU]), and medication order review (Frontier Community Health Integration Project, Telehealth, 2014).

Questions related to IT for public health in rural areas include:

- What is the role of telehealth in public health?
- What impact is distance learning having on the skills of rural public health professionals?
- What are the costs and infrastructure implications of ensuring access to IT in rural areas?
- How can IT be used to fill the gaps in epidemiology and surveillance capacity in rural health departments?

RESEARCH HIGHLIGHTS

Defining Rural Areas: Old and New Classifications

Old System (Before Census 2000)

Metropolitan (metro) areas:

- Cities of 50,000 or more residents *or*
- Urbanized areas of 50,000 or more residents and total area population of 100,000 or more

Nonmetropolitan (nonmetro) areas:

- All counties not classified as metropolitan

New Core-Based System (Starting with Census 2000)

Metropolitan (metro) areas:

- Central counties with 50,000 or more residents, regardless of total area population; includes outlying counties with 25% or more of the employed population commuting daily

Micropolitan (micro) areas:

- Central counties with one or more urban clusters of 10,000–50,000 persons; includes outlying counties with 25% or more of the employed population commuting daily

Noncore areas:

- All counties not meeting the new "metro" or "micro" classification are classified as "outside core-based statistical areas."

Data from Slifkin RT, Randolph R, Ricketts TC: The changing metropolitan designation process and rural America, *J Rural Health* 20(1):1–6, 2004.

Performance Standards in Rural Public Health

The National Public Health Performance Standards Program (NPHPSP) was a collaborative effort, organized through the CDC, whose mission is to improve the quality of public health practice and the performance of local public health systems by providing and evaluating standards of performance.

The NPHPSP utilized the "10 Essential Public Health Services" to establish three assessment instruments that can be used by local and state public health systems for evaluation and improvement. Standards describe an optimal level of performance by public health systems, which include all public, private, and voluntary entities that contribute to activities directed toward public health in an assessment area. The assessment can be used to improve collaborations among key public health partners, educate participants about public health, strengthen the network of public health partners, identify strengths and weaknesses, and provide benchmarks for public health practice improvements (CDC, 2012a).

In 2012, the Public Health Act and Prevention and Public Health Fund were created as part of the Patient Protection and Affordable Care Act (Public Law 111-148). With this law and allocation of resources, the National Public Health Improvement Initiative—part of the CDC's larger effort to increase the performance management capacity of public health departments to ensure that public health goals are effectively and efficiently met—was born. The focal point of this work will be to strengthen the public health infrastructure so as to improve health outcomes. Research questions that need to be addressed in rural areas may focus on the extent to which state and local performance assessments outlined by NPHPSP have been carried out, as well as on the ability of rural public health systems to respond to needed changes to comprehensively address essential services. Additionally, rural areas may benefit from research examining resource constraints and the need to expand partnerships to address essential services that may be difficult to provide in isolated populations.

Leadership and Workforce Capacity for Rural Public Health

In 2003, the NAM published results of a project intended to improve our understanding of what is needed to prepare the public health workforce for the twenty-first century (Gebbie et al., 2003). Workforce capacity challenges cited by the NAM report include globalization, which increases travel and allows for distribution of emerging and reemerging diseases (e.g., HIV and AIDS, tuberculosis, hepatitis B, malaria, cholera, diphtheria, and Ebola virus); advances in scientific and medical technologies that challenge the public health workforce in areas of ethics, data security, and communication; and demographic transformations that require new skills and services as our population ages and becomes more diverse.

The CDC's Public Health Improvement Initiative (CDC, 2012b) aims to accelerate public health accreditation readiness activities; to provide additional support for performance management and improvement practices; and to develop, identify, and disseminate innovative and evidence-based policies and practices. This program supports the *Healthy People 2020* focus area of addressing public health infrastructure. Cross-jurisdictional (state, local, tribal, territorial, regional, community, and border) collaboration is encouraged to increase the impact of limited resources, to improve efficiency, and to leverage other related health reform efforts and projects. This initiative suggests that

an initial strategy should be to monitor workforce composition and conduct research to validate methodology for public health worker enumeration.

Interaction and Integration of Community Health Systems, Managed Care, and Public Health

The evolution of managed care into rural environments has limited the safety-net role of some local health departments to provide primary care by preventing fee-for-service reimbursement and contracting care to networks of providers or organizations. This statement is especially true for Medicaid managed care, which serves the same population of people who traditionally receive primary care services through local public health departments. As Hurley et al. (2002) note, Medicaid's importance for rural areas is likely to grow as broader health care developments, such as declining inpatient use of rural hospitals and reductions in Medicare reimbursement, provoke more interest in using the Medicaid system to support threatened rural infrastructure.

Consequently, the administration of the Medicaid program will increasingly seek the cost savings promised by managed care, and the role of rural public health departments may increasingly narrow into areas that are currently without any type of reimbursement. For this reason, Berkowitz et al. (2002) argue that finding ways to integrate public health into rural primary care at the community level will become more and more important. Many questions will have to be answered by additional research. What factors are associated with successful integration of public health and managed care in rural environments? What capacity do rural health departments have for contracting arrangements with MCOs? What are the effects of local public health and managed care contracts on direct provision of services?

NEW MODELS OF HEALTH CARE DELIVERY FOR RURAL AREAS

In recent years, several innovative pilot projects have been implemented to address care delivery in rural areas. The Frontier Community Health Integration Project, authorized by the Public Health Service Act and guided by the Medicare Improvements to Patients and Provider Act of 2008, is testing new models of care delivery to frontier areas in critical access hospitals and through the use of telemedicine. Four frontier states have been identified: Alaska, Montana, North Dakota, and Wyoming. A frontier area is defined as a county with six or fewer people in a square mile and a daily hospital census of five or less (Frontier Community Health Integration Project, 2014.). The telehealth application can include home monitoring and electronic ICU services; other applications include remote medication review by a pharmacist and consultation by a specialist at a distance. Payment for these services varies by third-party payer, and distinct challenges in credentialing providers and leveraging technology exist.

ⓔ EVOLVE WEBSITE

http://evolve.elsevier.com/Nies/community
- NCLEX Review Questions
- Case Studies

BIBLIOGRAPHY

Agency for Healthcare Research and Quality: *Patient Centered Medical Home Resource Center*. Available to: https://pcmh.ahrq. gov/page/defining-pcmh.

Agency for Healthcare Research and Quality: *Coordinating Care in the Medical Neighborhood: Critical components and Available Mechanisms*, 2011. Downloaded March 25, 2017 from https://pcmh.ahrq. gov/sites/default/files/attachments/coordinating-care-in-the-medical-neighborhood-white-paper.pdf.

Aldwin C, Gilmer D: *Health, Illness, and Optimal Aging: biological and Psychosocial Perspectives*, ed 2, New York, Springer Publishing.

American Association of Colleges of Nursing: *Joint Statement on Academic Progression for Nursing Students and Graduates,* 2012. Downloaded March 25, 2017 from http://www.aacn.nche.edu/ aacn-publications/position/joint-statement-academic-progression.

American Academy of Family Practitioners: *Rural practice, keeping physicians in (position paper)*. Available from: <http://www. aafp.org/online/en/home/policy/policies/r/ruralpracticekeep.html>.

Alker J, Mancini T, Heberlein M: *Uninsured children 2009-2011: charting the nation's progress*. Available from: <http://ccf. georgetown.edu/wp-content/uploads/2012/10/Uninsured-Children-2009-2011.pdf>.

Allender JA, Rector C, Warner KD: *Community health nursing: promoting and protecting the public's health*, 7th ed, Philadelphia, 2010, Lippincott Williams & Wilkins.

Alterman T, Steege A, Petersen M, et al.: Ethnic, racial, and gender variations in health among farm operators in the United States, *Ann Epidemiol* 18(3):179–186, 2008.

American Academy of family practitioners: *Rural Practice, keeping physicians (position paper)*, 2014. Available from: <http://www. aafp.org/about/policies/all/rural-practice-paper.html>.

Artnak K, McGraw R, Stanley V: Health care accessibility for chronic illness management and end-of-life care: a view from rural America, *J Law, Med & Ethics* 39(2):140–155, 2011.

Bailey J: *The Top 10 rural issues for health care reform: a series examining health care in rural America*. Available from: <http:// files.cfra.org/pdf/Ten-Rural-Issues-for-Health-Care-Reform.pdf>.

Baldwin LM, Hollow WB, Casey S, et al.: Access to specialty health care for rural American Indians in two states, *Rural Health* 24(3):269–278, 2008.

Barnett JC, Vornovitsky MS: *Health Insurance Coverage 2015*, 2016. Available from: https://www.census.gov/content/dam/Census/ library/publications/2016/demo/p60-257.pdf.

Becker G, Gates RJ, Newsom E, et al.: Self-care among chronically ill African Americans: culture, health disparities, and health insurance status, *Am J Public Health* 94(12):2066–2073, 2004.

Berkowitz B, Ivory J, Morris T: Rural public health: policy and research opportunities, *J Rural Health* 18(Suppl):186–196, 2002.

Bigbee J: The uniqueness of rural nursing, *Nurs Clin North Am* 28:131–144, 1993.

Bishaw A: *Poverty 2010 and 2011, American Community Service Briefs*, 2012. Available from: <http://www.census.gov/prod/ 2012pubs/acsbr11-01.pdf>.

Bishop B: *Poverty rate jumps in rural America*, 2009. Available from: <http://www.dailyyonder.com/poverty-rate-jumps-rural-america/2009/11/23/2466>.

Blanchard BW: Guide to Emergency Management and Related Terms, Definitions, Concepts, Acronyms, Organizations, Programs, Guidance, Executive Orders, and Legislation: A Tutorial on Emergency Management, Broadly Defined, Past and Present, October 22, 2018. Available from: https://training.fema.gov/ hiedu/docs/terms%20and%20definitions/terms%20and% 20definitions.pdf.

Bolin J, Gamm LG: Access to quality health services in rural areas: insurance. In *Rural Healthy People 2010: a Companion Document to Healthy People*, Vol. 1. College Station, TX, 2010, The Texas A&M University System Health Science Center, School of Rural Public Health, Southwest Rural Health Research Center.

Bolin J, Bellamy G: *Rural Healthy People 2020* (n.d.) Available from: https://sph.tamhsc.edu/srhrc/docs/rhp2020.pdf.

Branas CC, MacKenzie E, Williams JC, et al.: Access to trauma centers in the United States, *JAMA* 293(21):2626–2633, 2005.

Branas CC, Nance MD, Elliott MR, et al.: Urban-rural shifts in intentional firearm death: different causes, same results, *Am J Public Health* 94(10):1750-1755, 2004.

Braum S: *Where do states stand on private coverage of telemedicine?* 2013. Available from: <http://medcitynews.com/2013/05/where-do-states-stand-on-private-coverage-of-telemedicine-check-out-this-map/>.

Braveman P: Social conditions, health equity, and human rights, *Health Hum Rights* 12(2):31–48, 2010.

Bryant D: *Challenges of rural emergency management*, Homeland1 News, 2009. Available from: <http://www.home-land1.com/print.asp?act=print&vid=480917>.

Bureau of Health Professions: *Changing demographics: implications for physicians, nurses, and other health workers*. Available from: <ftp://ftp.hrsa.gov/bhpr/nationalcenter/changedemo.pdf>.

Bureau of Labor Statistics: *Number of Fatal Work Injuries 1992-2011, 2012a*. Available from: <http://www.bls.gov/iif/oshwc/ cfoi/cfch0010.pdf>.

Bureau of Labor Statistics: *National Census of Fatal Occupational Injuries in 2012 (Preliminary Results)*, 2012b. Available from: <http://www.bls.gov/news.release/pdf/cfoi.pdf>.

Bureau of Primary Health Professions, 2016. Available from: https:// bphc.hrsa.gov/.

Bureau of Primary Health Care: *Migrant and seasonal farmworker enumeration profiles study*. Available from: <http://bphc.hrsa. gov/migrant/Enumeration/EnumerationStudy.htm>.

Canadian Association for Parish Nursing Ministry: *Definition of parish nurses*. Available at: http://capnm.ca/fact_sheet.htm.

Castillo G, Alexander J: Injury and violence prevention in rural areas. In Gamm L, Hutchison L, editors: *Rural Healthy People 2010: a companion document to Healthy People*, College Station, TX, 2010, The Texas A&M University System Health Science Center, School of Rural Public Health, Southwest Rural Health Research Center. <www.srph.tamhsc.edu/ centers/rhp2010>.

Catholic Health Association of the United States: Improving the Lives of Older Adults through Faith Community Partnerships: Healing Body, 2016. Mind and Spirit.

Cawthorne A: The Not-So-Golden Years Confronting Elderly Poverty and Improving Seniors' Economic Security, 2010. Available from: <http://www.americanprogress.org/wp-content/uploads/issues/ 2010/09/pdf/not_so_golden_years.pdf>.

Centers for Disease Control: *Health Disparities and Inequalities, Equity Health-Minority Health*. <https://www.cdc.gov/minority-health/chdireport.html>.

Centers for Disease Control: *Rural Americans at higher risk of death from five leading causes*. Available from: https://www.cdc.gov/ media/releases/2017/p0112-rural-death-risk.html.

Centers for Disease Control and Prevention: *Health, United States, 2007, with chartbook of trends in the health of Americans.* Available from: <http://www.cdc.gov/nchs/data/hus/hus07.pdf>.

Centers for Disease Control and Prevention: *Health, United States, 2008, with chartbook on trends in the health of Americans.* Available from: <http://www.cdc.gov/nchs/data/hus/hus08.pdf>.

Centers for Disease Control and Prevention: *Health, United States, 2011, with a special feature on socioeconomic status and health.* Available from: <http://www.cdc.gov/nchs/data/hus/hus11.pdf#091>.

Centers for Disease Control and Prevention: *Behind international rankings of infant mortality: how the United States compares with Europe (NCHS Brief no. 23),* 2009a. Available from: <http://www.cdc.gov/nchs/data/databriefs/db23.htm>.

Centers for Disease Control and Prevention: *Mammography use.* Retrieved from: <http://www.cdc.gov/nchs/data/health_policy/mammography.pdf>.

Centers for Disease Control and Prevention: *National Public Health Performance Standards Program.* Available from: <http://www.cdc.gov/nphpsp/index.html>.

Centers for Disease Control and Prevention: *PPHF National Public Health Improvement Initiative.* Available from: <http://www.cfda.gov/?s=program&mode=form&tab=step1&id=64d3ba3bc-07bea2d79d07bf7650ba066>.

Centers for Disease Control and Prevention: *Injury Center. Violence Prevention. National suicide statistics at a glance: trends in suicide rates among persons ages 10 years and older, by sex, United States, 1991–2009,* 2013. Available from: <http://www.cdc.gov/violenceprevention/suicide/statistics/trends01.html>.

Centers for Disease Control and Prevention: *National Center for Health Statistics: HHS issues report on community health in rural, urban areas (HHS News),* 2001. Available from: <http://www.cdc.gov/nchs/pressroom/01news/hus01.html>.

Centers for Disease Control and Prevention: *NIOSH Program Portfolio. Occupational health disparities: occupational safety and health risks.* Available from: <http://www.cdc.gov/niosh/programs/ohd/risks.html>.

Coen Buckwalter K, Lindsey Davis L, Wakefield BJ, et al.: Telehealth for elders and their caregivers in rural communities, *Fam Commun Health* 25(3):31–40, 2002.

Cutler D, Lleras-Muney A: *NBER Working Paper Series, Education and Health Evaluating health theories and evidence,* 2006. Available from: <http://www.nber.org/papers/w12352.pdf?new_window=1>.

Daniels N, Kennedy BP, Kawachi I: Why justice is good for our health: the social determinants of health inequalities, *Daedalus* 128:215–251, 1999.

DeHaven M, Hunter I, Wilder L, et al.: Health programs in faith-based organizations: are they effective? *Am Public Health* 94(6):1030–1036, 2004.

DeNavas-Walt C, Proctor B, Smith J: *Income, poverty and health insurance coverage in the United States in 2011.* Available from: http://www.census.gov/prod/2012pubs/p60-243.pdf.

Elliott MR, Ginsburg KR, Winston FK: Unlicensed teenaged drivers: who are they, and how do they behave when they are behind the wheel? *Pediatrics* 122(5):994–1000, 2008. Farm Worker Fund. *Innovative outreach practices report.* Available from: http://www.farmworkerhealth.org/docs/IOPR2006.pdf.

Farrigan T, Parker T: *The concenteration of poverty is a growing rural problem.* Available from: <http://www.ers.usda.gov/amber-waves/2012-december/concentration-of-poverty.aspx>.

Federal Register Annual Update of the HHS Poverty Guidelines. Available from: https://www.federalregister.gov/documents/2017/01/31/2017-02076/annual-update-of-the-hhs-poverty-guidelines.

Ferrer RL: Pursuing equity: contact with primary care and specialist clinicians by demographics, insurance, and health status, *Ann Fam Med* 5(6):492–502, 2007.

Frontier community health integration project: *White Paper #2 Case study on Frontier Telehealth,* 2014. Available from: <http://www.raconline.org/new-approaches/pdf/case-study-on-frontier-telehealth.pdf>.

Gamm LD, Hutchison L: Rural Healthy People 2010: evolving interactive practice, *Am J Public Health* 94(10):1711–1712, 2004. Also available from: <http://www.pubmedcentral.nih.gov/articlerender.fcgi?artid=1448522>.

Gebbie K, Rosenstock L, Hernandez L, et al.: *Who will keep the public healthy? Educating public health professionals for the 21st century.* Washington, DC, 2003, The National Academies Press.

Gordon D: *Provider Shortage Threatens Rural Primary Care,* 2014. Available from: http://www.beckershospitalreview.com/hospital-physician-relationships/provider-shortage-threatens-rural-primary.html.

Hale NL: *"Rural Public Health Systems: Challenges and Opportunities for Improving Population Health,"* AcademyHealth. October 2015. Downloaded on March 25, 2017 at http://www.academyhealth.org/files/AH_Rural%20Health%20brief%20final2.pdf.

Hanrahan N, Hartley D: Employment of advanced-practice psychiatric nurses to stem rural mental health workforce shortages, *Psychiatr Serv* 59(1):109–111, 2008.

Health Resources and Services Administration: *Rural health research programs.* https://www.hrsa.gov/ruralhealth/research/.

HealthyPeople.gov: Home. Available from: <http://www.healthypeople.gov/2020/default.aspx>.

Healthy People 2020, *Disparities,* 2010. Available from: <http://www.healthypeople.gov/2020/about/DisparitiesAbout.aspx>.

Holder KA, Fields A, Lofquist D: *Rurality Matters,* 2016. Available from: https://www.census.gov/newsroom/blogs/random-samplings/2016/12/rurality_matters.html.

Hoyer DL, Kung HC, Smith BL: *Deaths: preliminary data for 2003 (National Vital Statistics Report vol. 53 no. 15).* Hyattsville, MD, National Center for Health Statistics.

HRSA, *Medicare rural hospital flexibility grant program,* n.d. Available from: <http://www.hrsa.gov/ruralhealth/about/hospitalstate/medicareflexibility_.html>.

Hsia R, Shen Y: Possible geographical barriers to trauma center access for vulnerable patients in the United States: an analysis of urban and rural communities, *Arch Surg* 146(1):46–52, 2011. <https://doi.org/10.1001/archsurg.2010.299>.

Hurley RE, Crawford H, Praeger S: Medicaid and rural health care, *J Rural Health* 18 (Suppl):164–175, 2002.

Hutchison L, Blakely C: Substance abuse: trends in rural areas. In *Rural People 2010.* Available from: <http://sph.tamhsc.edu/centers/rhp2010/11Volume2substanceabuse.pdf>.

Institute of Medicine: *Quality through collaboration: the future of rural health care,* Washington, DC, 2005, National Academy Press.

Johnson AO, Mink MD, Harun N, et al.: Violence and drug use in rural teens: national Prevalence estimates from the 2003 youth risk behavior survey, *J School Health* 10(78):554–561, 2008.

Jones C, William K, Parker T: Population dynamics are changing the profile of rural areas, *Amber Waves* 5(2):30–35, 2007.

Jones CA, Parker TS, Ahearn M, et al.: *Health status and health care access of farm and rural populations (ERS Report Summary)*, 2009. Available from: <http://www.ers.usda.gov/media/155449/eib57_reportsummary_1_.pdf>.

Kaiser Family Foundation: *State health facts.* Available from: <http://www.statehealthfacts.org/>.

Kandel W: *Rural Hispanics at a glance (Economic Information Bulletin No. EIB-8 2005)*, 2003 Available from: <http://www.ers.usda.gov/publications/eib8/>.

Kosman, Susan: *Nurse Residencies: Building a Better Future for patients and Nurses*, 2011. Available at: http://www.rwjf.org/en/culture-of-health/2011/10/nurse-residencies-building-a-better-future-for-patients-and-nurses.html.

Kulbok P, Thatcher E, Park E, et al.: Evolving public health nursing roles: focus on community participatory health promotion and prevention, *Online J Issues in Nurs* 17(2), 2012. Available from: <http://www.nursingworld.org/MainMenuCategories/ANAMarketplace/ANAPeriodicals/OJIN/TableofContents/Vol-17-2012/No2-May-2012/Evolving-Public-Health-Nursing-Roles.html>.

Lee H, Winters C: Testing rural nursing theory: perceptions and needs of service providers, *Online J Rural Nurs Health Care* 4(1):51–63, 2004. Available from: <http://www.rno.org/journal/issues/Vol-4,/issue-1/Lee_article.htm>.

Levy J: *In US, uninsured rate drops to 12.9%*, 2015. Available from: http://www.gallup.com/poll/180425/uninsured-rate-sinks.aspx.

Malecki E: Digital development in rural areas: potentials and pitfalls, *J Rural Studies* 9(2):201–214, 2003.

Mathews T, MacDorman M: Infant mortality statistics from the period linked birth/infant death data set, *Natl Vital Stat Rep* 62(8):2010, 2013.

McClelland S, Steel S, Marsh L, et al.: *Dimensions in health: a sample of rural and global health issues*, 2010. Available from: http://hdl.handle.net/1928/11329.

Medicaid.gov: *Telemedicine.* Available from: <http://www.medicaid.gov/Medicaid-CHIP-Program-Information/By-Topics/Delivery-Systems/Telemedicine.html>.

Miller, Geneva. *Lay Caregivers.* Theworldlink.com. Posted article May 26, 2015. Available at: http://theworldlink.com/lifestyles/thrive/lay-caregivers-hb/article_bd2d484e-8f27-5783-93d3-5d8752186159.html.

Molanari D, Jaiswal A, Hollinger-Forrest T: Rural Nurses: lifestyle Preferences and Education Perceptions, *Online J Rural Nurs Health Care* 11(2):16–26, 2011. Available from: <http://rnojournal.binghamton.edu/index.php/RNO/article/view/27>.

National Advisory Committee on Rural Health and Human Services: *Rural Implications of Changes to the Medicare Hospice Benefit: A Policy Brief* (August, 2013). Available at: https://www.hrsa.gov/advisorycommittees/rural/publications/nacrhhshospicebrief.pdf.

National Center for Education Statistics: Available from: https://nces.ed.gov/programs/coe/indicator_tla.asp.

National Center for Farmworker Health: *Farmworker occupational health and safety fact sheet.* Available from: <http://www.ncfh.org/docs/fs-Occ%20Health.pdf>.

National Conference of State Legislatures: *Closing the Gaps in the Rural Primary Care Workforce.* Available from: http://www.ncsl.org/research/health/closing-the-gaps-in-the-rural-primary-care-workfor.aspx.

National Institute for Occupational Safety and Health (NIOSH): *Agricultural Safety.* Available from: https://www.cdc.gov/niosh/topics/aginjury/default.html.

National Rural Health Association: *Mental health in rural America: what's different about rural healthcare*, n.d. Available from: <http://www.ruralhealthweb.org/go/left/about-rural-health/what-s-different-about-rural-health-care>.

National Rural Healthcare Association: *Burrows, Elizabeth, Suh Ryung, and Hamann,* Danielle. 2012. National Rural Healthcare Association Policy Brief. Available from: https://www.ruralhealthweb.org/getattachment/Advocate/Policy-Documents/HealthCareWorkforceDistributionandShortageJanuary2012.pdf.aspx?lang=en-US.

National Rural Health Association: *what's different about rural health care?* 2014. Available from: <http://www.ruralhealthweb.org/go/left/a bout-rural-health/what-s-different-about-rural-health-care>.

Newkirk V: 2014. Available from: http://kff.org/uninsured/issue-brief/the-affordable-care-act-and-insurance-coverage-in-rural-areas/.

North Dakota State University: *Center for Rural Health.* https://ruralhealth.und.edu/what-we-do/research.

Office of Management and Budget: *Metropolitan and micropolitan statistical areas main.* Available from: <http://www.census.gov/population/www/metroareas/metroarea.html>.

Office of Minority Health: *Infant mortality and African Americans.* Available from: <http://minorityhealth.hhs.gov/templates/content.aspx?ID=3021>.

Patterson D: Parish nurse scope and standards of practice, *American Nurses Today* 5(12), 2010. Available at: https://www.american-nursetoday.com/parish-nursing-reclaiming-the-spiritual-dimensions-of-care-2/. Accessed February 13, 2018.

Peek-Asa C, Zwerling C, Stallones L: Acute traumatic injuries in rural populations, *Am J Public Health* 94(10):1689–1693, 2004.

Rasheed MN, Rasheed JM: Rural African American older adults and the black helping tradition, *J Gerontol Social Work* 41:137–150, 2003.

Reschovsky JD, Staiti A: Access and quality of medical care in urban and rural areas: does rural America lag behind? *Health Affairs* 24(4):1128–1139, 2005.

Ricketts TC: Education of physician assistants, nurse midwives, and nurse practitioners for rural practice, *J Rural Health* 4(6):537–543, 2008.

Robinson LR, Holbrook JR, Bitsko RH, et al.: Differences in health care, family, and community factors associated with mental, behavioral, and developmental disorders among children aged 2–8 years in rural and urban areas—United States, 2011–2012, *MMWR Surveill Summ* 66(No. SS-8):1–11, 2017. DOI: https://doi.org/10.15585/mmwr.ss6608a1.

Rosenblatt RA, Casey S, Richardson M: Rural-urban differences in the public health workforce: local health departments in 3 Western states, *Am J Public Health* 92(7):1102–1105, 2002.

Rosenthal K: What rural nursing stories are you living? *Online J Rural Nurs Health Care* 5(1), 2005. Available from: <http://www.rno.org/journal/issues/Vol-5/issue-1/Rosenthal_article.htm>.

Rural Assistance Center: *What is rural?* n.d. Available from: <http://www.raconline.org/topics/what-is-rural/>.

Rural Information Center Health Service: *Rural health statistics.* Available from: www.nal.usda.gov/ric/.

Rural Health Information Hub: *Rural Health Disparities,* 2014. Available from: https://www.ruralhealthinfo.org/topics/rural-health-disparities.

Sanford JT, Townsend-Rocchiccioli J: The perceived health of rural caregivers, *Geriatr Nurs* 75(3):145–148, 2004.

Scharff KE: The distinctive nature and scope of rural nursing practice: philosophical bases. In Lee HJ, editor: *Conceptual basis for rural nursing*, New York, 1998, Springer.

Sigma Theta Tau International: *Facts on the nursing shortage*, n.d. Available from: <http://www.nursingsociety.org/MEDIA/Pages/shortage.aspx>.

Slifkin RT, Randolph R, Ricketts TC: The changing metropolitan designation process and rural America, *J Rural Health* 20(1):1–6, 2004.

Sorrell J: Ethics: the patient protection and affordable care act: ethical perspectives in 21st century health care, *Online J Issues Nurs* 18(1), November 09, 2012. Available from: http://www.nursingworld.org/MainMenuCategories/ANAMarketplace/ANAPeriodicals/OJIN/Columns/Ethics/Patient-Protection-and-Affordable-Care-Act-Ethical-Perspectives.html.

The Westberg Institute: *Definition of parish nurses*. Available at: http://www.parishnurses.org/.

Thorngren J: Rural mental health: a qualitative inquiry, *J Rural Commun Psychol* E6(2):1–6, 2003. Available from: <http://muwww-new.marshall.edu/jrcp//JRCP_E6_2_Thorngren.htm>.

Thrall T: Rural recruitment, *Hosp Health Netw* 81(12):45–48, 2007.

University of Minnesota: *Rural Health Research Center*. http://rhrc.umn.edu/.

U.S. Census Bureau: *Overview of Race and Hispanic Origin: 2010; Census Briefs*. Available from: <http://www.census.gov/prod/cen2010/briefs/c2010br-02.pdf>.

U.S. Census Bureau: *Income, poverty, and health insurance coverage in the United States*, 2011a. Available from: <http://www.census.gov/hhes/www/poverty/data/incpovhlth/2011/index.html>.

U.S. Census Bureau: *Income, poverty and health insurance coverage in the United States*, 2011b; correction to Table A. Available from: <http://www.census.gov/newsroom/releases/archives/income_wealth/cb12-172.html>.

U.S. Census Bureau, U.S. Census Bureau: *Small area income and poverty estimates*. Available from: <http://www.census.gov/did/www/saipe/>.

U.S. Census Bureau: *Metropolitan and Micropolitan. Metropolitan and Micropolitan Statistical Areas Main*. Available from: <https://www.census.gov/population/metro/>.

U.S. Department of Agriculture: *State Fact Sheets: United States*, Updated July 11, 2011. Available from: www.ers.usda.gov/StateFacts.US.HTM.

U.S. Department of Agriculture Economic Research Service: *Rural Economy and Population: Population Overview*. https://www.ers.usda.gov/topics/rural-economy-population/population-migration/.

U.S. Department of Agriculture Economic Research Service: *Poverty Overview*. Available from: https://www.ers.usda.gov/topics/rural-economy-population/rural-poverty-well-being/poverty-overview/.

Department of Agriculture: *Population and Migration Overview*. https://www.ers.usda.gov/topics/rural-economy-population/population-migration/- -p. 4.

U.S. Department of Agriculture; Economic Research Service: *Measuring what is rural*. Available from: <http://www.ers.usda.gov/Briefing/rurality/Whatisrural>.

U.S. Department of Agriculture: *Economic Research Service*. Rural America at a Glance: 2016 Edition. Available from: https://www.ers.usda.gov/webdocs/publications/eib162/eib-162.pdf?v=42684.

U.S. Department of Agriculture; Economic Research Service: *Rural income, poverty, and welfare: poverty geography*. Available from: <http://webarchives.cdlib.org/sw1rf5mh0k/http://www.ers.usda.gov/Briefing/IncomePovertyWelfare/PovertyGeography.htm>.

U.S. Department of Agriculture; Economic Research Service: *Employment & education: rural education*. Available from: <http://www.ers.usda.gov/topics/rural-economy-population/employment-education/rural-education.aspx>.

U.S. Department of Agriculture Economic Research Service: *Immigration and the Rural Workforce*. Available from: https://www.ers.usda.gov/topics/in-the-news/immigration-and-the-rural-workforce.aspx#Hispanic.

U.S. Department of Agriculture, Economic Research Service: *Rural economy & population*. Available from: <http://www.ers.usda.gov/Emphases/Rural/>.

U.S. Department of Agriculture; Economic Research Service: *Rural income, poverty, and welfare: poverty demographics*. Available from: <http://webarchives.cdlib.org/sw1rf5mh0k/http://www.ers.usda.gov/Briefing/IncomePovertyWelfare/PovertyDemographics.htm>.

U.S. Department of Agriculture; Economic Research Service: *Rural labor and education: farm labor*. Available from: <http://www.ers.usda.gov/topics/rural-economy-population/employment-education/rural-education.aspx>.

U.S. Department of Agriculture; Economic Research Service: *The concentration of poverty is a growing rural problem*. Available from: <http://www.ers.usda.gov/amber-waves/2012-december/concentration-of-poverty.aspx>.

U.S. Department of Agriculture; Economic Research Service: *Farm labor: background*. Available from: <http://www.ers.usda.gov/topics/farm-economy/farm-labor/background.aspx>.

U.S. Department of Agriculture; Economic Research Service: *Immigration and the Rural Workforce*, 2013c. Available from: <http://www.ers.usda.gov/topics/in-the-news/immigration-and-the-rural-workforce.aspx#.U12qyKLwnWc>.

U.S Department of Agriculture; Economic Research Service: *Farm Workers Background*, 2013d. Available from: <http://www.ers.usda.gov/topics/farm-economy/farm-labor/background.aspx>.

U.S. Department of Agriculture, Economic Research Service: *Rural poverty & well-being: Geography of Poverty*. Available from: <http://www.ers.usda.gov/topics/rural-economy-population/rural-poverty-well-being/geography-of-poverty.aspx>.

U.S. Department of Agriculture; National Institute of Food and Agriculture: *Agricultural systems overview*. Available from: https://www.ers.usda.gov/data-products/ag-and-food-statistics-charting-the-essentials/ag-and-food-sectors-and-the-economy.aspx.

U.S. Department of Health and Human Services; Health Resources and Services Administration: *Emergency medical services in frontier areas: volunteer community organizations*. Available from: <ftp://ftp.hrsa.gov/ruralhealth/FrontierEMS.pdf>.

U.S. Department of Health and Human Services: *Office of Disease Prevention and Health Promotion*. Available from: <http://www.healthypeople.gov/>.

U.S. Department of Health and Human Services; Health Resources and Services Administration, Maternal and Child Health Bureau: *The health and well-being of children in rural areas: a portrait of the nation, 2011-2012*, Rockville, MD, 2015, U.S. Department of Health and Human Services.

van Exel J, de Graaf G, Brouwer W: Give me a break! Informal caregiver attitudes towards respite care, *Health Policy* 88(1):73–87, 2008.

Vernig B, Moscovice I, Durham S, et al.: Do rural elders have limited access to medicare hospice services, *J Am Geriat Soc* 52(5):731–735, 2004.

Weinert C, Long KA: Understanding the health care needs of rural families, *Fam Relat* 36:450–455, 1987.

Weisbecker A: *Local health departments hit hard by budget woes*. Food Safety News (May 6, 2010). Available from: <http://www.foodsafetynews.com/2010/05/local-health-departments-hit-hard-by-budget-woes/>.

Williams M, Andrews J, Zanni K, et al.: Rural nursing: searching for the state of the science, *Online J Rural Nurs Health Care* 2(12): 102–117, 2012.

Zahner SJ, Corrado SM: Local health department partnerships with faith-based organizations, *J Public Health Manag Pract* 10(3): 258–265, 2004.

Ziller E, Lenardson J, Coburn A: Health care access and use among the rural uninsured, *J Health Care Poor Underserved* 23(3): 1327–1345, 2012.

25

Populations Affected by Mental Illness

Meredith Troutman-Jordan*

OUTLINE

OBJECTIVES

Upon completion of this chapter, the reader will be able to do the following:

1. Explain the concept of mental health and discuss the importance of mental health promotion in special populations.
2. Discuss the historical context for contemporary community-based mental health care.
3. Describe biological, social, and political factors associated with mental illness.
4. Illustrate the impact of natural and human-made disasters on mental health.
5. Describe some of the most common types of mental illnesses encountered in community settings.
6. Discuss the problem of suicide and recognize suicide warning signs.
7. Describe different types of evidence-based treatment for mental disorders, including use of psychotropic medications, community case management, and crisis intervention.
8. Describe the role of mental health nurses in the community.

KEY TERMS

2008 Mental Health Parity and Addiction Equity Act
Affordable Care Act (ACA)
Agoraphobia
anorexia nervosa
anosognosia
anxiety disorders
Assertive Community Treatment
attention deficit disorder
attention deficit/hyperactivity disorder
bipolar disorder
bulimia nervosa

case management
Community Mental Health Centers Act
co-occurring
comorbidity
Crisis Intervention Team
Deinstitutionalization
Depression
generalized anxiety disorder
major depression
mental health
mental health consumer

mental illness
obsessive-compulsive disorder
panic disorder
phobia
posttraumatic stress disorder
psychotropic/psychotherapeutic medications
schizophrenia
severe emotional disorder
severe mental illness
stigma

---

* The author would like to acknowledge the contribution of Kim Jardine-Dickerson, who wrote this chapter for the previous edition.

Mental health refers to the absence of mental disorders and includes emotional, psychological, and social well-being. It affects how we think, feel, and act (USDHHS, 2017). Mental illness consists of a major disturbance in an individual's thinking, feelings, or behavior that reflects a problem in mental function and causes distress or disability in social, work, or family activities (American Psychiatric Association, 2015). Other effects of mental illnesses include disruptions of daily function and lifestyles. This in turn may result in incapacitating personal, social, and occupational impairment, as well as premature death.

Mental health can be affected by numerous factors, such as biological and genetic vulnerabilities, acute or chronic physical dysfunction, environmental conditions, and stressors. Twenty-first-century community mental health care necessitates comprehensive mental health services, as well as inpatient, outpatient, home-based, school, and community-based programs for individuals, families, and populations at need. Threats such as vulnerability, poverty, homelessness, and the cost and limited accessibility of community mental health care can be pervasive. Whether populations live in rural or urban settings, people need mental health services. Community mental health care exists throughout all levels of prevention and can be designed to supplement and decrease the need for more costly inpatient mental health care delivered in hospitals. The mental health of a population is a reflection of a community as a whole, and community mental health professionals work with populations at risk such as homeless veterans, families, children, and the elderly.

About 25% of all U.S. adults have a mental illness (CDC, 2013b), and nearly 50% of U.S. adults will experience at least one mental illness during their lifetime (CDC, 2013c). Mental illness is a significant public health problem affecting not only the person with mental illness but also their family, friends, schoolmates, work colleagues, and others. Mental illness is associated with lower use of health care, reduced adherence to treatment therapies for chronic diseases, and higher risks of adverse health outcomes. The costs of mental health care can be estimated much the way that other health care costs are determined. There are significant studies that look at co-occurring mental illness and chronic diseases such as cardiovascular disease, diabetes, obesity, asthma, epilepsy, and cancer. There is increased co-occurring use of tobacco products and abuse of alcohol in mental illness populations (SAHMSA, 2016). Rates for intentional and unintentional injuries are higher among people with a mental illness than in the general population (van der Westhuizen et al., 2014). The knowledge that many mental illnesses can be managed successfully offers hope, and increasing access to and use of mental health treatment services could substantially reduce the associated morbidity. There are evidence-based practice (EBP) models consisting of community-based programs of intervention, education, and collaboration. Continual monitoring of mental illness is critical in providing appropriate organizations the data required to assess the need for mental and behavioral health services and to inform the population of the provision of those services.

The Affordable Care Act (ACA) builds on the 2008 Mental Health Parity and Addiction Equity Act (Substance Abuse and Mental Health Services Administration [SAHMSA], 2017) to extend federal parity protections to 62 million Americans with mental illnesses (USDHHS, Office of the Assistant Secretary for Planning and Evaluation, 2013). This parity law aims to ensure that when coverage for mental health and substance use conditions is provided, it is generally comparable to coverage for medical and surgical care. The ACA builds on the parity law by requiring coverage of mental health and substance use disorder benefits for millions of Americans who currently lack these benefits.

More than ever, community mental health nurses and interdisciplinary community teams face multiple challenges, such as complex patient comorbidity, lack of resources, competent mental health professional workforce and law enforcement, physical facility inadequacies, and the stigma of mental illness. The purpose of this chapter is to describe critical issues that affect the mental health of individuals, families, groups, and special populations and to explore the potential influences and advocacy issues that nurses can be involved with. The chapter depicts issues that affect individuals, families, groups, and populations and explores promising EBP programs and educational models utilized in community mental health.

Severe mental illness (SMI) is a diagnosis applied to any adult who currently or at any time during the past year has had a diagnosable mental, behavioral, or emotional disorder with moderate, severe, or extreme functional behavior in specific lifestyle areas. These mental health disorders of persons 18 years of age or older present emotional or behavioral functioning that is so impaired as to interfere substantially with their capacity to remain in the community without supportive treatment or services of a long-term or indefinite duration. SMI disability can be severe and persistent, associated with very high unemployment rates and disproportionate vulnerability, leading to homelessness, stigma, and victimization (Drake and Whitley, 2014). Support for various models of care is mixed. There is some evidence to suggest that intensive case management is effective in ameliorating many outcomes relevant to people with severe mental illness (Dieterich et al., 2017).

OVERVIEW AND HISTORY OF COMMUNITY MENTAL HEALTH: 1960 TO THE PRESENT DAY

The National Institute of Mental Health (NIMH) initially developed a Community Mental Health Center (CMHC) program in the 1960s. CMHCs were designed to provide comprehensive services for people with mental illness, locate these services closer to home, and provide an umbrella of integrated services for catchment areas of 125,000 to 250,000 people. These centers were intended to provide prevention, early treatment, and continuity of care in communities, promoting social integration of people with mental health needs. In 1963 President John F. Kennedy signed the Community Mental Health Centers Act (CMHCA), which resulted in deinstitutionalization of inpatients and the closing of mental institutions (NIMH, 2017). As a result, patients with SMI were released into communities too often without supporting community services. Further cuts in housing and other services throughout the 1980s resulted in a growing population of homeless individuals.

TABLE 25.1	Community Mental Health Movements from 1960 to the Present Day	
1960	Blue Ribbon Panel report *Action for Mental Health*	Recommendations for intensive care of acutely ill mental patients and community mental health clinics
1963	Community mental health clinics legislation	Community mental health centers in some urban communities
1960s	Deinstitutionalization	Discharged mentally ill from state hospitals, patients returned to communities with inadequate resources (i.e., finances, housing, health care, supportive employment)
1981	Mental Health Block Grant, as part of the Omnibus Reconciliation Act	States develop comprehensive mental health plans for persons with serious mental illness
1986	State Mental Health Planning Act	
1999	U.S. Surgeon General's Report on Mental Health	Acknowledging mental illness as a disease
2008	Mental Health Parity and Addiction Equity Act of 2008	Insurance coverage for mental health and substance use conditions
2010	Affordable Care Act	Builds on the Mental Health Parity and Addiction Equity Act of 2008 to extend federal parity protections to 62 million Americans

A landmark work—the 1999 *Surgeon General's Report on Mental Health*—defined mental health as a state of successful performance of mental function that results in productive activities, fulfilling relationships with others, and an ability to adapt to change and cope with adversity.

Table 25.1 provides a snapshot of the development of community-based mental health interventions from the 1960s to present day.

Deinstitutionalization Cause and Effects

Deinstitutionalization is the release of hospitalized inpatients, especially mental health patients, from an institution for placement and care in the community. Between 1955 and the mid-1980s, the number of patients in state facilities fell from 560,000 to 155,000 as patients were moved to the communities. The United States now has 37,679 state psychiatric beds, down about 13% since 2010 (Treatment Advocacy Center, 2016), even though national deinstitutionalization began gaining momentum in the 1950s (Shen and Snowden, 2014). This national movement was led by concerns over civil rights issues and the perceived conditions of the state institutions. These questions and concerns led courts throughout the country to limit involuntary institutionalization and to set minimum standards for care in institutions. Although there was great success in moving people out of mental hospitals, there were not sufficient community resources, such as adequate housing, supported employment, community mental health professional workforce, and other community mental health care services, available to meet the needs of patients coming back to communities. What followed was an evolution in the structure, practice, experiences, and purposes of community mental health care in the United States. The CMHCA of 1964 provided federal support for mental health services (National Council for Behavioral Health, 2015). The act supported measures to implement facilities to care for those who were mentally retarded and to construct CMHCs.

After passage of the act, individuals with serious mental illness were returned to families and communities who were often ill prepared to care for them, and funding did not follow the change in policy. Too many individuals with mental illness found themselves homeless, in shelters, or in prisons or jails. There was a critical need for more effective mental health treatment, improvements in the social welfare system, and provision of community support for this population, and shortly thereafter, the federal government recommended linking community mental health services with informal community support services to improve treatment options.

Present-Day Community Mental Health Reform

Mental health reform works toward monitoring federal legislation, administration activity, and public education initiatives. Such reform policies make community mental health a national priority and establish early access, recovery, and quality in mental health services as quality standards in our nation's mental health care delivery systems. There is unprecedented agreement in Congress on the need for mental health reform. Consequently, several bills, each of which the National Alliance for Mental Illness (NAMI) supports, have been introduced.

Currently pending measures include one measure in the House of Representatives (H.R. 2646), the Helping Families in Mental Health Crisis Act of 2015, and a second bill in the Senate (S. 2680), the Mental Health Reform Act of 2016. Both the Mental Health Reform Act of 2016 (S. 2680) and the Helping Families in Mental Health Crisis Act of 2015 (H.R.-2646) will improve integration and program coordination across federal agencies that serve people living with mental illness, improve integration of mental and physical health care, promote early intervention in the treatment of psychosis and use of evidence-based interventions, and provide resources for suicide prevention (NAMI, 2017b).

Medicalization of Mental Illness

The American Psychiatric Association's (APA) *Diagnostic and Statistical Manual of Mental Disorders, Fifth Edition* (DSM-5; APA, 2017a) has supported the medicalization of mental illness and has helped put mental disorders on parity with other diseases. The DSM-5 is an evidence-based manual that is useful to clinicians in helping them accurately diagnose mental disorders (APA, 2017a). With mental health parity, schizophrenia, depression, and substance abuse may be treated as vigorously as diabetes, heart disease, or cancer. There is hope that federal laws barring health insurers from imposing lower coverage limits on mental health services than they do on other medical treatments will change. The aim of the medicalization movement was to create an optimistic therapeutic ideology and to remove the stigma attached to mental illness by lessening perceptions of personal responsibility (Pattyn et al., 2013). Medicalization of mental illness involves a comprehensive perspective which recognizes biopsychosocial causal attributions and applies the disease view to facilitate treatment recommendations.

Brain Neuroimaging, Genetics, and Hope for New Treatments

Brain imaging scans, also called *neuroimaging scans,* are being used more and more to help detect and diagnose a number of medical disorders and illnesses. Brain scans alone, however, cannot be used to diagnose a mental disorder such as autism, anxiety, depression, schizophrenia, or bipolar disorder (Berretta et al., 2015). Currently, the main use of brain scans for mental disorders is in research studies to learn more about the disorders. In many instances, researchers use neuroimaging to study healthy brain development and the effects of mental illnesses or the effects of mental health treatments on the brain.

 ACTIVE LEARNING

Locate the National Alliance for Mental Illness (NAMI) and Suicide Prevention Action Network chapters in your community. What services do these agencies offer? How might those services be helpful in the community mental health nursing role?

 HEALTHY PEOPLE 2020: **MENTAL HEALTH AND MENTAL DISORDERS**

Healthy People 2020 is a collaboration among federal, state, and territorial governments and other organizations to set national disease prevention and health promotion objectives (Healthypeople.gov, 2017a, 2017b; 2017c). The *Healthy People 2020* box lists several objectives that cover issues related to mental health. Major mental health objectives target decreasing suicides, reducing teen suicide attempts and eating disorders, and reducing the number of persons with major depressive episodes. There are objectives for treatment expansion and providing adequate community resources for adults, children, and families struggling with mental illnesses.

FACTORS INFLUENCING MENTAL HEALTH

Although treatment of mental disorders has dramatically improved, the cause of most mental illnesses is not well understood. Research has identified a number of biological and sociological factors that contribute to mental health and mental illness. Some of these factors are discussed here.

Biological Factors

For centuries, mental illnesses were viewed as conditions that needed to be contained in institutions. Neuroscience research has provided a better understanding of the biology of mental illnesses; however, many questions remain unanswered.

 HEALTHY PEOPLE 2020

Objectives Related to Mental Illness and Health

Mental Health Status Improvement
MHMD–1: Suicide
MHMD–2: Adolescent suicide attempts
MHMD–3: Eating disorders
MHMD–4: Major depressive episodes

Treatment Expansion
MHMD–5: Mental health treatment provided in primary care facilities
MHMD–6: Treatment for children with mental health problems
MHMD–7: Juvenile justice facility screening
MHMD–8: Employment of persons with serious mental illness
MHMD–9: Treatment of adults with mental health disorders
MHMD–10: Treatment for co-occurring substance abuse and mental disorders
MHMD–11: Depression screening by primary care providers
MHMD–12: Receipt of mental health services among homeless adults

From HealthyPeople.gov: *Healthy People 2020: topics & objectives: mental health and mental disorders, 2017.* https://www.healthypeople.gov/2020/topics-objectives/topic/mental-health-and-mental-disorders/objectives.

Biological factors associated with mental illness include genetic factors, neurotransmission, and abnormalities of brain structure and functioning.

Genetic Factors

Genetic expressions, combined with neurochemical and metabolic changes and environmental insults, may result in the display of mental disorder characteristics. Genetic testing and counseling offer promise for understanding the complexities associated with gene variation, brain structure, and the physiological response to information processing (Kohlmann et al., 2015). There is evidence of predisposition to mental illnesses in families, suggesting that people who have a family member with a mental illness are more likely to experience one themselves. Experts believe that some mental illnesses are linked to abnormalities in many genes, not just one. People may inherit a susceptibility to a mental illness and do not necessarily go on to have a mental illness. Mental illnesses more likely occur from the interaction of genetic predisposition and other factors, such as stress, substance abuse, and traumatic events. These factors can influence, trigger, or exacerbate an illness in a person who has an inherited susceptibility to it.

Abnormalities of Brain Structure and Functioning

Evidence indicates that structural brain abnormalities can be related to some mental illnesses, such as schizophrenia, depression, and Alzheimer disease. As the science of neuroimaging evolves, a more refined view of the role of brain structure and functioning is unfolding. For example, neuroimaging studies are beginning to explain the role of different central nervous system structures in regulating the hypothalamic-pituitary-adrenal axis that controls responses to stress (Bonaz and Bernstein, 2013; Lucassen et al., 2014).

Although a number of theories on the etiology of mental disorders have been developed, information is insufficient to establish a definitive biological cause for mental illness. Scholars have concluded that mental disorders are multifactorial and complex. The important point for public health nurses to understand is that mental illnesses have a strong biological basis, much like other chronic conditions such as diabetes and heart disease, but that other factors are highly influential.

Social Factors

Some community occurrences and phenomena, such as school shootings, public bombings, bullying, domestic violence, and other tragic events, have identified critical gaps in the need for public education, advocacy, and treatment of mental illness (Schildkraut and Elasass, 2016). Throughout history, the symptoms of mental illness have been perceived as permanent, dangerous, frightening, and shameful. People with a diagnosis of mental illness have been described as lazy, idle, weak, immoral, irrational, and too often criminal. On the basis of these characterizations and assumptions, many people with a diagnosis of mental illness have experienced widespread social rejection, leading to isolation, more social stigma (Corrigan et al., 2014) (see Clinical Example 25.1), and delay or avoidance of seeking treatment (Clement et al., 2015).

Clinical Example 25.1

Michael Nye, a photographer, spent hundreds of hours photographing and taping illness narratives of individuals living with serious mental illness. Viewing his photographs and listening to the accounts of those living with these conditions are valuable experiences for nurses who care for this population (http://michaelnye.org/fineline/index.html). Han and Oliffe (2016) reviewed the use of photovoice in mental illness in several qualitative studies. In these, participants described feelings of loneliness, being marginalized, and their support care needs to build self-confidence.

Another social concern is the tendency of communities to make use of prisons rather than psychiatric hospitals as a solution to the "mental health problem." Though the United States has only 5% of the world's population, it has nearly 25% of its prisoners—about 2.2 million people (APA, 2014). Incarcerated individuals are more likely than people in the general population to have mental health problems and addictions. Many of these individuals lack access to treatment for these problems outside of jails and prisons.

Over half of all inmates experience a mental health problem, and 16% to 24% of them exhibit serious mental illness (with rates even higher among women), compared with 5% to 7% in the community (Dumont et al., 2013). Prisons are woefully unprepared to provide adequate care to the mentally ill. To help address this problem, in 2008, Senate Bill S.2304, the Mentally Ill Offender Treatment and Crime Reduction Reauthorization and Improvement Act, was signed into law. This bill provided grants aimed at improving the mental health treatment provided to criminal offenders with a mental illness. Other related initiatives have focused on establishing specialty courts or problem-solving courts. There may be mental health courts in communities to address the needs of the community and those who are charged with a criminal offense and also experience a mental illness (Mental Health America, 2017b).

Gender, Racial, and Sexual Orientation Disparities

Racial and ethnic minorities are growing rapidly in the United States. The NIMH's Office for Research on Disparities and Global Mental Health (ORDGMH) (2017) is active in reducing mental health disparities. ORDGMH collects local and global mental health disparities data, including movements of populations, global economic relationships, and communication technologies. Culturally diverse groups often bear a disproportionately high burden of disability due to mental disorders. For example, in schizophrenia and mood disorders, there is a high probability of misdiagnosis because of differences in how African Americans express symptoms of emotional distress (Schwartz and Blankenship, 2014).

Because of the lack of access in their communities, Hispanic Americans use mental health services far less than other ethnic and racial groups. Yet 17.4% of the U.S. population identifies as Hispanic or Latino (over 8.6 million people), of whom over 15% had a diagnosable mental illness in the past year (Mental Health America, 2017a). This population also constitutes the largest group of uninsured in the United States. American Indian and Alaska Natives also experience higher rates of mental disorders compared with the overall population. These groups experience far greater psychological distress and are at greater risk for mental disorders such as depression, substance abuse, anxiety, and posttraumatic stress disorder (PTSD). In some American Indian groups, the rates of alcoholism and illicit drug use disorders are much higher than the U.S. average. Of note, lifetime percentages of depression reveal ethnic differences: 6.52% among whites, 4.57% among blacks, and 5.17% among Hispanics (CDC, 2016b).

Although a majority of gay, bisexual, and other men who have sex with men (MSM) have good mental health, there are MSM populations at greater risk for mental health problems. Homophobia, stigma, and discrimination have negative effects on the health of MSM, lesbians, and other sexual minorities. The lesbian, gay, bisexual, and transgendered (LGBT) community are at increased risk for a number of mental health problems. LGBT individuals regularly face discrimination from society at large and sometimes from family, coworkers, or classmates (NAMI, 2017a). Research has provided evidence of sexual orientation disparities across a number of mental disorders, including depression, anxiety, attention-deficit, bipolar, bulimia, panic attacks, and obsessive-compulsive disorders. Findings also suggest differences in mental health between gay/lesbian and bisexual women, indicating worse mental health status among bisexual women than both heterosexual and lesbian women (Przedworski et al., 2015).

Natural and Human-Made Disasters and Mental Illness

Natural and human-made disasters, such as hurricanes, floods, violence, terrorism, war, and economic crises, are profound stress-inducing events that can lead to mental illness. For

From U.S. Department of Health and Human Services, Office of the Surgeon General and National Action Alliance for Suicide Prevention: *2012 National Strategy for Suicide Prevention: Goals and Objectives for Action*, Washington, DC, 2012, Author.

BOX 25.1   2012 National Strategy for Suicide Prevention

- Create supportive environments that promote healthy and empowered individuals, families, and communities
- Enhance clinical and community preventive services
- Promote the availability of timely treatment and support services
- Improve suicide prevention surveillance collection, research, and evaluation

example, researchers reported high levels of PTSD among survivors of Hurricane Katrina, which devastated New Orleans in 2005. Community mental health nurses must be prepared not only to respond to the mental health needs of a community during a disaster but also to maintain vigilance in caring for survivors many years thereafter.

PTSD is highly prevalent among combat veterans returning from war. The condition is associated with extreme anxiety that can result in suicide. Male veterans in communities are twice as likely to die by suicide as their civilian counterparts (NIMH, 2013). During 2014, there were 53 suicides among active duty members of the Navy, 60 in the Air Force, 122 in the Army, and 34 in the Marine Corps (U.S. Department of Defense [DoD], 2015b). Throughout the U.S. military, there was a slight increase in the overall number of suicides from the second quarter of 2014 compared with the second quarter of 2015 (70 to 71), and a total increase from 2013 (254) to 2014 (273) (U.S. DoD, 2015a). Early intervention is key to prevention and treatment. The *2015 Department of Defense Strategy for Suicide Prevention* was released by the U.S. Surgeon General and U.S. DoD (2015c) (Box 25.1).

Political Factors

Political factors can dramatically influence how mental disorders are managed. One significant factor in the politics of mental illness is parity in health care coverage—that is, the equal access to health care for physical and mental illnesses. Historically, health insurance companies have provided less access to treatment for mental disorders than for physical disorders. Since 2008, when the Paul Wellstone and Pete Domenici Mental Health Parity and Addiction Equity Act was enacted, there are laws requiring health insurance to cover treatment for mental illness on the same terms and conditions as physical illness. Although this legislation was a victory for mental health, there has been inconsistency in how it has moved forward.

Health care disparities have become a key issue in public health policy discussions. As previously mentioned, members of ethnic minority groups have less access to mental health services than do their white counterparts. Compared with whites, minorities are less likely to seek mental health care, and black individuals are more likely to have an episode needing acute psychiatric care. This greater acute mental health care use raises concerns over monitoring of their treatment (Lê Cook et al., 2014).

MENTAL DISORDERS ENCOUNTERED IN COMMUNITY SETTINGS

The influence of untreated mental illness on communities and their social structure has been vastly understated. SAHMSA (2016) reports an estimated 43.6 million (18.1%) Americans 18 years and older experienced some form of mental illness, and in the past year, 20.2 million adults (8.4%) had a substance use disorder. Of these, 7.9 million people had both a mental disorder and substance use disorder. Mental illness is one of the leading causes of disability in the United States, affecting roughly 43 million (or 1 in 5) Americans, and mental illness accounts for more than 10% of the disease burden worldwide, ranking it second, after all forms of cardiac disease (NIMH, 2017c). In the United States, the economic impact of behavioral health conditions, including lost earnings/productivity and health and treatment expenses, is estimated to be nearly $500 billion per year (SAHMSA, 2014).

Because most mental illnesses are identified and managed in community settings, it is essential that public health nurses be familiar with frequently occurring mental disorders. There is a need for screening, referring, and follow-up for people with mental health problems in order to meet these mental health needs (SAHMSA, 2014).

Overview of Selected Mental Disorders

The *DSM*-V (APA, 2017) classifies mental illnesses and outlines diagnostic criteria for more than 300 disorders. Children with mental disorders are often referred to as children with severe emotional disorder (SED). SED disturbance suggests broad ranges of behaviors that might result in classification of a student with SED as eligible for special education. A child with SED may demonstrate emotional disturbance with hallucinations; may have a very short attention span; may hurt others physically; may destroy property; or may have severe presentations of depression, anger, or fear. Among students with SED, externalizing behaviors such as acting out are significantly more prevalent than internalizing behaviors such as withdrawal or depression.

Schizophrenia

Schizophrenia is the most severe and most profound of all mental illnesses; it is chronic, and globally, it affects about 1.1% of the population (Brain and Behavior Research Foundation, 2017; NIMH, 2017). The effect of this condition on the community is enormous in terms of social and economic burden. To the individual and families affected by schizophrenia, the impact is incalculable. The affected person may present with positive symptoms, including hallucinations, delusions, disorganized thinking and speech, and bizarre behavior, or with negative symptoms, such as flat affect, poor attention, lack of motivation, apathy, lack of pleasure, and lack of energy. Onset typically occurs during late adolescence and early adulthood in males and somewhat later in females. There is an increased risk for alcohol use, depression, suicide, and diabetes among persons with schizophrenia. These factors compound the problems associated with living with a psychotic disorder.

BOX 25.2 Symptoms of Depression

- Persistent sad, anxious, or "empty" feelings
- Feelings of hopelessness or pessimism
- Feelings of guilt, worthlessness, or helplessness
- Irritability, restlessness
- Loss of interest in activities or hobbies once pleasurable, including sex
- Fatigue and decreased energy
- Difficulty concentrating, remembering details, and making decisions
- Insomnia, early-morning wakefulness, or excessive sleeping
- Overeating or appetite loss
- Thoughts of suicide, suicide attempts
- Aches or pains, headaches, cramps, or digestive problems that do not ease even with treatment

From National Institute of Mental Health: *Depression* (NIH Publication No. 11-3561), Rockville, MD, 2000, Revised 2011, Author.

RESEARCH HIGHLIGHTS

Measuring Mental Illness–Related Stigma Imposed by Health Care Providers

Knowing that mental illness–related stigma can lead to low rates of seeking help, lack of access to care, undertreatment, and social marginalization, Kassam and associates (2012) developed the *Opening Minds Scale for Health Care Providers* (OMS-HC) and tested the tool on 787 health care providers/trainees. The OMS-HC provides hope in demonstrating that it that can be utilized in evaluating programs, with goals to reduce mental illness–related stigma imposed by health care providers.

Data from Kassam A et al.: The development and psychometric properties of a new scale to measure mental illness related stigma by health care providers: the Opening Minds Scale for Health Care Providers (OMS-HC), *BMC Psychiatry* 12:62, 3–12, 2012.

Among people diagnosed with schizophrenia, an estimated 20% to 40% attempt suicide; between 5% and 13% actually succeed (Thompson and Hollister, 2016). Approximately 50% of patients with schizophrenia may have **anosognosia** (Treatment Advocacy Center, 2017), an impaired awareness of illness, so they may not recognize that they are ill (Torrey, 2017). This impaired awareness of illness affects approximately 50% of individuals with schizophrenia (Treatment Advocacy Center, 2017). Anosognosia contributes to noncompliance with medications and treatment.

Treatment for schizophrenia must be intensive and generally involves hospitalization (initially), antipsychotic medications, and psychotherapy/counseling. Long-term follow-up by mental health professionals is necessary to monitor medication compliance and to watch for side effects and complications, which may be severe and life threatening, and to evaluate the patient's ability to integrate into the community.

Depression

Depression is the most frequently diagnosed and one of the most disabling mental illnesses in the United States. Depression affected approximately 16.1 million American adults, or about 6.7% of the U.S. population age 18 and older, in the past year (NIMH, 2017). The disorders include major depressive disorder, dysthymic disorder, and bipolar disorders. Depression often co-occurs with serious physical disorders, such as heart attack, stroke, diabetes, and cancer. At any point in time, 3% to 5% of adults suffer from major depression; the lifetime risk is about 17% (Anxiety and Depression Association of America, 2016). Although effective treatments exist, most people with depressive illness—almost 65%—do not seek help (Pratt and Brody, 2014). Having a family or personal history of depression, childhood trauma, serious or chronic illness, traumatic or stressful events such as physical or sexual abuse, the death or loss of a loved one, a difficult relationship, or financial problems are among the risk factors for depression (Mayo Clinic, 2017). Health education for patients with depression should include risk factor identification as well as when and how to obtain treatment. Symptoms of depression are listed in Box 25.2.

Depression in Children and Adolescents. The incidence of depression in children is 0.9% in preschool-age children, 1.9% in school-age children, and 4.7% in adolescents (Healthy Place, 2016). According to the NIMH (2017) 2.7% of children ages 8 to 15 have been diagnosed with depression ,and as of 2015, an estimated 3 million adolescents aged 12 to 17 in the United States had at least one major depressive episode in the past year. This number represented 12.5% of the U.S. population aged 12 to 17. A family history of depression is a major risk factor for childhood depression. Other associated factors that may increase the risk of depression in children and adolescents are a history of verbal, physical, or sexual abuse; frequent separation from, or loss of, a loved one; poverty; mental retardation; attention-deficit hyperactivity disorder; hyperactivity; and chronic illness.

Treatment for depression includes pharmacological therapy, psychotherapy, behavior therapy, electroconvulsive therapy, or a combination of these (Moreland and Bonin, 2017; NIMH, 2017). In general, the most effective first-line treatment is a combination of antidepressant medication and psychotherapy.

Bipolar Disorder

Bipolar disorder refers to a group of mood disorders that manifest as changes in mood from depression to mania. The depressed phase manifests as symptoms seen in major depressive disorder. The manic phase is characterized by a persistent abnormally elevated or irritable mood, impaired judgment, flight of ideas, pressured speech, grandiosity, distractibility, excessive involvement in goal-directed activities, spending few hours sleeping, and impulsivity. These symptoms may co-occur with psychotic features such as hallucinations and delusions. Persons with bipolar disorder are at increased risk for alcohol and substance abuse as well as suicide. The presence of bipolar disorder often results in poor occupational and social functioning.

Management of bipolar disorder must be ongoing and should involve close monitoring. Treatment generally involves use of mood-stabilizing medication, often in combination with antipsychotic and antidepressant therapy (NIMH, 2016). When working with persons with bipolar disorder, nurses need to monitor symptoms and response to psychopharmacological treatment.

Anxiety Disorder

Anxiety disorders are a group of conditions characterized by feelings of persistent or potentially debilitating apprehension. Anxiety disorders affect around 15% of people during their lifetime (CDC, 2016). They may be attributed to the genetic makeup and life experiences of the individual. Some of the more commonly encountered anxiety disorders are generalized anxiety disorder, panic disorder (sometimes accompanied by agoraphobia), social anxiety disorder, phobias, obsessive-compulsive disorder (OCD), and PTSD (Anxiety and Depression Association of America, 2016c). They are discussed briefly here.

Generalized Anxiety Disorder.
Generalized anxiety disorder (GAD) is characterized by chronic, unrealistic, and exaggerated worry and tension about one or more life circumstances lasting 6 months or longer (Anxiety and Depression Association of America, 2016c). Approximately half of cases of GAD begin in childhood or adolescence, and the disorder is more common in women than in men. Symptoms of GAD include trembling, twitching, muscle tension, headaches, irritability, sweating or hot flashes, dyspnea, and nausea (Anxiety and Depression Association of America, 2016c; NIMH, 2016). Periods of increasing symptoms are usually associated with life stressors or impending difficulties. GAD is probably the most underdiagnosed mental disorder.

Panic Disorder.
Approximately 2.7% American adults have panic disorder in a 12-month period (NIMH, 2017). **Panic disorder** can occur at any age, but it most often begins in young adulthood (average age, 18 to 45 years, with an average onset of 24 years) (Memon and Welton, 2016). A panic attack consists of a period of intense fear that develops abruptly and unexpectedly. Typically, the patient experiences tachycardia; dyspnea; dizziness; chest pain; nausea; numbness or tingling of the hands and feet; trembling or shaking; sweating; choking; or a feeling that he or she is going to die, go crazy, or do something uncontrolled. It can be extremely frightening. A diagnosis of panic disorder is made when attacks occur with some degree of frequency or regularity.

As the disorder evolves, the anxiety attacks become increasingly frequent and severe, and anticipatory anxiety (fear of having a panic attack) develops. During this phase, events and circumstances associated with the attack may be selectively avoided, leading to phobic behaviors. Thus the client's life may become progressively constricted.

As the avoidance behavior intensifies, the client begins to withdraw further to avoid being in places or situations from which escape may be difficult or embarrassing or in which help may be unavailable in the event of a panic attack (e.g., church, elevators, movie theaters). The fear of being in these situations or places can lead to **agoraphobia** (literally, fear of the marketplace or open places). Individuals with agoraphobia frequently progress to the point that they cannot leave their homes without experiencing anxiety.

Nearly half of people diagnosed with depression are also diagnosed with an anxiety disorder (Anxiety and Depression Association of America, 2016b). Cognitive-behavioral treatment and short-course benzodiazepine therapy are used to treat panic disorder.

Phobias.
A **phobia** is an irrational fear of something (an object or situation), and nearly 11% of the U.S. population—about 25,000,000 people—may suffer from a phobia during their lifetime (Remedy Health, 2016). Adults with phobias realize that their fears are irrational, but facing the feared object or situation might bring on severe anxiety or a panic attack. Although phobias may begin in childhood, they usually first appear in adolescence or adulthood.

Social phobia, or social anxiety disorder, is a persistent and intense fear of, and compelling desire to avoid, something that would expose the individual to a situation that might be humiliating and embarrassing (NIMH, 2017). It has a familial tendency and may be accompanied by depression or alcoholism. The most common social phobia is a fear of public speaking. Other examples include being unable to urinate in a public bathroom and not being able to answer questions in social situations. Most people with social phobias can be treated with cognitive-behavioral therapy and medication.

Simple phobias involve a persistent fear of, and compelling desire to avoid, certain objects or situations. Common objects of phobias are spiders, snakes, dogs, cats, and situations such as flying, heights, and closed-in spaces. The person often recognizes that the fear is unreasonable but avoids the situation or endures it with intense anxiety. Systematic desensitization and normal exposure are the most effective treatments for simple phobias.

Obsessive-Compulsive Disorder.
Obsessive-compulsive disorder is characterized by anxious thoughts and rituals that the individual has difficulty controlling. The person with OCD feels compelled to engage in some ritual to avoid a persistent frightening thought, idea, image, or event. *Obsessions* are recurrent thoughts, emotions, or impulses that cannot be dismissed. *Compulsions* are the rituals or behaviors that are repeatedly performed to prevent, neutralize, or dispel the dreaded obsession. When the individual tries to resist the compulsion, anxiety increases. Common compulsions include hand washing, counting, checking, and touching (WebMD, 2017). Most individuals recognize that what they are doing is senseless but are unable to control the compulsion. About 1% of Americans are afflicted with OCD, which often appears in the teenage years or early adulthood (NIMH, 2017). Depression and other anxiety disorders often accompany OCD. Behavioral therapy and medication aimed at reducing accompanying symptoms have been found to be helpful.

Posttraumatic Stress Disorder.
Posttraumatic stress disorder is a debilitating condition that follows a shocking, scary, or dangerous event. It affects about 3.5% of U.S. adults (NIMH, 2016). Individuals with PTSD have recurring, persistent, frightening thoughts and memories of their ordeal. The event may involve "shell shock" or "battle fatigue" common to war veterans, a violent attack, serious accident, or natural disaster or having witnessed a mass destruction or injury, such as an airplane crash. Sometimes the individual is unable to recall an important aspect of the traumatic event. The highest incidence of PTSD occurs among combat-experienced military personnel.

People with PTSD repeatedly relive the trauma in the form of nightmares or disturbing recollections or flashbacks during the day, resulting in sleep disturbances, depression, feelings of detachment or emotional numbness, or being easily startled. They may avoid places or situations that bring back memories (e.g., a woman raped in an elevator may refuse to ride in elevators), and anniversaries of the event are often very difficult. PTSD occurs at all ages and may be accompanied by depression, substance abuse, and/or anxiety. It usually begins within 3 months of the trauma, and the course of the disorder varies. Some individuals recover within 6 months; the condition becomes chronic in others. Infrequently, the illness does not manifest until years after the traumatic event. Treatment includes antidepressants and antianxiety medications and psychotherapy. Support from family and friends can be very beneficial.

Eating Disorders

Eating disorders—anorexia nervosa and bulimia nervosa—are increasingly prevalent in the United States. In the United States, 20 million women and 10 million men suffer from a clinically significant eating disorder at some time in their life (National Eating Disorder Association [NEDA], 2016).

Anorexia affects about 0.9% of females and 0.3% males in their lifetimes (NIMH, 2017). As many as 0.6% U.S. adults have a lifetime prevalence of bulimia.

Most clients with a diagnosis of eating disorders are white; however, the reason may be socioeconomic factors rather than race. Anorexia and bulimia are often triggered by developmental milestones (e.g., puberty, first sexual contact) or another crisis (e.g., death of a loved one, ridicule over weight, starting college).

Bulimia nervosa refers to binge eating: recurrent and frequent episodes of eating unusually large amounts of food and feeling a lack of control over the eating. This binge eating is followed by a type of behavior that compensates for the binge, such as purging (e.g., vomiting, excessive use of laxatives or diuretics), fasting, and/or excessive exercise (NIMH, 2017). For example, a person with bulimia might eat an entire pie, half a cake, or a half-gallon of ice cream at one sitting. Snacking throughout the day is not considered bingeing. To lose or maintain weight, the person with bulimia practices purging, which usually involves self-induced vomiting, caused by gagging, using an emetic, or simply mentally willing the action. Laxatives, diuretics, fasting, and excessive exercise may also be employed to control weight.

Bulimia nervosa typically begins in adolescence or during the early 20s, usually in conjunction with a diet. High school and college students, as well as members of certain professions that emphasize weight and/or appearance (e.g., dancers, flight attendants, cheerleaders, athletes, actors, models), are at risk. The condition may lead to electrolyte imbalance, resulting in fatigue, seizures, muscle cramps, arrhythmias, and decreased bone density. Vomiting can damage the esophagus, stomach, teeth, and gums.

The person with anorexia nervosa becomes obsessed with a fear of fat and with losing weight. Anorexia nervosa often develops as a fairly gradual decrease in caloric intake. However, the decrease continues until the person is consuming almost nothing. Anorexia usually begins in early adolescence (12 to 14 years is the most common age group) and may be limited to a single episode of dramatic weight loss within a few months, followed by recovery, or may last for many years. Recently, the DSM-5 introduced three changes to the criteria defining anorexia nervosa: the weight loss criterion was revised, fear of weight gain does not need to be verbalized if behaviors interfering with weight gain can be observed, and amenorrhea was no longer required. Another revision in the DSM-5 is the introduction of a body mass index–based severity rating) (Mustelin et al., 2016).

Risk factors for eating disorders are perfectionism, low self-esteem, stress, poor coping skills, sexual/physical abuse, poor self-image, dependency on others' opinions and deference to others' wishes, and being emotionally reserved. In response to the severely decreased caloric intake, the body tries to compensate by slowing down body processes. In many instances, blood pressure, pulse, and respiration rates slow and thyroid activity diminishes. Electrolyte imbalance can become very severe. Other symptoms are mild anemia, joint swelling, and reduced muscle mass. Anorexia nervosa can be life threatening and has a mortality rate of 5% to 21%.

Treatment for eating disorders involves long-term nutrition counseling, psychotherapy, and behavior modification. Hospitalization may be required for clients with serious complications. Self-help groups and support groups can be very beneficial for both the client and the family.

Nurses need to be aware of the resources available at the American Academy of Child and Adolescent Psychiatry, which has a section for families and youth. Such knowledge is important, as community health nurses assess the social influences that contribute to the condition.

Attention-Deficit Hyperactivity Disorder

Two of the most common conditions encountered by nurses who work with children in community settings are attention deficit/hyperactivity disorder (ADHD) and attention deficit disorder (ADD). About 10.2% of school-age children ages 5 to 17 in the United States have been diagnosed with ADHD (CDC, 2016). Behaviors that might indicate ADHD/ADD usually appear before age 7 years and are often accompanied by related problems, such as learning disability, anxiety, and depression. The three major characteristics of ADHD/ADD are inattention, hyperactivity, and impulsivity.

The cause of ADHD/ADD is not known. Although there are familial tendencies to develop attention disorders, it is important to note that they are not caused by minor head injuries, birth complications, food allergies, too much sugar, poor home life, poor schools, or too much television watching. Maternal substance use and abuse (e.g., alcohol, cigarettes, cocaine) may affect the brain of the developing baby and produce symptoms of ADHD/ADD later in life. This possibility, however, accounts for only a small percentage of those affected.

Although parents may notice symptoms and signs, it is often teachers who recognize the behaviors consistent with attention deficit disorders and suggest referral for assessment and treatment (NIMH, 2013). Experts caution that diagnosis of attention disorders should be made after a comprehensive physical, psychological, social, and behavioral evaluation and should not be based solely on anecdotal reports from parents or teachers.

TABLE 25.2	Suicide Warning Signs: "Is Path Warm"
Ideation	Does the person state that he or she is having thoughts of suicide?
Substance abuse	Is the person demonstrating increased use of alcohol or drugs?
Purposelessness	Does the person state that he or she feels as if there is no purpose in his or her life?
Anxiety	Is the person demonstrating anxiety-related behaviors such as talking about being overly worried about things, ruminating, difficulty concentrating, or exhibiting increased psychomotor agitation?
Trapped	Does the person state that he or she feels trapped, that there is no way out of the current situation except to die?
Hopelessness	Does the person state that he or she feels hopeless? Is the person able to describe something to look forward to?
Withdrawal	Is the person withdrawing from others such as family and friends? Is the person isolating?
Anger	Is the person demonstrating uncontrolled anger? Is the person acting with rage or seeking revenge?
Recklessness	Is the person engaged in risk-taking behaviors? Is the person acting as if he or she "doesn't care" or isn't thinking about the consequences of the risk-taking behavior?
Mood changes	Is the person experiencing dramatic mood changes?

From American Association of Suicidology: *Know the warning signs of suicide*, 2017. http://www.suicidology.org/resources/warning-signs. Contact information: American Association of Suicidology 5221 Wisconsin Ave. NW 2nd Floor Washington, DC 20015-2032 Phone (202) 237-2280, Fax (202) 237-2282. www.suicidology.org info@suicidology.org.

The evaluation should rule out other possible reasons for the behavior (e.g., emotional problems, poor vision or hearing, physical problems) and should include input from teachers, parents, and others who know the child well. Intelligence and achievement testing may also be performed to rule out or identify a learning disability.

Symptoms of ADHD/ADD are typically managed through a combination of behavior therapy, emotional counseling, and practical support. Use of medication is now becoming increasingly commonplace in the management of ADHD/ADD. It is very important, however, that children with attention disorders and their families understand that medication does not cure the disorder; it just temporarily controls symptoms.

Stimulants have been shown to be successful in treating attention disorders. The most commonly used medications are methylphenidate (Ritalin, Concerta, etc.) and amphetamines (e.g., Dexedrine, Adderall). Appetite suppression and poor sleep are common side effects.

Suicide

There are approximately 1 million deaths by suicide per year throughout the world. The American Foundation for Suicide Prevention (2017) reported there were 44,193 deaths by suicide in the United States in 2015. Men die by suicide 3.5 times more often than women, and white males accounted for 7 of 10 suicides in 2015. On average, in the United States, there are about 121 suicides per day (AFSP, 2017). Of concern, suicide is the third leading cause of death among those aged 15 to 24 years, but the highest rate of suicide occurs in males older than 65 years. Finally, white males older than 85 years are particularly vulnerable.

Historically, risk and protective factors have been used to identify those at highest risk for suicide. The American Association of Suicidology (AAS) (2017) has recommended recognition of warning signs as more relevant than risk and protective factors in preventing death by suicide. The AAS has organized the warning signs according to the easily remembered mnemonic, IS PATH WARM (Table 25.2). Warning signs that indicate acute risk for suicidality may be observed in individuals who are threatening to hurt or kill themselves, attempting to

identify access to lethal weapons or other means that could result in death, or communicating about dying when these thoughts or actions are out of the ordinary for them.

Risk factors include previous suicide attempts, mental illness, substance abuse, and barriers to accessing mental health treatment. Protective factors that may decrease the risk of suicide include appropriate mental health care, easy access to treatment, community support, and continuing support from medical and mental health care providers. Box 25.3 lists protective factors and risk factors that all community health nurses should recognize, and Box 25.4 provides warning signs of suicide.

Thus, it is important that all public health nurses become familiar with assessing for suicide warning signs and accessing appropriate resources. Nurses should refer the person exhibiting suicide warning signs to a mental health clinic or provider as soon as possible. This may involve taking emergency action by calling the local emergency services number in the community and staying with the person until help arrives. Table 25.3 provides a list of suicide information resources.

IDENTIFICATION AND MANAGEMENT OF MENTAL DISORDERS

Early identification, appropriate treatment, and rehabilitation can significantly reduce the duration and level of disability associated with mental disorders and decrease the possibility of relapse. Interventions to promote mental health and decrease mental disorders include focusing on decreasing stressors and/or increasing the capacity of the individual to cope with stress. Other interventions include the use of pharmacological agents and psychosocial interventions such as strengthening interpersonal, psychological, and physical resources through counseling, support groups, and psychoeducation.

The accessibility of mental health service is pivotal in promoting and maintaining health. Decreased funding for services, managed care limitations on mental health coverage, and the inequality of coverage by the insurance industry have caused downsizing or forced closure in the traditional places of treatment, such as CMHCs and community hospitals. Consequently, the accessibility to community mental health services has

BOX 25.3 Suicide: Protective Factors and Risk Factors

Protective Factors

- Effective clinical care for mental, physical, and substance abuse disorders
- Easy access to a variety of clinical interventions and support for help seeking
- Family and community support (connectedness)
- Support from ongoing medical and mental health care relationships
- Skills in problem solving, conflict resolution, and nonviolent ways of handling disputes
- Cultural and religious beliefs that discourage suicide and support instincts for self-preservation

Risk Factors

- Family history of suicide
- Family history of child maltreatment
- Previous suicide attempt(s)
- History of mental disorders, particularly clinical depression
- History of alcohol and substance abuse
- Feelings of hopelessness
- Impulsive or aggressive tendencies
- Cultural and religious beliefs (e.g., belief that suicide is noble resolution of a personal dilemma)
- Local epidemics of suicide
- Isolation, a feeling of being cut off from other people
- Barriers to accessing mental health treatment
- Loss (relational, social, work, or financial)
- Physical illness
- Easy access to lethal methods
- Unwillingness to seek help because of the stigma attached to mental health and substance abuse disorders or to suicidal thoughts

Adapted from Substance Abuse and Mental Health Services Administration, National Suicide Prevention Lifeline: *Risk factors for suicide,* n.d. http://www.suicidepreventionlifeline.org/learn/riskfactors.aspx.

BOX 25.4 Warning Signs of Suicide

Seek help as soon as possible by contacting a mental health professional or by calling the National Suicide Prevention Lifeline at 1-800-273-TALK if you or someone you know exhibits any of the following signs:

- Threatening to hurt or kill oneself or talking about wanting to hurt or kill oneself
- Looking for ways to kill oneself by seeking access to firearms, available pills, or other means
- Talking or writing about death, dying, or suicide when these actions are out of the ordinary for the person
- Feeling hopeless
- Feeling rage or uncontrolled anger or seeking revenge
- Acting reckless or engaging in risky activities—seemingly without thinking
- Feeling trapped—like there's no way out
- Increasing alcohol or drug use
- Withdrawing from friends, family, and society
- Feeling anxious, agitated, or unable to sleep or sleeping all the time
- Experiencing dramatic mood changes
- Seeing no reason for living or having no sense of purpose in life

From Suicidepreventionlifeline.org: *When it seems like there is no hope, there is help* (Brochure CMHS-SVP-0141), 2006. http://www.cbp.gov/linkhandler/cgov/careers/benefits_employees/frc/suicide_prevention/suicide_prevention_materials/prevention_brochure.ctt/prevention_brochure.pdf.

TABLE 25.3 Suicide Prevention and Referral Resources

National Suicide Prevention Lifeline	1-800-273-TALK (8255) www.suicidepreventionlifeline.org/
American Association of Suicidology	www.suicidology.org/home
Suicide Prevention Resource Center	www.sprc.org/
Suicide Awareness Voices of Education	www.save.org/
Suicide Prevention: A Resource Manual for the Army	http://www.armyg1.army.mil/dcs/docs/ Suicide%20Prevention%20Manual.pdf
Veterans Crisis Line	1-800-273-8255 Text to 838255 www.veteranscrisisline.net/ChatTermsOfService.aspx?account=Veterans%20Chat
American Foundation for Suicide Prevention	www.afsp.org/
Local emergency resource	Dial 911

become an issue of significant concern. In addition, the symptoms of mental illness often interfere with an individual's ability to access services. Alterations in thoughts and perceptions, anxiety, and decreased energy are common symptoms of mental illness, all of which interfere with negotiating the complex systems that currently surround the provision of mental health services. This section describes actions that may be taken by community health nurses to identify mental illness and outlines potential treatment options.

Identification of Mental Disorders

Whether the nurse is working in a physician's office, a community clinic, a school, or home health and hospice, occupational health, or other setting, recognition of signs and symptoms that might indicate a mental disorder is an important component of practice. More than ever, public health nurses work in collaboration with crisis housing agencies and school district managers for homeless families. In these situations, the nurse should continue to assess for other signs and symptoms that might indicate a mental disorder and should be prepared to intervene when they are observed.

Often, the assessment process includes direct questioning or observation. At other times, a standardized assessment tool or questionnaire might be employed. Figs. 25.1 and 25.2 contain examples of instruments that are available to elicit information about symptoms of anxiety or depression. Whenever using these or other screening tools, the nurse should be prepared in advance to intervene on the basis of assessment data. Often, this intervention incorporates referral to other health professionals for further assessment, testing, counseling, treatment, and follow-up by all health professionals involved.

Evidence-Based Practice Management of Mental Disorders

The website of the SAMHSA National Registry of Evidence Based Programs and Practices lists EBP programs and interventions that demonstrate positive outcomes in community mental

During the Past Week	Rarely or None of the Time (Less than 1 Day)	Some or a Little of the Time (1-2 Days)	Occasionally or a Moderate Amount of the Time (3-4 Days)	Most or All of the Time (5-7 Days)
1. I was bothered by things that don't usually bother me.	0	1	2	3
2. I did not feel like eating; my appetite was poor.	0	1	2	3
3. I felt that I could not shake off the blues even with the help of my family or friends.	0	1	2	3
4. I felt that I was just as good as other people.	3	2	1	0
5. I had trouble keeping my mind on what I was doing.	0	1	2	3
6. I felt depressed.	0	1	2	3
7. I felt everything I did was an effort.	0	1	2	3
8. I felt hopeful about the future.	3	2	1	0
9. I thought my life had been a failure.	0	1	2	3
10. I felt fearful.	0	1	2	3
11. My sleep was restless.	0	1	2	3
12. I was happy.	3	2	1	0
13. I talked less than usual.	0	1	2	3
14. I felt lonely.	0	1	2	3
15. People were unfriendly.	0	1	2	3
16. I enjoyed life.	3	2	1	0
17. I had crying spells.	0	1	2	3
18. I felt sad.	0	1	2	3
19. I felt that people disliked me.	0	1	2	3
20. I could not get "going."	0	1	2	3

FIG. 25.1 Center for Epidemiologic Studies depression scale. Interpretation: A total score of 22 or higher is indicative of depression when the scale is used in primary care. (From Radloff LS: The CES-D scale: a self-report depression scale for research in the general population, *Appl Psychol Meas* 1: 385–401, 1977. Copyright 1977, West Publishing Company/Applied Psychological Measurement, Inc.)

health. The goals of treatment for mental illness are to reduce symptoms, improve occupational and social functioning, develop and strengthen coping skills, and promote behaviors to improve the individual's life. Crisis housing programs, supportive employment programs, Assertive Community Treatment (ACT) team models, Crisis Intervention Team (CIT) models, psychotropic medication management programs, community case management programs, mobile crisis units, Cognitive Behavioral Intervention for Trauma in Schools programs, and many more are listed. Basic approaches to the treatment of mental disorders are detailed at the SAMHSA website (www.samhsa.gov/nrepp).

Psychotropic or Psychotherapeutic Medications

Psychotropic/psychotherapeutic medications treat symptoms of mental illness. The appropriateness of psychopharmacological

Rank	Life Event	Mean Value	Rank	Life Event	Mean Value
1	Death of spouse	100	23	Son or daughter leaving home	29
2	Divorce	73	24	Trouble with in-laws	29
3	Marital separation	65	25	Outstanding personal achievement	28
4	Jail term	63	26	Wife begins or stops work	26
5	Death of close family member	63	27	Begin or end school	26
6	Personal injury or illness	53	28	Change in living conditions	25
7	Marriage	50	29	Change in personal habits	24
8	Fired at work	47	30	Trouble with boss	23
9	Marital reconciliation	45	31	Change in work hours or conditions	20
10	Retirement	45	32	Change in residence	20
11	Change in health of family member	44	33	Change in schools	20
12	Pregnancy	40	34	Change in recreation	19
13	Sex difficulties	39	35	Change in church activities	19
14	Gain of new family member	39	36	Change in social activities	18
15	Business readjustment	39	37	Mortgage or loan less than $10,000	17
16	Change in financial state	38	38	Change in sleeping habits	16
17	Death of close friend	37	39	Change in number of family get-togethers	15
18	Change to different line of work	36	40	Change in eating habits	15
19	Change in number of arguments with spouse	35	41	Vacation	13
20	Mortgage over $10,000	31	42	Christmas	12
21	Foreclosure on mortgage or loan	30	43	Minor violations of the law	11
22	Change in responsibilities at work	29			

Life Crisis Categories and LCU Scores*

No life crisis	0-149
Mild life crisis	150-199
Moderate life crisis	200-299
Major life crisis	300 or more

*The LCU score includes those life event items experienced during a 1-year period.

FIG. 25.2 Social readjustment rating scale. *LCU,* Life change unit(s). (From Holmes TH, Rahe RH: The social readjustment rating scale, *J Psychosom Res* 11:213–217, 1967.)

agents and their prescribed regimen depends on the diagnosis, side effects, and client response. Some of the psychotropic medications prescribed are classified as antipsychotics, antidepressants, mood stabilizers, anticonvulsants, antianxiety agents, and hypnotics. Information about medication profiles and treatment regimens often changes as new information becomes available, so nurses should be aware of up-to-date medication information. Excellent resources include Medline (https://medlineplus.gov/druginformation.html) or private sources (www.rxlist.com).

Psychotherapy

Psychotherapy refers to a process of discovery that helps alleviate troubling emotional symptoms and assists individuals in returning to a healthy life (APA, 2017). In nursing, psychotherapy is an intervention used predominantly by psychiatric/mental health nurse practitioners. Psychotherapy involves the use of a professional, therapeutic relationship and the application of psychotherapy theories and best practices to change a client's attitudes, feelings, beliefs, defenses, personality, and behaviors. Therapy approaches vary among schools of psychotherapy and with the nature of the client's problem. Psychotherapy is often used in conjunction with medication to treat many mental disorders. Various types of psychotherapy include the following (NIMH, 2016):

- *Individual therapy* focuses on the client's current life and relationships within the family, social, and work environments.
- *Family therapy* involves problem-solving sessions with members of a family.
- *Couples therapy* is used to develop the relationship and minimize problems through understanding how individual conflicts are expressed in the couple's interactions.
- *Group therapy* involves a small group of people with similar problems who, with the guidance of a therapist, discuss individual issues and help one another with problems.
- *Play therapy* is a technique used for establishing communication and resolving problems with young children.
- *Cognitive-behavioral therapy* may be used in individual, family, couples, or group therapy. The goal is to identify and correct distorted thought patterns that can lead to troublesome feelings and behaviors.
- *Behavioral therapy* uses learning principles to change thought patterns and behaviors systematically; it is used to encourage the individual to learn specific skills to obtain rewards and satisfaction.

Psychotherapy may be short term or long term, depending on the nature of the problem and the availability of resources.

COMMUNITY-BASED MENTAL HEALTH CARE

Over the past several decades, a number of initiatives have directed toward improving and promoting community-based care of those with mental illness. One of those initiatives is the ACA. The ACA contained one of the largest expansions of mental health and substance use disorder coverage in a generation and requires that most individual and small employer health insurance plans cover mental health and substance use disorder services (MentalHealth.gov, 2017). Mental and behavioral health services are recognized as essential health benefits. Consequently, the ACA stipulated that all plans must cover behavioral health treatment, such as psychotherapy and counseling; mental and behavioral health inpatient services; and substance abuse treatment (HealthCare.gov, 2017). Similarly, preexisting mental and behavioral health conditions are covered, and spending limits aren't allowed. Marketplace plans also cannot deny one coverage or charge more on the basis of any preexisting condition, including mental health and substance use disorder conditions. Parity protections now exist for mental health services.

Marketplace plans must provide certain "parity" protections between mental health and substance abuse benefits, on the one hand, and medical and surgical benefits, on the other. As a rule, this means limits applied to mental health and substance abuse services cannot be more restrictive than limits applied to medical and surgical services.

ETHICAL INSIGHTS

Valuing Human Beings

A study by Eriksen and colleagues (2012) demonstrates how users of mental health services describe and make sense of their meetings with other people. Acknowledging and valuing one other is an essential human characteristic that promotes individual dignity and vulnerability in relationships. The group utilized the Interpretative Phenomenological Analysis to explore peoples' relationship to the world and how they make sense of their life experiences. Participants represented people living with mental health problems who depended on others for support and help in their everyday lives. Participants often would report the process "to be recognized" as a phenomenon in their life. To be recognized as a human being and be recognized as a human being struggling with a chronic mental health problem was helpful in their struggle in *self-preservation*. Mental health professionals may be challenged to recognize the struggle of the person with an SMI. Mental health professionals can be helpful and instrumental in health promotion with SMI populations.

In an earlier initiative, the Center for Mental Health Services (CMHS) was formed in the early 1990s to improve prevention and mental health treatment services for all Americans. The CMHS helps states improve and increase the quality and range of treatment, rehabilitation, and support services for people with mental health problems, their families, and their communities (SAMHSA, 2014).

BOX 25.5 Key Features of the Assertive Community Treatment (ACT) Program

- Psychopharmacological treatment
- Individual supportive therapy
- Mobile crisis intervention
- Hospitalization
- Substance abuse treatment
- Behaviorally oriented skill teaching
- Supported employment
- Support for resuming education
- Collaboration with families and assistance to clients with children
- Direct support to help clients obtain legal and advocacy services

One of the programs promoted by the CMHS is the Community Support System. The Community Support System uses case management strategies to comprehensively provide care for those with SMI. Components of the Community Support System include client identification and outreach, mental health treatment, crisis response service, health and dental care, housing, income support and entitlement, peer support, family and community support, rehabilitation services, and protection and advocacy. The case management approach serves to link the service system to the client and to coordinate their service received (National Center for Biotechnology Information [NCBI], 2017).

The Assertive Community Treatment (ACT) model is another example of a community-based initiative to help meet the needs of those with mental illness. ACT, which has been in existence since the late 1960s, has become the exemplar of community mental health treatment models. The program moves the traditional 24-hour treatment model of acute care setting into the community and serves people with mental illness in a highly individualized fashion (NAMI, 2013). The ACT model provides supportive therapy, mobile crisis intervention, psychiatric medications, hospitalization, education, and skill teaching for consumers and their families. Currently, seven states and the District of Columbia have statewide ACT programs, and many more have at least one pilot project (NAMI, 2013). Box 25.5 gives additional details about ACT programs.

The CIT program originates from the Memphis Model, an educational and advocacy training program (NAMI, 2017c). The Memphis Police Department joined with the Memphis Chapter of the NAMI, mental health providers, the University of Memphis, and the University of Tennessee in organizing, training, and implementing a specialized unit. CIT programs partner with mental health consumers and family members, mental health professionals, and advocacy organizations. Law enforcement personnel are trained in developing a more intelligent, understandable, and safe approach to mental crisis events. (See Box 25.6 for the core elements of the CIT.)

Specialty courts—also called *treatment courts, accountability courts,* and *problem-solving courts*—deal with a number of problem areas within the criminal justice system. These specialty courts can deal with adult, juvenile, users, and family drug problems; mental health disorders; military veterans; and people found to be driving under the influence of alcohol or drugs. These programs incorporate assessment and screening to

BOX 25.6 Core Elements of Crisis Intervention Teams (CITs) Ongoing Elements

1. Partnerships: law enforcement, advocacy, mental health
2. Community ownership: planning, implementation, and networking
3. Policies and procedures

Operational Elements
1. CIT: officer, dispatcher, coordinator
2. Curriculum: CIT training
3. Mental health receiving facility: emergency services

Sustaining Elements
1. Evaluation and research
2. In-service training
3. Recognition and honors
4. Outreach: developing CIT in other communities

From the University of Memphis, School of Urban Affairs and Public Policy, Department of Criminology and Criminal Justice, CIT Center CIT International, Dupont R, Cochran S, Pillsbury, S: Crisis Intervention Team core elements, 2006. http://www.citinternational.org/resources/Pictures/CoreElements.pdf. Accessed May 1, 2018.

examine problematic behavior due to mental health problems and substance abuse. Specialty courts provide education regarding mental and substance use disorders and medication monitoring and drug testing.

ROLE OF THE COMMUNITY MENTAL HEALTH NURSE

More than ever, there are opportunities for the community mental health nurse to make a difference. For the psychiatric–mental health nurse there are EBP models of care providing promising outcomes in communities. Application of the nursing process can be facilitated to help special populations affected by mental illness in the community. There are challenges to the effective provision of mental health services in the community, such as accessibility, disparity, and cost. In spite of multiple challenges, the role of a community mental health nurse can be extremely rewarding and filled with personal satisfaction (Gerber, 2017).

Community mental health nursing roles are multidimensional (e.g., participant in mental health courts, veterans courts, other specialty or problem-solving courts; educator, researcher, collaborator, consultant, case manager, content expert, administrator, activist, politician, advocate, initiator, evaluator, grant writer, practitioner, and coordinator). Mental health nurses serve on ACT, CIT, community case management, mobile crisis, and crisis housing coordination teams. Community mental health nurses as educators and activists dispel myths, provide accurate information about mental illness, and influence policy and legislation advocating for those with mental illness.

As practitioner and coordinator, the nurse works directly with individuals, groups, and families. Besides intervening to assist consumers in controlling or alleviating the symptoms of mental illness, the practitioner and coordinator also helps the consumer "navigate" the segmented web of agencies and other service providers. A list of organizations that advocate for mental health is shown in Table 25.4. Community mental health nurses not only take action to solve an immediate problem but also plan and intervene to ensure safety, continuity, and quality of care for consumers. Therefore the practitioner and coordinator roles require skills in anticipating and evaluating the actions of other providers and communicating with consumers, families, rehabilitation services, and government or social agencies.

Within this aspect of community mental health nursing, individual-, family-, and community-level crises are anticipated and prevented or, failing these, contained. For example, as practitioners and coordinators, nurses might organize people taking psychotropic medications to share experiences about interacting with a psychiatrist, managing side effects of medications, and enhancing their coping strategies. Such a proactive stance may help prevent problems that lead clients to discontinue medications and the consequences of such actions. In the practitioner and coordinator roles, community mental health nurses work toward matching consumers and families with culturally appropriate and sensitive providers to achieve the "best fit."

TABLE 25.4 Organizations That Promote Education and Advocate for Mental Health

Resource	Services	Contact Information
Substance Abuse and Mental Health Services Administration (SAMHSA)	Programs, policies, information and data, contracts, and grants Vision: Behavioral health is essential for health, prevention works, treatment is effective, people can recover from mental illness diagnosis and substance abuse	http://www.samhsa.gov/
National Alliance on Mental Illness (NAMI)	Consumer education regarding various mental health disorders, medication and treatment, research, public policy issues; links to find support at state and local level, including support groups and online discussion groups; tips for becoming politically involved in mental health public policy issues	http://www.nami.org/
Mental Health America (MHA)	Inform, advocate, and enable access to quality behavioral health services for all Americans	http://www.mentalhealthamerica.net/
National Institute of Mental Health (NIMH)	Education on mental health topics and research Vision: Understanding and treatment of mental illnesses through basic and clinical research, paving the way for prevention, recovery, and cure	http://www.nimh.nih.gov/index.shtml
Depression and Bipolar Support Alliance	Education on depression and bipolar disorder; online discussion and support groups; assistance in finding treatment resources	http://www.dbsalliance.org
National Education Alliance for Borderline Personality Disorder	Education about borderline personality disorder and treatment	www.borderlinepersonalitydisorder.com/

Continued

TABLE 25.4 Organizations That Promote Education and Advocate for Mental Health—cont'd

Resource	Services	Contact Information
Obsessive-Compulsive Foundation	Education about obsessive-compulsive and anxiety disorders and treatment	www.ocfoundation.org/
Postpartum Support International	Education and resource information for individuals experiencing symptoms of prenatal or postpartum mood or anxiety disorders	http://postpartum.net/
U.S. Department of Veteran Affairs National Center for PTSD	Public and professional sections for education and training materials, as well as information and tools to help with assessment and treatment	http://www.ptsd.va.gov/
Brain and Behavior Research Foundation, formerly called National Association for Research on Schizophrenia and Depression (NARSAD)	Alleviating the suffering caused by mental illness by awarding grants that will lead to advances and breakthroughs in scientific research	http://bbrfoundation.org/
National Council for Community Behavioral Healthcare	Behavioral health care, holistic approach to meet needs of the individuals and families	www.thenationalcouncil.org/cs/home

CASE STUDY Application of the Nursing Process

Client With Mental Illness

Joseph Green, a divorced 57-year-old veteran of Operation Iraqi Freedom, was discharged from the hospital with a referral to cardiac rehabilitation. Joseph has a ventricular pacemaker that was inserted 2 years ago. Last week he was brought into the emergency department for failure of the pacemaker. He was experiencing syncope and hypotension. His pacemaker was corrected and he was discharged back into the community, where he is currently living at a men's shelter.

Joseph has a history of a congestive heart failure, depression, alcoholism, chronic obstructive pulmonary disease, traumatic brain injury, and PTSD. He has prescriptions for citalopram, carvedilol, and an Advair inhaler. He admits to being noncompliant at times with taking his prescriptions. He has access to health care services from the nearest Veterans Administration (VA) medical center, which is 350 miles away. He takes a Disabled American Veterans (DAV) van to the medical center once or twice a month where he fills his prescriptions and sees mental health counselors. There is cardiac rehabilitation at the center, but Joseph does not want to go as often as the VA doctors have recommended. Joseph has no income and cooks meals at the men's shelter for his room and board. Because he cannot drink alcohol at the shelter, he has been abstinent for 9 months. He smokes a pack of cigarettes daily when he has cigarettes.

Joseph has difficulty sleeping most nights and awakens from nightmares. He was diagnosed with major depression and PTSD 5 years ago and reports having suicidal thoughts occasionally. He has been estranged from his grown children for several years. He has a sister living in the same city and his relationship with her is strained. The ACT team makes visits to the shelter to assist other men, and Joseph has inquired how to become a consumer of ACT services. There is a local veterans' support group at the Veterans of Foreign Wars (VFW) building that Joseph and others from the shelter go to several nights a week.

Assessment

On his first trip to the VA medical center after his recent discharge, the outpatient clinic nurse notes that Joseph was noncompliant with his mediations only 2 days the previous week. He reports that he is not depressed, and he denies having suicidal thoughts. He has had no syncope or chest palpations.

Diagnosis

Individual

- History of mental illness (depression, PTSD, and alcoholism)
- Difficulty following treatment regimen
- Less-than-adequate social skills
- Poor self-worth
- History of suicidal ideation

Family and Social Relationships

- Inability to communicate with family members effectively
- Jeopardy of recurring homelessness

Planning

Planning for Joseph is primarily through collaboration in the community where he resides at the men's shelter. His relationships with others at the shelter and the VFW are important. The staff at the men's shelter are familiar with the VA's homeless program information: 1-877-4AID-VET (1-877-425-3838) and http://www.va.gov/HOMELESS/for_homeless_veterans.asp.

The men's shelter also supports Joseph by helping him get to the DAV van when he has an appointment at the VA medical center. The shelter offers chaplain services and also utilizes the community CIT law enforcement officers at times to help talk with residents when they are experiencing stress or need de-escalation of their behavior. A CIT officer who is a veteran stops in once in a while to see the men as a proactive visit.

Individual

Long-Term Goal

- Joseph will progress with community supportive services and relationships with people.

Short-Term Goals

- Joseph will remain medication compliant.
- Joseph will remain abstinent from alcohol.

Family and Social Relationships

Long-Term Goals

- Safe housing
- Compliance with medications
- Sobriety
- Case management with ACT team and VA

Short-Term Goals

- Working with shelter staff and ACT team
- Sobriety
- Compliance with medications

Intervention

The staff at the men's shelter meet with Joseph regularly to evaluate compliance with medications. The staff also will know when his appointments are at the VA

Client With Mental Illness

in order to plan transportation on the DAV van. The relationships that Joseph has with other veterans are helpful in a support milieu.

Individual

- Joseph has agreed to work with the staff at the shelter in a team effort to keep him in safe housing. He has agreed to work with the ACT team, VA case management, and his Alcoholics Anonymous (AA) community.

Family and Social Relationships

- Joseph will continue to work with VA case management, the ACT team, and the staff at the shelter.
- He will call his sister weekly.

Evaluation

Joseph verbalized understanding of the importance of safe housing, the ACT team intervention, and social relationships with VA peers and AA peers. He also agreed to call his AA or VA contact when needed if he is

beginning to feel agitated or wanting to isolate himself. The ACT team will consistently contact Joseph and be available on weekends. Joseph has agreed to give permission for the ACT team to report his status to the VA case managers.

Levels of Prevention

Primary

- Maintaining housing at shelter
- Assisting Joseph with compliance with medications

Secondary

- Encouraging maintenance of social relationships (shelter staff, other veterans, AA peers) and relationship with sister

Tertiary

- Monitoring of medical health status and psychological health status
- Group therapy at AA meetings and the VA medical center

SUMMARY

Like all other aspects of nursing, community mental health nursing is developing, applying, and utilizing EBP models of community treatment, such as ACT, community case management, or CIT. The twenty-first-century community mental health multidisciplinary team approaches can promote improvement in the identification of and care for those with mental illness. Improved information and EBP may result in greater understanding of the factors that contribute to mental disorders and lead to more effective treatment.

As discussed in this chapter, the vast majority of individuals with diagnosable mental disorders are found in the community, and many, if not most, never seek professional help. The framework for community mental health nursing presented in this chapter should prove useful in improving the lives of individuals, families, and groups of people with mental illness. Further, it is hoped that all nurses will become advocates for the mentally ill and will support social and political change to improve the mental health of all.

? ACTIVE LEARNING

1. Reflect on your personal experience interacting with individuals with mental illness. What thoughts or feelings did these experiences produce? What are several issues that nurses can advocate for in caring for this special population?

2. List five topics or issues for which the community mental health nurse can facilitate individual, family, or group education in the community.

ⓔ EVOLVE WEBSITE

http://evolve.elsevier.com/Nies/community

- NCLEX Review Questions
- Case Studies

BIBLIOGRAPHY

American Association of Suicidology: *Know the warning signs of suicide*, 2017. Available at: http://www.suicidology.org/resources/warning-signs.

American Foundation for Suicide Prevention: *Suicide statistics*. Available at: https://afsp.org/about-suicide/suicide-statistics/, 2017.

American Psychiatric Association: *Understanding mental disorders: your guide to DSM-5*. Available at: https://www.psychiatry.org/patients-families/understanding-mental-disorders, 2015.

American Psychiatric Association: *Diagnostic and statistical manual of mental disorders*, ed 5, Arlington, VA, 2017a, American Psychiatric Publishing.

American Psychiatric Association: *DSM-V: Frequently asked questions*. Available at: http://www.psychiatry.org/psychiatrists/practice/dsm/feedback-and-questions/frequently-asked-questions, 2017b.

American Psychological Association: Incarceration nation: the United States leads the world in incarceration, *Monitor on Psychology* 45(9):56, 2014.

American Psychological Association: *Understanding psychotherapy and how it works*. Available at: http://www.apa.org/helpcenter/understanding-psychotherapy.aspx, 2017.

Anxiety and Depression Association of America: *Depression*. Available at: https://www.adaa.org/understanding-anxiety/depression# Depression, 2016a.

Anxiety and Depression Association of America: *Facts and statistics*. Available at: https://www.adaa.org/about-adaa/press-room/facts-statistics, 2016b.

Anxiety and Depression Association of America: *Generalized anxiety disorder (GAD)*. Available at: https://www.adaa.org/understanding-anxiety/generalized-anxiety-disorder-gad. Accessed February 20, 2017, 2016c.

Berretta S, Heckers S, Benes F: Searching human brain for mechanisms of psychiatric disorders. Implications for studies on schizophrenia, *Schizophr Res* 167:91–97, 2015.

Bonaz B, Bernstein C: Brain-gut interactions in inflammatory bowel disease, *Gastroenterology* 144(1):36–49, 2013.

Brain and Behavior Research Foundation: *Schizophrenia.* Available at: http://bbrfoundation.org/schizophrenia, 2017.

Centers for Disease Control and Prevention (CDC): Mental health surveillance among children – United States, 2005-2011, *MMWR* 62(2):1–35, 2013a. Available at: http://www.cdc.gov/mmwr/preview/mmwrhtml/su6202a1.htm?s_cid=su6202a1_w.

Centers for Disease Control and Prevention (CDC): *Mental illness among U.S. adults.* Available at: https://www.cdc.gov/mentalhealth surveillance./, 2013b.

Centers for Disease Control and Prevention (CDC): *CDC report: 'Nearly 50% of U.S. Adults will develop at least one mental illness'.* Available at: www.cnsnews.com/news/article.cdc-nearly-50-us-adults-will-develop-at-least-one-mental-illness, 2013c.

Centers for Disease Control and Prevention (CDC): *Suicide: facts at a glance.* Available at: http://www.cdc.gov/ViolencePrevention/pdf/Suicide_DataSheet-a.pdf, 2015.

Centers for Disease Control and Prevention (CDC): *Attention deficit hyperactivity disorder (ADHD).* Available at: https://www.cdc.gov/nchs/fastats/adhd.htm, 2016a.

Centers for Disease Control and Prevention (CDC): *Burden of mental illness.* Available at: https://www.cdc.gov/mentalhealth/basics/burden.htm, 2016b.

Clement S, Schauman O, Graham T, et al.: What is the impact of mental health-related stigma on help-seeking? A systematic review of quantitative and qualitative studies, *Psychol Med* 45(1):11–27, 2015.

Corrigan P, Druss B, Perlick D: The impact of mental illness stigma on seeking and participating in mental health care, *Psychol Sci Public Interest* 15(2):37–70, 2014.

Department of Health and Human Services (USDHHS): *Healthy People 2020.* Available at: http://www.healthypeople.gov/2020/. Accessed March 25, 2017.

Dieterich M, Bergman C, Khokhar H, et al.: *Intensive case management for people with severe mental illness.* Available at: www.cochrane.org/CD007096/SCHIZ_intensive-case-management-people-severe-mental-illness, 2017.

Drake R, Whitley R: Recovery and severe mental illness: description and analysis, *Can J Psychiatry* 59(5):236–242, 2014.

Dumont D, Allen S, Brockman B, et al.: Incarceration, community health, and racial disparities, *J Health Care Poor Underserved* 24(1):78–88, 2013.

Eriksen KA, Sundfor B, Karlsson B, et al.: Recognition as a valued human being: perspectives of mental health service users, *Nursing Ethics* 19(3):357–368, 2012.

ExploreHealthCareers.org: *Public health nurse.* Available at: https://explorehealthcareers.org/career/nursing/public-health-nurse/, 2017.

Gerber L: Community health nursing: a partnership of care, *Nursing* 42(1), 2017. Available at: http://www.nursingcenter.com/journalarticle?Article_ID=1287272.

Han B, Oliffe J: Photovoice in mental illness research: a review and recommendations, *Health: An Interdisciplinary Journal for the Social Study of Health, Illness and Medicine* 20(2):110–126, 2016.

Healthy Place: *Depression in children: Causes and treatment of childhood depression.* Available at: http://www.healthyplace.com/depression/children/depression-in-children-causes-treatment-of-child-depression/. Accessed March 25, 2017, 2016.

Healthcare.gov: *Read the affordable care act.* Available at: https://www.healthcare.gov/where-can-i-read-the-affordable-care-act/. Accessed March 25, 2017, 2017.

HealthyPeople.gov: *Healthy people 2020: topics & objectives: mental health and mental disorders.* Available at: https://www.healthypeople.gov/2020/topics-objectives/topic/mental-health-and-mental-disorders/objectives. Accessed March 25, 2017, 2017.

HealthyPeople.gov: *About healthy people.* Available at: https://www.healthypeople.gov/2020/About-Healthy-People. Accessed March 07, 2017, 2017a.

HealthyPeople.gov: *Federal interagency workgroup.* Available at: https://www.healthypeople.gov/2020/about/history-development/Federal-Interagency-Workgroup. Accessed March 07, 2017, 2017b.

Kassam A, Papish A, Modgill G, et al.: The development and psychometric properties of a new scale to measure mental illness related stigma by health care providers: the opening minds scale for health care providers (OMS-HC), *BMC Psychiatry* 12(62):3–12, 2012.

Kohlmann W, Champine M, Colona S: *Communicating genetic test results to patients and their families.* Available at: https://am.asco.org/communicating-genetic-test-results-patients-and-their-families. Accessed March 07, 2017, 2015.

Lê Cook B, Zuvekas S, Carson N, et al.: Assessing racial/ethnic disparities in treatment across episodes of mental health care, *Health Services Res* 49(1):206–229, 2014.

Lucassen P, Pruessner J, Sousa N, et al.: Neuropathology of stress, *Acta Neuropathologica* 127(1):109–135, 2014.

Mayo Clinic: *Depression: risk factors.* Available at: http://www.mayoclinic.org/diseases-conditions/depression/basics/risk-factors/con-20032977. Accessed March 07, 2017, 2017.

Memon M, Welton R: *Panic disorder: epidemiology.* Available at: http://emedicine.medscape.com/article/287913-overview#a5. Accessed March 07, 2017, 2016.

Mental Health America: *Latino/Hispanic communities and mental health.* Available at: http://www.mentalhealthamerica.net/issues/latinohispanic-communities-and-mental-health. Accessed March 07, 2017, 2017a.

Mental Health America: *Position statement 53: mental health courts.* Available at: http://www.mentalhealthamerica.net/positions/mental-health-courts. Accessed March 12, 2017, 2017b.

MentalHealth.gov: *Health insurance and mental health services.* Available at: https://www.mentalhealth.gov/get-help/health-insurance/. Accessed March 07, 2017, 2017.

Moreland C, Bonin L: Patient education: depression treatment options for children and adolescents (beyond the basics), *Uptodate*, 2017. Available at: https://www.uptodate.com/contents/depression-treatment-options-for-children-and-adolescents-beyond-the-basics. Accessed March 12, 2017.

Mustelin L, Silén Y, Raevuori A, et al.: The DSM-5 diagnostic criteria for anorexia nervosa may change its population prevalence and prognostic value, *J Psychiat Res* 77:85–91, 2016.

National Alliance on Mental Illness: *Assertive community treatment (ACT).* Available at: http://www.nami.org/Template.cfm?Section=ACT-TA_Center&Template=/TaggedPage/TaggedPageDisplay.cfm&TPLID=4&ContentID=28611. Accessed March 12, 2017, 2013.

National Alliance on Mental Illness: *Depression.* Available at: http://www.nami.org/Learn-More/Mental-Health-Conditions/Depression. Accessed March 12, 2017, 2017a.

National Alliance on Mental Illness: *Mental health reform.* Available at: http://www.nami.org/Learn-More/Mental-Health-Public-Policy/Mental-Health-Reform. Accessed March 12, 2017, 2017b.

National Alliance for the Mentally Ill: *What is CIT ?* Available at: http://www.nami.org/Law-Enforcement-and-Mental-Health/What-Is-CIT. Accessed March 12, 2017, 2017c.

National Center for Biotechnology Information: *Chapter 2 - applying case management to substance abuse treatment.* Available at: https://www.ncbi.nlm.nih.gov/books/NBK64857/. Accessed March 12, 2017, 2017.

National Council for Behavioral Health: *Community mental health act.* Available at: https://www.thenationalcouncil.org/about/national-mental-health-association/overview/community-mental-health-act/. Accessed March 12, 2017, 2015.

National Eating Disorder Association (NEDA): *What are eating disorders ?* Available at: https://www.nationaleatingdisorders.org/get-facts-eating-disorders. Accessed March 12, 2017, 2016.

National Institute of Mental Health: *Neuroimaging and mental illness: a window into the brain: frequently asked questions about brain scans.* Available at: http://www.nimh.nih.gov/health/publications/neuroimaging-and-mental-illness-a-window-into-the-brain/neuroimaging-faq.pdf. Accessed March 12, 2017.

National Institute of Mental Health: *Psychotherapy.* Available at: http://www.nimh.nih.gov/health/topics/psychotherapies/index.shtml. Accessed March 12, 2017, 2016.

National Institute of Mental Health: *Alliance for research progress: February 8, 2013 meeting.* Available at: http://www.nimh.nih.gov/outreach/alliance/alliance-report-february-2013/alliance-for-research-progress-february-8-2013-meeting.shtml. Accessed March 12, 2017, 2013.

National Institute of Mental Health, National Institute of Mental Health: *Panic disorder among adults,* n.d. Available at: http://www.nimh.nih.gov/statistics/1PANIC_ADULT.shtml. Accessed March 12, 2017.

National Institute of Mental Health: *Anxiety disorders.* Available at: https://www.nimh.nih.gov/health/topics/anxiety-disorders/index.shtml. Accessed March 12, 2017, 2016.

National Institute of Mental Health: *Bipolar disorder.* Available at: https://www.nimh.nih.gov/health/topics/bipolar-disorder/index.shtml. Accessed March 12, 2017, 2016.

National Institute of Mental Health: *PTSD.* Available at: https://www.nimh.nih.gov/health/statistics/prevalence/file_148029.pdf. Accessed March 12, 2017, 2016.

National Institute of Mental Health: *The NIH almanac.* Available at: https://www.nih.gov/about-nih/what-we-do/nih-almanac/national-institute-mental-health-nimh. Accessed March 12, 2017, 2017.

National Institute of Mental Health: *Antidepressant medications for children and adolescents: information for parents and caregivers.* Available at: https://www.nimh.nih.gov/health/topics/child-and-adolescent-mental-health/antidepressant-medications-for-children-and-adolescents-information-for-parents-and-caregivers.shtml. Accessed March 12, 2017, 2017a.

National Institute of Mental Health: *Any disorder among children.* Available at: https://www.nimh.nih.gov/health/statistics/prevalence/any-disorder-among-children.shtml. Accessed March 12, 2017, 2017b.

National Institute of Mental Health: *Any mental illness (AMI) among U.S. adults.* Available at: https://www.nimh.nih.gov/health/statistics/prevalence/any-mental-illness-ami-among-us-adults.shtml. Accessed March 12, 2017, 2017c.

National Institute of Mental Health: *Eating disorders among adults - anorexia nervosa.* Available at: https://www.nimh.nih.gov/health/statistics/prevalence/eating-disorders-among-adults-anorexia-nervosa.shtml. Accessed March 12, 2017, 2017d.

National Institute of Mental Health: *Eating disorders among adults - bulimia nervosa.* Available at: https://www.nimh.nih.gov/health/statistics/prevalence/eating-disorders-among-adults-bulimia-nervosa.shtml. Accessed March 12, 2017, 2017e.

National Institute of Mental Health: *Major depression among adolescents.* Available at: https://www.nimh.nih.gov/health/statistics/prevalence/major-depression-among-adolescents.shtml. Accessed March 12, 2017, 2017f.

National Institute of Mental Health: *Major depression among adults.* Available at: https://www.nimh.nih.gov/health/statistics/prevalence/major-depression-among-adults.shtml. Accessed March 18, 2017, 2017g.

National Institute of Mental Health: *Panic disorder among adults.* Available at: https://www.nimh.nih.gov/health/statistics/prevalence/panic-disorder-among-adults.shtml. Accessed March 18, 2017, 2017h.

National Institute of Mental Health: *Schizophrenia.* Available at: https://www.nimh.nih.gov/health/statistics/prevalence/schizophrenia.shtml. Accessed March 18, 2017, 2017i.

National Institute of Mental Health: *Social anxiety disorder: more than just shyness.* Available at: https://www.nimh.nih.gov/health/publications/social-anxiety-disorder-more-than-just-shyness/index.shtml. Accessed March 18, 2017, 2017j.

National Institute of Mental Health: *Obsessive compulsive disorder among adults.* Available at: https://www.nimh.nih.gov/health/statistics/prevalence/obsessive-compulsive-disorder-among-adults.shtml. Accessed March 18, 2017, 2017k.

National Institute of Mental Health: *Office for research on disparities and global mental health (ORDGMH).* Available at: https://www.nimh.nih.gov/about/organization/gmh/index.shtml. Accessed March 18, 2017, 2017.

Pattyn E, Verhaeghe M, Sercu C, et al.: Medicalizing versus psychologizing mental illness: what are the implications for help seeking and stigma? A general population study, *Soc Psychiatry Psychiatr Epidemiol* 48(10):1637–1645, 2013.

Pratt L, Brody D: *Depression in the U.S. household population, 2009-2012,* NCHS Data Brief No. 172, 2014. Available at: https://www.cdc.gov/nchs/products/databriefs/db172.htm. Accessed March 18, 2017.

Przedworski J, VanKim N, Eisenberg M, et al.: Mental disorders and distress by sexual orientation: results of the minnesota college student health survey, *Am J Prev Med* 49(1):29–40, 2015.

Remedy Health Communities.com: *Phobias.* Available at: http://www.healthcommunities.com/phobias/overview-of-phobia.shtml. Accessed March 18, 2017, 2016.

SAHMSA: *Screening and referral in integrated health systems.* Available at: https://www.samhsa.gov/health-care-health-systems-integration/screening-referral. Accessed March 18, 2017, 2014.

SAHMSA: *Co-occurring disorders.* Available at: https://www.sahmsa.gov/disorders/co-occurring. Accessed March 18, 2017, 2016.

SAHMSA: *Implementation of the mental health parity and addiction equity act (MHPAEA).* Available at: https://www.samhsa.gov/health-financing/implementation-mental-health-parity-addiction-equity-act. Accessed March 23, 2017, 2017.

Schildkraut J, Elsass H: *Mass shootings: media, myths, and realities,* Santa Barbara: ABC-CLIO, 2016.

Schwartz R, Blankenship D: Racial disparities in psychotic disorder diagnosis: a review of empirical literature, *World J Psych* 4(4): 133–140, 2014.

Shen G, Snowden L: Institutionalization of deinstitutionalization: a cross-national analysis of mental health system reform, *Int J Ment Health Syst* 8(47), 2014. http://doi.org/10.1186/1752-4458-8-47. Accessed March 23, 2017.

Substance Abuse and Mental Health Services Administration (SAMSHA): *State and local government partnerships.* Available at: https://www.samhsa.gov/state-local-government-partnerships. Accessed March 23, 2017, 2014.

Substance Abuse and Mental Health Services Administration (SAMSHA): *Mental and substance use disorders.* Available at: https://www.samhsa.gov/disorders. Accessed March 23, 2017, 2016.

Surgeon General and US DHHS: *Department of Defense strategy for suicide prevention.* Available at: www.dspo.mil/Portals/113/Documents/TAB%20B%20-%20DSSP_FINAL%20USD%20PR%20SIGNED.PDF. Accessed March 23, 2017, 2017.

Thompson E, Hollister B: Schizophrenia and suicide attempts: findings from a representative community-based Canadian sample, *Schizophr Res Treatment*, 2016. Article ID 3165243, 11 pages. Available at: https://doi.org/10.1155/2016/3165243. Accessed March 23, 2017.

Torrey D: *Impaired awareness of illness: anosognosia.* Available at: http://mentalillnesspolicy.org/medical/anosognosia-studies.html. Accessed March 23, 2017, 2017.

Treatment Advocacy Center: *Going, going, gone; Trends and consequences of eliminating state psychiatric beds,* 2016. Available at: http://www.treatmentadvocacycenter.org/evidence-and-research/studies. Accessed March 23, 2017. Accessed March 25, 2017

Treatment Advocacy Center: *Anosognosia.* Available at: http://www.treatmentadvocacycenter.org/key-issues/anosognosia. Accessed March 23, 2017, 2017.

U.S. Department of Defense: *Suicide prevention and awareness.* Available at: http://www.defense.gov/home/features/2012/0812_suicide-prevention/. Accessed March 23, 2017, 2015a.

U.S. Department of Defense: Defense Suicide Prevention Office, *Department of defense quarterly suicide report calendar year 2015 2nd Quarter,* 2015b. Available at: www.dspo.mil/Portals/113/Documents/DoD%20Quarterly%20Suicide%20Report%20CY2015%20Q2.pdf. Accessed March 23, 2017.

U.S. Department of Defense: *Strategy for suicide prevention.* Available at: www.dspo.mil/.../TAB%20B%20-%20DSSP_FINAL%20USD%20PR%20SIGNED.PDF. Accessed March 25, 2017, 2015c.

U.S. Department of Defense: *Suicide event report: calendar year 2014 annual report.* Available at: http://www.dspo.mil/Prevention/Data-Surveillance/DoDSER-Annual-Reports/. Accessed March 25, 2017, 2015d.

U.S. Department of Health and Human Services; Office of the Assistant Secretary for Planning and Evaluation: *Affordable care act expands mental health and substance use disorder benefits and federal parity protections for 62 million Americans.* Available at: https://aspe.hhs.gov/report/affordable-care-act-expands-mental-health-and-substance-use-disorder-benefits-and-federal-parity-protections-62-million-americans. Accessed March 25, 2017, 2013.

U.S. Department of Health and Human Services; Office of the Surgeon General and National Action Alliance for Suicide Prevention: *National strategy for suicide prevention: goals and objectives for action,* Washington, DC, 2012, Author.

USDHHS/SAMHSA: *Behavioral health, United States.* Available at: http://www.samhsa.gov/data/2012BehavioralHealthUS/Index.aspx. Accessed March 25, 2017, 2012.

USDHHS.gov: *What is mental health?* Available at: https://www.mentalhealth.gov/basics/what-is-mental-health/. Accessed March 25, 2017, 2017.

van der Westhuizen C, Wyatt G, Williams J, et al.: *Prevalence and predictors of mental disorders in intentionally and unintentionally injured emergency centre patients.* Available at: https://www.ncbi.nlm.nih.gov/pmc/articles/PMC41700144/. Accessed March 25, 2017, 2014.

WebMD: *Obsessive-compulsive disorder.* Available at: http://www.webmd.com/mental-health/obsessive-compulsive-disorder#1. Accessed March 25, 2017, 2017.

World Health Organization: *Suicide.* Available at: http://www.who.int/mediacentre/factsheets/fs398/en/. Accessed March 25, 2017, 2017.

26

Communicable Disease

Deanna E. Grimes

OBJECTIVES

Upon completion of this chapter, the reader will be able to do the following:

1. Review principles related to the occurrence and transmission of infection and infectious diseases.
2. Describe the three focus areas in *Healthy People 2020* objectives that apply to infectious diseases.
3. Describe the chain of transmission of infectious diseases.
4. Apply the chain of transmission to describing approaches to control infectious disease.
5. Review types of immunity, including herd immunity.

6. Review principles of immunization, and specify the immunization recommended for all age groups in the United States.
7. Describe the legal responsibility for control of communicable diseases in the United States.
8. Describe the chain of transmission and control for priority infectious disease.
9. Identify nursing activities for control of infectious diseases at primary, secondary, and tertiary levels of prevention.

KEY TERMS

acquired immunity	host	portal of entry
active immunity	immunity	portal of exit
agent	immunization	primary vaccine failure
antigenicity	incidence	quarantine
carriers	incubation period	reservoir
case	indirect transmission	resistance
cold chain	infection	secondary vaccine failure
communicable disease	infectious disease	subclinical infection
communicable period	infectivity	susceptible
control	isolation	toxigenicity
direct transmission	latency	universal precautions
elimination	multicausation	vaccination
endemic	natural immunity	Vaccine Adverse Event Reporting
environment	notifiable infectious diseases	System (VAERS)
epidemic	outbreak	Vaccine Information Statements
eradication	pandemic	(VISs)
fomites	passive immunity	vectors
herd immunity	pathogenicity	virulence

Throughout history, epidemics have been responsible for the destruction of entire groups of people. Despite amazing advances in public health and health care, control of communicable diseases continues to be a major concern of health care providers. The emergence of new pathogens, the reemergence of old pathogens, and the appearance of drug-resistant pathogens are creating formidable challenges in the United States and worldwide.

Despite global eradication campaigns, malaria and other vectorborne diseases and life-threatening gastrointestinal infections continue to cause significant morbidity and mortality in the developing world. Although the incidence rate of tuberculosis (TB) has been declining, in 2015 there were an estimated 10.4 million new cases of TB worldwide, with 1.4 million people dying from the disease (World Health Organization [WHO], 2016). To add to the world's growing infectious disease burden, human immunodeficiency virus (HIV) and acquired immunodeficiency syndrome (AIDS) continue to spread worldwide, as evidenced by the estimate that 36.7 million adults and children were living with HIV/AIDS globally at the end of 2015. Although new HIV infections have been declining slowly since 2001, there were approximately 2.1 million new infections worldwide in 2015 (UNAIDS, 2016).

Great strides have been made in the United States with respect to vaccine-preventable diseases, yet segments of the population remain unimmunized or underimmunized. Both measles and pertussis can be prevented with a vaccine, and indigenous measles had been virtually eliminated in the United States, with only 43 cases reported in 2007 (CDC, 2012). This number has varied yearly since then, increasing from 63 cases in 2010 to 667 cases in 2014 (CDC, 2017). These cases mainly have occurred in outbreaks among populations unimmunized because of philosophical or religious preferences (CDC, 2016). Pertussis incidence has also gradually increased, rising from 10,500 cases in 2007

to almost 33,000 cases in 2014 (CDC, 2016). Cases of hepatitis A, B, and C have been significantly reduced since the 1990s through administration of vaccines for hepatitis A and B and testing of the blood supply for hepatitis C. Yet these diseases persist. Treatable sexually transmitted diseases (STDs), such as gonorrhea, *Chlamydia*, and syphilis, are still occurring at significant rates. Gonorrhea declined until 2009 but has steadily increased since then (CDC, 2016). *Chlamydia,* the most commonly reported bacterial disease in the United States, reached 1,441,789 cases in 2014 (CDC, 2016), although some of this increase is thought to be the result of improved screening for the infection. Rates of primary and secondary syphilis also have increased to an all-time high in 2014 (CDC, 2016).

In the United States, there have been significant accomplishments in preventing foodborne and waterborne infections through environmental sanitation. The incidence, however, of vectorborne infections, such as Lyme disease, Rocky Mountain spotted fever, St. Louis encephalitis, West Nile encephalitis, and Zika, appears to be increasing. Furthermore, although the advent of effective antiretroviral treatment for AIDS in the mid-1990s briefly slowed the incidence of AIDS diagnosis, about 30,000 new cases were reported yearly between 2008 and 2011 in the United States. Approximately 36,000 new HIV infections were diagnosed in the United States during 2014 (CDC, 2016).

Probably one of the most profound failures in infectious disease control in the United States and elsewhere is that the successes are not equally distributed in the general population. Infectious diseases continue to be differentially distributed by income and ethnic groups, and the poor and minorities continue to experience the greater burden.

Although there has been marked improvement, infectious and communicable diseases persist. Scientific discoveries about the infectious etiology of stomach ulcers, coronary artery

BOX 26.1 Antimicrobial-Resistant Pathogens by Priority

Urgent Threats (Potential to Become Widespread)
- Clostridium difficile (CDIFF)
- Carbapenem-resistant Enterobacteriaceae (CRE)
- Neisseria gonorrhoeae (cephalosporin resistant)

Serious Threats (May Become Urgent if Incidence Increases)
- Multidrug-resistant Acinetobacter
- Drug-resistant Campylobacter
- Fluconazole-resistant Candida
- Extended-spectrum Enterobacteriaceae (ESBL)
- Vancomycin-resistant Enterococcus (VRE)
- Multidrug-resistant Pseudomonas aeruginosa
- Drug-resistant nontyphoidal Salmonella
- Drug-resistant Salmonella serotype Typhi
- Drug-resistant Shigella
- Methicillin-resistant Staphylococcus aureus (MRSA)
- Drug-resistant Streptococcus pneumoniae
- Drug-resistant Tuberculosis

Concerning (Serious Conditions With Multiple Therapeutic Options Currently)
- Vancomycin-resistant *Staphylococcus aureus*
- Erythromycin-resistant Group A *Streptococcus*
- Clindamycin-resistant Group B *Streptococcus*

Data from Centers for Disease Control and Prevention: *Diseases/pathogens associated with antimicrobial resistance,* 2017. https://www.cdc.gov/drugresistance/biggest_threats.html; and Heymann DL, editor: *Control of communicable diseases manual,* ed 20, Washington, DC, 2015, American Public Health Association.

BOX 26.2 Centers for Disease Control and Prevention List of Potential Bioterrorism Agents and Diseases by Priority Category

Category A
Highest priority; easily transmitted with high mortality and social disruption:
- Anthrax (Bacillus anthracis)
- Botulism (botulinum toxin)
- Plague (Yersinia pestis)
- Smallpox (variola virus)
- Tularemia (Francisella tularensis)
- Viral hemorrhagic fevers (Ebola, Lassa, and Marburg viruses)

Category B
Moderately easy to disseminate; high morbidity with low mortality:
- Brucellosis (*Brucella* spp.)
- Epsilon toxin of *Clostridium perfringens*
- Food safety threats:
  - Salmonellosis (*Salmonella* spp.)
  - *Escherichia coli* 0157:H7
  - Shigellosis (*Shigella* spp.)
- Glanders (*Burkholderia mallei*)
- Melioidosis (*Burkholderia mallei*)
- Psittacosis (*Chlamydia psittaci*)
- Q fever (*Coxiella burnetii*)
- Ricin toxin
- Staphylococcal enterotoxin B
- Typhus fever (Rickettsia prowazekii)
- Viral encephalitis (alphaviruses)
- Water safety threats:
  - Cholera (*Vibrio cholerae*)
  - *Cryptosporidium parvum*

Category C
Emerging pathogens that could be engineered for mass dissemination because of availability and ease of production and dissemination

Modified from Centers for Disease Control and Prevention 2017: https://emergency.cdc.gov/agent/agentlist.asp https://emergency.cdc.gov/bioterrorism/surveillance.asp and *Bioterrorism overview.* https://www.emergency.cdc.gov/bioterrorism/pdf/bioterrorism_overview.pdf

disease, and cervical cancer, for example, suggest that infectious agents may be responsible for more morbidity and mortality than previously recognized. New concerns include the rapid proliferation of drug-resistant organisms (Box 26.1) and the threat that deadly pathogens may be weaponized by terrorists (Box 26.2). Other threats are emerging infectious diseases, those diseases for which the incidence in humans has increased within the past two decades or threatens to increase in the near future. For more information, see the Centers for Disease Control (CDC), National Center for Emerging Zoonotic Infectious Diseases website at https://www.cdc.gov/ncezid/.

This chapter provides nurses with the knowledge necessary to help control infectious diseases. The terms *communicable disease* and *infectious disease* are synonymous and will be used interchangeably.

♥ COMMUNICABLE DISEASE AND *HEALTHY PEOPLE 2020*

The U.S. Department of Health and Human Services program *Healthy People 2020* contains several hundred objectives to improve health; these are organized into 38 topic areas. Three of the topic areas (Immunization and Infectious Diseases, Sexually Transmitted Diseases, and HIV) are specific to infectious diseases. These objectives have been used to evaluate national prevention and control efforts and can guide local prevention and control efforts. The *Healthy People 2020* box lists examples of objectives for immunizations and infectious diseases, objectives related to STDs, and a few of the objectives covering HIV/AIDS. These lists suggest strategies for prevention and control of infectious diseases. Additional information, including baseline and target data for all objectives, can be found on the *Healthy People 2020* website: www.healthypeople.gov/2020/topicsobjectives2020.

HEALTHY PEOPLE 2020

Communicable Disease

Topic Area—Immunization and Infectious Diseases. Retrieved from: https://www.healthypeople.gov/2020/topics-objectives/topic/immunization-and-infectious-diseases/objectives (Website updated 5/01/17)

IID-1: Reduce, eliminate or maintain elimination of cases of vaccine preventable diseases

IID-2: Reduce early-onset group B streptococcal disease

IID-3: Reduce meningococcal disease

IID-4: Reduce invasive pneumococcal infections

IID-5: Reduce outpatient visits for ear infections where antibiotics were prescribed to young children

IID-6: Reduce outpatient visits where antibiotics were prescribed for the sole diagnosis of the common cold

IID-7 to IID-11: Achieve and maintain effective vaccination coverage levels for universally recommended vaccines among children and adolescents

IID-12: Increase the percentage of children and adults who are vaccinated annually against seasonal influenza

IID-13: Increase the percentage of adults who are vaccinated against pneumococcal disease

IID-14: Increase the percentage of adults who are vaccinated against zoster (shingles)

IID-15: Increase hepatitis B vaccine coverage among high-risk populations (hemodialysis patients, men who have sex with men, health care personnel, and injection drug users)

IID-16: Increase the scientific knowledge on vaccine safety and adverse events

IID-17: Increase the percentage of providers who have had vaccination coverage levels among children in their practice population measured within the past year

IID-18: Increase the percentage of children under 6 years of age whose immunization records are in a fully operational, population-based information system

IID-19: Increase the number of states collecting kindergarten vaccination coverage data according to CDC minimum standards

IID-20: Increase the number of reporting areas that have 80% of adolescents with two or more age-appropriate immunizations recorded in an immunization information system

IID-21: Increase the number of states that use electronic data from rabies animal surveillance to inform public health prevention programs

IID-22: Increase the number of public health laboratories monitoring influenza virus resistance to antiviral agents

IID-23 to IID-26: Reduce hepatitis A, hepatitis B, and hepatitis C in all populations

IID-27: Increase the proportion of persons aware they have a hepatitis C infection

IID-28: Increase the proportion of persons who have been tested for hepatitis B virus within minority communities experiencing health disparities

IID-29 to IID-30: Reduce TB; increase treatment completion rate

IID-31: Increase the percentage of contacts to sputum smear-positive TB cases who complete treatment after being diagnosed with latent tuberculosis infection (LTBI) and initiated treatment for LTBI

IID-32: Increase the proportion of culture-confirmed TB patients with a positive nucleic acid amplification test result reported with 2 days of specimen collection

IID-33: Increase the proportion of adults with TB who have been tested for HIV

Topic Area—Sexually Transmitted Diseases. Retrieved from: https://www.healthypeople.gov/2020/topics-objectives/topic/sexually-transmitted-diseases/objectives (Website updated 5/01/17)

STD–1-2: Reduce the proportion of adolescents and young adults with *Chlamydia trachomatis* infections

STD-3-4: Increase the proportion of sexually active females who are screened for genital *Chlamydia*

STD-5: Reduce the proportion of females aged 15 to 44 years who have ever required treatment for pelvic inflammatory disease

STD-6: Reduce gonorrhea rates

STD-7: Reduce sustained domestic transmission of primary and secondary syphilis

STD-8: Reduce congenital syphilis

STD-9: Reduce the proportion of females with human papillomavirus (HPV) infection

STD-10: Reduce the proportion of adults with genital herpes infection due to herpes simplex type 2

Topic Area—Human Immunodeficiency Virus (HIV). Retrieved from: https://www.healthypeople.gov/2020/topics-objectives/topic/hiv/objectives (Website updated 5/01/17)

HIV-1 to HIV-3: Reduce new HIV infection, transmission, and diagnosis among adolescents and adults

HIV-4 to HIV-7: Reduce new cases of acquired immunodeficiency syndrome (AIDS) among all adolescents and adults

HIV-8: Reduce perinatally acquired HIV and AIDS

HIV-9: Reduce the proportion of persons with a diagnosis of stage 3 HIV (AIDS) within 3 months of diagnosis of HIV infection

HIV-10: Increase the proportion of HIV-infected adolescents and adults who receive HIV care and treatment consistent with current standards

HIV-11: Increase the proportion of persons surviving more than 3 years after a diagnosis with AIDS

HIV-12: Reduce deaths from HIV infection

HIV-13: Increase the proportion of persons living with HIV who know their serostatus

HIV-14: Increase the proportion of adolescents and adults who have been tested for HIV in the past 12 months

HIV-15: Increase the proportion of adults with TB who have been tested for HIV

HIV-16: Increase the proportion of substance abuse treatment facilities that offer HIV/AIDS education, counseling, and support

HIV-17: Increase the proportion of sexually active persons who use condoms

HIV-18: Reduce the proportion of men who have sex with men who reported unprotected anal sex in the past 12 months

HIV-19: Increase the proportion of person who are linked to HIV medical care within 3 months of HIV diagnosis

HIV-20: Increase the proportion of persons with an HIV diagnosis who had at least one HIV medical care visit in each 6-month period of the 24-month measurement period, with a minimum of 60 days between medical visits

HIV-21: Increase the proportion of persons with an HIV diagnosis in medical care who were prescribed antiretroviral therapy

HIV-22: Increase the proportion of persons with an HIV diagnosis in medical care with a viral load <200 copies/mL at the last test during the 12-month measurement period

HIV-23: Reduce the proportion of persons with an HIV diagnosis receiving HIV services who were homeless in the 12-month measurement period

PRINCIPLES OF INFECTION AND INFECTIOUS DISEASE OCCURRENCE

Nurses in all settings must be aware of potential threats related to communicable diseases and be prepared to intervene (see Ethical Insights box). To help prepare nurses for this responsibility, biological and epidemiological principles inherent in infection and infectious disease occurrence are reviewed and major terms defined in this section.

Nurse's Responsibility Regarding Communicable Diseases

Rapid proliferation of drug-resistant organisms, bioterrorism, and emerging infectious diseases are all concerns that have great implications for nursing practice. Every nurse should be knowledgeable about recognizing, reporting, preventing, and controlling infectious diseases. Infectious disease control can no longer be limited to the jurisdiction of the public health department or the hospital infection control nurse; it is every nurse's responsibility.

Multicausation

During the early years of medical and nursing history, science promulgated cause-and-effect theories of disease that relied on specifying one cause for each disease. Today, it is understood that disease etiology is complex and multicausal. Infectious diseases are the result of interaction among the human host, an infectious agent, and the environment that surrounds the human host where transmission can occur. This interaction is pictured in the epidemiological triangle of agent, host, and environment described in Chapter 5. The principle of multicausation emphasizes that an infectious agent alone is not sufficient to cause disease; the agent must be transmitted within a conducive environment to a susceptible host. Of special note, nurses are part of the environment and, consequently, must maintain their own up-to-date immunization status and must practice optimum infection control.

Spectrum of Infection

Not all contact with an infectious agent leads to infection, and not all infection leads to an infectious disease. The processes, however, begin in the same way. An infectious agent may contaminate the skin or mucous membranes of a host but not invade the host. Or it may invade, multiply, and produce a subclinical infection (unapparent or asymptomatic) without producing overt symptomatic disease. Or the host may respond with overt symptomatic infectious disease. Infection, then, is the entry and multiplication of an infectious agent in a host. Infectious disease and communicable disease refer to the pathophysiological responses of the host to the infectious agent manifesting as an illness. When the disease is diagnosed in a person, the occurrence would be considered a case. Once infectious agents replicate in a host, they can be transmitted from the host irrespective of the presence of disease symptoms. Some persons become carriers and continue to shed the infectious agent without any symptoms of the disease.

Stages of Infection

An infectious agent that has invaded a host and found conditions hospitable will replicate until it can be shed from the host. This period of replication before shedding is called the *latent period,* or latency. The communicable period, or communicability, follows latency and begins with shedding of the agent. The incubation period is the time from invasion to the time when disease symptoms first appear. Frequently the communicable period begins before symptoms are present. Understanding the distinctions among these terms is important in controlling transmission. These stages of infection are depicted in Fig. 26.1.

Spectrum of Disease Occurrence

The principles covered to this point apply to individuals and their acquisition of infections and infectious diseases. Control of infectious diseases in a population requires identifying and monitoring the occurrence of new cases (incidence) in a population. Some infectious diseases are endemic and occur at a consistent, expected level in a geographic area. Such is the case with some STDs and with TB. An outbreak is an unexpected occurrence of an infectious disease in a limited geographic area during a limited period. Outbreaks of pertussis and salmonellosis, for example, are not uncommon. An epidemic is an unexpected increase in occurrence of an infectious disease in a geographic area over an extended period. Epidemics are defined relative to the infectious agent and the history of the disease in the area. One case of smallpox anywhere would constitute an epidemic, whereas 1000 new cases of gonorrhea would not be considered an epidemic in an area where gonorrhea is common. A pandemic is a steady occurrence of a disease, or an epidemic, that covers a large geographic area or is evident worldwide. In July 2009, for example, the WHO designated the occurrence of H1N1 influenza as a pandemic.

CHAIN OF TRANSMISSION

Transmission is frequently conceptualized as a chain with six links, all connected, as in Fig. 26.2. Each of the links (infectious agent, reservoir, portal of exit, mode of transmission, portal of entry, and host susceptibility) represents a different component that contributes to transmission. The chain of transmission and its elements are summarized in Table 26.1.

Infectious Agents

Because the process of transmission is different for every infectious agent, one might envision a different configuration of the chain and its links for each infectious agent and infectious disease that exist. Infectious agents act differently, depending on their intrinsic properties and interactions with their human host. For example, an agent's size, shape, chemical composition, growth requirements, and viability (ability to survive for extended periods) have an impact on transmission and the type of parasitic relationship it establishes with its host. These characteristics determine the classifications of different agents (e.g.,

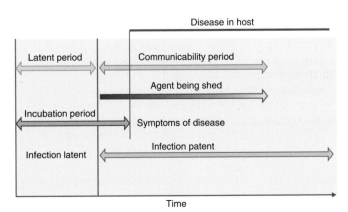

FIG. 26.1 Stages of infection. (From Grimes DE: *Infectious diseases*, St Louis, 1991, Mosby.)

prions, viruses, bacteria, fungi, and protozoa), and knowing the classification is helpful in understanding how specific agents are transmitted and produce disease. Also important are how the agent interacts with its host and its mode of action in the body. For example, it may kill cells, like *Mycobacterium tuberculosis,* or interfere with circulation, like the spirochete that causes syphilis. Or maybe it produces a toxin (**toxigenicity**) as does *Clostridium botulinum,* or stimulates an immune response in the host (**antigenicity**), as does rubella virus. Other considerations for understanding the action of agents are their power to invade and infect large numbers of people (**infectivity**), their ability to produce disease in those infected with the agent (**pathogenicity**), and their ability to produce serious disease in their hosts (**virulence**). If we apply the preceding concepts to the chickenpox virus, we see that it has high infectivity, high pathogenicity, and very low virulence. On the other hand, *M. tuberculosis* has low infectivity and low pathogenicity but high virulence if untreated. Smallpox virus is high on all three concepts. Last, one must consider how adaptable an agent is to its human host and whether the agent changes, or mutates, over time, as HIV does.

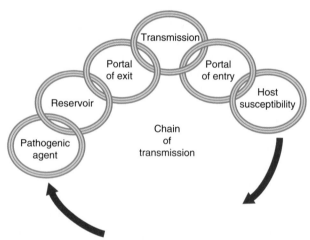

FIG. 26.2 Chain of transmission. (From Grimes DE: *Infectious diseases,* St Louis, 1991, Mosby.)

Reservoirs

The environment in which a pathogen lives and multiplies is the **reservoir**. Reservoirs can be humans, animals, arthropods, plants, soil, water, or any other organic substance. Some agents have more than one reservoir. Knowing the reservoirs for infectious agents is important, because in some cases, transmission can be controlled by eliminating the reservoir, such as eliminating the standing water where mosquitoes breed.

Portals of Exit and Entry

Agents leave the human host through a **portal of exit** and invade through a **portal of entry**. Portals of exit include respiratory secretions, vaginal secretions, semen, saliva, lesion exudates, blood, and feces. Portals of entry are associated with the portal of exit and include the respiratory passages, mucous membranes, skin and blood vessels, oral cavity, and the placenta.

Modes of Transmission

Direct transmission is the immediate transfer of an infectious agent from an infected host or reservoir to an appropriate portal of entry in the human host through physical contact, such as a touch, bite, kiss, or sexual contact. Direct projections of mucous secretions by droplet spray to the conjunctiva or mucous membranes of the eye, nose, or mouth during coughing, sneezing, or laughing are also considered direct transmission. Direct person-to-person contact is responsible for the transmission of many communicable diseases (e.g., STDs, influenza).

Indirect transmission is the spread of infection through a vehicle of transmission outside the host. These may be contaminated fomites or vectors. **Fomites** can be any inanimate objects, materials, or substances that act as transport agents for a microbe (e.g., water, a telephone shared by many, or a contaminated tissue). The infectious agent may or may not reproduce on or in the fomite. Substances such as food, water, and blood products can provide indirect transmission through ingestion and intravenous transfusions. Botulism is an example of an indirectly transmitted foodborne enterotoxin disease.

TABLE 26.1	**Chain of Transmission**	
Link of the Chain	**Definition**	**Factor(s)**
Infectious agent	An organism (virus, rickettsia, bacteria, fungus, protozoan, helminth, or prion) capable of producing infection or infectious disease	Properties of the agent: morphology, chemical composition, growth requirements, and viability; interaction with the host: mode of action, infectivity, pathogenicity, virulence, toxigenicity, antigenicity, and ability to adapt to the host
Reservoir(s)	The environment in which a pathogen lives and multiplies	Humans, animals, arthropods (bugs), plants, soil, or any other organic substance
Portal(s) of exit	Means by which an infectious agent is transported from the host	Respiratory secretions, vaginal secretions, semen, saliva, lesion exudates, blood, and feces
Mode(s) of transmission	Method whereby the infectious agent is transmitted from one host (or reservoir) to another host	*Direct:* Person to person *Indirect:* Implies a vehicle of transmission (biological or mechanical vector, common vehicles or fomites, airborne droplets)
Portal(s) of entry	Means by which an infectious agent enters a new host	Respiratory passages, mucous membranes, skin, percutaneous new host space, mouth, and through the placenta
Host susceptibility	The presence or absence of resistance to an infectious agent	Biological and personal characteristics (e.g., gender, age, genetics), general health status, personal behaviors, anatomical and physiological lines of defense, immunity

Vectors can be animals or arthropods, and they can transmit through biological and mechanical routes. The mechanical route involves no multiplication or growth of the parasite or microbe within the animal or vector. Such is the case when a housefly carries gastrointestinal agents from raw sewage to uncovered food. Biological transmission occurs when the parasite grows or multiplies inside the animal, vector, or arthropod. Examples of diseases spread by this method of transmission include arthropodborne diseases such as malaria, hemorrhagic fevers, and viral encephalitis. Transmission from a vector to the human host usually occurs through a bite or sting. Such is the case with the mosquito vector that transmits St. Louis encephalitis and West Nile and Zika viruses.

Fecal-oral transmission can be direct or indirect. It can occur indirectly through the ingestion of water that has been fecally polluted or through consumption of contaminated food. Direct transmission occurs through engagement in oral sexual activity. Poliovirus and hepatitis A are spread through fecal-oral routes.

Airborne transmission occurs mainly through dissemination of microbial aerosols and droplet nuclei (small residues that result from evaporation of droplets of fluid from an infected host). The time frame in which an airborne particle can remain suspended greatly influences the virility and infectivity of the organism. The size of the particle can also determine how long it remains airborne and how successful it will be at penetrating the human lung. Aerosols are extremely small solid or liquid particles that may include fungal spores, viruses, and bacteria. Droplet nuclei, such as the spray from sneezing or coughing, may make direct contact with an open wound or with a mucous membrane, or they may be inhaled into the lung. TB is spread through inhalation of contaminated droplets.

Host Susceptibility

Not all humans are equally susceptible to, or at risk for, contracting an infection or development of an infectious disease. Biological and personal characteristics play an important role. Just as the young are at greater risk for diphtheria, older adults are at greater risk for bacterial pneumonia. Further, a fetus is at greater risk for harm from the Zika virus than is the pregnant woman. General health status is important, as evidenced by the increased risk for gastrointestinal parasites in children living in poverty. Personal behaviors certainly influence susceptibility, as does the presence of healthy lines of defense. The immune system and immunization status play important roles in the increased number of infections in unimmunized and immunocompromised persons.

BREAKING THE CHAIN OF TRANSMISSION

Picture a situation in which one of the links in the chain of transmission is broken (see Fig. 26.2). Breaking just one link of the chain at its most vulnerable point is, in fact, what is done to control transmission of an infectious agent. Of course, where the chain is broken depends on all of the factors that have just been discussed—characteristics of the agent, its reservoir, portals of exit and entry, how the agent is transmitted, and susceptibility of the host.

Controlling the Agent

Controlling the agent is an area in which technology and medical science have been extremely effective. Inactivating an agent is the principle behind disinfection, sterilization, and radiation of fomites that may harbor pathogens. Antiinfective drugs, such as antibiotics, antivirals, antiretrovirals, and antimalarials, play important roles in controlling infectious diseases. Not only do they permit recovery of the infected person, but they also play a major role in preventing transmission of the pathogens to another. The first step in preventing transmission of TB and syphilis is to treat the infected person with antibiotics. Early treatment of an HIV infection with antiretrovirals suppresses the virus and thus has the potential to reduce transmission and to improve the health status of the infected person (The INSIGHT Study Group, 2015).

Eradicating the Nonhuman Reservoir

Common nonhuman reservoirs for pathogens in the environment include water, food, milk, animals, insects, and sewage. Treating or eliminating them is an effective method of preventing replication of pathogens and thus preventing transmission.

Controlling the Human Reservoir

Treating infected persons, whether they are symptomatic or not, is effective in preventing transmission of pathogens directly to others. Quarantine is an enforced isolation or restriction of movement of those who have been exposed to an infectious agent during the incubation period; this is another method of controlling the reservoir. Quarantine was used effectively during the outbreak of severe acute respiratory syndrome (SARS) in 2003, when some hospitals required that their staff exposed to patients with SARS remain at the hospital until proven to be symptom-free at the end of the incubation period.

Controlling the Portals of Exit and Entry

The transmission chain may be broken at the portal of exit by properly disposing of secretions, excretions, and exudates from infected persons. Additionally, isolation of sick persons from others and requiring that persons with TB wear a mask in public can be effective.

The portal of entry of pathogens also can be controlled by using barrier precautions (masks, gloves, condoms); avoiding unnecessary invasive procedures, such as indwelling catheters; and protecting oneself from vectors, such as mosquitoes. In response to the risk of exposure to bloodborne pathogens (e.g., HIV, hepatitis B, and hepatitis C) the CDC developed a set of guidelines, called universal precautions, to prevent transmission of diseases found in blood and other body fluids. These guidelines were developed because infected people may be asymptomatic and have no knowledge of their conditions; therefore health care workers must assume that every patient is infectious and must protect themselves, other health care workers, and other patients.

Improving Host Resistance and Immunity

Many factors, such as age, general health status, nutrition, and health behaviors, contribute to a host's resistance, or ability to ward off infections. Immunity, however, is an incredible defense against infection. There are several kinds of immunity, each providing resistance in different ways to different pathogens.

TABLE 26.2	Types of Acquired Immunity		
Type of Immunity	**How Acquired**	**Example**	**Duration of Resistance**
Natural			
Active	Natural contact and infection with the antigen	Acquiring measles	May be temporary or permanent
Passive	Natural contact with antibody trans-placentally	Infant born with temporary antibodies to measles	Temporary or through colostrum and breast milk
Artificial			
Active	Inoculation of antigen	Tetanus vaccine to stimulate production of antibodies to tetanus	May be temporary or permanent
Passive	Inoculation of antibody or antitoxin	Injection of tetanus antitoxin to an unimmunized person	Temporary

Modified from Grimes DE: Infectious diseases. In Thompson JM et al., editors: *Mosby's clinical nursing*, St Louis, 1991, Mosby.

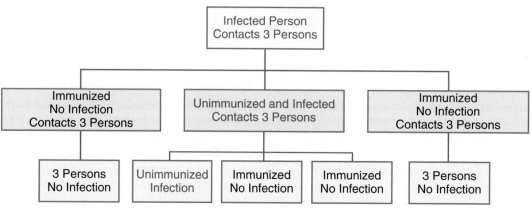

Herd Immunity: 66% immunized (10/13 or 77%) protected

FIG. 26.3 Example of herd immunity.

Natural immunity is an innate resistance to a specific antigen or toxin. **Acquired immunity** is derived from actual exposure to the specific infectious agent, toxin, or appropriate vaccine. There are two types of acquired immunity: active and passive. **Active immunity** occurs when the body produces its own antibodies against an antigen, from either infection with the pathogen or introduction of the pathogen in a vaccine. **Passive immunity** is the temporary resistance that has been donated to the host either through transfusions of plasma proteins, immunoglobulins, or antitoxins or transplacentally (from mother to fetus). Passive immunity lasts only as long as these substances remain in the bloodstream. Types of acquired immunity with examples are summarized in Table 26.2.

When administered according to established guidelines and protocols, vaccines provide acquired immunity in most cases. However, there are exceptions. **Primary vaccine failure** is the failure of a vaccine to stimulate any immune response. It can be caused by improper storage that may render the vaccine ineffective, improper administration route, or exposure of a light-sensitive vaccine to light. Additionally, seroconversion never occurs in some immunized persons, either because of failure of their own immune system or for some other unknown reason. **Secondary vaccine failure** is the waning of immunity after an initial immune response. It often occurs in patients with immunosuppression and in those who have undergone organ transplantation in whom the immune memory is essentially destroyed.

Herd immunity is a state in which those not immune to an infectious agent are protected if a certain proportion (generally considered to be 80%) of the population has been vaccinated or is otherwise immune (Fig. 26.3). This effect applies only if those who are immune are distributed evenly in the population. This is especially true for the transmission of diseases, such as diphtheria, that are found only in the human host and that have no invertebrate host or other mode of transmission. Without the presence of a susceptible population to infect, the organism will be unable to live because the vast majority of the population is immune.

PUBLIC HEALTH CONTROL OF INFECTIOUS DISEASES

Most human diseases (e.g., cancer or diabetes) can be classified as personal health problems. Individuals with personal health problems can be treated by the health care system one person at a time. By contrast, infectious diseases are categorized as public or community health problems. Because of their potential to spread and cause community-wide or worldwide emergencies, infectious diseases require organized, public efforts for their prevention and control.

Such organized public efforts are under the jurisdiction of official public health agencies at local, state, national, and international levels. Each government unit obtains its powers through a complex array of laws. It is important to remember that in areas of health within a state, state laws usually prevail over federal law. The reason for this hierarchy is that the U.S. Constitution did not address health and the Tenth Amendment reserved power to the states over all issues not addressed in the Constitution (Schneider, 2006). Historically, states have accepted this responsibility. For example, all states have laws addressing infectious disease control, such as what diseases must be reported and who has authority to implement quarantines. Every state has a board of health and a department of health to implement state laws.

The CDC is the national public health entity responsible for infectious disease control across the states. It has responsibility for monitoring infectious diseases and for supporting local and state governments to control outbreaks and epidemics if such assistance is needed. Although there are many aspects of public health control of infectious diseases, only three are presented here: common control terminology, reporting diseases, and preventing diseases by vaccination.

Terminology: Control, Elimination, and Eradication

Control of a communicable disease is, by definition, the reduction of incidence (new cases) or prevalence (existing cases) of a given disease to a locally acceptable level as a result of deliberate efforts (Dowdle, 1999). The World Health Organization's (WHO) Expanded Programme on Immunizations is a global attempt to control morbidity and mortality for many vaccine-preventable diseases, with each country adapting these guidelines as necessary. An example of control of pertussis would be to achieve 80% immunization coverage of children against pertussis.

Elimination of a communicable disease occurs when it is controlled within a specified geographic area, such as a single country, an island, or a continent, and the prevalence and incidence of the disease is reduced to near zero. Elimination is the result of deliberate efforts, but continued intervention measures are required (Dowdle, 1999). Such would be the case if no new cases of polio were reported in the United States during the year after an aggressive immunization campaign. Localized elimination of a vaccine-preventable condition, however, does not suggest eradication of the condition. Continued vaccination is still necessary.

The International Task Force for Disease Eradication defines eradication as reducing the worldwide incidence of a disease to zero as a function of deliberate efforts, without a need for further control measures (Dowdle, 1999). Eradication is possible under certain conditions. Criteria for assessing eradicability are listed in Box 26.3.

Smallpox was eradicated in 1977, and the virus now exists only in storage in laboratories. Many factors contributed to the successful eradication of the disease, including the mode of transmission, the isolated geographic distribution of the infection, the ease of administration of the freeze-dried vaccine, the establishment of an effective surveillance system, the increase in national and international political will, and tremendous community participation.

Defining and Reporting Communicable Diseases

Standardized definitions of diseases are necessary for public health monitoring and surveillance throughout all levels of government. Diseases are defined and classified according to confirmed cases, probable cases, laboratory-confirmed cases, clinically compatible cases, epidemiologically linked cases, genetic typing, and clinical case definition. Once defined, disease occurrences can be compared across time, populations, and geographic areas, and appropriate control efforts can be implemented.

BOX 26.3 Criteria for Assessment of Disease Eradicability

Criteria for assessment of the possibility of disease eradication include the following:

- Human host only; no host in nature
- Easy diagnosis; obvious clinical manifestations
- Limited duration and intensity of infection
- Natural lifelong immunity after infection
- Highly seasonal transmission
- Availability of vaccine, curative treatment, or both
- Substantial global morbidity and mortality rates
- Cost-effectiveness of campaign and eradication
- Integration of eradication with additional public health variables
- Eradication is preferred over use of control measures only

From Centers for Disease Control and Prevention: Recommendations of the international task force for disease eradication, *MMWR Morb Mortal Wkly* Rep 42:1–38, 1993; and Dowdle WR: The principles of disease elimination and eradication, *MMWR Morb Mortal Wkly Rep* 48(Suppl 1):23–27, 1999.

The CDC is responsible for monitoring communicable disease in the United States. Along with the Council of State and Territorial Epidemiologists, the CDC has designated notifiable infectious diseases, meaning that health care providers who encounter cases of these diseases must report them to, or notify, the local or regional health department. These notifiable diseases are listed in Box 26.4.

Because state health departments have the responsibility for monitoring and controlling communicable diseases within their respective states, they determine which diseases will be reported within their jurisdictions. Although not all nationally notifiable diseases are reportable in every state or territory, some states have notifiable disease lists that are longer than the CDC's list. All health professionals are advised to check the websites of their state health departments for specifics about reporting laws in their states. The processes for reporting also vary by state, and this information usually is available on the state health department's website. Generally, providers are encouraged to report cases of infectious diseases to their local or regional health departments, who then report to the state and to the CDC.

The CDC publishes a weekly list of notifiable diseases reported by region, state, and nation in *Morbidity and Mortality Weekly Report* (MMWR). MMWR can be found in medical libraries, local health departments, infection control departments in hospitals and medical centers, and on the Internet at https://www.cdc.gov/mmwr/index.html.

? ACTIVE LEARNING

1. Subscribe to the e-mail Listserv to receive *Morbidity and Mortality Weekly Report* (www.cdc.gov/mmwr).
2. Attend an immunization clinic at your local health department to observe a nurse screening children for immunizations.
3. Obtain and evaluate health education materials regarding childhood immunizations from your local health department.
4. Log on to your state health department website to learn about the process of reporting notifiable diseases in your state. Who is responsible for the reporting process? To whom do they report, what information is reported, and how often are diseases reported?

BOX 26.4   Infectious Diseases Designated as Notifiable at the National Level, 2011

- Anthrax
- Arboviral neuroinvasive and nonneuroinvasive diseases: California serogroup virus disease, Chicungunya virus disease, Eastern equine encephalitis, Powassan virus disease, St. Louis encephalitis, West Nile virus disease, and Western equine encephalitis
- Babesiosis
- Botulism (foodborne, infant, wound, and other)
- Brucellosis
- Campylobacteriosis
- Chancroid
- *Chlamydia trachomatis*, genital infections
- Cholera
- Coccidioidomycosis
- Congenital syphilis
- Cryptosporidiosis
- Cyclosporiasis
- Dengue virus infections (dengue, denguelike illness, severe dengue)
- Diphtheria
- Ehrlichiosis/anaplasmosis (*Anaplasma phagocytophilium, Ehrichia chaffeensis, Ehrlichia ewingii*, undetermined human ehrlichiosis/anaplasmosis)
- Giardiasis
- Gonorrhea
- *Haemophilus influenzae*, invasive disease
- Hansen disease (leprosy)
- Hantavirus infection
- Hantavirus pulmonary syndrome
- Hemolytic uremic syndrome, postdiarrheal
- Hepatitis A, acute
- Hepatitis B, acute and chronic
- Hepatitis B, perinatal virus infection
- Hepatitis C, acute and chronic
- HIV infection
- Influenza-associated pediatric mortality
- Invasive pneumococcal disease
- Legionellosis
- Leptospirosis
- Listeriosis
- Lyme disease

- Malaria
- Measles
- Meningococcal disease
- Mumps
- Novel influenza A virus infections
- Pertussis
- Plague
- Poliomyelitis, paralytic
- Poliovirus infection, nonparalytic
- Psittacosis
- Q fever (acute and chronic)
- Rabies (animal and human)
- Rubella
- Rubella, congenital syndrome
- Salmonellosis
- Severe acute respiratory syndrome–associated coronavirus (SARS-CoV) disease
- Shiga toxin–producing *Escherichia coli* (STEC)
- Shigellosis
- Smallpox
- Spotted fever rickettsiosis (formerly Rocky Mountain spotted fever)
- Streptococcal toxic-shock syndrome
- Syphilis (all stages)
- Tetanus
- Toxic shock syndrome (other than streptococcal)
- Trichinellosis (trichinosis)
- Tuberculosis
- Tularemia
- Typhoid fever
- Vancomycin-intermediate *Staphylococcus aureus* (VISA)
- Vancomycin-resistant *Staphylococcus aureus* (VRSA)
- Varicella (morbidity and death)
- Vibriosis
- Viral hemorrhagic fevers (Crimean–Congo hemorrhagic fever virus, Ebola virus, Lassa virus, Lujo virus, Marburg virus, New World Arenaviruses [Guanarito, Machupo, Junin, and Sabia viruses])
- Yellow fever
- Zika virus disease and infection (all stages)

From Centers for Disease Control and Prevention: Infectious diseases designated as notifiable at the national level during 2017. https://wwwn.cdc.gov/nndss/conditions/notifiable/2017/infectious-diseases

---

VACCINES AND INFECTIOUS DISEASE PREVENTION

This section contains comprehensive information on vaccines and vaccine-preventable diseases. Diseases for which there are vaccines are listed in Box 26.5. Recommended vaccination schedules for selected groups are available on the CDC website, which is listed in Table 26.3 along with other resources.

Vaccines: A Word of Caution

As with other areas of health care, information and recommendations on immunizations and vaccine usage change regularly. Therefore health care providers should seek the most current information on the CDC website. Recommendations, policies, and procedures concerning international immunization practices are determined by the WHO. In the United States,

national governance is provided by the American Academy of Pediatrics Committee on Infectious Diseases and the U.S. Public Health Service Advisory Committee on Immunization Practices (ACIP). Occasionally these agencies differ in their recommendations.

Precautions must be taken when giving any immunization. The most recent recommendations—which immunizations to give; to whom they should be given; how they should be given; and how they are to be transported, stored, and administered—can be obtained from the CDC.

The CDC produces Vaccine Information Statements (VISs) that explain the benefits and risks of a vaccine to vaccine recipients, their parents, or their legal representatives. Federal law requires that VISs be handed out before each dose whenever certain vaccinations are given. VISs can be downloaded from the Internet at http://www.cdc.gov/vaccines/hcp/vis/index.html.

BOX 26.5   Vaccine-Preventable Diseases

- Anthrax
- Chickenpox (varicella)
- Diphtheria
- Flu (Influenza)
- *Haemophilus influenzae* type b (Hib)
- Hepatitis A
- Hepatitis B
- Human papillomavirus (HPV)
- Japanese encephalitis (JE)
- Measles
- Meningococcal disease
- Mumps
- Pertussis
- Pneumococcal disease
- Poliomyelitis
- Rabies
- Rotavirus
- Rubella
- Shingles (herpes zoster)
- Smallpox
- Tetanus
- Tuberculosis
- Typhoid fever
- Yellow fever

From Centers for Disease Control and Prevention: *Recommended vaccines by disease,* 2016. https://www.cdc.gov/vaccines/vpd/vaccines-diseases.html

TABLE 26.4   Available Vaccines by Type

Type	Description
Live Attenuated	
Viral	Measles, mumps, rubella, oral polio, vaccinia, yellow fever, and varicella
Bacterial	*BCG* (bacille Calmette-Guérin)
Recombinant	Oral typhoid
Inactivated	
Viral	Influenza, polio, rabies, and hepatitis A
Bacterial	Typhoid, cholera, and plague
Subunit (fractional)	Influenza, acellular pertussis, typhoid VI, and Lyme disease
Toxoid	Diphtheria and tetanus
Recombinant	Hepatitis B and human papilloma virus (HPV)
Conjugate polysaccharide	*Haemophilus influenzae* type b and pneumococcal 7-valent
Pure polysaccharide	Pneumococcal 23-valent, meningococcal, and *Haemophilus influenzae* type b

From Centers for Disease Control and Prevention: *Epidemiology and prevention of vaccine-preventable diseases.* Hamborsky J, Kroger A, Wolfe S, eds. 13th ed. Washington, DC, Public Health Foundation, 2015.

TABLE 26.3   Resources for Recommended Vaccine Schedules for Selected Population Groups

Children/adolescents age 18 years or younger	http://www.cdc.gov/vaccines/schedules/hcp/child-adolescent.html
Adults	http://www.cdc.gov/vaccines/schedules/hcp/adult.html
Travelers	http://www.cdc.gov/travel/destinations/list
Pregnant and breastfeeding women	www.cdc.gov/vaccines/pubs/preg-guide.htm
Health care workers	https://www.cdc.gov/vaccines/adults/rec-vac/hcw.html
Specific health conditions	www.cdc.gov/vaccines/spec-grps/conditions.htm
Other special groups	www.cdc.gov/vaccines/spec-grps/default.htm

Types of Immunizations

Immunization is a broad term used to describe a process by which active or passive immunity to an infectious disease is induced or amplified. Immunizing agents can include vaccines, immune globulins, or antitoxins. **Vaccination** is a narrower term referring to the administration of a vaccine or toxoid to confer active immunity by stimulating the body to produce its own antibodies.

Vaccines can be prepared in several ways. They may be suspensions in a variety of solutions; protected with preservatives, stabilizers, or antibiotics; or mixed with adjuvants, which are used to increase immunogenicity. Vaccines can be live and attenuated (with the virulence reduced), or they may be killed or inactivated (with the virulence removed), leaving only the antigenic property necessary to stimulate the human immune system to produce antibodies. Types of inactivated vaccines include toxoids and polysaccharide vaccines. Inactivated conjugate vaccines, containing chemically linked polysaccharides and proteins, and genetically engineered "recombinant" vaccines are also now being administered. Inactivated vaccines can be fractions or subunits or whole "killed" bacteria or viruses. Immune globulins and antitoxins are solutions that contain antibodies from human or animal blood and are introduced into a patient to provide passive protection without initiating the immune system to produce an immunogenic response. Table 26.4 presents information on types of available vaccines.

Vaccine Storage, Transport, and Handling

Vaccines should be safely stored, transported, and handled at all times to ensure their efficacy. A **cold chain** is a system used to ensure that vaccines are kept at a designated temperature from the time they are manufactured until they are used for vaccination. Failing to maintain the cold chain and exposing the vaccines to higher or lower temperatures than recommended may result in loss of potency and vaccine failure. Several methods are available for ensuring that the appropriate temperature has been maintained throughout vaccine transport and storage. These include liquid crystal thermometers, dial thermometers, recording thermometers, digital thermometers, ice pack indicators, shipping indicators that change color if the temperature exceeds or falls below the recommended level, freeze-watch indicators, and cold chain monitors. Vaccine storage and handling information can be obtained at https://www.cdc.gov/vaccines/hcp/admin/storage/toolkit/storage-handling-toolkit.pdf.

Vaccine Administration

The efficacy of a vaccine can be adversely affected if it is not administered appropriately. Information on the correct dosage can be found on the package insert. If more than one vaccine is being administered simultaneously, different anatomical sites should be used. Additionally, it is important to follow the same safety procedures one would use to administer any intramuscular or subcutaneous injection (i.e., use sterile technique, use the correct size needle, avoid injecting in a blood vessel, and dispose of the needle and syringe properly).

Vaccine Spacing

Wherever possible, all children should be age-appropriately immunized and their immunization status kept up to date according to current recommendations. The same applies to adolescents, adults, persons with chronic illness, pregnant women, health care workers, and international travelers.

The number of injections for any one immunobiological substance should be administered according to recommendations of the ACIP. An interruption in the schedule does not require that the entire series begin again. However, if vaccines are administered at less than the recommended intervals, they should not be counted as part of the primary series of immunization. Completion of the primary vaccine series and receiving periodic booster doses as recommended are necessary to ensure protective levels of immunity. Additional information is available at www.CDC.gov/vaccines.

Vaccine Hypersensitivity and Contraindications

Minor and common side effects may include redness and/or pain at the injection site and mild fever. Although adverse reactions are not common after immunization, they can occur in some individuals. These reactions can be to vaccine components such as eggs, egg proteins, antibiotics, preservatives, and adjuvants. Patient allergies should be considered before administration of specific vaccines. For additional precautions and contraindications, refer to the vaccine package insert and the latest instructions from the CDC at https://www.cdc.gov/vaccines/hcp/acip-recs/general-recs/contraindications.html.

Mild illness with or without low-grade fever is not a contraindication to vaccination. However, vaccination should be postponed in cases of moderate or severe febrile illness to avoid any confusion between a vaccine side effect and an unknown underlying cause.

Pregnancy is not a contraindication to immunization using inactivated vaccines, antitoxins, or immune globulins. However, pregnant women should avoid live vaccines, including those for measles-mumps-rubella (MMR), varicella, and yellow fever, unless the risk of infection is very high (see the link to guidelines for vaccinating pregnant women in Table 26.3).

Immunocompromised patients should not receive live vaccines; however, MMR can be administered to asymptomatic HIV-infected people, and varicella can be given to people with humoral immunodeficiency and some HIV-asymptomatic people as determined by their physician. Killed or inactivated vaccines can be given, but they may not produce an optimal antibody response (see the link to guidelines for vaccinating specific groups of people in Table 26.3).

Vaccine Documentation

Legal documentation of vaccinations is important for both the individual and the provider for future administration and follow-up of hypersensitivity reactions. Both individual and provider immunization records should be maintained. The health care provider is responsible for maintaining accurate records, including patient name; dates immunized; vaccine type; vaccine manufacturer; vaccine lot number; date of the VIS; and the name, title, and address of the person administering the vaccine. VISs can be downloaded from http://www.cdc.gov/vaccines/hcp/vis/index.html.

Vaccine Safety and Reporting Adverse Events and Vaccine-Related Injuries

No drug is perfectly safe or effective, and vaccines are no exception. They are biological rather than chemical, and when introduced into the human biological system, they can and do produce a variety of responses, both positive and negative. Furthermore, vaccines are administered to healthy people; they are given to prevent illness and not treat it; and they are given to far greater numbers of people than other pharmaceuticals.

Public concern regarding the health risks associated with vaccines has increased as the risk of contracting the diseases has declined. For example, wild polio virus has been eliminated in the United States, yet between 1979 and 1997 cases of poliomyelitis were reported in the United States in association with use of the oral, live virus vaccine. The health risk of the oral vaccine exceeded that of the risk of the disease. This led to a change in vaccine policy from the use of the live oral vaccine to the inactivated polio vaccine (IPV) (CDC, 1999). Likewise, whole cell pertussis vaccine has been changed to an acellular pertussis vaccine because of the adverse side effects, most notably convulsions, associated with the whole cell vaccine.

To enable monitoring of actual and potential vaccine-related problems, health care providers must report specific postvaccination "adverse events" to the Vaccine Adverse Event Reporting System (VAERS). Information and reporting forms are available at www.cdc.gov/vaccinesafety/Activities/vaers.html.

The National Vaccine Injury Compensation Program reviews all VAERS reports and provides assistance for individuals and families who experience a vaccine-related injury, including disability and death.

 ACTIVE LEARNING

Log on to the website of an advocacy group against immunizations to understand the messages that they are communicating to the public.

VACCINE NEEDS FOR SPECIAL GROUPS

Recommendations on immunizations and schedules for vaccination are routinely updated and published by the CDC on its website. Practitioners are encouraged to check regularly for updates. Travelers can obtain the most current recommendations from the CDC through its telephone hotline, 1-800-CDC-info (1-800-232-4636), or at its website: http://wwwnc.cdc.gov/travel.

HEALTHY PEOPLE 2020 FOCUS ON IMMUNIZATION AND INFECTIOUS DISEASES

Healthy People 2020 objectives, discussed earlier in this chapter, detailed three topic areas for infectious diseases. Immunization and Infectious Diseases (IID), as listed in the *Healthy People 2020* table, highlights vaccine-preventable and other priority infectious diseases, excluding STDs and HIV. This section provides tables summarizing the chain of transmission and control of such conditions. Table 26.5 covers childhood vaccine–preventable diseases, excluding hepatitis, which is summarized in Table 26.6. Table 26.7 summarizes tuberculosis. For more information see the *Healthy People 2020* website: www.healthypeople.gov/2020/topicsobjectives2020.

HEALTHY PEOPLE 2020 FOCUS ON SEXUALLY TRANSMITTED DISEASES

STDs include the more than 25 infectious organisms that are transmitted primarily through sexual activity. STDs, even those for which treatment exists, continue to be a major public health problem. The rates of STDs in the United States are among the highest in the industrialized world, approaching those in some developing countries. Indeed, an estimated 20 million cases of STDs occur each year in the United States, almost half of them in persons aged 15 to 24 years (CDC, 2016).

Concern over the persistence and increases in STDs led those formulating the *Healthy People 2020* objectives to create a topic area specific to STDs (https://www.healthypeople.gov/2020/topics-objectives/topic/sexually-transmitted-diseases/objectives). For easy reference, the chain of transmission and control of STDs addressed in the *Healthy People 2020* objectives is presented in Table 26.8. The CDC regularly updates STD treatment guidelines, which are available on the its website.

 ## *HEALTHY PEOPLE 2020* FOCUS ON HIV/AIDS

No other infection or infectious disease in recent history has inflicted as much destruction and pain on individuals, families, and communities and created as many challenges for health care professionals as HIV/AIDS. Indeed, HIV stands out as the one condition that touches nurses everywhere. HIV affects persons of every age, ethnicity, socioeconomic status, gender, and occupation. Eventually, HIV/AIDS has an impact on every organ and function of the human body. Every nurse, regardless of area of practice, will eventually care for someone with HIV infection. Currently, there is no cure or vaccine, although early treatment with antiretroviral therapy has shown signs of effectively reducing transmission of the HIV virus (The INSIGHT START Study Group, 2015). Due to the worldwide spread of HIV, it is not surprising that *Healthy People 2020* objectives have an entire topic area specific to HIV/AIDS (https://www.healthypeople.gov/2020/topics-objectives/topic/hiv/objectives).

⚑ RESEARCH HIGHLIGHTS

Human Papilloma Virus Immunization

Humans are subject to infection from more than 100 human papilloma viruses (HPVs). HPV infects skin and mucous membrane cells and is transmitted by direct contact. Pathogenic HPV has been recovered from fingertips, nails, breast tissue, sinonasal areas, nipples, and hair follicles. In addition, it has been found in 6.5% of the oral cavities of a random sample of Americans and can readily be transmitted from infected mothers to their children during childbirth and by touch after birth. The vast majority of HPVs are not pathogenic, but a small number are known to be oncogenic. Two—HPV 16 and HPV 18—are known to be causative agents for cancers of the cervix, vulva, vagina, anus, penis, and oropharynx; they may also contribute to prostate and breast cancer. In addition, HPV 6 and HPV 11 are known to cause genital warts.

Two vaccines that protect against oncogenic HPVs have been approved for use in the United States. One of the vaccines, Cervarix, protects against HPV 16 and 18, and Gardasil protects against HPV 6, 11, 16, and 18. Currently, the CDC recommends that both boys and girls between 11 and 12 years of age be immunized against HPV. For those who did not receive the vaccine at these ages, it can be administered up to age 26 for females and age 21 for males (CDC, 2015). Although widespread HPV vaccine use in other countries has proved to be extremely effective, less than a third of young adolescent males and less than half of adolescent females in the United States had received the recommended three doses in 2015. Uptake of the vaccine in the United States has been poor for several reasons, including cost, parental concerns that children will become sexually active, concerns about the safety of the vaccine, lack of understanding of the nature of transmission of HPV, and failure of health professionals to promote and adhere to the recommendations.

Research has shown that girls who were vaccinated did not have higher rates of pregnancy or STD than did those who were not vaccinated. Unfortunately, many health professionals are not aware of the widespread nature of HPV, its association with certain cancers, or of the vaccine and its safety. Some health

professionals have viewed the transmission of HPV as occurring only during sex and have not allayed parental concerns about potential increases in sexual behavior or the safety of the vaccine. Education is critical, because research shows that young women are three times more likely to undergo immunization if it is strongly recommended by their health care providers. Furthermore, even partial immunization, both at the individual level and within a community, has been very effective in reducing overall prevalence of HPV through the effects of herd immunity.

Implications for Nurses

1. Nurses need to educate patients and others that HPV is not only sexually transmitted, but can be transmitted by other means.
2. Nurses can be central to reduction of a number of cancers by encouraging widespread use of the HPV vaccine for both males and females as recommended by the CDC.

Further Reading

Centers for Disease Control and Prevention: *HPV vaccination coverage data.* https://www.cdc.gov/hpv/hcp/vacc-coverage.html. Accessed February 09, 2018.

Centers for Disease Control and Prevention: *HPV vaccine information for clinicians 2016.* https://www.cdc.gov/hpv/hcp/need-to-know.pdf. Accessed February 09, 2018.

Centers for Disease Control and Prevention: *National, Regional, State, and Selected Local Area Vaccination Coverage Among Adolescents Aged 13-17 Years-United States, 2015.* https://www.cdc.gov/mmwr/volumes/65/wr/mm6533a4.htm. Accessed February 09, 2018.

Centers for Disease Control and Prevention: Vaccine safety: human papillomavirus (HPV) vaccine. Updated 2017. http://www.cdc.gov/vaccinesafety/Vaccines/HPV/index.html. Accessed February 09, 2018.

Grimes RM, Benjamins LJ, Williams KL: Counseling about the HPV vaccine: desexualize, educate, and advocate, *J Pediatr Adolesc Gynecol* 26(4):243, 2013.

TABLE 26.5 Chain of Transmission and Control: Childhood Vaccine–Preventable Diseases

	Chickenpox	Diphtheria	Pertussis	Tetanus	Polio
Occurrence	Worldwide and universal in all populations, primarily in children	Rare where immunization rates are high; affects unimmunized children under 15 yr and adults whose immunity has waned	Worldwide and common in children; declined with immunization; some outbreaks in recent years in U.S. adults whose immunity has waned	Worldwide; occurs sporadically and affects all ages; more common in agricultural areas and among parenteral drug users; rare in areas with high immunization rates	Worldwide before immunization; is now rare in countries with adequate immunization rates
Etiological agent(s)	Human (alpha) herpesvirus 3 (varicella zoster virus)	Corynebacterium diphtheriae, of gravis, mitis, or intermedius biotypes	Bordetella pertussis	Clostridium tetani (an anaerobic pathogen)	Poliovirus types 1, 2, and 3; all are paralytogenic
Reservoir	Humans	Humans	Humans	Intestines of humans and animals	Humans, particularly children with subclinical infections
Transmission	Direct and indirect contact with droplets from respiratory passage or vesicle fluid; extremely contagious	Direct or indirect contact with exudates from mucous membrane lesions of infected person or carrier; raw milk has served as a vehicle	Direct contact with droplets from respiratory passages	Tetanus spores enter body through a wound (usually puncture wound) contaminated with soil and feces; necrotic tissue favors the growth of the anaerobic bacillus	Direct and indirect contact with respiratory discharges and feces; fecal-oral route more common than respiratory transmission
Incubation period	14–16 days; range 2–3 wk; prolonged in immunocompromised persons	2–5 days; occasionally longer	9–10 days; range 6–20 days	10 days; range 3–21 days; rarely, several months	7–14 days; range 3–35 days
Communicability period	1–2 days before onset of rash to 5 days after lesions have crusted	Until bacilli have disappeared from discharges and lesions (usually 2 wk); effective antibiotic therapy interferes with shedding; a carrier may transmit for 6 mo	Highly communicable during early catarrhal and coughing stages; gradually decreasing until week 3; communicability is negligible after 5 days with effective antibiotic therapy	Not transmitted directly	Highly communicable during first days after onset of symptoms; virus is in throat secretions within 36 hr and in feces 72 hr after infection; remains 1 wk in throat and 6 wk in feces
Susceptibility and resistance	General population not previously infected or vaccinated are at risk; can be severe or fatal in adults and immunocompromised persons	General unimmunized population are at risk; infants born of immune mothers have passive immunity for 6 mo; recovery from disease or asymptomatic infection usually confers lifetime immunity; immunization confers prolonged, but not lifetime, immunity	General unimmunized population are at risk; unimmunized children under 5 yr are most susceptible; no passive immunity from mother; disease confers prolonged, but not lifetime, immunity	General unimmunized population are at risk; active immunity from tetanus toxoid persists for 10 yr; tetanus immune globulin confers temporary immunity; infants born to immune mothers are protected at birth; active disease does not confer lifetime immunity	General unimmunized population is at risk; active immunization confers lifetime immunity; disease or subclinical infection confers type-specific lifetime immunity
Prevention and control	Two-dose vaccination of children: first dose between 12 and 15 mo. of age; second dose between 4 and 6 yr (see Table 26.3)	After initial immunization with diphtheria-pertussis-tetanus vaccine (DPT), immunization with diphtheria toxoid boosters every 10 yr (see Table 26.3)	Childhood immunization with DPT (see Table 26.3) Immunization with whole cell vaccine prophylaxis with a 7-day course of erythromycin should be given to all exposed persons, including health care workers, regardless of vaccination status	Active immunization with tetanus toxoid boosters every 10 yr, and as prophylaxis after penetrating injuries for those whose last booster was more than 10 yr ago	Active immunization with inactivated polio virus (IPV) in childhood as recommended (see Table 26.3)

TABLE 26.5 Chain of Transmission and Control: Childhood Vaccine–Preventable Diseases—cont'd

	Chickenpox	Diphtheria	Pertussis	Tetanus	Polio
Disease manifestations	Sudden mild fever and malaise, rash, or both; rash is progressive, changing from maculopapular to vesicular and then forming a crust or scab; lesions tend to be more numerous on covered parts of the body; can be on all mucous membranes and are highly pruritic; complications are more common in persons over 15 yr old, infants under 1 yr old, and immunocompromised persons; virus can persist in a dormant state in sensory nerve endings and can reactivate, causing herpes zoster, or shingles	Acute onset; usually affecting the upper respiratory tract. Lesions are caused by the release of a cytotoxin and manifest as a patch or patches of inflammation surrounding a grayish membrane; complications may result in severe swelling of the neck, thrombocytopenia, neuritis, and myocarditis	Pertussis (whooping cough) begins with an upper respiratory cough and proceeds to a paroxysmal stage of coughing, often ending in vomiting; paroxysmal stage may last 1–2 mo or longer; complications include seizures, pneumonia, encephalopathy, and death	Tetanus (lockjaw) is an acute neurological illness caused by an anaerobic bacterium that produces an exotoxin in the portal of entry in the human host; tetanus causes gradually worsening neurological symptoms, including painful muscle contractions and spasms frequently resulting in death	Symptoms may range from inapparent illness to severe paralysis or death
Diagnosis	By symptoms	Bacteriological culture of nasal and throat secretions and from lesions	Bacteriological culture of nasal or throat secretions	History of injury plus clinical symptoms; bacterium is rarely found in wound cultures	Isolation of the virus from fecal or oropharyngeal specimens
Treatment	Antiviral drugs within 1 wk of exposure may modify severity; varicella-zoster immune globulin administered within 96 hr of exposure can modify or prevent the disease	Single dose of equine antitoxin followed by a full course of antibiotic therapy	Treatment with antibiotics reduces the period of infectivity and may lessen the severity of the disease if given before the paroxysmal stage	Tetanus antitoxin or tetanus immune globulin (TIG), preferably human; supportive care	Supportive care
Report to local health authority?	Yes	Yes	Yes	Yes	Yes

Continued

TABLE 26.5 Chain of Transmission and Control: Childhood Vaccine–Preventable Diseases—cont'd

	Measles	Mumps	Rubella	H. Influenza B	Pneumonia	Influenza
Occurrence	Worldwide; endemic and epidemic occurrences where immunization rates are low; still a major killer of children worldwide	Worldwide; incidence decreasing where immunization rates are high; one third of infected persons have subclinical infections	Worldwide and endemic where immunization rates are low; epidemics occur every 5–9 yr; primarily a disease of children	Worldwide; most common in children 2 mo to 5 yr of age; rare with widespread immunization	Worldwide; most common in children 2 mo to 3 yr of age, the elderly, and immunocompromised adults	Worldwide; in pandemics, epidemics, localized outbreaks, and sporadic cases
Etiological agent(s)	Measles virus, a paramyxovirus	Mumps virus, a paramyxovirus	Rubella virus	*H. influenzae* serotype B (Hib)	*Streptococcus pneumoniae*	Three types of influenza virus (A, B, and C), each with many subtypes
Reservoir	Humans	Humans	Humans	Humans	Humans (often found in respiratory passages of healthy persons)	Humans; some mammals and birds suspected as sources of new subtypes
Transmission	Direct or indirect contact with nasal or throat secretions of infected person; highly communicable	Direct contact with saliva (airborne or droplets) from infected person	Direct or indirect contact with nasopharyngeal secretions of infected person; transplacental transmission leads to congenital rubella syndrome (CRS)	Direct or indirect contact with droplets of nasopharyngeal secretions of infected person	Direct or indirect contact with droplets of nasopharyngeal secretions of infected person	Airborne spread
Incubation period	10 days until fever; 14 days until rash; range 7–18 days	16–18 days; range 14–25 days	14–17 days; range 14–21 days	Unknown; probably 2–4 days	Unknown; probably 1–4 days	1–3 days
Communicability period	1 day before the prodromal period to 4 days after appearance of the rash	2 days before to 4 days after onset of parotitis; but the range can be 7 days before to 15 days after onset; can be transmitted by persons with subclinical infections	7 days before to 4 days after onset of rash; highly communicable; infants with CRS may shed virus for months after birth	Variable as long as organisms are in nasopharynx; noncommunicable within 24–48 hr after onset of effective antibiotic therapy	As long as organism is found in nasopharynx; may be prolonged in immunocompromised persons	3–5 days from clinical onset in adults; up to 7 days in children
Susceptibility and resistance	General population who has not had disease or immunization is at risk; lifetime immunity after illness; infants of mothers who have had the disease are protected for 6–9 mo; infants of immunized mothers have variable level of passive antibody; length of immunity following immunization is unknown	Lifetime immunity develops after subclinical or clinical illness	General unimmunized or previously uninfected population is at risk; lifetime immunity after illness; infants born to immune mothers are protected for 6–9 mo; long-term immunity following immunization	General unimmunized or previously uninfected population is at risk; immunity acquired transplacentally, by infection, and by immunization	General population is probably at risk; immunity is acquired transplacentally, from prior infection, or from immunization	General population is at risk; infection and immunization produces immunity to only one subtype of the virus

	Measles	Mumps	Rubella	H. Influenza B	Pneumonia	Influenza
Prevention and control	Active immunization with live, attenuated measles vaccine (see Table 26.3)	Active immunization with live, attenuated mumps virus vaccine (see Table 26.3)	Active immunization with live, attenuated rubella virus vaccine in childhood (see Table 26.3); immunity in adolescent girls should be ensured	Active immunization with Hib conjugate vaccine (see Table 26.3)	Pneumococcal conjugate vaccine (PCV) for infants and children; pneumococcal polysaccharide vaccine (PPV) for high-risk groups (see Table 26.3)	Active immunization yearly prior to influenza season
Disease manifestations	Acute-onset fever of 101°F or higher, cough, coryza, conjunctivitis, Koplik spots on the buccal mucosa, and a red rash lasting longer than 3 days that begins on the face and becomes generalized; measles can progress into severe complications, including pneumonia, encephalitis, and death	Acute-onset fever and painful swelling of the salivary and parotid glands; may be asymptomatic; complications range from meningoencephalitis to permanent hearing impairment and orchitis in postpubescent males, but rarely sterility	Maculopapular rash and postauricular, occipital, and posterior cervical lymphadenopathy; children are usually relatively asymptomatic, but adults may experience fever, headache, and malaise; rare complications include encephalitis and thrombocytopenia; congenital defects in fetuses of pregnant women who are infected	Hib can affect multiple organ systems, resulting in meningitis, epiglottitis, otitis media, pneumonia, arthritis, and cellulitis, with symptoms associated with those conditions; complications are serious and include septic arthritis, life-threatening airway obstruction, fulminating infection, and death	Acute-onset symptoms of meningitis or pneumonia	Acute-onset dry cough, fever, headache, myalgia, sore throat, and other generalized symptoms; symptom severity depends on the subtype of the virus; complications include pneumonia, otitis media, meningitis, Reye's syndrome, and death
Diagnosis	Tissue culture of nasopharyngeal secretions and serological testing	Isolation of virus from oral and throat spray, urine, and cerebrospinal fluid	Serological testing	Identification of organisms in blood or cerebrospinal fluid	Isolation of the organism from the blood or other sterile body site	Isolation of virus from nasal or pharyngeal secretions, serological testing, antigen detection, gene amplification, and rapid diagnostic test
Treatment	Supportive care	Supportive care	Supportive care	10-14 days of antibiotics	Antibiotics	Antiviral drugs started within 48 hr of onset of symptoms
Report to local health authority?	Yes	Yes	Yes	Yes	Epidemics only	Epidemics only

Modified from Grimes DE, Grimes KA, Zack CM: Infectious diseases. In Thompson JM et al., editors: *Mosby's clinical nursing*, ed 5, St. Louis, 2002, Mosby; with data from Heymann DL, editor: *Control of communicable diseases manual*, ed 20, Washington, DC, 2015, American Public Health Association; and from Centers for Disease Control and Prevention: Advisory Committee on Immunization Practices (ACIP) recommended immunization schedules for persons aged 0 through 18 years and adults aged 19 years and older—United States, 2017. https://www.cdc.gov/vaccines/schedules/index.html.

TABLE 26.6 Chain of Transmission and Control: Hepatitis

	Hepatitis A	Hepatitis B	Hepatitis C	Hepatitis D	Hepatitis E
Occurrence	Worldwide; sporadic and epidemic with cyclic recurrence; outbreaks in institutions where sanitation is poor	Worldwide; endemic; highest in young adults, homosexually active men, persons engaging in unprotected sex, injection drug users, health care and public safety workers	Worldwide; directly related to prevalence of injection drug use in the population, HCV in the donated blood supply, and lack of use of parenteral precautions in health care	Worldwide; occurs epidemically and endemically in population at risk for HBV infection; declining in areas where chronic carriers of HBsAG	Epidemic and sporadic cases, particularly in developing countries; highest in young adults; rare in children or the elderly
Etiological agent(s)	Hepatitis A virus (HAV)	Hepatitis B virus (HBV); made up of a core antigen, HBcAG, and a surface antigen, HBsAG; HBV has at least eight different genotypes	Hepatitis C virus (HCV), which has 6 genotypes and 100 subtypes	Hepatitis delta virus (HDV), which consists of a coat of HBsAG and an internal antigen, the delta antigen	Hepatitis E virus (HEV)
Reservoir(s)	Humans and captive primates	Humans and possibly captive primates	Humans; virus has been transmitted experimentally to chimpanzees	Humans; virus can be transmitted experimentally to chimpanzees and to woodchucks	Humans and nonhuman primates, pigs, chickens, and cattle
Transmission	Person-to-person by fecal-oral route; contaminated food, water, shellfish, etc.	Direct and indirect contact with blood and serum-derived fluids; sexual contact; perinatal	Parenteral; sexual and perinatal transmission are less likely to occur	Similar to that of HBV; must co-infect with HBV	Person-to-person by fecal-oral route; contaminated food or water
Incubation period	28–30 days; range 15–50 days	60–90 days; range 45–180 days	6–9 wk; range 2 wk to 6 mo	2–8 wk	26–42 days; range 15–64 days
Communicability period	Latter half of incubation period to 1 wk after onset of jaundice	During incubation period and throughout clinical course of disease; carrier state may persist for years	Virus persists indefinitely	Throughout acute and chronic disease	Unknown; virus has been detected in stools 14 days after onset of symptoms and 4 wk after ingestion of contaminated food or water
Susceptibility and resistance	General population is at risk; usually affects children and young adults; probable lifetime immunity after infection	General population is at risk; disease is mild in children; lifetime immunity follows infection if antibody to HBV develops and test for HBV is negative	General population is at risk; degree of immunity after infection is not known	All persons susceptible to HBV or who have an HBV infection and are coinfected with HDV	Unknown
Prevention and control	Eliminate common sources of infection with sanitation; improve hygienic practices and hand washing; cook shellfish; immunize high-risk groups or persons in high-risk situations with HAV vaccine; for postexposure: administer vaccine and immune globulin (IG) within 2 wk; use universal precautions	Routinely immunize infants, children, and high-risk groups (see Table 26.3); at birth give HBIG and Hep B vaccine to infants born to HBsAg-positive mothers, followed by additional vaccine doses at 1 and 6 months of age; immunize persons exposed to HBV; test all donated blood for HBV antigen; practice safe sex; use universal precautions	Apply HBV control measures except immunization; no vaccine exists at this time, and IG does not prevent HCV infection	Apply HBV prevention and control measures; however, HBIG, IG, and hepatitis B vaccine do not prevent HDV infection in those already infected with HBV	No vaccine; IG not effective; sanitation appears to be the only effective measure of prevention

Disease manifestations	Acute-onset fever, anorexia, malaise, dark urine, and jaundice, usually lasting 2 mo; has a very low fatality rate and, although rare, can last up to 6 mo	Insidious onset that ranges from asymptomatic illness to generalized nonspecific symptoms, such as anorexia, nausea, and vomiting followed by jaundice and occasionally resulting in fulminant fatal hepatitis	Like HBV, has an insidious onset; symptoms vary from completely asymptomatic (80%) to the rare fulminating, fatal disease; mild symptoms are same as those for HBV; chronic hepatitis develops in 75%–85% of those who are acutely ill	Abrupt onset with range of symptoms similar to those of HBV; always associated with HBV infection, either coinfection or as a suprainfection in persons with chronic hepatitis B	Clinical course similar to that of HAV; no chronic form
Diagnosis	Serum antibodies (anti-HAV) detectable 5–10 days postexposure	Presence in sera of HBsAG, anti-HBsAG (antibodies), HBcAG and anti-HBcAG, HBeAG and anti-HBeAG	Presence of serum antibodies to HCV (anti-HCV) and HCV RNA. Tests to detect antibodies do not distinguish between acute, chronic, and resolved infection	Presence of serum antibodies to HDV (anti-HDV)	Exclusion of other causes of hepatitis, particularly HAV; presence of serum antibodies, anti-HEV; presence of HEV RNA in feces and serum
Treatment	Supportive care	Supportive care	Treatment depends on genotype. Genotype 1 is treated with boceprevir or telaprevir with pegylated- interferon plus ribavirin. Other genotypes are currently treated with pegylated interferon plus ribavirin	Pegylated- interferon	Supportive care; pegylated; interferon and/or ribavirin
Report case to local health authority?	Yes	Yes	Yes	Yes	Yes

Modified from Grimes DE, Grimes KA, Zack CM: Infectious diseases. In Thompson JM et al., editors: *Mosby's clinical nursing*, ed 5, St. Louis, 2002, Mosby; with data from Heymann DL, editor: *Control of communicable diseases manual*, ed 20, Washington, DC, 2015, American Public Health Association; and from Centers for Disease Control and Prevention, Vaccines, 2017. Available at: https://www.cdc.gov/vaccines/vpd/index.html.

TABLE 26.7 Chain of Transmission and Control: Tuberculosis

TUBERCULOSIS

Occurrence	Worldwide; tuberculosis (TB) cases have declined in the United States since 1993; multidrug-resistant cases continue to be reported; most newly reported cases in the United States occur in foreign-born, immunosuppressed, homeless, and disadvantaged persons or are a reactivation of a latent infection in older age groups and those with chronic diseases; in areas of world with high incidence of new transmission cases occur in working-age adults, children, and disadvantaged populations
Etiological agent	*Mycobacterium tuberculosis*; less often *Mycobacterium bovis* or *Mycobacterium africanum*
Reservoir	Humans; diseased cattle for *M. bovis*
Transmission	Inhalation of airborne droplets from the sputum of persons with active disease; children rarely transmit TB because they do not cough forcefully; infrequently by ingestion or skin penetration

	Infection (New or Latent)	Active Disease (Case)
Incubation period	2–10 wk	Anytime during one's lifetime
Communicability period	Not communicable unless there are viable bacilli in the sputum	As long as bacilli are in sputum; may be communicable for years in inadequately treated persons
Susceptibility and resistance	Anyone, such as health care workers, family members, or the institutionalized, working or living in close contact with a person who has active disease can become infected	Vulnerable persons such as children and persons who are older than 65 years, have chronic diseases or compromised immune systems, are malnourished, etc.
Prevention and control	Perform skin testing in high-risk groups (e.g., health care workers), and treat those with new infections to prevent progression to active disease; routine skin testing, particularly of children, is no longer recommended in United States; bacille Calmette-Guérin (BCG) vaccine is still used in some parts of the world	Promptly identify, diagnose, and treat those with active disease; ensure compliance with treatment; initiate respiratory isolation until sputum is clear of bacilli; have patient wear a mask; examine close contacts of TB cases and treat, if infected
Disease manifestations	Initial infection goes unnoticed; 5%–10% of infected persons eventually have active disease, 50% of those within the first 2 yr	Onset of active disease can occur immediately after an initial infection or after a variable latency period for untreated persons; disease onset is usually insidious, with fever, night sweats, and weight loss; cough with pulmonary disease; extrapulmonary symptoms correspond with the location of disseminated bacilli and lesions
Diagnosis	TB skin test reaction and/or blood tests (interferon-gamma release assays); immunosuppressed persons may have a negative skin test reaction due to anergy. Skin test results: 5-mm induration = positive for the immunosuppressed and close contacts with active cases; 10 mm induration = positive for infections <2 yr and persons with high-risk conditions; 15 mm induration = positive for all low-risk persons	10%–20% of those with active disease have a negative skin test reaction; demonstration of acid-fast bacilli in stained smears of sputum or other body fluids; isolation of organism from cultured specimen; radiological evidence of TB in lungs or elsewhere
Treatment	Treat with isoniazid (INH) for 6–9 mo for all new/latent infections to prevent progression to active disease; treat HIV-infected persons with INH in combination with antiretrovirals	Treat with combination of antimicrobial drugs to which the strain of *Mycobacterium* is susceptible, such as isoniazid (INH), rifampin (RIF), pyrazinamide (PZA), and ethambutol (EMB), for 6–12 mo or until sputum cultures are negative; monitor adherence to therapy carefully because nonadherence is increasing drug resistance
Report to local health authority?	No	Yes

Data from Heymann DL, editor: *Control of communicable diseases manual*, ed 20, Washington, DC, 2015, American Public Health Association; and Centers for Disease Control and Prevention: Tuberculosis—United States, 2016, *MMWR Morb Mortal Wkly Rep* 66(11):289–309, 2017. Available at https://www.cdc.gov/mmwr/volumes/66/wr/pdfs/mm6611a2.pdf.

TABLE 26.8　Chain of Transmission and Control: Sexually Transmitted Diseases (STDs)

	Gonorrhea	Chlamydia Trachomatis	Syphilis	Genital Herpes	Warts, Human Papilloma Virus (HPV) Infection
Occurrence	Worldwide; highest in males and females 15–30 yr old	Worldwide; most prevalent STD; continues to increase	Worldwide and increasing; highest in males and females 20–30 yr old	Worldwide and increasing; highest in males and females 15–30 yr old	Worldwide; most common STD (see Research Highlights box)
Etiological agent	*Neisseria gonorrhoeae*, the gonococcus	*Chlamydia trachomatis*	*Treponema pallidum*	Herpes simplex virus (HSV) types 1 and 2	HPV, which has 100 types
Reservoir	Humans	Humans	Humans	Humans	Humans
Transmission	Contact with exudates from mucous membranes of infected persons; usually by direct sexual contact, although the pathogens can be transmitted during childbirth	Contact with exudates from mucous membranes of infected persons; usually by direct sexual contact, although the pathogens can be transmitted during childbirth	Direct sexual contact with infectious exudates from lesions; transplacental; blood transfusion early in infection of donor	Direct contact with secretions from mucous membranes and lesions; transplacental	Direct contact with infected skin and mucous membranes; autoinoculation; during childbirth
Incubation period	2–7 days	7–10 days	3 wk; range 10 days to 3 mo	2–12 days	2–3 mo; range 1–20 mo
Communicability period	Months if untreated	Unknown	When moist lesions are present during the primary and secondary stages, generally 1 yr	During and up to 7 wk after primary lesions; transient shedding of virus occurs in absence of lesions for years	Unknown, probably as long as lesions persist
Susceptibility and resistance	General population is at risk; antibodies are not protective against reinfection	General population is at risk; no acquired immunity	General population is at risk; however, only 30% of exposures lead to infection; some immunity develops over time	General population is at risk; immune response does not prevent recurrence	General population is at risk; immunosuppressed persons are more susceptible
Prevention and control	Safer sexual practices; detect and treat cases and contacts; test pregnant women for infection and treat			Safer sexual practices; cesarean delivery if lesions are present during late pregnancy	Routinely immunize females and males aged 11–12 yr against HPV, with "catch-up" vaccination for females 13–26 yr; HPV vaccination may be recommended for some males aged 9–26 yr; safer sexual practices

Continued

TABLE 26.8 Chain of Transmission and Control: Sexually Transmitted Diseases (STDs)—cont'd

	Gonorrhea	Chlamydia Trachomatis	Syphilis	Genital Herpes	Warts, Human Papilloma Virus (HPV) Infection
Disease manifestations	*Males:* urethritis with purulent discharge from anterior urethra *Females:* mucopurulent cervicitis, often asymptomatic; 20% progress to endometritis, salpingitis, and pelvic peritonitis Both genders may have pharyngeal or anorectal infections, depending on their sexual practices; individuals are frequently coinfected with *N. gonorrhoeae* and *C. trachomatis*	*Males:* urethritis with purulent discharge from anterior urethra *Females:* mucopurulent cervicitis, often asymptomatic; 20% progress to endometritis, salpingitis, and pelvic peritonitis Both genders may have pharyngeal or anorectal infections depending on their sexual practices; individuals are frequently coinfected with *N. gonorrhoeae* and *C. trachomatis*	*Primary:* moist lesion appearing within 3 wk at area of contact *Secondary:* symmetrical maculopapular rash in 4–6 wk *Latency:* indefinite time, no symptoms *Tertiary:* late lesions of bone, viscera, central nervous system (CNS), and cardiovascular system	Local, primary, vesicular lesions, period of latency and recurring, localized lesions; lesions start at area of contact but may spread to surrounding tissues or be disseminated in body, even to the CNS; other disease symptoms depend on extent of dissemination	Skin and mucous membrane lesions that are circumscribed, hyperkeratotic, and of varying sizes and shapes; certain types of HPV, specifically 16 and 18, have been found to be associated with cancer of the cervix, vulva, anus, penis, vagina, and oropharynx; HPV 16 and 18 account for more than 70% of these cancers
Diagnosis	Gram staining of discharges, bacteriological cultures, or tests that detect gonococcal nucleic acid	Failure to detect *N. gonorrhoeae* in discharges from symptomatic persons; mononuclear antibody tests of discharges	Serological testing of blood and cerebrospinal fluid, if indicated	Detection of cell changes in tissue scrapings or biopsy specimens; isolation of virus from lesions or other affected tissue; serological tests	Visualization of the lesion; excision and histological examination of the lesion
Treatment	Treat with antibiotics, preferably with single dose, intramuscular antibiotics, such as ceftriaxone; treatment depends on extent of infection; follow-up testing is recommended	Treat with antibiotics such as single-dose azithromycin or 7 days of doxycycline; advisable to treat for gonorrhea and chlamydia concurrently	Treat with antibiotics; treatment differs with stage of the disease	Treatment with antivirals; treatment varies depending on area of lesions and whether they are disseminated	Removal of the warts by freezing with liquid nitrogen or other chemical; treatment of cancers
Report to local health authority?	Yes	Yes	Yes, including congenital syphilis	No	No

Modified from Grimes DE, Grimes KA, Zack CM: Infectious diseases. In Thompson JM et al., editors: *Mosby's clinical nursing*, ed 5, St. Louis, 2008, Mosby; with data from Heymann DL, editor: *Control of communicable diseases manual*, ed 20, Washington, DC, 2015, American Public Health Association; from Centers for Disease Control and Prevention: *HPV vaccine*, 2009. Available from www.cdc.gov/vaccines/vpd-vac/hpv/default.htm#vacc; and from Centers for Disease Control and Prevention: *Sexually transmitted diseases (STD): human papillomavirus (HPV)*, n.d. Available from http://www.cdc.gov/std/hpv/; and from Centers for Disease Control and Prevention: *Sexually transmitted diseases treatment guidelines, 2015*. Available from https://www.cdc.gov/mmwr/pdf/rr/rr6403.pdf.

HIV, a retrovirus, is the organism that causes the syndrome known as AIDS. After initial infection and a possible flulike illness during the first few weeks, the disease is typically asymptomatic for months to years. In most cases the infected person does not know that he or she is infected and continues to transmit the virus to others. HIV usually manifests gradually as conditions that result from inadequate immune system function as the virus slowly attacks the body's immune system. Over time, the body loses its ability to fight illnesses, and opportunistic infections occur and become recurrent. A standardized case definition for AIDS was specified by CDC in 1993. An updated case definition for AIDS as well as revised classifications for HIV infection can be found at http://www.cdc.gov/hiv/statistics/recommendations/. The critical elements for both HIV and AIDS are summarized for easy reference in Table 26.9.

HIV infection is defined by laboratory criteria, generally based on detection of HIV antibodies and/or p24 antigen. Molecular tests for DNA or RNA may be added to identify presence of the virus. Further information on testing for HIV can be found at http://www.cdc.gov/hiv/testing/index.html.

Treatment for HIV and AIDS is complex and changes frequently. Of note, recent research suggests that early treatment is preferred as a way of controlling transmission of the virus and preventing symptoms of AIDS (INSIGHT START Study Group, 2015). The U.S. Food and Drug Administration has approved many drugs for HIV infection and AIDS-related conditions. At present there are six classes of antiretroviral drugs, each corresponding to different mechanisms whereby HIV invades the cells of the immune system. Current information on treatment is always available from the CDC. One source is the HIV/AIDS Treatment Information Service at www.aidsinfo.nih.gov.

Exposure of health care personnel to HIV, although rare, remains a concern for the CDC and health care workers. The CDC continues to update recommendations for postexposure prophylaxis for occupational exposures. These guidelines are among the many that can be downloaded from the CDC's website. Additional resources include a postexposure hotline for clinicians, the PEPline, at 1-888-448-4911, which is available 24 hours a day, 7 days a week.

Before the development of effective antiretroviral therapies in the late 1990s, reported cases of AIDS provided a good indicator of the progression of the epidemic. With effective treatment, persons with HIV infection have taken longer to progress to having AIDS, and the incidence of AIDS has declined. This change has given the false impression that the epidemic was coming under control. Reporting cases of HIV infection has been incomplete and has varied by state. In 2011, all states reported HIV infection as well as AIDS cases (CDC, 2013).

Eradication of HIV/AIDS depends on development of a vaccine and the infrastructure necessary to vaccinate populations at risk worldwide. Neither possibility is foreseen in the near future. Given that reality, control of HIV/AIDS currently depends on preventing transmission of the virus. One current approach is to successfully treat those who are infected to lower their viral load, thus lowering their risk of transmitting the virus. Problems with adherence to the therapy are interfering with the "treatment as prevention" approach.

 ACTIVE LEARNING

Log on to the CDC website to obtain the most recent guidelines for treating persons with HIV/AIDS, STDs, or TB.

PREVENTION OF COMMUNICABLE DISEASES

All practicing nurses have a role in primary, secondary, and tertiary prevention of communicable diseases. Examples of appropriate interventions are reviewed here and in Table 26.10.

Primary Prevention

Primary prevention of communicable diseases involves measures to prevent transmission of an infectious agent and to prevent pathology in the person exposed to an infection. All of the activities described in the section on breaking the chain of transmission are primary prevention activities. Immunization is primary prevention. Changing the behaviors that lead to exposure to a pathogen is primary prevention. See Tables 26.5 through 26.9 for primary preventions specific to the conditions listed in those tables.

Secondary Prevention

Secondary prevention consists of activities to detect infections early and effectively treat persons who are infected. These actions prevent not only progression of the infectious disease but also transmission of the pathogen to others. Reporting infectious diseases, investigating contacts, notifying partners, finding new cases, and isolating infected people also are examples of secondary prevention.

Tertiary Prevention

Tertiary prevention includes activities involved in caring for persons with an infectious disease to ensure that they are cured or that their quality of life is maintained. Perhaps the most important part of the treatment process is to ensure that people take their antimicrobial agents completely and effectively. In a time of increased resistance to pathogens, helping patients adhere to a drug regimen is critical. Additionally, caregivers should be taught to protect themselves and their environment by using appropriate precautions when caring for an infected family member.

TABLE 26.9   Chain of Transmission and Control: Human Immunodeficiency Virus/Acquired Immunodeficiency Syndrome (HIV/AIDS)

	HIV/AIDS
Occurrsence	Worldwide estimates in 2015: about 36.7 million persons were living with HIV; 2.1 million new infections in 2015 and 1.1 million deaths. Since the start of the epidemic, approximately 78 million people have become infected with HIV
Etiological agent	HIV is a retrovirus with two serologically and geographically distinct types (HIV-1 and HIV-2); HIV-1 makes up 90%–95% of the world's cases; it may be more pathogenic, lead to more rapid disease progression, and have higher mother-to-infant transmission than HIV-2 does; multiple subtypes (sometimes called *clades*) have been identified for both HIV-1 and HIV-2
Reservoir	Humans; HIV may have evolved from a chimpanzee virus
Transmission	Direct person-to-person through unprotected sexual contact or from mother to fetus or mother to infant (during birth or by breastfeeding) Indirect through contact of abraded skin or mucous membranes with infected blood or body fluids, injection of contaminated blood or fluids, use of contaminated needles, or transplantation of organs from infected person

	HIV Infection	AIDS
Incubation period	1–3 mo before antibodies are detectable	<1 yr to 15 yr; may be longer with effective antiretroviral therapy
Communicability period	Presumed to be <10 days after infection and lasting throughout life; may be highest in early infection when viral load is highest, and again later when clinical status worsens	
Susceptibility and resistance	General population is at risk; increased risk for infection with untreated ulcerative STDs and in uncircumcised males; evidence that some persons are less susceptible because of chemokine-receptor polymorphisms; very small percentage of infected persons do not progress to AIDS, for an unknown reason	
Prevention and control	Practice universal precautions and safer sex; treat pregnant women with antiretrovirals to prevent transmission to fetus; teach infected women to avoid breastfeeding; treat drug users and provide needle exchange programs for injection drug users; treat STDs to decrease chance of acquisition of HIV through sores on mucous membranes; maintain a safe blood supply; encourage autologous blood transfusions, when possible Early treatment of HIV-infected persons suppresses the virus enough to decrease risk of transmission to others	Adherence to effective antiretroviral therapy delays progression to AIDS; prophylactic treatment for opportunistic infections delays onset of conditions associated with AIDS diagnosis
Disease manifestations	Within several weeks an infected person experiences an acute, self-limiting illness lasting for 1–2 wk with symptoms that mimic other conditions (fever, rash, pharyngitis, myalgia, lymphadenopathy, and malaise); although immune deficiency may progress, the person may be without further symptoms for years	Progressive immune deficiency and increasing susceptibility to life-threatening infections and cancers in untreated populations
Diagnosis	*Early after infection:* the p24 and polymerase chain reaction blood tests identify the presence of viral nucleic acids *Within 1–3 mo after infection:* serologic tests (enzyme-linked immunosorbent assay, western blot) identify antibodies to HIV in the blood; a more rapid test is now available to detect antibodies in saliva.	A standardized case definition for AIDS was specified by the CDC in 1993 An updated case definition for AIDS and revised classifications for HIV infection can be found in the CDC document cited in the "Resources" portion
Treatment	Treatment with antiretroviral drugs to suppress the virus, not eradicate it Currently six classes of drugs are available: nucleoside reverse transcriptase inhibitors, nonnucleoside reverse transcriptase inhibitors, protease inhibitors, integrase inhibitors, fusion inhibitors, and CCR5 antagonists; each attacks a different target in the reproduction process of the virus; current treatment strategies use at least three drugs from at least two classes Requires almost perfect adherence to regimen because development of drug-resistant HIV is common Current guidelines recommend early treatment to suppress the virus to prevent transmission and treatment as pre-exposure prophylaxis (PrEP) for high-risk persons	
Report to local health authority?	Yes in all states	Yes in all states

Resources for Information on HIV/AIDS

Case Definition:
CDC definition (http://www.cdc.gov/hiv/pdf/statistics_HIV_Case_Def_Consult_Summary.pdf) **OR** *2016 UNAIDS Report on the Global AIDS Epidemic* (http://www.unaids.org)
Testing: www.cdc.gov/hiv/testing
Treatment: www.aidsinfo.nih.gov
Treatment as prevention and pre-exposure prophylaxis: https://www.cdc.gov/hiv/guidelines/index.html

Data from Heymann DL, editor: *Control of communicable diseases manual,* ed 20, Washington, DC, 2015; and UNAIDS: *Fact sheet, global HIV statistics 2016.* Available at http://www.unaids.org/en/resources/documents/2016/Global-AIDS-update-2016.

TABLE 26.10 Examples of Primary, Secondary, and Tertiary Prevention Activities for Control of Infectious Diseases at the Individual and Population Levels

Infectious Disease	Individual	Population
Primary Prevention		
Sexually transmitted disease	Teach safe sex practices. Provide education and access to HPV vaccine.	Place condom machines in accessible areas in places where young adults congregate.
Diseases caused by blood-borne pathogens	Teach barrier precautions to all health care workers. Teach injecting drug users about dangers of sharing needles.	Provide an adequate supply of gloves and sharps containers in patient care areas. Initiate citywide needle exchange programs and methadone programs.
Vaccine-preventable diseases	Ensure that all children who come to the clinic have age-appropriate immunizations.	Work with community groups to cosponsor immunization clinics in areas where immunization rates are low. Work to counteract parental fears of vaccines. Educate on the value and safety of HPV vaccine.
Hepatitis A, gastrointestinal infections	Teach safe food-handling practices in the home.	Require as part of the licensing of restaurants that food handlers take a course in safe food handling.
Hepatitis A and B	Provide immune globulin after exposure to hepatitis A or B.	Mandate immunization of health care workers for hepatitis A and B.
Secondary Prevention		
STDs	Screen and treat for all STDs.	STD partner notification program
Tuberculosis	Screen close contacts of persons with TB. Treat persons with a recent skin test "conversion" (from negative to positive).	Initiate a program of yearly testing of health care workers for TB. Provide treatment to all with recent skin text conversions free of charge at their workplace.
HIV/AIDS	Provide testing and treatment for HIV in local clinics. Monitor patient adherence to antiretroviral therapy	Educate public about the concept of treatment as both prevention and pre-exposure prophylaxis
Meningitis	Provide immunization and chemoprophylaxis to persons exposed to meningitis.	Provide immunization and chemoprophylaxis to all students in a school following an exposure.
Tertiary Prevention		
Tuberculosis	Provide therapy for persons with active TB. Teach patients to take all doses of prescribed antibiotics, and monitor adherence.	Initiate a directly observed therapy (DOT) program in the community shelters and jails. Initiate community education campaigns about the problem of drug resistance associated with incomplete antibiotic use.

CASE STUDY   Application of the Nursing Process

Employee With a Communicable Disease

Adrienne Zack is the employee health nurse for a large city hospital. On a recent workday, she saw Beverly Yancy, a staff nurse in the newborn nursery of the hospital, who presented to the employee health clinic with a productive cough, wheezing, low-grade fever, chills, and fatigue lasting more than 1 month. Beverly stated that she had been treating her symptoms with over-the-counter antihistamines, cough suppressants, and antipyretics. When weighed in the clinic, Beverly was surprised that she had lost 10 lb since she was weighed last. She told Adrienne that she has no history of asthma or lung disease.

Beverly's employee health record revealed that she had had a positive tuberculin skin test (TBST) reaction of 15-mm induration when she was screened 11 years earlier for employment at the hospital. A chest radiograph at that time showed no evidence of TB. Because Beverly was without TB symptoms at the time of employment and declined to take isoniazid (INH) for treatment of the latent tuberculosis infection (LTBT), she believed that the positive TBST reaction was the result of having received bacille Calmette-Guérin (BCG) vaccination at birth in the Philippines. Furthermore, she has had no symptoms during her annual symptom screen by the employee health clinic.

A chest x-ray showed suspicious areas indicating that Beverly most likely had active, infectious pulmonary TB. The diagnosis was confirmed when a sputum smear examination was positive for acid-fast bacilli (AFB). On the basis of the timing of Beverly's symptoms, Adrienne determined that Beverly's disease probably has been communicable for 3 months.

Diagnosis

Individual
- Active TB
- Potential for spread of TB to close contacts

Family
- Potential for undiagnosed TB

Community
- At risk for exposure to TB

Planning

M. tuberculosis (MTB) is transmitted by airborne droplets of sputum from persons with active disease who cough or otherwise discharge respiratory droplets into the air. Health care workers are at risk for TB infection because of frequent exposure to patients with active disease. Beverly could not have been infected by the newborns in the nursery where she worked. Most likely she was exposed to TB before her screening 11 years previously. The skin test reaction of 15-mm induration suggested a latent TB infection rather than a BCG vaccination at birth. Latent TB infection can become active TB disease at any time. In this case, latency lasted more than 11 years.

Health care workers, like anyone with active TB, can transmit the infection to close contacts such as coworkers, high-risk patients, and personal

continued

Employee With a Communicable Disease

contacts. Newborns and children younger than 2 years are at high risk for acquiring TB infection and for progressing to TB disease. Such contacts must be found, screened, and treated as soon as possible. The incubation period for a detectable infection is 2 to 10 weeks after exposure. Recent contacts whose skin test results are negative now should be retested in 2 to 3 months.

Goals

Individual

Short-Term Goals

- Beverly will begin her course of medications immediately.
- Beverly will take short-term disability and will not return to work until her sputum culture results are negative and she is cleared by the employee health clinic.

Long-Term Goals

- Beverly will complete her course of medications as directed.
- Beverly will provide sputum cultures and undergo chest x-ray examination at 3, 6, and 9 months and will be free of evidence of active TB.

Family

Short-Term Goals

- All of Beverly's family members will be tested for TB within 3 days.
- Any family member testing positive will be started on a course of medication as recommended by the health department and his or her health care provider.

Long-Term Goal

- All family members will be retested in 6 months.

Community (Hospital)

Short-Term Goals

- Beverly's coworkers will be tested for TB within 3 days.
- The parents of all of Beverly's patients from the past 3 months will be contacted to encourage that they be tested and have their babies tested.
- Any contact or patient testing positive will be started on a course of medications as recommended by the local health department and his or her health care provider.

Long-Term Goal

- All contacts will be retested in 6 months.

Intervention

TB must be reported to local public health authorities, who are responsible for control of TB in the community. Control relies on identifying and adequately treating all active TB cases and those with latent infections. The public health department will investigate Beverly's contacts inside and outside the hospital during the previous 3 months. This process will identify and treat persons, including the discharged newborns, to whom Beverly might have transmitted MTB. Adrienne and the other health clinic employees may be asked to assist with screening hospital workers exposed to Beverly and providing education about treatment.

TBST reactions are determined to be positive under the following conditions:

1. Induration of 5 mm in persons with HIV infection, those in close personal contact with someone with active TB, or persons who have fibrotic chest radiographs.
2. Induration of 10 mm in other high-risk persons, such as injecting drug users and persons with chronic disease or other causes of immune suppression and those from countries or communities where TB prevalence is high.
3. Induration of 15 mm for anyone who does not meet the preceding criteria.

All persons with a positive skin test reaction should be tested for active disease. Those for whom AFB are identified in a stained smear of sputum,

mycobacteria are isolated from a cultured specimen, or there is radiological evidence of TB must be treated for active disease with a combination of drugs according to protocols established by the CDC.

Multidrug-resistant TB is an ever-increasing problem. Of active TB cases, 1% to 2% are now resistant to all available drugs. Patients must be helped to meticulously adhere to the prescribed regimen. Studies have demonstrated that health care workers are as poor as the general public at adhering to long-term drug therapy.

Persons with a recent "conversion" to a positive TBST result should undergo treatment for latent TB according to CDC protocols. Such treatment reduces lifetime risk that a latent infection will progress to active disease. Persons taking INH should be taught the symptoms of side effects to the drug, including hepatotoxicity, peripheral neuropathy, and central nervous system (CNS) changes.

Teaching should include the following information:

- The importance of isolating oneself from contact with others and wearing a mask in public until sputum is clear of bacilli—around 4 to 8 weeks with effective treatment.
- Proper discharge of sputum and materials contaminated with sputum.
- Drug therapy must be continued uninterrupted for the designated period even after sputum tests are negative for bacilli.
- Drug toxicity and side effects must be reported to the physician immediately. These include, but are not limited to, the following:
  - *INH:* Hepatotoxicity, peripheral neuropathy, CNS changes
  - *Ethambutol:* Reduced visual acuity with inability to see the color green
  - *Streptomycin:* Rash, fever, malaise, vertigo, deafness, gastrointestinal disturbance, CNS changes
  - *Pyrazinamide:* Hypersensitivity, hepatotoxicity, gastrointestinal disturbances, renal failure
  - *Rifampin:* Red-orange urine, hepatotoxicity, CNS symptoms
  - *Ethionamide:* Gastrointestinal disturbance and symptoms of hepatotoxicity
  - *Cycloserine:* CNS effects
- Sputum must be reexamined monthly until it tests negative for bacilli, then every 3 months for the duration of therapy.

Evaluation

Beverly and anyone else with active TB can return to work when the results of AFB testing of three sputum smear specimens collected 8 to 24 hours apart, at least one of which is an early morning specimen, are negative. Adrienne will refer to the CDC's latest guidelines for preventing transmission of TB in health care settings, available at www.cdc.gov/tb/topic/infectioncontrol/default.htm and will update the hospital's infection control plan in accordance with the guidelines.

Levels of Prevention

Primary

- Educate health care workers and others about TB infection and disease.
- Educate staff on airborne precautions and the proper use of respiratory protection.
- Design and implement signage throughout the hospital to remind staff and patients about respiratory hygiene, cough etiquette, and hand hygiene.

Secondary

- Establish regular screening of health care workers for positive skin test conversions.
- Establish mechanisms for detection, referral, and treatment of staff with latent TB infections and with active TB.
- Implement procedures for rapid detection and treatment of patients with active TB.
- Coordinate efforts with the local health department.

Tertiary

- Monitor medication compliance and follow-up testing.

SUMMARY

This chapter presents the challenges of infectious diseases that face all nurses. It reviews principles that are the foundation for the occurrence, transmission, and control of infectious diseases and applies those principles to infectious diseases that are emphasized in the *Healthy People 2020* objectives. Most important, because nurses will be affected by infectious diseases wherever they practice, resources from which any nurse can obtain up-to-date information on any infectious disease at any time are included.

EVOLVE WEBSITE

http://evolve.elsevier.com/Nies/community
- NCLEX Review Questions
- Case Studies

BIBLIOGRAPHY

Centers for Disease Control and Prevention: Recommendations of the advisory committee on immunization practices: revised recommendations for routine poliomyelitis vaccination, *MMWR Morb Mortal Wkly Rep* 48(27):590, 1999.

Centers for Disease Control and Prevention: Measles—United States, 2011, *MMWR Morb Mortal Wkly Rep* 61(15):253–257, 2012.

Centers for Disease Control and Prevention: *final pertussis surveillance report*, 2012. Available from: www.cdc.gov/pertussis//reporting.html.

Centers for Disease Control and Prevention: Diagnoses of HIV infection in the United States and dependent areas, 2011, *HIV Surveillance Report vol 23*, 2013. Available from: http://www.cdc.gov/hiv/topics/surveillance/resources/reports.

Centers for Disease Control and Prevention: *2011 sexually transmitted diseases surveillance*, 2016. Available from: www.cdc.gov/std/stats11/default.htm.

Centers for Disease Control and Prevention 2016: *Diagnoses of HIV infection in the United States and dependent areas*. HIV Surveillance Report, 2014. Available from: http://www.cdc.gov/hiv/topics/surveillance/resources/reports.

Centers for Disease Control and Prevention: *Sexually Transmitted Diseases Treatment Guidelines*, 2015. Available from: https://www.cdc.gov/mmwr/pdf/rr/rr6403.pdf.

Centers for Disease Control and Prevention: National, regional, state, and selected local area vaccination coverage among adolescents aged 13-17 years—United States, 2015, *MMWR Morb Mortal Wkly Rep* 65:850–858, 2016.

Centers for Disease Control and Prevention: *Advisory Committee on Immunization Practices (ACIP) recommended immunization schedules for persons aged 0 through 18 years and adults aged 19 years and older—United States*, 2016. https://www.cdc.gov/vaccines/vpd/index.html.

Centers for Disease Control and Prevention: Tuberculosis—United States, 2016, *MMWR Morb Mortal Wkly Rep* 66(11):289–309, 2017. Available at https://www.cdc.gov/mmwr/volumes/66/wr/pdfs/mm6611a2.pdf.

Centers for Disease Control and Prevention: *Vaccines*, 2017. Available at: https://www.cdc.gov/vaccines/vpd/index.html.

Centers for Disease Control and Prevention: *Infectious diseases designated as notifiable at the national level during 2017*, Retrieved from: https://wwwn.cdc.gov/nndss/conditions/notifiable/2017/infectious-diseases.

Centers for Disease Control and Prevention: *National Center for Emerging Zoonotic Infectious Diseases*, 2017. At https://www.cdc.gov/ncezid/.

Dowdle WR: The principles of disease elimination and eradication, *MMWR Morb Mortal Wkly Rep* 48(Suppl 1):23–27, 1999.

HealthyPeople.gov: *Healthy People 2020: Topics & objectives*. Available from: www.healthypeople.gov/2020/topicsobjectives2020/.

HealthyPeople.gov: *Healthy People 2020: Topics & objectives: HIV.* Available from: https://www.healthypeople.gov/2020/topics-objectives/topic/hiv/objectives.

HealthyPeople.gov: *Healthy People 2020: Topics & objectives: Immunization and infectious diseases.* Available from: https://www.healthypeople.gov/2020/topics-objectives/topic/immunization-and-infectious-diseases/objectives.

HealthyPeople.gov: *Healthy People 2020: Topics & objectives: Sexually transmitted diseases.* Available from: https://www.healthypeople.gov/2020/topics-objectives/topic/sexually-transmitted-diseases/objectives.

Heymann DL, editor: *Control of communicable diseases manual*, ed 20, Washington, DC, 2015, American Public Health Association.

Schneider MJ: *Introduction to public health*, ed 2, Boston, 2006, Jones and Bartlett.

The INSIGHT STUDY Group: Initiation of Antiretroviral Therapy in Early Asymptomatic HIV Infection, *New England Journal of Medicine* 373:795–807, 2015.

UNAIDS: *Global AIDS Update 2016*, 2016. Available at: http://www.unaids.org/en/resources/documents/2016/Global-AIDS-update-2016.

World Health Organization : Global tuberculosis report 2016. Available from: http://www.who.int/tb/publications/global_report.

Substance Abuse

*Meredith Troutman-Jordan**

OBJECTIVES

Upon completion of this chapter, the reader will be able to do the following:

1. Discuss the historical trends and current conceptualizations of the cause and treatment of substance abuse.
2. Describe the current social, political, and economic aspects of substance abuse.
3. Describe the ethical and legal implications of substance abuse.
4. Detail the typical symptoms and consequences of substance abuse.
5. Identify issues related to substance abuse in various populations encountered in community health nursing practice.
6. Apply nursing care standards related to patients with substance abuse problems.

KEY TERMS

Abstinence
Addiction
Alcoholics Anonymous
case management
co-occurring disorders
delirium tremens
detoxification

dual diagnosis
harm reduction
initiation
Intensive Outpatient Treatment
Intervention
mutual help groups
National Institute on Drug Abuse

professional enablers
social consequences
substance abuse
Substance Abuse and Mental Health Services Administration
substance abuse treatment
War on Drugs

---

* The author would like to acknowledge the contribution of Kim Jardine Dickerson, who revised this chapter for the previous edition.

Perhaps no other health-related condition has as many far-reaching consequences in contemporary Western society as substance abuse. These consequences include a wide range of social, psychological, physical, economic, and political problems. Drug abuse and addiction have negative consequences for individuals, families, and communities. Estimates of the total overall costs of substance abuse in the United States, including productivity and health- and crime-related costs, exceed $700 billion annually (NIDA, 2015). This figure includes approximately $193 billion for illicit drugs, $295 billion for tobacco, and $224 billion for alcohol. These numbers in dollars do not describe the extent of public health and safety implications (SAMHSA, 2016; Wilkinson et al., 2016). Some of these critical implications are family disintegration, loss of employment, failure in school, domestic violence, and child abuse.

Excessive alcohol use led to approximately 88,000 deaths and 2.5 million years of potential life lost annually in the United States from 2006 to 2010, shortening the lives of those who died by an average of 30 years. Moreover, excessive drinking was responsible for 1 in 10 deaths among working-age adults aged 20 to 64 years (CDC, 2016). Roughly 15.5 million people were dependent on or abused alcohol alone, with some 100,000 people dying each year in the United States as a result (CDC, 2016).

The **social consequences** of substance abuse include its role in crime, need for money to buy substances, specific theft of drugs, and irreversible health consequences/disabilities that can result from use. Many offenders commit crimes while under the influence of drugs, alcohol, or both. In state and federal correctional facilities, 32% of state prisoners and 26% of federal prisoners said they had committed their current offense while under the influence of drugs. Among state prisoners, drug offenders (44%) and property offenders (39%) reported the highest incidence of drug use at the time of the offense; among federal prisoners, drug offenders (32%) and violent offenders (24%) were the most likely to report drug use at the time of their crimes (U.S. Department of Justice, 2017).

Alcohol and drugs are implicated in an estimated 80% of offenses leading to incarceration in the United States (National Council on Alcoholism and Drug Dependence, 2017). Nearly 50% of jail and prison inmates are clinically addicted, 80% of offenders abuse drugs or alcohol, and approximately 60% of individuals arrested for most types of crimes test positive for illegal drugs at arrest (National Council on Alcoholism and Draug Dependence, 2017).

All aggregates in society are potentially affected by substance abuse problems. Infants exposed in utero to alcohol, amphetamines, or opiates are at risk for withdrawal syndromes and later developmental problems. Indirect social effects of substance abuse include relationship conflicts, divorce, job loss/lack of employment, spousal and child abuse, and child neglect.

In the past, alcoholism and drug addiction were considered problems of the urban poor; society and most health professionals virtually ignored them. Substance abuse problems now pervade all levels of U.S. society, and awareness has increased. Community health nurses must be knowledgeable about substance abuse because it is a problem that frequently intertwines with other medical and social conditions.

This chapter focuses on helping community health nurses recognize substance abuse in their clients and in the larger community. It reviews historical trends, the causes of substance abuse, the most common symptoms of these disorders, and treatment options. The chapter also suggests nursing interventions appropriate for assisting those with substance-related problems in a community context.

ETIOLOGY OF SUBSTANCE ABUSE

Substance abuse has an impact on virtually every aspect of individual and communal life, and many institutions and academic fields have addressed it. Several theories attempt to explain the cause and scope of the problem and offer solutions. Some theories address individual, physiological, spiritual, and psychological factors. Others deal with social influences involving family, ethnicity, race, access to drugs, environmental stressors, economics, political status, culture, and sex roles. Most theories suggest that a combination of factors is the underlying impetus for substance abuse.

Although previous research studies have suggested a link between genetics and alcoholism, there is growing evidence that genetic variations may contribute to the nature of alcoholism within families. Individual and environmental factors also contribute to an increased risk for alcohol abuse. On the individual level, a person's inherited sensitivity to alcohol is a predictor for the development of alcohol abuse. Two broad personality dimensions are also associated with an increased risk for alcohol abuse. Impulsivity and ease of disinhibition add to risks for substance abuse (Vrieze et al., 2013; Wardell et al., 2016). Proneness to anxiety and depression are also risks (Kenney et al., 2015; Miozzo et al., 2014), and these comorbidities are not well understood. Alcohol expectancies (i.e., beliefs about anticipated consequences of drinking) are also a predictor of alcohol abuse. If one expects a certain effect, such as relief, one is more likely to feel it after use of a drug. The satisfied expectancies may set up neural pathways that are interpreted as pleasurable.

Medical models of alcoholism and other substance abuse conditions may not provide an understanding of commonalities among addictive behaviors (e.g., excessive drinking, gambling, eating, drug use, and sexual behavior). Cross-addiction, or multidrug use, is more prevalent now than in the past, and more studies point to the presence of both automatic and nonautomatic factors in physiological and psychological dependence. Specific biological medical models are giving way to multicausal models.

In the biopsychosocial model, risk factors interact with protective factors to develop a predisposition toward drug or alcohol use (University of Florida Department of Psychology, 2017). This predisposition is then influenced by exposure to the substance, availability, and the experiential interpretation of the drug experience (e.g., pleasant or unpleasant). Continued availability of the substances and a social support system that enables or supports their use is also necessary. These factors combine to determine whether addiction develops and is maintained.

HISTORICAL OVERVIEW OF ALCOHOL AND ILLICIT DRUG USE

During the twentieth century, fluctuations in the use of alcohol and illicit drugs were influenced by shifts in public tolerance and political and economic trends. In general, alcohol use gained more social acceptance than other drug use. Alcohol consumption in the United States was higher during World Wars I and II and decreased during Prohibition and the Great Depression. During the late 1960s and early 1970s, many states lowered the legal drinking age from 21 to 18 (NIAA, 2013). Consequently, the number of alcohol-related traffic fatalities among young people increased. In response to these outcomes, beginning in the early 1980s individual states increased the drinking age to 21 (NIAA, 2013). Then, in 1984, Congress passed legislation that would withhold federal highway construction funds from any state that had not adopted a minimum legal drinking age of 21. Thus, by 1988, all states had adopted age 21 as the minimum legal drinking age; alcohol-related traffic deaths among young drivers then declined (NIAA, 2013). The prevalence of underage alcohol use, daily alcohol use, and binge drinking also declined since 1982.

The decline in alcohol consumption through the 1990s and into the twenty-first century is attributed to less tolerant national attitudes toward drinking, increased societal and legal pressures and actions against drinking and driving, and increased health concerns among Americans. The identification of, and response to, driving under the influence of alcohol or another drug is an example of a shift in thinking from addiction as the primary concern to other problems linked with, for example, alcohol use. These problems are thus termed *substance-related problems* and have become a significant community concern.

Public attitudes and governmental policies also have influenced the history of illicit drug use. Although nineteenth-century physicians prescribed morphine for a large variety of ailments, the discovery of the addictive properties of cocaine and opiates led to increased governmental regulation at the beginning of the twentieth century. The Harrison Narcotic Act of 1914 and subsequent laws lessened the medical profession's control over the use of addictive drugs (Ling, 2016); the legislation specified that the physician could prescribe these drugs only in the course of general practice and not to maintain an addiction. This limitation on the physician's power to prescribe and dispense addictive drugs and restrictions on the importation of narcotics limited the supply of these drugs until the 1950s and 1960s (PBS, 2014). At that time, an increase in illegal drug trafficking caused heroin use to proliferate, particularly in inner cities.

By the 1970s, drugs were increasingly available. During this period, a counterculture population, composed largely of young people, focused their efforts on enhancing social justice, ending the Vietnam War, and lessening "repressive" sexual mores; many conceptualized drug use as a way to liberate the mind. Marijuana use occurred in communal, social settings; alcohol use was less favored because it was associated with the "establishment" the young people were critiquing

(PBS, 2014). Consequently, the use of hallucinogens, cannabis, and heroin spread beyond urban drug subcultures to the general population. Alarmed by the social and personal problems inherent in this change, the public grew less tolerant of drug use, and prevention and treatment programs were given more attention and resources. After peaking in 1979, illicit drug use decreased among most segments of the population throughout the 1980s, reaching a low in the early 1990s. The Anti-Drug Abuse Acts of 1986 and 1988 increased funding for treatment and rehabilitation, and also stiffened penalties for drug offenses (Sterling, 2014); the 1988 act created the Office of National Drug Control Policy. The director, referred to as the "drug czar," is responsible for coordinating national drug control policy.

To combat concerns about the physical, social, and psychological impacts of drug abuse and dependence, federal drug policy has emphasized law enforcement and interdiction—the War on Drugs—to reduce the supply. Trends have shown renewed interest in prevention and treatment efforts to decrease the amount of illicit drug use in society and to lessen its impact (SAMHSA, 2016d). Federal drug control spending increased from $21.7 billion in fiscal year 2007 to approximately $30.6 billion in allocated funding in fiscal year 2016, and spending in these two programs went from $8.4 billion in fiscal year 2007 to $14.7 billion allocated in fiscal year 2016 (ONDCP, 2016; SAMHSA, 2016d).

There are numerous federal resources that nurses and other health care professionals need to be familiar with. For instance, there is the National Institute on Drug Abuse (NIDA) (http://www.drugabuse.gov/). NIDA's mission is to lead the United States in research on drug abuse and addiction. Its strategic goals address substance abuse as a complex disease and underlying causes. The institute works with research programs in basic, clinical, and translational science, including genetics, functional neuroimaging, social neuroscience, medication and behavioral therapies, prevention, and health services. There are four strategic goals: identify the biological, environmental, behavioral, and social causes and consequences of drug use and addiction across the life span; develop new and improved strategies to prevent drug use and its consequences; develop new and improved treatments to help people with substance use disorders achieve and maintain a meaningful and sustained recovery; and increase the public health impact of NIDA research and programs (NIDA, 2017). NIDA gathers data on health disparities related to drug addiction and its many effects. The institute has many education programs encompassing criminal justice, medical, and educational systems. It continues to promote research addressing nicotine addiction, HIV/AIDS, and emerging trends, as well as training and dissemination of science-based information on drug abuse.

The Substance Abuse and Mental Health Services Administration (SAMHSA), builds and sustains programs, policies, information and data, contracts, and grants with the intent of helping the nation act on the knowledge that promotes behavioral health treatment through all levels of prevention. SAMHSA promotes programs that work with military families as well as justice systems (SAMHSA, 2017).

PREVALENCE, INCIDENCE, AND TRENDS

The growing recognition of the widespread effects of substance abuse has initiated extensive collection of data by multiple agencies. This section describes selected statistics and current trends. The U.S. National Survey on Drug Use and Health is an annual survey conducted by SAMHSA that estimates the prevalence of illicit drug and alcohol use in the United States. Findings from a 2015 report include the following (SAMHSA, 2017).

Alcohol

A reported 138.3 million Americans aged 12 or older were current drinkers of alcohol in the 2015 survey. Of greatest concern, perhaps, is the prevalence of occasions of heavy drinking—five or more drinks in a row at least once in the prior 2-week period—which was reported by 4% of eighth graders, 11% of tenth graders, 17% of twelfth graders, 32% of college students, and 32% of young adults surveyed in 2015. Of these, 66.7 million persons aged 12 or older participated in binge drinking. Heavy drinking was reported by 6.5% of the population aged 12 or older, or 17.3 million people. Among young adults aged 18 to 25 in 2015, the rate of binge drinking was 39%. The rate of current alcohol use among youths aged 12 to 17 was 9.6% (2.4 million adolescents) in 2015. About 1.4 million (5.8%) adolescents age 12 to 17 were past-month binge alcohol users in 2015. Thus around 1 in 17 adolescents aged 12 to 17 in 2015 were current binge drinkers.

There were an estimated 7.7 million underage (aged 12 to 20) drinkers in 2015, including 5.1 million binge drinkers and 1.3 million heavy drinkers (drinking more than three times weekly). From 2007 through 2015 alcohol use continued its trend of decline, reaching historic lows, including significant declines in binge drinking in 2015 for tenth- and twelfth-grade students.

Twenty percent of youth aged 12 to 20 years drink alcohol, and 13% reported binge drinking in the past 30 days in 2015 (Center for Behavioral Health Statistics and Quality, 2016). College students' level of binge drinking in 2015 was 32%, down slightly from their 1993 (and 2008) level of 40%. The level among noncollege peers was 24% in 2015 (and 30% in 2012)—down from 34% in 1993 (Miech et al., 2016). In 2015, about 7.7 million people aged 12 to 20 reported drinking alcohol in the *past month,* including 5.1 million who reported binge alcohol use and 1.3 million who reported heavy alcohol use, however (SAHMSA, 2016).

Excessive drinking is responsible for more than 4300 deaths among underage youth annually (Sacks et al., 2015). Perhaps most alarming, nearly half of teens (44%) do not see a "great risk" in drinking five or more drinks nearly every day, and there is low social disapproval from peers; only 34% strongly disapprove of "teens your age getting drunk" (Partnership for Drug-Free Kids, 2016).

Young people rarely drink alone. Nearly 80% of those drinking underage in 2013 were with two or more people the last time they drank (Center for Behavioral Health Statistics and Quality, 2015).The National Institute on Alcohol Abuse and Alcoholism (2015) has found that alcohol use by a friend makes it very likely that a young person already is using alcohol or might start drinking.

Alcohol use by young people often occurs in a home setting. In 2013, 52% of 12- to 20-year-olds who drank reported that they last drank in someone else's home, and 34% reported that the drinking occurred in their own home (Center for Behavioral Health Statistics and Quality, 2015).

Illicit Drug Use

An estimated 27.1 million Americans aged 12 or older were current (past-month) illicit drug users, meaning they had used an illicit drug during the month before the survey interview (SAMHSA, 2016a). Illicit drugs included marijuana, cocaine (including crack), heroin, hallucinogens, inhalants, and prescription-type psychotherapeutics (pain relievers, tranquilizers, stimulants, and sedatives) used nonmedically. The rate of current illicit drug use among persons aged 12 or older in 2015 (10.1%) (SAHMSA, 2016a) was slightly greater than the rate in 2010 (8.9%). Further findings are as follows:

- Marijuana was the most commonly used illicit drug. In 2015, there were 22.2 million current users, or 8.3% of the population age 12 and older. The proportion of people age 12 or older who were current marijuana users in 2015 was similar to the proportion in 2014, but it was higher than the percentages from 2002 to 2013 (SAHMSA, 2016a).
- About 329,000 people age 12 or older (0.1% of the population age 12 and older) were current heroin users in 2015 (SAHMSA, 2016a). Despite the dangers associated with heroin, its use has increased in recent years; estimated current heroin use in 2015 among people aged 12 or older was higher than the estimates in most years between 2002 and 2009, but it was similar to the estimates between 2010 and 2014 (SAHMSA, 2016a).
- Hallucinogens had been used in the past month by 1.2 million persons (0.5%) aged 12 or older in 2015. (In 2015, the National Survey on Drug Use and Health estimate of any hallucinogen use was expanded to include the use of ketamine, DMT/AMT/"Foxy," and *Salvia divinorum.* Because of this change, estimates of hallucinogen use in 2015 are not compared with estimates in prior years.) (SAHMSA, 2016a).
- Due to the changes that were made to the prescription drug questions in 2015, a new baseline started in 2015 for all prescription drug measures. The four categories of prescription drugs (pain relievers, tranquilizers, stimulants, and sedatives) cover numerous medications that currently are or have been available by prescription.
- In 2015, 6.4 million persons (2.4%) aged 12 or older had used prescription-type psychotherapeutic drugs nonmedically in the month before the survey. These estimates were higher than the estimates in 2011 (6.1 million or 2.4%).
- In 2015, approximately 897,000 people aged 12 or older were current users of methamphetamine (MA) (0.9 million people), about 0.3% of the population aged 12 or older. About 13,000 adolescents aged 12 to 17 (about 0.1% of adolescents) were current MA users in 2015. About 128,000 adults aged 18 to 25 in 2015 used MA in the past month (about 0.4% of young adults). In 2015, an estimated 757,000 adults aged 26 or older used MA (0.4% of this age group).

- Among youths aged 12 to 17, the 2015 illicit drug use rates were 2.2 million (8.8% adolescents).
- The rate of current marijuana use among youths aged 12 to 17 decreased slightly, to 7%, down from 7.4% in 2009. Rates in 2010 were 7.4% and in 2011 were 7.9%.
- The rate of current use of illicit drugs among young adults aged 18 to 25 increased from 21.4% in 2011 to 22.3% in 2015. This proportion corresponds to about 7.8 million young adults in 2015 who were current users of illicit drugs.
- In 2015, an estimated 492,000 persons aged 12 to 17 misused psychotherapeutic drugs in the past month; about 1 in 50 adolescents (2.0%) were current misusers of psychotherapeutic drugs. An estimated 1.8 million adults ages 18 to 25 (5.1% of young adults) were current misusers of psychotherapeutic drugs. There were 4.1 million adults aged 26 or older (2.0% of adults in this age group) who were current misusers of psychotherapeutic drugs (SAHMSA, 2016a).
- Among adults aged 50 to 64, the rate of illicit drug use increased from 2.7% to 6.0% in 2013; for those ages 50 to 54, the rate increased from 3.4% to 7.9% in 2013. Among those aged 55 to 59, the rate of current illicit drug use increased from 1.9% in 2002 to 5.7% in 2013. In those aged 60 to 64, the rate of current illicit drug use increased from 1.1% in 2003 and 2004 to 3.9% in 2013 (USDHHS, 2014).
- Among unemployed adults aged 18 or older in 2013, 18.2% were current illicit drug users, which was higher than the 9.1% of those employed full time and 13.7% of those employed part time. However, most illicit drug users were employed. Of the 22.4 million current illicit drug users aged 18 or older in 2013, 15.4 million (68.9%) were employed either full or part time (USDHHS, 2017).
- In 2013, 9.9 million persons aged 12 or older reported having driven under the influence of illicit drugs during the past year. This corresponds to 3.8% of the population aged 12 or older, which was similar to the rate in 2012 (3.9%). Across age groups, the rate of driving under the influence of illicit drugs in 2013 was highest among young adults aged 18 to 25 (10.6%); this rate for young adults was lower than the rate in 2012 (11.9%) (USDHHS Substance Abuse and Mental Health Services Administration, 2017).

Among persons aged 12 or older in 2012 to 2013 who used pain relievers nonmedically in the past 12 months, 53.0% obtained the drug they used most recently from a friend or relative for free; 10.6% bought the drug from a friend or relative, and another 21.2% reported that they obtained the drug through a prescription from one doctor. An annual average of 4.3% people got pain relievers from a drug dealer or other stranger, and 0.1% bought them on the Internet (USDHHS Substance Abuse and Mental Health Services Administration, 2017).

Nonmedical Use of Prescription-Type Psychotherapeutics

Nonmedical use and abuse of prescription drugs constitute a serious public health problem in this country. An estimated 52 million people (20% of those aged 12 and older) have used prescription drugs for nonmedical reasons at least once in their lifetimes. The NIDA Monitoring the Future (MTF) survey (2016a) found that nonmedical use of prescription narcotic drugs has been declining among college students, since reaching a high in 2006 of 8.8% annual prevalence (that is, any use in the prior 12 months). By 2015, 3.3% of college students reported using any narcotic drug in the past 12 months without medical supervision (NIDA, 2016). As of 2015, 38% of college students said they had used marijuana in the prior 12 months, up from 30% in 2006, though daily use has declined since 2014; 4.3% (about 1 in every 22) college students now report daily marijuana use.

As of 2015, 4.4% high school seniors reported past-year nonmedical use of the prescription pain reliever hydrocodone (Vicodin), 3.7% reported abusing oxycodone (OxyContin), 7.7% reported use of amphetamines, and 7.5% reported misuse of Adderall—making these medications among the drugs most commonly abused by adolescents (Miech et al., 2016). There are three classes of the most commonly abused prescription drugs: opioids, central nervous system depressants, and stimulants. There has been a significant increase in the lifetime nonmedical use of pain relievers (2 million individuals, or 0.8% people, aged 12 years and older), specifically Vicodin, codeine, OxyContin, and Percocet (Miech et al., 2016).

Hallucinogen, Inhalant, and Heroin Use

Hallucinogen drugs cause hallucinations by disrupting the interactions of nerve cells and the neurotransmitter serotonin. There are profound distortions of perceptions of reality. People may see things, hear sounds, and feel sensations that seem real but do not exist. Some hallucinations may also produce emotional changes in behavior. There may be changes in mood, hunger sensations, body temperature, sexual behavior, and muscle coordination.

LSD (D-lysergic acid diethylamide), which was discovered in 1938 and is manufactured from lysergic acid, has unpredictable psychological effects, "trips" that may last 12 hours. Some doses of LSD may cause delusions and hallucinations. LSD may be sold in tablets, capsules, or, occasionally, liquid form; thus it is usually taken orally. The drug is often added to absorbent paper, which is then divided into decorated pieces, each equivalent to one dose. Behavior of someone using LSD may manifest as psychosis. There may be other symptoms, such as increases in body temperature, heart rate, and blood pressure; sleeplessness; and loss of appetite (NIDA, 2016a, 2016b). Fortunately, availability of LSD has recently been at or near the lowest levels ever recorded by the MTF survey (ongoing since 1975), although 2015 brought slight, nonsignificant increases in tenth and twelfth graders (Miech et al., 2016).

Peyote is a small, spineless cactus in which the principal active ingredient is mescaline. The peyote cactus has been used by natives in northern Mexico and the southwestern United States as a part of religious ceremonies. Tops (buttons) of the peyote cactus are cut from the roots and dried, then are chewed or soaked in water to produce an intoxicating liquid. Extracts are bitter and may be prepared into a tea by boiling the cacti for several hours. A hallucinogenic dose of mescaline is about 0.3 to 0.5 grams, and its effects last about 12 hours (NIDA, 2015).

Psilocybin (4-phosphoryloxy-*N,N*-dimethyltryptamine), also known as *magic mushrooms,* is obtained from certain types of mushrooms that are indigenous to tropical and subtropical regions of South America, Mexico, and the United States. Mushrooms containing psilocybin are available fresh or dried and are typically taken orally. They may be brewed as a tea or added to other foods to mask their bitter flavor. Hallucinatory effects may appear within 20 minutes of ingestion and may last up to 6 hours (NIDA, 2015).

PCP (phencyclidine) was developed in the 1950s as an intravenous anesthetic for surgery but was never approved for human use because of problems during clinical studies, including intensely negative psychological effects. PCP is a white crystalline powder that is readily soluble in water or alcohol. It can also be mixed easily with dyes and is often sold on the illicit drug market in a variety of tablet, capsule, and colored powder forms that are normally snorted, smoked, or orally ingested. PCP has a distinctive bitter chemical taste. When smoked, it is often applied to a leafy material such as mint, parsley, oregano, or marijuana. Depending on concentration and route of ingestion, its effects can last approximately 4 to 6 hours (Drugs.com, 2017; NIDA, 2015.

Approximately 0.5% of individuals aged 12 to 17 years abuse inhalants (SAMHSA, 2016). Inhalants can be found in many products readily available in the home or workplace. Spray paints, markers, glues, and cleaning fluids contain volatile substances that have psychoactive properties when inhaled. They can be used especially, but not exclusively, by young children and adolescents. Most often these substances produce a rapid high that resembles alcohol intoxication, resulting in a loss of sensation and even unconsciousness. Serious and irreversible effects include hearing loss, limb spasms, central nervous system or brain damage, and bone marrow damage. Inhaling high concentrations of these substances may result in death from heart failure or suffocation.

In 2015, about 329,000 (or 0.3 million) people aged 12 or older were current heroin users. Regarding past-year use, 0.3% of people aged 12 or older in 2015 had used heroin, which represents about 828,000 people. It is estimated that about 23% of individuals who use heroin become dependent on it. An opioid drug, heroin is synthesized from morphine. Heroin usually is a white or brown powder or a black sticky substance, known as *black tar heroin*. Injection of drugs like heroin brings about the highest risk of contracting HIV and hepatitis C. These diseases are transmitted through contact with blood or other bodily fluids, which can occur through the sharing of needles or other injection drug use equipment. Hepatitis C is the most common bloodborne infection in the Unites States. HIV can also be contracted during unprotected sex, which drug use makes more likely. There is close association between drug abuse and the increase of infectious diseases.

Gender Differences

In general, higher proportions of males than females are involved in illicit drug use, especially heavy use, and overall, more males than females abuse prescription drugs in all age groups except those 12 to 17 years old. Females in this age group exceed males in the nonmedical use of all psychotherapeutics, including pain relievers, tranquilizers, and stimulants (Miech et al., 2016). There are no appreciable gender differences in

2015 among eighth graders in their use of hallucinogens, LSD, MDMA, salvia, cocaine, crack, other cocaine, heroin, Vicodin, Ritalin, Adderall, MA, bath salts, or Rohypnol. The levels of use of inhalants, alcohol, flavored alcoholic beverages, and the frequency of being drunk are slightly higher among females in eighth grade. By tenth grade use among boys catches up and in some cases surpasses use among girls on many of these drugs, as use increases faster among boys than among girls with age (Miech et al., 2016).

Demographics

Demographic correlates show some regional, racial, and gender differences and changes over the past few years. For example, people living in the West continue to have the highest percentage of past-month illicit drug use, at 11.56%, compared with 8.83% for those in the Midwest, 9.61% for those in the Northeast, and 7.95% for those in the South (SAMHSA, 2013a). Additionally, rates of current illicit drug use vary significantly among major racial/ethnic groups. Among those age 12 or older, blacks and individuals from other racial and ethnic groups were equally likely to need treatment for substance use in the past year; 9.1% of blacks (2.6 million persons) and 9.3% of persons from other racial and ethnic groups (20.4 million persons) needed treatment for illicit drug or alcohol use (SAMHSA, 2013b). Although blacks were less likely than persons from other racial and ethnic groups to need treatment for alcohol use (6.8 vs. 7.8%), they were more likely to need treatment for illicit drug use (4.1 vs. 3.0%). (SAMHSA, 2013b). Visit the SAMHSA data website, at https://www.samhsa.gov/data/node/20, for more information about substance abuse trends and statistics.

Trends in Substance Use

Research has revealed that problems associated with substance abuse may or may not relate to classically or clinically defined dependence or addiction. Many people are turning to recovery before they have developed physiological dependence. Thus many in the field have begun to differentiate between use and misuse (*misuse* being interchangeable with *abuse*), and these terms now appear in the literature. This section describes significant trends in substances that are being abused and discusses substance abuse among special populations.

Healthy People 2020 and Substance Abuse

The U.S. Department of Health and Human Services (USDHHS) set goals and objectives related to substance abuse in *Healthy People 2020* (HealthyPeople.gov, 2017). *Healthy People 2020*'s overarching goals for all Americans are attaining high-quality, longer lives with more prevention opportunities in preventable disease, disability, injury, and premature death. Positive directions in achieving health equity, eliminating disparities, and improving the health of all groups are much more possible today. With ideas to create social and physical environments that promote good health for all, more communities are working together in health promotion education and programs. *Healthy People 2020*'s mission encompasses promoting quality of life, healthy development, and healthy behaviors across all life stages. The use of harmful substances is indirectly and directly related to all of the leading health indicators (i.e., tobacco use, alcohol and other drug abuse, physical activity, overweight and obesity, mental health, injury and violence, environmental quality, responsible sexual behavior, immunization, and access to health care). The *Healthy People 2020* box presents selected objectives and targets from *Healthy People 2020* related to substance abuse.

 HEALTHY PEOPLE 2020

Selected Proposed Objectives for Substance Abuse

Policy and Prevention
- Reduction of proportion of adolescents who report they rode during the previous 30 days with a driver who had been drinking alcohol
- Increase the proportion of adolescents never using substances
- Increase the proportion of adolescents who disapprove of substance abuse
- Increase the proportion of adolescents who perceive great risk associated with substance abuse
- Increase the number of drug and other specialty courts
- Increase the number of states with mandatory ignition interlock laws for first-time and repeat driving offenders

Screening and Treatment
- Increase number of admissions to substance abuse treatment for injection drug use
- Increase the proportion of persons who need alcohol and/or illicit drug treatment and received specialty treatment for abuse or dependence in the past year
- Increase the proportions of persons referred for follow-up care of alcohol problems, drug problems after diagnosis, or treatment of one of those conditions in a hospital emergency department
- Increase the number of Level I and Level II Trauma Centers and primary care settings that implement evidence-based alcohol screening and brief intervention

Epidemiology and Surveillance
- Reduce cirrhosis death
- Reduce drug-induced deaths
- Reduce past-month use of illicit substance abuse
- Reduce the proportion of persons engaging in binge drinking of alcoholic beverages
- Reduce proportion of adults who drank excessively in the past 30 days
- Reduce average annual alcohol consumption
- Decrease the rate of alcohol-impaired driving fatalities
- Reduce steroid use among adolescents
- Reduce the past-year nonmedical use of prescription drugs
- Reduce the number of deaths attributed to alcohol
- Reduce the proportions of adolescents who use inhalants

From HealthyPeople.gov: *Healthy People 2020: Substance abuse.* https://www.healthypeople.gov/2020/topics-objectives/topic/substance-abuse. Accessed April 6, 2018.

Methamphetamine

MA has evolved as the most widely produced controlled substance in the United States. It is appearing in mass quantities, in part because of the ease with which the fertilizer anhydrous ammonia can be converted into MA, which has attracted more individuals to this clandestine business. Illegal street forms of the drug, often called *crank, crystal,* or *meth,* are available as a powder that can be injected, inhaled, or taken orally. In addition, a smokable form, known as *ice* or *glass,* is widely available. "Methamphetamine users often begin with intranasal or oral use and progress to intravenous use, and occasionally smoking" [National Highway Traffic Safety Administration, 2017]).

The pleasurable effects of MA are due to the release of high levels of dopamine in the brain, leading to increased energy, a sense of euphoria, and greater productivity. Short-term effects are increased heart rate, insomnia, excessive talking, excitation, and aggressive behavior. Prolonged use results in tolerance and physiological dependence. MA has multiple negative effects for users, their families, and communities. It appears to damage the brain in ways that are different from, and more severe than, damage from using other drugs. Negative consequences range from anxiety, convulsions, and paranoia to brain damage.

MA user profiles represent the most common categories reported by officials and treatment professionals: high school and college students and college athletes; and white, blue-collar workers and men and women in their 20s and 30s who are jobless (Rehab International, 2017). Meth abuse occurs across rural and urban boundaries. Usage is divided equally among both women and men. Past-year use of MA has been declining steadily since it was first added to the ongoing nationwide MTF survey in 1999 (Miech et al., 2016). Use of MA among adolescents was at or near historic low levels, and among eighth-, tenth-, and twelfth-grade students the proportion reporting use in the past year was 0.5%, 0.8%, and 0.6%, respectively. Since its 1999 peak prevalence, use of MA has declined more than 80% in all grades (Miech et al., 2015). In 2015, 897,000 individuals 12 or older reported past-month use of MA; about 13,000 of these were age 12 to 17 and 128,000 were aged 18 to 25, and about 757,000 were age 26 or older (Bose et al., 2017).

The impact of MA abuse on communities, families, and social networks is considerable. Reported use is highest among 20- to 29-year-olds. This group often has young children, putting these children at risk for abuse and neglect. Furthermore, exposure to combustible secondhand fumes puts children at risk for not only complications related to primary ingestion but also fatalities and injuries related to the highly combustible nature of the chemicals used in manufacture of the drug.

Steroids

Anabolic steroids are synthetic variants of the male sex hormone testosterone. The proper term for these compounds is *anabolic-androgenic steroids.* They can build muscle and are said to be androgenic, referring to increased male sexual characteristics. These steroids are taken orally, injected into the muscles, or applied topically. Doses taken may be 10 to 100 times higher than the doses prescribed to treat medical conditions (NIDA, 2016b). Steroids taken continuously can decrease the body's responsiveness to the drugs, increasing tolerance as well as causing the body to stop producing its own testosterone. Evidence suggests that steroid use among adolescents is decreasing (Miech et al., 2016). In 2015, in its annual survey used to assess drug use among our nation's teens, MTF found that 0.5% of eighth graders, 0.7% of tenth graders, and 1.7% of twelfth graders had used anabolic steroids during the previous year (NIDA, 2016b). Steroid use is more common in athletes and other individuals willing to risk potential and irreversible health consequences to build muscle. There are other more potentially fatal risks, including blood clots, liver damage, premature cardiovascular changes, and increased cholesterol (NIDA, 2016b).

Evidence also points at behavioral changes leading to an increased potential for suicide and aggressive and risky behaviors among steroid users. Collaborative treatment programs that monitor both psychological and physical issues, including options to inject the drug, are necessary to combat steroid abuse.

Anabolic steroids do not cause the same high as other drugs. But use of this type of steroid can lead to addiction. Steroid use may persist despite the physical problems and negative effects on social relationships that it causes. Steroid abusers typically spend large amounts of time and money obtaining the drug. Individuals who abuse steroids often experience withdrawal symptoms when they stop using them, including mood swings, fatigue, restlessness, loss of appetite, insomnia, reduced sex drive, and steroid cravings. One of the most dangerous withdrawal symptoms is depression. Persistent depressive symptoms can sometimes lead to suicide attempts. Research has found that some steroid abusers turn to other drugs, such as opioids, to counteract the negative effects of steroids (NIDA, 2015a).

ADOLESCENT SUBSTANCE ABUSE

Youth are a particularly susceptible aggregate for substance abuse. Drug use is highest among individuals in their late teens and 20s; in 2013, 22.6% of people ages 18 to 20 reported using an illicit drug during the past month (NIDA, 2015a).

Of all of the drugs used by adolescents, cigarettes have some of the highest levels of daily use. The percentages of teens who reported using one or more cigarettes per day in the last 30 days were 1.3%, 3.0%, and 5.5% in grades 8, 10, and 12, respectively (Miech et al., 2016). Youth (ages 12 to 20) binge and heavy drinking rates in 2015 (13.4% and 3.3%, respectively) were higher than rates in 2010 (7.8% and 1.7%, respectively) (NIAAA, 2017). It is noteworthy, however, that this significant decline in adolescent smoking and use of smokeless tobacco has decelerated sharply (Miech et al., 2016). Cigarettes are still highly available to the young, and concerned groups continue to monitor advertising that targets new potential smokers, such as youth and women.

The 2015 National Survey on Drug Use and Health measured perceived risk as the percentage of youth reporting that there is great risk in the substance use behavior (SAMHSA, 2015). The percentage aged 12 to 17 years who perceived great risk in smoking marijuana once or twice a week decreased from 47.5% in 2010 to 40.6% in 2015 (SAMHSA, 2015). Studies demonstrated that from 2002 to 2008, almost half of 12- to 17-year-old respondents reported in 2010 that it would be fairly easy or very easy to obtain marijuana. This number is consistent, at 46%, in 2015. Most of the movement in teen substance use has been in a downward direction, but generally the declines have been marginal (NIDA, 2010c).

With nearly half of teens trying marijuana before they graduate, there is definitely skepticism about the drug's danger. There is research that marijuana use during adolescence has the potential to set young people up for a cascade of life-altering events, impeding their success and hindering them from fulfilling their potential. Teens too often do not believe this to be true. The MTF survey of drug use has for years demonstrated a steady drop in the number of middle- and high-school students who think occasional or even regular marijuana users risk harming themselves physically or in other ways. With this

declining perception comes the risk of increasing use. Among twelfth graders in 2015, 12% reported using marijuana daily for at least a month at some point in their lives; this is twice as high as the 6.0% reporting current daily use (Miech et al., 2015).

In order to effectively plan for the present and future needs of the community, the community health nurse needs the most current overall perspective. Information on the prevalence, incidence, and trends in the amount and types of substance abuse at the general, state, and local levels is readily available on the Internet. As harmful, illicit substances come in and out of vogue, particularly among young people, the community health nurse must develop a good understanding of drug culture, terminology, and differing signs and symptoms.

CONCEPTUALIZATIONS OF SUBSTANCE ABUSE

Conceptualizations of substance abuse and dependence have changed over the years, often for political and social reasons rather than for scientific reasons. Some conceptualizations focus on the phenomenon of addiction, which is manifested by compulsive use patterns and the onset of withdrawal symptoms when substance use is abruptly stopped. Other views focus on the problems resulting from the substance use itself, regardless of whether an addictive pattern is present. Problematic consequences of substance use include intoxication, psychological dependence, relational conflicts, employment or economic difficulties, legal difficulties, and health problems. For example, addiction need not be present for individuals to experience legal consequences of illicit drug use, such as driving while intoxicated or alcohol- or drug-related domestic violence.

Drawing fine distinctions among ideas of dependence, addiction, and abuse concerning substance use may seem irrelevant if there is evidence that the substance use has become problematic. Indeed, the DSM-5 Substance-Related Disorders Work Group recommendations for *Diagnostic and Statistical Manual of Mental Disorders, Fifth Edition* (DSM-5) revisions included combining abuse and dependence criteria into a single substance use disorder based on consistent findings from over 200,000 research participants (Hasin et al., 2014), dropping legal problems and adding craving as criteria, adding cannabis and caffeine withdrawal syndromes, aligning tobacco use disorder criteria with other substance use disorders, and moving gambling disorders to the chapter formerly reserved for substance-related disorders. General concerns for the group "included whether to retain the division into two main disorders (dependence and abuse), whether substance use disorder criteria should be added or removed, and whether an appropriate substance use disorder severity indicator could be identified (p. 834)." It is also becoming increasingly evident that specific interventions may be needed for each separate addictive problem (e.g., overeating and gambling). Moreover, in each specific group, there is wide individual diversity.

Definitions

Traditional conceptualizations of substance use focus solely on alcohol and illicit street drugs. Other conceptualizations include prescription medications such as tranquilizers and analgesics. In eating disorders such as bulimia and compulsive overeating,

TABLE 27.1 Classification of Commonly Used and Abused Substances

Substance	Desired Effect(s)	Possible Withdrawal Symptoms
Central Nervous System Depressants		
Alcohol	Euphoria, disinhibition, and sedation	Anxiety, irritability, seizures, delusions, hallucinations, and paranoia
Barbiturates	Euphoria and sedation	Restlessness, tremors, and anxiety
Sedative-hypnotics (e.g., benzodiazepines [Rohypnol])	Sedation and amnesia	Insomnia, anxiety, restlessness, and tremors
Tranquilizers (e.g., GHB [gamma-hydroxybutyrate], the "date rape" drug)	Depress consciousness	Confusion, psychosis, agitation
Central Nervous System Stimulants		
Amphetamines (e.g., methamphetamine)	Euphoria, hyperactivity, omnipotence, insomnia, and anorexia	Depression, apathy, lethargy, and sleepiness
Cocaine	Increased sense of energy and alertness	Depression and anxiety
Nicotine	Calmness, concentration	Restlessness and agitation
Caffeine	Concentration, energy	Restlessness and agitation
Narcotics-opioids	Euphoria and sedation	Restlessness, pain, and agitation
Codeine	Euphoria and sedation	Anxiety, irritability, agitation, runny nose, watery eyes, chills, sweating, nausea and vomiting, diarrhea, tremors, and yawning
Meperidine and acetaminophen (e.g., Demerol)	Euphoria and sedation	Restlessness, pain, and agitation
Hydromorphone (e.g., Dilaudid)	Euphoria and sedation	Restlessness, pain, and agitation
Fentanyl	Euphoria and sedation	Restlessness, pain, and agitation
Heroin	Euphoria and sedation	Restlessness, pain, and agitation
Methadone	Euphoria and sedation	Restlessness, pain, and agitation
Morphine	Euphoria and sedation	Restlessness, pain, and agitation
Opium	Euphoria and sedation	Restlessness, pain, and agitation
Oxycodone (e.g., Percodan)	Euphoria and sedation	Restlessness, pain, and agitation
Hallucinogens		
Mescaline	Hallucinations, illusions, and heightened awareness	Depression
LSD	Hallucinations, illusions, and heightened awareness	Depression
PCP (phencyclidine) (e.g., ketamine)	PCP: violent dissociative and anesthetic effect Ketamine: agitation, confusion, psychosis, (including delusions and hallucinations), loss of motor skills, rage, nausea, decrease in respiratory and cardiac functions, insomnia, tremors, hearing loss, fatigue	Depression
STP (2,5-dimethoxy-4-methylamphetamine) and MDMA (methylenedioxymethamphetamine [i.e., Ecstasy])	Hallucinations, illusions, and heightened awareness	Depression
Psilocybin (e.g., mushrooms)	Hallucinations, illusions, and heightened awareness	Depression
Cannabis		
Marijuana	Hallucinations, illusions, and heightened awareness	Depression
Hashish and THC (tetrahydrocannabinol)	Hallucinations, illusions, and heightened awareness	Depression
Inhalants		
Gasoline	Euphoria	Restlessness, anxiety, and irritability
Toluene acetate	Euphoria	Restlessness, anxiety, and irritability
Cleaning fluids	Euphoria	Restlessness, anxiety, and irritability
Airplane cement	Euphoria	Restlessness, anxiety, and irritability
Amyl nitrate	Euphoria	Restlessness, anxiety, and irritability

Modified from Faltz B, Rinaldi J: *AIDS and substance abuse: a training manual for health care professionals*, San Francisco, 1987, Regents of the University of California.

food is viewed as the abused substance. Table 27.1 shows a classification scheme for commonly used substances.

In addition to varying in their abuse potential, substances vary in their degree of potential harm to those who use them and to others in the immediate environment. Tobacco is an example of a substance that is unsafe to the smoker and to those who inhale secondhand smoke. Those who abuse alcohol may also harm others by driving under its influence, and its lowering of inhibitions may foster violent activities in some users (e.g., child or partner abuse).

The American Psychiatric Association (APA), in the DSM-5, no longer uses the terms *substance abuse* and *substance dependence*. Rather, it refers to substance use disorders, which are defined as mild, moderate, or severe to indicate the level of severity, which is determined by the number of diagnostic criteria met by an individual (Hasin et al., 2014). The presence of 2 or more of 11 criteria now indicate substance use disorder: hazardous use; social/interpersonal problems related to use; neglected major roles to use; legal problems; withdrawal (but not for inhalant or hallucinogen disorders); tolerance; used larger amounts/longer; repeated attempts to quit/control use; much time spend using; physical/psychological problems related to use; and activities given up to use (Hasin et al., 2014). The APA (2017) focused on the following psychoactive substances that affect the nervous system: alcohol, amphetamines, caffeine, cannabis, cocaine, hallucinogens, inhalants, tobacco, opioids, phencyclidine, sedatives, and hypnotics or anxiolytics. Substance use disorders can also be categorized as being in early remission (≥3 to <12 months without meeting substance use disorders criteria, except craving) and sustained remission (≥12 months without meeting substance use disorders criteria, except craving) (Hasin et al., 2014). A diagnosis of substance use disorder indicates a maladaptive pattern of substance use that is manifested as recurrent and significant adverse consequences related to repeated use of a substance. These adverse consequences include failure to fulfill major role obligations, repeated use in physically hazardous situations, multiple legal problems, and recurrent social and interpersonal problems.

The criteria for the diagnosis of dependence include a cluster of cognitive, behavioral, and physiological symptoms that indicate continued use of the substance despite significant substance-related problems. A criteria count is used (from 2 to 11) as an overall severity indicator, with 2 to 3 being mild, 4 to 5 being moderate, and 6 or more being severe. A pattern of repeated, self-administered use results in tolerance, withdrawal, and compulsive drug-taking behaviors, which are frequently accompanied by a craving or strong desire for the substance. This craving then motivates the user to be preoccupied with supply, money to purchase drugs, and getting through time between periods of use, all of which take up mental energy—effort that is diverted from work or school and from connectedness to significant others. This process is how the use becomes problematic and how others around the user become confused and eventually often feel rejected, hurt, ignored, angry, or even responsible for the user's behavior.

SOCIOCULTURAL AND POLITICAL ASPECTS OF SUBSTANCE ABUSE

Within community settings, substance-related problems are not always easy to identify. For example, the consequences of the sale and use of crack cocaine in an inner-city, African American neighborhood may be apparent through media attention. The traffic of these drugs into the middle classes, on the other hand, is less easily recognized. The increasing tendencies of elderly persons to rely on alcohol and other, even illicit, drugs may be shocking to some nurses. It can be understood contextually, however, and may be the result of multiple factors, such as isolation, fears, uncontrolled chronic pain, anxiety, and sleep disturbances. Nurses must incorporate sociocultural and political dimensions into caring for clients in the community. Nurses must also possess knowledge that is useful in countering media stereotypes and allows them to model a more holistic, multifaceted approach to prevention and management of substance abuse.

Although there are subcultural and regional variations, drinking norms of the dominant culture in the United States are relatively permissive. Traditional ethnic ceremonial and symbolic substance use patterns vary significantly. As acculturation occurs, however, cultural definitions of "appropriate" use of alcohol and drugs have been dulled, leaving a void regarding social expectations. Subcultural groups such as gay, lesbian, bisexual, and transgender persons have often had a social center that was a bar, and alcohol use was historically a way of demonstrating and celebrating differentiation from a more repressive majority. These cultural conditions create ambiguity in clearly determining when a substance abuse problem exists. Furthermore, each subculture may define abuse differently. It can be theorized that stigmatized minorities might be under more stress, and perhaps more likely to use substances, but this cannot be assumed in any individual case.

Substances are also given economic value and are bought and sold as commodities in a variety of social arenas, both legal and illegal. The ways in which drugs, including nicotine, medications, and alcohol, are produced and distributed among the various segments of the population are determined largely by economic, cultural, and political conditions.

COURSE OF SUBSTANCE-RELATED PROBLEMS

There is no predictable course of addictive illness and no "addictive personality type." When habitual use is well established, behaviors may be clinically visible and similar; this observation has led to assumption of a singular, addiction-prone personality. However, not everyone who initiates drug or alcohol use progresses to dependence or displays associated behaviors. Because the path from initiation to dependency is multidimensional, the context of client and community experiences is key to understanding and responding to problems encountered. Nurses need to take a comprehensive health and substance use history and place it in a context of cultural, historical, family, and social factors. Neither addiction nor dependency is a unitary phenomenon with a single isolated cause; rather, it is the result of interactions among a host of variables.

A variety of screening sand assessment tools are available (NIDA, 2014). It is important to consider the person, substance, and the context (Patrick et al., 2016). The person assessment involves demographic information, medical history, comorbidities, and known perceptions and meanings the individual displays. The drug assessment consists of the qualities of the substance itself, physiopharmacological effects, pattern of use, availability, and toxicity. Context assessment should cover family, social, employment, legal, cultural, and economic contingencies.

The progression from initiation to continuation, transition to abuse, and, finally, addiction and dependency varies. Individuals often describe a progression that began with initiation through social interactions. For some, the substance and setting are reinforcing and prime the individual for a pattern of use. For others, the experience is unpleasant enough to prevent further use. It cannot be assumed, however, that an unpleasant initiation will always be preventive. In the case of stimulants, such as MA, the drug produces such strong feelings of euphoria, alertness, control, and increased energy that future use is enticing, especially when the drug is easily accessible.

The continuation stage of substance abuse is a subsequent period in which substance use persists but does not appear to be detrimental to the individual. In stimulant abuse, continued use often occurs in a binge pattern. Individuals are able to exercise some control over use, but use becomes more frequent. Neither the individual nor the social network views use during this stage as problematic.

A critical point is the transition stage from substance use to substance abuse. It may be evident to both the user and his or her social network that the use of the substance is having adverse effects. During this stage, users begin to use more often and in more varied settings. Rationalizations that deny the seriousness and consequences of the substance use are commonly constructed during this stage.

The research on correlates and antecedents of substance abuse points to a variety of personal and social motivations. For many young people, motivators are the attraction of a rebellious subculture, peer pressure, and nationwide fads. Considerable research exists on the self-medication aspects of individuals with comorbid mental illnesses. Once the addiction is established, unpleasant physical and emotional withdrawal symptoms are strong motivators to continue use. Abstinence in the stimulant abuser can result in symptoms such as depression, lethargy, and anhedonia (i.e., inability to feel pleasure). The depression experienced by the user when not using stimulants is contrasted with the recalled euphoria produced by the use of the drug. These factors, coupled with associated cues, help initiate the cycle of binge use, with increased craving and continued self-administration to relieve symptoms. Brain imaging techniques have demonstrated that abuse of drugs such as cocaine and amphetamine produce immediate and long-lasting physical changes that are likely to contribute to the maintenance of dependency. Nurses can learn more about this research from the NIDA's web page on addiction science, at http://www.drugabuse.gov/related-topics/addiction-science.

The development of addiction or dependency is marked by changes in both behavior and cognition. There is a growing focus on the substance and a narrowing of interests, social activities, and relationships. The process of becoming dependent or addicted requires the individual to deny or ignore evidence or

TABLE 27.2	Typical Course of Addictive Illness: Stages in Continuum from Initiation to Dependency
Stage	**Characteristics**
Initiation	First use of the substance
	Exposure frequently occurs through family or friends
Continuation	Continued, more frequent use of substance
	Usually social use only, with no detrimental effects
Transition	Beginning of change in total consumption, frequency, and occasions of use
	More than just social use, with beginning of loss of control
Abuse	Adverse effects and consequences of substance use
	Rationalizations for continued use and denial of adverse effects present in user and significant others
	Unsuccessful attempts at control of use
Dependency and addiction	Physical or psychological dependency, or both, on the substance; marked by behavioral and cognitive changes
	Preoccupation with the substance and its procurement, despite negative consequences
	Narrowing of interests, social activities, and relationships to only those related to the substance use

information that may challenge the behavior or the rationalization of the behavior. There is a preoccupation with the substance and its procurement during this stage, even in the face of negative consequences. Table 27.2 outlines the stages in the process of stimulant addiction.

LEGAL AND ETHICAL CONCERNS RELATED TO SUBSTANCE ABUSE

For the past 30 years, the United States has pursued a drug policy based on prohibition and the active application of criminal sanctions against the use and sale of illicit drugs. During this time, the number of criminal penalties for drug offenses has climbed to 1.5 million offenses. This increase in drug-related imprisonment is a result of harsher enforcement policies and longer mandatory sentences for possession of smaller quantities of drugs. Although some individuals are in prison for violent crimes (Drugwarfacts.org, 2016) or major drug trafficking, many drug offenders are arrested for small-scale drug deals made to support their personal use (Drugwarfacts.org, 2016); nearly 50% (92,000 prisoners) of sentenced federal prisoners on September 30, 2015 (the most recent date for which federal offense data are available) were serving time for drug offenses

Alcohol use and abuse are different issues because the possession and sale of alcoholic beverages is illegal only if the individual involved is a minor. Concerns arise when individuals are intoxicated during work, while driving, or in situations that may affect the welfare of others. Legal penalties have increased for driving under the influence of alcohol because groups such as Mothers Against Drunk Driving have influenced legislation (Box 27.1).

One area that has also received the attention of the legal system is the use by pregnant women of substances known to increase risks to their fetuses in terms of future long-term developmental and behavioral problems (Box 27.2). Pregnant addicts

BOX 27.1   Drunk Driving

In 2010, the rate of alcohol-impaired driving fatalities per 100,000 population was 3.2, representing a significant 20-year decrease (65% since 1982). For every 100,000 people in the United States in 2010, 1.2 people were killed in a drunk driving fatal crash in 2015, a rate that has declined 49% over the past decade. Alcohol-impaired driving fatalities accounted for 29% of the total vehicle traffic fatalities in 2015. The rate of drunk driving fatalities per 100,000 population has decreased 49% nationally and 68% among those younger than 21 years. These improved statistics are positive indicators of the gains being made to fight drunk driving. According to the National Highway Traffic Safety Administration, 35,092 people died in traffic crashes in 2015 in the United States. Among the people killed in these drunk driving crashes, 67% were in crashes in which at least one driver in the crash had a blood alcohol content (BAC) of .15 or higher.

Source: Foundation for Advancing Alcohol Responsibility: *Drunk driving fatalities*. https://responsibility.org/get-the-facts/research/statistics/drunk-driving-fatalities/

BOX 27.2   Substance Abuse and Pregnancy

Use of a drug, alcohol, or tobacco by a pregnant woman, thereby exposing her developing fetus to the substance, can have potentially deleterious and even long-term effects on the exposed child. Smoking during pregnancy can increase risks of stillbirth, infant mortality, sudden infant death syndrome, preterm birth, respiratory problems, slowed fetal growth, and low birth weight. Alcohol use during pregnancy can lead to the development of fetal alcohol spectrum disorders, characterized by low birth weight and enduring cognitive and behavioral problems. Prenatal use of opioids and other drugs may cause a withdrawal syndrome in newborns called *neonatal abstinence syndrome (NAS)*. These infants are at greater risk of seizures, respiratory problems, feeding difficulties, low birth weight, and even death. There are evidence-based treatments for pregnant women (and their babies), including medications. Methadone maintenance combined with prenatal care and a comprehensive drug treatment program can improve many of the detrimental outcomes associated with untreated maternal heroin abuse. However, newborns exposed to methadone during pregnancy still require treatment for withdrawal symptoms. A medication option for opioid dependence, buprenorphine, has been shown to produce fewer NAS symptoms in babies than methadone, resulting in shorter infant hospital stays. In general, it is important to closely monitor women who are trying to quit drug use during pregnancy and to provide treatment as needed.

Data from National Institute on Drug Abuse: *Principles of drug addiction treatment: a research-based guide,* ed 3, 2012b. NIH Publication No. 12–4180.

have been imprisoned and forced into treatment, and their children have been removed from their custody after birth. Many treatment providers and patient advocates view this approach as punitive and counterproductive to assisting these women and their children. There is concern that such sanctions may prevent addicted women from seeking treatment for fear of legal consequences.

Military veterans are an aggregate also deserving quality **substance abuse treatment** (Health.mil, 2017; Tollison et al., 2012). The U.S. Department of Veterans Affairs (VA) can address the following areas in substance abuse: screenings for alcohol or tobacco use, outpatient counseling, intensive outpatient treatment, marriage and family counseling, self-help groups, and drug substitution therapies.

 ACTIVE LEARNING

Locate resources in your community that help veterans with substance abuse.

MODES OF INTERVENTION

Correlating with the numerous theories about substance abuse is the wide variety of **intervention** strategies incorporating all levels of prevention. National, state, and local legislative measures have attempted to limit access to potentially addictive pharmaceuticals and illicit street drugs. The growing social demand for smoke-free environments in public buildings, restaurants, airplanes, and similar areas exemplifies how perceptions of tobacco and its risks have changed over the past 50 years. Alcohol taxes, zoning schemes for liquor outlets, a legal drinking age, and legal sanctions on driving while intoxicated are other examples of community efforts to prevent or contain substance abuse.

Media campaigns provide public service communications about the risks of substance abuse and the availability of treatment for these problems. However, these efforts must have culturally relevant and realistic goals. Some have proved to be quite successful. The Partnership for a Drug-Free America conducted an antiinhalant media campaign. Several goals of *Healthy People 2020* are reduction of the proportion of adolescents who report they rode, during the previous 30 days, with a driver who had been drinking alcohol and increases in the proportions of adolescents who have never used substances, who disapprove of substance abuse, and who perceive great risk associated with substance abuse. Educational programs administered through schools and penal institutions have been developed, but evaluation and evidence of success or failure of the interventions have been sporadic. National organizations such as the Partnership for a Drug-Free America and NAMI have national, state, and local chapters and affiliates that support community education, research, and support.

Prevention

The principles of prevention are paramount in community nursing practice. Primary prevention in the community includes working with other providers to perform a needs assessment. This process identifies high-risk situations and potential problems that threaten the integrity of the community and its inhabitants—in particular, what factors in the community are encouraging initiation of substance abuse, how effective school- and community-based programs are, and what political issues in the community may be influencing resource allocation.

On the federal level, primary prevention efforts have been overshadowed by the ongoing "War on Drugs." A significant amount of fiscal resources has been allocated to law enforcement, interdiction, crop eradication, and harsh, punitive laws to prosecute drug users and manufacturers. Debate continues at both the state and federal levels regarding the cost–benefit ratio of drug legalization or decriminalization. Supporters argue that legalization and decriminalization would lead to a reduction in crime and would move the drug problem out of the realm in which it is regarded as the moral failure of individuals toward more humane treatment approaches. For example as of 2017, 26 states and the District of Columbia have now laws broadly legalizing marijuana in some form (Governing, 2017).

There is no question that substance abuse is a costly medical, social, and legal problem. Until society can effectively deal with the serious effects of two lethal but legal drugs, alcohol and nicotine, there will be an argument for adding further sanctions that is difficult to accept and justify. Other preventive efforts at government and private levels include community-based programs, training of health professionals, faith-based initiatives, volunteer consumer groups, organized sports programs, and employer programs.

The secondary prevention role of the community health nurse involves screening and finding resources and solutions specific to the particular community. It is important for the community health nurse to be aware of the evidence base for certain programs and to modify or discard those programs that have not proved successful over time.

Screening tools such as the CAGE (Ewing, 1984) test are brief and simple and allow health providers to talk about substance abuse by incorporating relevant questions into the interview and history of any client. A positive response to any of the CAGE questions does not constitute a diagnosis of alcohol or drug dependence, but it should raise suspicion and mandate further investigation.

Prevention efforts should be specific to aggregates rather than directed at the general public. The Clinical Institute Withdrawal Assessment (CIWA) is a continual assessment protocol commonly utilized in the medical setting that helps patients transition through alcohol withdrawal with less risk of delirium tremens and other medical problems (Sen et al., 2017). The CIWA focuses on common withdrawal symptoms, such as nausea and vomiting, anxiety, paroxysmal sweats, tactile disturbances, tremors, agitation, orientation, auditory disturbances, and headaches.

Prevention efforts focusing on minority groups such as African Americans have been only marginally successful. A possible reason is that such treatment programs fail to incorporate culturally sensitive and appropriate interventions and strategies. The demand for a culturally specific approach is evidence that previous approaches, and the assumptions that underlie them, are insufficient for understanding and explaining the etiology of substance abuse among members of minority groups. Successful prevention efforts are usually not focused solely on alcohol and drug abuse, but are appropriately matched with cultural traditions, respect the values of clients, and are grounded in partnership with communities (Blume, 2016).

Treatment

Substance abuse problems are socially defined and frequently attributed to sufferers who do not recognize their substance use as a problem. Furthermore, the substance abuse treatment system has increasingly taken on social welfare and criminal justice tasks. In this sense, substance abuse differs from many other health-related problems. Most states have laws pertaining to involuntary treatment of substance abusers. Employers and families are often enlisted to assist or coerce the identified client into accepting treatment. This aspect of substance abuse as a health concern raises some crucial questions for health care providers in terms of the encroachment of therapeutic interventions on individual rights to privacy, informed consent, and self-determination.

On the individual level, those providing substance abuse treatment should take into consideration the cultural and educational background and resources of the person, the attitudes of significant others, the degree of invasiveness of the effects of the substance use, and the existence of alternatives. Interventions have been developed to assist some individuals in achieving moderation. Additionally, some research has shown that a small percentage of individuals who recognize a harmful pattern of substance use are able to stop using the substance or to achieve a controlled, nonpathological pattern of use. There are those who, because they experience an important life change, such as graduating from college or getting married, appear to change from excessive alcohol use to social alcohol use.

Nevertheless, people exhibit serious problems related to their use of substances and are usually not able to stop or control their use without outside intervention. Research on identified problem drinkers' ability to return to social alcohol use is still inconclusive. Consequently, most scientists and health care providers advocate abstinence as a cornerstone of recovery.

Abstinence is difficult to maintain on a long-term basis. Therefore an important area of continuing research is relapse prevention (i.e., a behavioral approach that aims to prepare the client for the relapse situation in the hope of preventing it or minimizing its impact on recovery). Relapse prevention models can be applied to alcohol, drug, and behavioral addictive problems (e.g., overeating and compulsive gambling) and can have either controlled use or abstinence as their goal. In relapse prevention, relapses are reframed as learning opportunities, and the client makes plans for coping with negative mood states, meeting the challenge of craving, and stopping a relapse quickly if it should occur.

Inpatient and outpatient are the two main types of treatment programs for substance abuse. Each of these programs may or may not include a detoxification component. Treatment programs also differ in the following ways: they may be voluntary or compulsory and pharmacologically based or drug free. In general, although treatment is intricately tied to the concept of recovery, disciplinary philosophy guides specific treatment approaches. There are a variety of treatment approaches and models, which are sometimes contradictory. The treatment models vary by such factors as the composition of staff and the philosophical approach (i.e., social vs. psychological vs. medical models) to substance abuse problems.

Inpatient treatment isolates individuals from the external world and provides an opportunity to focus only on substance abuse issues. Outpatient treatment is appropriate for those who do not require such structure and protection, those with strong supportive social networks and high levels of motivation, and those who need to continue working while in recovery.

The severity of the individual's alcohol or drug problems and pertinent cultural factors determine the necessity and type of treatment. Therefore the assessment process is of primary importance and begins with an accurate social and medical history. The history taking begins with more general questions about lifestyle, employment, relationships, and self-perception. This general line of questioning permits the development of a therapeutic relationship with the client.

A therapeutic relationship based on trust is essential to collecting information about sensitive issues such as drug and alcohol use. The assessment should then proceed to determining risky behavior patterns and stressors. The interviewer assesses dietary practices; prior health problems; allergies; hospitalizations, including psychiatric disorders; and family history of similar problems, including drug- and alcohol-related problems. This general line of questioning can be followed by more specific questions about harmful behaviors, such as smoking, drinking, and illicit drug use. This ordering of questions progresses from the more socially sanctioned behaviors to more "socially disapproved" behaviors and from the general to the more specific. Positive responses to questions about drug and alcohol use should be probed in a nonjudgmental, direct way and treated as "routine" in health care encounters.

A physical examination is another valuable tool in evaluating the client for potential or actual alcohol and drug problems. Although at-risk clients may not have physical signs of alcohol and drug problems and may even deny obvious consequences of such, certain physical findings warrant further investigation. Complaints such as vague, nonspecific abdominal pain; insomnia; depression; chronic fatigue; back pain; chronic anxiety; refractory hypertension; and night sweats require more intensive investigation. Consistent and heavy users of MA commonly experience extensive and rampant tooth decay, known as *meth mouth,* due to the acidic nature of the drug. Although laboratory tests may not yield clues to drug or alcohol use, certain laboratory findings (e.g., abnormal liver function), in the absence of other etiological agents, may raise the index of suspicion.

Intervention strategies frequently begin with information about the effects of alcohol and drugs and a discussion of the solutions to substance abuse–related problems. This initial educational approach can defuse frequently encountered barriers to intervention, such as shame, guilt, fear, and the client's erroneous perceptions regarding risks. Presenting information and solutions in a nonjudgmental and clear manner may help minimize defensiveness. Reframing interventions within the context of health maintenance or health promotion and education minimizes the sense of stigma.

Ambivalent clients may respond to education and decide to abstain from substances or seek treatment. Other clients, however, even when confronted with legal, financial, physical, and psychological consequences of substance abuse, may resist treatment offers. Therefore the clinician must continue to work with clients and involve important members of their social network to remove internal and environmental barriers and move clients toward readiness for change and treatment. Potential discrimination in group settings and logistical problems, such as lack of child care, may be barriers to treatment.

Much of the effort for substance abuse treatment has been invested in detoxification, residential, and outpatient treatment programs. Secondary problems related to drug and alcohol abuse are intoxication, overdose, and withdrawal. Overdose may be accidental or intentional and requires acute interventions to stabilize the client. As a client advocate, the community health nurse can be an important ally in ensuring that adequate follow-up is conducted for those admitted to emergency departments for overdose. Detoxification is best described as a short-term treatment intervention designed to manage acute withdrawal from the substance. It involves medical management to reduce the adverse side effects of the substance and help stabilize the client. It may be performed on an inpatient or outpatient basis, depending on the substance and severity of dependence.

Addressing acute withdrawal symptoms is of utmost importance in detoxification. The cocaine abuser may experience extreme depression with suicidal ideation. Withdrawal from central nervous system depressants, including alcohol, produces the most life-threatening medical consequences, including anxiety, tremors, delirium, convulsions, and possible death, unless medically managed. Symptoms of withdrawal from narcotics, although less life threatening, are temporarily disabling and painful; they include chills, sweating, cramps, and nausea. Such feelings may cause the individual who is withdrawing from treatment to begin the cycle of abuse again. Detoxification is one of the most crucial periods in the recovery process. Clinicians should be aware of the level of services offered in any detoxification program in order to make appropriate referrals.

Outpatient and inpatient treatment programs vary, but they usually include group and individual therapy and counseling, motivational interviewing, family counseling, education, and socialization into 12-step mutual self-help groups. Many programs are integrating psychotherapy, such as cognitive-behavioral therapy, with pharmacotherapy. The medications used are discussed more fully in the next section. Other strategies are hypnosis, occupational therapy, confrontation, assertiveness training, blood alcohol level discrimination training, and other behavior modification approaches. Relapses are common; therefore the most effective treatment programs incorporate some form of relapse prevention as a part of the healing process.

Therapy that involves the family has proved to be most effective in aiding recovery. Family and social contacts can be helped to initiate change in the abuser, to aid in recovery, and to assist in maintenance of treatment gains. A well-known family involvement motivational technique is the Johnson Institute Intervention, which involves a confrontation of the abuser with guidance from therapists (Intervention Support, 2017). A less coercive version is called A Relational Sequence for Engagement (Association of Intervention Specialists, 2014), whereby significant others are educated and coached over time. Another effective strategy is Community Reinforcement and Family Training (CRAFT) (Center for Motivation and Change, 2014). With this approach, a concerned significant other is trained in techniques such as positive reinforcement, identification of dangerous situations, and stress reduction. The television network HBO made a video called "Getting an Addict into Treatment: The CRAFT

BOX 27.3 Guidelines for Drug Abuse Treatment

- Drug addiction is a brain disease that affects behavior.
- Recovery from drug addiction requires effective treatment, followed by management of the problem over time.
- Treatment must last long enough to produce stable behavioral changes.
- Assessment is the first step in treatment.
- Tailoring services to fit the needs of the individual is an important part of effective drug abuse treatment for criminal justice populations.
- Drug use during treatment should be carefully monitored.
- Treatment should target factors that are associated with criminal behavior.
- Criminal justice supervision should incorporate treatment planning for drug-abusing offenders, and treatment providers should be aware of correctional supervision requirements.
- Continuity of care is essential for drug abusers reentering the community.
- A balance of rewards and sanctions encourages prosocial behavior and treatment participation.
- Offenders with co-occurring drug abuse and mental health problems often require an integrated treatment approach.
- Medications are an important part of treatment for many drug-abusing offenders.
- Treatment planning for drug-abusing offenders who are living in or reentering the community should include strategies to prevent and treat serious, chronic medical conditions, such as HIV/AIDS, hepatitis B and C, and tuberculosis.

From National Institute on Drug Abuse: *Principles of drug abuse treatment for criminal justice populations: a research-based guide*, 2014. http://www.drugabuse.gov/sites/default/files/podat_cj_2012.pdf.

BOX 27.4 Criteria for Measuring Effectiveness of Substance Abuse Treatment Programs

- Number of days abstinent
- Number of days without negative consequences of substance use
- Employability or work attendance
- Self-image improvement
- Spouse's assessment of client's functionality
- Regular attendance at 12-step group meetings
- Compliance with follow-up appointments
- Absence of overt psychiatric symptoms such as depression and anxiety
- Self-reports of progress
- Evidence of personal satisfaction and growth

Approach". NIDA (2012b) published a research-based guide to drug addiction treatment. Important points from this publication are listed in Box 27.3.

Treatment programs have been unprepared for the influx of users of MA and the unique problems associated with its use. Prolonged MA use may lead to serious acute psychotic disorders with intensive physical and psychological withdrawal characterized by protracted anhedonia and dysphoria and accompanied by severe craving. Currently, there are no medications to reverse overdoses of MA and no reliable drugs to treat the paranoia and psychosis associated with it. Complications of treatment include high dropout rates, severe behavioral and psychotic states, and severe craving. Various treatments for MA abuse and addiction are being tried, with mixed results. The effect of MA on brain functioning suggests a need for longer treatment plans. The most promising is a long-term comprehensive case-study approach, using home visits and assisting with transportation and emergency fund provision. Although evidence-based psychosocial treatments (including cognitive-behavioral therapy) are available for the treatment of MA, there are no Food and Drug Administration–approved medications for this substance use disorder.

Studies show that clients respond favorably to treatment for MA use, but because of the multiple dimensions, it is a very challenging problem. Women with MA problems who have young children require a higher level of care. Specifics may include an environment of security and safety with social and emotional support (New Beginnings, 2016). Because many abusers lack a supportive environment, the potential for relapse is high. Also,

because of MA addicts' typical inability to recognize the problematic nature of their use, combined drug court and outpatient treatment strategies are being developed.

Having a substance abuse problem does not mean that all problems are attributable to the addiction. Many substance-abusing clients also have other psychiatric problems (e.g., schizophrenia, depression, bipolar affective disorder, dissociative disorder, posttraumatic stress disorder). The coexistence of both a mental health and a substance use disorder is referred to as *co-occurring disorders*, formerly known as *dual diagnoses* (SAMHSA, 2016). In cases with compounding problems, specialized attention involving a case management approach is warranted.

Research demonstrates that treatment for substance abuse can be more effective than no treatment, but evaluation of treatment alternatives requires establishing appropriate criteria to measure effectiveness (Sobell et al., 2013).). Examples of criteria that have been used are shown in Box 27.4. It is clear that treatment programs vary and that certain programs will be more culturally appropriate and therefore more effective than others for particular aggregates of individuals.

Pharmacotherapies

In the search for successful treatment of those susceptible to drug and alcohol problems, several pharmacotherapeutic adjuncts to formalized treatment have been developed. Medications include drugs used to assist in the initiation and maintenance of abstinence, drugs used as substitutes for illegal drug use, and drugs used to treat comorbidities. This section discusses pharmacotherapies that providers currently use. Good clinical judgment and patient motivation should guide the use of any pharmacotherapy, and therapy should be combined with psychosocial support.

Pharmacotherapeutics are used in detoxification, stabilization, and maintenance; as antagonists; and as treatment for coexisting disorders. Clinically, it is considered better to prevent withdrawal symptoms with medication than to wait for symptoms to appear. Methadone is the treatment of choice in withdrawal from heroin and other opiates. As a detoxification agent, methadone is dispensed over an 8-day period in a tapering dose. Dosage depends on the severity of opiate withdrawal symptoms present. A widely used example of the use of medication for long-term stabilization is methadone maintenance. The client is prescribed daily administration of a long-acting opioid (methadone) as a substitute for the illicit use of opiates (typically heroin). A large body of research confirms its effectiveness in treatment retention and in reduction of risks such as HIV (http://www.drugabuse.gov/publications/drugfacts/heroin).

However, there are continuing varying philosophical opinions about abstinence versus sanctioned use in the debate over the use of methadone. Methadone maintenance is more controversial because the individual remains dependent on the drug. It is dispensed under medical supervision as part of a treatment program. Maintenance may minimize or abate illegal activity, eliminate the infection hazards of injection drug use, reduce the social disruption typically seen with opiate use, and facilitate increased levels of functioning. A myth about maintenance programs is that methadone produces a euphoric "high" and is therefore merely a legal substitute for heroin.

Naltrexone is a long-acting narcotic antagonist traditionally used as an adjunct in the treatment of opiate dependence. It blocks the effects of opiates via competitive binding, but it does not block the effects of other substances, such as benzodiazepines, cocaine, and alcohol (SAMHSA, 2016a). Studies indicate that naltrexone is also effective in reducing craving, rates of relapse to alcohol, and severity of alcohol-related problems.

Buprenorphine is an opioid agonist-antagonist that has been used in the treatment of opiate-dependent clients and those with concurrent cocaine dependence (NIDA, 2017b). Buprenorphine does not produce severe withdrawal on abrupt cessation of its use, giving it an advantage over methadone. Its antagonist component helps reduce the possibility of lethal overdose. Clinical studies support the use of buprenorphine in reducing the frequency of heroin and cocaine self-administration.

Use of disulfiram (Antabuse) to promote cessation of alcohol abuse (NIH, 2016) is rare today because of serious safety issues. A select group (i.e., those who are relapse prone, those who have supportive networks, and those who have histories of abstinence) may benefit from its short-term use. Requests for disulfiram should not be granted in the absence of treatment and supportive relationships. Disulfiram, when combined with alcohol, produces the classic disulfiram ethanol reaction (DER) (i.e., flushing, tachycardia, nausea, headache, chest tightness, and chest pain). The DER is thought to be the result of a disturbance in alcohol metabolism. The response, which typically begins within minutes after alcohol consumption, is dose dependent and highly variable. Significant risks of the DER are cardiovascular symptoms of tachycardia, hypotension, dysrhythmia, and shock. Preexisting cardiac disease is an absolute contraindication to disulfiram. Emergency treatment of the DER is symptomatic.

Benzodiazepines are considered effective tools for alcohol withdrawal because they decrease the likelihood of seizures and delirium (Sachdeva et al., 2015). Acamprosate (calcium acetyl homotaurine; Campral) has been used successfully in Europe over the past decade and was approved for use in the United States in 2004 (USDHHS, 2015). The main efficacy is in reducing frequency of drinking and maintenance of abstinence. Acamprosate reduces glutamatergic transmission and neuronal

---

BOX 27.5   Basic Tenets of 12-Step Programs

- Admission of defeat and surrender to a higher power
- Inventory of past shortcomings and strengths
- Spiritual practices (e.g., prayer and meditation)
- Willingness to change
- Making amends
- Extension of this process into daily life

---

hyperexcitability during withdrawal from alcohol. This drug has a low incidence of side effects, but should be used under the care of a physician and prescribed cautiously in patients with liver or kidney problems.

Mutual Help Groups

Mutual help groups are associations that are voluntarily formed, are not professionally dominated, and operate through face-to-face supportive interaction focusing on a mutual goal. Many mutual help groups exist, and they are usually organized by recovering substance abusers or those recovering from compulsive behavior patterns. The first mutual help group was Alcoholics Anonymous (AA) (AA, 2017), founded in 1935. Initially, a small group of male alcoholics found a way to stay sober "one day at a time" through meeting regularly with others like themselves. The early AA members developed 12 steps to guide the recovery process, which are summarized in Box 27.5.

As a nonprofessional ongoing source of assistance, AA is viewed as an invaluable resource to the community. However, not all of those with alcohol problems find AA comfortable, culturally relevant, and socially supportive. Because of the realities of social discrimination and regional variation in customs, AA should not be considered a universal form of assistance for alcohol problems. Predominantly in large cities, women and members of racial, ethnic, religious, or sexual preference minority groups with alcohol problems have formed their own AA groups and other mutual help organizations for support in recovery.

Other 12-step programs have developed through the adaptation of AA's approach to similar addictive problems. Narcotics Anonymous, Gamblers Anonymous, Debtors Anonymous, Cocaine Anonymous, Overeaters Anonymous, and Sex and Love Addicts Anonymous are examples. Because they became organized more recently than AA, these groups may not be as well known or as widely available, and they may not exhibit as much diversity among their membership as AA. Children, partners, and close associates of substance abusers have also founded self-help groups, such as Al-Anon, Codependents Anonymous, and Adult Children of Alcoholics. Although these groups initially had a predominance of female members, the trend is moving toward participation by equal numbers of men and women.

AA meetings are not standardized. Customs shaping the actual format and sequence of the meeting vary according to region, group size, ethnic and sex composition, and other cultural variations of the members. In general, 12-step meetings follow one of the following formats:

- Uninterrupted talks by one or more speakers about "what it was like, what happened, and what it is like now."

TABLE 27.3 Modes of Intervention for Substance Abuse

Level	Intervention
Individual and family levels	Education
	Treatment: detoxification, inpatient, outpatient, and residential
	Mutual help groups (e.g., Alcoholics Anonymous, Narcotics Anonymous, Cocaine Anonymous, Al-Anon)
Community level	Law enforcement measures to limit access to and distribution of addictive substances (e.g., street drugs)
	Alcohol taxes and zoning schemes for liquor outlets
	Legal drinking age and legal sanctions on driving while intoxicated
	Educational programs at schools and penal institutions
	Television and radio public service communications concerning the risks of substance abuse and the availability of treatment
State and federal levels	Formation of national associations such as the National Council on Alcoholism and Drug Dependence
	Establishment of federal research entities such as the National Institute on Drug Abuse and the National Institute on Alcohol Abuse and Alcoholism to centralize research, education, and treatment efforts
	Specialty courts/problem-solving courts (drug courts, veteran courts)

- Each person at the meeting being given the opportunity to speak briefly during discussion.
- A combination of the first two options.
- Meetings either closed or open to the general public.

At least two mutual help groups have developed in response to their founders' negative experiences in AA or their failure to succeed in AA. Women for Sobriety was organized in 1976 to replace or augment AA for women; it addresses women's needs to overcome depression, guilt, and low self-esteem (Women for Sobriety, 2016). Secular Sobriety Groups were organized to meet the needs of individuals who are unable to accept the concept of, or to depend on, a "higher power" in their recovery from alcohol problems. Other mutual help groups that do not follow the 12 steps are available for a variety of addictive problems. AA does not require dues or fees, but some groups, such as Weight Watchers, require monetary commitment. Other groups, such as Recovery Incorporated, have more professional involvement. Any of these groups could be a resource for selected people with substance abuse problems.

To be effective, interventions for substance abuse must take place at multiple levels and must involve a number of individuals, activities, policies, and substances. Table 27.3 summarizes some of the many interventions available for substance abuse at various levels.

Harm Reduction

New approaches reflecting a changing view of drug and alcohol addiction have been proposed for substance use problems that are not amenable to traditional approaches. Some of these have been grouped under the general term harm reduction. Harm reduction consists of individual and collective approaches to the treatment of substance use that are not primarily aimed at complete abstinence from all substances. Instead, incremental change is sought, which involves elimination of the more harmful effects of substance use through behavior and policy modifications. Harm reduction is a process rather than a static approach or an end in itself. It is used in various ways, depending on the context and the needs of individual clients (Harm Reduction Coalition, 2017).

Harm reduction strategies remain controversial, although some see them as evidence of a paradigm shift with the potential to significantly improve treatment results. They are often the only options that will preserve a therapeutic relationship when people continue to use or drink problematically. An early example of harm reduction is the substitution of methadone for heroin. Although they are still using an opiate, individuals taking methadone can be functional without getting high and without the need to engage in criminal activity for drugs. Harm reduction psychotherapy aims to support the process of self-transformation through empathetic resonance, raising awareness of harm, setting goals, and understanding the multiple meanings of the substance. Harm reduction has been used in response to alcohol, illicit drugs, and tobacco use. In the case of alcohol, harm reduction might involve decreasing the number of drinks, decreasing the number of days in which drinking occurs, or avoiding drinking when driving.

On a community level, harm reduction may include attempts to legislate for decreased access to alcohol or raising the legal age for drinking. More controversial public health projects aimed at harm reduction are legalization of some illicit drugs and needle exchange programs. Needle exchange programs have had some success, and although they may not lead the intravenous drug user to abstinence, they do, in fact, serve to break the link in the deadly chain of exposure to and transmission of AIDS.

Viewed from a community health perspective, harm reduction involves planned social and policy changes. "Harm reduction is a movement for social justice built on a belief in, and respect for, the rights of people who use drugs" (Harm Reduction Coalition, 2017). Although harm reduction strategies are not usually sanctioned by lay support systems (e.g., 12-step groups), they can have an important impact. Community health nurses using harm reduction strategies can help reduce drug- and alcohol-related social problems by advocating for programs that "bridge the gap" for those who cannot immediately reach the goal of abstinence.

? ACTIVE LEARNING

1. Attend a local AA, Narcotics Anonymous, or Cocaine Anonymous meeting, and share impressions with classmates.
2. Visit a local treatment center that provides detoxification, inpatient, or outpatient treatment, and determine the center's treatment philosophy and the types of services it provides to patients and their families.

SOCIAL NETWORK INVOLVEMENT

Family and Friends

The social network of the substance abuser either can be highly influential in helping the individual alter behavior or can aid and abet the substance abuser in self-destruction. There is evidence for both positive and negative effects of social support in either mitigating or supporting the behaviors of substance abusers (Alcoholrehab.com, 2017). Evidence suggests that particularly among adolescents and young adults, substance use and abuse often occur in the context of social interactions. Adolescents may use alcohol and other substances as social lubricants during an often-troubled developmental period. Family treatment is considered essential because of the potential for enabling behavior. In addition, the family has suffered the effects of substance abuse emotionally, socially, economically, physically, and spiritually. The family's wounds must be acknowledged and treated in order for the substance abuser to return to an environment supportive of recovery.

A user's social network may play a role in allowing the substance abuse to continue. Spouses may call to work to report that their partner is "sick" or may remain silent after discovering evidence of abuse. Complex community and family interactions that serve to promote certain behaviors are commonly known as *codependency* and *enabling*. The boundaries between the nonaddicted family members and addict waver, with the result that the excessive substance-abusing behavior is covered up or excused. Social network members may compensate for the fact that the student is absent from school, the car payment is late, or an important appointment is canceled or forgotten. These distress signals are common but often go unrecognized because periods of use are often interspersed with periods of abstinence. This behavior reinforces the individual's, and often the significant other's, perceived sense of control over the substance use. There are mutual help groups for addressing codependency that are founded on the principles of AA and provide opportunities to discuss the issues germane to the alcoholic or addicted family system or network. Families participating in treatment should also be encouraged to participate in these mutual help groups.

Codependency cannot be concretely defined the same way in each culture. Cultural groups vary in the degree to which individuals are expected to anticipate the needs of others and care for them. The danger in applying a rigid definition of codependency in all cases is that it might unfairly and inappropriately label it as a disease in some cultures that value interdependency over individualism.

Through development of a therapeutic relationship and comprehensive assessment, the community nurse should identify the important members of the social network for each client and the ways in which these individuals provide support for the client. The nurse must also recognize that the concept of family refers not only to nuclear families but also to alternative family systems. Whatever the constellation of family, significant others should be included in the treatment and intervention. Substance abuse, addiction, and recovery do not occur in a vacuum, and many relapses are precipitated by interpersonal conflicts.

Effects on the Family

Substance abuse has been called a *family disease* because it affects the entire family system and holds potential adverse psychological and physical consequences for the family members in addition to the abuser. Family theorists view families, whether the traditional nuclear form or an alternative, as social systems that try to stay in balance (Wright and Leahy, 2013). Professionals may see families as either functional or dysfunctional, depending on how well they fulfill the social tasks expected of them by society. Substance-abusing families are frequently observed to be dysfunctional in clinical terms. However, cultural and political factors should also be considered, because families may have developed these patterns for historical reasons rather than as the effects of substance abuse.

A functional family system is open and flexible and allows its members to be themselves. In the nuclear family model, the parents model intimacy for the children, differences are negotiated, boundaries are defined and maintained, and communication is consistent and clear. In functional family systems, whether the traditional nuclear family or other nontraditional forms, there is trust, individuality, and accountability among family members. All family members are able to have their needs met in a reasonable way.

On the other hand, dysfunctional families are closed systems with fixed, rigid roles. In the case of substance abuse, a major purpose of the system is to deny the substance abuse of the affected family member and keep it a "shameful" family secret. Generally, ego boundaries between the family members are weakened or nonexistent, with enmeshment of the members and an intolerance of individual differences. Rules are rigid and communication is unbalanced; the dynamics are either always conflicting or always superficially pleasant. Children may become involved in a "role reversal" in which they act as caretakers of their parents.

When one or more family members are substance abusers, family functions revolve around the substance abuser and accommodate or compensate the abuser's behavior (Low, 2017). The individual needs of other family members are often unmet. Denial is central to a "dysfunctional" family system. The spouse of the substance abuser may gradually take over the latter's role, functions, and control of the family. The children are cast into various roles in their struggle for survival in this environment and to maintain the family.

Children from dysfunctional families often carry these roles and coping mechanisms into adult life, with many becoming substance abusers or partners of substance abusers. Children of alcoholics also have a higher risk for many other behavioral and emotional problems (NIAAA, 2012). Frequently, they have difficulties with intimacy and parenting. Many have lifelong emotional problems, such as depression and anxiety, and physical illnesses often associated with these conditions (e.g., ulcers, colitis, migraine headaches, and eating disorders). However, alcoholism is not determined only by the genes inherited from one's parents; more than one half of all children of alcoholics do not become alcoholic (NIAAA, 2012). Some offspring exhibit thriving and resilient behavior. Using a strength-based approach, the community health nurse can work with resiliency factors (Xie, 2013).

In addition to psychological burdens that substance abuse places on families, there are the financial burdens related to medical costs, loss of income from job difficulties or unemployment, and the financial losses attributable to divorce. Furthermore, spousal violence and child abuse and neglect are strongly associated with substance abuse.

Professional Enablers

Health care professionals can also contribute to the initiation and continuation of substance abuse and dependency in various ways, becoming professional enablers. One obvious way is the physician's role in prescribing psychoactive medications. The medical model advocates the treatment of symptoms with medication. The relief of pain, anxiety, and insomnia is not an exception. The addictive potential of narcotic analgesics and antianxiety agents is often ignored if quick symptom relief is the main goal. Long-term goals for the treatment of medical problems and nonmedication management of pain and anxiety are more thoughtful approaches. However, undermedication or refusal to use "addictive" medicines can lead susceptible clients to self-medicate with illegal drugs or alcohol.

Physicians and nurses are often the first to see the physical effects of substance abuse and are in an excellent position to intervene. By focusing on the health consequences of substance abuse, they can form trusting relationships, provide information, and refer patients to the appropriate treatment. Too often, this opportunity is missed because the health care professional is reluctant to bring up this taboo subject. This reluctance may be based on professionals' inability to examine their own drinking or drug-taking behaviors, or those of significant others, or on concerns about negative responses from clients.

In the past, many psychiatrists and psychotherapists have focused on the reasons the client uses substances rather than on the dependency itself. The assumption was that insight would lead to a change in behavior. This approach has usually not proved to be effective, especially if the psychiatrist is concurrently prescribing other potentially addictive antianxiety medications or hypnotics. Complete abstinence from all mood-altering medication is a model for preventing the cross-addiction common in substance abusers (i.e., substituting one substance for another, such as a benzodiazepine for alcohol). Exceptions to this approach are patients with serious medical conditions requiring pain medication and those who also have a second psychiatric disorder that requires medication (i.e., schizophrenia, depression, bipolar affective disorder). The recovering substance abuser often needs support when he or she must take medication for these psychiatric conditions, because others may criticize the use of any medication and place the patient in a difficult situation.

Caregivers have become more aware of signs of client substance abuse. Some providers are willing to begin therapy with a nonabstinent client under the stipulation that, if therapeutic gains are not made, the client will be referred for treatment or the caregiver will withdraw services. Clients who lack social support may succeed using this strategy, which allows the formation of a trusting relationship before taking the leap to abstinence. Clinical wisdom and research continue to point toward more tailored, individualized approaches to substance abuse.

VULNERABLE AGGREGATES

When viewed from a community perspective, substance abuse problems clearly affect some populations more severely than others. Some groups are more susceptible to experiencing substance abuse problems, may tend to deteriorate more quickly in the process, or may have fewer sources of support for recovery. These groups, termed *vulnerable aggregates,* require special attention in terms of prevention, intervention, and rehabilitation strategies.

Current resources for prevention, treatment, and mutual support may not be flexible enough to meet the needs of various vulnerable aggregates who are at risk of experiencing substance abuse problems and are often excluded or alienated from services by policies, provider attitudes, economic constraints, and social isolation. This section describes the issues of substance abuse with several vulnerable aggregates, including adolescents, the elderly, women, and racial and ethnic minorities.

Hispanic youth may have positive recovery outcome with family intervention programs such as "the Familia Adelanate Program" (National Network to Eliminate Health Disparities, 2017). This program looks at and works with HIV prevention, risk, and family intervention.

Preadolescents and Adolescents

Why do young people use drugs? It is clear that drug and alcohol use among adolescents is a pervasive problem with many devastating consequences. The trend data in some aspects are undoubtedly worse for adolescents than for adults. The teenage years may be a turbulent time for some because of the necessary developmental tasks of discovering their own unique identity, learning how to form intimate relationships, and developing autonomy. Currently, this maturing is accomplished in a confusing era in which the cultural status of adolescents is undefined. Today's teenagers are an increasingly independent subculture with more money available than any time before, yet they have not attained full adult status.

The teenage years may be a time of experimentation, searching, confusion, rebellion, poor self-image, alienation, and insecurity. There is no such thing as the typical adolescent substance abuser, and there are multiple theories of causation for the abuse. Researchers have concluded that adolescent drug use is a symptom and not the cause of maladjustment. Those with significant difficulty are usually using substances as coping mechanisms.

Studies have identified various predictors of adolescent substance abuse. For example, use of legal substances (e.g., tobacco, alcohol) almost always precedes use of illegal drugs. Familial risk factors include childhood maltreatment (abuse and neglect), parental or familial substance abuse, marital status of parents, level of parental education, parent–child relationships, familial socioeconomic status, and child perception that parents approve of their substance use (Whitesell et al., 2013). Social factors include deviant peer relationships, popularity, bullying, and association with gangs. Individual risk factors commonly identified in the literature and discussed are attention-deficit hyperactivity disorder and depression (Whitesell et al., 2013). The younger the age at initiation, the greater the probability of prolonged and accelerated substance use. Other contributing factors are the feeling of powerlessness and selling drugs as a viable economic solution to poverty. Subculture theory describes the status and power that charismatic leaders have to influence members of peer groups. In drug-using peer groups, such leaders have influence over inexperienced drug users and acculturate them into the drug scene. Thus it is crucial that communities work to maintain strong family and social bonds.

The community health nurse can play an important part in advocating for these vulnerable children and educating teachers on the vital importance of maintaining a validating, nonjudgmental attitude toward these students.

It is especially important that families are supported in the community. Substance abuse is less likely in families who give clear messages and have open communication and more likely in families in which parents are alcoholic, condemning, overly demanding, or overly protective. Committed family involvement helps retain the adolescent in treatment. However, it must be remembered that many well-functioning families have children who succumb to substance abuse.

There is positive outcome with wraparound recovery programs (National Wraparound Initiative, 2017). Wraparound programs take a team approach, with children, parents, counselors, and other invested team members involved in the adolescent's successful recovery through abstinence, education, and life skills. Families whose teenagers are substance abusers also may experience significant community rejection and judgmental attitudes.

The preadolescent years are a particularly vulnerable time for initiation into and subsequent problematic substance use. When drug use escalates in adolescents, it can have devastating, long-lasting consequences. There is a strong relationship between adolescent behavior problems, such as aggressiveness, delinquency, and criminal activity, and heavy alcohol use between the ages of 12 and 17 years.

Escalating use of substances enhances the risk of school and social failure, criminal activities, violent behavior, sexual risk taking, sexual violence, depression, suicide, and unintended injuries. Primary prevention for adolescents is typically focused on education aimed toward complete abstinence, which some say is unrealistic. Education plays an important role. A striking feature is the strong inverse relationship between perceived risk and drug use. Historically for all drugs, with no change in drug availability, when students perceive a drug as harmful, fewer students actually use it. However, marijuana use has remained steady among eighth, tenth, and twelfth graders because of the lessening of perceived risks (NIDA, 2016).

Responsible media efforts can bring about change, but only with accompanying parental and community efforts. Early detection of predisposing factors, such as underlying psychiatric illness, is important. Other strategies are providing structured clubs and organizations and facilitating school success, career skills, family communication skills, and conflict resolution. Secondary prevention is targeted at inpatient and outpatient treatment and harm reduction.

However, almost as important as intervention and treatment is recognizing when treatment is unnecessary. Not all drug use requires therapy, nor is it even desirable. Not all young drug users are antisocial or mentally unstable, nor should they be labeled as such. Most will develop a responsible philosophy concerning substance use if given support and opportunity.

Elderly

Elderly men and women are considered vulnerable to substance abuse problems because of diminished physiological tolerance, increased use of medically prescribed drugs, and cultural and social isolation. One estimate is that up to 60% of elderly patients entering acute medical wards are active alcoholics (Alcoholism-guide.org, 2017).

Misuse of prescription drugs may be the most common form of drug abuse among the elderly. As of 2014, prescription drug misuse or abuse was increasing among people in their 50s (NIDA, 2015b). SAMHSA (2012) projects that misuse of prescription medications by older adults will increase 100% from 2001 to 2020. In addition, data from the VA Hospital System suggest that elderly patients may be prescribed inappropriately high doses of benzodiazepines.

Women

Since the 1970s, much attention has been turned to substance abuse problems in women. Evidence is mounting that alcohol use and abuse affect women much differently from how they affect men. Women absorb and metabolize alcohol differently, partly because of body composition differences and the production of less gastric alcohol dehydrogenase in women (Center for Substance Abuse Treatment, 2015). Specific aggregates of women may be more severely affected by substance abuse problems, including those from minority groups, those with low or no income, and those of the working classes. The increased risk stems from economic, social, and cultural factors.

Lesbians are another aggregate of women in whom substance abuse may be associated with marginalization and should be understood within the diversity of lesbians individually and culturally. This issue is especially heightened in periods when homosexuality is demonized through media, churches, and legislation linking homosexuality with pathology and when lesbians and gays are denied the right to marry (e.g., civil unions, partner benefits).

Women who were abused as children are more susceptible to substance abuse problems in adolescence and adulthood than are nonabused women. They also face many more distressing consequences in substance abuse treatment and recovery. Disclosure of abuse in group treatment contexts or 12-step meetings is risky. In some cases, women are told to compartmentalize the abuse issues and speak only of addiction. In other cases, women are told that if they do not disclose in a group, they will fail in their recovery program (Center for Substance Abuse Treatment, 2015). However, many current-day treatment programs designed for women now routinely address interpersonal violence in individual and group settings, leaving disclosure up to the client.

Drug-dependent women report frequent physical and medical problems, many related to their reproductive systems (Center for Substance Abuse Treatment, 2015). Women tend to experience symptoms of alcoholic hepatitis and cirrhosis sooner than men because they metabolize alcohol at a different rate. They also have higher blood alcohol levels relative to body weight and higher mortality rates from heavy drinking (Center for Substance Abuse Treatment, 2015).

Excessive alcohol use, especially binge drinking, during pregnancy continues to have long-term developmental consequences in the newborn (Center for Substance Abuse Treatment, 2015). Cocaine use during pregnancy is associated with increased risk of spontaneous abortion, premature delivery, and abruptio placentae (Cain et al., 2013). Infants who have been addicted to cocaine in utero are often delivered prematurely, have low birth weights, have smaller head circumferences, and are shorter in length than babies born to mothers who do not use cocaine (Behnke and Smith, 2013; Cain et al., 2013. Long-term learning disabilities, behavioral problems, mental retardation, and physical handicaps are other potential consequences associated with children of cocaine-using mothers (Center for Substance Abuse Treatment, 2015).

Getting the pregnant woman into treatment and managing her withdrawal are frequently problematic. The woman's fear of punitive legal actions complicates the process. Additionally, the addiction itself often interferes with obtaining adequate prenatal care. If addiction is linked with risky sexual behavior or sexual assault, there is an increased risk of contracting HIV and hepatitis viruses, which can infect the infant; testing should be recommended.

Ethnocultural Considerations

Community health nurses need to be culturally competent and aware of certain ethnocultural vulnerabilities and differing perspectives when considering treatments for individuals with substance abuse. Data on African Americans, Hispanics, and Native Americans suggest an increased risk for substance abuse in these groups (Chartier and Caetano, 2017; Substance Abuse and Policy Research Program, 2017). However, the usual ethnic/racial categories in research do not take into account the distinctions within each category. Consequently, there are limited data, especially about middle-class minorities. Creating another stereotype might undermine prevention and treatment strategies. However, it is true that, under the strain of poverty, underemployment, decreased job opportunities, macro-level and micro-level aggression, and ongoing racism, some members of these aggregates find the relief in using substances, which numb the "social pain" caused by their environments. Racial and ethnic minorities are overrepresented among the economically disenfranchised. Limited financial resources may limit alternatives to public treatment settings, which are often understaffed, underfunded, and filled to capacity and have long waiting lists. The privatization of treatment has further decreased access to treatment.

Theories of stress, social causation, and oppressed status support the belief that discrimination and racism are factors in the generation of mental illness and alcohol and drug problems in members of racial and ethnic minorities. Socioeconomic, political, and historical realities have encouraged some minorities to enter into the illegal drug trade as a means of economic survival. In working with ethnic and racial minorities, health care professionals must recognize the sociopolitical and socioeconomic factors that form the context of substance use, abuse, and dependency. These same factors will have an impact on seeking help, treatment, and outcome. In one study, black and Hispanic

> ### BOX 27.6 Barriers to Treating Substance Abuse and Addiction Problems in African Americans
>
> - Weekend drinking as a reward
> - Ongoing sociocultural violence
> - Use of substances to escape the emotional pain caused by racism
> - Poverty, underemployment, and unemployment
> - Prevalence of both drugs and liquor stores within the community
> - Cultural and community disintegration, which has altered traditional values and behaviors
> - Allure and economic rewards of selling drugs
> - Inadequate social support system for recovery
> - Internalized racism harming the self-concept, along with anger and frustration
> - Greater likelihood of being arrested than treated (three to six times more than whites)
> - Limited role models
> - Inability to "change people and places" as advocated by 12-step programs

individuals were 3.5 to 8.1 percentage points less likely than whites to complete treatment for alcohol and drugs, and Native Americans were 4.7 percentage points less likely to complete alcohol treatment. Completion disparities for blacks and Hispanics were largely explained by differences in socioeconomic status and, in particular, by greater unemployment and housing instability (Saloner and LêCook 2013). Recovery for minority groups might be contextually and experientially different from that for whites, just as the environment that contributed to the initial abuse was different. Community health nurses will be better positioned to work with diverse individuals if they are aware of treatment disparities and obstacles for minority groups.

During periods of slavery, alcohol was used as a reward, and it was seen as a way to cope. The value themes for this aggregate are a oneness with nature and spirituality, the importance of extended family, a present orientation, and a spiral concept of time. Barriers to treating African Americans with substance abuse or addiction problems are listed in Box 27.6.

Myths about certain ethnicities must be critically examined. Native Americans, for example, fight the stereotype of the drunken, once-noble warrior. However, alcohol as the predominant drug of choice does pose a threat to this population, particularly among youth and young adults. Native American adolescents use drugs and alcohol earlier and with more devastating consequences than other groups (NIH, 2014). From 2009 to 2012, 56.2% of Native American eighth graders and 61.4% of those in tenth grade had used marijuana, compared with 16.4% of eighth graders and 33.4% of tenth graders in the MTF survey. American Indian students' annual heroin and OxyContin use was about two to three times higher than the national averages in those years (NIH, 2014). Evidence for a biological predisposition is conflicting, and many stop drinking when they reach adulthood and their sense of family and social responsibility increases. Interventions for this group must involve long-term outreach that gains respect from the community.

Studies have identified that social support has a positive effect on treatment and outcome. Without this support, the individual

BOX 27.7 Intervention Approaches for Working with People From Diverse Cultures

- Show respect for another culture's values and identity
- Improve your ability to connect with your target community
- Increase the relevance of your actions
- Decrease the possibility of unwanted surprises
- Increase the involvement and participation of members of other cultural groups
- Increase support for your program by those cultural group members, even if they don't participate or get directly involved
- Build future trust and cooperation across cultural lines—which should raise the prospects for more successful interventions in the future.

From Work Group for Community Health and Development, University of Kansas: *The community toolbox*, chapter 19, section 4: adapting community interventions for different cultures and communities, 2016. http://ctb.ku.edu/en/tablecontents/sub_section_main_1163.aspx.

completing treatment may return to the original social environment, undermining any gains made within the treatment setting. Environmental cues and conditioned reinforcement for continued drug and alcohol use may be extremely powerful. The individual may return to an environment of nonsupport, characterized by continued use by important members of the individual's social network. The individual needs a well-coordinated aftercare program that addresses these issues.

The treatment of ethnic and racial minority aggregates poses special challenges related to the individuals seeking treatment. Treatment providers must recognize that these vulnerable aggregates will encounter a host of barriers that will make treatment and long-term recovery extremely difficult. For example, providers should understand the effect of rituals, holidays, music, and customs and how they can hinder progress. Providers who work from the public health perspective of "thinking upstream" will examine larger, macro-level issues that increase the susceptibility of at-risk populations to alcohol and drug problems. Box 27.7 presents helpful information on working with people from diverse cultures.

Other Aggregates

Substance abuse is the most common psychopathological problem in the general population. Within this category is a smaller aggregate of people with one or more psychiatric diagnoses in addition to substance abuse; this situation is referred to as **dual diagnosis**. Roughly 50% of individuals with severe mental disorders are affected by substance abuse; 37% of alcohol abusers and 53% of drug abusers also have at least one serious mental illness. And of all people diagnosed as mentally ill, 29% abuse either alcohol or drugs (NAMI, 2017). This may be less readily identified by health care providers, who may fail to recognize that the two problems may coexist. Treatment of the individual with a dual diagnosis is complicated when the individual must take prescribed psychotropic medications. As previously mentioned, it may be perceived as prescription drug abuse or as the substitution of one addiction for another. Special attention and flexibility are needed to meet the needs of the dual diagnosis aggregate, and such strategies are still in the developmental phase.

In assessing the risks for substance abuse and the extent of its impact on the community, nurses must be aware that are there frequently several bases for the vulnerability in an individual or group. The adolescent, the low-income Hispanic male, the lesbian African American mother receiving public assistance, and the Native American family living on reservation land are all facing multiple sources of vulnerability that contribute to an increased potential for substance abuse.

Special attention must be paid to the impact of sexually transmitted diseases (STDs) (e.g., HIV, herpes, genital warts, and syphilis) and their relationship to substance abuse. Substance abusers are at increased risk of STDs, including HIV, in the following ways:
- Substances may cloud judgment, leading to high-risk sexual practices involving the exchange of body fluids (e.g., sex without the use of appropriate barriers such as condoms).
- Intravenous drug use may involve the sharing of hypodermic needles.
- Chronic substance use (e.g., of alcohol, heroin, amphetamines, nicotine, and cocaine) impairs the immune system and facilitates infection by HIV or by other pathogens that increase the chances of HIV infection.
- Substance abuse may hasten physical and mental deterioration from the condition of seropositivity to an AIDS diagnosis and, eventually, the terminal phase of the disease.
- Chronic substance abusers generally have few supportive relationships available to them in the process of coping with the hardships that accompany severe and chronic illnesses.
- People facing a stigmatizing, terminal, debilitating illness, in themselves or in a significant other, are more prone to experiencing substance abuse problems in an attempt to cope with distress.

ETHICAL INSIGHTS
Ethical Issues Related to Substance Abuse

Ethical issues regarding substance use and abuse relate to behaviors of the user/abuser that present a risk to the self, coworkers, or the public. A nurse who diverts medication from a patient, thereby depriving the patient of pain relief, is acting both unethically and illegally. Other ethical areas of concern include property theft or damage and the general welfare of others. The National Council of State Boards of Nursing (NCSBN) (2011) observed that when nurses have untreated addiction problems, there is always the possibility of compromised safety to patients, due to impaired judgment, slower reaction time, drug diversion from patients, and patient neglect. Nurses who are living in addiction have more options than ever with assessment and treatment that may not necessarily end their professional careers. Currently 37 states offer some form of substance abuse treatment program to direct nurses to treatment, monitor their reentry into work, and continue their licensure according to the NCSBN (Thomas and Siela, 2011).

Finally, substance abuse among health care professionals cannot be ignored. Physicians, nurses, dentists, and pharmacists are vulnerable to substance abuse; alcohol or narcotic use is most common (DrugRehab.com, 2017). Health care professionals are assumed to be "immune" to dependency because they are knowledgeable about medications. However, their increased access to drugs, belief in pharmaceutical solutions, and work-related stress increase their risk for substance abuse. Typically, they gain access to drugs through their work settings by diverting medications for their own use or by abusing drugs obtained by prescription. State regulatory boards discover the abuse by these health care professionals after drug theft or when the effects of the substance abuse impair professional functioning.

Community health nurses should be especially vigilant about this possibility because colleagues are working in isolation and episodes of incompetence may not be easily observed. Most states have rehabilitation programs for health care professionals that consist of treatment and monitoring. They are allowed to retain their professional licenses during treatment. Despite their usually favorable recovery rate, it is difficult to get this population into treatment because they exhibit denial and shame related to their substance abuse. However, the threatened loss of their professional license to practice may be a good motivator to break through denial of the problem and encourage them to seek treatment.

 ACTIVE LEARNING

Visit a treatment program for women, and determine how the particular needs of this population are assessed and addressed.

NURSING PERSPECTIVE ON SUBSTANCE ABUSE

Nurses have encountered substance abuse in clients whose health problems are clearly related to alcohol abuse, such as cirrhosis of the liver, heart disease, neurological syndromes, and nutritional deficits. Unfortunately, alcohol problems were often not addressed in these health encounters in the past because of the stigma of alcoholism and a lack of effective treatments. The nursing literature did not clearly address substance abuse as a nursing problem until the late 1960s and did not address it as a significant problem until the 1970s. Before the 1970s, substance abuse was usually viewed as a moral problem or, if it involved illicit drugs, as a legal problem.

Since the 1970s, nursing has become more involved in the spectrum of compulsive behavior problems, including substance abuse. A specialized organization, the International Nurses Society on Addictions (IntNSA; at http://www.intnsa .org/), has been established with the philosophy that alcohol abuse and other drug abuse; eating disorders; sexual and relational addiction; and compulsive gambling, working, and spending are closely related behavior patterns. There is a tendency in society to deal with substance abusers in stigmatizing, devaluing, coercive, and punitive ways. Negative attitudes are ubiquitous in our culture. As part of the larger culture, nurses may reflect these attitudes and have difficulty providing care to these individuals. The moral view of substance abuse implies that individuals choose to become sick, injured, or addicted.

Strong negative feelings that conflict with nursing's humanistic stance may also stem from personal experiences. Being the emotionally or physically abused spouse or child of a substance abuser can have lasting effects on a nurse's attitude toward substance-abusing clients. The nurse who uses alcohol or drugs to relieve stress or to self-medicate a dysphoric state may overidentify with the client and deny the severity of the client's substance abuse.

Frequently, substance abusers are difficult clients in health care settings. When intoxicated, they may be raucous, uncooperative, and antisocial. When not intoxicated, they may exhibit none of these negative behaviors, or they may be manipulative and demanding, using flattery or intimidation to hide drug-seeking behavior. Nurses may initially be warm and understanding, but once aware of manipulative attempts, they may have difficulty maintaining an accepting, nonjudgmental attitude. Realizing that recovery from substance abuse often comes very slowly can help nurses feel less pressured to get patients into treatment and more able simply to raise consciousness by presenting the facts about addictive illness and leaving the decision making to the client.

Nursing Interventions in the Community

The problem of substance abuse is so widespread that it affects every community and its inhabitants to varying degrees. Hence, the community health nurse is often involved with substance abusers or their significant others. Substance abuse nursing interventions with clients and their caregivers are necessary to ensure the success of other health interventions. Ignoring substance abuse problems frequently leads to lack of progress and clients' inability to perform needed health practices. This situation is especially frustrating for the community health nurse and other professionals who have collaborated on a comprehensive plan to allow an individual with a serious health problem to remain at home and avoid placement in an institution.

There are many ways in which community health nurses can assist individuals, families, and groups experiencing substance abuse problems. Community health nurses may be the first to identify or suspect an alcohol or drug problem in the clients and families with whom they are working. Nurses in all care contexts should routinely assess substance use patterns when performing client histories. The client history is a critical assessment and screening tool that can identify those at risk. Using current knowledge and theories about substance abuse etiology and risk factors should help identify those individuals predisposed to alcohol and drug use.

The community health nurse can be alert to environmental cues in the home that indicate substance abuse, such as empty liquor and pill bottles. An indication of prescription medication abuse is the patient's involvement with several physicians from whom narcotic analgesics and tranquilizers are obtained. This type of assessment can help with case finding and treatment referral, although the individual may have denied the existence of a substance abuse problem initially.

Denial of substance abuse or dependence may range from completely blocked awareness of the problem to partial disavowal of the detrimental effects of the substance use and abuse. One of the primary tasks for intervention and treatment with the substance-dependent individual is to increase the individual's awareness of the problem. Family and significant others can assist with this process by being more honest and direct with the individual about the detrimental effects of the substance abuse. Before this occurs, the significant others must overcome their own denial of the problem and its associated shame and guilt. Referrals to community education programs on substance abuse and dependence and mutual help groups such as Al-Anon and Narcotics Anonymous are helpful interventions for families and significant others.

The community health nurse may also involve the social network in getting the client into treatment. Although individuals who are forced to enter treatment may not be willing to admit the severity of the abuse, they can still benefit from exposure to the treatment program and eventually begin recovery. Experiencing serious health consequences related to dependency may constitute "hitting bottom" for the individual. This experience may also break through denial or collusion on the part of the family.

The trust that develops in a caring nursing relationship can support disclosure of substance abuse problems and decrease denial in the client or family members. A realistic and positive attitude toward the person with substance abuse can provide families with hope. Community health nurses must have knowledge of available community resources. One of the primary roles of the community health nurse in helping substance abusers is to facilitate contact with helping agencies such as local treatment programs or mutual help groups. Collaboration with the client's physician is helpful should medical detoxification be necessary. Community health nurses should assume a validating, nonjudgmental position toward the whole family and should avoid being confrontational so as not to fan the fires of resistance. It is imperative that nurses ascribe a noble intention to their substance-abusing clients and families and avoid negativity and preaching.

Other traditional community health nursing roles and interventions also are appropriate to use with substance abusers. Examples follow:

- Health teaching regarding addictive illness and addictive effects of different substances
- Advocating that evidence-based practice treatment works in special populations through problem-solving courts (drug courts), specialized adolescent treatment, and other community case management programs

- Providing direct care for abuse-related and dependence-related co-occurring medical problems
- Educating clients and families about problems related to substance abuse
- Collaborating with other disciplines to ensure continuity of care
- Coordinating health care services for the client to prevent prescription drug abuse and avoid fragmentation of care
- Providing consultation to nonmedical professionals and lay personnel
- Facilitating care through appropriate referrals and follow-up
- Knowing how to refer to community resources working with substance abuse, mental health, and other issues

Nursing Care Standards Related to the Patients With Substance Abuse Problems

Utilization of the nursing process is critical to quality care of patients with substance abuse problems. Nurses must know how to develop therapeutic alliances with the patient and family to develop trust and rapport. There is no single treatment appropriate for all individuals, and in the development of health teaching for clients, evidence-based models meeting the needs for many specific populations may be chosen. Evidence demonstrates that effective treatment must address the multiple holistic needs of the individual. Ongoing assessment is critical for continual assessment in treatment planning and services. Knowledge, skills, and attitudes of the behavioral health workforce must be adequate. More success is noted when patients remain in treatment for adequate periods and when individual and group counseling and other behavioral therapies are utilized. Medications are an important element of treatment for many patients, especially when combined with counseling and other behavioral therapies. Nurses must have the knowledge of treatment in co-occurring mental health disorders and substance use disorders. Addiction recovery usually is a long-term process and frequently requires multiple episodes of treatment.

❓ ACTIVE LEARNING

1. Learn about problem-solving courts in your community.
2. Contact mental health services or substance abuse treatment services at the county or city level, and obtain a list of local treatment and education resources.

CASE STUDY Application of the Nursing Process
Client With an Alcohol Abuse Problem and Hepatitis C

Kate Gray, 29 years old, was having abdominal pain, nausea, and vomiting. She was admitted to the hospital thorough the emergency department. After 3 days she was discharged and referred to a community clinic and public health department. Kate has been diagnosed with hepatitis C and alcoholism. She weighs 115 pounds. She is taking a multivitamin, cimetidine for symptoms of gastroesophageal reflux disease, gabapentin for chronic pain, and Atarax for pruritus. She had abdominal pain and a low-grade fever on discharge from the hospital. Her appetite is poor, and she often is nauseated. She becomes fatigued easily. She agrees to comply with discharge planning from the hospital. She is unemployed and recently started Medicaid benefits.

Kate's drug use history is as follows: marijuana use starting at age 16, alcohol use starting at age 20, MA use at age 26; she has been injecting the drug for 2 years. She was arrested 4 months ago for drug use and mandated to participate in a community felony drug court. She has been abstinent from marijuana and MA since her arrest. However, 2 weeks ago she violated probation by drinking and received 3 days in jail for probation violation. She has two daughters ages 6 and 8. Her children live with their father in the same city.

Assessment
Individual

The drug court team nurse practitioner sees Kate 2 days after discharge. Kate is still struggling with fatigue and poor appetite. She is afebrile. The nurse

continued

Client With an Alcohol Abuse Problem and Hepatitis C

practitioner will follow her through drug court. When participating in drug court, Kate will attend **Intensive Outpatient Treatment (IOT)** and Narcotic Anonymous (NA) meetings. She has an NA sponsor.

Family
Kate will meet with her daughters weekly for family therapy through drug court. She meets with her husband, daughters, and pastor weekly for family counseling. Kate's husband attends NA meetings. He has been clean and sober for 1 year. He also is on felony probation and has recently graduated from drug court. He works as a mechanic. Their daughters have safe and adequate housing with their father.

Community
Drug court firmly assists with keeping individuals in treatment long enough for it to work while supervising them closely. Participants are held accountable by the drug court judge for meeting their obligations to the court, society, themselves, and their families. Participants are regularly and randomly tested for drug use. Kate is required to appear in court frequently so that the judge may review her progress and reward her for doing well or sanction her when she does not live up to drug court obligations.

Diagnosis
Individual
- Altered gastrointestinal and hepatic status secondary to hepatitis C and alcoholism pain
- Poor nutritional status
- Inadequate coping related to substance abuse history
- Need for patient education regarding hepatitis C, alcoholism, and addiction

Family
- Inadequate knowledge about addictive disease and effects of alcoholism, MA abuse, and polysubstance abuse
- Inadequate knowledge of treatment approaches available for alcohol abuse and the recovery process
- Family dysfunction secondary to poor communication and denial of addiction in client

Community
- Need for understanding of the prevalence of alcohol abuse problems in the community and adverse health effects of alcohol consumption
- Inadequate knowledge in community agencies that assist alcohol abusers (e.g., local AA and counselors) regarding the need to make home visits and provide services

Planning
Planning for Kate and her family's care involves collaboration among her family, her case management team through drug court, probation services, her pastor, and other community treatment resources. Case management health promotion teaching, counseling, support, and advocacy are the main approaches used to directly assist the client and her family. Indirect approaches involve networking with community agencies, collaboration, and communication networks.

Individual
Short-Term Goals
- Kate will follow her posthospitalization IOT attendance, drug court, and case management.
- Kate will be compliant with her medications.

Long-Term Goals
- Kate will continue to be clean and sober.
- Kate's health status will improve and/or stay at optimal health status as indicated by stabilization of weight and optimal pain control.
- Kate will complete drug court.

Family
Short-Term Goals
- Kate's family will continue family therapy.
- Communication will improve between Kate, her husband, and children.

Long-Term Goals
- Family recovery in abstinence and sobriety

Community
Long-Term Goals
- NA meetings and sponsorship
- Successful completion of and release from probation
- Optimal health status

Intervention
Individual
- Nurse practitioner appointments weekly initially to monitor the client's medication issues or problems as related to maintaining abstinence, gastrointestinal and hepatic functioning, medication compliance, and nutritional status
- Health promotion and patient/family education regarding addiction, hepatitis C, and alcoholism
- Patient teaching about the client's medications, their effects and side effects, and the necessity of following recommended dosing schedules

Family
- Continued support for Kate and her family through early recovery
- Health promotion and education to the family on the course and treatment of addiction and other medical problems associated with Kate's medical diagnosis
- Nonjudgmental support and advocacy

Community
- List of local and national referral resources for clients with substance abuse problems made available to the drug court team and physicians, with a particular focus on resources providing services for drug court participants
- Educating community stakeholders about drug courts, NA and other 12-step programs, and community case management
- Collaboration with community organizations that provide outreach for other individuals and families living with addiction

Evaluation
Individual
Kate was very compliant with drug court, IOT, NA meetings, and following medical treatment.

Family
Kate's family joined her in drug court graduation. Kate continues outpatient drug court once weekly, NA meetings, and family therapy.

CASE STUDY Application of the Nursing Process—cont'd

Client With an Alcohol Abuse Problem and Hepatitis C

Community

Drug court case management will follow through with compliance in IOP attendance, NA meeting compliance, family therapy compliance, and other treatment obligations.

Levels of Prevention

Primary

- Health teaching to individuals and groups on the risk factors, early symptoms, and adverse health and social consequences of substance abuse; the addictive disease process; and available treatment services
- Need to gear educational approaches to the more vulnerable aggregates

Secondary

- Screening and earlier treatment approaches aimed at minimizing health and social consequences of substance abuse
- Involvement of physicians, nurses, and other health care professionals in various community health care settings in this process

Tertiary

- More direct approaches, such as case management, IOT, family therapy, and NA meeting with sponsorship. Goals are to halt the physiologically damaging effects of hepatitis C and alcoholism in Kate's abstinence and sobriety.
- Frequent use of medications to treat the symptoms of substance abuse–related disorders or as part of aversion therapy (e.g., disulfiram)
- Services provided by medical practitioners, treatment services, and mutual help organizations generally advocate abstinence from the substance and improving the individual's health status

This case study illustrates the complexity of substance abuse and **co-occurring disorders**. There is hope in treatment through problem-solving courts. Substance abuse affects patients and their families. Now more than ever, substance abuse may be treated through case management involving multidisciplinary team members. In sobriety, the social situation, living situation, or social acquaintances must change to maintain long-term recovery. However, with patience, persistence, and a caring, nonjudgmental attitude, the nurse can often be effective in helping clients with substance abuse problems attain recovery and improve their health status.

■ SUMMARY

This chapter provides an overview of the complex, multifaceted phenomenon of substance abuse and its manifestations in the community. The focus is on social, economic, political, and health-related aspects of substance abuse. In addition, the concept of substance abuse is related to the more general concept of addictive behaviors, not just those related to drug or alcohol abuse.

From the review of the various etiological theories, it is clear that there is no one causative factor in the development of substance abuse. Consequently, one treatment approach does not apply to all substance abusers. Multiple factors as well as issues specific to vulnerable aggregates, such as women, adolescents, the elderly, and people of color, must be considered in the development of intervention plans and strategies and in the evaluation of outcomes. Resources for prevention and intervention at the individual, family, and community levels are outlined here and should be familiar to nurses practicing in the community.

ⓔ EVOLVE WEBSITE

http://evolve.elsevier.com/Nies/community

- NCLEX Review Questions
- Case Studies

BIBLIOGRAPHY

Alcoholics Anonymous: *Historical data: The birth of A.A. and its growth in the U.S./Canada*, 2017. Available at: http://www.aa.org/pages/en_US/historical-data-the-birth-of-aa-and-its-growth-in-the-uscanada. Accessed April 01, 2017.

Alcoholism-guide.org: *Alcoholism and the elderly*, 2017. Available at: http://www.the-alcoholism-guide.org/alcoholism-and-the-elderly.html. Accessed April 01, 2017.

Alcoholrehab.com: *Positive social support*, 2017. Available at: http://alcoholrehab.com/alcohol-rehab/positive-social-support/. Accessed April 01, 2017.

American Psychiatric Association: *Diagnostic and statistical manual of mental disorders, DSM-5*. 5th ed, Arlington, Va, 2013, APA Publishing.

American Psychiatric Association: *Substance-related and addictive disorders*, 2017. Available at: http://dsm.psychiatryonline.org/doi/abs/10.1176/appi.books.9780890425596.dsm16. Accessed March 29, 2017.

Association of Intervention Specialists: *What is ARISE?*, 2014. Available at: http://www.associationofinterventionspecialists.org/arise-gains-more-ground/. Accessed April 01, 2017.

Behnke M, Smith V: Prenatal substance abuse: short- and long-term effects on the exposed fetus, *Pediatrics* 131(3):e1009–e1024, 2013, https://doi.org/10.1542/peds.2012-3931.

Blume A: Advances in substance abuse prevention and treatment interventions among racial, ethnic, and sexual minority populations, *Alcoh Res: Curr Rev* 38(1), 2016. Available at: https://www.arcr.niaaa.nih.gov/arcr381/article05.htm. Accessed April 01, 2017.

Bose J, Hedden S, Lipari R, et al.: *Key substance use and mental health indicators in the United States: results from the 2015 National Survey on Drug Use and Health*, 2017. Available at: https://www.samhsa.gov/data/sites/default/files/NSDUH-FFR1-2015/NSDUH-FFR1-2015/NSDUH-FFR1-2015.htm#fig1. Accessed March 29, 2017.

Cain M, Bornick P, Whiteman V: The maternal, fetal, and neonatal effects of cocaine exposure in pregnancy, *Clin Obstet Gynecol* 56(1):124–132, 2013. https://doi.org/10.1097/GRF.0b013e31827ae167.

Center for Behavioral Health Statistics and Quality: *Behavioral health trends in the United States: Results from the 2014 National Survey on Drug Use and Health* (HHS Publication No. SMA 15-4927, NSDUH Series H-50). Rockville, MD, 2015, Substance Abuse and Mental Health Services Administration.

Center for Behavioral Health Statistics and Quality: *2015 National Survey on Drug Use and Health: Detailed Tables*, Rockville, MD, 2016, Substance Abuse and Mental Health Services Administration.

Centers for Disease Control: *Fact Sheets—Alcohol Use and Your Health*, 2016. Available at: http://www.cdc.gov/alcohol/fact-sheets/alcohol-use.htm. Accessed March 26, 2017.

Center for Motivation and Change: *What is CRAFT*, 2014. Available at: http://motivationandchange.com/outpatient-treatment/for-families/craft-overview/. Accessed April 01, 2017.

Center for Substance Abuse Treatment: *Substance Abuse Treatment: Addressing the Specific Needs of Women. Treatment Improvement Protocol (TIP) Series 51. HHS Publication No. (SMA) 09-4426*, Rockville, MD, 2015, Substance Abuse and Mental Health Services Administration.

Chartier K, Caetano R: *Ethnicity and health disparities in alcohol research*, 2017. Available at: https://pubs.niaaa.nih.gov/publications/arh40/152-160.htm. Accessed April 01, 2017.

DrugRehab.com: *Doctors and addiction*, 2017. Available at: https://www.drugrehab.com/addiction/doctors/. Accessed April 2, 1027.

Drugs.com: *PCP (Phencyclidine)*, 2017. Available at: https://www.drugs.com/illicit/pcp.html. Accessed March 28, 2017.

Drugwarfacts.org: *Prisons, Jails, and People Arrested for Drugs*, 2016. Available at: http://www.drugwarfacts.org/cms/Prisons_and_Drugs#sthash.OajBAhra.dpbs. Accessed March 31, 2017.

Ewing J: Detecting alcoholism. The CAGE questionnaire, *JAMA* 252(14):1905–1907, 1984, https://doi.org/10.1001/jama.1984.03350140051025. 6471323.

Governing: *Governing data: State marijuana laws in 2017 map*, 2017. Available at: http://www.governing.com/gov-data/state-marijuana-laws-map-medical-recreational.html. Accessed April 01, 2017.

Harm Reduction Coalition: *Principles of harm reduction*, 2017. Available at: http://harmreduction.org/about-us/principles-of-harm-reduction/. Accessed April 01, 2017.

Hasin D, O'Brien C, Auriacombe M, et al.: DSM-5 criteria for substance use disorders: recommendations and rationale, *Am J Psychiat* 170(8):834–851, 2014.

Health.mil: *That guy campaign*, 2017. Available at: https://health.mil/Military-Health-Topics/Conditions-and-Treatments/Substance-Abuse/Getting-Help/That-Guy-Campaign. Accessed April 01, 2017.

HealthyPeople.gov: *Substance abuse*, 2017. Available at: https://www.healthypeople.gov/2020/topics-objectives/topic/substance-abuse. Accessed March 28, 2017.

Intervention Support: *Johnson Model Intervention*, 2017. Available at: http://www.interventionsupport.com/intervention-techniques/johnson-model/. Accessed April 01, 2017.

Jesse S, Bråthen G, Ferrara M, et al.: Alcohol withdrawal syndrome: mechanisms, manifestations, and management, *Acta Neurol Scand* 135:4–16, 2017. https://doi.org/10.1111/ane.12671.

Kenney S, Jones RN, Barnett NP: In *J Youth Adolesc*, 44. 2015, pp 1884–1897. https://doi.org/10.1007/s10964-015-0311-3.

Ling W: A perspective on opiod pharmacotherapy: where we are and how we got there, *J Neuroimmune Pharmacol* 11(3):394–400, 2016.

Low M: *Substance abuse and the impact on the family system*, 2017. Available at: http://www.rehabs.com/pro-talk-articles/substance-abuse-and-the-impact-on-the-family-system/. Accessed April 01, 2017.

Miech RA, Johnston LD, O'Malley PM, et al.: *Monitoring the Future national survey results on drug use, 1975–2015: Volume I, Secondary school students*, Ann Arbor, 2016, Institute for Social Research, The University of Michigan. Available at: http://www.monitoringthefuture.org//pubs/monographs/mtf-vol1_20152.pdf.

Miozzo R, Bienvenu O, Eaton W, et al.: *Prevalence and Comorbidity of Alcohol Dependence, Depression, and Anxiety Disorders in their Association with the Serotonin Transporter Gene*, Worcester, Mass, 2014, Poster presentation, UMass Center for Clinical and Translational Science Research Retreat, held on May 20, 2014 at the University of Massachusetts Medical School.

National Alliance on Mental Illness (NAMI): *Dual diagnosis*, 2017. Available at: http://www.nami.org/Learn-More/Mental-Health-Conditions/Related-Conditions/Dual-Diagnosis. Accessed April 02, 2017.

National Council of State Boards of Nursing: *Substance Abuse Disorder in Nursing*, 2011. Available at: https://www.ncsbn.org/substance-use-in-nursing.htm. Accessed April 02, 2017.

National Council on Alcoholism and Drug Dependence: *Alcohol, drugs and crime*, 2017. Available at: https://www.ncadd.org/about-addiction/alcohol-drugs-and-crime. Accessed March 26, 2017.

National Highway Traffic Safety Administration: *Drug and human performance fact sheets: methamphetamine (And Amphetamine)*, 2017. Available at: https://one.nhtsa.gov/people/injury/research/job185drugs/methamphetamine.htm. Accessed March 28, 2017.

National Institutes of Health: *Antabuse-disulfiram tablet*, 2016. Available at: https://dailymed.nlm.nih.gov/dailymed/drugInfo.cfm?setid=f0ca0e1f-9641-48d5-9367-e5d1069e8680. Accessed April 01, 2017.

National Institute on Alcohol Abuse and Alcoholism: *A family history of alcoholism: Are you at risk?* 2012. Available at: https://pubs.niaaa.nih.gov/publications/familyhistory/famhist.htm. Accessed April 01, 2017.

National Institute on Alcohol Abuse and Alcoholism: *Underage drinking*, 2013. Available at: https://report.nih.gov/NIHfactsheets/ViewFactSheet.aspx?csid=21. Accessed March 26, 2017.

National Institute on Alcohol Abuse and Alcoholism: *Alcohol screening and brief intervention for youth: A practitioner's guide. (NIH Publication No. 11–7805)*, Rockville, MD, 2015, National Institutes of Health.

National Institute on Alcohol Abuse and Alcoholism: *Alcohol Facts and Statistics*, 2017. Available at: https://www.niaaa.nih.gov/alcohol-health/overview-alcohol-consumption/alcohol-facts-and-statistics. Accessed March 29, 2017.

National Institute on Drug Abuse: *Hallucinogens and Dissociative Drugs: Common Hallucinogens and Dissociative Drugs*, 2015. Available at: https://www.drugabuse.gov/publications/research-reports/hallucinogens-dissociative-drugs/what-are-dissociative-drugs. Accessed March 28, 2017.

National Institute on Drug Abuse: *Commonly abused drug charts*, 2016a. Available at: https://www.drugabuse.gov/drugs-abuse/commonly-abused-drugs-charts#LSD. Accessed March 28, 2017.

National Institute on Drug Abuse: *What are anabolic steroids?* 2016b. Available at: https://www.drugabuse.gov/publications/drugfacts/anabolic-steroids. Accessed March 29, 2017.

National Institute on Drug Abuse: *What are hallucinogens?* 2016c. Available at: https://www.drugabuse.gov/publications/drugfacts/hallucinogens. Accessed March 28, 2017.

National Institute on Drug Abuse: *Screening, assessment, and drug testing resources*, 2014. Available at: https://www.drugabuse.gov/nidamed-medical-health-professionals/tool-resources-your-practice/additional-screening-resources. Accessed March 31, 2017.

National Institute on Drug Abuse: *Strategic plan national institute on drug abuse*, NIH Publication Number, 2010c, pp 10–6119.

National Institute on Drug Abuse: *Principles of drug addiction treatment: a research-based guide*, ed 3, NIH Publication No, 2012b, pp 12–4180.

National Institute on Drug Abuse: *Nationwide trends*, 2015a. Available at: https://www.drugabuse.gov/publications/drugfacts/nationwide-trends. Accessed March 29, 2017.

National Institute on Drug Abuse: *Trends and statistics*, 2015b. Available at: https://www.drugabuse.gov/related-topics/trends-statistics. Accessed March, 25 2017.

National Institute on Drug Abuse; National Institutes of Health: *U.S. Department of Health and Human Services: Monitoring the Future 2016 Survey Results*, 2016a. Available at https://www.drugabuse.gov/related-topics/trends-statistics/infographics/monitoring-future-2016-survey-results. Accessed March, 28 2017.

National Institute on Drug Abuse: *What are anabolic steroids?* 2016b. Available at: https://www.drugabuse.gov/publications/drugfacts/anabolic-steroids. Accessed March 29, 2017.

National Institute on Drug Abuse: *2016-2020 NIDA Strategic Plan*, 2017. Available at: https://www.drugabuse.gov/about-nida/strategic-plan/strategically-supporting-conducting-basic-clinical-research. Accessed March 26, 2017.

National Institute on Drug Abuse: *Buprenorphine*, 2017b. Available at: https://archives.drugabuse.gov/drugpages/buprenorphine.html. Accessed April 01, 2017.

National Institutes of Health: *Substance use in American Indian youth is worse than we thought*, 2014. Available at: https://www.drugabuse.gov/about-nida/noras-blog/2014/09/substance-use-in-american-indian-youth-worse-than-we-thought. Accessed April 01, 2017.

National Network to Eliminate Health Disparities: *Familia Adelante: Multi-risk reduction behavioral health prevention for Latino youth and families*, 2017. Available at: http://nned.net/familia-adelante. Accessed April 01, 2017.

National Wraparound Initiative: *What is wraparound?* 2017. Available at: http://nwi.pdx.edu/wraparound-basics/#whatisWraparound. Accessed April 01, 2017.

New Beginnings: *The single parent's guide to addiction recovery*, 2016. Available at: http://www.newbeginningsdrugrehab.org/drug-addiction/the-single-parents-guide-to-addiction-recovery/. Accessed April 01, 2017.

Office of National Drug Control Policy (ONDCP): *Progress toward Some National Drug Control Strategy Goals, but None Have Been Fully Achieved*, 2016. Available at: www.gao.gov/assets/680/677235.pdf. Accessed March 26, 2017. Available from: <http://www.whitehouse.gov/ondcp>.

Partnership for Drug-Free Kids: *Underage drinking: What you should know*, 2016. Available at http://drugfree.org/parent-blog/underage-drinking-know/. Accessed March 27, 2017.

Patrick M, Schulenberg J, Maggs J, et al.: Substance use and peers during adolescence and the transition to adulthood: Selection, socialization, and development, In: Scher K, editor: *Oxford handbook of substance use and substance use disorders*, volume 1, p. 526, 2016.

PBS: A social history of America's most popular drugs, *Frontline*, 2014. Available at: http://www.pbs.org/wgbh/pages/frontline/shows/drugs/buyers/socialhistory.html. Accessed March 26, 2017.

Rehab International: *Crystal Meth Addiction Statistics*, 2017. Available at: http://rehab-international.org/crystal-meth/addiction-statistics. Accessed March 29, 2017.

Sacks J, Gonzales K, Bouchery E, et al.: 2010 National and state costs of excessive alcohol consumption, *Am J Preventive Med* 49(5):e73–e79, 2015.

Sen S, Grgurich P, Tulolo A, Smith-Freedman A, et al.: A symptom-triggered benzodiazepine protocol utilizing SAS and CIWA-Ar scoring for the treatment of alcohol withdrawal syndrome in the critically ill, *Annals of Pharmacother* 51(2):101–110, 2017.

Sobell L, Sobell M, Ward E: *Evaluating alcohol and drug treatment effectiveness*, New York, 2013, Pergamon Press.

Sterling E: *Drug laws and snitching: A primer*, PBS Frontline, 2014. Available at: http://www.pbs.org/wgbh/pages/frontline/shows/snitch/primer/. Accessed March 26, 2017.

Sachdeva A, Choudhary M, Chandra M: *Alcohol withdrawal syndrome: Benzodiazepines and beyond*, 2015. Available at: https://www.ncbi.nlm.nih.gov/pmc/articles/PMC4606320/. Accessed April 01, 2017.

Substance Abuse and Mental Health Services Administration: *Specific populations and prescription drug misuse and abuse*, 2012. Available at: https://www.samhsa.gov/prescription-drug-misuse-abuse/specific-populations. Accessed April 01, 2017.

Substance Abuse and Mental Health Services Administration: *National Survey on Drug Use and Health; United States*, 2013a. Available at: https://www.samhsa.gov/data/sites/default/files/NSDUHsaeSpecificStates2013/NSDUHsaeSpecificStates2013.htm. Accessed March 28, 2017.

Substance Abuse and Mental Health Services Administration: *Need for and receipt of substance abuse treatment among Blacks*, 2013b. Available at: https://www.samhsa.gov/data/sites/default/files/NSDUH124/NSDUH124/sr124-african-american-treatment.htm. Accessed March 28, 2017.

Substance Abuse and Mental Health Services Administration: *Results from the 2015 National Survey on Drug Use and Health: Detailed Tables*, 2015. Available at: https://www.samhsa.gov/data/sites/default/files/NSDUH.../NSDUH-DetTabs-2015.pdf. Accessed March 29, 2017.

Substance Abuse and Mental Health Services Administration: *Key substance use and mental health indicators in the United States: results from the 2015 National Survey on Drug Use and Health*, 2016a. Available at: https://www.samhsa.gov/data/sites/default/files/...2015/...2015/NSDUH-FFR1-2015.pdf. Accessed March 27, 2017.

Substance Abuse and Mental Health Services Administration: *Naltrexone*, 2016b. Available at: https://www.samhsa.gov/medication-assisted-treatment/treatment/naltrexone. Accessed April 01, 2017.

Substance Abuse and Mental Health Services Administration: *SAMHSA's strategic initiatives*, 2016c. Available at: https://www.samhsa.gov/about-us/strategic-initiatives. Accessed March 26, 2017.

Substance Abuse and Mental Health Services Administration: *The Center for Behavioral Health Statistics and Quality Report*, 2016d. Available at: https://www.samhsa.gov/data/sites/default/files/report_2716/ShortReport-2716.html. Accessed March 27, 2017.

SAHMSA: *SAHMSA's Efforts to Support Veterans and Military Families*, 2017. Available at: https://www.samhsa.gov/veterans-military-families/samhsas-efforts. Accessed March 26, 2017.

SAHMSA: *National Survey on Drug Use and Health*, 2017. Available at: https://nsduhweb.rti.org/respweb/homepage.cfm##. Accessed March 26, 2017.

Saloner B, LêCook B: Blacks and Hispanics less likely than Whites to complete addiction treatment, largely due to socioeconomic factors, *Health Aff* 32(1):135–145, 2013.

Substance Abuse and Policy Research Program: Key results: Racial and ethnic disparities in substance abuse treatment, 2017. Available at: http://saprp.org/knowledgeassets/knowledge_results.cfm?KAID=11. Accessed April 01, 2017.

Thomas C, Siela D: The impaired nurse: Would you know what to do if you suspected substance abuse?, *Am Nurse Today* 6(8), 2011. Available at: http://www.medscape.com/viewarticle/748598_8. Accessed April 02, 2017.

Tollison SJ, Henderson RC, Baer JS, et al.: Next steps in addressing the prevention, screening, and treatment of substance use disorder in active duty and veteran operation enduring freedom and Operation Iraqi Freedom populations, *Mil Med* 177(8):39–46, 2012.

University of Florida Department of Psychology: *Chapter 1 UF/Psychology*, 2017. Available at: www.psych.ufl.edu/~steh/PSY4930/Treatment%20of%20abuse.ppt. Accessed March 26, 2017.

U.S. Department of Health and Human Services, 2013 U.S. Department of Health and Human Services: *Substance abuse and mental health services administration center for behavioral health statistics and quality. Results from the 2013.*

National Survey on Drug Use and Health: *Summary of National Findings.* Available at: https://www.google.com/url?sa=t&rct=j&q=&esrc=s&source=web&cd=1&ved=0ahUKEwi8q4TB1obTAhVDQiYKHYq7CFYQFggcMAA&url=https%3A%2F%2Fwww.samhsa.gov%2Fdata%2Fsites%2Fdefault%2Ffiles%2FNSDUHresultsPDFWHTML2013%2FWeb%2FNSDUHresults2013.pdf&usg=AFQjCNEoXS5CSBa-XwhdFZQT7QzQT1xg4A

U.S. Department of Health and Human Services: *Results from the 2013 National Survey on Drug Use and Health: Summary of National Findings*, 2014. Available at: https://www.samhsa.gov/data/sites/default/files/NSDUHresultsPDFWHTML2013/Web/NSDUHresults2013.htm#2.10. Accessed March 27, 2017.

U.S. Department of Health and Human Services Substance Abuse and Mental Health Services Administration: *Results from the 2013 National Survey on Drug Use and Health: Summary of National Findings*, 2017. Available at: https://www.samhsa.gov/data/sites/default/files/NSDUHresultsPDFWHTML2013/Web/NSDUHresults2013.htm#2.10. Accessed March 27, 2017.

U.S. Department of Health and Human Services: *TIP 49 Incorporating Alcohol Pharmacotherapies into Medical Practices*, 2015. Available at: store.samhsa.gov/shin/content/SMA13–4380/SMA13-4380.pdf - 820k - 2015-09-25 -. Accessed April 01, 2017.

U.S. Department of Justice: *Drugs and Crime Facts*, 2017. Available at: https://www.bjs.gov/content/dcf/duc.cfm. Accessed March 26, 2017.

Vrieze S, McGue M, Miller M, et al.: Three mutually informative ways to understand the genetic relationships among behavioral disinhibition, alcohol use, drug use, nicotine use/dependence, and their co-occurrence: twin biometry, GCTA, and genome-wide scoring, *Behavior Genetics* 43(2):97–107, 2013.

Wardell J, Quilty L, Hendershot C: Impulsivity, working memory, and impaired control over alcohol: A latent variable analysis, *Psychol Addictive Behav* 30(5):544–554, 2016.

Whitesell M, Bachand A, Peel J, et al.: Familial, social, and individual factors contributing to risk for adolescent substance use, *J Addict* 9, 2013, https://doi.org/10.1155/2013/579310.

Wilkinson S, Yarnell S, Radhakrishnan R, et al.: Marijuana legalization: Impact on physicians and public health, *Ann Rev Med* 67:453–466, 2016.

Women for Sobriety: *Women for Sobriety*, 2016. Available at: http://www.womenforsobriety.org/beta2/. Accessed April 01, 2017.

Wright L, Leahy M: *Nurses and families : a guide to family assessment and intervention*, Philadelphia, 2013, F.A. Davis.

Xie H: Strengths-based approach for mental health recovery, *Iran J Psychiatry Behav Sci* 7(2):5–10, 2013.

Violence

Ginette G. Ferszt*

OBJECTIVES

Upon completion of this chapter, the reader will be able to do the following:
1. Describe the concepts of interpersonal and community violence.
2. Identify factors that influence violence.
3. Identify populations at risk for violence and the role of public health in dealing with the epidemic of violence.
4. Describe the role of the nurse in primary, secondary, and tertiary prevention of violence.

KEY TERMS

abusive head trauma
bullying
child maltreatment
date rape drugs
dating violence
elder abuse
emotional abuse

hate crimes
human trafficking
intentional injuries
interpersonal violence
intimate partner violence
neglect
physical abuse

prison violence
sexual abuse
stalking
terrorism
violence
workplace violence
youth-related violence

Violence is a serious national public health problem that affects all ages from the very young to the very old. Violent deaths, however, only tell part of the problem. Although many victims of violence survive, they, their families, and their friends often have permanent emotional and physical scars. Violence occurs around the world on a daily basis, as evidenced by the nightly newscast and stories on the Internet. For example:

April 1999: In Columbine High School, Littleton, Colorado, 13 killed by two teenagers who then committed suicide.
September 11, 2001: 2974 people from 90 different countries killed when 19 terrorists hijacked four planes and intentionally crashed two of them into the World Trade Center's twin towers, the third into the Pentagon, and the fourth in an empty field in Pennsylvania.
April 2007: 32 killed, 15 wounded at Virginia Tech University in Blacksburg, Virginia, by a student who then committed suicide—the deadliest school shooting in U.S. history.

* The author would like to acknowledge the contributions of Cathi A. Pourciau and Elaine C. Vallette, who revised this chapter for the previous edition.

November 2009: 13 killed, 42 injured at a military base in Fort Hood, Texas, by a U.S. Army psychiatrist.

January 2011: 6 killed, including a 9-year-old girl, and 12 injured, including Congresswoman Gabrielle Giffords, at a political meeting in Tucson, Arizona.

July 2012: 12 killed, 58 injured during a midnight showing of the movie *Batman: The Dark Knight* in Aurora, Colorado.

December 2012: 20 students and 7 adults killed, 2 wounded, at Sandy Hook Elementary School in Newtown, Connecticut—the second deadliest school shooting in U.S. history.

April 2013: 3 killed and an estimated 264 injured when two men set two pressure-cooker bombs at the finish line of the Boston Marathon.

September 2013: 12 killed and 3 injured in a Navy Yard complex in Washington, DC, by a man who was then shot by police.

December 2015: 14 killed and 22 injured at a regional center in San Bernadino, California. The perpetrators—husband and wife—were later killed by police.

June 2016: 49 killed and 58 injured in a night club in Orlando, Florida, by a man who was killed by the police.

October 2017: 58 killed and 851 injured when a 64-year-old man fired on a crowd of concert-goers in Las Vegas.

February 2018: 17 people killed and 17 more wounded at Marjory Stoneman Douglas High School in Parkland, Florida.

Although the preceding list shows well-publicized acts of extreme violence, violence occurs every day in communities across the country. The woman who is beaten and killed by her husband, the cousins who are kidnapped and murdered by a neighbor, the infant who is shaken to death by his mother, the young woman who is gang raped, the children who are sexually abused, and the coworkers who are killed by a disgruntled former employee are all examples of the violence that occurs with alarming frequency.

The purpose of this chapter is to explore the influence of violence from a public health perspective as it relates to individuals and communities. It includes discussions of the effects of violence in terms of homicides and suicides, the direct influence of violence on individuals and communities, public health interventions to reduce violence, the roles and responsibilities of the community health nurse in dealing with those experiencing violence, and measures to increase awareness of violence in the workplace. An in-depth look at the causes, effects, interventions, and measures to increase awareness of violence is presented.

OVERVIEW OF VIOLENCE

The World Health Organization (WHO) defines **violence** as "the intentional use of physical force or power, threatened or actual against oneself, another person, or against a group or community, which either results in or has a high likelihood of resulting in injury, death, psychological harm, maldevelopment, or deprivation" (WHO, 2017). In the field of public health, injuries from violence are referred to as **intentional injuries**. Violence threatens the health and well-being of people of all ages across the globe. Worldwide, 1.6 million people lose their lives annually as a result of violence. In 2014, close to 15,809 people were the victims of homicide in the United States alone (CDC, 2016).

The reasons for the high rate of violence in societies are complex. Universally recognized factors that contribute to violence include the following:

1. Poverty, unemployment, economic dependency
2. Substance abuse
3. Mental illness
4. Media influence
5. Access to firearms
6. Political and/or religious ideology
7. Intolerance and ignorance

HISTORY OF VIOLENCE

Violence is a global problem. From prehistoric times humans have dealt violently with other humans. In the Bible, Cain killed his brother Abel out of jealousy and anger. Throughout history, sporting events often resulted in death for the audience's pleasure, such as the gladiator events in Rome. Infanticide, or the killing of unwanted newborn children, has been practiced throughout history. For example, a female, a twin, sickly, or deformed child was often left to die of exposure. Children, especially firstborn children, were often sacrificed for religious reasons. Infanticide was not condemned until early in the fifth century; however, this did not protect children in many societies.

Throughout the ages, corporal punishment has been used as a means of controlling children. Biblical reference to corporal punishment has often been used as justification for some types of child abuse. To some parents, "spare the rod and spoil the child" (Proverbs 13:24) implies an imperative to abusively discipline an errant child. The idea of "beating some sense into him" was considered necessary to ensure that a lesson was learned. In 1874, the first legal protection against child abuse in the United States was created when the Society for the Prevention of Cruelty to Animals intervened to protect an 8-year-old girl. As a result of the notoriety associated with this case, the New York Society for the Prevention of Cruelty to Children was organized in 1875 (The New York Society for the Prevention of Cruelty to Children, 2016).

Even nursery rhymes that adults read to small children seem to condone violence against them. Consider the following Mother Goose nursery rhyme:

> *There was an old woman who lived in a shoe,*
> *She had so many children she didn't know what to do,*
> *She gave them some broth without any bread,*
> *And whipped them all soundly and sent them to bed.*
> **(Mother Goose Nursery Rhymes, 2000, pp. 195–196)**

Wife beating was legal in the United States until 1824. Wives were seen as their husbands' chattel and could be beaten for such offenses as "nagging too much." In fact, the common phrase "rule of thumb" was derived from English law that allowed a man to beat his wife with a cane no wider than his thumb. Biblical interpretation of "wives be subject to your husband" (Ephesians 5:22) still provides some men with a faulty rationalization for wife beating. Some cultures and religions still allow, and even support, abuse of wives.

The silence that long surrounded domestic violence is derived from a historical perspective of women as their husbands' property. The problem of assault against women was not explored in America until the Civil Rights Movement of the 1960s. In fact, marital rape was not considered an offense in the United States until 1980. In the last three decades, additional cultural issues have surfaced regarding domestic abuse that includes female circumcision and genital mutilation, abuse between gay partners, and the realization that men are also victims of domestic violence.

Elder abuse is also a continuing problem. The problem is of greater magnitude now because people are living longer, resulting in increased numbers of dependent and vulnerable adults. Elder abuse frequently goes undetected because of a lack of awareness on the part of health care professionals and society. The exact prevalence of elder abuse is unknown because reporting is not mandatory in all states.

INTERPERSONAL VIOLENCE

Homicide and Suicide

In the United States, homicide claimed the lives of 15,695 individuals in 2015; over 10,000 deaths involved the use of firearms. Of note, almost 80% of the murder victims were male and 90% of the offenders were male. When race of the murder victims could be determined, 53% were black, 44% were white, and 2.8% were other races. Approximately 50% of victims were killed by someone they knew (Federal Bureau of Investigation [FBI], 2017a). Statistics related to homicide and age groups are quite astonishing. In 2014, homicide was the third leading cause of death for age groups 1 to 4 and 15 to 34. It was the fourth cause of death for 5- to 9-year-olds and the fifth leading cause of death for 10-to-14 and 35-to-44 age groups. Notably, 37% of female murder victims are killed by an intimate partner (CDC, 2016).

Suicide is also a serious problem in the United States, and its incidence keeps rising at an alarming rate. In 2013, there were more than 41,000 deaths as a result of suicide in the United States. Indeed, more people died from suicide than from motor vehicle accidents. Although females have more suicidal thoughts than males, males commit suicide four times more often than females. The most commonly used method for suicide for males is firearms (56.9%), and poisoning (i.e., intentional ingestion of drugs or medications) is the most common for women (34.8%) (CDC, 2016). In 2014, suicide was the second leading cause of death for age groups 10 to 34, and the fourth for age groups 35 to 54. Suicide rates vary considerably within different population subgroups. Socioeconomic status, employment, occupation, sexual orientation, and gender identity are all factors that are related to suicide. For example, the rates of suicide were highest among whites. In 2013, suicide rates were 11.7 per 100,000 for American Indians/Alaska Natives, 6.0 per 100,000 for Asians/Pacific Islanders, 5.3 per 100,000 for Hispanics, and 5.4 per 100,000 for African Americans (Substance Abuse and Mental Health Services Administration [SAMHSA], 2015).

Nurses have an important role in identifying individuals who are at risk for suicide. Risk factors for suicide include:

1. History of depression or other psychiatric disorders
2. Alcohol and/or substance abuse
3. Physical illness
4. Past history of attempted suicide
5. Past history of violence
6. Age
7. Environmental stressors

Refer to Chapter 25 for further discussion on suicide.

Intimate Partner Violence

Intimate partner violence (IPV) is a serious public health problem that affects the lives of millions of people in the United States (CDC, 2014). IPV is defined as violence that occurs between two people in a close relationship, usually spouses, former spouses, and dating partners. According to the CDC (2014), in the United States almost 12 million women (3 in 10) and men (1 in 10) are victims of rape, physical violence, or stalking by an intimate partner each year.

IPV includes four different types of behavior: physical violence (hitting, kicking, or another type of physical force), sexual violence (forcing a partner to take part in a sex act without their consent), psychological aggression (verbal and unwanted attention and contact by a partner with the intent to harm and control another person), and stalking, which will be discussed later in this chapter. IPV is often repetitive, progressive, and escalates in frequency and severity. Because many people are afraid to report IPV to the police, family, or friends, it is hard to capture the exact incidence of this type of violence. IPV has been reported in all types of relationships: women against women in lesbian relationships, men against men in homosexual relationships, and women against men. Box 28.1 presents commonly held myths about IPV.

IPV crosses all ethnic, racial, socioeconomic, and educational lines. The CDC has identified a number of factors that increase the risk of being a victim of IPV: the perpetrator often has a past history of being violent or aggressive, seeing or being a victim of violence as a child, using drugs and/or consuming large amounts of alcohol, and unemployment or other life events that cause stress. Victims of IPV have reported serious negative health outcomes. Physical injuries can include bruising, welts, internal bleeding, disabilities, head trauma, and even death. Victims can also be traumatized and experience depression, chronic pain, sleep difficulties, and a range of other serious mental health problems. IPV can also lead to long-term consequences, including physical injury, poor mental health, and chronic physical health problems. For some people, IPV results in hospitalization, disability, or even death. Previous research indicates that victimization as a child or adolescence can increase the likelihood that victimization will occur in adulthood (CDC, 2014).

BOX 28.1   Common Myths Associated with Intimate Partner Violence

- It occurs only in poor, uneducated, minority households.
- It is a private family matter (vs. a societal problem).
- It only occurs in heterosexual relationships.
- Victims deserve the abuse.
- Victims can change the abusers' behavior.
- Abusers will stop the abuse on their own without professional intervention.

In order to cope with their suffering, victims may use various substances, drink alcohol, and/or have risky sex.

Societal awareness of IPV during pregnancy is a relatively recent phenomenon; the mention of abuse during pregnancy began to appear in the literature in the 1980s. The image of a woman being battered during pregnancy shatters the idealized image of pregnancy as a time of nurturing and protection. All pregnant women should be routinely screened for abuse. Common signs of IPV in pregnancy are delay in seeking prenatal care, unexplained bruising or damage to breasts or abdomen, use of harmful substances (cigarettes, alcohol, drugs), recurring psychosomatic illnesses, and lack of participation in prenatal education. Violence during pregnancy can result in hemorrhage, spontaneous abortion, stillbirths, preterm deliveries, and fetal fractures (CDC, 2014). Indeed, pregnancy may increase stress within the family and provoke the first instances of battering. It is estimated that one in six pregnant women have been abused by a partner (March of Dimes, 2017).

🔍 RESEARCH HIGHLIGHTS

Physical Dating Violence From Middle to High School

A study led by a professor at the University of Georgia examined the association of physical dating violence with relationship quality and acceptability of aggression. The study showed "that the kids who were involved in dating violence are consistently involved in dating violence and this violence starts early." The study began while the sample of students were in the sixth grade and followed them through the twelfth grade. Close to a third of study participants report abusive relationships, and this cycle increases over time. "Bad dating experiences, particularly those related to physical violence, are associated with a plethora of negative experiences such as anxiety, depressed moods, suicidal thoughts, alcohol and drug abuse, lower educational achievement and poor relationships with parents," the researchers observed.

Data from Orpinas P, Hsieh HL, Song X, et al: Trajectories of physical dating violence from middle to high school; association with relationship quality and acceptability of aggression. *J Youth Adolesc* 42(4): 551–565, 2012.

Sexual Assault

Every 98 seconds an American is sexually assaulted, and every 8 minutes the victim is a child. Nine out of every 10 sexual assaults occur in females and are perpetrated by someone they know. The majority occur at or near the victims' homes (Rape, Abuse & Incest National Network, 2016). Women may report that they were subjected to forced intercourse when they were ill or had recently given birth. They also report forced anal intercourse and other violent sexual acts. Box 28.2 includes considerations for working with victims of IPV.

To address the underreporting and underprosecution of adult sexual assaults, communities throughout the United States have implemented a model using the Sexual Assault Nurse Examiner (SANE). These specially trained nurses provide comprehensive psychological, medical, and forensic services for sexual assault. SANE nurses often work collaboratively with community-based victim advocates assuring continuity of support over time.

The Domestic Abuse Intervention Project (2011) in Duluth, Minnesota, has developed a wheel of violence that depicts how men who batter gain and maintain control over their female

---

BOX 28.2 Considerations for Working with Victims of Violence

1. Working with victims of intimate partner violence (IPV):
   - Establish rapport and trust.
   - Deal with issues of confidentiality honestly.
   - Provide current information regarding shelters and sources of support.
   - Recognize and accept that clients may "choose" to stay in an abusive relationship.
2. Working with victims of child abuse:
   - Protect the well-being of the child; this is the primary obligation of health care providers.
   - Report child abuse; it is a legal and ethical obligation in all states.
   - Establish rapport and trust; this may take time.
   - Remain objective when dealing with suspected family members.
3. Working with victims of elder abuse:
   - Establish rapport and trust; this may take time.
   - Report elder abuse; it is an ethical obligation for health care providers and a legal obligation in most states.
   - Remember that competent adults have the right to make decisions about their own care, even if it means staying in an abusive situation.
   - Support efforts to create respite programs and support groups for caregivers.
4. Advocating for the rights of vulnerable populations, which is the responsibility of all health care professionals:
   - Support research on effective interventions for violence prevention and reduction.
   - Lobby for a decrease in media violence.
   - Support community efforts to increase resources for victims of violence.
   - Lobby for effective regulation of firearms and cyberstalking.

---

partners. The Power and Control Wheel was developed by documenting women's experience of being battered within an intimate relationship. The Power and Control Wheel is therefore not a generic, genderless tool to understand domestic violence. Figure 28.1 depicts the Power and Control Wheel, "a helpful tool in understanding the overall pattern of abusive and violent behaviors that are used by a batterer to establish and maintain control over his partner. Very often, one or more violent incidents are accompanied by an array of these other types of abuse." The organization has also developed other wheels that focus on domestic abuse that include equality, abuse of children and nurturing children. The Post Separation Wheel is the newest put out by the DAIP and that focuses on the tactics used by men when there partner leaves and they share children.

Dating violence, which has become a national concern, refers to abusive, controlling, or aggressive behavior in an intimate relationship that can take the form of emotional, verbal, physical, or sexual abuse. Dating violence occurs in all types of relationships. A national survey from 2011 "found that 23% of females and 14% of males who ever experienced rape, physical violence, or stalking by an intimate partner, first experienced some form of partner violence between 11 and 17 years of age" (CDC, 2016).

Teens may not be aware of what constitutes an unhealthy relationship. They may think that teasing and name calling are a "normal" part of a relationship. However, these behaviors can become abusive and develop into more serious forms of violence. Unhealthy, abusive, or violent relationships can have severe consequences and short- and long-term negative effects on developing teens.

A number of national initiatives have developed to address teen dating violence. For example, the CDC's dating violence prevention initiative seeks to reduce dating violence and increase healthy relationships in high-risk urban communities through comprehensive, multisector prevention.

Dating violence can involve the use of date rape drugs, also known as *predator drugs,* such as gamma-hydroxybutyrate (GHB), flunitrazepam (Rohypnol), and ketamine, to reduce inhibitions and promote anesthesia or amnesia in the victim. GHB is odorless and colorless and can easily be made at home. Instructions are available in libraries and on the Internet, possibly explaining the drug's rapid rise in popularity. Although illegal in the United States, it has become available in many nightclubs, where it is sold in clear liquid form. GHB has been touted as an aphrodisiac and an anesthetic. It is actually a depressant that slows down the respiratory system and has been responsible for numerous overdoses. When mixed with alcohol, it can be deadly.

Flunitrazepam, which is classified as a benzodiazepine, has been compared with methaqualone (Quaalude), the "love drug" of the 1960s and 1970s. Like GHB, flunitrazepam is not legal in the United States, but many reports have been received of its use at fraternity parties, college gatherings, and in bars. Two other drugs in the benzodiazepine family, alprazolam (Xanax) and clonazepam (Klonopin), are also used as date rape drugs. The ability to provide a quick, cheap high with long-lasting effects may explain their popularity. When they are combined with alcohol, serious side effects, including death, have been reported.

Ketamine (ketamine hydrochloride) is an anesthetic used primarily in veterinary practice. It causes a lost sense of time and problems with memory. Another drug that is becoming more common as a date rape drug is carisoprodol (Soma), a prescription muscle relaxant and central nervous system depressant.

Studies have also linked alcohol, "a hallmark of college campus social life," with dating violence. Substance abuse is often implicated in sexual assaults on college campuses. Alcohol contributes to sexual assault because it impairs the ability to think clearly, lowers inhibitions, and impairs the ability to evaluate an unsafe situation.

Stalking is a pattern of repeated and unwanted attention, contact, harassment, or any type of conduct directed at a person that instills fear. Like IPV, stalking is a crime of power and control. Types of stalking include unwanted phone calls, waiting at places for the victim, leaving unwanted items such as flowers and gifts, posting information or spreading rumors about the victim, messaging through the Internet or cell phone (cyberstalking), damaging the victim's property, following the victim, obtaining personal information about the victim, and making direct or indirect threats to the victim's family or friends. During a 1-month period an estimated 14 in every 1000 persons age 18 or older are victims of stalking. Nearly two in four stalking victims knew their offender in some capacity, and approximately one in four victims reported some type of cyberstalking such as email or instant messaging (Office of Justice Programs, Bureau of Justice Statistics, 2016).

BOX 28.3 Bullying

Bullying includes repeated harmful acts and a real or perceived imbalance of power. Often underreported, bullying creates a climate of fear. Bullying can be physical, verbal, or psychological/relational bullying or cyberbullying.

- Physical bullying involves assault, intimidation, and/or destruction of property.
- Verbal bullying includes threats and name calling.
- Psychological/relational bullying can include all of the first two categories and is distinguished by the power imbalance between the victim and the bully.
- Cyberbullying consists of targeting the victim online.

Modified from U.S. Department of Justice, Office of Justice Programs: *OJP factsheet,* 2011. http://www.ojp.usdoj.gov/newsroom/factsheets/ojpfs_bullying.html.

Bullying

Bullying has been described as a form of youth violence and is defined as any "unwanted aggressive behavior by another youth or group of youths who are not siblings or current dating partners that involve an observed or perceived power imbalance" (CDC, 2016). Bullying is often repeated multiple times or is highly likely to be repeated. Types of bullying include physical threats, hitting, tripping, verbal teasing, and spreading rumors (Box 28.3). We've seen an increase in bullying with the use of technology that occurs through email, chat rooms, messaging, cell phones, and even posting videos on websites. In 2015, 20% of high school students reported being bullied on school property and 16% reported being bullied electronically. An increasing concern is the number of suicides occurring as a result of bullying (CDC, 2016).

To address the complex issues of bullying in schools, it has been recommended that a common school vision and culture that promote a safe and supportive learning environment be developed. Education of the whole school community, which includes school staff, students, parents, and their families, must be integrated to reduce the incidence of bullying (Pearce, Cross, Monks, Waters & Falconer, 2011).

Child Maltreatment

Child maltreatment includes all kinds of abuse and neglect of someone under 18 years of age. Children are maltreated more often by parents, family members, caregivers, clergy, coaches, and teachers. Maltreatment is more commonly seen in families who are under a great deal of stress; are living in poverty or isolation; or when a family member has a history of violence, uses substances, or has a mental illness. Children who increase caregiver burden—for example, children who have a disability (mental retardation, mental illness, and chronic physical illness)—or are under the age of 4 are at higher risk for being maltreated (CDC, 2016).

In 2014, there were more than 702,000 victims of confirmed cases of child maltreatment in the United States (CDC, 2016). The fatality rate for boys was slightly higher than that of girls, and infants less than 1 year old accounted for 21.7% of nonfatal maltreatment cases, followed by 12.9% of children who were 1 year old.

The four types of child maltreatment are:

- Neglect
- Physical abuse

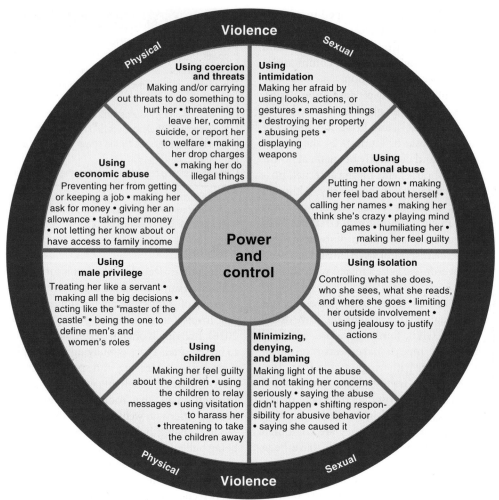

FIG. 28.1 Power and Control Wheel. (Developed by the Domestic Abuse Intervention Project, 206 West Fourth Street, Duluth, MN 55806. Used with permission.)

- Emotional abuse
- Sexual abuse

Although each state is responsible for providing definitions of child abuse and neglect, there is general consensus of what is included under each category.

Neglect is the failure of the responsible person to provide basic needs such as shelter, food, clothing, education, and access to medical care; permitting the child to use drugs/alcohol; and inattention to the child's emotional needs (Child Welfare Information Gateway, 2013). Failure to provide a nurturing environment for a child to thrive, learn, and develop and to provide for the health needs of a child is also considered neglect. Examples of emotional neglect include failure to cuddle and/or physically stimulate a newborn, failure to give positive feedback, failure to pay attention to the overall emotional needs of a child, and failure to show affection. It is important to be nonjudgmental when assessing a child for neglect. Poverty and cultural values may contribute to child neglect. Nurses can play a pivotal role in assessing the family's need for information or assistance. In some states abandonment is also considered a form of neglect. This occurs when the parents' identity or whereabouts are unknown and the child has been left alone where the child can suffer serious harm.

Physical abuse is intentional physical injury inflicted on a child by another person who has responsibility for the child. Injuries can range from minor bruises to severe fractures or death as a result of beating, kicking, stabbing, choking, burning, biting, throwing, or hitting with a hand, stick, strap, or other object. Spanking or paddling is not considered abuse as long as it does not cause bodily injury to the child. These types of injuries are considered abuse, regardless of whether the caregiver intended to hurt the child (Child Welfare Information Gateway, 2013).

Parents who abuse often have unreasonable expectations of their children and may misinterpret children's behavior as threats to their parental self-esteem and need to control. Patterned injuries may give some clue as to how the child was injured. A child who touches a light cord or light plug might be beaten with it, producing a looped or linear pattern. A child who plays with matches or the stove might have his or her hand placed in the flame. A crying child or a child who talks back might have hot pepper sauce poured into his or her mouth or might be suffocated with a pillow.

Abusive head trauma/inflicted traumatic head injury, also known as *shaken baby syndrome,* is a leading cause of death from

TABLE 28.1 Physical and Behavioral Indicators of Child Abuse and Neglect

Physical Indicators	Behavioral Indicators
Physical Abuse	
Unexplained bruises and welts in various stages of healing that may form patterns	Wary of adult contact
Unexplained burns by cigars or cigarettes or immersion burns (e.g., socklike, glove-like, or on buttocks or genitalia)	Apprehensive when other children cry
	Constantly on alert
Burns in the shapes of objects	Exhibiting extremes of behavior; aggressive or passive and withdrawn, or overly friendly to strangers
Rope burns	
Unexplained lacerations or abrasions	Frightened of parents
Unexplained fractures in various stages of healing; multiple or spiral fractures	Afraid to go home
Unexplained injuries to mouth, lips, gums, eyes, or external genitalia	
Physical and Emotional Neglect	
Hunger	Begging or stealing food
Poor hygiene	Alone at inappropriate times or for prolonged periods
Poor or inappropriate dress	Delinquent behavior
Lack of supervision for prolonged periods	Stealing
Lack of medical or dental care	Arriving early to and departing late from school
Constant fatigue, listlessness, or falling asleep in class	Lack of affection
Sexual Abuse	
Difficulty in walking or sitting	Exhibiting negative self-esteem
Torn, stained, or bloody underwear	Exhibiting inability to trust and function in intimate relationships
Genital pain or itching	Exhibiting cognitive and motor dysfunctions
Bruises in or bleeding from the external genitalia, vaginal, or anal area	Exhibiting deficits in personal and social skills
Sexually transmitted disease	Exhibiting bizarre, sophisticated, or unusual sexual behavior or knowledge
Drug and alcohol abuse	Delinquent or runaway behavior
Developmental delays	Exhibiting suicide ideation
	Reporting sexual assault
Emotional Abuse	
Failure to thrive	Exhibiting behavior extremes from passivity to aggression
Lag in physical development	Exhibiting habit and conduct disorders (e.g., antisocial behavior and destructiveness)
Speech disorders	
Developmental delays	Exhibiting neurotic traits
	Attempting suicide

abuse in the United States. Most victims are between 3 and 8 months of age. In this form of abuse, violent shaking of the infant causes trauma at the junction of the brainstem and spinal cord that can result in death. Serious and permanent brain damage may occur, with results such as cerebral palsy, seizures, severe retardation, blindness, hearing loss, speech and learning difficulties, problems with memory and attention, and developmental delays. Children with special needs or other medical conditions, including colic or gastroesophageal reflux disease; multiple siblings; and families living in poverty are at greater risk. In 70% of abusive head trauma cases, a male is the perpetrator (KidsHealth, 2017).

Emotional abuse, also called *psychological abuse,* is a pattern of behavior that negatively affects a child's self-worth and/or emotional development. This type of abuse may include constant criticism, rejection, and withholding love, affection, and support (Child Welfare Information Gateway, 2013). The child may demonstrate a substantial impairment in behavior, such as being overly compliant or passive, being very aggressive, or being inappropriately adult or infantile. Emotionally abused children frequently do not progress at a normal rate of physical, intellectual, or emotional development. Emotional abuse usually occurs

in the home, is not witnessed by others, and is therefore difficult to prove. Impairment in behavior may also occur in children who are not abused; therefore identification of emotional abuse is difficult.

Sexual abuse involves activities by a parent or caregiver that include fondling a child's genitals, incest, rape, sodomy, exploitation through prostitution, or production of pornographic material (Child Welfare Information Gateway, 2013). The incidence of sexual exploitation of children by Internet pedophiles has increased in recent years. Most research has focused on girls as victims of sexual abuse, but boys are also targets. In such cases, the male victim may refrain from reporting abuse because he is ashamed or because cultural values expect males to be assertive and capable of self-defense.

Child maltreatment can have serious long-term effects. Although physical wounds may heal, the child's ability to cope with life's challenges can be impaired. Childhood trauma may affect the nervous system and development of the immune system, putting the child at a higher risk for health problems as adults. The child may delay reporting the abuse for months or years because it may take that long for him or her to feel safe. Table 28.1 describes physical and behavioral indicators of child abuse and neglect.

All states mandate that health care providers and teachers report suspected child abuse. Reporting child abuse may be one of the hardest things a nurse will ever have to do, but may be one of the most rewarding when an abused child is removed from an unsafe and harmful situation.

Elder Abuse

Elder abuse is any form of mistreatment that results in harm or loss to an older person. It occurs in community settings, including private homes, nursing homes, and long-term care facilities. Unfortunately we do not know the exact numbers of elders who suffer from abuse and neglect. However, it is estimated that 4% to 6% of the elderly are abused (National Committee for the Prevention of Elder Abuse [NCPEA], 2017). Elders are often hesitant to report their abuse due to fear of retribution, shame, and social and physical isolation. Signs of elder abuse may be missed by health care professionals due to a lack of awareness and of adequate training (National Center on Elder Abuse [NCEA], 2016). Elders at risk for being abused include those in poor physical or mental health; those dependent on others for physical or financial support; and those who are confused, depressed, or socially isolated.

According to the NCPEA types of abuse and neglect of older adults are categorized as follows:

- Physical abuse (purposeful infliction of physical pain or injury or unnecessary physical or drug-induced restraints).
- Psychological-emotional abuse (verbal assault, threats, provoking fear, or isolation).
- Sexual abuse (unwanted sexual contact or taking pornographic pictures).
- Neglect (withholding of personal care, food, or medications; intimidation; humiliation; abandonment). Self-neglect is the failure of the elder who is competent to provide for one's own essential needs.
- Financial exploitation (theft or misuse of money or property).
- Health care fraud and abuse (charging for services not delivered or Medicare/Medicaid fraud).

Elder abuse tends to escalate in incidence and severity. When an older adult cannot care for himself or herself because of the physical or mental infirmities of age, what happens to that person may depend on whether relatives can provide care, or whether the person has financial resources to obtain care in his or her own home, a retirement home, or a residential care facility. Caregivers are often adult children or other relatives. The generation of individuals currently in their 40s, 50s, and 60s is often called the "sandwich generation" because they are caring for their children at the same time they are providing care for their aging parents. As parents age, the role reversal is often painful and demanding for both the elder and the caregiver.

Care of an aging parent requires sacrifice and commitment. As parents age, they may become more physically and cognitively impaired, increasing the likelihood of abuse. Elders who were themselves abusers are more likely to be abused by their caregivers. Older adults may undergo changes in personality that make it difficult for their adult children to care for them. They may need to be lifted, which may be difficult for someone with limited strength. They may need assistance walking, toileting, or eating that requires time the caregiver may not have. There is also an intimacy in caring for a parent that the caregiver may not be comfortable with. All of these factors cause stress, which can be associated with abuse—especially in families in which violence is a response to stress.

The needs of the older adult may exceed the family's ability to meet them. In many ways, helpless older adults are in the same vulnerable position as children because they are dependent on others for care. The population of the United States is aging, and by 2020, the number of adults older than 65 years is expected to account for 15% of the population (NCEA, 2017). Recognition of physical and behavioral indicators helps the professional become aware of possible abusive situations. None is conclusive in itself; however, each alerts the professional to the need for careful and complete assessment. Even though nurses are required to report instances of elder abuse, they may be reluctant to do so because assessment is not always conclusive. However, if there is a question of possible abuse, it must be reported to the appropriate authorities for further investigation. The state of New York took the lead in passing legislation with its "Granny's Law," which stiffened the penalties for assaults on elders. Table 28.2 lists the indicators of possible abuse of older adults.

 ACTIVE LEARNING

Investigate professional responsibilities relative to reporting abuse, neglect, or violence in your state. Share findings with classmates.

COMMUNITY VIOLENCE

The United States is one of the most violent countries in the industrialized world. Every day we hear about some community, region, or state that has been affected by violent crime. Community violence may not affect everyone directly, but it affects all indirectly. In contrast to interpersonal violence, which affects only one or two individuals, community violence usually occurs suddenly and without warning and can potentially destroy entire segments of the population. Community violence includes workplace violence, youth violence, gang-related violence, hate crimes, and terrorism.

Workplace Violence

Workplace violence is another serious safety and health issue. In 2014, nearly 2 million Americans reported having been victims of workplace violence. Homicide is currently the fourth leading cause of fatal occupational injuries in the United States. According to the U.S. Department of Labor, of the 4679 fatal workplace injuries that occurred in the United States in 2014, 403 were workplace homicides. Violence in the workplace includes threats of physical violence, physical assaults such as rape and homicide, muggings, verbal and written threats, and bullying (U.S. Department of Labor, Bureau of Labor Statistics, 2016).

Workplace violence tends to be more common in some service-oriented work environments, including health care. In the health care field, frequent areas for the occurrence of

TABLE 28.2 Indicators of Possible Elder Abuse or Neglect

Abuse

Physical Indicators	Emotional/Behavioral Indicators
Bruises, black eyes, welts, lacerations, and rope marks	Being emotionally upset or agitated
Bone and skull fractures	Being extremely withdrawn and noncommunicative or nonresponsive
Open wounds, cuts, punctures, untreated injuries in various stages of healing	Unusual behavior usually attributed to dementia (e.g., sucking, biting, rocking)
Sprains, dislocations, and internal injuries/bleeding	Sudden change in behavior
Signs of being subjected to punishment and signs of being restrained	Elder's report of being verbally or emotionally mistreated
Laboratory findings of medication overdose or underutilization of prescribed drugs	
Report of being hit, slapped, kicked, or mistreated	
The caregiver's refusal to allow visitors to see an elder alone	
Unexplained sexually transmitted disease	
Elder's sudden change in behavior	
Elder's report of sexual assault	

Neglect

Physical Indicators	Financial Indicators (Material Exploitation)
Dehydration, malnutrition, untreated bedsores, and poor personal hygiene	Sudden changes in bank account or banking practice (e.g., unexplained withdrawal of large sums of money, inclusion of additional names on an elder's bank signature card)
Unattended or untreated health problems	Unauthorized withdrawal of the elder's funds using the elder's automatic teller machine card
Hazardous or unsafe living conditions/arrangements (e.g., improper wiring, no heat, or no running water)	Abrupt changes in a will or other financial documents (e.g., power of attorney)
Unsanitary and unclean living conditions (e.g., dirt, fleas, lice, soiled bedding, fecal/urine smell, inadequate clothing)	Unexplained disappearance of funds or valuables
Elder's report of being mistreated or neglected	Bills unpaid despite the availability of adequate financial resources
Abandonment (desertion of an elder at a hospital, nursing facility, or other similar or public places or institutions)	Elder's signature being forged for financial transactions or for the titles of his or her possessions
	Sudden appearance of previously uninvolved relatives interested in the elder's affairs and possessions
	Unexplained sudden transfer of assets to a family member or someone outside the family
	The provision of services that are not necessary
	Report of financial exploitation

Modified from Administration on Aging/National Center on Elder Abuse: *Elder Abuse* https://ncea.acl.gov/faq/index.html

violence include emergency departments, psychiatric units, geriatric units, and waiting rooms. Nurses and nursing assistants who work directly with patients are often at risk. Nurses who work in public health roles are not immune to violence because their work may bring them in direct contact with individuals prone to violent behavior. Delivery drivers, public service workers, people who work where alcohol is served, and law enforcement are also at higher risk for workplace violence.

Examples of risk factors for workplace violence include:

- Working in high-crime areas
- Working alone or isolated
- Availability of drugs at the worksite
- Low staffing levels
- Poorly lit parking areas and corridors
- Long waits for service
- Inadequate security
- Increasing numbers of people who use substances
- Access to firearms

Violence also negatively affects the workplace, resulting in low morale, increased job stress and turnover, reduced trust of management and/or coworkers, and hostile work environments.

Youth-Related Violence

Violence is taking a toll on American youth. It is the third leading cause of death for young people ages 10 to 24. In 2014, there were 4300 homicides of young people ages 10 to 24. This is an average of 13 victims each day. The following factors may increase the risk of becoming a perpetrator of youth violence: prior history of violence; drug, alcohol, and tobacco use; poor family functioning; poor grades in school; associating with delinquent peers; and poverty in the community (CDC, 2016) (see Table 28.3).

Youth-related violence is more concentrated in minority communities and inner cities, putting a disproportionate burden on these communities. Violence is a complicated and multilayered problem. Adolescents and children increasingly use violence to settle disputes. Children are often not taught peaceful ways of resolving differences and learn by what they observe at home, on television, in movies, and through video games. Consequently, schools have become a common site for violence. See Chapter 30 for more information on violence in schools.

TABLE 28.3	**Risk Factors for Youth-Related Violence**
Individual Risk Factors	Involvement with drugs, alcohol, or tobacco
	Antisocial beliefs and attitudes
	Low IQ
	History of violent victimization
	History of early aggressive behavior
	Attention deficits, hyperactivity, or learning disorders
	Poor behavioral control
	Deficits in social, cognitive, or information-processing abilities
	Exposure to violence and conflict in the family
	High emotional distress
	History of treatment of emotional problems
Community Risk Factors	Diminished economic opportunities
	High concentration of poor residents
	High level of family disruption
	Low levels of community participation
	Socially disorganized neighborhoods
	High level of transiency
Family Risk Factors	Poor family functioning
	Low emotional attachment to parents or caregivers
	Low parental education and income
	Parental substance abuse or criminality
	Poor monitoring and supervision of children
	Harsh, lax, or inconsistent disciplinary practices
	Authoritarian child-rearing attitudes
Peer/Social Risk Factors	Association with delinquent peers
	Involvement in gangs
	Social rejection by peers
	Lack of involvement in conventional activities
	Poor academic performance
	Low commitment to school and school failure

Data from Centers for Disease Control and Prevention, National Center for Injury Prevention and Control, Division of Violence Prevention: *Youth violence: risk and protective factors*, 2013. www.cdc.gov/ViolencePrevention/youthviolence/riskprotectivefactors.html.

Gangs

Gangs are increasingly responsible for crimes and violence throughout the United States. In 2015, it was estimated that approximately 1.4 million members are criminally active in the United States and Puerto Rico with 33,000 violent street gangs, motorcycle gangs, and prison gangs. Gangs use violence to control neighborhoods and increase their illegal money-making activities, which include robbery, fraud, drug and gun trafficking, prostitution, and human trafficking. To address this national problem the National Gang Intelligence Center was established in 2005 (FBI, 2017a).

Reasons that young people give for joining gangs include the belief that gangs will protect them, peer pressure, the need for respect, and a sense of belonging.

Prison Violence

The United States has one of the world's highest incarceration rates. At the end of 2015, an estimated 6,741,400 persons were supervised by U.S. adult correctional systems (U.S. Department of Justice [DOJ], 2015). This number includes federal and state prisons, jails, and community corrections facilities. Women accounted for 7% (105,000 prisoners) of the sentenced federal and state prison population. The prison population is relatively young, as only about 11% were age 55 or older and 2% were age 65 or older. State prisons had jurisdiction over an estimated 1000 prisoners age 17 or younger in 2015.

Violence also occurs within prison walls among prisoners or between inmates and prison staff. Types of prison violence include murder, manslaughter, forcible rape, theft, and aggravated assault. The public and the judicial system have expressed little sympathy for this population for a variety of reasons, including indifference, disbelief, and denial. Little research exists to reflect the long-term effects on these victims or on society when they are released. See Chapter 32 for more information on forensic and correctional nursing.

Human Trafficking

Human trafficking is a global problem and public health issue both domestically and internationally. It is considered a modern-day form of slavery involving the illegal trade of people for exploitation. Human trafficking is the third largest criminal activity in the world. Threats, the use of force, coercion, abduction, fraud, and abuse of power are all methods used by human traffickers to obtain some type of labor or commercial sex act. Some common ways that girls and women become victims of trafficking include the following: abduction, meeting traffickers in advertising modeling jobs, responding to ads to work or study abroad, seeking the help of smugglers to get into the United States, sold to traffickers by a parent or intimate partner, or promises of marriage or education or a better life (United Nations Office on Drugs and Crimes, 2017; U.S. Institute Against Human Trafficking, 2017).

Every year, millions of men, women, and children are trafficked in countries around the world, including the United States. It is estimated that human trafficking generates many billions of dollars of profit per year, second only to drug trafficking as the most profitable form of transnational crime. Human trafficking is a hidden crime, as victims rarely come forward to seek help because of language barriers, fear of the traffickers, and/or fear of law enforcement. Health care providers are in a unique position to identify victims of trafficking and provide important physical and psychosocial care. Common health problems among trafficking victims include anxiety, depression, cigarette burns, complications from unsafe abortion, fractures, pelvic pain, sexually transmitted diseases, oral health problems, unhealthy weight loss, and unwanted pregnancy (Dovydaitis, 2010).

There are a number of barriers that can prevent victims from disclosing even to health care professionals. Because many victims are undocumented, they may be afraid that they will be deported. If the victim is a minor, the provider has a legal responsibility to phone child protective services. Organized crime is heavily involved in sex trafficking, so victims may be afraid that their families will be harmed (Dovydaitis, 2010).

Despite these potential barriers, it is important for nurses to become knowledgeable about this population in order to effectively respond if they do come in contact with a victim who is seeking health care.

Hate Crimes

Hate crimes are crimes in which the offender is motivated by factors such as an individual's race, sexual orientation, religious beliefs, ethnic background, or national origin. Hate crimes may include murder, sexual or physical assault, harassment, attacks on homes or on places of worship, or vandalism. Because hate crimes attack an individual's identity, the emotional effects are compounded. It is estimated that only 44% of hate crimes are reported. In 2015, 5850 hate crimes were reported in the United States (FBI, 2017b).

Terrorism

Terrorism has been present throughout history. The Department of Defense (2017) defines terrorism as "the unlawful use of violence or threat of violence to instill fear and coerce governments or societies. Terrorism is often motivated by religious, political, or other ideological beliefs and committed in the pursuit of goals that are usually political." All terrorist acts include at least three key elements: violence, fear, and intimidation. Nurses need to be prepared for terrorism in whatever form it takes, from an explosion at a local refinery to an act that affects an entire region or country, such as biological, chemical, or nuclear incidents. Mental and physical health issues remain a nursing concern for the victims, responders, and the community long after the act has occurred. See Chapter 29 for a more detailed discussion of terrorism.

FACTORS INFLUENCING VIOLENCE

Controversy surrounds the factors that influence violence in today's society. Three of them are easy access to firearms, the impact of media, and mental illness. These will be discussed briefly.

Firearms

Approximately 270 million privately owned firearms exist in the United States, and more than 1 million new handguns are sold in the United States annually. The United States ranks number one in privately owned guns among 179 countries, and statistics indicate that firearms are the weapon of choice in homicides in the United States. Of the nearly 15,696 murders in the United States in 2013, 71.5% were committed with firearms (U.S. DOJ, 2015).

Although some persons suggest that firearms provide protection, substantial evidence indicates that firearms increase the likelihood of homicide or, even more commonly, suicide (Weinberger et al, 2015). It is important for health care professionals to be comfortable speaking with their patients in a nonjudgmental manner about firearms, provide patients with factual information about firearms relevant to their health and the health of those around them, fully answer their patients' questions, and advise them on safe gun protection.

The cost of gun violence is staggering. The direct cost of violence related to firearms in the United States is in millions of dollars annually. Indirect costs, including loss of productivity, mental health treatment, rehabilitation, and legal and judicial costs, add even more. Heated discussions regarding firearms occur daily between opponents and proponents of gun control. Even the underlying meaning of the Second Amendment of the Constitution, "the right to bear arms," is argued.

Media

Media violence is prevalent and is accessible to all age groups. It includes exposure to and participation in violent video games, music and music videos that depict rape or violence, and virtual violence that allows subscribers to harm or kill victims. Television and movies often depict people being tortured or killed in such graphic detail that may make it hard for children and adults to distinguish between reality and fantasy. Media violence has become more pronounced and graphic in nature. There is concern in the public health community that repeated exposure to media violence leads to emotional desensitization to real-life violence.

Mental Illness

A general consensus exists that severe mental illness (SMI) increases the risk of violence. The media's portrayal of people with mental illness committing violence adds to the belief that a great deal of violence is committed by people with SMI. However, there is little population-level evidence that supports the notion that individuals diagnosed with mental illness are more likely than anyone else to commit gun crimes. The connections between mental illness and gun violence are less causal and more complex than current U.S. public opinion and legislative action allow. It is undeniable that persons who have shown violent tendencies should not have access to weapons that could be used to harm themselves or others. However, notions that mental illness caused any particular shooting or that advance psychiatric attention might prevent these crimes are more complicated than they often seem (Metzl and MacLeish, 2015).

After the violence in Newtown, Connecticut, there has been an increased push for legislation to fund public health strategies that identify and treat mental illness across the country. This is especially important because the budget crisis in the United States has forced many states to eliminate or reduce the availability of mental health services. See Chapter 25 for a more in-depth discussion of mental illness.

🔍 ACTIVE LEARNING

1. Call a child abuse center in the community and ask what services they provide.
2. Call a battered women's shelter and determine the procedure for securing shelter placement for a battered victim and her children.
3. Visit a respite center for the elderly and observe the clients and the activities that are provided. Observe behaviors that would contribute to stress in the caregiver.
4. Find out what support groups exist in the community for older adult caregivers.
5. Read your local newspaper for 1 month and clip articles that deal with violence and gun control. Determine how many individuals were killed or injured during that period. How many of the deaths and injuries were gun related?
6. Look up the laws that relate to the reporting of child and elder abuse in your area.

VIOLENCE FROM A PUBLIC HEALTH PERSPECTIVE

Dealing with violence has traditionally been the U.S. criminal justice system's responsibility. However, because violence is also a public health epidemic, efforts are being made to prevent and manage it using public health strategies and community approaches such as church groups, community groups, and local, state, and federal governments. Violence, as discussed previously, has a tremendous influence on morbidity and mortality rates and health care resources. The public health system is challenged to go beyond its traditional programs to include prevention and management of violence. As is true with most public health problems, many interrelated factors must be addressed.

Healthy People 2020 and Violence

Violence was one of the areas addressed by *Healthy People 2000* and again in *Healthy People 2010* and *Healthy People 2020*. Several objectives regarding violence and abuse prevention have been established. The *Healthy People 2020* box lists a few of these (*Healthy People*, 2017). These objectives are intended to target causes of violence and abuse, improve national data collection and analysis, provide input for legislative funding, facilitate research efforts, and concentrate public health efforts on models that demonstrate effectiveness.

Many of the *Healthy People 2020* objectives are difficult to achieve because of complex barriers. These include lack of comparable data sources and standardized definitions, as well as inadequate resources to establish consistent tracking systems and fund prevention programs.

HEALTHY PEOPLE 2020

Objectives Related to Injury and Violence Prevention

IVP–29: Reduce homicides.
IVP–30: Reduce firearm-related deaths.
IVP–31: Reduce nonfatal firearm-related injuries.
IVP–32: Reduce nonfatal physical assault injuries.
IVP–33: Reduce physical assaults.
IVP–34: Reduce physical fighting among adolescents.
IVP–35: Reduce bullying among adolescents.
IVP–36: Reduce weapon carrying by adolescents on school property.
IVP–37: Reduce child maltreatment deaths.
IVP-38: Reduce nonfatal child maltreatment.
IVP-41: Reduce nonfatal intentional self-harm injuries.
IVP-42: Reduce children's exposure to violence.
IVP-43: Increase the number of states and the District of Columbia that link data on violent deaths from death certificates, law enforcement, and coroner and medical examiner reports to inform prevention efforts at the state and local levels.

From HealthyPeople.gov: *Healthy People 2020: Topics & objectives: injury and violence prevention, 2012*. http://www.healthypeople.gov/2020/topicsobjectives2020/objectiveslist.aspx?topicId=24. Accessed Feb 20, 2018

PREVENTION OF VIOLENCE

The nurse who cares for people experiencing violence must be a skilled clinician who is knowledgeable about both the problem

BOX 28.4   Safety Issues for the Community Health Nurse

Plan Ahead
- Know the area you are visiting.
- Schedule the visit ahead of time and get the correct address, directions, and information about who will be in the home.
- Tell the office where you will be and check in regularly.
- Carry a cell phone, possibly a pager, and a small amount of money.
- Dress for function and mobility and wear a name tag. Avoid any provocative clothing.
- Ensure that the vehicle you drive is in good repair, has a full gas tank, and has emergency equipment. Always carry two sets of car keys.

Approaching the Home
- Notice the environment, animals, fences, activity, possible indicators of crime, and places you could go for assistance if necessary.
- Walk with confidence and maintain a professional attitude.
- Listen for signs of fighting before knocking. If you hear sounds of fighting, leave!
- Do not enter a home if you suspect an unsafe situation.

In the Home
- Be aware of who is in the home and what is going on. If angry people are in the home, use your professional and social skills. Do not expect the client to protect you.
- Note the exits and sit between the client and an exit of the home. Be prepared to leave quickly if the situation changes suddenly.
- If someone in the home is violent, leave and call 911.

Handling a Tight Situation
- Do not show fear; control your breathing.
- Speak calmly and in a soothing manner. Be assertive but not aggressive.
- Repeat the reason for your visit and find a reason to leave.

Leaving the Home
- Take all of your belongings and keep your car keys in your hand.
- Watch for cars following you when you leave. Do not stop. If you feel that you are in danger, go to the nearest police station or well-lighted business and ask for help.
- Trust your instincts. Never forget your own safety.

Modified from Oregon Public Health Association, Public Health Nursing Section, Seattle–King County Department of Public Health, and Washington State Public Health Association: *Public health nursing domestic violence protocol* [booklet], Seattle, WA, and Salem, OR, 1993, Authors.

and available community resources. Box 28.4 presents tips regarding safety issues for a community health nurse. A considerable body of knowledge has been developed about trends in violence. Table 28.4 provides the components of a comprehensive program to reduce violence in individuals and the community.

Primary Prevention

The goal of primary prevention is to stop violence, abuse, or neglect before it occurs. Education plays a major part in primary prevention and may include life-skills training such as parenting and family wellness, anger management, and/or conflict resolution. Professionals should increase their awareness of violence and identification of cases. The nurse can work in or with the community to educate citizens about the problem of violence, potential causes of violence, and available community services.

TABLE 28.4 Examples of Prevention Strategies to Reduce Violence for Individuals and Communities

Individuals	Community
Primary Prevention—Goal: Promotion of Optimal Parenting and Family Wellness	
Life-skills training in schools, churches, and communities	Community education concerning violence
Education of children, adolescents, and adults on methods of conflict resolution	Reduction of media violence
Parenting classes in hospitals, schools, and other community agencies	Development of community support services such as crisis lines, respite care for families with dependent members, shelters for battered women and their children, and development and vigorous enforcement of antistalking measures, including cyberstalking
Mental health services for all age groups	
Training for professionals in early detection of violence	
	Handgun safety education
Secondary Prevention—Goal: Diagnosis of and Service for Families in Stress	
Nursing assessment for evidence of violence in all health care settings	Education of all health professionals in assessment of violence and possible protocols for dealing with victims
A safety plan for victims	List of hospital emergency departments and trauma centers with 24-hour response
Knowledge of legal options	Reporting of different types of abuse
Shelter referral for victims	Coordination with medical authorities
Social services for individuals or families	Coordination with voluntary and social service agencies for provision of services
Referral to self-help groups in the community	Death review teams to review deaths from injury, especially in infants and children
Referral to appropriate community agencies	Public authority involvement by police, district attorneys, and courts
	Epidemiological tracking and evaluation of violence
Tertiary Prevention—Goal: Reeducation and Rehabilitation of Violent Families	
Empowerment strategies for battered women	Foster homes, shelters, and care for dependents
Professional counseling services for individuals	Public authority involvement
Parenting reeducation (i.e., formal training in child rearing)	Follow-up care for known cases of abuse, neglect, or violence
Counseling services for individuals and families	
Self-help groups	

Primary prevention must begin at a community level, helping change attitudes about abuse and violence. Primary prevention focuses on stopping the transgenerational aspect of abuse, starting with young children and continuing throughout the life span. Mentoring and peer programs can be designed to promote healthy relationships and decrease conflict. For example, parenting is one of the most difficult jobs that individuals will undertake, yet there is a widespread myth that parenting "comes naturally." Classes for parents should focus on physical care of the infant, including ways to soothe and manage a "fussy" baby, the effect of fatigue on new parents, the need for support, and the fears and questions of new parents. Nurses in the hospital have little time to help new parents learn basic newborn care before discharge. Some hospitals and public health agencies provide follow-up to parents to ensure that they can adequately care for their newborn. This support is especially given to all persons deemed to be high risk for infant abuse, including teenage mothers, mothers without support, or women with a history of spousal abuse.

Secondary Prevention

The goal of secondary prevention is to assess, diagnose, and treat victims and perpetrators of violence. Consideration of the safety of the potential victim is critical.

Secondary prevention begins with assessment. For example, consistent assessment of women during health care visits will increase case finding and provide opportunities for early intervention that is particularly crucial during pregnancy. Women should be interviewed in private when asked about abuse. Questions should be asked in a matter-of-fact way, and the health care provider should not show shock or dismay at the response.

Victims, once identified, must be offered resources to increase their safety. However, all victims may not be ready or able to leave the situation, and available options must be explored. Victims should have knowledge of legal options and how to access them. The nurse must be ready to intervene when the abuse involves a child or someone who is cognitively impaired. Some states have developed protocols for nurses who deal with victims of violence. Review of these protocols can help the nurse become familiar with the questions to ask and suggestions that should be made to help the victim develop a safety plan.

Another example of secondary prevention involves screening for abuse in the elderly that should occur at every health care visit. Elder abuse remains underreported across the United States; therefore routine screening can facilitate early intervention. Nurses can help raise professional and community consciousness of elder abuse by participating in political activities to create or strengthen mandatory reporting laws and funding of support groups.

The nurse should work with family members or caregivers who provide care for the elderly to promote healthier relationships. Helping the caregiver deal with stress by finding respite care, a home health aide, or counseling may help. Documentation is crucial in meeting medical-legal requirements. The nurse should record observations accurately and refrain from opinions and interpretations because this documentation may be used in court proceedings.

The problem of violence cannot be managed by nurses alone, but rather in combination with other professionals, including physicians, child and adult protective services providers, social workers, clergy, and police. This interdisciplinary approach leads to optimal outcomes. Public health surveillance is important in obtaining accurate numbers of intentional injuries for individuals. Death review teams can analyze records to determine whether an injury was intentional or unintentional.

Tertiary Prevention

Tertiary prevention is aimed at rehabilitation of individuals, families, groups, or communities and includes both victims and perpetrators of violence. Rehabilitation may take months or even years, depending on the situation. For example, the September 11, 2001, attack on the United States disrupted thousands of lives and changed the country's sense of security. This attack affected everyone in the country, not just those in the immediate vicinity. After all these years, the effects continue. The nurse must be able to work in conjunction with a variety of mental health professionals and social service agencies to provide coordinated care. The nurse may have also been a victim and may be experiencing many of the same problems as those he or she is trying to help. Self-care and recognition of the nurse's own limitations or needs are critical.

 ACTIVE LEARNING

Using the telephone directory or computer search engine, find three public or private agencies in the community that provide help for victims of violence. Make a list of the telephone numbers and post copies of it in public areas.

CASE STUDY   Application of the Nursing Process

Intimate Partner Violence

Karen, 36 years old, comes to the neighborhood clinic where you are the nurse. She is obviously distraught and is holding her head down when she enters the exam room. As you are getting her vital signs, she lifts her head and you notice multiple bruises on her face, around her left eye, and on her left cheek and the right side of her neck. She sees you looking at her and she begins to cry. You ask her what happened and she tells you that her boyfriend hit her two nights ago. As you question her further, you find out that she is divorced, has custody of her two children, a boy age 8 and a daughter age 3, and is unemployed. Her ex-husband lives three states away, about an 8-hour drive. She has been with the current boyfriend about 6 months and they have been living together about 3 months. He hit her repeatedly the night before last after he came home upset about a problem at work. The attack ended as abruptly as it started. He apologized repeatedly, hugged her, and left the house. Her children were in bed and did not witness the abuse. She took the children to a friend's house and then went to an after-hours clinic for treatment. While she was at the after-hours clinic, the police were notified, and she pressed charges against her boyfriend. He was arrested later that night and she subsequently filed a restraining order against him.

After further discussion, she tells you that this is not the first time he has hit her; that it has happened twice before, always after something has upset him. She then states that she knows he loves her and that he would not deliberately hurt her—that she must have done something to make him angry. She feels that he does really love her and she regrets having him arrested and filing the restraining order. She felt as if she had no choice once the clinic personnel and the police urged her to do something. He is now in the county jail, and she is considering going to the police station and dropping the charges. She does admit, however, that she is afraid about how angry he is going to be once he gets out.

You tell her about the cycle of domestic violence and how it repeats itself. You give her information about local shelters and explain that abusers usually do not stop their cycle of violence on their own, but only after counseling and support. You also tell her that she may be in danger of serious harm and even death if she stays with him. You recommend that she leave where she is living, take her children with her, and talk with an attorney before doing anything about the legal situation.

One month later, Karen again appears in your clinic. She tells you that she did leave home and take her two children to her ex-husband's house. She also states that the boyfriend is still in county jail, that she did not drop the restraining order, and that she has moved in with her boyfriend's mother. She visits him every Sunday afternoon and talks to him once a week on the phone. His mother refuses to speak with him.

Assessment

The following are the summary assessment points:

- The boyfriend has a history of IPV—duration unknown.
- Karen is a stay-at-home mom, with two children under the age of 9 years, who currently live with their father in another state.
- Karen does not have close family in the area.
- Karen does not believe that she is in danger.
- Karen believes she lacks employable skills.
- The boyfriend's abuse is aggravated by problems at work.

Diagnoses

- Potential for severe injury or death related to abuse
- High risk for emotional trauma from dysfunctional family dynamics
- High risk for loss of children

Planning
Short-Term Goals

- Boyfriend will be referred for anger management classes once released.
- Strategies will be identified to help Karen regain her children.
- A safe setting will be identified for Karen and the children.

Long-Term Goals

- Karen will be free of IPV.
- Karen will enter individual counseling.
- Boyfriend will enter counseling.

Intervention
Individual

Karen was assessed for injuries, and none were found to be life threatening. She was given a referral for counseling at the local counseling center where a community health nurse works. She was also given locations and numbers for local shelters. She did leave the charges against her boyfriend standing and decided not to drop the restraining order.

Karen agreed to enter counseling and continues to live with her boyfriend's mother until other arrangements can be made. She decided to leave her children at her ex-husband's house until she feels more secure about her situation. Karen has spoken with the community health nurse at the local counseling center. The nurse's goals are centered on Karen's ongoing physical and emotional well-being.

During these visits the nurse was able to engage Karen in conversation regarding her future and that of her children. Karen indicated that this most recent episode of violence had frightened her and caused her to question the wisdom

CASE STUDY Application of the Nursing Process—cont'd

Intimate Partner Violence

of her decision to stay with her boyfriend. Her boyfriend was found guilty of domestic abuse and was released after 2 months with a probation period of 2 years and mandatory anger management classes. She and her ex-husband are discussing child care arrangements and the possibility of her moving closer to him where she should be able to find work.

Community

The community health nurse arranged to speak at the monthly breakfast meeting of community pastors where she presented an informational program on IPV. Within 3 weeks she received speaking invitations from four of the nine churches represented at the meeting. The first of the programs will take place in the next month. In two of the churches, "mother's day out" (a partial day of babysitting) services are available to church members, and after an appeal from the community health nurse, one of the churches has expressed a willingness to open its program to nonchurch members.

Evaluation
Individual and Community

You and the community health nurses jointly focused on safety as a priority of care for Karen. The visit to the after-hours clinic and the medical personnel's call to the police started the chain of events. Karen's injuries created an opportunity for the community health nurse to maintain contact and provide psychosocial support. During visits the nurse was able to speak openly with Karen and offer options to enhance her coping skills. One of the local pastors has encouraged Karen to focus on both her children and her own future.

Karen came back into the clinic where you are working and seems healthier. She states that she is going to move to the same area where her ex-husband is

living and will be reconciled with her children. Karen also says that her ex-husband agreed to help her find employment in the area. Her boyfriend continues to fulfill the requirements of his probation, and he acknowledges that this will be an ongoing recovery process.

Levels of Prevention
Primary
Goal: Promote safety and prevent violence.
- Encourage contact with friends in the neighborhood and at church.
- Provide services of the community health nurse.
- Provide community education programs about anger management.
- Provide community education programs about IPV.

Secondary
Goal: Assess for signs of IPV.
- Facilitate health care for treatment of injuries.
- Provide both physical and psychosocial support.
- Provide referral for anger management.
- Provide individual and family counseling.
- Provide a 24-hour abuse hotline number.

Tertiary
Goal: Promote development of healthy family dynamics.
- Encourage continued use of community resources.
- Encourage community involvement with other young families.
- Provide community education programs on the cycle of violence.

SUMMARY

Violence is a major public health issue in the United States and affects individuals across the life cycle. Morbidity and mortality statistics indicate that violence is epidemic in many communities. Whether it occurs at home, in the neighborhood, or at school, violence affects countless numbers of individuals. The influence of media, easy access to and proliferation of firearms, and mental illness in the United States are considered contributing factors to violence. The cycle of violence will persist if not broken. The abuser is also a victim, and the ultimate victim is society, which must care and pay for the results of violent acts.

There are a wealth of resources that nurses can use to broaden their knowledge of the different types of violence and address best practices for preventing, detecting, and intervening in a timely way. For example, there are free online video training resources for health providers dealing with screening for IPV and effective communication strategies that promote therapeutic conversations

with women who experience IPV (Health Cares About IPV, 2015). A number of elder abuse screening tools are available from the NCEA (2016) website. Screening tools for human trafficking, including guidelines and victim identification, are available on the Vera Institute of Justice website (2014). The National Domestic Violence Safety Hotline has excellent resources that nurses can use to help women develop safety plans and legal information that can be discussed with women.

Violence is a public health epidemic, and national objectives for reducing it have been identified. The core public health functions of needs assessment and surveillance, policy development, and assurance are useful methods of combating this epidemic. The literature describes interventions that focus on the three levels of prevention. The need for continued research in violence should be a funding priority at the local, state, and national levels. The reality of violence has been validated. Everyone is affected.

EVOLVE WEBSITE

http://evolve.elsevier.com/Nies/community
- NCLEX Review Questions
- Case Studies

BIBLIOGRAPHY

Centers for Disease Control and Prevention: *CDC Helps Prevent Global Violence*, July 12, 2016. Available from: <https://www.cdc.gov/violenceprevention/globalviolence/index.html>.

Centers for Disease Control and Prevention: National center for health statistics, *Assault and homicide*, Oct. 6, 2016. Available from: <http://www.cdc.gov/nchs/fastats/homicide.htm>.

Centers for Disease Control and Prevention: Prevalence and characteristics of sexual violence, stalking, and intimate partner violence victimization — National Intimate Partner and Sexual Violence Survey, *United States*, 2011. September 5, 2014, Available from: <https://www.cdc.gov/mmwr/preview/mmwrhtml/ss6308a1.htm>.

Centers for Disease Control and Prevention: *Understanding bullying*, Fact Sheet, 2016. Available from: <www.cdc.gov/violenceprevention/pdf/bullying_factsheet.pdf>.

Centers for Disease Control and Prevention: *Understanding intimate partner violence*, Fact Sheet, 2014. Available from: <https://www.cdc.gov/violenceprevention/pdf/ipv-factsheet.pdf>.

Centers for Disease Control and Prevention: *Violence prevention. CDC prevents global violence*, July 12, 2016. Available from: <https://www.cdc.gov/violenceprevention/globalviolence/index.html>.

Centers for Disease Control and Prevention: *Violence prevention. Child abuse and neglect prevention*, May 25, 2016. Available from: <www.cdc.gov/violenceprevention/childmaltreatment/>.

Centers for Disease Control and Prevention: *Violence prevention, Elder abuse*, July 14, 2016. Available from: <https://www.cdc.gov/violenceprevention/elderabuse/index.html>.

Centers for Disease Control and Prevention: Violence prevention, *National suicide statistics*, July 19, 2016. Available from: <https://www.cdc.gov/violenceprevention/suicide/statistics/index.html>.

Centers for Disease Control and Prevention: Violence prevention, *Teen dating violence*, July 21, 2016. Available from: <https://www.cdc.gov/violenceprevention/intimatepartnerviolence/teen_dating_violence.html>.

Centers for Disease Control and Prevention: Youth violence, *Facts at a glance*, 2016. Available from: <www.cdc.gov/violenceprevention/pdf/yv-datasheet.pdf>.

Centers for Disease Control and Prevention: Child maltreatment, *Facts at a glance*, 2014. Available From <https://www.cdc.gov/violenceprevention/pdf/childmaltreatment-facts-at-a-glance.pdf>.

Child Welfare Information Gateway: *What is child abuse and neglect? Recognizing the signs and symptoms*, July 2013. Available from: https://www.childwelfare.gov/pubpdfs/whatiscan.pdf.

Department of Defense: *DOD dictionary of military and associated terms*, March, 2017. Available from: <www.dtic.mil/doctrine/new_pubs/dictionary.pdf>.

Domestic Abuse Intervention Program: *Wheel gallery*, 2011. Available from: http://www.theduluthmodel.org/index.htm.

Dovydaitis t: Human trafficking: The role of the health care provider, *J of Mid and Women's Health* 55(5):462–467, 2010.

Federal Bureau of Investigation: *2015 Crime in the United States*, 2017a. Available from: https://ucr.fbi.gov-/hate-crime/2015/topic-pages/incidentsandoffenses_final.

Federal Bureau of Investigation: *What we investigate. Hate crimes*, 2017b. Available from: https://www.fbi.gov/investigate/civil-rights/hate-crimes#Definition.

Health Cares About IPV: *Intimate partner violence screening and counseling toolkit*, 2015. Available from: <http://www.healthcaresaboutipv.org/getting-started/training-resources/>.

HealthyPeople.gov: *Healthy people 2020: topics & objectives*, March 31, 2017. Available from: <www.healthypeople.gov/2020/topics-objectives/topic/injury-and-violence-prevention/objectives>.

KidsHealth: *Abusive head trauma (shaken baby syndrome)*, 2017. Available from: <http://kidshealth.org/en/parents/shaken.html#>.

March of Dimes: Abuse during pregnancy. Available from: <http://www.marchofdimes.org/pregnancy/abuse-during-pregnancy.aspx>

Metzl JM, MacLeish KT: Mental Illness, mass shootings and the politics of American firearms, *Am J Public Health* 105(2):240–249, 2015.

Mother Goose nursery rhymes, Bath, England, 2000, Robert Frederick Publishing.

National Center on Elder Abuse: *Research. Statistics/Data*, 2017. Available from: https://ncea.acl.gov/whatwedo/research/statistics.html#population.

National Center on Elder Abuse: *Elder abuse screening tools for health care professionals*, 2016. Available from: <http://eldermistreatment.usc.edu/wp-content/uploads/2016/10/Elder-Abuse-Screening-Tools-for-Healthcare-Professionals.pdf?.

National Committee for the Prevention of Elder Abuse, 2017. Available from. <http://www.preventelderabuse.org/elderabuse/>.

Office of Justice Programs: Bureau of justice statistics, *Correctional populations in the United States*, 2015. Available from: <https://www.bjs.gov/index.cfm?ty=pbdetail&iid=5870>.

Office of Justice Programs: Bureau of justice statistics, *Stalking*, February 17, 2016. Available from: <https://www.bjs.gov/index-.cfm?ty=tp&tid=97>3.

Pearce N, Cross D, Monks H, Waters S, Falconer S: Current evidence of best practice in whole-school bullying intervention and its potential to inform cyberbullying interventions, *J of Psychologists and Counselors in Schools* 21(1):1–21, 2011.

Rape, Abuse, & Incest National Network: *Statistics*, 2016. Available from: <www.rainn.org/statistics>.

Substance Abuse and Mental Health Services Administration (SAMHSA): *Suicide and Race*, July 28, 2015. Available from: <https://blog.samhsa.gov/2015/07/28/suicide-and-race/#.WNrAWLhKYfw>.

The National Domestic Violence Hotline: What is safety planning? Available from <http://www.thehotline.org/help/path-to-safety/#types>.

The New York Society for the Prevention of Cruelty to Children, 2016. Available from. <www.nyspcc.org>.

United Nations Office on Drugs and Crimes. (UNODG): *Human Trafficking FAQ's*, 2017. Available from: <https://www.unodc.org/unodc/en/human-trafficking/faqs.html?>.

U.S. Department of Justice: Bureau of Justice Statistics, *Prisoners in 2015*, Dec, 2016. Available from: <https://www.bjs.gov/content/pub/pdf/p15.pdf>.

U.S. Department of Labor/ Bureau of Labor Statistics: *Occupational Injuries*, 2016. Available from: https://www.bls.gov/news.release/cfoi.nr0.htm.

U.S. Institute Against Human trafficking [usiaht]: *Human Trafficking in the US*, 2017. Available from: <http://usiaht.org/the-problem>.

Vera Institute of Justice: Screening for human trafficking, *Guidelines for Administering the Trafficking Victim Identification Tool*, June 2014. Available from: <http://archive.vera.org/sites/default/files/resources/downloads/human-trafficking-identification-tool-and-user-guidelines.pdf>.

Weinberger SE, Hoyt DB, Lawrence HC, et al.: Firearm-related injury and death in the United States: a call to action, *Ann Intern Med* 162:513–516, 2015.

World Health Organization: *Health topics. Violence*, 2017. Available from: <http://www.who.int/topics/violence/en/>.

Natural and Manmade Disasters

Elda G. Ramirez*

OBJECTIVES

Upon completion of this chapter, the reader will be able to do the following:

1. Identify the types of disasters.
2. Discuss the characteristics of disasters.
3. Describe the stages of a disaster.
4. Discuss the stages of disaster management.
5. Describe the roles of federal, state, local, and volunteer agencies involved in disaster management.
6. Identify potential bioterrorist chemical and biological agents.
7. Discuss the impact of disasters on a community.
8. Describe the role and responsibilities of nurses in relation to disasters.

KEY TERMS

American Red Cross
direct victim
disaster
disaster triage
displaced persons
Federal Emergency Management
   Agency
first responders
frequency
imminence

indirect victim
mass casualty
mitigation
multiple casualty
natech (natural-technological) disaster
National Incident Management System
National Response Framework
Office of Emergency Management
Predictability
Preventability

refugees
resource map
risk map
shelter in place
terrorism
U.S. Department of Homeland
   Security
weapon of mass destruction

Communities throughout the world experience an emergency or disaster incident of one kind or another almost daily. The media tracks events based on magnitude of disaster and effect on the community it serves. These events may be sensationalized, depending on the number of dead or injured, the amount of devastation or damage to the area involved, and how much the event has disrupted normal activities within the community.

The health of a community can be affected significantly by disasters. Hurricanes Harvey, Sandy, Katrina, and Rita are examples of how communities and their hospitals, clinics, nursing homes, and other health care facilities are directly affected by a disaster. During Katrina and Rita, both of which occurred in 2005, access to health care was impeded by physical barriers, such as road closures due to flooding, inadequate numbers of first responders, and limited transportation for search and rescue.

*The author would like to acknowledge the contribution of Edith B. Summerlin, who wrote this chapter for the previous edition.

Patients were evacuated from one hospital to another, sometimes more than once. Medical and nursing personnel, medicines, and needed supplies were unavailable, scarce, or depleted because of the increased demand. Temporary shelters and health care services were established in schools, churches, and a variety of other facilities throughout the area. The wind damage and extensive flooding from Hurricane Katrina resulted in panic for food, water, and rescue in the Gulf Coast regions between New Orleans, Louisiana, and Biloxi, Mississippi. First responders and rescue teams were overwhelmed in their attempts to reach the victims. The same was experienced during Hurricane Sandy, which devastated New York and New Jersey in 2012.

The evacuation of Houston, Texas, and the surrounding coastal area because of Hurricane Rita created severe traffic jams, many lasting 18 to 20 hours, so travelers needed water, food, and gasoline before they reached shelter. As a result, many people suffered from dehydration and urinary tract infections. In addition, Hurricane Rita occurred during a period of record heat, and many travelers became victims of heat exhaustion caused by the high temperature and humidity.

The lessons learned from these events resulted in changes in disaster plans that made a significant difference in how subsequent hurricanes were managed. In September 2017 Hurricane Harvey became the costliest natural disaster in U.S. history, after the release of more than 50 inches of rainfall in Houston, Texas, and surrounding areas. One third of the city of Houston was under water, and only 82 people lost their lives.

Hurricanes, tornadoes, floods, wildfires, and industrial accidents occur yearly in some parts of the United States. Fires in California in the month of October 2017 burned 245,000 acres and destroyed 8900 homes, and 42 people lost their lives. Communities then must deal with ash and other health hazards postburn. Further, in recent years, terrorist attacks have become more common. The bombings of the World Trade Center in New York City in 1991 and the bombing of the Alfred P. Murrah Federal Building in 1995 occurred two decades ago, but the combined terrorist attacks on the Twin Towers of the World Trade Center in New York City, the Pentagon in Washington, DC, the plane hijacking and crash in Pennsylvania in 2001, the Boston Marathon bombings in 2013, and the Orlando nightclub shooting in 2016 indicate that the potential is ever present. Additionally, terrorist attacks occur all over the world on an almost daily basis, and concerns about potential terrorist attacks have increased the focus on what needs to be done in terms of prevention/mitigation, preparedness, response, and recovery—not only in the event of terrorist attacks but also in the event of disasters of all kinds (Federal Bureau of Investigation [FBI], 2017).

Because of the recognition of the need to be prepared, programs have been created to address the national, state, and local management of disasters. President George W. Bush established the U.S. Department of Homeland Security (DHS) in March 2003 and put into place the National Incident Management System (NIMS) the following year. The NIMS provides a systematic, proactive way for all levels of governmental and nongovernmental agencies to work seamlessly to prevent, protect against, respond to, recover from, and prevent the effects of disasters (Federal Emergency Management Agency [FEMA], 2017a). Local Citizen Corps Councils have been established throughout the country to give volunteers an opportunity to support local fire, law enforcement, emergency medical services, and community public health efforts and to contribute to the four stages of emergency management: prevention, preparedness, response, and recovery (Ready.gov, 2017).

Efforts to prepare for disasters have also been significantly enhanced at the state level. In 2003, for example, the Texas Legislature passed a bill requiring nurses to attend a continuing education program related to bioterrorism. Further, the Ready Texas Nurses Emergency Response System (Ready Texas Nurses) was created to allow mobilization of volunteer nurses to support communities in times of crisis or disaster. Similar actions are occurring throughout the country.

Nurses have both a personal and a professional role in relation to disasters. Nurses' personal role is to develop a disaster plan for work, home, and family. Disaster kits for survival in each of these settings should be prepared. Professionally nurses are uniquely positioned to provide valuable information for the development of plans for disaster prevention, preparedness, response, and recovery for the facilities in which they are employed as well as the communities in which they live. Nurses, as team members, can cooperate with health and social representatives, government bodies, community groups, and volunteer agencies in disaster planning and preparedness programs (e.g., drills). Using their knowledge of nursing, public health, and cultural-familial structures, as well as their clinical skills and abilities, nurses can actively assist with or participate in all aspects and stages of an emergency or disaster, regardless of the setting in which the event may occur. Disaster nursing requires the application of basic nursing knowledge and skills in difficult environments with scare resources and changing conditions.

DISASTER DEFINITIONS

A **disaster** is any event that causes a level of destruction, death, or injury that affects the abilities of the community to respond to the incident using available resources. Emergencies differ from disasters, in that agencies, communities, families, or individuals can manage emergencies using their own resources. But a disaster event, depending on the characteristics of the disaster, may be beyond the ability of the community to respond and recover from the incident using its own resources. Disasters frequently require assistance from outside the immediate community, both for management of resulting issues and for recovery.

Some disasters (e.g., a house fire) may affect only a few persons, whereas others (e.g., a hurricane) can affect thousands. A **mass casualty** event is one in which 100 or more individuals are involved; a **multiple casualty** event is one in which more than 2 but fewer than 100 individuals are involved. A casualty can be classified as a direct victim, an indirect victim, a displaced person, or a refugee. A **direct victim** is an individual who is

BOX 29.1 Types of Disasters

Natural Disasters
- Avalanches
- Blizzards
- Communicable disease epidemics
- Droughts, wildfires
- Earthquakes, tsunamis
- Hailstorms
- Heat waves
- Hurricanes
- Tornadoes, cyclones
- Volcanic eruptions

Manmade Disasters
- Terrorism
- Civil unrest (riots)
- Explosions, bombings
- Fires
- Structural collapse (bridges)
- Floods, mudslides
- Toxic or hazardous spills
- Mass transit accidents
- Pollution
- Wars

immediately affected by the event; the **indirect victim** may be a family member or friend of the victim or a first responder. Displaced persons and refugees are special categories of direct victims. **Displaced persons** are those who have to evacuate their homes, schools, or businesses as a result of a disaster; **refugees** are a group of people who have fled their homes or even their country as a result of famine, drought, natural disaster, war, or civil unrest.

TYPES OF DISASTERS

Disasters are identified as natural, manmade, or a combination of both. A **natech (natural-technological) disaster** is a natural disaster that creates or results in a widespread technological problem. An example of a natech disaster is an earthquake that causes structural collapse of roadways or bridges, which, in turn, leads to downed electrical wires and subsequent fires. Another example is a chemical spill resulting from a flood. Types of natural disasters and manmade disasters are listed in Box 29.1.

The American Public Health Association identified types of disasters and their consequences (Landesman and Burke, 2017). Types of disasters are blizzards, cold waves, heavy snowfalls, cyclones, tornadoes, drought, earthquakes, floods, heat waves, thunderstorms, volcanic eruptions, wildfires, manmade and technological events, explosions or blasts, and epidemics. It was noted in the report that injury or death from the disaster in question may be direct or indirect. For example, injuries from hurricanes occur because people fail to evacuate or take shelter, do not take precautions in securing their property despite adequate warning, and do not follow guidelines on food and water safety or injury prevention during recovery.

Drowning, electrocution, lacerations or punctures from flying debris, and blunt trauma from falling trees or other objects are some of the morbidity concerns. Heart attacks and stress-related disorders also occur. In addition, injuries may occur from activities in the recovery phase, for example, from use of chain saws or other power equipment or from animal, snake, or insect bites.

Americans are familiar with most of the disasters listed in Box 29.1, but terrorism was largely unknown or unheeded before the bombing of the Alfred P. Murrah Federal Building in Oklahoma City in 1995. The U.S. Code of Federal Regulations defines **terrorism** as violent acts or acts dangerous to human life that appear to be intended to intimidate or coerce the civilian population or to influence the policy or conduct of a government (18 U.S. CFR § 2331, 1992). The FBI is charged with the responsibility for investigating terrorism-related matters in the United States and internationally. According to the Central Intelligence Agency (2013), terrorism "is premeditated, politically motivated violence perpetrated against noncombatant targets by sub-national groups or clandestine agents." International terrorism involves the territory or the citizens of more than one country (p. 1).

Specific incidents of terrorism include the September 11, 2001, terrorist attacks; bombing of the Alfred P. Murrah Federal Building, 1995; the nerve gas (sarin) attack in the Tokyo subway in March 1995, which killed 12 and injured more than 6000 people; the bombing of the commuter train in Spain in March 2004, which killed 191 people; the suicide bombings in the London transport system in July 2005, which killed 52 commuters and four terrorists; the shooting and bombing attacks in the financial district of Mumbai, India, in November 2008, which killed more than 170; an attack in a Paris theater and nearby neighborhoods in November 2015 that resulted in 137 deaths and injured 368, and a vehicle attack in Nice, France, in July 2016 that killed 86 and injured 434.

In the United States since 2015, there have multiple terrorist attacks. In December 2015, 14 people were killed in a mass shooting at a health center in San Bernardino, California; in June 2016, 49 people were killed and 58 wounded in a nightclub in Orlando, Florida; and in October 2017, 8 people died in New York City when a man drove a rented truck down a crowded bike path.

Concerns now are increasingly focused on weapons of mass destruction. **Weapon of mass destruction** refers to any weapon that is designed or intended to cause death or serious bodily injury through release, dissemination, or impact of toxic or poisonous chemicals, or their precursors; any weapon involving a disease organism; or any weapon that is designed to release radiation or radioactivity at a level dangerous to human life. Biological organisms considered to be potential weapons of mass destruction are shown in Box 29.2, and chemicals that are potential weapons of mass destruction are listed in Table 29.1. Chemical warfare agents are classified as nerve agents, vesicants, pulmonary agents, and cyanides (formerly "blood agents"). These tables also include information about the lethality, treatment, and impact related to each.

BOX 29.2 Bioterrorism Agents/Diseases

Category A

High-priority agents include organisms that pose a risk to national security because they:

- Can be easily disseminated or transmitted from person to person
- Result in high mortality rates and have the potential for major public health impact
- Might cause public panic and social disruption
- Require special action for public health preparedness

Agents/Diseases

- Anthrax (Bacillus anthracis)
- Botulism (Clostridium botulinum toxin)
- Plague (Yersinia pestis)
- Smallpox (Variola major)
- Tularemia (Francisella tularensis)
- Viral hemorrhagic fevers (filoviruses [e.g., Ebola, Marburg]) and arenaviruses [e.g., Lassam, Nacgyoi])

Category B

Second-highest-priority agents include those that:

- Are moderately easy to disseminate
- Result in moderate morbidity rates and low mortality rates
- Require specific enhancements of CDC's diagnostic capacity and enhanced disease surveillance

Agents/Diseases

- Brucellosis (Brucella species)
- Epsilon toxin of Clostridium perfringens
- Food safety threats (e.g., Salmonella species, Escherichia coli 0157:H7, Shigella)

Category C

Third-highest-priority agents include emerging pathogens that could be engineered for mass dissemination in the future because of:

- Availability
- Ease of production and dissemination
- Potential for high morbidity and mortality rates and major health impact

Agents

- Emerging infectious diseases such as Nipah virus and hantavirus

Data from National Center for Environment Health (NCEI): http://www.cdc.gov/nceh/; Agency for Toxic Substances and Disease Registry (ATSDR): http://www.atsdr.cdc.gov/; and National Center for Injury and Violence Prevention and Control (NCIPC): http://www.cdc.gov/injury/.

TABLE 29.1 Chemical Agents of Mass Destruction

Chemical Agent	Lethality	Treatment	Impact
Sarin (nerve agent)	High	Move to fresh air; wash skin; drugs have limited effectiveness	Likely nerve agent; chemicals needed to produce are banned by International Chemical Weapons Convention
VX (nerve agent)	Very high	Move to fresh air; wash skin; drugs have limited effectiveness	Not likely weapon; difficult to manufacture
Tabun (nerve agent)	High	Move to fresh air; wash skin; drugs have limited effectiveness	Easy-to-manufacture nerve agent; likely agent to be used
Chlorine (pulmonary agent)	Low	Move to fresh air; wash skin; no antidote	Readily available; likely agent because of availability; breaks down with water
Hydrogen cyanide (blood agent)	Low to moderate	Move to fresh air; wash skin; some drugs mitigate effects	Industrial product; some chemicals used to produce it are banned; likely agent because of availability

Modified from Cieslak TJ, Eitzen EM: Bioterrorism: agents of concern, *J Public Health Manag Pract* 6(4):19–29, 2000.

BOX 29.3 Characteristics of Disasters

- Frequency
- Predictability
- Preventability
- Imminence
- Scope and number of casualties
- Intensity

CHARACTERISTICS OF DISASTERS

Several characteristics have been used to describe disasters (Box 29.3). These characteristics are interdependent and therefore important to consider in plans for managing any disaster event. Each is discussed briefly.

Frequency

Frequency refers to how often a disaster occurs. Some disasters occur relatively often in certain parts of the world. Terrorist activities are occurring on an almost daily basis in Iraq and elsewhere in the world. Other examples are hurricanes, which occur with variable frequency between the months of June and November in the Northern Hemisphere, and earthquakes, which occur periodically throughout the world. In the United States, earthquakes are generally considered to be a West Coast problem, but 45 states and territories are at moderate to high risk for an earthquake, and earthquakes have occurred in every region of the country (DHS, 2016a). Other disasters, such as volcanic eruptions, are far less frequent and are geographically limited to certain regions.

Predictability

Predictability relates to the ability to determine when and whether a disaster event will occur. Some disasters, such as floods, may be predicted in the spring through monitoring of the snowmelt. Weather forecasters can predict when conditions are right for the development of tornadoes; these generally occur between April and June, but they may occur at any time of the year or as secondary results of hurricanes. Weather forecasters can predict hurricanes with increasing accuracy. Other disasters (e.g., fires and industrial explosions) may not be predictable at all.

Preventability/Mitigation

Mitigation refers to actions taken to reduce loss of life and property by lessening the impact of disasters. It means taking action now—before the next disaster—to reduce human and financial consequences (FEMA, 2017b). Preventability assumes that all disasters are not inevitable and steps can be taken to prevent them. Some disasters (e.g., hurricanes, tornadoes, and earthquakes) are not preventable, whereas others can be easily controlled, if not prevented entirely. For example, flooding can be controlled or prevented through construction of dams or levees or deepening bayous.

Primary prevention is aimed at preventing the occurrence of a disaster or limiting consequences when the event itself cannot be prevented (mitigation). Primary prevention occurs in the nondisaster and predisaster stages. The *nondisaster stage* is the period before a disaster occurs, and the *predisaster stage* is the time when a disaster is pending. Preventive actions during the nondisaster stage include assessing communities to determine potential disaster hazards; developing disaster plans at local, state, and federal levels; conducting drills to test the plan; training volunteers and health care providers; and providing educational programs of all kinds.

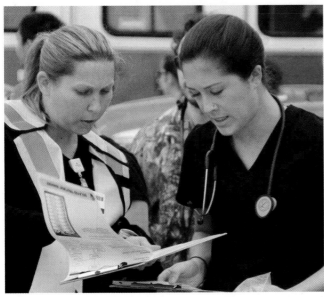

Two emergency nurses in "incident command" for a mass casualty drill in the nondisaster stage.

Risk maps and resource maps are developed to aid in planning. A **risk map** is a geographic map of an area that is analyzed for the impact of a potential disaster on the population and buildings in the area that would be involved (e.g., an area in a flood plain, an area covered if a nuclear explosion would occur, an area involved in an explosion of an industrial site) (Fig. 29.1). A **resource map** is a geographic map that outlines the resources that would be available in or near the area affected by a potential disaster (e.g., potential shelter sites, potential medical sources, and location of equipment that might be needed) (Fig. 29.2).

The disaster plan is initiated predisaster, or when a disaster is imminent. Primary prevention actions during this stage include notifying the appropriate officials, warning the population, and advising what response to take (e.g., voluntary or mandatory evacuation).

Secondary prevention strategies are implemented once the disaster occurs. They are actions aimed at preventing further injury or destruction. Safety is considered before search and rescue.

Tertiary prevention focuses on recovery of the community—that is, restoring the community to its previous level of functioning and its residents to their maximum functioning. Tertiary prevention is aimed at preventing a recurrence or minimizing the effects of future disasters through debriefing meetings to identify problems with the plan and make revisions.

Nurses should be involved in all stages of prevention and related activities. In order to respond effectively, personally, and professionally during different types of disasters, nurses need to know (1) what kind of disasters threaten their communities, (2) what injuries to expect from different disaster scenarios, (3) evacuation routes, (4) locations of shelters, and (5) warning systems. They must be able to educate others about disasters and how to prepare for and respond to them. Finally, nurses need to keep up to date on the latest recommendations and advances in lifesaving measures (e.g., basic first aid, cardiopulmonary resuscitation [CPR], and use of automated external defibrillators).

Imminence

Imminence is the speed of onset of an impending disaster and relates to the extent of forewarning possible and the anticipated duration of the incident. Weather forecasters can tell when a hurricane may be developing days ahead of its expected arrival and can give the time of arrival, the general direction it will take, and an approximate location for its landing and forward movement. Hurricanes, however, are subject to other weather variables and can change direction and intensity several times before making landfall. A warning for a hurricane means it will reach landfall in 24 hours or less, whereas a watch means it will reach landfall in 24 to 36 hours. A warning for tornadoes means to take shelter immediately, and a watch means to stay alert for possible tornadoes.

Some disastrous incidents (e.g., wildfires, explosions, and terrorist attacks) have no warning time. Bioterrorist attacks are generally silent, and the first awareness may be days or even weeks after exposure. For example, individuals exposed to a pathologic agent (e.g., anthrax, smallpox) may arrive at health care facilities at various times and to various providers, making diagnosis and early treatment difficult. Nurses and medical personnel need to know the signs and symptoms of biological, chemical, radiation, and nuclear exposure in order to identify the nature of the threat, report the problem to the Centers for Disease Control and Prevention (CDC), and then treat and control the spread of both biological and chemical agents (see Box 29.2 and Table 29.1).

Scope and Number of Casualties

The *scope* of a disaster indicates the range of its effect. The scope is described in terms of both the geographic area involved and the number of individuals affected, injured, or killed. From a health care perspective, the location, type, and timing of a disaster event are predictors of the types of injuries and illnesses that might occur. For example, the October 1989 earthquake in San Francisco occurred while people were on their way to work. Overall, more than 60 people died from a multitude of causes, including a motorcycle officer who was killed after the collapse of a freeway, 16 people who were killed by building collapses, 5 who died as a result of falls, and 9 who died of heart attacks.

In contrast, the earthquake and tsunami in December 2004 killed more than 174,000 people in South Asia, Southeast Asia, and East Africa; most died of drowning (CDC, 2017). Another example of the horribly destructive power of earthquakes is the

FIG. 29.1 Community risk map.

Haitian quake of 2010, which resulted in the death of more than 160,000 people and displacement of more than a million.

Hurricanes generally affect a large geographic area. Nevertheless, they may cause few, if any, deaths if sufficient preventive measures are taken. The scope of Hurricane Katrina in September 2005 covered all of New Orleans; most of south Louisiana; and parts of Florida, Alabama, and Mississippi. Hurricane Rita, only a few days later, struck New Orleans again as well as south Louisiana and much of eastern Texas. Remarkably, despite the widespread destruction caused by these storms, the number of dead from Katrina was more than 1300, and the number of dead from Hurricane Rita was 58, including 23 elders who were killed in a bus accident while evacuating. As mentioned previously, Hurricanes Sandy (2012) and Harvey (2017) were much more destructive but resulted in many fewer deaths. Much of the improvement in loss of life can be attributed to better preparation and timely notifications, allowing for evacuations.

Intensity

Intensity is the characteristic describing the level of destruction and devastation of the disaster event. Factors contributing to the amount of damage from a disaster event such as a hurricane are the distance from the zone of maximum winds, how exposed the location is, building standards, vegetation type, and resultant flooding. Parts of New Orleans were under water from the primary effects (storm surge and rain) and secondary effects (levee failure) of Hurricane Katrina. Some buildings and homes were completely destroyed, and others were left in terrible condition by flooding and wind damage.

Various hurricane and tornado scales have been developed on the basis of wind intensity and predicted level of destruction. The Fujita Tornado Intensity Scale, developed in 1971, categorized each tornado by its intensity and the area involved. In 1992, Fujita updated the scale to include an estimate of F-scale damage. The new scale, the Enhanced Fujita Scale (EF Scale), implemented in the United States on February 1, 2007, is still a set of wind estimates (not measurements) based on types of structural damage. The estimates vary with the height of apparent damage above the ground and exposure (National Oceanic and Atmospheric Administration, 2017).

Hurricanes have been categorized since 1975 with use of the Saffir-Simpson Hurricane Scale, which includes sustained wind intensity, storm surge ranges, and flooding references. On an

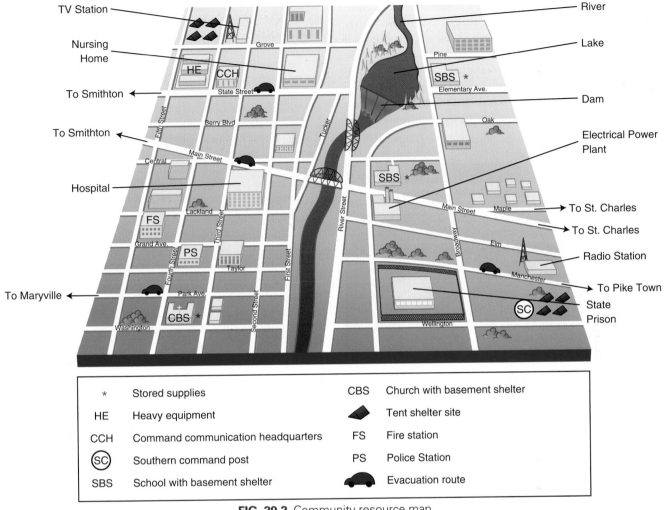

FIG. 29.2 Community resource map.

*	Stored supplies	CBS	Church with basement shelter
HE	Heavy equipment		Tent shelter site
CCH	Command communication headquarters	FS	Fire station
SC	Southern command post	PS	Police Station
SBS	School with basement shelter		Evacuation route

BOX 29.4 The Saffir-Simpson Hurricane Wind Scale

- *Category 1* (74–95 mph): Very dangerous winds will produce some damage.
- *Category 2* (96–110 mph): Extremely dangerous winds will cause extensive damage.
- *Category 3* (111–129 mph): Devastating damage will occur.
- *Category 4* (130–156 mph): Catastrophic damage will occur.
- *Category 5* (157 mph or higher): Catastrophic damage will occur.

Data from National Oceanic and Atmospheric Administration National Weather Service, National Hurricane Center: *Saffir-Simpson hurricane wind scale*, 2017. http://www.nhc.noaa.gov/aboutsshws.php.

experimental basis for the 2009 tropical cyclone season, the storm surge ranges and flooding references were removed for each of the five categories (Box 29.4) because storm surge information is inaccurate. For example, Hurricane Ike in 2008 was a category 2 hurricane but had a storm surge at Galveston, Texas, equivalent to a category 4 to 5 storm surge, and Hurricane Katrina in 2007 was a category 3 hurricane with a storm surge equivalent to a category 5. The scale was revised in 2012 and is now called the *Saffir-Simpson Hurricane Wind Scale*. The new scale does not include storm surge, rainfall-induced floods, and tornadoes (National Oceanic and Atmospheric Administration, 2017).

? ACTIVE LEARNING

Assess the community where you live for potential disasters that could result in mass casualties. What disasters are predictable? Are there measures that can be taken to prevent or minimize injuries, death, or destruction?

DISASTER MANAGEMENT

When one is aware of the types and characteristics of disasters, the question then becomes: What can be done to prevent/mitigate, prepare for, respond to, and recover from disasters? Disaster management requires an interdisciplinary, collaborative team effort and involves a network of agencies and individuals to develop a disaster plan that covers the multiple elements necessary for an effective plan. Communities can respond more quickly, more effectively, and with less confusion if the efforts needed in the event of a disaster have been anticipated and plans for meeting them identified. The result of planning is that more lives are saved and less property is damaged. Planning ensures that resources are available and that roles and responsibilities of all personnel and agencies, both official and unofficial, are delineated.

Nurses need to know their personal, professional, and community responsibilities. They should realize that conflicts may arise between their personal and professional responsibilities if they have not been considered and planned for in advance (see the Ethical Insights box). Also, nurses may be direct or indirect victims and may even be displaced persons as a result of a disaster event. Recognizing this possibility, nurses need to plan, prepare, practice, and teach their family and significant others how to respond.

ETHICAL INSIGHTS

Deciding Whether to Care for Family or Care for Patients

During a disaster, a nurse might face an ethical dilemma because of competing responsibilities to self, family, employer, and patients. For example, a nurse who is a single parent with young children and has a limited support system may be forced to decide between her responsibility to care for her children and a mandate to report to work to care for patients. Choosing may result in loss of employment or danger to the children. Potential conflicts such as this should be considered and discussed and decisions made in conjunction with the employer before a disaster event.

Local, State, and Federal Governmental Responsibilities

Local Government

The local government is responsible for the safety and welfare of its citizens. Emergencies and disaster incidents are handled at the lowest possible organizational and jurisdictional level. Police, fire, public health, public works, and medical emergency services are the **first responders**, responsible for incident management at the local level. Local officials and agencies are responsible for preparing their citizens for all kinds of emergencies and disasters and for testing disaster plans with mock drills. They manage events during an incident by carrying out evacuation, search and rescue, and maintaining public health and public works responsibilities. Local communities should have contingency operation plans for multiple disaster situations and for various aspects of the plan. For example, landline telephone service and cell phone service may not work because of being restricted for emergency use only or damage to the infrastructure, so other forms of communication need to be available.

In an incident other than a biological, chemical, radiation, or nuclear event, in most cases, it is the 911 communication center or the fire or police department that gets the initial message. The emergency communication center then communicates the incident to the other first responders and the director of the **Office of Emergency Management**, who determines what others may be needed (e.g., ambulances, other officials, and voluntary group representatives). Local hospitals are notified of the incident and the predicted nature of impending casualties. The hospitals may begin to receive victims via private automobiles who have not been triaged at the site of the incident. According to the CDC, a hospital can assess the expected number of victims that it may receive by counting the number that arrive within the first hour and doubling it.

BOX 29.5 Guidelines for Early Detection of Biochemical Terrorist Incidents

- A rapidly increasing disease incidence (within hours or days) in a normally healthy population.
- An unusual increase in the number of people seeking care, especially with fever, respiratory, or gastrointestinal complaints.
- An endemic disease rapidly emerging at an uncharacteristic time or in an unusual pattern.
- Clusters of patients arriving from a single locale.
- Large numbers of rapidly fatal cases—patients who die within 72 hours after admission to the hospital.
- Any patient presenting with a disease that is relatively uncommon and has bioterrorism potential (e.g., pulmonary anthrax, smallpox, or plague).

From Chettle C: Recognizing bioterrorism: nurses on the frontline, *NurseWeek* 6:29–30, 2001.

For a biological or chemical terrorist incident, the process is very different. First responders generally are not involved. Rather, nurses and doctors in health care facilities may be the first to suspect that a biological or chemical agent has been released into the community. Box 29.5 lists the guidelines for detecting biochemical incidents. If any of these instances occur in a health care provider setting, the suspicion should be immediately reported to the infection control department, the administration of the facility, or both. Each setting should post near the telephone the numbers to be called if a biochemical incident (whether internal or external) is suspected. These numbers should include those of the CDC Bioterrorism Emergency Response, the CDC Hospital Infections program, and the U.S. Army Medical Research Institute of Infectious Diseases (Chettle, 2001).

The Office of Emergency Management involves representatives from all official and unofficial agencies in developing the community disaster plan; developing scenarios to test the plan through drills; and assessing the scope, intensity, and number of casualties once an incident has occurred in order to initiate the proper response. For those events that are not within the abilities of the local community or in the event of a terrorist-type incident, higher-level agencies and resources must be requested and will become involved.

State Government

When a disaster overwhelms the local community's resources, the state's Department or Office of Emergency Management is called for assistance. Before such an event, state officials provide technical support for prevention, preparedness, response, and recovery. State officials visit local officials to assist and assess local emergency management plans, promote and conduct workshops and training courses, help with training exercises, advise and support local government officials, and are on scene at disaster events to facilitate coordination of state resources and to disseminate information. In some cases, the National Guard may be called in to aid the community. When the scope of the event is so great that local and state resources are not adequate to meet the needs, the state calls on the federal government; at that point, the president may declare the incident a "national disaster." Once the president declares a national disaster, federal aid is made available. The **National Response Framework** is the core operational

> **BOX 29.6 Operational and Support Components that Make Up the Department of Homeland Security**
>
> United States Citizenship and Immigration Services (USCIS)
> United States Customs and Border Protection (CBP)
> United States Coast Guard (USCG)
> Federal Emergency Management Agency (FEMA)
> Federal Law Enforcement Training Center (FLETC)
> United States Immigration and Customs Enforcement (ICE)
> United States Secret Service (USSS)
> Transportation Security Administration (TSA)
> Directorate for Management
> National Protection and Programs Directorate
> Domestic Nuclear Detection Office
> Science and Technology Directorate
> Office of Health Affairs
>
> U.S. Department of Homeland Security: *Operational and support components*, 2017. https://www.dhs.gov/operational-and-support-components.

> **BOX 29.7 Federal Emergency Management Agency Recommendations for Basic Disaster Supplies Kit**
>
> - Three-day supply of nonperishable food
> - Three-day supply of water—one gallon of water per person, per day
> - Portable, battery-powered radio or television and extra batteries
> - Flashlight and extra batteries
> - First aid kit and manual
> - Sanitation and hygiene items (moist towelettes and toilet paper)
> - Matches and waterproof container
> - Whistle
> - Extra clothing
> - Kitchen accessories and cooking utensils, including a can opener
> - Photocopies of credit and identification cards
> - Cash and coins
> - Special needs item, such as prescription medications, eye glasses, contact lens solution, and hearing aid batteries
> - Items for infants, such as formula, diapers, bottles, and pacifiers
> - Other items to meet your unique family needs
> - If you live in a cold climate, you must think about warmth. Be sure to include one complete change of clothing and shoes per person, including:
>   - Jacket or coat
>   - Long pants
>   - Long-sleeve shirt
>   - Sturdy shoes
>   - Hat, mittens, and scarf
>   - Sleeping bag or warm blanket (per person)
>
> https://www.ready.gov/build-a-kit

plan for domestic incident management for an all-hazards response. It describes best practices for managing incidents "that range from the serious but purely local, to large-scale terrorist attacks or catastrophic natural disasters" (DHS 2016a).

Federal Government

U.S. Department of Homeland Security. As previously mentioned, the U.S. Department of Homeland Security was established in March 2003 to realign the existing federal departments, agencies, groups, and organizations into a single department focused on protecting the American people and their homeland.

There are five homeland security missions: (1) prevent terrorism and enhance security; (2) secure and manage U.S. borders; (3) enforce and administer immigration laws; (4) safeguard and secure cyberspace; and (5) ensure resilience to disasters (DHS, 2016b).

The organizational structure of the DHS has several divisions, and within each of these divisions are multiple offices and centers, listed in Box 29.6.

The DHS established its Homeland Security Advisory System to build a comprehensive and effective communication structure for disseminating threat information to public safety officials and the public at large. The previous color-coded threat level system has been replaced with the National Terrorism Advisory System. "The system provides timely, detailed information to the public, government agencies, first responders, airports and other transportation hubs, and the private sector" (DHS, 2017). The threat alert indicates whether there is an elevated threat (no specific information about timing or location) or imminent threat (impending or very soon). DHS (2017) has published a public guide with recommended steps that individuals, communities, businesses, and governments can take to help prevent, mitigate, or respond to the threat.

FEMA (2017c) has published an in-depth guide for citizen preparedness, *Are You Ready?* The focus of the contents is on how to prepare, practice, and maintain emergency plans that indicate what must be done before, during, and after a disaster. The guide explains how to prepare disaster supplies sufficient in quantity for individuals and families to survive (Box 29.7).

Additionally, *Are You Ready?* lists specific natural hazards, technological hazards, and terrorism incidents with detailed information on what to do in each incident (Box 29.8). Nurses could use this guide in developing educational programs and disaster plans related to natural and manmade disasters to which individuals, families, or communities may be exposed.

The DHS has presented a national preparedness goal. The goal is "a secure and resilient nation with the capabilities required across the whole community to prevent, protect against, mitigate, respond to, and recover from the threats and hazards that pose the greatest risk." The risks cited include natural disaster, pandemic, chemical spills, terrorist attacks, and cyberattacks. The plan identifies and elaborates on the "core capabilities" and target necessary to achieve preparedness across five mission areas: prevention, protection, mitigation, response, and recovery (DHS, 2016c). Thirty-one core capabilities needed to achieve the goal have been identified where they most logically fit. Materials to enhance the capabilities are available from the DHS.

The Federal Emergency Management Agency. The Federal Emergency Management Agency became part of DHS in 2003. FEMA's mission is to support citizens and first responders to ensure that as a nation, everyone works together to build, sustain, and improve the capacity to prepare for, protect against, respond to, recover from, and mitigate all hazards. In 2006, President George W. Bush signed into law the Post-Katrina Emergency Reform Act (PL 109-295). The act significantly reorganized FEMA, giving it substantial new authority to remedy gaps that became apparent in the response to Hurricane Katrina in 2005 (FEMA, 2017b).

BOX 29.8 What to Do in Different Types of Emergencies

Biological Attack

- Move away quickly.
- Wash with soap and water.
- Contact authorities.
- Listen to the media for official instructions.
- Seek medical attention if you become sick.

Nuclear Blast

- Do not look at the flash or fireball—it can blind you.
- Take cover behind anything that might offer protection.
- Lie flat on the ground and cover your head. If the explosion is some distance away, it could take 30 seconds or more for the blast to hit.
- Take shelter as soon as you can, even if you are many miles from ground zero—where the attack occurred; radioactive fallout can be carried by the winds for hundreds of miles. Remember the three protective factors: distance, shielding, and time.

Chemical Attack

- If you are instructed to remain in your home or office building, you should:
  - Close doors and windows and turn off all ventilation, including furnaces, air conditioners, vents, and fans.
  - Seek shelter in an internal room and take your disaster supplies kit.
  - Seal the room with duct tape and plastic sheeting.
  - Listen to your radio for instructions from authorities.
- If you are caught in or near a contaminated area, you should:
  - Move away immediately in a direction upwind of the source.
  - Find shelter as quickly as possible.

Radiation Dispersion Device Event
Outdoors

- Seek shelter indoors immediately in the nearest building.
- If appropriate shelter is not available, move as rapidly as is safe upwind and away from the location of the explosive blast. Then seek appropriate shelter as soon as possible.
- Listen for official instructions and follow directions.

Indoors

- If you have time, turn off ventilation and heating systems, and close windows, vents, fireplace dampers, exhaust fans, and clothes dryer vents. Retrieve your disaster supplies kit and a battery-powered radio, and take them to your shelter room.
- Seek shelter immediately, preferably underground or in an interior room of a building, placing as much distance and dense shielding as possible between you and the outdoors where the radioactive material may be.
- Seal windows and external doors that do not fit snugly with duct tape to reduce infiltration of radioactive particles. Plastic sheeting will not provide shielding from radioactivity or from blast effects of a nearby explosion.
- Listen for official instructions, and follow directions.

Explosions

- If there is an explosion, you should:
  - Get under a sturdy table or desk if things are falling around you.
  - When they stop falling, leave quickly, watching for obviously weakened floors and stairways.
  - As you exit from the building, be especially watchful of falling debris.
  - Leave the building as quickly as possible. Do not stop to retrieve personal possessions or make phone calls.
- Do not use elevator. Once you are out:
  - Do not stand in front of windows, glass doors, or other potentially hazardous areas.
  - Move away from sidewalks or streets to be used by emergency officials or others still exiting the building.
- If you are trapped in debris:
  - If possible, use a flashlight to signal your location to rescuers.
  - Avoid unnecessary movement so you don't kick up dust.
  - Cover your nose and mouth with anything you have on hand. (Dense-weave cotton material can act as a good filter. Try to breathe through the material).
  - Tap on a pipe or wall so rescuers can hear where you are.
  - If possible, use a whistle to signal rescuers.
  - Shout only as a last resort. Shouting can cause a person to inhale dangerous amounts of dust.

Modified from Federal Emergency Management Agency: *Are you ready? An in-depth guide to citizen preparedness*, 2004. https://www.fema.gov/pdf/areyouready/areyouready_full.pdf.

Puerto Rican survivors of Hurricane Maria meet with FEMA and U.S. Small Business Administration officials inside a baseball stadium serving as a disaster recovery center, October 2017. (Photo by Stephen Shepard.)

The close-knit community of Breezy Point, New York, lost more than 100 homes to fire during Hurricane Sandy. FEMA is providing ongoing support and resources to the Queens, New York community. (Photo by Andre R. Aragon/FEMA.)

Centers for Disease Control and Prevention. After the rescue of survivors has been accomplished, the Department of Health and Human Services and sometimes the CDC conducts surveillance to ensure that clean drinking water, food, shelter, and medical care are available for those affected. Whether CDC's involvement is necessary depends on the type of disaster. For example, floods pose risks of contaminated water (e.g., cholera) and food supplies (e.g., *Escherichia coli*); loss of shelter leaves people vulnerable to heat or cold and other environmental hazards (e.g., insects); and earthquakes create traumatic injuries (e.g., broken bones, head injuries) that will need to be addressed.

Public Health System

The public health system's mission is the promotion of health, prevention of disease, and protection from threats to health. *Public health system* is a broad term used to describe all of the governmental and nongovernmental organizations and agencies that contribute to the improvement of the health of populations. Public health agencies are the primary agencies for the health and medical responses to disaster incidents and therefore are a part of the initial response activities.

Public health officials provide advice and assistance to other public officials on environmental and health matters. Preparedness includes surveillance and reporting of suspicious illnesses (e.g., signs and symptoms of biological agents, foodborne diseases, and communicable diseases) in the community by physicians and nurses in local health care facilities or private offices and clinics. Public health officials then have the responsibility of detecting outbreaks, determining the cause of illness, identifying the risk factors for the population, implementing interventions to control the outbreak, and informing the public of the health risks and preventive measures that need to be taken. These activities relate both directly and indirectly to the 10 essential public health services described in Chapter 1.

📋 NURSING CARE GUIDELINES

Role of Nurses in Disaster

Role of Nurses in Disaster "When disaster strikes, nurses form the backbone of our nations' health care response" (RWJF, 2016). Indeed, as Deputy Surgeon General, Rear Admiral, Sylvia Trent-Adams, PhD, RN, noted: "Nurses play an essential role in our nation's ability to prepare for, respond to, and recover from disasters." A new report from the Robert Wood Johnson Foundation highlights how nurses contributed to saving lives during three of the country's recent disasters: the Ebola outbreak, the Joplin, Missouri tornado, and Hurricane Sandy. The report describes how nurses worked within disaster teams to meet both immediate and long-term care needs.

Review the report (the link is provided at the end) to recognize the importance of nurses being prepared to respond during multiple types of disasters and to be encouraged by the leadership of nurses during very challenging circumstances.

https://www.rwjf.org/content/dam/farm/reports/issue_briefs/2016/rwjf429036

American Red Cross

The American Red Cross (ARC or Red Cross) is not a governmental agency. It is, however, chartered by Congress to provide disaster relief. The ARC works in partnership with FEMA; DHS; the CDC; and other local, state, and federal agencies to provide and manage needed services (ARC, 2017).

The ARC is primarily a volunteer organization with chapters in all 50 states, Puerto Rico, the Virgin Islands, and the Pacific Rim; its national headquarters is in Washington, DC. Disaster Services is only one of the programs that this agency provides. Others are International Services; Biomedical Services; Armed Forces Emergency Services; and Health, Safety, and Community Services.

The Red Cross places great emphasis on preparedness and participates with communities in developing and testing their disaster plans, maintaining and training personnel for disaster response, and responding during an actual emergency or disaster. The ARC publishes many pamphlets and educational materials to help individuals, families, neighborhoods, schools, and businesses prepare for potential disasters. The key actions the agency recommends are (1) identify potential disaster events, (2) create a disaster plan for sheltering in place or for evacuation, (3) assemble a disaster supplies kit, and (4) practice and maintain the plan. The disaster plan should include an emergency communications plan, a predetermined meeting place for family members or significant others, and plans for care of pets in the event that evacuation is required.

The Red Cross disaster response efforts focus on meeting the immediate disaster-related needs of affected people and providing support services to the emergency rescue and recovery workers (ARC, 2012). The disaster response functions are to provide health services, mental health services, family services, and mass care and to inquire about family well-being. Mass care involves feeding, sheltering, providing basic first aid, bulk distribution, and a Disaster Welfare Information system (ARC, 2012).

❓ ACTIVE LEARNING

- Find out who is responsible for disaster management in your community. What plans are in place for warning people and for communicating which actions to take in the event of a disaster? Are the people aware of these plans?
- Interview the person or persons in the ARC responsible for disaster services in your area. What is the role of their disaster nurses? What are the requirements to become a disaster nurse for the ARC?
- Speak with police and fire department personnel about their responsibilities during a disaster. Do their roles during a disaster differ from their roles on a day-to-day basis? Do they have special teams and plans for biological, chemical, nuclear, or radiological incidents?

DISASTER MANAGEMENT STAGES

Prevention Stage

The first stage in disaster management occurs before a disaster is imminent and is also known as the *nondisaster stage*. Potential disaster risks should be identified and risk maps created (see Fig. 29.1). The population demographics and vulnerabilities, as well as the community's capabilities, should be analyzed. Primary prevention measures include educating the public regarding what actions to take to prepare for disasters at the individual, family, and community levels. Furthermore, on the basis of the assessment of potential risks, the community must develop a plan for meeting the potential disasters identified.

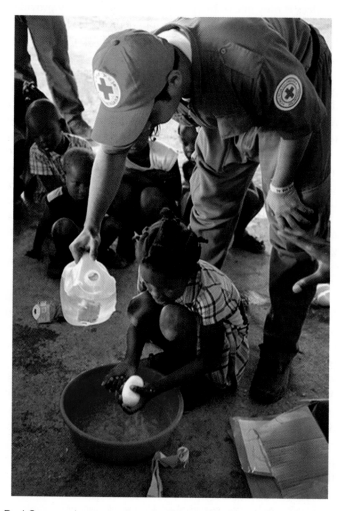

Red Cross volunteers share health and hygiene messages with young earthquake survivors. (Photo by Bonnie Gillespie/American Red Cross.)

With regard to bioterrorist attacks, prevention means that health care providers need to be knowledgeable about the biological and chemical agents that might be used. In addition, health care providers must be able to recognize the signs and symptoms of the various biological and chemical agents that have been recognized as potential threats and must know what to do in the event of exposure for themselves and others. As mentioned, unlike other disasters, biochemical terrorist threats may be identified only when events raise suspicions of health care providers rather than by first responders at a particular site.

Early identification of ill or exposed persons, rapid implementation of preventive therapy, special infection control considerations, and collaboration or communication with the public are essential in controlling the spread of cases. Hospitals need to identify rooms that can be converted into isolation units to meet the demand. Nurses must be instructed in decontamination and reminded of isolation techniques that might be needed, depending on the biological agent. Volunteers and professionals must remain current in first aid, CPR, and advanced lifesaving procedures.

Preparedness and Planning Stage

Individual and family preparedness involves training in first aid, assembling a disaster emergency kit, establishing a predetermined meeting place away from home, and making a family communication plan. Recommendations for what needs to be included in each of these activities are available from many sources (e.g., ARC, DHS, and FEMA). These are guidelines, and each individual and each family must modify the preparations to meet their personal needs. Nurses need to have plans and survival kits for work, family, and evacuation.

Although there will be some variation according to the individual community's needs, all community disaster plans should address the following elements: authority, communication, control, logistical coordination of personnel, supplies and equipment, evacuation, rescue, and care of the dead. The plan should indicate who has the power to declare that there is a disaster and who has the power to initiate the disaster plan.

Authority should be designated by the title of the person; it should not specify a person by name. Backup positions should also be identified in the event the first individual is not available. Every individual should be equally informed about the role and responsibilities that go with this authority. A clear chain of authority for carrying out the plan is critical for its successful implementation. Authority may change, depending on whether the disaster is natural or manmade, and change of authority should be addressed in the plan.

Communication is recognized as a very significant problem during disasters. Misinformation and misinterpretation can occur when communication is ineffective. Reliance on telephone systems or cell phones should not be the sole planned means of communicating because these may not work or the systems might be overwhelmed. The communication section of the disaster plan should address how the authority figure will be notified of the disaster, how the emergency management team members will be notified, how the community residents will be warned about the incident, and what actions to take. This section needs to address how communication between relief workers and authorities will be maintained. Also, it should include information on the role of the media in keeping people informed and in letting people know what assistance and supplies are needed.

The analysis of the population that was completed during the nondisaster stage should identify groups that need special attention as to how they will be notified. These people should be noted in advance and plans developed to meet the varied needs of these vulnerable groups. Such groups include those who speak different languages; are homeless or poor;

are without television or other means of communication; and are in institutions such as prisons, nursing homes, day care settings, or schools. Effective communication during a disaster must be credible, current, and authoritative and must give some indication of future events.

The *logistical* section should specify where supplies and equipment are located or where additional supplies and equipment can be obtained, where they will be stored or found, and how they will be transported to the disaster site (see Fig. 29.2). Essential *human resources* (e.g., emergency and disaster specialists, officials of governmental and voluntary agencies, engineers, weather specialists, and community leaders) should be identified and where they will be located together determined. The plan should include information about transportation for *evacuation and rescue* (particularly taking into account vulnerable groups), documentation and record keeping, and plans for evaluation of the success or failure of the plan.

A disaster plan is a dynamic entity. Planning is a continuous process, and the plan changes with circumstances and when gaps are identified during drills or from actual disaster incidents. The plan should set realistic expectations of effects and needs, should be brief and concise, and should establish priorities and timelines for actions. It should also follow the disaster planning principles listed in Box 29.9.

For a plan to be effective, it must be tested with different disaster scenario drills. The more times realistic scenarios are created to test the plan in actual practice sessions, and not just with tabletop or paper drills, the more problems with the plan will be identified and solutions for those problems found. Without practice drills, a plan may have many unrecognized faults, and as a result, many more individuals may be harmed and communities damaged when an actual disaster occurs.

Response Stage

The response stage begins immediately after the disaster incident occurs. The community preparedness plans that have been developed are initiated. If a disaster occurs, people should remain calm and exert patience, follow the advice of local emergency officials, and listen to the radio or television for news and instructions. If people nearby are injured, one should give first aid, seek help, and check the area for dangerous hazards. Those at home should shut off any damaged utilities, confine or secure pets, call family contact(s), and check on neighbors, especially the elderly or disabled.

The plan may call for people to shelter in place or to evacuate, or for search and rescue to begin. If the only response needed is to shelter in place, people need to know what to do if they are at home, at work, at school, or in their vehicles.

Shelter in Place

The ARC has provided explicit instructions for individuals and families to be followed when told by authorities to "shelter in place" in the event of a disaster. Table 29.2 shows these guidelines.

If local authorities issue a shelter-in-place communication, instructions that address what actions to take if at home, at work, at school, or in a vehicle should be followed. For example, during a disaster such as hazardous gas emission from an industrial plant, anyone at home, at a business, or in a public building may be instructed to go inside and follow home or work shelter-in-place recommendations (i.e., close doors, turn off fans and air conditioning, bring children and pets inside, and stay inside until "all clear" has been called).

BOX 29.9   Disaster Planning Principles

1. Measures usually taken are not sufficient for major disasters.
2. Plans should be adjusted to people's needs.
3. Planning does not stop with development of a written plan.
4. Lack of information causes inappropriate responses by community members.
5. People should be able to respond with or without direction.
6. Plans should coordinate efforts of the entire community, so large segments of the citizenry should be involved in the planning.
7. Plans should be linked to surrounding areas.
8. Plans should be general enough to cover all potential disaster events.
9. As much as possible, plans should be based on everyday work methods and procedures.
10. Plans should specify a person's responsibility for implementing segments by position or title rather than by name.
11. Plans should develop a record-keeping system before a disaster occurs regarding:
    - Supplies and equipment
    - Records of all present at any given time (to account for everyone and to identify the missing)
    - Identification of victims and deceased, conditions and treatment documented, and to which facility victims are sent
12. Backup plans need to be in place for the following:
    - Disruption of telephone and cell phone lines
    - Disruption of computer data (should be downloaded weekly and stored off-site)
    - Protecting essential public health functions (e.g., vital records and communicable disease data)

A FEMA mobile disaster recovery unit travels around the state of Georgia to offer assistance in the aftermath of Hurricane Matthew. (Photo by Gary Petty/FEMA.)

TABLE 29.2 Shelter-in-Place Instructions

Location	Instructions
Home	Bring children and pets indoors immediately; close and lock all outside doors and windows; close the window shades, blinds, or curtains; turn off fans, heating, ventilation, or air conditioning system, and close the fireplace or woodstove damper; get the disaster supplies and make sure the radio is working; take everyone, including pets, into an interior room with no or few windows and shut the door; if instructed to seal the room, use duct tape and plastic sheeting (e.g., heavy-duty plastic garbage bags) to seal all cracks around the door into the room; keep the phone handy in case it is needed to report a life-threatening condition; keep listening to the radio or television until told all is safe or told to evacuate (do not evacuate unless instructed to do so).
Day care centers and schools	Close the school; activate the school's emergency plan and follow reverse evacuation procedures to bring students, faculty, visitors, and staff indoors; have all children, staff, and visitors take shelter in preselected rooms that have phone access, stored disaster supply kits, and, preferably, access to a bathroom; shut the doors and lock all windows and doors; if it is not possible for a person to monitor the telephone and the school has voice mail or an automated attendant, change the recording to indicate that the school is closed and that students and staff are remaining in the building until authorities say it is safe to leave; turn off heating, ventilating, and air conditioning systems; if children have cell phones, allow them to use them to call a parent or guardian to let them know that they have been asked to remain in school until further notice and that they are safe; one teacher or staff member in each room should write down the names of everyone in the room and call the designated contact to report who is in that room; everyone should stay in the room until school officials announce that all is safe or say everyone must evacuate.
Work	Close the office or business, making any customers, clients, or visitors in the building aware that they need to stay until the emergency is over; close and lock all windows, exterior doors, and any other openings to the outside; a knowledgeable person should use the building's mechanical systems to turn off all heating, ventilating, and air conditioning systems (systems that automatically provide for exchange of inside air with outside air, in particular, need to be turned off, sealed, or disabled); turn on call-forwarding or alternative telephone answering systems or services; if there is danger of explosion, close any window shades, blinds, or curtains; go to a predetermined sheltering room(s), and when everyone is in, shut and lock the doors; monitor radios or TVs for updates until you are told all is safe or you are told to evacuate.
Vehicle	If close to home, workplace, or a public building, go there immediately and go inside. If unable to get indoors quickly and safely, stop the vehicle in the safest place possible (e.g., stop under a bridge or in a shady spot to avoid being overheated); turn off the engine and close windows and vents; if possible, seal the heating, ventilating, and air conditioning vents with duct tape or anything else you may have available; listen to the radio periodically for updated advice and instructions; stay in place until you are told it is safe to get back on the road, and follow the directions of law enforcement officials.

Modified from American Red Cross: *Shelter-in-place during a chemical or radiation emergency*, 2006. www.redcross.org/preparedness/cdc_english/Sheltering.asp#howdo.

Between February 8 and March 9, 2010, 125,000 earthquake survivors in Port-au-Prince, Haiti, were vaccinated against measles, diphtheria, pertussis, and tetanus. (Photo by Bonnie Gillespie/American Red Cross.)

Evacuation

Each community should have established evacuation routes for the residents to use if evacuation from the area is necessary. In some instances, mandatory evacuation may be implemented. However, there are always some individuals who will not leave their homes for any number of reasons (e.g., fear of vandalism, denial of the potential extent of the disaster, pride in home and belongings). Education of residents as to the potential damage,

deaths, and injuries that will be incurred from the potential disasters that may affect their community needs to be accomplished during the preparedness stage and not when evacuation is ordered. In some extreme cases, it may be necessary for hospitals and other facilities, such as nursing homes, to evacuate patients. This procedure requires significant advance planning, because health practitioners must determine how to move seriously ill, and even critically ill, people and coordinate transportation and placement for their disposition to safe facilities.

Search and Rescue

Before search and rescue begin, safety must be considered. In some instances, if a criminal action is suspected as part of the disaster, law officials will be among the first to respond in order to secure the area and possibly gather evidence. While the area is being checked and then cleared of potential threats, a staging area can be set up at or near the site of the incident to direct on-site activities. Search for and rescue of victims can begin once clearance is given, a disaster triage area is established, and an emergency treatment area is set up to provide first aid until transportation for victims to hospitals or health care facilities for treatment can be coordinated (Fig. 29.3).

Staging Area

The staging area is the on-site incident command station. Disaster responders should report to this area to "check in" so that

FIG. 29.3 Areas of operation of disaster response.

Initial triage and rescue area

Treatment and transportation/ evacuation area

Incident command staging area

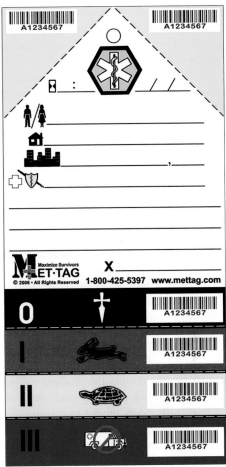

FIG. 29.4 Disaster triage tag. (From METTAG: *The original medical emergency triage tag*, 2006. http://www.mettag.com. Reprinted with permission.)

everyone is accounted for and can be given an assignment. This arrangement allows for the most effective use of the skills and abilities of those responding. No one should go to the disaster site unless directed to do so by the staging area commander. The staging area is also where the authority rests for decisions as to the need for additional resources to manage the disaster incident. Such resources include construction equipment to move building materials; rescue dogs to locate humans who are buried in the debris; and more fire, police, or medical personnel.

Disaster Triage

Triage is identifying and separating individuals quickly according to injury severity and treatment needed. Disaster triage focuses on sorting the greatest number of people as fast as possible. Triage performed at the site and again at the treatment area is very different from triage that is routinely conducted in the emergency department. The focus of **disaster triage** is to do the greatest good, for the greatest number, in the shortest time. One triage system that is used by first responders is START. START stands for "simple triage and rapid treatment." This system describes what to do when first arriving at a multiple casualty or mass casualty incident. Disaster triage of an injured person should occur in less than 1 minute. This system also describes how to use people with minor injuries to help. As a decision is made regarding the status of an individual, the person is labeled with a colored triage tag (Fig. 29.4).

Green on the triage tag is for the walking wounded or those with minor injuries (e.g., cuts and abrasions) who can wait several hours before they receive treatment; yellow is for those with systemic but not yet life-threatening complications who can wait 45 to 60 minutes (e.g., simple fractures); red is considered top priority or immediate and is for those who have life-threatening conditions but who can be stabilized and have a high probability of survival (e.g., amputations); black is for the deceased or for those whose injuries are is so extensive that nothing can be done to save them (e.g., multiple severe injuries).

A new classification of victim, those who are contaminated, will require a hazmat (for "hazardous materials") tag. To assess an individual within the 1-minute guideline, the START system uses three characteristics. First, respiration is checked; if the rate is more than 30 per minute, the individual is tagged red or immediate. If the rate is fewer than 30 per minute, the assessor moves to the second step, *perfusion*. The assessor pinches the nail bed and observes the reaction. Color should return to normal within

2 seconds; if it takes longer, the person is tagged red or immediate. The third step is checking mental status. If the person is able to answer a question, he or she is tagged yellow; the person not able to answer a question is tagged red or immediate. By doing these steps, the individual responsible for triage can very quickly assess an individual and decide which color tag fits his or her condition. Furthermore, the steps are easy to remember with the mnemonic "30—2—can do," in which "30" is the number of respirations, "2" is the number of seconds needed to check for perfusion, and "can do" relates to checking mental status.

After triage, victims are moved to the treatment area where their condition is checked again. First aid may be provided there until transportation is available. Ambulances, helicopters, buses, or all three may be used to transport the victims to various hospitals or health care facilities. Some victims, such as those in the surrounding area that may have been affected by the incident, may even go by private vehicle to a hospital or medical facility. This process may go on for days as it did in the September 11, 2001, incidents; the 2005 tsunami in South Asia; and Hurricanes Katrina, Rita, Sandy, and Harvey. Search and rescue eventually will be called off, and the recovery stage will begin.

While search and rescue are going on, other agencies (e.g., public health agencies) are surveilling for threats such as contaminated water, vectors, and air quality. They also disseminate data on what has been found and relate health information to officials, the media, and the public as appropriate. Designated agencies gather epidemiological information as to the occurrence and distribution of health-related events associated with the disaster, describe factors contributing to health-related effects, and assess the needs of populations and facilities. They then allocate resources and work to prevent further adverse health problems that might result from the disaster. For example, after Hurricane Katrina, public health officials administered tetanus and hepatitis A immunizations to rescuers and victims. In the aftermath of Hurricane Harvey, first responders and some of the victims of the flood were exposed to stagnant water and developed life-threatening infections. Resources were allocated to offer protection to those supporting relief efforts such as gloves and other protective gear.

Although triage of individuals exposed to chemical warfare agents is basically the same as for any multiple or mass casualty incident, it poses special challenges. For these events, the triage area is set up in the "hot zone" to assist in determining priorities for resuscitation, decontamination, pharmacological therapy, and site evacuation. Only specially trained emergency personnel who are familiar with chemical agents and the use of personal protection equipment should triage victims of a chemical agent. The same triage categories can be assigned to these victims.

Psychological triage presents the challenge of determining who most needs help and deciding what interventions will help. Mental health disorders related to disasters include anxiety disorders, exacerbation of existing substance abuse problems, somatic complaints, depression, and later, posttraumatic stress disorder (PTSD). Risks for PTSD include living through dangerous events or traumas; having a history of mental illness; getting hurt; seeing people hurt or killed; feeling horror, helplessness, or extreme fear; having little or no social support after the event; and dealing with extra stress after the event, such as loss of a loved one, pain and injury, or loss of a job or home. Research has identified four keys to gauging the mental health impact of such events, any two of which may result in severe, lasting, and pervasive psychological effects. The key factors are (1) extreme and widespread property damage; (2) serious and ongoing financial problems; (3) high prevalence of trauma in the form of injuries, threat to life, and loss of life; and (4) when human intent caused the disaster. In addition, panic during the disaster, horror, separation from family, and relocation or displacement are factors that may play a part in psychological impairment. Nurses need to evaluate an individual's risk to self or others.

Box 29.10 is a list of positive coping strategies for survivors in the event of a disaster.

Community Responses to a Disaster
Heroic Phase

The classic four phases of a community's reaction to a disaster are the heroic phase, honeymoon phase, disillusionment phase, and reconstruction phase. During the heroic phase, nearly everyone feels the need to rush to help people survive the disaster. Medical personnel may work hours without sleep, under very dangerous and life-threatening conditions, in order to take care of their patients. Medical personnel may help out in areas with which they are not familiar and have no experience. Disaster Medical

---

BOX 29.10 Positive and Maladaptive Coping Strategies

Positive Coping Strategies
- Relaxation methods (muscular relaxation, deep breathing, meditation)
- Exercise in moderation.
- Talking to another person for support
- Getting adequate rest
- Positive distracting activities
- Trying to maintain a normal schedule (if appropriate)
- Scheduling pleasant activities
- Eating healthy meals
- Taking breaks
- Spending time with others
- Keeping a journal
- Participating in a support group
- Seeking counseling

Maladaptive Coping Strategies
- Use of alcohol or drugs to cope
- Social isolation and withdrawal
- Extreme avoidance of thinking or talking about the event
- "Workaholism"
- Anger or violence

From VA National Center for PTSD: *Psychosocial treatment of disaster-related mental health problems*, 2010. https://www.ptsd.va.gov/professional/pages/handouts-pdf/Psychosocial_Treatment.pdf.

Assistance Teams, consisting of professional and paraprofessional medical personnel, provide emergency relief during a disaster and may travel long distances to help out in one. This was illustrated by the thousands of people who volunteered to help in the immediate aftermaths of September 11 and Hurricanes Katrina and Rita.

Honeymoon Phase

Individuals who have survived the disaster gather together with others who have simultaneously experienced the same event; this is known as the *honeymoon phase*. People begin to tell their stories and review over and over again what has occurred. Bonds are formed among victims and health care workers. Gratitude is expressed for being alive.

Disillusionment Phase

When time has elapsed and a delay in receiving help or failure to receive the promised aid has not occurred, feelings of despair arise. Medical personnel and other first responders may begin to experience depression due to exhaustion from many long days of long hours. Depression may set in as a result of knowledge about what has happened to the community, friends, and family. People realize the way things were before the disaster is not the way things are now and may never be again. They recognize that many things are different and much needs to be done to adjust to the current situation.

Reconstruction Phase

Once the community has restored some of the buildings, businesses, homes, and services and some sense of normality is returning, feelings of despair subside. Counseling support for victims and helpers may need to be initiated to help people recover more fully. During this phase, people begin to look to the future.

NATURAL AND MANMADE DISASTERS

The devastation of the tsunami that occurred in Indonesia in December 2004. (Copyright Associated Press.)

Many homes and vehicles were destroyed in a wildfire in Santa Rosa, California, in October 2017. (Photo by Dominic Del Vecchio/FEMA.)

The remaining section of the World Trade Center, New York, City, is surrounded by a mountain of rubble after the September 11, 2001, terrorist attacks. (Photo by Bri Rodriguez/FEMA News Photo.)

CDC personnel in Sierra Leone teach the proper use of personal protective equipment (PPE) for those working with Ebola patients. (Photo by CDC.)

FEMA disaster survivor assistance team members are "boots on the ground," passing out information after tornado devastation in Alabama, 2014.

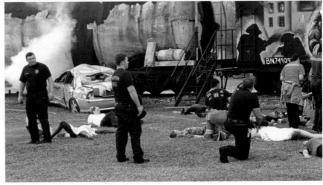

Houston Fire Department cadets and nursing students as victims and providers for a mass casualty drill.

DISASTER RELIEF: HURRICANE HARVEY, AUGUST/SEPTEMBER 2017

When Hurricane Harvey hit the Gulf Coast in late August 2017, more than 30,000 evacuees from the area sought shelter—the vast majority in the Houston metropolitan area. Two huge shelters and many smaller shelters were set up to accommodate those displaced, and the needs, as was documented in the media, were massive.

- More than 1 million relief items were distributed.
- More than 3.1 million meals and snacks were served.
- Immediate financial assistance was offered to nearly 320,000 severely affected households.
- More than 98,000 health and mental health contacts were made.
- More than 413,000 people stayed in overnight shelters.

Faculty, staff, and students from the University of Texas Health Science Center at Houston (UT-Houston), personnel from the city and county health departments, and local emergency medical services personnel were joined by thousands of volunteers to care for these disaster victims. Indeed, doctors, nurses, and other health care providers came from across Texas and the Gulf Coast area and from as far away as California, Arizona, Illinois, and New York to help. To care for the health needs of the evacuees, a clinic was established in the George R. Brown Convention Center. The clinic was modeled after army field hospitals, with a command center, triage areas, and various clinics. There were sections for trauma and acute care, adult medical care, women's/gynecological care, and pediatric care, as well as an area for people with mental health concerns. A full-service pharmacy was also set up.

The "Cajun Navy" (civilian boat owners from across the region and even beyond) rescued thousands of stranded people during Hurricane Harvey, September 1, 2017. (Photo courtesy Scott McEwen.)

This is the morning after Hurricane Harvey. Most Houston streets were flooded, leading to many water rescues.

People waiting to get supplies during Hurricane Harvey.

Floodwaters from Hurricane Harvey reached higher than this street sign. (Photo courtesy Scott McEwen.)

Continued

A collection of donated supplies at a Houston church to assist residents with cleanup. (Photo courtesy Scott McEwen.)

In many neighborhoods, homes were completely destroyed and families were forced to discard all their belongings. Flooded houses had to be taken down to the studs/framing with all appliances, cabinets, sheetrock, and windows removed. Massive piles of debris lined the streets. Houston, Texas, September 2, 2017. (Photo courtesy Scott McEwen.)

Supplies for evacuees at the George R. Brown Convention Center.

Salvation Army volunteers distribute food to survivors of Hurricane Harvey, September 8, 2017. (Photo by Steve Zumwalt/FEMA.)

Community-based donation site in one neighborhood hard-hit by Harvey, September 2, 2017. (Photo courtesy Scott McEwen.)

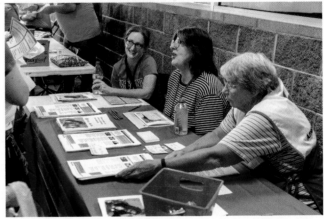

Red Cross volunteers distribute information to survivors of Hurricane Harvey, September 16, 2017. (Photo by Steve Zumwalt/FEMA.)

DISASTER RELIEF: HURRICANE HARVEY, AUGUST/SEPTEMBER 2017—cont'd

FEMA representatives offer relief to a family of survivors, September 16, 2017. (Photo by Steve Zumwalt/FEMA.)

A disaster recovery center in a downtown Houston mall, September 20, 2017. (Photo by Steve Zumwalt/FEMA.)

TABLE 29.3	Common Responses to a Traumatic Event
Cognitive	• Poor concentration • Confusion • Disorientation • Indecisiveness • Shortened attention span • Memory loss • Unwanted memories • Difficulty making decisions
Emotional	• Shock • Numbness • Feeling overwhelmed • Depression • Feeling lost • Fear of harm to self and/or loved ones • Feeling nothing • Feeling abandoned • Uncertainty of feelings • Volatile emotions
Physical	• Nausea • Lightheadedness • Dizziness • Gastrointestinal problems • Rapid heart rate • Tremors • Headaches • Grinding of teeth • Fatigue • Poor sleep • Pain • Hyperarousal • Jumpiness
Behavioral	• Suspicion • Irritability • Arguments with friends and loved ones

TABLE 29.3	Common Responses to a Traumatic Event—cont'd
	• Withdrawal • Excessive silence • Inappropriate humor • Increased/decreased eating • Change in sexual desire or functioning • Increased smoking • Increased substance use or abuse

From Centers for Disease Control and Prevention: *Coping with a traumatic event: information for health professionals*, 2005. https://www.cdc.gov/masstrauma/factsheets/professionals/coping_professional.pdf.

Common Reactions to a Disaster

The reactions by individuals to a disaster vary. Table 29.3 lists some of the more commonly encountered emotional, cognitive, physical, and interpersonal reactions to a disaster that anyone may experience.

Posttraumatic Stress Disorder

The reactions mentioned usually resolve in 1 to 3 months after the disaster event, but, in some cases, may lead to PTSD. PTSD is a psychiatric disorder that can occur after an individual experiences or witnesses a life-threatening event, such as a disaster. Men and women, adults and children, and all socioeconomic groups can experience PTSD. People who have the disorder often relive the experience through nightmares and flashbacks. The social and psychological symptoms mentioned in Table 29.3 can be severe enough and last long enough to significantly impair a person's daily life. If PTSD occurs in conjunction with related disorders (e.g., depression, substance abuse, and other problems of physical and mental health), the situation becomes more complicated. Individuals experiencing PTSD require medical attention (National Institute of Mental Health, 2016).

❓ ACTIVE LEARNING

1. What social and cultural factors need to be considered in disaster planning in your community? Are there vulnerable populations with special needs (e.g., homeless, imprisoned, mobility impaired)? If evacuation of the community is mandated, have plans for evacuation of these groups been made?
2. Create an emergency plan for yourself, your family, or both. What factors would you consider in deciding whether to stay or leave your home? If evacuation were mandated, what important documents and mementos would you need to take with you?
3. What emergency supplies does your health care facility have available in the event of a disaster? What provisions have been made available for vulnerable patients when there is no electricity? How would patients be evacuated from the facility to safe shelters?

CASE STUDY   Application of the Community Assessment Process

Coastal City: Preparedness for Disaster

Assessment

Deer Park, Texas, is a city 20 miles east of Houston, Texas. The population is approximately 32,000 people. The majority of the people are white (80.8%) and Hispanic (15.2%). The median age of the population is 34.7 years, and the median income $61,334. Eighty-nine percent of the population older than 25 years has a high school diploma or higher education degree. The unemployment rate is 5.6%. The city consists of residential homes, apartment complexes, and retail and service businesses. There are nine schools and several churches of all denominations. Many AM and FM radio stations and TV broadcast stations are available to the Deer Park area.

The Federal Communications Commission (FCC) has developed the Emergency Alert System to warn of any emergency (nuclear attack, hurricane, tornado, flood, or chemical release). The FCC has designated KTRH 740 AM as the station for the Houston area. The city has a volunteer fire department (5 full-time employees) and a city police department (55 full-time employees). The city government consists of a mayor, city council, and city manager. The city has two emergency committees: the Community Awareness and Emergency Response Committee and the Local Emergency Planning Committee.

There are no hospitals in Deer Park. The closest hospitals are 6 to 7 miles away and take 20 minutes to reach. The closest level 1 trauma center is 15 miles away, and the nearest adult care burn center is 20 miles away; the pediatric burn center is in Galveston, Texas, which is about 45 miles away.

The city is also the home of the Shell Deer Park Chemical Plant and the Shell Deer Park Refining Company. The company processes 3% of the nation's oil supply into gasoline. The Shell plants are located on 1500 acres in the Houston Ship Channel. Shell employs approximately 1100 people and 2200 contract workers. The chemical plant and the refining company have their own fire stations, an internal railroad, docks and transportation networks, small medical facilities (one physician and four nurses, 7 days a week, 24 hours a day), first responder teams, two ambulances, and a vehicle that can handle 30 casualties.

Diagnosis
Individual
Because of Deer Park's location on the Gulf Coast and the presence of the Shell Deer Park Refining Company and Shell Deer Park Chemical Plant, the residents are at risk for injury or death due to hurricane disasters and potential industrial incidents from either accidental or terrorist causes.

Family
The families of Deer Park are at risk for losing their homes, separation from family members, and having to evacuate from their homes either temporarily or permanently due to hurricane damages or industrial accidents.

Community
The community of Deer Park is at risk for destruction of buildings and city public works due to hurricane disasters and potential explosions from either accidental or terrorist causes.

Planning
Disaster Management
Deer Park is in the storm surge zone, requiring its residents to evacuate when a category 1 hurricane is predicted to land in or within a 100-mile radius of the Deer Park area. The media sources available to the Deer Park area or the city officials are to give instructions about supplies and equipment to have ready and when to leave. Only one evacuation route is available to the community.

A survey was conducted during the nondisaster stage to identify vulnerable groups that would need help in evacuating.

Individual
Vulnerable individuals who would need to have special consideration for evacuation are the very young (4000 individuals between birth and 10 years), the elderly (2110 individuals aged 65 years and over), and families below the poverty level (1200). It was determined that more than 7000 individuals might need some form of transportation in order to evacuate.

Long-Term Goal
- Residents will have a disaster kit prepared according to ARC and FEMA guidelines.

Short-Term Goals
- Residents will follow officials' instructions for sheltering in place or evacuation.
- Vulnerable individuals will know what to do in the event of an evacuation order or shelter-in-place announcement.

Family
Long-Term Goal
- Family members will continually update their family disaster plans according to family dynamics.

Short-Term Goals
- Families will have a disaster plan in place for communicating.
- Families will have a disaster kit in place to accommodate each family member for a period of at least 3 days.

Community
Long-Term Goals
- Additional evacuation routes will be identified for area residents.
- Central meeting locations will be identified for those needing transportation assistance for evacuation.

Short-Term Goal
- School buses will be used for evacuation of vulnerable individuals and families who need transportation.
- Other sources must be identified that could be called upon to provide transportation.

Coastal City: Preparedness for Disaster

- School bus drivers should be able to include their family members on the buses with others being evacuated so the drivers will not have to worry about their families.
- If all individuals follow instructions, there should be no injuries to or deaths of Deer Park residents from a hurricane or related storm surge. Homes may be damaged or destroyed, but no lives should be lost. With the help of local, state, and possibly federal agencies, the community should recover.

Long-Term Goal

- City officials will continually update the community disaster plan as gaps are identified and keep the residents informed as the plan changes.

Onsite Management

The following figure summarizes the disaster plan in place for the Deer Park Shell plants for handling any industrial accident that occurs on their property.

Shell has annual drills with the Harris County's Emergency Management and Channel Industries Mutual Aid organization to evaluate emergency response. This group is Shell's direct link to support in the event of a disaster. Many buildings on Shell property can serve as shelters, and no visitor or employee is allowed on the property without having a "safe shelter map" in his or her possession. If an explosion occurs that is confined to the property, and only minor casualties result, the resources available should be sufficient to manage the disaster.

Shell has developed a buffer zone between the plants and the city of Deer Park. However, if fumes were to escape as a result of the explosion, a shelter-in-place warning would be issued for Deer Park residents through a specific six-sound message system. Chemical products that are used and that might potentially escape are benzene, toluene, solvent xylene, isoprene butadiene, sulfur, phenol, hydrogen sulfide, and asbestos. Citizens would be advised about actions to take according to the chemical released. Most plants have also installed dedicated fiber-optic telephone lines so that the city and industry can stay in touch even when normal phone circuits are overloaded or out of service.

Community and Local Response Preparedness

Deer Park's police and fire dispatchers have been trained on how to handle calls from industries about a chemical release and how to quickly activate the city's emergency warning systems. The local emergency planning committee has adopted a leveled community awareness and emergency response system to categorize the severity of each chemical release. Level 1 is information only, level 2 is standby alert, and level 3 is full emergency condition, with sheltering in place required. The final level is "all clear." Deer Park has a website featuring Wally Wise Guy, who gives instructions to the citizens about what to do if a shelter-in-place emergency is issued.

The local emergency planning committee hired a consulting group to study the impact of toxic substances on the community to ensure that shelter-in-place procedures are adequate for protecting the residents. The consulting group recommended that each home in the region have a shelter-in-place kit containing 2- to 3-inch–wide masking tape, plastic film or sheets, towels or sheets for sealing under doors, battery-powered radio and extra batteries, flashlight and extra batteries, and bottled water stored inside a designated shelter-in-place room.

The Deer Park Communications Subcommittee works with others to develop detailed procedures on how to notify and warn the public of a chemical release. The city and local industry have invested in six state-of-the-art systems to provide reliable and redundant warning to homes, schools, businesses, and visitors. Siren-type alarms have been mounted on utility poles throughout the city. This system is used only for chemical emergencies, not for tornadoes, hurricanes, or other types of emergencies. In addition, the city has contracted with First Call Interactive Network, an automated telephone notification network that can ring the telephones of homes and businesses in the immediate danger area to give prerecorded instructions about what to do.

Evaluation
Individuals and Families

- Before a hurricane, all residents will have been evacuated.
- All vulnerable individuals and families will have been evacuated to shelters.
- All residents will know and respond to shelter-in-place warnings as indicated by the siren-type alarm system in place.

Community

- City officials will evaluate and continually update the community disaster plan as gaps are identified.
- Community residents will remain informed and prepared.

The city of Deer Park and the Deer Park Shell plants have detailed plans for prevention, preparedness, and response in the event of an industrial accident. In that event, evaluation of the plan will take place to identify gaps and make appropriate changes. A plan needs to be in place for hurricane preparedness of the plants to avoid industrial accidents, and the plan evaluated for effectiveness. Drills are conducted to test their industrial accident plans; they provide training of personnel; they have identified sites for shelters both on Shell property and in the city; and they have elaborate notification and warning systems in place.

Areas that need to be enhanced include readily available city health resources (lack of a nearby trauma hospital or burn center to care for the types of injuries that would occur). Plans for preparing the plants for hurricanes and evacuation need to be developed and made available to the workers.

Prevention
Primary

- Perform periodic education of area residents regarding warning systems in place and appropriate response to take should they be implemented.
- Perform periodic review of plans in response to changing demographics.

Secondary

- Check credentials of first responders for currency.
- Screen first responders for training needs and preparedness to take action during disasters.

Tertiary

- Institute building codes that will reduce the amount of damage to infrastructures.

Recovery Stage

The recovery stage begins when the danger from the disaster has passed and all local, state, and federal agencies are present in the area to help victims rebuild their lives and the community restore public services. Cleanup of the damage and repair of homes and businesses begin. Evaluation and revision of the disaster plans based on lessons learned from the experience are made. Understanding the financial impact on the community and agencies involved is essential in developing future public health policy.

Research is needed on all aspects of prevention, preparedness, response, and recovery stages of disasters. Research is also needed on the education and training needs of first responders, health care providers, and community populations. Nurse researchers, in partnership with researchers from other disciplines, can play a significant role in conducting research on disaster management.

■ SUMMARY

Communities, now more than ever, need to be aware of potential disasters that may affect their residents. Comprehensive disaster plans need to be developed at all levels of government and by all communities, families, and individuals. Having disaster plans in place increases the likelihood of an effective response, resulting in saved lives and minimized destruction to the community.

Nurses have a role in and contribution to make at every stage of disaster management. Nurses need to have personal and professional plans in place for any disaster. All medical personnel must keep their credentials current and must learn the signs and symptoms of exposure to weapons of mass destruction so that they will recognize people who may have been exposed. They should learn what injuries may be sustained from various disasters and know which types of disasters are most likely to affect their communities so that disaster triage and treatment can save lives. Finally, they must take drills in their respective health care facilities seriously. The more prepared the population and health care providers are for all kinds of disasters, the fewer lives will be lost.

ⓔ EVOLVE WEBSITE

http://evolve.elsevier.com/Nies/community
- NCLEX Review Questions
- Case Studies

BIBLIOGRAPHY

18 U.S. Code § 2331 – *Definitions*. 1992.

American Red Cross (ARC): *Our Federal Charter*, 2017. Available from: http://www.redcross.org/about-us/who-we-are/history/federal-charter.

American Red Cross (ARC): *Disaster service program review, Fiscal year 2011*, 2012. Available from: http://www.redcross.org/what-we-do/disaster-relief/2011-disaster-relief-program. http://www.red-cross.org/images/MEDIA_CustomProductCatalog/m8540111_Disaster-Relief-Program-Review-2011.pdf, 2012.

Centers for Disease Control and Prevention: *Emergency preparedness and response*, 2017. Available from: http://emergency.cdc.gov/disasters/. https://emergency.cdc.gov/, 2017.

Central Intelligence Agency: *Terrorism FAQs*, 2013. Available from: http://www.cia.gov/about-cia/faq/index/html. https://www.cia.gov/news-information/cia-the-war-on-terrorism/terrorism-faqs.html, 2013.

Chettle C: Recognizing bioterrorism: nurses on the frontline, *Nurse Week* 6:29–30, 2001.

Federal Bureau of Investigation: *What we investigate: terrorism*, 2017. Available from: https://www.fbi.gov/investigate/terrorism. Accessed December, 01 2017.

Federal Emergency Management Agency: *National incident management system*, 2017a. Available from: http://www.fema.gov/about-national-incident-management-system. https://www.fema.gov/national-incident-management-system, 2017a.

Federal Emergency Management Agency: *What is mitigation?*, 2017b. Available from: https://www.fema.gov/what-mitigation.

Federal Emergency Management Agency: *Post-Katrina Emergency Management Reform Act*, 2017b. Available from: https://emilms.fema.gov/is230c/fem0101200.htm.

Federal Emergency Management Agency: *Are you ready?*, 2017c. Available from: https://www.fema.gov/pdf/areyouready/areyouready_full.pdf.

Landesman LY, Burke RV: *Landesman's public health management of disasters: The practice guide*, ed 4, Washington, DC, 2017, American Public Health Association.

National Institute of Mental Health: *Post-traumatic stress disorder (PTSD)*, 2016. Available from: http://www.nimh.nih.gov/. https://www.nimh.nih.gov/health/topics/post-traumatic-stress-disorder-ptsd/index.shtml, 2016.

National Oceanic and Atmospheric Administration: National Weather Service, National Hurricane Center, *Saffir-Simpson hurricane wind scale*, 2017. Available from: http://www.nhc.noaa.gov/aboutsshws.php.

Ready.gov: *Citizen Corps*, 2017. Available at https://www.ready.gov/citizen-corps.

U.S. Department of Homeland Security: *National response framework*, ed 3, . Available from. https://www.fema.gov/media-library-data/1466014682982-9bcf8245ba4c60c120aa915abe74e15d/National_Response_Framework3rd.pdf, 2016a.

U.S. Department of Homeland Security: *Our Mission*, 2016b. Available from: https://www.dhs.gov/our-mission.

U.S. Department of Homeland Security: *National preparedness goal*, 2016c. Available from: https://www.dhs.gov/national-preparedness-goal.

U.S. Department of Homeland Security: *National Terrorism Advisory System*, 2017. Available from: https://www.dhs.gov/national-terrorism-advisory-system.

30

School Health

Christina N. DesOrmeaux*

OBJECTIVES

Upon completion of this chapter, the reader will be able to do the following:

1. Discuss how *Healthy People 2020* can be used to shape the care given in a school health setting.
2. Identify and discuss the eight components of a comprehensive school health program.
3. Recognize the major stressors that can negatively affect an adolescent's mental and physical health.
4. Identify common health concerns of school-age children and associated health interventions.
5. Explore the various roles of the nurse in the school setting.
6. Be familiar with the standards according to which school nurses practice.
7. Cite several resources available to the school nurse.

KEY TERMS

Early and Periodic Screening, Diagnosis, and Treatment
emergency care plan
Family Educational Rights and Privacy Act
Health Insurance Portability and Accountability Act of 1996

individualized health care plan
Individuals With Disabilities Education Act of 1990
Public Law 99-142
school emergency plan
school health
school nurse

school-based health centers
Shattuck Report
Youth Risk Behavior Surveillance System

According to the Centers for Disease Control and Prevention (CDC) (2016), the healthy development of children and adolescents is influenced by many societal institutions, and after the

family, the school is the primary institution responsible for the development of young people in the United States. The school environment is also a key setting in which students' behaviors and ideas are shaped. Just as schools are critical to preparing students academically and socially, they are also vital partners in helping young people take responsibility for their health and adopting health-enhancing attitudes and behaviors that can last a lifetime (CDC, 2017).

*The author would like to acknowledge the contributions of Cathi A. Pourciau and Elaine C. Vallette, who revised this chapter for the previous edition.

BOX 30.1 Youth at Risk

- Every day nearly 3200 young people start smoking (CDC, 2015).
- Daily participation in high school physical education classes dropped from 42% in 1991 to 27.1% in 2013 (CDC, 2017).
- Seventy-five percent of young people do not eat the recommended number of servings of fruits and vegetables.
- Marijuana use among young people increased from 15% in 1991 to 46% in 2015.

From National Institute on Drug Abuse: *National survey of drug use and health*, 2015. https://www.drugabuse.gov/national-survey-drug-use-health

TABLE 30.1 Racial and Ethnic Breakdown of Uninsured Children in the United States in the Year 2012

Race	Number	Percentage
White	2.9 million	38.8
Hispanic	2.7million	38.1
Black	1.0 million	14.2
Asian and Pacific Islander	306,000	4.3

Data from Children's Defense Fund: *The state of America's children*, 2014. http://www.childrensdefense.org/library/state-of-americas-children/2014-soac.pdf.

Academic success and healthy children and youth are closely intertwined. It is impossible to achieve success in school without maximizing the health of the students. School-age children and adolescents face increasingly difficult challenges related to health. Many of today's health challenges are different from those of the past and include behaviors and risks linked to the leading causes of death such as heart disease, injuries, and cancer. Examples of behaviors that often begin during youth and increase the risk for serious health problems are the use of tobacco, alcohol, and drugs; poor nutritional habits; inadequate physical activity; irresponsible sexual behavior; violence; suicide; and reckless driving (Box 30.1).

In the United States, approximately 55.6 million children attend school every day (National Center for Educational Statistics, 2016). Their presence creates a unique opportunity for school nurses to have a positive impact on the nation's youth. The primary providers of health services in schools are school nurses, and there are approximately 73,000 registered nurses working in schools in the United States (U.S. Department of Health and Human Services [USDHHS], Health Services and Resources Administration, 2010).

School nursing is a specialized practice of professional nursing that advances the well-being, academic success, and lifelong achievement and health of students. To that end, school nurses facilitate positive student responses to normal development; promote health and safety, including a healthy environment; intervene with actual and potential health problems; provide case management services; and actively collaborate with others to build student and family capacity for adaptation, self-management, self-advocacy, and learning (NASN, 2017). The National Association of School Nurses (NASN) recommends one school nurse for every 750 students in the general population, one for every 225 students in mainstreamed special education populations, and one for every 125 severely chronically ill or developmentally disabled students; however, caseloads vary widely, depending on mandated functions, socioeconomic status of the community, and service delivery model (NASN, 2015).

More than 21% of the nation's children live in poverty (National Center for Children in Poverty, 2017). Poverty is defined as an annual income below $24,339 for a family of four (U.S. Census Bureau, 2017). Decreased or inferior health care has been linked to serious health problems, resulting in an increase in absenteeism that may be correlated with failure in school. The school nurse can effectively manage many complaints and illnesses, allowing these children to return to or remain in class.

Indeed, on a daily basis, school nurses see students with a variety of complaints. Increasing numbers of children are being seen in the school setting because they lack a source of regular medical care. According to the Children's Defense Fund (2014), nearly 9.2 million U.S. children, or 1 in 11, do not have health insurance. This is a decrease from the nearly 12 million in previous years. Table 30.1 illustrates the racial and ethnic breakdown of uninsured children in the United States in the year 2012. Poor academic performance is strongly correlated with the uninsured status of youth, and conversely, acquisition of health insurance leads to an improvement in school performance. Through education, counseling, advocacy, and direct care across all levels of prevention, the nurse can improve the immediate and long-term health of this population.

There is a need for mental and physical health services for students of all ages to improve both their academic performance and their sense of well-being. This chapter provides an overview of school health and the role of the nurse in the provision of health services and health education. It also offers an in-depth look at the components of a successful school health program and the major health problems of today's youth.

HISTORY OF SCHOOL HEALTH

Before 1840, education of children in the United States was uncoordinated and sparse. In 1840, Rhode Island passed legislation that made education mandatory, and other states soon followed. In 1850, a teacher and school committee member, Lemuel Shattuck, spearheaded the legendary report that has become a public health classic. This report, known as the Shattuck Report, has had a profound impact on school health because it proposed that health education was a vital component in the prevention of disease.

Public health officials and others soon realized that schools played an important part in the prevention of communicable disease. When smallpox broke out in New York City in the 1860s, health officials were faced with trying to implement a widespread prevention program. They chose to target the schools and began vaccinating children. This experience led to the 1870 requirement that all children be vaccinated against smallpox before entering school (Allensworth et al., 1997).

At that time, schools were frequently poorly ventilated and lacked fresh air, effectively spreading diseases among the children. Late in the nineteenth century, a practice of inspecting schools began to identify children who were ill and exclude them until it was deemed they were no longer infectious. Soon thereafter, compulsory vision examinations became a requirement to identify children who might have difficulty in school. In 1902, New York City hired the first nurses to help inspect children, educate families, and ensure follow-up treatment. Within a few years the renowned nurse Lillian Wald was able to show that the presence of school nurses could reduce absenteeism by 50%. By 1911, more than 100 cities were using school nurses, and by 1913, New York City employed 176 school nurses (Allensworth et al., 1997).

As they became more comfortable in their positions, early school nurses began to take on more active roles in the assessment of children, treatment of minor conditions, and referral for more serious problems. In addition to identification, treatment, and exclusion for communicable diseases and screening for problems that might affect learning, other issues quickly became part of school nurses' practice. In the early part of the twentieth century the temperance movement led schools to teach children about the effects of alcohol and tobacco. Also early in the twentieth century, "gymnastics" was introduced in schools in an effort to promote physical activity. World War I was a pivotal point for school health services, and the call for a national effort to improve the health of schoolchildren emerged. In 1918 the National Education Association joined forces with the American Medical Association (AMA) to form the Joint Committee on Health Problems and publish the report *Minimum Health Requirements for Rural Schools*. This group also called for the coordination of health education programs, medical supervision, and physical education. By 1921 nearly every state had laws that required physical and health education in schools. Additionally, fire drills became part of safety education programs introduced during and after World War I (Allensworth et al., 1997).

Even though emphasis was placed on health services in schools, barriers still existed. Many schools and cities were unwilling to take on the task of providing primary health care for all children. The idea that schools should simply identify and refer problems to physicians was a common practice backed by the AMA. By the 1920s, medical services and preventive health services were clearly separated in the public health arena and in the schools, thereby largely supported by each state, which focused more attention on "health education." The federal government did not get involved with school health until the passage of the National School Lunch Program in 1946. The School Breakfast Program was implemented 30 years later (Allensworth et al., 1997).

There was no impetus to change the direction of school health programs until the 1960s and 1970s. During these decades there was increasing publicity about children living in poverty and the move to mainstream children with disabilities. These two issues, along with an increase in the number of children of immigrants, contributed to changes in school health programs.

During the 1960s the first nurse practitioner training programs opened and made the inclusion of primary care services in schools possible. In 1976 the first National School Conference, supported by the Robert Wood Johnson Foundation, was held in Galveston, Texas. After this conference a variety of school health service models began to emerge with new partnerships and ideas created to provide the most comprehensive health care services for school-age children. In addition, the Education for the Handicapped Act in 1975 mandated that all children, regardless of disabilities, have access to educational services.

The 1980s and 1990s saw several measures aimed at improving the health of schoolchildren. The Drug-Free Schools and Community Act was implemented in 1986 to fight substance abuse through education and was expanded in 1994 to include violence prevention measures. During this period, the Centers for Disease Control and Prevention (CDC), Division of Adolescent and School Health, began funding state education agencies to develop and implement programs aimed at alcohol and tobacco use, physical education, and the reduction of sexually transmitted diseases (STDs) and HIV infection among the nation's youth. Also, the federal government encouraged states to use part of their maternal and child block grant monies to fund school-based health centers.

The No Child Left Behind Act (NCLB) was signed into law by President Bush in 2002. As part of the NCLB, the Safe and Drug Free Schools and Communities Act (SDFSC) became effective that same year. SDFSC supports programs that focus on prevention of school violence and illegal use of alcohol, tobacco, and drugs. This legislation promotes the involvement of parents and communities in efforts and resources to create a safe and drug-free environment in order to enhance student academic achievement.

The Patient Protection and Affordable Care Act was signed into law March 23, 2010, by President Obama. Under this act, an initial 95 million dollars was awarded to 278 school-based health centers (SBHCs) as part of a capital program to create new sites and expand existing services in 2011. In 2012, an additional 14.5 million dollars was awarded to 45 SBHCs for expansion of services in medically underserved areas (USDHHS, 2013). See the later discussion of SBHCs.

School health services vary widely among states and school districts. There continues to be a lack of coordination among providers, with no single agency responsible for tracking services. Recognizing that there are differences among schools in the United States and that important health information must be delivered to children and adolescents, the USDHHS addressed many related issues in the *Healthy People 2020* program. Objectives targeting children and adolescents are written for diverse areas, including physical activity, sex education and HIV prevention, nutrition, smoking prevention, injury prevention, and school absences related to asthma. The *Healthy People 2020* box lists a few of these objectives related to school health.

SCHOOL HEALTH SERVICES

The School Health Policies and Programs Study describes school health services as a "coordinated system that ensures a continuum of care from school to home to community health care provider and back" (Allensworth et al., 1997, p. 153). School health services goals and objectives vary from state to

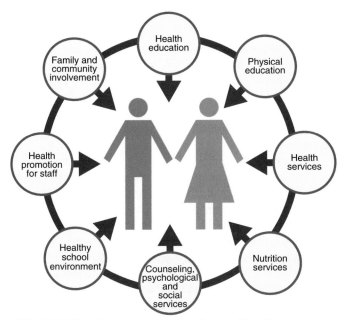

FIG. 30.1 The eight components of school health programs.

state, community to community, and school to school. These differences reflect wide variations in student needs, community resources, funding sources, and school leadership preferences. Many organizations, such as the American School Health Association and NASN, are involved in the care and welfare of school-age children and have compiled and adopted definitions, standards, and statistics related to school health.

According to the School-Based Health Alliance (2014), there are 2315 SBHCs located in 49 out of 50 states, including the District of Columbia. Most SBHCs are staffed with a nurse, a nurse practitioner, or physician assistant. The following services provided in these centers typically include first aid, medication administration, and preventive screenings (vision, hearing, scoliosis, and acanthosis nigricans). Nearly all schools maintain health records on students and, at a minimum, monitor immunization status per federal and state laws. Most authorities agree that comprehensive school health programs should have the following eight components (Fig. 30.1): health education; physical education; health services; nutrition services; counseling, psychological, and social services; healthy school environment; health promotion for staff; and family and community involvement.

 HEALTHY PEOPLE 2020

Selected Objectives for School Health

AH-5.6: Decrease school absenteeism among adolescents due to illness or injury.
AH-8: Increase the proportion of adolescents whose parents consider them to be safe at school.
DH-14: Increase the proportion of children and youth with disabilities who spend at least 80% of their time in regular education programs.
EMC-1: (Developmental) Increase the proportion of children who are ready for school in all five domains of healthy development: physical development, social and emotional development, and approaches to learning, language, and cognitive development.

 HEALTHY PEOPLE 2020—cont'd

Selected Objectives for School Health

EMC-4: Increase the proportion of elementary, middle, and senior high schools that require school health education.
ECBP-5: Increase the proportion of the nation's elementary, middle, and senior high schools that have a full-time registered school nurse–to-student ratio of at least 1:750.
EH-16: Increase the proportion of the nation's elementary, middle, and high schools that have official school policies and engage in practices that promote a healthy and safe physical school environment.
FP-12: Increase the proportion of adolescents who received formal instruction on reproductive health topics before they were 18 years old.
IID-10: Maintain vaccination coverage levels for children in kindergarten.
IVP-27: Increase the proportion of public and private schools that require students to wear appropriate protective gear when engaged in school-sponsored physical activities.
MHMD-6: Increase the proportion of children with mental health problems who receive treatment.
NWS-10: Reduce the proportion of children and adolescents who are considered obese.
NWS-2: Increase the proportion of schools that offer nutritious foods and beverages outside of school meals.
OH-1: Reduce the proportion of children and adolescents who have dental caries in their primary or permanent teeth.
PA-4: Increase the proportion of the nation's public and private schools that require daily physical education for all students.
RD-5.1: Reduce the proportion of children aged 5 to 17 years with asthma who miss school days.
SA-18: Reduce steroid use among adolescents.
TU-3: Reduce the initiation of tobacco use among children, adolescents, and young adults.
V-2: Reduce blindness and visual impairment in children and adolescents age 17 and under.

From HealthyPeople.gov: *Healthy People 2020: Topics & objectives.* www.healthypeople.gov/2020/TopicsObjectives2020/default.aspx Accessed: February 21, 2018.

Health Education

An objective of *Healthy People 2020* sets a goal that middle, junior, and senior high schools provide health education courses in priority areas. The CDC (2016) identified the following six high-risk behaviors, utilizing the Youth Risk Behavior Surveillance System (YRBSS), as needing to be targeted in health education courses:

1. Alcohol and drug use
2. Injury and violence (including suicide)
3. Tobacco use
4. Poor nutrition
5. Lack of physical activity
6. Sexual behavior that results in STDs or unwanted pregnancies

These problems and behaviors are preventable and often coexist. They also lead to both social and educational problems that contribute to our nation's high dropout and unemployment rates and crime statistics.

The National Health Education Standards were established to promote positive health behaviors for students in all grades (CDC, 2016). These standards give educators, administrators, and policy makers a framework for developing and designing

BOX 30.2   **Purposes of the Youth Risk Behavior Survey System**

- Determine the prevalence of health risk behaviors.
- Assess whether health risk behaviors increase, decrease, or remain the same over time.
- Examine the co-occurrence of health risk behaviors.
- Provide comparable data among subpopulations of youth.
- Provide comparable national, state, territorial, tribal, and local data.
- Monitor progress toward achieving the *Healthy People 2020* objectives and other program indicators.

From Kann L, McManus T, Harris WA, et al.: Youth risk behavior surveillance—United States, 2015, *MMWR Surveill Summ* 65(No. SS-6):1–174, 2016.

health education programs in schools. The standards are written to promote personal, family, and community health in students, targeting grades 2, 5, 8, and 12. The standards provide a guide for curricula development in health education and specify that the students will (1) comprehend concepts related to health promotion and disease prevention to enhance health; (2) analyze the influence of family, peers, culture, media, technology, and other factors on health behaviors; (3) demonstrate the ability to access valid information, products, and services to enhance health; (4) demonstrate the ability to use interpersonal communication skills to enhance health and avoid or reduce health risks; (5) demonstrate the ability to use decision-making skills to enhance health; (6) demonstrate the ability to use goal-setting skills to enhance health; (7) demonstrate the ability to practice health-enhancing behaviors and avoid or reduce health risks; and (8) demonstrate the ability to advocate for personal, family, and community health.

In 1990, to learn more about high-risk behaviors among youth, the CDC (2016) instituted the **Youth Risk Behavior Surveillance System**. The YRBSS survey is conducted every 2 years among selected high school students throughout the United States in both private and public schools. Box 30.2 lists the purposes of the YRBSS. Reports from the survey provide valuable information that can help improve health education programs in schools.

Injury Prevention

Injury prevention should be taught early in schools, and the information should be age appropriate. For example, bicycle safety, including the importance of wearing a helmet and the proper use of backpacks, must be stressed beginning in elementary schools. Safety on the schoolyard and playground is also important for this age group, because approximately 200,000 children per year are injured on playgrounds in the United States (U.S. Consumer Product Safety Commission, 2009). Motor vehicle safety should be included in programs for adolescents who are beginning to drive. These motor vehicle safety programs should include the hazards of distracted driving (e.g. cell phones, texting), which are issues affecting all drivers.

Sports safety is particularly important among adolescents as participation in sports continues to grow, especially among girls. More than 3.5 million children younger than 14 years receive medical treatment in emergency rooms each year for sports-related injuries (Safe Kids USA, 2011). Injuries occur most commonly on playgrounds, on athletic fields, and in gymnasiums. Orthopedic injuries (e.g., strains, sprains, fractures, and dislocations), dental injuries, neurological problems (e.g., traumatic brain injury [TBI] and concussion), ophthalmic injuries, cuts, abrasions, and bruises are frequently seen. TBI accounts for more 20,000 of these injuries and continues to be a significant concern for health care providers and school nurses (Cheng et al., 2016).

Use of proper equipment should be mandatory for children and adolescents participating in sports activities. Fitted mouth guards, shin guards, pads, helmets, and other protective gear should be required to prevent injury. Regular hydration and frequent rest periods should be required to prevent heat-related illnesses, especially during hot weather. Effective warm-up and cool-down exercises should be encouraged to prevent muscle strain. Schools that participate in aquatic sports should include pool safety. The school nurse has a unique opportunity to work with the athletic staff to promote these kinds of policies.

The sports physical is a good time for the school nurse to counsel the student about the risk of health problems related to physical activity. This is also an appropriate setting for the nurse to question girls about menstrual irregularities and to ask all students about their eating behaviors, feelings about their weight, and history of musculoskeletal injuries. The nurse can use this setting to teach the importance of stretching exercises to help prevent injuries.

Many school districts have school safety committees that make recommendations for sports-related safety. These committees collect data on injuries, develop safety inspection policies, and plan staff training and student education related to school environmental factors. Nurses are vital members of school health teams and committees from instituting injury prevention programs to injury response on the athletic field.

Tobacco Use

For the past several decades, major concerns have been raised about long-term health problems associated with adolescents' use of tobacco, alcohol, and illegal substances. There is an increased likelihood that these youthful abusers will ultimately engage in other high-risk behaviors. Adolescent smoking has been closely correlated with alcohol use and other drugs. Smoking by young people can cause serious health problems, such as heart disease; chronic lung disease; and cancers of the lung, pharynx, esophagus, and bladder. Factors that have been associated with youth tobacco use include low economic status, peer pressure, smoking by parents, a perception that tobacco use is the norm, low levels of academic achievement, exposure of advertising, and history of aggressive behavior such as membership in gangs (CDC, 2016).

Although there has been improvement over the last decades, smoking remains a major problem in this country and is the single leading preventable cause of death in the United States. Cigarette smoking has declined significantly, but the usage of other forms of tobacco has emerged; this includes electronic cigarettes, hookah, pipes, bidis, flavored tobacco, and smokeless tobacco (CDC, 2016). Prevention should be a priority in youth because 9 out of 10 cigarette smokers first tried smoking by 18 years of age (USDHHS, 2014). Of continued concern, it is estimated that more than 25% of high school students in 2015 used some form of tobacco (CDC, 2016). Further, an estimated 3200 youth under the age of 18 try their first cigarette each day, with an additional 2100 youth becoming daily smokers (USDHHS, 2014). White high school students have the highest rate of consumption of tobacco in various forms, at 24.0%, followed by Hispanics at 23.9%, and blacks at 21.0%. Finally, percentage rates for any tobacco product usage are 20.3% in females and 30.0% in males (CDC, 2016).

Substance Abuse

The use of alcohol and other drugs is associated with problems in school, injuries, violence, and motor vehicle deaths. All 50 states and the District of Columbia have outlawed the sale of alcohol to anyone under the age of 21, yet it is still the most commonly used and abused drug among children and adolescents. In 2014, statistics show that 33% of 15-year-olds and 60% of 18-year-olds had tried alcohol; thus use increased in frequency as youths progressed in school (Substance Abuse and Mental Health Services Administration, 2016). Furthermore, approximately 17.7% of high school students reported they had five or more drinks of alcohol in a row within a couple of hours at least 1 day within the last 30 days (CDC, 2016). Additionally, almost 32.8% reported having had at least one drink of alcohol during the last 30 days (CDC, 2015). Alcohol use is more prevalent among Hispanics (34.4%) and whites (35.2%) than blacks (23.8%) (CDC, 2015).

The most commonly used illicit drug in the United States is marijuana. In 2015, 38.6% of young people reported using marijuana one or more times in their lives (CDC, 2015). A new disturbing trend is the use of synthetic marijuana as known as *K2, Spice, fake weed, King Kong, or Moon Rocks,* with 9.2% of high school students reporting its use in 2015 (CDC, 2015).

The use of other illegal drugs in high school students includes cocaine (5.2%), hallucinogenics (6.4%), Ecstasy (5.0%), inhalants (7.0%), heroin (2.1%), methamphetamine (3.0%), steroids (3.5%), and prescription drugs (opioids, depressants, or stimulants) (16.8%) (CDC, 2015). Of significant concern is the growing abuse of prescription drugs. Opioids (e.g., Vicodin or OxyContin), depressants or antianxiety medications (e.g., Valium or Xanax), and stimulants (e.g., Ritalin or Adderall) are the most commonly abused. Many times students obtain these drugs from other family members who have been prescribed the medication or from the illegal sale on the streets or through the Internet.

The use of anabolic steroids has decreased somewhat among high school students, declining from 3.6% in 2011 to 3.0% in 2015, but the issue should remain a concern to school health nurses because of the number of athletes who abuse the drugs (CDC, 2015). Many athletes believe that anabolic steroids will produce an increase in strength and muscle mass and enhance their performance. There are more than 100 different types of anabolic steroids, and all require a prescription. Abuse or improper use of anabolic steroids can result in severe problems, including renal impairment or failure; liver

---

BOX 30.3   Teen Pregnancy

- The U.S. teen birth rate is one of the highest among developed countries.
- 249,078 babies were born to teenagers aged 15 to 19 in 2014.
- Black and Hispanic youth have a disproportionately high rate of teen pregnancy.
- Teen mothers are less likely to complete high school.
- Teen mothers are more likely to be single parents and to live in poverty.
- Birth rates among teenagers vary substantially from state to state.

Data from Centers for Disease Control and Prevention: *About teen pregnancy,* 2016. https://www.cdc.gov/teenpregnancy/about/

---

cancer; cardiovascular problems such as high blood pressure and elevated cholesterol levels; and sexual changes such as testicular shrinkage, clitoral enlargement, and accelerated puberty (National Institute on Drug Abuse, 2016.

Sex Education

A number of objectives of *Healthy People 2020* address issues of human sexuality and prevention of pregnancy, STDs, and HIV. These issues are important for the nurse working with older children and adolescents.

Many teens become sexually active at an early age, and despite recent declines, pregnancy rates continue to be high (Box 30.3). Data obtained from the YRBSS reveals a decrease from 47.4% in 2011 to 41.2% in 2015 of adolescents in grades 9 through 12 who have had sexual intercourse (CDC, YRBSS, 2016).

Sex education in the school setting is a controversial topic. Opponents of sex education believe that parents have the responsibility for teaching this content to their children. Laws in certain states prohibit or dramatically limit sex education in public schools. However, 24 states and the District of Columbia mandate that public schools teach sex education (National Conference of State Legislatures, 2016). Proponents argue that for many children sex education will not be addressed in the home. If this information is not taught in schools, children may receive inadequate or incorrect information from peers, media, or other sources. Contrary to some concerns, there is no research that concludes that sex education in the schools increases sexual activity. According to the Future of Sex Education Initiative (2012), the following seven topics are considered fundamental to a comprehensive sex education curriculum: anatomy and physiology, puberty and adolescent development, identity (sexual orientation), pregnancy and reproduction, STDs and HIV, healthy relationships, and personal safety. School nurses have been caught in the center of this controversy but historically have advocated for education on normal human sexuality that encourages discussion in an objective, nonjudgmental manner and in which students are free to ask questions and receive correct answers.

Tattoos and Body Piercings

Tattoos and body piercings are a form of self-expression and attention-seeking behavior. Their popularity has risen dramatically in the last decade. The procedures are often done at home, on the streets, or in parlors where sterile technique and safety precautions are not practiced. Both hepatitis C and methicillin-resistant *Staphylococcus aureus* have been linked to tattoos and body piercings. This fact presents an opportunity for the school nurse to teach students the importance of making healthy decisions on whether to have such procedures done and, if so, under what conditions they will be performed.

Dental Health

One of the most common complaints of school-age children is dental caries. There are numerous contributing factors, including poor oral hygiene, lack of fluoridated water, and lack of funds or insurance for dental care. More than half of children have dental caries by the time they are 8 years of age. This disease is more common in lower-income children, and approximately 66% of those between the ages of 12 and 19 have had tooth decay. Untreated cavities can greatly affect a child's quality of life and cause pain, absence from school, and decreased self-worth (CDC, 2015). Proper brushing of teeth should be taught along with good nutritional habits and the importance of regular dental checkups. Children should also be taught the relationship between high-sugar foods and dental caries.

Physical Education

One of the major objectives of *Healthy People 2020* is improvement of health and fitness through regular physical activity. Children today are less active than children in the past. Daily enrollment in physical education classes among high school students dropped from 42% in 1991 to 29% in 2013 (CDC, 2013). Children are becoming more sedentary as a result of increased use of computers and television and decreasing requirements for physical education. It was reported in 2011 that 31% of high school children used a computer 3 or more hours a day and 32% watch television 3 or more hours a day (CDC, 2012).

A sedentary lifestyle is associated with obesity, hypertension, heart disease, and diabetes. Studies show that people who are active have a better quality of life and outlive those who are inactive. Habits in childhood are likely to continue into adulthood, making it imperative that children are taught the importance of being physically active at a young age. Studies also show that children and adolescents who are physically active have increased self-confidence and self-esteem and decreased anxiety, stress, and depression. Regular physical activity helps build and maintain healthy bones and muscles.

Physical education should focus on activities that children can continue into their adult years, such as walking, swimming, biking, and jogging. The educational content should change as the child ages. For example, what may appeal to a young child, such as playing on the playground with friends, is different from what motivates an adolescent, such as competitive sports and aerobic exercise. The CDC has made 10 recommendations for the promotion of lifelong physical activity (Box 30.4).

Health Services

Health care provided in schools includes preventive services such as immunizations and health screenings. This component of a comprehensive school health program may also involve emergency care, management of acute and chronic health conditions, appropriate referrals, health counseling, education about healthy lifestyles, and medication administration.

BOX 30.4 Guidelines for School Programs: Promoting Healthy Eating and Physical Activity

- Use a coordinated approach to develop, implement, and evaluate healthy eating and physical activity policies and practices.
- Establish school environments that support healthy eating and physical activity.
- Provide a quality school meal program and ensure that students are offered only appealing, healthy food and beverage choices outside the school meal program.
- Implement a comprehensive physical activity program with quality physical education as the cornerstone.
- Implement health education that provides students with the knowledge, attitudes, skills, and experiences needed for healthy eating and physical activity.
- Provide students with health, mental health, and social services to address healthy eating, physical activity, and related chronic disease prevention.
- Partner with families and community members in the development and implementation of healthy eating and physical activity policies, practices, and programs.
- Provide a school employee wellness program that includes healthy eating and physical activity services for all school staff members.
- Employ qualified persons and provide professional development opportunities for physical education; health education; nutrition services; and health, mental health, and social services staff members, as well staff members who supervise recess, cafeteria time, and out-of-school-time programs.

From Centers for Disease Control and Prevention: School health guidelines to promote healthy eating and physical activity, *MMWR Recomm Rep* 60(RR-5):1–76, 2011. www.cdc.gov/mmwr/pdf/rr/rr6005.pdf.

Immunizations

Immunizations are a vital component of routine health care, providing long-lasting protection against many diseases. Vaccine-preventable deaths are at record-low levels. Many communicable diseases have been reduced by more than 99% as a result of immunizations. Undervaccination of children, especially those in large urban areas, is a concern because of the potential for disease outbreaks.

All states now require proof of immunization status or evidence of immunity before a child can enter school. Certain exceptions based on religious and philosophical beliefs or medical contraindications may apply. The school nurse plays an important role in verifying compliance with immunization requirements and in educating children and parents about the benefits of immunization. See the CDC website (https://www.cdc.gov/vaccines/schedules/hcp/index.html) for current immunization schedules.

Health Screenings

Many children in the United States are not appropriately screened for certain treatable conditions. Impaired vision and hearing can result in poor academic performance, slowed emotional development, and stress-related disorders. Early identification and treatment of these problems is highly effective and less costly. Vision and hearing screenings are provided at most schools according to a schedule set by the state or school district. These screenings usually occur upon a child's initial entry to school and at least once during elementary, middle, and high school. Children and adolescents may need to be screened more often on the basis of family history, developmental delays, recurrent ear infections, or exposure to loud noise.

Vision screening is required in most states, with referrals as needed. The standard Snellen vision chart is the usual screening tool. Screening for strabismus is a nursing responsibility, and this condition must be identified and treated early to prevent amblyopia. If left untreated, amblyopia may result in loss of vision. Referral to an eye specialist is a critical component of all abnormal eye examination results.

Scoliosis or postural screening should be done to identify spinal deviations in an effort to prevent secondary problems. Spinal problems may lead to cosmetic, functional, or emotional problems. Scoliosis screening in the school consists primarily of a visual inspection of the back. The American Academy of Pediatrics and the American Academy of Orthopedic Surgeons recommend screening of all girls at 10 and 12 years and boys once at either 13 or 14 years (Hresko et al., 2015).

The assessment of high blood pressure during childhood is important in identifying children who have hypertension and who will benefit from early intervention and follow-up. Vascular and end-organ damage from hypertension can begin in early childhood. Periodic blood pressure measurements are inexpensive and should be performed routinely for all children. Other periodic screenings may be mandated by various state or district regulations. These include body mass index (BMI) (height and weight) and dental screenings.

The Children's Health Insurance Program is a national program designed for children of families who earn too much money to qualify for Medicaid but cannot afford the high cost of health insurance. Medicaid-eligible children are guaranteed access to comprehensive health care services and routine dental examinations. Medicaid created the **Early and Periodic Screening, Diagnosis, and Treatment** (EPSDT) service because of the large number of uninsured children. EPSDT, a comprehensive child health program for the uninsured under the age of 21, includes health education and periodic screening. Services provided under the EPSDT program are often performed through the public health offices in each state, but may occur in community health clinics and schools. Screening services must include a comprehensive health and developmental history, an unclothed physical examination, immunizations and laboratory testing that are age appropriate, and lead toxicity screenings (Centers for Medicare and Medicaid Services, 2017).

Emergency Care

Schools are a common site of injuries ranging from minor scrapes, bruises, and fractures, to more severe life-threatening events such seizures, head injuries, severe asthma attacks, and mass casualty incidents. Injuries may occur in school buildings or classrooms or during physical education classes or athletic events. Emergencies can include natural events, such as hurricanes, tornadoes, and earthquakes, or manmade disasters, such as hazardous material spills, fires, and acts of terror. Basic first aid equipment should be available in all schools. The school nurse must be knowledgeable about standard first aid and certified in cardiopulmonary resuscitation and use of an automated external defibrillator. The school nurse must also be responsible for the development of a school emergency plan that provides school staff with a guide to facilitate quick response in case of a student or school emergency.

Care of the Ill Child

The school nurse is responsible for monitoring the health of all students. For students with acute or chronic illnesses, administration of medications or treatments may be necessary. The nurse is often required to assess an ill child to determine the type of illness or health problem and develop a management plan. Two commonly encountered chronic illnesses are asthma and diabetes.

In 2014, 8.6% of U.S. children younger than 18 years had asthma, which was most prevalent among poor children (16.4%) and non-Hispanic black children (18.4%) (CDC, 2014). Asthma is one of the most common chronic childhood conditions, causing more than 4.6 million people to miss more than 1 day of school or work (CDC, 2011). Because asthma is so prevalent, it is recommended that school-based support exists for children who have it. Actions undertaken by some schools across the country include immediate access to asthma medications, development and implementation of asthma action plans, and student and staff education on asthma. An assessment tool has been developed to determine how well schools assist children with asthma (Box 30.5). Answers to all the questions in the assessment tool should be "yes." "No" answers indicate that students may not be in an environment conducive to asthma control.

According to the American Association of Diabetes Educators (AADE, 2016), diabetes is prevalent in school-age children, affecting around 190,000 people younger than 20 years. Most cases of diabetes in this cohort is type 1, but type 2 diabetes is being diagnosed with increasing frequency in children. Type 2 diabetes in youth is projected to increase by 49% in the next 40 years, and the number of children diagnosed with type 1 diabetes is expected to increase 23%. The figures are disproportionately larger in minority populations. Childhood obesity and the decline in physical activity are considered major factors in this development (American Diabetes Association [ADA], 2012). In general, teachers are inadequately prepared to care for children with diabetes and must rely on the school nurse. Children should be able to participate in their care to the extent that they are able (ADA, 2012). With the growing number of children who have diabetes, it is imperative that the nurse recognize the signs and symptoms of hypoglycemia and hyperglycemia in order to assist children in the monitoring of glucose levels and the administration of insulin or glucagon. The ADA has specific recommendations based on age, as shown in Box 30.6.

Medication Administration

Administration of medications is a service provided almost universally by school districts across the country. The use of medications by school-age children has increased over the last several years, allowing many children to attend school despite serious health problems.

Medication administration in the schools is a serious undertaking. Issues facing the school nurse include safety, monitoring of both therapeutic and side effects, proper documentation, confidentiality, and ongoing communication with the student and family. Only those medications considered necessary are administered at school.

BOX 30.5 How Asthma-Friendly Is Your School? Checklist

Children with asthma need proper support at school to keep their asthma under control and be fully active. Use the following questions to find out how well your school assists children with asthma.

☐ Yes ☐ No Is your school free of tobacco smoke at all times, including during school-sponsored events and on school buses?

☐ Yes ☐ No Does the school maintain good indoor air quality? Does it reduce or eliminate allergens and irritants that can make asthma worse? Check if any of the following are present:
    ☐ Cockroaches
    ☐ Dust mites (commonly found in humid climates in pillows, carpets, upholstery, and stuffed toys)
    ☐ Mold
    ☐ Pets with fur or feathers
    ☐ Strong odors or fumes from art and craft supplies, pesticides, paint, perfumes, air fresheners, and cleaning chemicals

☐ Yes ☐ No Is there a school nurse in your school all day, every day? If not, is a nurse regularly available to help the school write plans and give the school guidance on medicines, physical education, and field trips for students with asthma?

☐ Yes ☐ No Can children take medicines at school as recommended by their doctor and parents? May children carry their own asthma medicines?

☐ Yes ☐ No Does your school have a written, individualized emergency plan for teachers and staff in case of a severe asthma episode (attack)? Does the plan make clear what action to take under different emergency situations such as fire, weather, or lock-down? Whom to call? When to call?

☐ Yes ☐ No Does someone teach school staff about asthma, asthma action plans, and asthma medicines? Does someone teach all students about asthma and how to help a classmate who has it?

☐ Yes ☐ No Can students actively participate in physical education class and recess? (For example, do students have access to their medicine before exercise? Can they choose modified or alternative activities when medically necessary?)

If the answer to any question is "no," students in your school may be facing obstacles to asthma control. Uncontrolled asthma can hinder a student's attendance, participation, and progress in school. School staff, health professionals, and parents can work together to remove obstacles and promote students' health and education.

From National Heart, Lung, and Blood Institute, National Asthma Education and Prevention Program, NAEPP School Asthma Education Subcommittee: *How asthma friendly is your school?* 2008. www.nhlbi.nih.gov/health/public/lung/asthma/friendly.pdf

---

BOX 30.6 Expectations of the Child With Diabetes

Toddler and Preschool Age
- The child should be able to determine which finger to prick.
- The child can usually choose an injection site.
- The child is generally cooperative.

Elementary School Age
- The child should be able to assist in all diabetes tasks at school.
- The child is usually able to perform his or her own fingerstick glucose monitoring.
- The child can administer his or her own insulin with supervision.
- The child is usually able to let an adult know when he or she is experiencing a hypoglycemic episode.

Middle School and High School Age
- The child should be able to perform self-monitoring of blood glucose.
- Most children should be able to administer their own insulin with supervision; adolescents should be able to administer insulin without supervision.
- All children may need assistance with blood glucose testing when the glucose level is low.

Data from American Diabetes Association: Diabetes care in the school and day care setting, *Diabetes Care* 35:S76–S80, 2012.

The following guidelines from NASN (2017) should be included in school medication policies:
- Delegation (including training and supervision of unlicensed assistive personnel)
- Medication orders
- Prescription and over-the-counter medications
- Proper labeling, storage, disposal, and transportation of medication
- Documentation of medication administration
- Rescue and emergency medications
- Off-label medications and investigational drugs
- Complementary and alternative medications
- Psychotropic medications and controlled substances
- Medication doses that exceed manufacturer's guidelines
- Student confidentiality

Medications commonly given in schools include analgesics and antipyretics (e.g., acetaminophen [Tylenol] or ibuprofen [Advil]), antacids, antitussives, anticonvulsants, antiemetics and antidiarrheals, antifungals, antihistamines, and antibiotics. Medications used to treat attention-deficit hyperactivity disorder (ADHD) are among the most commonly administered. In a report released in 2015, 9.5% of children in the United States between 4 and 17 years were diagnosed with ADHD, and this number appears to be increasing (Pastor, 2015).

Alternative and complementary medicine includes practices and products outside the realm of conventional medicine. Medication administration policies should exist that reflect local and state laws that address these products. The request for the administration of any of these medications provides the nurse with an excellent health teaching opportunity.

School nurses must be aware of medications that are being self-administered on school grounds and must provide education as needed to both children and parents. Rescue medications such as albuterol for asthma or an EpiPen for a child with a severe allergic reaction must be administered quickly to affect asthma symptoms, and the nurse must be familiar with its expected effects to properly assist the child who needs it. It is now legal in all 50 states for students to carry and self-administer asthma medications (NASN, 2017).

TABLE 30.2 Overview of Increase in Number of Students With Disabilities*

Type of Disability	1976–1977	1990–1991	2000–2001	2009–2010	2013–2014
All disabilities	8.3	11.4	13.3	13.1	12.9
Specific learning disabilities	1.8	5.2	6.1	4.9	4.5
Speech or language impairments	2.9	2.4	3.0	2.9	2.7
Developmental delays	—	—	0.4	0.7	0.8
Emotional disturbance	0.6	0.9	1.0	0.8	0.7
Hearing impairment	0.2	0.1	0.2	0.2	0.2
Orthopedic impairments	0.2	0.1	0.2	0.1	0.1
Other health impairments	0.3	0.1	0.6	1.4	1.6
Visual impairments	0.1	0.1	0.1	0.1	0.1
Multiple disabilities	—	0.2	0.3	0.3	0.3
Autism and related disorders	—	—	0.2	0.8	1.1

*Children age 3 to 21 years served in federally supported programs for the disabled by type of disability: selected years 1976– 1977 through 2013–2014.
From National Center for Education Statistics: *NCES fast facts: students with disabilities,* 2016. https://nces.ed.gov/fastfacts/display.asp?id=64

Children With Special Health Needs

In 1976, Public Law 99-142 was enacted, giving all students, including those who are severely handicapped, the right to public education in the least restrictive environment possible, regardless of mental or physical disabilities. The Education for All Handicapped Children Act of 1973 and the subsequent Individuals with Disabilities Education Act (IDEA) of 1990 enhanced the opportunities for children previously served in acute care and long-term care settings to have access to public education. Children affected by these laws include those who are hearing impaired, mentally challenged, multihandicapped, orthopedically impaired, "other" health impaired (e.g., chronic or acute health problems such as a heart condition or epilepsy), seriously emotionally disturbed, speech impaired, visually handicapped, or who have a specific learning disability.

The development of health care services and technology has enabled students whose conditions may have prevented them in the past from leaving an institution or controlled environment to attend public school. Many of these children need nursing services of varied types (e.g., tube feedings, suctioning, catheterization) to continue their progression in school. Public Law 94-142 requires school nurses to screen or identify children in need of special education and related services and to participate in the development of an interdisciplinary individualized education program (IEP) that includes educational goals and specific services to be provided. The nurse is also responsible for the development of an individualized health care plan (IHP) for all students requiring continuous nursing management while at school. Table 30.2 gives an overview of the increase in the number of students with disabilities.

Student Records

Health records are maintained for all students according to individual school district policy. At a minimum, student health records should include immunization status, pertinent history, results of screenings and examinations, and IHPs. The Family Educational Rights and Privacy Act, a strong privacy protection act, protects student education and health records. Student health records should be afforded the same level of confidentiality as that given to clients and patients in other settings (i.e., sharing confidential information with others without approval is considered unethical and improper except in emergency situations).

The Health Insurance Portability and Accountability Act of 1996 (HIPAA) was instituted in 2003. A major component of HIPAA is ensuring confidentiality of personal health information. Public schools that provide health care services fall under HIPAA regulations. Private schools that do not receive federal funding but engage in HIPAA-related activities are also governed by this act.

Delegation of Tasks

Not every school has a full-time nurse available on site. A nurse may be assigned to three or four schools, resulting in delegation of certain tasks to unlicensed personnel. Each state's Nurse Practice Act stipulates which procedures may be delegated. The responsibility for assessment, diagnosis, goal setting, and evaluation may never be delegated. When tasks are delegated, the nurse must provide appropriate education, written procedures, and ongoing supervision and evaluation of the caregivers.

Nutrition

School-age children are undergoing periods of rapid growth and development and have complex nutritional needs. They must eat a variety of foods to meet their daily requirements. Diets should include a proper balance of carbohydrates, protein, and fat, with sufficient intake of vitamins and minerals. Children and adolescents share a well-known preference for junk food (Box 30.7), and their diet is often high in fat and sugar and frequently consists of fast-food items, such as hamburgers and French fries, instead of fruits and vegetables. Skipping meals, especially breakfast, and eating unhealthy snacks contribute to poor childhood nutrition. Identifying nutritional problems, counseling, and making appropriate referrals are important in the school setting. The school nurse should consider cultural influences on diet when teaching students and assessing their nutritional status.

Poor nutritional status is closely associated with poverty. Federally funded programs such as the School Breakfast Program and National School Lunch Program were initiated to ensure that all children have access to these meals during the school day.

Eating Disorders

It is imperative that the school nurse recognize the association between feelings of inadequacy and unhealthy eating practices in adolescents and young people. These self-perceptions begin early in life; therefore education and counseling must begin in elementary school. Prevention should concentrate on eliminating misconceptions surrounding nutrition, dieting, and body composition and should stress optimal health and personal performance. Outside influences such as social media, celebrity admiration, commercials, and advertisements make this a serious problem.

School nurses must also be aware of eating disorders and related risk factors. Anorexia, bulimia, and binge eating are the three most common eating disorders, and anorexia is ranked number three in terms of chronic disorders in adolescents (NIMH, 2016). *Binge eating* is defined as recurrent, out-of-control eating of large amounts of food whether a person is hungry or not. *Anorexia* is a severely restricted intake of food based on an extreme fear of weight gain. Literature has shown that anorexia is multifactorial, seen primarily in females, and often correlated with family dysfunction or a history of sexual abuse. *Bulimia* is a form of anorexia characterized by a chaotic eating pattern with recurrent episodes of binge eating followed by purging. Health consequences of eating disorders may include reduction of bone density, severe dehydration, tooth decay, and potentially fatal electrolyte imbalances.

Female Athlete Triad. The "female athlete triad" is a syndrome consisting of eating disorders, amenorrhea, and osteoporosis. Pressure to attain a particular body shape or weight considered desirable in a selected sport may put the female athlete at risk for development of this disorder. The triad is a complex problem with psychological and physiological factors. It can result in menstrual irregularities, premature osteoporosis, and decreased bone mineral density; if taken to the extreme, it can become life threatening.

Obesity

Obesity is the fastest-rising public health concern in the nation and will likely overtake tobacco use as the single leading preventable cause of death. The obesity rate has more than doubled in children and tripled in adolescents over the past three decades. Today one in five school-aged children (ages 6 to 19) are considered obese (CDC, 2016). Statistics show that obese children and adolescents are more likely to become obese adults. Obesity and its prevention or treatment must be of concern to the school nurse (CDC, 2013).

Although many of the underlying causes of obesity are not well understood, several contributing factors have been identified; they include reduced access to and affordability of nutritious foods, decreased physical activity, and cultural and genetic influences. Obesity is associated with development of diabetes, dyslipidemia, hypertension, and other disorders, such as osteoarthritis, sleep apnea, different cancers, and cholelithiasis.

In addition, obesity may result in social and quality-of-life impairment, and obese children often have low self-esteem and may be labeled by their peers and ridiculed (CDC, 2013). The school nurse should determine the BMI for all adolescents. A BMI greater than the eighty-fifth percentile for age and gender indicates the need for further assessment and referral. To be successful, the treatment of obesity must begin early and must be multifaceted. Some of the solutions include improved health education related to nutrition and dietary behavior, increased physical activity and physical education programs, healthier school environments, and better nutrition services.

Nutritional Education Programs

Nutritional education is essential and must include parents, teachers, and the child. Children need to know the basics of good nutrition, how to make healthy snack choices, and the importance of balancing physical activity with food intake. Obesity, dental caries, anemia, and heart disease can be reduced or prevented with proper education and lifestyle changes. In addition, all adolescents and school-age children should receive counseling regarding intake of saturated fat.

The United States Department of Agriculture (USDA) Food and Nutrition Service (FNS) provide nutritional education for food service educators, professionals, parents, and child care providers. The USDA and FNS have a number of resources, including *MyPlate,* Team Nutrition, Let's Move, and SNAP-Ed Connection. These programs focus on healthy nutritional choices and health promotion and disease prevention topics in school and child care settings. Comprehensive school-based nutrition programs and services should be provided to all students. The ultimate goal of these efforts is that children will make healthy nutritional choices both inside and outside the school setting.

Counseling, Psychological, and Social Services

The mental health of a child or adolescent is affected by physical, economic, social, psychological, and environmental factors. Children, like adults, often hide problems from others. They may see problems as a sign of weakness or as a lack of control. Children may also be trying to protect themselves or someone they love and so do not seek help, with tragic results. Promotion of mental health and reduction or removal of threats to mental health is important to children and adolescents. This can be an enormous challenge for school nurses as mental health is difficult, yet essential, to assess.

Children and teens often struggle with depression, substance abuse, conduct disorders, self-esteem issues, suicidal ideation, eating disorders, and underachievement or overachievement. They may also have to cope with physical or mental abuse, chronic health conditions, or pregnancy. Common warning signs of stress in children are presented in Box 30.8. Drugs and alcohol can enter a child's life as early as elementary school. Many children live in single-parent households with little social or economic support. They may not have enough to eat or a safe, warm place to sleep, yet are expected to come to school each day ready to learn. Services aimed at helping children cope with these problems are often lacking or too costly for many families.

ETHICAL INSIGHTS

An Ethical Dilemma: What Would You Do?

You are working as the school nurse in a rural high school when Grace, a 15-year-old female student, enters the clinic. Grace appears very worried, and, after several hesitant starts, she begins to cry and tells you that she is sexually active with a 17-year-old senior. She goes on to tell you that she has missed her last period and that her home pregnancy test result was positive. She states that she is afraid to tell her parents because she feels that they will be very disappointed in her and because she is afraid of what her father will do. She asks you where she can go to get an abortion. You speak with Grace for quite a while and encourage her to speak with her parents. She leaves the clinic a little more composed and promises you that she will think about what you have said. The next day Jenny, Grace's mother, comes into the clinic and asks to speak with you. She confides that she is worried about Grace and asks whether you know what is going on with her child. What would you do in this situation?

Although maintaining confidentiality and a professional relationship respectful of the student's wishes is vital, state laws and school district policies determine what a school nurse may do, and in some cases is required to do, when providing care to minor children. In order to deal with personal and sensitive information such as described here, the school nurse should be well versed in relevant laws and policies and should follow them. When in doubt, contact a supervisor.

BOX 30.8 Warning Signs of Stress

- Problems eating or sleeping
- Use of alcohol or other substances (e.g., sedatives, sleep enhancers)
- Problems making decisions
- Persistent anger or hostile feelings
- Inability to concentrate
- Increased boredom
- Frequent headaches and ailments
- Inconsistent school attendance

BOX 30.9 Truths About Adolescent Suicides

- Most adolescents who attempt suicide are ambivalent and torn between wanting to die and wanting to live.
- Any threat of suicide should be taken seriously.
- Warning signs usually precede a suicide attempt; they may include depression, substance abuse, decreased activity, isolation, and appetite and sleep changes.
- Suicide is more common in adolescents who are dealing with bisexuality or homosexuality without support or in a hostile school environment.
- Education concerning suicide does not lead to an increased number of attempts.
- Females are more likely to consider or attempt suicide, and males are more likely to complete a suicide attempt.
- One suicide attempt is more likely to result in a subsequent attempt.
- Sixty percent of completed suicides in children and adolescents are committed with guns.
- Most adolescents who have attempted or completed suicide have not been diagnosed as having a mental disorder.
- Suicide affects all socioeconomic groups.

BOX 30.10 Possible Signs of Abuse and Neglect

Physical Abuse
- Has unexplained burns, bites, bruises, black eyes, or broken bones
- Is wary of adult contact
- Appears frightened of parents or other relatives and cries when it is time to go home

Neglect
- Is frequently absent from school
- Steals food or money
- Lacks adequate medical or dental care
- Appears dirty or disheveled or is underweight
- Does not have proper seasonal clothing

Sexual Abuse
- Has difficulty walking or sitting
- Reports new onset of nightmares or bedwetting
- Refuses to change into gym attire or participate in physical activities
- Runs away from home
- Becomes pregnant or has a sexually transmitted disease

Emotional Abuse
- Exhibits changes in behavior, such as acting out or extreme passivity
- Exhibits delay in either physical or emotional development
- Has attempted suicide
- Exhibits inappropriate adult or infantile behavior

Data from Child Information Gateway: *What is child abuse and neglect? Recognizing the signs and symptoms*, 2013. https://www.childwelfare.gov/pubs/factsheets/whatiscan.cfm.

The nurse or teacher may be the only stable adult in a child's life who will listen without being judgmental. Therefore one of the most important roles of the school nurse is to act as counselor. Children may come to the school nurse with various vague complaints, such as recurrent stomachaches, headaches, and history of sexually promiscuous behavior, and the nurse must look beyond the initial complaint to identify underlying problems.

Major depressive disorders often have their onset in adolescence and are associated with an increased risk of suicide. In 2014 suicide was the second leading cause in both the 10- to 14-year and 15- to 19-year age groups (CDC, 2014). Suicide attempts are more common than completed suicides. A 2015 survey of students in grades 9 through 12 showed that 8.0% attempted suicide in the preceding year and 17% seriously considered suicide (CDC, 2015). The nurse and other school personnel must be on the alert for suicide clusters that are often known to follow a successful suicide. Adolescents may approach school nurses and other school professionals for help before a suicide attempt. The call for help may be subtle and not recognized as such. Therefore it is important for the school nurse to be cognizant of the warning signs associated with suicide and to recognize and refer at-risk adolescents to appropriate mental health professionals (Box 30.9).

Unfortunately, a large number of children are victims of abuse. Physical and psychological abuse and neglect are usually a result of many interacting factors, such as poverty, social isolation, and drug and alcohol abuse. School nurses and other school personnel are mandated to report suspected cases of child maltreatment and neglect. The nurse must be alert to subtle changes in behavior or physical appearance that may point to abuse. Box 30.10 outlines some of the signs and symptoms of child maltreatment.

In cases of child abuse or neglect, the school nurse may help the child learn problem solving, coping mechanisms, and steps to build self-esteem. The role of the nurse may extend outside the school campus. The nurse may need to work closely with families and social services to develop an appropriate health plan for a particular child.

Healthy School Environment

A healthy school environment is one in which distractions are minimized and that is free of physical hazards and psychological health risks. The NASN believes that all students and staff have an inherent right to learn and work in a healthy school environment and that the school nurse can "assess the learning environment for risk factors, educate the community on the impact of environmental exposure, and advocate for the need to address environmental pollution issues" (NASN, 2014).

Violence

Violence is a major public health problem because it threatens the health and well-being, both physical and psychological, of many children and adolescents. According to the U.S. Department of Justice, Bureau of Justice Statistics (2016), during the 2014 school year, students were victims of 850,100 nonfatal victimizations at school, including 363,700 thefts and 486,400 violent crimes. Further, during the 2012–2013 school year, 31 homicides occurred at school in K–12 schools (CDC, 2016). In high school–aged youths, 7.8% of students reported they had been in a physical fight in the last year, and 5.6% stated that they did not attend school for one or more days because they felt unsafe (CDC, 2016).

In recent years, there have been a number of shootings and other acts of serious violence in schools. The CDC (2016) reported that 4.1% of children admitted to having carried a weapon at least 1 day out of the last 30 and that 6.0% had been threatened or injured with a weapon on school property within the last year. The school shooting at Columbine High School in Littleton, Colorado, in 1999 was probably the first time that people in this country realized how unsafe schools could be. More recently, the mass shooting, in Newtown, Connecticut, killed 20 children and six adults, making it the nation's worst K–12 school shooting.

School nurses and other school personnel should be aware of risk factors and signs that could indicate a tendency to violence. Factors common in those who commit violent acts in school include being male and having a history of being ostracized or bullied in school. Media influences such as movies and video games that desensitize the impact of violence are being studied more closely as a possible cause of increased violence among children and adolescents. Children involved in school shootings often have a need for instant gratification, have easy access to guns, and may have a history of discipline problems.

Although the number of students who commit violent acts is small, these random acts are frightening, and school officials struggle with ways to prevent their occurrence and to recognize the signs of troubled youth. Violence prevention programs should begin in elementary schools. Children who exhibit aggressive behavior in elementary school are more likely to exhibit antisocial and violent behavior as adolescents and adults. Programs should target stress management, conflict and anger resolution, and personal and self-esteem development. Nurses should use data collected through the YRBSS and other local data as a means of assessment when developing violence policies and prevention programs in the school and community. Additionally, nurses should initiate and participate in research that examines the complex developmental, social, and psychological factors surrounding violence.

Terrorism

Schools may not be the primary target in an act of terrorism, but they will be affected. Events following the September 11, 2001, terrorist attack illustrate potential problems facing schools, which may include fear and panic among students, teachers, and parents and anxiety among those directly affected.

Every school is expected to have an emergency management plan. In fact, many states mandate that schools develop plans to address the potential threat of a terrorist attack or natural or manmade disaster. School nurses must be prepared to act after any form of terrorism has occurred. The school nurse has an important role as a potential first responder in any emergency situation and should be an active participant in planning and policy development.

Health Promotion for School Staff

Although specific numbers vary, it is estimated that schools in the United States employ more than 5.5 million teachers and other employees. Health promotion programs at the work site have beneficial results, including positive effects on blood pressure control, daily physical activity, smoking cessation, stress management, and weight control. Staff who participate in health promotion programs increase their knowledge and positively change their attitudes and behaviors relative to smoking practices, nutrition, physical activity, stress, and emotional health. Health promotion programs improve morale, reduce job stress and absenteeism, and heighten interest in teaching health-related topics to students. School nurses play an important role in all levels of prevention through assessment, planning, intervention, and evaluation. The school nurse can assist the faculty and staff by giving workshops on exercise and nutrition, screening for increased blood pressure, and establishing weight management programs.

Family and Community Involvement

School nurses are often asked to provide health education to family, parents, and the community on a variety of topics, such as sexuality, STDs, health promotion, communicable diseases, and substance abuse. Health education in the community consists of programs that are designed to positively influence parents, staff, and others in matters related to health. School nurses are a resource in the community and can take a leadership role in developing programs that positively affect the community. School nurses may also serve as consultants and advocates for other community health programs.

Programs that engage the parents in school activities should be based on community needs and resources. Studies show that students who have parental support are more successful, experience less emotional distress, eat healthier, and are more actively engaged in learning. School nurses can promote parental involvement through the establishment of clear communication, involving parents as volunteers and including them in the planning of health-related events at schools. The nurse must also recognize that an increasing number of children are being raised in nontraditional families—single parents, grandparents, gay or lesbian couples, and interracial couples. When addressing issues with families, the nurse cannot let personal feelings alter the plan of care and must be aware that what worked with one family situation will not necessarily work for another.

School nurses need to understand the needs of families and how these needs may affect children in the school setting. The Annie E. Casey Foundation (AECF) looks at some of these key needs using the KIDS COUNT Index. The index looks at four domains that kids need in order to thrive: 1) economic well-being, 2) education, 3) health, and 4) family and community. Using these, the AECF measures the status of child well-being at both state and national levels. In 2016, Minnesota ranked first among all states in overall child well-being, with Mississippi coming in last (AECF, 2016). During the past 6 years, there has been progress in some of the domains of child well-being (health and education) but setbacks in others (economic well-being, family, and community).

Nurses should become adept at working in the public sphere by increasing their visibility and becoming skilled in working with the media and legislators. The media can be useful in assisting school nurses with health education advocacy.

? ACTIVE LEARNING

1. Explain how the *Healthy People 2020* objectives can be used to shape school-based health care.
2. Log on to one of the websites for school nurses such as http://www.school-nurse.com/ or https://www.nasn.org/ and review the many resources available.
3. Interview a member of the local school board about controversial subjects in health education (e.g., sex education).
4. Review the most common diseases and reported injuries in school-age children in your area. Develop a plan for how the school and the community can work together to decrease their incidence.
5. Interview the parents of several school-age children. Ask what health services they would like to see provided in the school setting.
6. Arrange with the principal of a local school to have a discussion session with children in a particular grade level. Ascertain what their eating habits are and then develop a class that can enhance healthy eating.

SCHOOL NURSING PRACTICE

School nursing is a specialty practice. School nurses need education in specific areas, such as growth and development, public health, mental health nursing, case management, program management, family theory, leadership, and cultural sensitivity, to effectively perform their roles. They must be prepared to work with children of all ages and cultures and under variable circumstances. The nurse must also keep abreast of issues affecting children and must participate in research that explores and expands the role. The school nurse's practice is relatively independent and autonomous, even though the school nurse functions as a member of an interdisciplinary team. For entry into school nursing, it is recommended that nurses hold a minimum of a bachelor's

degree. The school nurse must be able to identify and access professional development opportunities in order to maintain competency in the care of children and adolescents.

School nurses function in many roles. Among these are care provider, student advocate, educator, community liaison, and case manager. Additional skills needed by school nurses include the ability to supervise others, to practice relatively independently, and to delegate care. The American Nurses Association developed competencies relevant to school nurses and updated them in 2011. *School Nursing: Scope & Standards of Practice* (3rd ed) can be purchased at https://portal.nasn.org/members_online/members/viewitem.asp?item=S001&catalog=MAN&pn=1&af=NASN.

The school setting is a perfect place to conduct research on how children adapt to life transitions such as divorce, illness or death of a loved one, illness of either themselves or a peer, and domestic violence. The health-related behaviors of the young are a rich source of research opportunities. The school nurse must be aware of and interested in participating in different research studies.

⚡ RESEARCH HIGHLIGHTS
Research Priorities for School Nursing

The National Association of School Nursing (NASN) has identified critical areas for needed research in which there is no evidence supporting or identifying best practices and the cost-effectiveness of nursing practice in school (NASN, 2016). These critical areas are:

- Diabetes and Asthma: Determine the impact of school nurse interventions on students managing their chronic conditions in the school environment.
- Identified School Nurse–Sensitive Indicators: Determine the impact of school nurse interventions on issues such as attendance, medication administration accuracy, immunization rates, seat time, or health office visits.
- Cost–Benefits Analysis: Conduct analysis of the various interventions used by the school nurse with regard to prevention services, emergency room visits, student safety, and care coordination.
- Current Models of School Nurse Practice: Evaluate registered nurse (RN) practice on campus versus an RN managing multiple campuses and the impact(s) on student health, safety, and academics.

Additionally, Gordon and Barry (2006) surveyed 263 school nurses to identify what the nurses believed to be the top research priorities for the specialty. Ten areas were identified as being priority research topics. These priority areas, and examples for each, are presented here:

- Obesity/Nutrition: Nutrition and weight-loss counseling programs, eating disorders, obesity in children and teens, important of exercise
- Legal/Ethical Issues: Legal liability when delegating to nonmedical personnel, ethical issues related to children with Do Not Resuscitate orders, confidentiality, HIPAA mandates
- Emergencies: Emergency preparedness, administering epinephrine autoinjectors (EpiPens) in school, standing orders for emergencies
- Health Education: Effective curricula for health promotion on hot topics (drugs, sexual activity, nutrition, exercise)
- Absenteeism/Attendance: The school nurse's impact on student attendance, impact of absenteeism on educational success, strategies to decrease absenteeism
- Injuries: Playground safety, sports injuries
- Health Services: Funding of school health services by using matching reimbursement (Medicaid), access to health services for students and their families, benefits and cost-effectiveness of school health services

Data from Gordon SC, Barry CD: Development of a school nursing research agenda in Florida: a Delphi study. *J Sch Nurs* 22(2):114–119, 2006.

ACTIVE LEARNING

Attend a meeting of the school nurse association in your area. Identify the major pros and cons of being a school nurse. Look at factors such as working conditions, number of children assigned to each nurse, job functions, and job satisfaction.

SCHOOL-BASED HEALTH CENTERS

School-based health centers are one of the best ways to offer comprehensive health care services to school-age children and adolescents. It is important to note that the center or clinic works in collaboration with, but does not take the place of, the school nurse. The collaboration between the school nurse and the SBHC staff prevents fragmented care and duplication of services. SBHCs provide an interdisciplinary team approach with personnel such as nurse practitioners, social workers, psychologists, and physicians. Services provided in these centers include nutrition education, injury treatment, general and sports physicals, prescriptions, pregnancy testing, laboratory services, immunizations, gynecological examinations, medication dispensing, social work services, and management of chronic illnesses. Close

collaboration must exist within and among the community, the educational board, and the families for such a center to develop and flourish.

 ACTIVE LEARNING

1. Visit a comprehensive school-based clinic in your area. Discuss how the care given in this type of clinic differs from the care that a school nurse can provide. Review the protocols of both settings and see how they differ.
2. What is the cultural makeup of your local area? How should this knowledge influence the school nurses' practice?

FUTURE ISSUES AFFECTING THE SCHOOL NURSE

Our nation's youth are our greatest asset and our hope for the future. The school nurse's role must constantly evolve to meet the demands of this future hope. Issues that will face the school nurse of tomorrow include ethical dilemmas, use of telehealth, continued threat of school violence, threat of bioterrorism, new and emerging infectious diseases, and increase in antibiotic-resistant diseases. The school nurse will need to understand and appreciate the multicultural community in which he or she will practice.

CASE STUDY **Application of the Nursing Process**

Student With Lice

The nursing process is a systematic, organized approach to problem solving that nurses use when working with clients. It is neither fixed nor stagnant. It is a flexible process that allows for ongoing changes. This case study illustrates the use of the nursing process in a school setting.

Sandra Baker is a nurse at an elementary school in a small town. A second-grade teacher brought Carrie Broussard to the clinic and told Sandra that Carrie had been scratching her head all day and she was worried that Carrie might have an infection.

Assessment

Carrie was 7 years old. Her shoulder-length blond hair appeared neat and clean. When questioned by Sandra, Carrie replied that her head had been itching for 2 or 3 days, but she denied any pain or trauma. Sandra noted that Carrie did not have a fever or swollen lymph nodes, but examination of her scalp revealed multiple excoriated areas. Carrie's hair was examined with a Wood's light, and Sandra saw adult lice at the base of the hair follicles on the back of her head, near the nape of the neck. She also saw multiple nits. Sandra learned that Carrie had two brothers in the school and one sister who was a toddler at home.

On Carrie's initial visit to the clinic, Sandra assessed the following:
- Temperature
- Lymph nodes
- Scalp for any abnormal findings

Diagnosis
Individual
- Head lice

Family and Community (School)
- Potential for spread of infestation in both family and school
- Educational opportunity to prevent the spread of lice by teachers and family members

Planning

Sandra was familiar with the school district's policy that covers head lice in schoolchildren. According to the policy, the nurse must do the following:

Individual
Long-Term Goal
- Carrie's return to school after successful treatment

Short-Term Goals
- Contact Carrie's parents to tell them about the lice.
- Inform Carrie's parents that she must be picked up from school.
- Recommend treatment based on school protocol.
- Provide guidelines for returning to school.

Family and Community
Long-Term Goal
- Ensure that the teachers, staff, and family members have the necessary education relative to prevention and treatment of head lice.

Short-Term Goals
- Examine the hair of all other children in Carrie's class for lice, and treat each according to the school protocol.
- Check the hair of all siblings who attend the school for lice.
- Check the hair of all students in the siblings' classes if lice are identified.

Intervention
Family
Carrie's brothers, David and Paul, were brought to the clinic for examination. Both brothers had lice. Sandra contacted Mrs. Broussard, explained the situation to her, and requested that she come to the school to pick up her children. When Mrs. Broussard arrived at the school, Sandra gave her

continued

CASE STUDY　Application of the Nursing Process—cont'd

Student With Lice

written information on treatment and prevention of lice and showed her what nits and lice look like. Mrs. Broussard was also instructed to check other members of the family not attending this school, especially those who share hairbrushes, pillowcases, and towels, because all family members with lice must be treated or the lice would continue to be passed from member to member. Sandra also explained procedures for cleaning combs, brushes, bedding, and potentially contaminated clothing and toys. Finally, Mrs. Broussard was informed that the children could return to school the day after treatment.

It was obvious to Sandra that Mrs. Broussard was embarrassed. To ease her mind, Sandra carefully explained that head lice are highly contagious, are easily passed from child to child, and are not an indication of poor hygiene. Mrs. Broussard repeated the instructions and left with her three children.

Community

Sandra examined all of the students from each of the Broussard children's classes for head lice. From the three classes, she identified five more children with head lice and notified their parents. Those children had siblings in three additional classrooms and she repeated the procedure for each of them. At the end of the day, she had identified a total of 15 children with head lice and contacted all parents.

Sandra investigated whether the teachers and staff desired an information session on the transmission and spread of head lice because so many students

had lice. She discovered that it had been 2 years since this was done, and so she arranged a class for the coming week for the teachers and teachers' aides to learn how to identify and treat head lice.

Evaluation
Individual and Family

Mrs. Broussard brought Carrie, David, and Paul to school the following day, and on examination Sandra found their hair to be free of lice and nits. Mrs. Broussard expressed her appreciation for the nurse's help and nonjudgmental approach to the problem.

Community

Over the next 2 days, Sandra reexamined all of the children in the affected classrooms and found that the infected children had been successfully treated and that there were no new cases. New cases were not identified during the remainder of the semester. The teachers and staff gave her positive feedback about the head lice education class and asked for it to be repeated at the beginning of each school year.

Levels of Prevention and School Health

School nursing encompasses all three levels of prevention (i.e., primary, secondary, and tertiary), and all three may be practiced individually or concurrently. Table 30.3 lists examples of school nursing interventions for each of the three levels of prevention.

TABLE 30.3　Examples of Prevention and the Role of the Nurse in the School Setting

Example	Nurse's Role
Primary Prevention	
Nutrition education	Provide education to children and parent(s); consult with dietary staff
Immunizations	Provide for or refer to source(s) for immunizations; offer consultation for immunization in special circumstances
Safety	Provide safety education; inspect playgrounds and buildings for safety hazards
Health education	Teach healthy lifestyle education; develop health education curriculum for appropriate grade levels; provide health education to parents, faculty, and staff; develop suicide prevention and sex education programs
Secondary Prevention	
Screenings	Schedule routine screenings for scoliosis, vision and hearing problems, eating disorders, obesity, depression, anger, dental problems, and abuse
Case finding	Identify at-risk students
Treatment	Administer medications; develop individualized health plan; implement procedures and tasks necessary for students with special health needs; administer first aid
Home visits	Assist with family counseling and assess special and at-risk students
Tertiary Prevention	
Referral of student for substance abuse or behavior problems	Serve as an advocate; assist with resource referrals; assist parents, faculty, and staff; consult with neighborhood and law enforcement officials; initiate outreach programs
Prevention of complications and adverse effects	Follow-up and referral for students with eating disorders and obesity; participate with faculty and staff to reduce recurrence and risk factors; serve as a case manager
Faculty and staff monitoring	Follow-up for faculty and staff experiencing chronic or serious illness; follow-up of work-related injuries and accidents

▋ SUMMARY

Components of a comprehensive school health program have been clearly identified and discussed. Many of the *Healthy People 2020* objectives specifically relate to issues that can be addressed in the school setting. The role of the school nurse has changed dramatically since its inception and continues to evolve to meet the demands of school-age children, their parents, and the communities in which they live. School nurses continue to reduce the number of days and the frequency with which students miss school related to illness. They have become child advocates, counselors, health promoters and collaborators, educators, researchers, and resources in both the school and the community.

BIBLIOGRAPHY

Allensworth D, Lawson E, Nicholson L, Wyche J, editors: *Schools and health: our nation's investment*, Washington, DC, 1997, National Academies Press.

American Diabetes Association: Diabetes care in the school and day care setting, *Diabetes care* 35:S76–S80, 2012.

American Association of Diabetes Educators: *Management of children with diabetes in the school setting: AADE Position statement*, 2016. Available at <https://www.diabeteseducator.org/docs/default-source/practice/practice-resources/position-statements/diabetes-in-the-school-setting-position-statement_final.pdf>.

Centers for Disease Control and Prevention: *10 Leading cause of death by age group, United States-2014*, 2014. Available at <https://www.cdc.gov/injury/images/lc-charts/leading_causes_of_death_age_group_2014_1050w760h.gif>.

Centers for Disease Control and Prevention: *Had obesity*, 2016. Available at <https://www.cdc.gov/healthyschools/dataandstatistics.htm>.

Centers for Disease Control and Prevention: *HIV/STD prevention at a glance*, 2017. Available at <https://www.cdc.gov/healthyyouth/about/hivstd_prevention.htm>.

Centers for Disease Control and Prevention: *National health education standards*, 2016. Available at <https://www.cdc.gov/healthyschools/sher/standards/index.htm>.

Centers for Disease Control and Prevention: Nonfatal traumatic brain injuries related to sports and recreation activities among persons aged ≤19 years—United States, 2001–2009, *MMWR Morb Mortal Wkly Rep* 60(39):1337–1342, 2011.

Centers for Disease Control and Prevention: *Dental caries and sealant prevalence in children and adolescents in the United States, 2011–2012*, 2015. Available from: https://www.cdc.gov/nchs/products/databriefs/db191.htm.

Centers for Disease Control and Prevention: *School health guidelines*, 2017. Available at <https://www.cdc.gov/healthyschools/npao/strategies.htm>.

Centers for Disease Control and Prevention: *Suicide: facts at a glance*, 2015. Available at <https://www.cdc.gov/violenceprevention/pdf/suicide-datasheet-a.pdf>.

Centers for Disease Control and Prevention: *Summary health statistics: national health interview survey*, 2014. Available at <https://ftp.cdc.gov/pub/Health_Statistics/NCHS/NHIS/SHS/2014_SHS_Table_C-1.pdf>.

Centers for Disease Control and Prevention: *Teen pregnancy in the United States*, 2016. Available at <https://www.cdc.gov/teenpregnancy/about/>.

Centers for Disease Control and Prevention: *The case for coordinated school health*, 2015. Available from: <www.cdc.gov/healthyyouth/cshp/case.htm>.

Centers for Disease Control and Prevention: Tobacco use among middle and high school students—United States, 2011–2015, *Morb Mortal Wkly Rep* 65(14):361–367, 2016. Available at https://www.cdc.gov/mmwr/volumes/65/wr/mm6514a1.htm?s_cid=mm6514a1_w.

Centers for Disease Control and Prevention: *Trends in the prevalence of alcohol use National 1991-2015*, 2016. Available at https://www.cdc.gov/healthyyouth/data/yrbs/pdf/trends/2015_us_alcohol_trend_yrbs.pdf.

Centers for Disease Control and Prevention: *Trends in the prevalence of sexual behaviors and HIV testing national YRBS: 1991-2015*, 2016. Available at <https://www.cdc.gov/healthyyouth/data/yrbs/pdf/trends/2015_us_sexual_trend_yrbs.pdf.

Centers for Disease Control and Prevention: *Understanding school violence: fact sheet*, 2016. Available at <https://www.cdc.gov/violenceprevention/pdf/school_violence_fact_sheet-a.pdf>.

Centers for Disease Control and Prevention: Vital signs: asthma prevalence, disease characteristics, and self-management education—United States, 2001-2009, *MMWR Morb Mortal Wkly Rep* 60(17):547–552, 2011. Available from: <www.cdc.gov/mmwr/preview/mmwrhtml/mm6017a4.htm?s_cid=mm6017a4_w>.

Centers for Disease Control and Prevention: *Youth Risk Behavior Surveillance—United States, 2013*, *MMWR* 63(SS-4), 2014.

Centers for Disease Control and Prevention: *Youth risk behavior surveillance system (YRBSS) overview*, 2016. Available at <https://www.cdc.gov/healthyyouth/data/yrbs/overview.htm>.

Centers for Medicare & Medicaid Services: *Early and periodic screening, diagnostic, and treatment*, 2017. Available from: https://www.medicaid.gov/medicaid/benefits/epsdt/index.html.

Cheng TA, Bell JM, Haileyesus T, et al.: *Nonfatal playground-related traumatic brain injuries among children, 2001-2013*, Pediatrics publish0ed online, May 2, 2016. https://doi.org/10.1542/peds.2015-2721.R3.

Children's Defense Fund: *Child poverty in America 2014: state analysis*, 2014. Available at http://www.childrensdefense.org/library/poverty-report/child-poverty-in-america-2014-1.pdf.

Department of Justice Stats Zhang A, Musu-Gillette L, Oudekerk BA: Indicators of school crime and safety: 2015 (NCES 2016-079/NCJ 249758). National Center for Education Statistics, U.S. Department of Education, and Bureau of Justice Statistics, Office of Justice Programs, U.S. Department of Justice, 2016, Washington, DC.

Fryar CD, Carroll MD, Ogden CL: *Prevalence of overweight and obesity among children and adolescents: United States, 1963-1965 through 2011-2012*, Atlanta, GA, 2014, National Center for Health Statistics.

Future of Sex Education Initiative: *National sexuality education standards: core content and skills, K-12*, 2012. Available from: http://www.futureofsexed.org/documents/josh-fose-standards-web.pdf.

Hresko T, Talwalkar V, Schwend R: Position statement – screening for the early detection of idiopathic scoliosis in adolescents. SRS/POSNA/AAOS/AAP position statement. CDC. Youth risk behavior surveillance—United States, 2013, *MMWR* 63(SS-4), 2015.

National Assembly on School-Based Health Care: Core values. Available from: <www.nasbhc.org/site/ c.jsJPKWPFJrH/b.2663979/k.7566/Vision_Mission_Core_Value>.

National Association of School Nurses: *Role of the school nurse*, 2017. Available from: https://schoolnursenet.nasn.org/blogs/nasn-profile/2017/03/13/the-role-of-the-21st-century-school-nurse.

National Association of School Nurses: *Environmental health concerns in the school setting*, 2014. Available from: https://schoolnursenet.nasn.org/blogs/nasn-profile/2017/03/13/environmental-health-in-the-school-setting-the-role-of-the-school-nurse.

National Association of School Nurses: *Research priorities for school nursing*, 2016. Available at <https://www.nasn.org/Research/ResearchPrioritiesforSchoolNursing>.

National Association of School Nurses: *School nurse workload: staffing for safe care*, 2015. Available at <https://www.nasn.org/Policy Advocacy/PositionPapersandReports/NASNPositionStatements FullView/tabid/462/ArticleId/803/School-Nurse-Workload-Staffing-for-Safe-Care-Adopted-January-2015>.

National Association of School Nurses: *Medication administration in schools*, 2017. Available from: https://schoolnursenet.nasn.org/blogs/nasn-profile/2017/03/13/medication-administration-in-schools.

National Association of School Nurses: Self-administration of rescue inhalers for asthma in the school setting. Available from: https://www.nasn.org/PolicyAdvocacy/PositionPapersandReports/NASNIssueBriefsFullView/tabid/445/smid/853/ArticleID/122/Default.aspx

National Center for Children in Poverty: *Basic facts about low-income children*, 2017. Available at <http://www.nccp.org/topics/childpoverty.html>.

National Center for Education Statistics: *Fast facts: back to school statistics*, 2016. Available at <https://nces.ed.gov/fastfacts/display.asp?id=372>.

National Conference of State Legislatures: *State policies on sex education in schools*, 2016. Available at <http://www.ncsl.org/research/health/state-policies-on-sex-education-in-schools.aspx>.

National Institute on Drug Abuse: *Drugfacts: anabolic steroids*, 2016. Available from: <www.drugabuse.gov/publications/drugfacts/anabolic-steroids>.

National Institute on Drug Abuse: *National survey of drug use and health*, 2015. Available at <https://www.drugabuse.gov/national-survey-drug-use-health>.

National Institute of Mental Health: *Eating disorders*, 2016. Available at <https://www.nimh.nih.gov/health/topics/eating-disorders/index.shtml>.

Pastor Patricia N: QuickStats: percentage of children and adolescents aged 5–17 years with diagnosed attention-deficit/hyperactivity disorder (ADHD), by race and hispanic ethnicity—national health interview survey, United States, 1997–2014, *Morb Mortal Wkly Rep (MMWR)* 64(33):925–925, 2015. Available at <http://www.chadd.org/Understanding-ADHD/About-ADHD/Data-and-Statistics/General-Prevalence.aspx#sthash.eHxXPPHs.dpuf>.

Safe Kids USA: *Preventing injuries: at home, at play, and on the way, sport and recreation safety fact sheet*, 2011. Available from: <www.safekids.org/our-work/research/fact-sheets/sport-and-recreation-safety-fact-sheet.html>.

School-based Health Alliance: *National school-based health care census*, 2014. Available at: http://www.sbh4all.org/school-health-care/national-census-of-school-based-health-centers/.

Substance Abuse and Mental Health Services Administration: *2015 National survey on drug use and health (NSDUH). Table 2.19B: Alcohol Use in Lifetime, Past Year, and Past Month, by Detailed Age Category: Percentages, 2014 and 2015*, Rockville, MD, SAMHSA, 2016. Available at <http://www.samhsa.gov/data/sites/default/files/NSDUH-DetTabs-2015/NSDUH-DetTabs-2015/NSDUH-DetTabs-2015.htm#tab2-19b>.

The Annie E: *Casey Foundation: KIDS COUNT Data book: state trends in child well-being*, 2016. Available at <http://www.aecf.org/m/resourcedoc/aecf-the2016kidscountdatabook-2016.pdf>.

U.S. Census Bureau: *Poverty threshold*, 2017. Available at <https://www.census.gov/topics/income-poverty/poverty.html>.

U.S. Consumer Product Safety Commission: *Injuries and investigated deaths associated with playground equipment, 2001-2008*, 2009. Available at <https://www.cpsc.gov/PageFiles/108596/playground.pdf>.

U.S. Department of Agriculture Food and Nutrition Services: *Get involved: provide nutrition education*, 2017. Available at <https://www.fns.usda.gov/get-involved/provide-nutrition-education>.

U.S. Department of Education: *National Center for Education Statistics: Digest of Education Statistics, 2015 (NCES 2016-014), Chapter 2*, 2016. Available at <https://nces.ed.gov/fastfacts/display.asp?id=64>.

U.S. Department of Health and Human Services: *Preventing tobacco use among youth and young adults: a report of the surgeon general*, Atlanta: U.S. Department of Health and Human Services, Centers for Disease Control and Prevention, National Center for Chronic Disease Prevention and Health Promotion, Office on Smoking and Health, 2014. Available at https://www.cdc.gov/tobacco/data_statistics/sgr/50th-anniversary/index.htm.

U.S. Department of Health and Human Services: *The affordable care act and the school-based health center capital program*, 2013. Available from: https://aspe.hhs.gov/report/affordable-care-act-and-adolescents/school-based-health-centers.

U.S. Department of Health and Human Services: *The health consequences of smoking—50 years of progress: a report of the surgeon general*, Atlanta: U.S. Department of Health and Human Services, Centers for Disease Control and Prevention, National Center for Chronic Disease Prevention and Health Promotion, Office on Smoking and Health, 2014. Available at <https://www.cdc.gov/tobacco/data_statistics/sgr/50th-anniversary/index.htm>.

U.S. Department of Health and Human Services; Health Resources and Services Administration: *The registered nurse population: Initial findings from the 2008 national sample survey of registered nurses*, 2010. Available from: <http://bhpr.hrsa.gov/healthworkforce/rnsurveys/rnsurveyinital2008.pdf>.

Occupational Health

Bonnie Rogers

OBJECTIVES

Upon completion of this chapter, the reader will be able to do the following:

1. Describe the historical perspective of occupational health nursing.
2. Discuss emerging demographic trends that will influence occupational health nursing practice.
3. Identify the skills and competencies relevant to occupational health nursing.
4. Apply the nursing process and public health principles to worker and workplace health issues.
5. Discuss federal and state regulations that affect occupational health.
6. Describe a multidisciplinary approach for resolution of occupational health issues.

KEY TERMS

Ada Mayo Stewart
Americans With Disabilities Act
ergonomics
industrial hygiene

National Institute for Occupational Safety and Health
occupational health nursing
Occupational Safety and Health Administration

safety
toxicology
Workers' Compensation Acts

Occupational health nursing, a subspecialty of public health nursing, is defined by the American Association of Occupational Health Nurses (AAOHN) as the following:

Occupational and environmental health nursing [is] the specialty practice that focuses on preventive health care, and health restoration within the context of a safe and healthy environment. It includes the prevention of adverse health effects from occupational and environmental hazards and health promotion in general. The practice provides and delivers occupational and environmental health and safety

programs and services to clients. Nurses provide healthcare and make nursing decisions within the scope of practice determined by state law.

(AAOHN, 2015)

As depicted in Fig. 31.1, occupational health nursing derives its theoretical, conceptual, and factual framework from a multidisciplinary base. Elements of this multidisciplinary base include the following (Rogers, 1998, 2017):
Nursing science, which provides the context for health care delivery and recognizes the needs of individuals, groups, and

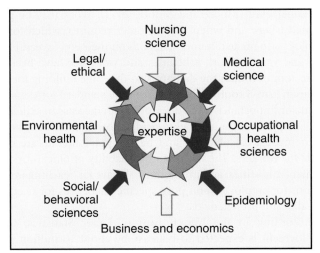

FIG. 31.1 Occupational health nursing knowledge domains. (From Rogers B: Occupational health nursing expertise, *AAOHN Journal* 46:477–483, 1998. Copyright Bonnie Rogers, 1998.)

populations within the framework of prevention, health promotion, and illness and injury care management, including risk assessment, risk management, and risk communication

Medical science specific to treatment and management of occupational health illness and injury, integrated with nursing health surveillance activities

Occupational health sciences, including **toxicology**, to recognize routes of exposure, examine relationships between chemical exposures in the workplace and acute and latent health effects such as burns or cancer and understand dose–response relationships; **industrial hygiene**, to identify and evaluate workplace hazards so control mechanisms can be implemented for exposure reduction; **safety**, to identify and control workplace injuries through active safeguards and worker training and education programs about job safety; and **ergonomics**, to match the job to the worker, emphasizing capabilities and minimizing limitations

Epidemiology, to study health and illness trends and characteristics of the worker population, investigate work-related illness and injury episodes, and apply epidemiological methods to analyze and interpret risk data to determine causal relationships and to participate in epidemiological research

Business and economic theories, concepts, and principles for strategic and operational planning, for valuing quality and cost-effective services and for management of occupational health and safety programs

Social and behavioral sciences, to explore influences of various environments (e.g., work and home), relationships, and lifestyle factors on worker health and determine the interactions affecting worker health

Environmental health, to systematically examine interrelationships between the worker and the extended environment as a basis for the development of prevention and control strategies

Legal and ethical issues, to ensure compliance with regulatory mandates and contend with ethical concerns that may arise in competitive environments

EVOLUTION OF OCCUPATIONAL HEALTH NURSING

The evolution of occupational health nursing in the United States has mirrored the societal changes in moving from an agrarian-based to an industrial-based economy and then, as we entered the twenty-first century, to a service-based economy. Occupational health nursing dates to the late 1800s with the employment of Betty Moulder and Ada Mayo Stewart (Parker-Conrad, 2002; Rogers, 2017).

A group of coal-mining companies hired Betty Moulder in 1888 to care for coal miners and their families (American Association of Industrial Nurses [AAIN], 1976). Seven years later, the Vermont Marble Company hired Ada Mayo Stewart to care for workers and their families. Stewart is often referred to as the first "industrial nurse," and her activities are well documented (Parker-Conrad, 1988). In 1897, Anna B. Duncan was employed by the John Wanamaker Company to visit sick employees at home; then, in 1899, a nursing service was established for employees of the Frederick Loeser department store in Brooklyn, New York (AAIN, 1976).

At the turn of the twentieth century, the industrial revolution was well under way, and the concept of health care for employees spread rapidly. Companies hiring industrial nurses in the early 1900s included the Emporium in San Francisco; Plymouth Cordage Company in Massachusetts; Anaconda Mining Company in Montana; Broadway Store in Los Angeles; Chase Metal Works in Connecticut; Hale Brothers in San Francisco; Filene's in Boston; Carson, Pirie, Scott in Chicago; Fulton Cotton Mills in Georgia; and Bullock's in Los Angeles (McGrath, 1946; Parker-Conrad, 1988). The cost-effectiveness of providing health care to employees achieved greater recognition, and by 1912, following implementation of workers' compensation legislation, 38 nurses were employed by business firms (McGrath, 1946; Parker-Conrad, 1988). The following year, a registry of industrial nurses was initiated, and in 1915, the Boston Industrial Nurses Club was formed; this group evolved into the Massachusetts Industrial Nurses Organization.

In 1916, the Factory Nurses Conference was organized. This group was open only to graduate, state-registered nurses affiliated with the American Nurses Association (ANA), and their efforts identified the industrial nurses' need to explore the uniqueness of this evolving specialty area (AAIN, 1976). More importantly, industrial nurses were practicing in single-nurse settings and recognized the benefit of uniting as a group for the purpose of sharing ideas with peers practicing in the same nursing arena. In 1917, the first educational course for industrial nurses was offered at Boston University's College of Business Administration.

During and after the Great Depression, many nurses lost jobs because employers and business managers viewed industrial nursing as a nonessential aspect of business (Felton, 1985, 1986). The focus of health care for employees again changed as a result of many factors, including the impact of the two world wars. During World War I, the government demanded health services for workers at factories and shipyards holding defense contracts. Demographics in the workplace were also dramatically different during World War II, because higher numbers of women entered the workforce. In 1942, the U.S. Surgeon General told an audience of nurses that the health conservation of the "industrial army" was the most urgent civilian need during the war (Felton, 1985).

From 1938 to 1943, the number of occupational health nurses increased by more than 10,000. In 1942, some 300 nurses from 16 states voted to create a national association for the specialty. Catherine R. Dempsey, a nurse at Simplex Wire and Cable Company in Cambridge, Massachusetts, was elected president of the national association. By 1943, approximately 11,000 nurses were employed in industry (AAIN, 1976).

Nine years later, members of AAIN voted to remain an independent, autonomous association rather than merge with the National League for Nursing or the ANA. In 1953, another important step was taken toward formalizing this specialty area of nursing practice when the *Industrial Nurses Journal* (now the *AAOHN Journal*) began publishing. In 1977, the organization changed its name to the AAOHN, reflecting a broader, more diverse scope of practice.

In the 1980s and 1990s, occupational health nursing rapidly increased its role in health promotion, policy development, management, and research while maintaining traditional occupational health nursing practice. In 1989, AAOHN developed its first research agenda, and in 1993, the Occupational Safety and Health Administration (OSHA) established the Office of Occupational Health Nursing, reenergizing the concept of occupational health into practice. In 1999, the AAOHN Foundation was established, and competencies in the specialty were delineated. In 2003, the 60-year-old Annual Joint Conference, the American Occupational Health Conference, was abolished by the physicians and nurses even though there was lack of consensus on this decision among the membership at large. Consequently, AAOHN held its first separate occupational health nursing conference in 2005. In the twenty-first century, the AAOHN continues to expand specialty borders, emphasizing the importance of occupational health concepts and population-based practice. National Institute for Occupational Safety and Health (NIOSH) Centers for Excellence to Promote a Healthier Workforce were established in 2006. In 2007 the first OHN Academic Certificate was established at the University of North Carolina School of Public Health. This led the way for the establishment of NIOSH-funded multidisciplinary academic certificate programs in 2015.

DEMOGRAPHIC TRENDS AND ACCESS ISSUES RELATED TO OCCUPATIONAL HEALTH CARE

At the beginning of the twenty-first century, sweeping transformations in industry are influencing the direction of occupational health nursing. These transformations include changing workforce demographics, rising health care costs, diversity of health care systems with the integration of managed care, influence of the world economy, shift in production from goods to services, and proliferation of advanced technologies. The focus of U.S. industry is moving away from large manufacturing facilities to smaller, service-based businesses, and other changes

are anticipated (Moore and Moore, 2014). Work may be performed where and when the customer requires, which forces employers to make different demands on their employees. Flexible and varying work schedules and worksites have become more common than the daily trek to the same building for the 40-hour, 9-to-5 routine that has been the standard for decades. Of major importance is the demand for an increase in skill level of all employees. The abilities to read, follow directions, perform mathematical calculations, and be computer literate are core skills for workers. The increasing availability of older workers, women, minorities, and immigrants all have far-reaching implications for employers and pose specific challenges for occupational health professionals.

According to the U.S. Bureau of Labor Statistics, total employment is expected to increase by about 10 million jobs from 2014 to 2024. Industries and occupations related to health care, personal care and social assistance, and construction are expected to have the fastest job growth. Service-producing industries are anticipated to produce nearly the greatest majority of the new jobs, with employment in health care–related occupations expected to grow fastest, followed by personal care and service, largely because an aging population will require more medical care. Furthermore, patients increasingly are seeking home care as an alternative to costly hospital or residential care stays (U.S. Bureau of Labor Statistics, 2015). These trends are important to understand because they have a direct impact on the national rate of economic growth, especially in the area of population-sensitive products such as food; automobiles; housing units; household goods; and services such as health care, education, and transportation. With expansion of each of these sectors, there are concomitant hazards.

Within the context of these evolving organizational trends, key characteristics include a focus on a shared vision, strategy, and long-term objectives in an environment composed of individuals working in teams. In contrast to the past, occupational health nurses have opportunities to work on cross-functional teams to shape decisions in areas such as benefits, research, safety, and legal matters. Specifically, occupational health nurses have opportunities to positively affect the transformation of the health care delivery system, establish policies within the managed care environment and within corporations, and assume leadership positions on legislative staffs and in governmental agencies.

Corporations have become driving forces in shaping the development of alternative approaches to health care. Rapidly rising health care costs have spawned a number of alternative approaches to providing health care, such as preferred provider organizations.

It is important that the occupational health nurse remain informed about the various health care options available to the workforce as rapid changes occur regarding corporate benefits. This issue is of particular importance when the nurse is considering the referral of an employee to a health resource. Participation in one of the managed care plans requires that treatment take place according to the organization's guidelines and within its health service delivery system. Managed care plans have nearly replaced traditional indemnity plans. Access to care is closely managed and often limited. As this trend continues, the role of the occupational health nurse will take on added importance. The nurse may be called upon to accept increasing responsibilities as a primary care provider as well as a tertiary care coordinator/case manager.

As businesses seek ways to maximize the value of the dollars they spend on health care services, occupational health nurses and other health professionals must validate the services they provide in order to demonstrate contributions to the health of the workforce and the company (Randolph et al., 2014). This must include a focus on cost-effectiveness and value to companies to demonstrate a return on the investment for quality health care.

OCCUPATIONAL HEALTH NURSING PRACTICE AND PROFESSIONALISM

As workplaces have continued to change over the past few decades, the role of the occupational health nurse has become even more diversified and complex (Rogers, 2012). Occupational health nurses work in a variety of settings including manufacturing such as meat packing, food production, battery manufacturing, and textiles; hospital employee health institutions; and service industries such as banking and government and academic centers. Often working as the only on-site health care professional, the occupational health nurse collaborates with workers, employers, and other professionals to identify health problems or needs, prioritize interventions, develop and implement programs, and evaluate services delivered. The occupational health nurse is in a unique and critical position to coordinate a holistic approach to the delivery of quality, comprehensive occupational health services. The Standards of Occupational and Environmental Health Nursing, the Code of Ethics, and AAOHN practice competencies guide the nurse.

AAOHN's Standards of Occupational and Environmental Health Nursing Practice form the basis of the profession's responsibilities and accountabilities (AAOHN, 2015). The 11 standard statements are listed in Table 31.1. For each standard, identifiable criteria are detailed that can be used to evaluate practice relative to the standard. Refer to the complete standards document from the AAOHN for this information.

Guided by an ethical framework made explicit in the AAOHN Code of Ethics, occupational health nurses encourage and enable individuals to make informed decisions about health care concerns (AAOHN, 2016) (Box 31.1). The occupational health nurse is a worker advocate and has the responsibility to uphold professional standards and codes. The occupational health nurse is also responsible to management, is usually compensated by management, and must practice within a framework of company policies and guidelines (Rogers, 2017). Ethical dilemmas arise because the nurse is loyal to both workers and management. Issues such as screening, drug testing, informing employees about hazardous exposures, and confidentiality of health information, which is integral and central to the practice base, often create ethical debates. As advocates for workers, occupational

TABLE 31.1	Standards of Occupational and Environmental Health Nursing
Standard I: Assessment	The occupational and environmental health nurse systematically assesses the health status of the client(s).
Standard II: Diagnosis	The occupational and environmental health nurse analyzes assessment data to formulate diagnoses.
Standard III: Outcome identification	The occupational and environmental health nurse identifies outcomes specific to the client(s) identification.
Standard IV: Planning	The occupational and environmental health nurse develops a goal-directed plan that is comprehensive and formulates interventions to attain expected outcomes.
Standard V: Implementation	The occupational and environmental health nurse implements interventions to attain desired outcomes identified in the plan.
Standard VI: Evaluation	The occupational and environmental health nurse systematically and continuously evaluates responses to interventions and progress toward the achievement of desired outcomes.
Standard VII: Resource management	The occupational and environmental health nurse secures and manages the resources that support occupational health and safety programs and services.
Standard VIII: Professional development	The occupational and environmental health nurse assumes accountability for professional development to enhance professional growth and maintain competency.
Standard IX: Collaboration	The occupational and environmental health nurse collaborates with the client(s) for the promotion, prevention, and restoration of health within the conduct of a safe and healthy environment.
Standard X: Research	The occupational and environmental health nurse uses research findings in practice and contributes to the scientific base in occupational and environmental health nursing to improve practice and advance the profession.
Standard XI: Ethics	The occupational and environmental health nurse uses an ethical framework for decision making in practice.

Data from American Association of Occupational Health Nurses: Standards of occupational and environmental health nursing, *AAOHN Journal* 60:151–157, 2012. Copyright American Association of Occupational Health Nurses. http://www.aaohn.org.

health nurses foster equitable and quality health care services and safe and healthy work environments.

Occupational health nurses make up the largest professional group providing health care services to employees in highly complex work environments. The roles of occupational health nurses are changing as a result of many factors, including rising health care costs, increased recognition of health effects associated with various exposures, emphasis on health promotion and wellness, health surveillance, women's issues, ergonomics, reproductive issues, company downsizing, trends in managed care, and multicultural workforces. Box 31.2 reflects this growth in scope of practice and outlines the occupational health nursing services currently mandated by state and federal regulations and those generally mandated by company policies.

ETHICAL INSIGHTS

Confidentiality of Employee Health Information

The occupational health nurse sometimes experiences ethical dilemmas because of dual responsibility to both the employer and the employees. In dealing with health information, the employee has the right to privacy; however, exceptions to legal protection of health information may require the nurse to provide health-related records without the worker's knowledge or consent. These exceptions are cases in which public benefit from disclosure outweighs loss of individual privacy. Specific circumstances include life-threatening emergencies; workers' compensation situations in which state regulations limiting information to carriers and/or employers are followed; examination for drug and alcohol testing in some circumstances; compliance with government regulations; OSHA-mandated surveillance and/or occupational injury or illness evaluations; and other situations as required by law (e.g., public health purposes, law enforcement, judicial proceedings, or court order).

From American Association of Occupational Health Nurses: *Position statement: confidentiality of employee health information*, 2016. http://aaohn.org/page/position-statements. Accessed February 21, 2018

BOX 31.1 American Association of Occupational Health Nurses Code of Ethics

I. The American Association of Occupational health Nurses (AAOHN) articulates occupational and environmental health nursing values, maintains the integrity of our specialty practice area and the nursing profession, and integrates principles of social justice into nursing and health policy.

II. The occupational and environmental health nurse (OHN) practices with compassion and respect for the inherent dignity, worth and unique attributes of every person. The occupational and environmental health nurse's (OHN) commitment is to the client, whether an individual, group, community or population.

IV. The occupational and environmental health nurse (OHN) promotes, advocates for, and protects the rights, health, and safety of the client.

V. The occupational and environmental health nurse (OHN) has authority, accountability, and responsibility for nursing practice; makes decisions; and takes action consistent with the obligation to prevent illness and injury, promote health, and provide optimal care.

VI. The occupational and environmental health nurse (OHN) owes the same duties to self and others, including the responsibility to promote health and safety, preserve wholeness of character and integrity, maintain competence, and continue personal and professional growth.

VII. The occupational and environmental health nurse (OHN), through individual and collective effort, establishes, maintains, and improves the ethical environment of the work setting and conditions of employment that are conducive to safe, quality health care.

VIII. Occupational and environmental health nurses (OHN) help advance the nursing profession and our specialty practice through research and scholarly inquiry, professional standards development, and the generation of nursing and health policy.

IX. The occupational and environmental health nurse (OHN) collaborates with other health professionals and the public to protect human rights, promote health, and reduce health disparities.

From American Association of Occupational Health Nurses: *AAOHN Code of Ethics and interpretive statements*, 2016. Available from: http://aaohn.org/p/cm/ld/fid=1350

According to the most recent National Nursing Workforce Survey, approximately 1% of the total nursing population practices in the occupational health field in the United States (Budden et al., 2016). Approximately 70% of these occupational health nurses work alone, making decisions about health and safety issues, influencing policy in health and safety, and planning and implementing myriad health programs. Nearly 70% of nurses practicing in occupational health are prepared at the baccalaureate level or higher, and 65% have been practicing in the field of occupational health for at least 6 years (AAOHN, 2013).

Meeting the needs of employees in smaller businesses is another important practice priority. The integration of occupational health and safety principles into the curricula of schools of nursing, engineering, and management is critical. Community health nurses may assume occupational health nursing roles; however, in order to do this they must be knowledgeable about the specialty area of occupational health nursing. Municipalities, smaller companies, visiting nurse associations, and home care agencies may provide opportunities for community health nurses to be involved in screening programs, health education activities, workplace hazard evaluations, and other occupational health–related activities.

The occupational health nurse's strengths are embedded in assessing, planning, implementing, and evaluating health programs for populations, creating plans for individuals, and health education activities for worker aggregates. Often, lack of understanding or misconceptions about the occupational health nurse's role have fostered the invisibility of the nurse, both within the nursing profession itself and within the business environment, thereby exacerbating the difficulties the nurses face in being the lone provider of health care for workers in many companies. Empowered, well-trained, educated occupational and environmental health nurses can help bring about crucial changes in the areas of primary, secondary, and tertiary prevention in occupational health.

In response to societal changes and historical events, the practice of occupational health nursing has changed dramatically, demanding a sophisticated knowledge base and problem-solving skills that are empirically grounded and multidisciplinary in nature (Rogers, 2017). For example, demographic changes with an aging population require more knowledge and skills about managing an aged workforce (Rogers et al., 2009). The roles and responsibilities of the occupational health nurse must be clearly articulated to lay people, managers, workers, union representatives, and colleagues in occupational health, nursing, and medicine to ensure that occupational health nursing can continue to positively affect workers' health, contribute to reducing health care costs, and foster reduction in health risks. Occupational health nurses must seize opportunities in areas such as program planning, research, and policy making during this era fraught with a health care system in crisis. Issues to be addressed and managed include nursing shortages in many areas of the country, dramatic changes in the business environment, employees' increasing awareness of workplace hazards, and the ever-increasing need to demonstrate the cost-effectiveness of occupational health nursing care and services (Towers Watson/National Business Group in Health, 2011).

Research is an integral component of occupational and environmental health nursing practice because it provides the basis for scientific discovery that improves practice. That National Occupational Research Agenda (National Institute

BOX 31.2 Occupational Health Nursing Services

Services Mandated by Federal and State Regulations

- Safe and healthful workplace
- Emergency medical response
- First aid responder selection and training
- First aid space, supplies, protocols, and records
- Designated medical resources for incident response
- Workers' compensation
- Confidentiality of medical records
- Compliance with medical record retention requirements
- Occupational Safety and Health Administration (OSHA) compliance
- Medical personnel requirement (29 *CFR* 1910.15)
- Injury and illness reporting and recording
- Accident and injury investigation
- Cumulative trauma disorder prevention
- Employee access to medical and exposure records
- Medical surveillance and hazardous work qualification
- Personal protective equipment evaluation and training
- Infection control
- Employee Right-to-Know Act notification and training
- Community Right-to-Know Act compliance
- Americans With Disabilities Act (ADA) compliance
- Rehabilitation Act: handicap, preplacement, fitness for duty evaluations, accommodations
- Department of Defense, Department of Transportation, Nuclear Regulatory Commission, and Drug-Free Workplace Act compliance
- Policy development
- Drug awareness education
- Drug testing and technical support
- Employee Assistance Program services
- Threat of violence and duty to warn
- Video display terminal (VDT) local regulations

- State and local public health regulations
- Nursing practice acts
- Board of Pharmacy and Drug Enforcement Agency regulations
- Continuing professional education required for licensure

Services Often Mandated by Company Policy

- Clinical supervision of on-site health services
- Health strategy development
- Health services standards
- Space, staffing, and operational standards
- Occupational illness and injury assessment, diagnosis, treatment, and referral
- Nonoccupational illness and injury assessment, diagnosis, treatment, and referral
- Disability and return-to-work evaluations and accommodations
- Impaired employee fitness-for-duty evaluation
- Preplacement evaluation and medical accommodation
- Handicap evaluation, placement, and accommodation
- Employee Assistance Program standards
- International health: travel, medical advisory, and immunizations
- Data collection and analysis
- Medical consultation
- Pregnancy placement in hazardous environments
- Professional education and development
- Audit and quality assurance

Optional Services

- Health education and health promotion
- Medical screening for early detection and disease prevention
- Physical fitness programs
- Allergy injection programs

---

for Occupational Safety and Health) first set the priorities for research in the occupational health field in 1996. Before that, in 1989, research priorities in occupational health nursing were first identified and published and were used as a model for the agenda (Rogers, 1989). They have been updated periodically to serve as the scientific basis to continue to build the body of knowledge in occupational and environmental health nursing for practice improvement and expansion (Box 31.3).

OCCUPATIONAL HEALTH AND PREVENTION STRATEGIES

Like the practice of all community health professionals, the occupational health nurse's practice is based on the concept of prevention. Promotion, protection, maintenance, and restoration of worker health are priority goals set forth in the definition of occupational health nursing. Prevention of exposure to occupational and environmental safety hazards and specific strategies for each level of prevention are described along with objectives from the *Healthy People 2020* program.

 Healthy People 2020 and Occupational Health

One topic area of *Healthy People 2020* concentrates on occupational safety and health (U.S. Department of Health and Human

BOX 31.3 Research Priorities in Occupational Health Nursing

- Effectiveness of primary health care delivery at the worksite
- Effectiveness of health promotion nursing intervention strategies
- Nature and effects of stress and workplace stressors on worker health
- Strategies that minimize work-related adverse health outcomes (e.g., respiratory disease)
- Health effects resulting from chemical exposures in the workplace
- Occupational hazards of health care workers (e.g., latex allergy and blood-borne pathogens)
- Factors that influence workers' rehabilitation and return to work
- Effectiveness of ergonomic strategies to reduce worker injury and illness
- Health effects resulting from the interaction between aging and workplace hazards
- Evaluation of critical pathways to effectively improve worker health and safety and enhance maximum recovery and safe return to work
- Evaluation of intervention strategies to improve worker health and safety
- Strategies for increasing compliance with or motivating workers to use personal protective equipment
- Emergency/pandemic preparedness in the workplace
- Impact of occupational health nursing interventions on workers' compensation claims

From American Association of Occupational Health Nurses: *Research priorities in occupational and environmental health nursing,* 2012. http://aaohn.org/page/aaohn-research-priorities

Services [USDHHS], 2017). Objectives from this priority area cover work-related injuries and deaths, repetitive-motion injuries, homicide, assault, lead exposure, skin disorders, stress, and hearing loss. In addition, objectives from other topic areas address issues related to occupational health and safety. The *Healthy People 2020* box lists objectives that deal with occupational health.

♥ HEALTHY PEOPLE 2020

Objectives for Some Areas of Occupational Health

ECBP-8: Increase the proportion of worksites that offer health promotion programs to employees

ENT-VSL-6: Increase the use of hearing protection devices

NWSS-7: Increase the proportion of worksites that offer nutrition or weight management classes or counseling

OSH-1: Reduce deaths from work-related injuries

OSH-2: Reduce nonfatal work-related injuries

OSH-5: Reduce deaths from work-related homicides

OSH-8: Reduce occupational skin diseases or disorders among full-time workers

OSH-9: Increase the proportion of employees who have access to workplace programs to prevent or reduce employee stress

OSH-10: Reduce new cases of work-related noise-induced hearing loss

PAF-12: Increase the proportion of employed adults who have access to and participate in employer-based exercise facilities and exercise programs

TU-13: Establish laws on smoke-free indoor air that prohibit smoking in public places and worksites

V-3: Reduce occupational eye injuries

From HealthyPeople.gov: *Healthy People 2020: topics & objectives,* 2017. http://healthypeople.gov/2020/topicsobjectives2020/. Accessed February 21, 2018

Prevention of Exposure to Potential Hazards

To prevent occupational and environmental safety hazards in the work environment, it is important to identify work-related agents and exposures that are potentially hazardous. These can be categorized as follows:

Biological-infectious hazards: Agents such as bacteria, viruses, fungi, and parasites that may be transmitted via contact with infected clients or contaminated objects or substances

Chemical hazards: Various forms of chemical agents, including medications, solutions, and gases, that interact with body tissues and cells and are potentially toxic or irritating to body systems

Enviromechanical hazards: Factors encountered in work environments that cause accidents, injuries, strain, or discomfort (e.g., poor equipment or lifting devices and slippery floors)

Physical hazards: Agents within work environments, such as radiation, electricity, extreme temperatures, and noise, that can cause tissue trauma through transfer of energy from these sources

Psychosocial hazards: Factors and situations encountered or associated with the job or work environment that create stress, emotional strain, or interpersonal problems

Table 31.2 provides examples of work-related exposures in each of these areas. Having a good understanding of the

TABLE 31.2 Types of Occupational Hazards and Associated Health Effects

Category	Exposures	Health Effects
Biological	Blood or body fluids	Bacterial, fungal, and viral infections (e.g., hepatitis B)
Chemical	Solvents	Headache and central nervous system dysfunction
	Lead	Central nervous system disturbances
	Asbestos	Asbestosis
	Acids	Burns
	Glycol ethers	Reproductive problems
	Mercury	Ataxia
	Arsenic	Peripheral neuropathy
Enviro-mechanical	Static or nonneutral postures	Musculoskeletal disorders
	Repetitive or forceful exertions	Back injuries
	Lighting	Headache and eye strain
	Shift work	Sleep disorders
	Electrical	Electrocution
	Slips and falls	Musculoskeletal conditions
	Struck by or against object	Injury
Physical	Noise	Hearing loss
	Radiation	Reproductive effects and cancer
	Vibration	Raynaud disease
	Heat	Heat exhaustion and heat stroke
Psychosocial	Stress	Anxiety reactions and a variety of physical symptoms
	Work–home balance	

nature of these hazards allows for the development of health promotion and prevention strategies to mitigate exposure risk.

Levels of Prevention and Occupational Health Nursing

Because occupational health nurses typically practice autonomously in their role as health care providers, their activities in primary, secondary, and tertiary prevention strategies are expected to assume an even more important role in the prevention and treatment of illness, injury, and chronic disease in the future. NIOSH has embarked on an initiative, Total Worker Health. Total Worker Health is defined as policies, programs, and practices that integrate protection from work-related safety and health hazards with promotion of injury and illness prevention efforts to advance worker well-being (NIOSH, 2017). This initiative is designed to integrate health protection and health promotion and is important for occupational health nurses to engage. Additional information can be found at https://www.cdc.gov/niosh/twh/totalhealth.html.

Primary Prevention

In the area of primary prevention, the occupational health nurse is involved in both health promotion and disease prevention. O'Donnell (2009) describes health promotion as follows:

FIG. 31.2 Occupational health nurses often perform "walk-throughs" in the workplace to look for potential hazards and maintain communication with workers to prevent illness and injury.

The art and science of helping people discover the synergies between their core passions and optimal health, enhancing their motivation to strive for optimal health, and supporting them in changing lifestyle to move toward a state of optimal health. Optimal health is a dynamic balance of physical, emotional, social, spiritual and intellectual health. Lifestyle change can be facilitated through a combination of learning experiences that enhance awareness, increase motivation, and build skills and most importantly, through creating opportunities that open access to environments that make positive health practices the easiest choice.

(p. iv)

Disease prevention, then, begins with recognition of a health risk, a disease, or an environmental hazard. This recognition is followed by measures to protect as many people as possible from harmful consequences of that risk.

The occupational health nurse uses a variety of primary prevention methods, with one-on-one interaction as an important strategy for evaluating risk reduction behavior for individuals. The occupational health nurse has daily contact with numerous employees for many reasons (e.g., assessment and treatment of episodic illness or injury, health surveillance); therefore this contact is an important method of promoting health. The phrase "seize the moment" aptly describes the opportunity that exists with every employee encounter.

Occupational health nurses plan, develop, implement, and evaluate aggregate-focused intervention strategies. The occupational health nurse plans and implements programs such as weight and cholesterol reduction, AIDS awareness, ergonomics training, and smoking cessation. Performing "walk-throughs" in the workplace on a regular basis, recognizing potential and existing hazards, and maintaining communications with safety and industrial hygiene resources to prevent illness and injury from occurring will continue to be critical work for the occupational health nurse (Levy et al., 2017) (Fig. 31.2).

For overall *health promotion*, the nurse may plan, implement, and evaluate a health fair, a multifaceted health promotion strategy that usually includes a number of community health resources to provide expertise on a wide range of health issues and community services. As part of an overall health and wellness strategy, the occupational health nurse may negotiate with the employer for an on-site fitness center or area with fitness equipment; if cost or space is prohibitive, the employer may choose to partially subsidize membership at a local fitness center (Rogers et al., 2018).

⚡ SAFETY ALERT

Violence has emerged as an important safety and health issue in the workplace. According to NIOSH, *workplace violence* is defined as a violent act, including physical assault, a threat of assault, harassment, intimidation, other threatening disruptive behavior, or homicide directed toward persons at work or on duty. The violent incident may threaten the safety of an employee, customer, or vendor; have an impact on an employee's physical or psychological well-being; or cause damage to company property. Violence can also involve an assault; an aggressive act of hitting, kicking, pushing, scratching; a sexual act or attempt, with or without a weapon; or any physical or verbal attacks or threats or bullying directed to a worker by a coworker, client, relative, customer, patient, or work-associated individual that arises during or as a result of the performance of duties and that results in death, physical injury, or mental harm.

Risk factors for workplace violence include working alone or in small numbers, exchanging money with the public, working late at night or during early-morning hours, having a mobile workplace such as taxi cab, working in high-crime areas, guarding valuable property or possessions, and dealing with violent people or volatile situations. Health care professionals, public service workers, law enforcement personnel, delivery drivers, and customer service agents are also at higher risk.

The occupational health nurse works collaboratively with others to develop and implement an effective violence prevention program. Responsibilities might include participating as a member of the threat assessment team, including representatives from senior management, operations, employees, security, finance, legal, human resources, and health and safety; identifying prevention and control strategies; assisting or providing guidance in dealing with difficult or disgruntled employees or customers; and coordination of care. The nurse also provides direct care and emotional support to the victimized worker and/or worker who witnessed the violent incident, including referral to employee assistance programs or other community agencies. In addition, the nurse assists the employee with return to work. Accurate and complete documentation of violence incidents is critical for preventing future incidents and for legal purposes.

Types of *nonoccupational programs* included in the area of primary prevention are cardiovascular health, cancer awareness, personal safety, immunization, prenatal and postpartum health, accident prevention, retirement health, stress management, and relaxation techniques. Occupational health programs could include topics such as emergency response, first aid and cardiopulmonary resuscitation training, right-to-know training, immunization programs for international business travelers, prevention of back injury through knowledge of proper lifting techniques, ergonomics, and other programs targeted to the specific hazards identified in the workplace (Burgel and Childre, 2012; Rogers et al., 2018).

Women's health and safety issues such as maternal-child health, reproductive health, breast cancer education and early detection, stress management, and work–home balance issues

TABLE 31.3	Work-Related Diseases and Injuries
Work-Related Disease(s) or Injury	**Example(s)**
Occupational lung disease	Cancer and asthma
Musculoskeletal injuries	Back, upper extremity, and musculoskeletal disorders
Occupational cancers	Leukemia, bladder, and skin
Trauma	Death, amputation, and fracture
Cardiovascular diseases	Hypertension and heart disease
Reproductive disorders	Infertility and miscarriage
Neurotoxic disorders	Neuropathy and toxic psychosis
Noise-induced hearing loss	Loss of hearing
Dermatological conditions	Chemical burns and allergies
Psychological disorders	Neurosis; alcohol or substance abuse

are very significant as more women have entered the workforce. Thirty percent of women currently in the workforce are between ages 16 and 44 years, and each year approximately 1 million infants are born to these women. Interest in workplace safety and the relationship to reproductive outcomes continues to grow as women of childbearing age enter the workplace in greater proportions than ever before.

The occupational health nurse can play a key role in the development and delivery of prenatal, postpartum, and childhood programs in the workplace. Of primary importance is the ability to serve as a change agent to initiate needed programs in the work environment. Employers must be educated regarding strategies not only to reduce health care costs for women and infants but also to improve the work environment for mothers. Women who believe their employers are interested in the well-being of themselves and their families are more apt to be productive and satisfied employees. The occupational health nurse can play a critical role in the shaping of supportive policies and practices to accommodate the needs of families, including flexible working hours, parental leave, and on-site child care (Rogers et al., 2018).

Members of *racial and ethnic minority* groups make up a large share of the labor force, and as the number of minority and ethnic workers in the workforce increases, so will the illnesses traditionally associated with these groups of workers (e.g., heart disease and stroke, hypertension, cancer, cirrhosis, and diabetes) (Rogers et al., 2018). In addition to basic health concerns for this population, available statistics indicate that minority workers have been disproportionately concentrated in some of the most dangerous work, and they are at greater risk for experiencing many of the leading occupation-related diseases and injuries. Table 31.3 illustrates examples of common occupational diseases and injuries.

The occupational health nurse may face challenges in developing programs that are culturally and linguistically appropriate. The occupational health nurse may be in an advocacy role to negotiate with the employer for changes in the work environment that will reduce or eliminate existing or potential occupational exposure to risk factors and assist with literacy efforts that can be offered at the worksite.

Finally, veterans of our uniformed services are being employed at noteworthy numbers as they return to civilian life. Occupational health nurses should be aware of health problems—both physical and mental—that are sometimes encountered among this aggregate. Nurses should ensure that information for education for potential and anticipated problems is readily available. Furthermore, they can collect and maintain resources for referral to help assist with the most serious issues.

Secondary Prevention

Secondary prevention strategies are aimed at early diagnosis, early treatment interventions, and attempts to limit disability. The focus at this level of prevention is on identification of health needs, health problems, and employees at risk.

As with primary prevention, the occupational health nurse uses a number of different secondary prevention strategies (Rogers, 2017). By providing direct care for episodic illness and injury, the occupational health nurse is afforded the opportunity to conduct assessments and provide treatment and referrals for a variety of physical and psychological conditions. The occupational health nurse can offer health screenings, which are designed for early detection of disease, at the worksite with relative ease and at minimal cost. Screenings may focus on vision, cancer, cholesterol, hypertension, diabetes, tuberculosis, and pulmonary function. Other types of screening, such as mammography, may be contracted with a vendor who uses mobile equipment.

Secondary prevention efforts provided by the occupational health nurse include *preplacement, periodic,* and *job transfer evaluations* to ensure that a worker is being placed or is continuing to work in a job that is safe for him or her (Rogers, 2017). The preplacement evaluation is performed before the worker begins employment in a new company or is placed in a different job (Fig. 31.3). The evaluation is a baseline examination that consists of a health history, an occupational health history, and a physical assessment that should target the type of work that the employee will be performing. For example, if the employee is going to be lifting materials in a warehouse, special attention should be paid to any history of musculoskeletal problems. Strength testing and range of motion should be performed for all muscle groups.

The preplacement examination may also include tests to determine specific organ functions that may be affected by exposure to existing agents in the employee's workplace. For example, if the employee is working with a chemical that is a known liver toxin, baseline liver function tests may be appropriate to determine the current health status of the liver and its ability to handle this specific chemical exposure. However, the preplacement examination must be carefully evaluated to ensure compliance with the Americans With Disabilities Act (ADA), which is discussed later in the chapter.

Periodic assessments usually occur at regular intervals (e.g., annual and biannual) and are based on specific protocols for those exposed to substances or irritants such as lead, asbestos, noise, and various chemicals. Examinations of individuals transferring to other jobs are critical to document any changes in health that may have occurred while the employee was working in a specific area or with a specific process. Such examinations are usually done to comply with OSHA regulations or NIOSH

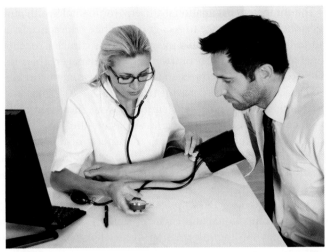

FIG. 31.3 Occupational health nurses may provide preemployment physical examinations or monitor health problems.

recommendations. (See **Resource Tool 30C** for an example of an OSHA screening and surveillance guide.) For full details of compliance requirements, OSHA standards must be consulted.

Activities must continue to focus on prevention and early detection by increasing awareness of the incidence of commonly occurring health conditions such as breast cancer and providing accessible and affordable screening programs. For example, it is estimated that in 2017 invasive breast cancer will be diagnosed in more than 252,000 women and that about 40,600 women will die of the disease each year, making breast cancer one of the most commonly diagnosed malignancies among women in the United States and the second leading cause of cancer death, after lung cancer (American Cancer Society, 2017). By detecting early malignancies, breast cancer screening reduces the mortality rate in women between ages 50 and 69 years. Mammography is the most effective method for detecting these early malignancies. The occupational health nurse is in an excellent position to play a key role in reducing morbidity and mortality associated with breast cancer. Increasingly, the occupational health nurse will be expected to document the return on investment for these and other related activities in the workplace.

Tertiary Prevention

On a tertiary level, the occupational health nurse plays a key role in the rehabilitation and restoration of the worker to an optimal level of functioning. Strategies include case management, negotiation of workplace accommodations, and counseling and support for workers who will continue to be affected by chronic disease and disability (Rogers, 2017; Rogers et al., 2009).

Disability management is complex, and the goal is to return the employee to gainful employment as soon as possible, but taking care to not reinjure the employee (AAOHN, 2012).

Knowledge of the workplace, the ability to negotiate with the employer for appropriate accommodations, early intervention, and comprehensive case management skills have been and will continue to be essential to the disabled employee's successful return to work. The process of returning an individual to work begins with the onset of injury or illness (Rogers, 2017; Rogers et al., 2009).

Regardless of whether an occupational or a nonoccupational condition is involved, the occupational health nurse is the center of case management (Levy et al., 2017). The nurse works closely with the primary care provider to monitor the progress of the ill or injured worker and to identify and eliminate potential barriers in the return-to-work process. The nurse has a comprehensive understanding of the workplace and of the physical requirements necessary for the employee to work. The physical demands analysis (Randolph and Dalton, 1989) is a useful tool for objectively assessing the physical demands of any job. (See **Resource Tool 30D**, Physical Demands Analysis.) Once the assessment is completed, the occupational health nurse can relay this information to community health professionals caring for the employee.

For workers needing special accommodations, the occupational health nurse can negotiate and facilitate those appropriate to the employee's health limitations (AAOHN, 2012). The nurse is often the driving force behind the employer's creation of a transitional duty pool. The goal of this type of program is to provide temporary work that is less physically demanding in nature than the employee's regular work. It facilitates the employee's return to the workplace earlier than if he or she was required to wait until after regaining full strength.

The occupational health nurse can monitor and support the health of employees returning to work who continue to experience adverse health effects of chronic disease. For example, the employee who is returning to work after sustaining a myocardial infarction may undergo blood pressure monitoring on a routine basis. Counseling regarding adjustment to normal work life and support for behavior modification (e.g., smoking cessation) also may be provided.

? ACTIVE LEARNING

1. A weight loss program was conducted during August. Ten people participated in the 6-week program. The total weight loss for the group was 185 pounds. The following chart indicates the weight loss for the individuals:

Weight before program (lb)	Weight after program (lb)
215	190
175	160
139	129
275	245
145	120
198	183
120	115
243	233
185	145
210	200

Is there a more effective way to show the results of the program? Assume a peer distributed this report for critique. Be creative, filling in any data, facts, figures, or other information that may be missing. Redesign a report to send to management.

2. Take an occupational history on five currently employed workers. Identify the occupation, associated job tasks, and potential health hazards. Describe control strategies that could minimize or eliminate the risk of adverse health effects.

3. Conduct a literature review to identify critical concepts in occupational health nursing, epidemiology, ergonomics, safety, industrial hygiene, and medicine, and describe how these disciplines work together to achieve optimal ends.

In addition, because the workforce is aging and because older workers are more prone to chronic disease, the occupational health nurse can implement and monitor treatment protocols and help workers live and work at their optimum comfort level while managing their diseases. Responsibilities for the care of elderly parents or significant others will influence the balance of work and home for older workers. The occupational health nurse's role as counselor, referral resource for workers, and consultant to management can influence future beneficial changes.

SKILLS AND COMPETENCIES OF THE OCCUPATIONAL HEALTH NURSE

Although clinical and emergency care remains an important tenet of occupational health nursing, the current and future practice must focus on a proactive approach with the goal of preventing illness and injury and promoting health. Therefore the occupational health nurse must possess competencies necessary to recognize and evaluate potential and existing health hazards in the workplace. Management and budgeting skills and knowledge of legal and regulatory requirements, toxicology, ergonomics, epidemiology, environmental health, safety, counseling, and health promotion and education are essential to meet the present and future demands of occupational health nursing practice.

Competencies in occupational and environmental health nursing have been outlined by AAOHN (2015) (Box 31.4). Each competency delineates comprehensive performance criteria at the competent, proficient, and expert levels. Each level is described here, followed by a description of occupational health nursing practice at that level.

Competent

At the "competent" level of practice, the nurse has gained confidence and his or her perception of the role is one of mastery and an ability to cope with specific situations. There is less of a need to rely on the judgments of peers and other professionals. Work habits tend to stress consistency rather than routine tailoring of care to encompass individual differences (Benner, 1984).

The competent occupational and environmental health nurse has sufficient experience to recognize a range of practice issues and to function comfortably in such roles as clinician, occupational health services coordinator, and case manager. This nurse follows company procedures and relies on assessment checklists and clinical protocols to provide treatment.

Proficient. The "proficient" nurse has an increased ability to perceive client situations as a whole on the basis of past experiences, focusing on the relevant aspects of the situation. The nurse is able to predict the events to expect in a particular situation and can recognize that protocols sometimes must be altered to meet the needs of the client (Benner, 1984).

Occupational and environmental health nursing example: A proficient occupational and environmental health nurse is able to quickly obtain the information needed for accurate assessment and move rapidly to the critical aspects of the problem. Structured goals are replaced by priority setting in response to the situation. The proficient nurse usually possesses sophisticated clinical or managerial skills in the occupational health setting.

Expert

The "expert" nurse has extensive experience and a broad knowledge base and is able to grasp a situation quickly and initiate appropriate action. The nurse has a sense of salience grounded in practice guiding actions and priorities (Benner, 1984).

Occupational and environmental health nursing example: Occupational and environmental health nurses at the expert level include those providing leadership in developing occupational and environmental health policy within an organization, those functioning in upper executive or management roles, those serving as consultants to business and government, and those designing and conducting significant research in the field.

Examples of Skills and Competencies for Occupational Health Nursing

As described, numerous skills and competencies are necessary for occupational health nursing practice. Examples of some of these are outlined here, according to four of the defined areas of competence.

- Manages total worker health independently and with other team members
  - Identifies hazards and exposures and recommends control strategies for their mitigation
  - Plans, implements, and evaluates occupational health and safety programs and services for the target populations
- Adheres to principles of professional nursing practice
  - Practices nursing ethically, competently, and within the legal scope of practice
  - Stays current with evidence-based occupational health nursing practice and interventions
- Demonstrates understanding of the business climate and its impact on the health of the community
  - Works with interdisciplinary teams to provide services to workforces and with those who provide disaster services in times of emergencies
  - Manages budgets

- Practices culturally appropriate, evidence-based nursing care within a licensed scope of practice
  - Gathers information related to occupational health history, conducts assessments, and informs decision making regarding fitness for duty and return to work (Fig. 31.3)
  - Provides education and counsels on strategies for risk identification and elimination

IMPACT OF FEDERAL LEGISLATION ON OCCUPATIONAL HEALTH

Legislation and associated activities have influenced the practice of occupational health in the United States. Table 31.4 presents a historical perspective of some of the major pieces of legislation that have had, and will continue to have, a direct impact on the general practice of occupational and environmental health nursing. The Occupational Safety and Health Act, Workers' Compensation Acts, and the ADA are highlighted here.

Occupational Safety and Health Act

The Occupational Safety and Health Act of 1970 was enacted 2 years after a major coal-mining disaster in West Virginia. The passage of this legislation came about because of concerns about workers' health, a burgeoning environmental awareness, union activities, and a greater knowledge about workplace hazards. The general duty clause of the act states that employers must "furnish a place of employment free from recognized hazards that are causing or likely to cause death or serious physical harm to employees" (OSHA, 1970). The act also identifies the roles of the various governmental agencies; provides for the establishment of federal occupational safety and health standards; and identifies a structure of penalties, fines, and sentences for violations of regulations. Under the act, any state has the right to implement its own occupational safety and health administration. The only requirement is that the state standards meet or exceed federal standards. Currently, 25 states and the Virgin Islands operate state occupational safety and health administrations. The following organizations were formed under the provisions of the act:

- Under the jurisdiction of the Department of Labor, the OSHA is responsible for promulgating and enforcing occupational safety and health standards.
- Under the jurisdiction of the USDHHS, NIOSH is responsible for funding and conducting research, making recommendations for occupational safety and health standards to OSHA, and for funding Occupational Safety and Health Education and Research Centers for the training of occupational health professionals.
- The Occupational Safety and Health Review Commission, which is appointed by the president, is responsible for advising OSHA and NIOSH regarding the legal implications of decisions or actions in the course of performing their duties.
- The National Advisory Committee on Occupational Safety and Health, which is also appointed by the president, is a group of consumers and professionals who are responsible

Year	Legislation
1836	First restrictive child labor law enacted (Massachusetts)
1877	State legislation passed requiring factory safeguards (Massachusetts)
1879	State legislation passed requiring factory inspections (Massachusetts)
1886	State legislation passed requiring reporting of industrial accidents (Massachusetts)
1910	State legislation passed requiring formation of an Occupational Disease Commission (Illinois)
1911	Workmen's Compensation Act passed (New Jersey)
1935	Social Security Act passed (state and federal unemployment insurance program)
1936	Walsh-Healey Act (federal legislation setting occupational safety and health standards for certain government contract workers)
1938	Fair Labor Standards Act (setting minimum age for child labor)
1948	All states now have Workers' Compensation Acts
1964	Civil Rights Act
1965	McNamara-O'Hara Act (extends protection of the Walsh-Healey Act to include suppliers of government services)
1966	Mine Safety Act (mandatory inspections and health and safety standards in mining industry)
1969	Coal Mine Health and Safety Act (mandatory health and safety standards for underground mines)
1970	Occupational Safety and Health Act
1970	Environmental Protection Agency established
1970	Consumer Protection Agency established
1972	Equal Employment Opportunity Act
1972	Noise Control Act
1972	Clean Water Act
1973	HMO Act
1973	Rehabilitation Act
1976	Toxic Substances Control Act
1976	Resources Conservation and Recovery Act
1977	Federal Mine Safety and Health Act
1990	Americans With Disabilities Act
1991	Bloodborne Pathogens Standard
1993	Family Medical Leave Act
1996	National Occupational Research Agenda (NIOSH) established
2000	Needlestick Safety and Prevention Act
2002	Recordkeeping Rule amended
2008	Genetic Information Nondiscrimination Act
2010	Patient Protection and Affordable Care Act

for making recommendations to OSHA and NIOSH regarding occupational health and safety.

- The National Commission on State Workers' Compensation Laws, appointed by the president as well, was tasked with studying the adequacy of state workers' compensation laws and making recommendations to the president on its findings. This commission's work ended as of October 30, 1972.

Since it was instituted, OSHA has promulgated occupational health and safety standards. These are published in the *Code of Federal Regulations* (CFR) and updated on a regular basis. Having access to the most recent publication of these standards is a crucial responsibility of the occupational health nurse.

The occupational health nurse must be knowledgeable of Title 29 of the *Code,* part 1910 (29 CFR 1910) (OSHA, 2014a), and other sections that apply to specific hazards in the workplace. For example, 29 CFR 1904 (OSHA, 2014b) pertains to OSHA's record-keeping requirements and mandates the employer's responsibility to keep records of work-related injuries, illnesses, and deaths. These records must be posted in the workplace for 1 month per year and made available for review by OSHA at any time. In many cases, the occupational health nurse has full responsibility for compliance with this standard.

OSHA has 10 regional offices throughout the United States. Inspectors are assigned to each region to enforce the standards and to provide consultation to industries. An OSHA inspection can be initiated in one of several ways. Each office plans a schedule of routine visits to the industries in their respective regions. In the past, funding has been an issue, and inspections have not taken place in the number or frequency originally intended. An inspection will occur if a major health or safety problem, such as a death, occurs at the worksite, or if three or more workers are sent to the hospital as a result of the same incident. Inspection also may occur by employer request. A request is not usually made unless the employer has an exemplary occupational health and safety program and wishes to participate in OSHA's voluntary inspection program. Inspection also may be initiated by an employee request if there is concern about a suspected hazardous condition. In this case, OSHA is mandated to respond, and it must keep the employee's name confidential at the employee's request. In the past, penalties for violations have been inconsequential, and sentences have rarely been served. However, events now indicate that fines have increased, and OSHA has made public its intention to criminally prosecute company executives for serious and willful violations.

In many organizations, the occupational health nurse is the interface with the OSHA inspector. This position requires the nurse to be knowledgeable about the potential hazards in the workplace and about the appropriate control measures designed to eliminate or minimize exposure. The nurse should know that employees or their union representatives have the right to accompany the OSHA investigators.

Workers' Compensation Acts

Workers' Compensation Acts are state mandated and state funded. Workers' compensation programs provide income replacement and pay for health care services for workers who sustain a work-related injury, temporary or permanent disability, or death. Workers' Compensation Acts also protect the employer if the compensation received by the employee precludes legal suits against the employer. Each state regulates its own workers' compensation program that is unique to that state. The employer can self-insure, contract with commercial insurance carriers, or purchase a policy with the state-operated insurance fund. Workers receive an average of 66% of their take-home pay before taxes as compensation. Some disabled workers and their families are eligible for other benefit programs, including old age, survivors, disability, and health insurance; supplemental security income; and any other disability arrangement that they may have purchased through the company or on an individual basis.

In an era of high health care costs and a propensity for injured workers to engage the services of lawyers to represent them in negotiating financial settlements, many employers are claiming that workers' compensation costs are crippling their ability to compete in an international marketplace. The occupational health nurse has a unique opportunity to support both the employee and employer in this arena. For the employee, the nurse may be the initial person to whom the work-related injury or illness is reported. Accurate assessment of the injury or illness and appropriate treatment are essential. Community resources must be identified to ensure that the injured worker is provided with high-quality health care and appropriate medical follow-up.

The occupational health nurse educates the employee regarding benefits under the Workers' Compensation Act and is often the one who files the claim. If the employee is unable to work for a period, the nurse provides case management support and remains in contact with the employee until they return to work. If the employer uses an insurance carrier, the nurse works closely with the claims adjuster to manage the case. The need for light duty or other workplace accommodations is determined before the employee's return. In most cases, the nurse facilitates this process with the employer.

For the employer, the occupational health nurse provides the expertise in early intervention and case management. The goal is to limit the worker's disability and provide an opportunity for early return to work through appropriate workplace accommodations. The desired outcome is a productive employee with optimum health and productivity, with reduced health care and workers' compensation costs.

Americans With Disabilities Act

The Americans With Disabilities Act, enacted by Congress in July 1990, is a comprehensive act that prohibits discrimination on the basis of disability. The core of this law requires employers to adjust facilities and practices for the purpose of making "reasonable accommodations" to enhance opportunities for individuals with disabilities. Employment provisions of this act began on July 26, 1992, for employers with 25 or more employees and were revised in July 1994 to include employers with 15 or more employees. Provisions regarding access to public transportation and accommodations became effective in January 1993.

The ADA defines disability as "physical or mental impairment that substantially limits one or more major life activities, having record of such an impairment, or being regarded as having such an impairment" (Kaminshine, 1991, p. 249). Physical or mental impairment guidelines are the same

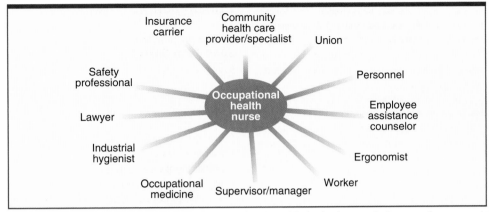

FIG. 31.4 The occupational health nurse's professional links in the workplace and community.

as those described by the Federal Rehabilitation Act and include "any physiologic disorder or condition, cosmetic disfigurement, anatomical loss affecting any of the major body systems, or any mental or psychological disorder" (Kaminshine, 1991, p. 249). Major life activities include caring for self, walking, seeing, hearing, and speaking. The ADA excludes conditions relating to sexual preference and gender identity, compulsive gambling, kleptomania, and pyromania. The ADA also denies protection for individuals who are currently involved in illegal drug use.

With regard to the ADA, the occupational health nurse has particular responsibility in two areas. The first involves the duty to provide or facilitate reasonable accommodations. This duty is facilitated by the nurse's familiarity with the physical requirements of jobs in the workplace. The second involves preplacement inquiries and health examinations. Preplacement health examinations will be permitted only if phrased in terms of the applicant's general ability to perform job-related functions rather than in terms of a disability and after a job offer has been made. The examination must be job related and consistently conducted for all applicants performing similar work.

As illustrated in this discussion of specific laws pertinent to occupational health, the legal context for occupational health nursing practice is broad and involves many arenas. The occupational health nurse must be knowledgeable about all laws and regulations that govern any industry in which the nurse provides health care to employees (e.g., laboratories, transportation, and utilities).

LEGAL ISSUES IN OCCUPATIONAL HEALTH

In recognition of the dynamic nature of occupational health nursing practice, coupled with the influences and impact of larger policy issues, the occupational health nurse must know the legal parameters of practice and must respond to legislative mandates that govern worker health and safety. Professionally, the occupational health nurse is primarily accountable to workers and worker populations and to the employer, the profession, and self (AAOHN, 2015). In particular, the occupational health

nurse must be aware of liability and legal issues related to the following:
- The employee–nurse relationship
- The employment capacity of the occupational health nurse
- Any acts of negligence

The employee–nurse relationship can be confusing when the employer hires the nurse to provide services to the employee. The concern is whether a professional relationship exists under the law or the relationship is based on a coworker status.

MULTIDISCIPLINARY TEAMWORK

As workplaces have become more complex, a diverse array of expertise has emerged in many functional and technical areas. To be successful, the occupational health nurse must recognize the need to work as part of an interdisciplinary team. The nurse may interact with occupational medicine professionals, industrial hygienists, safety and ergonomic professionals, employee assistance counselors, personnel professionals, and union representatives (Fig. 31.4). Community health professionals, insurance carriers, and other support agencies in the community are also critical links.

❓ ACTIVE LEARNING

A large automobile manufacturer needs a program designed to control respiratory disease among foundry workers. Workers in different areas of ferrous foundries are exposed to different respiratory hazards. The main problems are exposures to silica and formaldehyde. The corporation would like to develop a pilot program for one of its foundries that will then be applied to its other foundries. Health and industrial hygiene data will be collected. Both the corporation and the workers support the project, and both see the project as having the following three purposes:
- Detecting health effects in individuals who may benefit from intervention
- Determining the relationship of health effects with environmental exposures
- Identifying control strategies as appropriate

Outline a pilot program. Discuss the implications of discovering adverse health effects among current workers. Describe the roles of the occupational health nurse, physician, industrial hygienist, safety professional, manager, and employee.

Employee With Exposure to Chemicals

Leslie Johnston is a 23-year-old woman who was transferred by her employer into a job that required her to work with chemicals used in photolithography. Leslie became concerned when she noticed that the label on one of the pieces of equipment warned of possible adverse effects on reproduction. Because of her concern and related issues, she went to the on-site health clinic to talk with Peter Mitchell, the occupational health nurse.

Peter invited Leslie into his office to ask her questions and do a brief health history. Leslie reported that her health had been "excellent" until recently but that she had not felt well since transferring to her new position. She explained that she was newly married and thought she may be pregnant, but this was unconfirmed. She questioned whether her vague physical complaints (fatigue, headaches, occasional queasiness) might be related to working with chemicals, a pregnancy, or another reason.

Peter reassured Leslie that he had been employed at the company for 8 years, and he was aware that there were no restrictions in Leslie's work area for pregnant women. He pulled up her health file from his computerized database and gave her a set of health history forms to complete. He also had her read and sign several forms related to confidentiality and assured her that none of her health information would be shared with their employer without her consent.

Assessment

To obtain needed information, Peter:

- Completed general health and occupational health histories.
- Performed a modified physical assessment and discussed the symptoms Leslie was experiencing.
- Referred Leslie to her personal health care provider for further evaluation and to obtain a pregnancy test. (NOTE: In some cases, on-site clinics will be equipped for basic procedures such as this. If this is not a service provided by the occupational health nurse, referral must be made to the employee's health care provider. If the employee does not have one, referral must be made to an appropriate community health resource.) Peter encouraged Leslie to inform her supervisor and himself if the pregnancy test result was positive so they could adapt her assignments to her condition.
- Assessed Leslie's work area with an industrial hygienist to determine whether there might be problems, such as leaking equipment or problems with ventilation.
- Reviewed the most current industrial hygiene data appropriate to the area.

Diagnosis
Individual

- At risk for chemical exposure
- Vague physical complaints of unknown etiology
- Possible pregnancy
- At risk for possible adverse pregnancy outcomes
- Stress related to concern regarding possible exposure to harmful chemicals

Community

- Potential for exposure of employees to unsafe chemicals and/or working conditions

Planning

- Peter developed a plan of care based on Leslie's health history and concerns. Together they set the following goals:

Individual
Short-Term Goals

- Determine pregnancy status.
- Determine potential exposure levels and review side effects of chemicals.
- Determine reason for her vague physical complaints.
- Reduce stress experiences.

Long-Term Goals

- Ensure that the work environment is safe for future pregnancies (if Leslie is not pregnant at present).

- Collaborate with Leslie and her supervisor on possible work restrictions.

Community (Workplace)
Short-Term Goals

- Company personnel (e.g., the occupational health nurse, the industrial hygienist, and all others who are directly affected) will be knowledgeable in safe handling of all hazardous chemicals.
- All company policies regarding safety and exposure will be followed.

Long-Term Goals

- Policies on handling of chemicals and related information will be reviewed periodically as required by law.
- All employees who work with and around potentially hazardous chemicals will undergo periodic instruction and instruction in and confirmation of knowledge about proper procedures.
- Work areas will be monitored per policy for compliance with safe practices.
- There will be no incidents involving worker exposure to chemicals.

Intervention
Individual

Peter conducted a brief physical examination and did not identify any obvious physical abnormalities. Because Leslie's chief complaints were fatigue, occasional headaches, and queasiness, he encouraged her to make an appointment with her primary care provider or gynecologist for a more extensive workup and to assess for pregnancy.

With her permission, he called the industrial hygienist to counsel Leslie regarding the policies of the company, to explain what chemicals might potentially be hazardous, and to review procedures and restrictions. The hygienist also stated that he would send a team to Leslie's work area to take air samples, check lighting, and perform other tests to ensure there were no problems.

Community (Workplace)

The assigned industrial hygiene team sampled the environment for chemical exposure per established procedure. They also set up a plan to have the area more frequently observed pending the results of the tests. The hygienist assured Peter and Leslie that he would communicate any work restrictions or changes to the personnel department and Leslie's supervisor if needed.

Evaluation
Individual

After the meeting with Peter and the industrial hygienist, Leslie stated that she felt reassured. She agreed to make an appointment as soon as possible with her doctor for an evaluation and pregnancy test. She also agreed to inform Peter and her direct supervisor if she learned that she was pregnant.

Community (Workplace)

The industrial hygienist and his assistants performed several tests in close proximity to Leslie's work station; they found no abnormal readings, and all equipment was in good working order. Per agency policy and following OSHA regulations, they charted all findings and submitted reports.

Levels of Prevention
Primary

- Teach about chemicals, exposures, etc.
- Instruct about chemical avoidance.
- Remove employee from environment through work restrictions.

Secondary

- Assess employee for signs and symptoms.
- Assess work environment for exposure.
- Refer for evaluation of possible health problems as needed.

Tertiary

- Provide reproductive counseling.

SUMMARY

This chapter describes the evolution of occupational health nursing during its first century of practice. It also highlighted current and future demographics and business trends as they relate to this nursing specialty area. Aging workers, escalating health care costs, increasing numbers of women and minorities in the workforce, and the competitive international marketplace are key factors shaping occupational health nursing practice.

The occupational health nursing role is challenging and can have a tremendous impact on the quality and delivery of health care to workers and their families. Nurses working in occupational settings should have an excellent understanding of all levels of prevention and possess the skills and competencies outlined here.

For the community health nurse who works in other settings, such as home health, clinics, and schools, knowledge of occupational health nursing practice is also important. Many companies do not have on-site occupational health nurses and therefore must rely on community health nurses to support their occupational health and safety needs.

ⓔ EVOLVE WEBSITE

http://evolve.elsevier.com/Nies/community

- NCLEX Review Questions
- Case Studies

BIBLIOGRAPHY

American Association of Industrial Nurses: *The nurse in industry*, New York, 1976, Author.

American Association of Occupational Health Nurses: *Case management: the occupational and environmental health nurse role*, Chicago, 2012, Author.

American Association of Occupational Health Nurses: *Compensation and benefits study. Author*, Atlanta, GA, 2013, Author.

American Association of Occupational Health Nurses: Competencies in occupational and environmental health nursing, *AAOHN Journal* 55:442–447, 2015. Available from: <http://www.aaohn.org>.

American Association of Occupational Health Nurses: *AAOHN Code of ethics and interpretive statements*, 2016. Available from <www.aaohn.org>. Accessed April 04, 2017.

American Association of Occupational Health Nurses: *Standards of occupational and environmental health nursing*, 2015. Accessed April 04, 2017.

American Cancer Society: *Cancer statistics*, 2017. Available from: https://www.cancer.org/cancer/breast-cancer/about/how-common-is-breast-cancer.html.

Benner P: *From novice to expert: excellence and power in clinical nursing practice*, Menlo Park, CA, 1984, Addison-Wesley.

Budden JS, Moulton P, Harper KJ, et al.: The 2015 National Nursing Workforce Survey, *Journal of Nursing Regulation* 7(1S):S2–S90, 2016.

Burgel B, Childre F: The occupational health nurse as the trusted physician in the 21st century, *AAOHN J* 60:143–150, 2012.

Felton JS: The genesis of occupational health nursing: Part I, *Occup Health Nurse* 30:45–49, 1985.

Felton JS: The genesis of occupational health nursing: Part II, *AAOHN J* 34:210–215, 1986.

Kaminshine S: New rights for the disabled: the Americans With Disabilities Act of 1990, *AAOHN J* 39:249–251, 1991.

Levy BS, Wegman DH, Sokas R: *Occupational and environmental health*, ed 6, Philadelphia, 2017, Lippincott Williams & Wilkins.

McGrath BJ: *Nursing in commerce and industry*, New York, 1946, The Commonwealth Fund.

Occupational Health and Safety Administration (OSHA): Occupational Safety Act, 1970 (P.L. 91–596).

Moore P, Moore R: *Core curriculum for occupational and environmental health nursing*, ed 4, Chicago, 2014, AAOHN. https://www.osha.gov/pls/oshaweb/owadisp.show_document?p_table=OSHACT&p_id=3359.

Occupational Health and Safety Administration (OSHSA): Regulations (Standards – 29): 1910. 2014a. Available from: https://www.osha.gov/pls/oshaweb/owasrch.search_form?p_doc_type=STANDARDS&p_toc_level=1&p_keyvalue=1910

Occupational Health and Safety Administration (OSHSA): Regulations (Standards – 29): 1904. 2014b. Available from: https://www.osha.gov/pls/oshaweb/owasrch.search_form?p_doc_type=STANDARDS&p_toc_level=1&p_keyvalue=1904

O'Donnell M: Editor's notes: Definition of health promotion 2.0: embracing passion, enhancing motivation, recognizing dynamic balance, and creating opportunities, *Am J Health Promot* 24:Iv, 2009.

Parker-Conrad JE: A century of practice: occupational health nursing, *AAOHN J* 36:156–161, 1988.

Parker-Conrad JE: Celebrating our past, *AAOHN J* 50:537–541, 2002.

Randolph SA, Dalton PC: Limited duty work: an innovative approach to early return to work, *AAOHN J* 37:446–452, 1989.

Randolph S, Scully A, Bertsche P: Economic, political, and Business Factors. In Moore P, Moore R, editors: *Core curriculum for occupational and environmental health nursing*, ed 3, Chicago, 2014, AAOHN, pp 67–143.

Rogers B: Establishing research priorities in occupational health nursing, *AAOHN J* 37:493–500, 1989.

Rogers B: Occupational health nursing expertise, *AAOHN J* 46:477–483, 1998.

Rogers B: Nursing: an ethic of caring, *AAOHN J* 51:155–157, 2003.

Rogers B: *Occupational health nursing: Concepts and practice*, ed 3, Beverly, MA, 2017, In press. OEM Press.

Rogers B: Occupational and environmental health nursing: ethics and Professionalism, *AAOHN J* 60:177–182, 2012.

Rogers B, Franke J, Jeras J, et al.: The family medical leave act: implications for occupational health nursing, *AAOHN J* 57(6):239–250, 2009.

Rogers B, Randolph S, Mastrianno K: *Occupational health nursing guidelines for primary clinical conditions*, ed 5, Beverly, MA, 2018, In press. OEM Press.

Thompson M: Professional autonomy of occupational health nurses un the United States, *AAOHN J* 60:159–166, 2012.

Towers Watson/National Business Group on Health: *The road ahead: Shaping health care strategy in a post-reform environment: 16th Annual Employer Survey on Purchasing Value in Health Care*, 2011.

U.S. Bureau of Labor Statistics: *Employment Projections: 2014-24 Summary*, 2015. https://www.bls.gov/news.release/ecopro.nr0.htm.

U.S. Department of Health and Human Services: *Healthy People 2020*, 2017. www.healthypeople.gov.

32

Forensic and Correctional Nursing

*Stacy A. Drake**

OBJECTIVES

Upon completion of this chapter, the reader will be able to do the following:
1. Define forensic nursing.
2. Describe the specialties of forensic nurses.
3. Explain issues important to each of the subspecialty areas of forensic nursing.

4. Describe interventions and services forensic nurses perform.
5. Discuss factors affecting health and wellness in a correctional setting.

KEY TERMS

child abuse	forensic nurse death investigator	living forensics
coroner	forensic nurse examiner	medical examiner
correctional nursing	forensic nursing	nurse attorney
elder abuse	forensic psychiatric nurse	nurse coroner
forensic	legal nurse consultant	sexual assault nurse examiner

According to the Bureau of Justice Statistics National Crime Victimization Survey, in 2015 approximately 5 million violent crimes were reported; this was a slight decrease from the number of violent crimes in 2011 (U.S. Department of Justice/Bureau of Justice Statistics [USDOJ/BJS], 2015). These crimes ranged from vandalism and theft, to rape and sexual assault, to aggravated assault and murder. The estimated medical and productivity economic burdens of interpersonal and self-directed violence (suicide, homicide, child maltreatment, youth violence, intimate partner violence, and other assaults) are staggering. Because of the continued high prevalence of violence and violent crimes in society, health care professionals are recommended to identify and assess victims of interpersonal partner violence and provide proper care and referrals as needed. Indeed, screening for violence is now considered to be a minimum standard of care for all women, as is vigilance in looking for indications on when and where to screen for abuse among elders and vulnerable adults (U.S. Preventive Services Task Force [USPSTF], 2013).

The term forensic means "pertaining to the law, legal" (Lynch, 2011, p. 5). It refers to instances, activities, or information used in or suitable to courts of law. Health care providers, especially nurses, frequently care for both victims and perpetrators of crime, and they should be prepared to assess for indications of violence and abuse and to intervene as needed.

* The author would like to acknowledge the contribution of Angela Jarrell, who revised this chapter for the previous edition.

Forensic nursing is defined as "application of the nursing process to public or legal proceedings, and the application of forensic health care in the scientific investigation of trauma and/or death related to abuse, violence, criminal activity, liability, and accidents" (Lynch, 2011, p. 5). Forensic nursing combines the disciplines of nursing science, forensic science, medical science, sociology, and psychology with law enforcement and the criminal justice system. Recognized by the American Nurses Association (ANA), forensic nursing is growing nationally and internationally. The specialty of forensic nursing was officially recognized by the ANA in 1995, and the *Scope and Standards of Forensic Nursing Practice* was published in 1997 (ANA, 2014; Amar and Sekula, 2017)) and revised in 2009 (ANA, 2009). The International Association of Forensic Nurses (Price and Maguire, 2016), recognizing the need to provide accurate and reliable knowledge, skills, and scope of practice education to the new forensic nurse, endorsed the Core Curriculum for Forensic Nurses.

The International Association of Forensic Nurses (IAFN) explains that forensic nursing is the practice of nursing where the health and legal systems intersect (ANA, 2009). Thus the forensic nurse's role fills a gap between the health care system, the investigative process, and courts of law (Lynch, 2011).

Forensic nurses practice in multiple areas and settings of the health care and public health systems. Their responsibilities may include screening, assessment and documentation of injuries, and collection of evidence, and may also include expert witness testimony for victims and perpetrators across a variety of settings such as hospitals, community clinics, and death scenes. In addition to working with victims and perpetrators, forensic nurses may be involved in paternity disputes and cases involving workplace injuries, malpractice, transportation crashes, food or drug tampering (Fig. 32.1), and medical equipment defects (Lynch, 2011). The advanced forensic nurse or the graduate or doctoral prepared forensic nurse may assist in developing and implementing protocols and systems to help victims or perpetrators of violent occurrences, aid in research and policy changes, develop and supervise systems of care for complex health issues, and provide essential education to others (IAFN, 2004). The *Healthy People 2020* box lists some objectives related to this highly specialized practice area.

FIG. 32.1 A forensic nurse counting medications.

HEALTHY PEOPLE 2020
Objectives Related to Forensic Nursing

AH-11: Reduce adolescent and young adult perpetration of, and victimization by, crimes.

IVP HP2020-33: Reduce physical assaults.

IVP HP2020-38: Reduce nonfatal child maltreatment.

IVP HP2020-40: Reduce sexual violence.

IVP 2020-43: Increase the number of states that link data on violent deaths from death certificates, law enforcement, and coroner and medical examiner reports to inform prevention efforts at the state and local levels.

MHMD-HP2020-7: Increase the proportion of juvenile residential facilities that screen admissions for mental health problems.

SA HP2020-5: Increase the number of drug, driving while impaired, and other specialty courts in the United States.

SA HP2020-10: Increase the number of Level I and Level II trauma centers that implement evidence-based alcohol screening and brief intervention.

From HealthyPeople.gov: *Healthy People 2020: topics & objectives,* 2013. http://www.healthypeople.gov/2020/topicsobjectives2020/objectiveslist.aspx?topicId=24. Accessed February 21, 2018

SUBSPECIALTIES OF FORENSIC NURSING

The IAFN recognizes core specialties within forensic nursing (Box 32.1). Each of the subspecialties will be briefly discussed.

Sexual Assault Nurse Examiner

The sexual assault nurse examiner (SANE) is the most widely recognized subspecialty in forensic nursing. In the 1970s, emergency department (ED) registered nurses identified a special client population—sexual assault victims—who were not receiving the appropriate, compassionate care after a terrifying traumatic event (Ledray and Arndt, 1994). They observed that in many cases the staff did not know how to compassionately but objectively approach the sexual assault victim entering the ED; to properly assess, document, and collect evidence; or to provide testimony in a court of law. Therefore the SANE role was developed.

A SANE is a specially trained registered nurse who applies the nursing process during forensic examinations to victims or perpetrators of sexual assault. Recognizing cultural and developmental differences, as well as the impact of trauma of victims, the SANE assesses and documents detailed physical examination findings, collects forensic evidence related to a reported crime, and frequently testifies as an expert witness at subsequent trials (Office for Victims of Crime, 2017). SANEs are usually employed in EDs and community clinics dedicated to victims of interpersonal violence. SANEs may also be employed

BOX 32.1 Specialties of Forensic Nurses

- Sexual assault nurse examiner
- Nurse coroner and death investigator
- Legal nurse consultant and nurse attorney
- Forensic nursing educator and consultant
- Forensic psychiatric nurse
- Forensic nurse examiner
- Correctional nurse

to complete forensic examinations on deceased individuals for whom sexual assault is presumed.

If the client is medically stable, the SANE is responsible for conducting a thorough examination, including obtaining a history, performing the physical assessment, and collecting forensic evidence (Box 32.2). If the client is medically unstable, he or she will be assessed and stabilized by a provider before the forensic examination. Other responsibilities of the SANE are crisis intervention referral, pregnancy risk assessment and interception as needed, and client referral for additional support (Ledray, 2011).

A registered nurse caring for sexual assault victims may receive SANE certification offered through the IAFN. Both adult and pediatric certifications are available. The requirements for a registered nurse to be eligible for the SANE adult and/or pediatric certification examinations are that the nurse must (1) be in practice for a minimum of 2 years, (2) have successfully completed 40 hours of didactic instruction or academic course equivalent, and (3) demonstrate competency in sexual assault examinations (IAFN, 2015).

Medicolegal Death Investigation

According to Hanzlick (2007), there are four different types of death investigation: medicolegal, institution-based, private, and public health. Medicolegal death investigations are usually conducted to clarify the sudden, unexpected, and often nonnatural circumstances in which death occurred. Institution-based death investigations are usually those that occur in the hospital or nursing home setting. Private death investigations are family initiated and are focused on answering questions the family may have surrounding the death. Public health investigations are frequently conducted in cooperation with the medicolegal and/or are retrospective studies. An example of public health death investigation would be sudden unexpected infant deaths. The medicolegal death investigation system falls within the purview of the public health system as defined by the Centers for Disease Control and Prevention. One of the outputs of death investigation is death certificates. In the United States, medicolegal death investigation systems are characterized as medical examiner, coroner/justices of the peace, or mixed (Hanzlick, 2007; Lynch, 2011).

Typically, **medical examiners** are licensed physicians who are board certified in anatomic and forensic pathology (Hanzlick, 2007). Usually a medical examiner is appointed for an unspecified term and serves a county, district, region, or state as determined by law. The **coroners**/justices of the peace are usually elected laypersons; that is, persons who have little or no training in medicine or science who conduct medicolegal investigations and certify cause and manner of death. A mixed medicolegal system is a combination of medical examiner and coroners/justices of the peace systems, depending on state law (Hanzlick, 2007).

Most medicolegal death investigation agencies are responsible for issuing death certificates that state the cause and manner of death. These data are collected at city, county, state, and national levels and are used to determine the health of the nation and how best to allocate financial resources. The *cause of death* is the event that initiated the progression of events that ended in death (Lynch, 2011). The *manner of death* is categorization that relates to the conditions in which the cause of death occurred (Hanzlick, 2007). The National Association of Medical Examiners identifies five acceptable options for recording manner of death: natural, accident, suicide, homicide, and "undetermined" (Hanzlick et al., 2002).

Role of a Forensic Nurse Death Investigator

Typically the forensic nurse is employed in the medicolegal death investigation or public health setting. Forensic nurses enter the death investigation arena possessing knowledge of anatomy, physiology, pharmacology, growth and development, physical examination, and health history interviewing techniques, all of which are needed to conduct a comprehensive death investigation (Lynch and Koehler, 2011; Mitchell and Drake, 2017). In most cases related to a death scene investigation, investigators are police officers or homicide detectives—members of professions without medical knowledge. The **forensic nurse death investigator** (FNDI) evaluates the death scene from a holistic nursing perspective and might interpret the scene differently (Clinical Example 32.1 and Fig. 32.2). The requirements for being an FNDI vary; however, most employers ask for a minimum of 2 years of experience, preferably in the setting of critical care or emergency.

BOX 32.2 Type of Evidence Collected from a Victim of Sexual Assault

- Documentation of history of the event
- Documentation of injuries (photographic and written)
- All clothing worn at the time of incident
- Trace evidence (fiber, glass, soil, particulate matter)
- Biological evidence for DNA comparison (victim's blood or hair)
- Fingernail swabbing
- Swabs and smears (from the victim's mouth, vagina/penis, and anus)
- Pubic hair combings
- Evidence disbursement sheet
- Any additional evidence, as noted during examination (example: body piercings)

Data from Ferrell J, Caruso C: Sexual assault evidence recovery. In Lynch VA, Duval JB, editors: *Forensic nursing science*, ed 2, St Louis, 2011, Mosby pp. 144–154.

FIG. 32.2 A forensic nurse plans her day.

Clinical Example 32.1

A police officer entering a house observes several pools of blood located throughout the residence and discovers a deceased male, nude and lying in bed; the police officer suspects foul play or homicide. The FNDI entering the same death scene notices the same findings as the initial police officer, but also notes bloody emesis in the toilet, blood-soaked towels in the washing machine, and empty alcohol bottles in the trash. A preliminary examination of the decedent by the FNDI reveals ascites, jaundice, and multiple contusions on the body. Through communication with family members, the FNDI discovers the decedent was an alcoholic with many health problems; the FNDI suspects that he had ruptured esophageal varices. This suspicion was confirmed by an autopsy, and the manner of death was determined to be from natural causes rather than homicide, as initially believed.

Role of Nurse Coroner

In coroner systems in which the chief medicolegal death investigator is elected and often state laws do not have specific requirements of the office, nurses may decide to run for the position of coroner or nurse coroner. The nurse coroner is responsible for ensuring that appropriate measures are taken to perform death investigations and to certify death certificates. A nurse coroner's educational background and knowledge enables him or her to identify disease processes that the lay coroner may not recognize or may misinterpret as foul play, as in the preceding clinical example.

FNDIs and nurse coroners exhibit communication skills when dealing with grieving families. Nurses are given education in therapeutic communication and are able to practice those skills in any setting. They are acutely aware of the importance of using open-ended questions, listening attentively, and being fully present with family and friends. The use of these techniques allows family and friends to openly share the feelings and thoughts experienced with the death of a loved one (Potter and Perry, 2016). Additionally, nurses are guided by their nursing code of ethics (ANA, 2015). These codes cross all settings for the nurse and are the foundation for providing ethical values and obligations across the life span.

Nurse coroners and FNDIs may apply to become board certificated in death investigation through the American Board of Medicolegal Death Investigators (ABMDI). ABMDI requires applicants to (1) be certified at the Registry Level and in good standing for a minimum of 6 months, (2) have at least an associate's degree from a postsecondary institution recognized by a national educational accrediting agency, (3) be currently employed at an agency with the job responsibility to conduct scene investigations, and (4) have a minimum of 4000 hours of experience in the last 6 years (ABMDI, 2017). Once an investigator satisfies these requirements, he or she may take a standardized examination and become board certified as a Fellow of the ABMDI.

Legal Nurse Consultant and Nurse Attorney

Legal nurse consultants (LNCs) and nurse attorneys are nurses who provide assistance within the legal system using specialized nursing knowledge and expertise when interaction between law and health care quality and safety issues arise (Geissler-Murr and Moorhouse, 2006; Pagliaro and Cewe, 2013). Among many activities, LNCs evaluate, analyze, and render informed opinions on the delivery of health care and its outcomes, based on their area of expertise (American Association of Legal Nurse Consultants [AALNC], 2017). Many law firms hire LNCs to review and interpret medical records and charts, provide objective opinions based on standards of care, and possibly to testify in court as expert witnesses. A forensic nurse practicing as an LNC may apply for certification through the American Legal Nurse Consultant Certification Board (ALNCCB). The candidate must have (1) a current nursing license full and unrestricted, (2) a minimum of 5 years' experience as a registered nurse, and (3) evidence of 2000 hours of legal nurse consulting experience within the last 5 years (ALNCCB, 2017). Once the candidate meets these requirements, he or she may sit for a standardized examination, and once having passed the examination, he or she earns the Legal Nurse Consultant Certified credential.

Nurse attorneys are academically educated in both law and nursing. They may practice in health care, public health, or criminal or civil law, which would include malpractice cases. Malpractice cases may require participation of a nurse attorney on either the plaintiff's or the defendant's side, and may involve licensure disciplinary action or agency oversight (Collins and Halpern, 2005). Some practitioners have differing opinions regarding LNCs and nurse attorneys. They may be perceived as either defending the profession or prosecuting peers by testifying against professional colleagues. By providing services as experts and by testifying, nurses serving as legal consultants help hold accountable practitioners who are unsafe to the public. In contrast, meticulous practitioners who are wrongfully accused of negligence are defended by these nurses' actions.

According to the AALNC (2017), an LNC performs many different services and activities, as follows:

- Identify, organize, and analyze medical records and related materials
- Prepare chronologies or timelines of health care events
- Identify applicable standards of care
- Evaluate causation and damage issues
- Conduct literature research and summarize medical literature
- Evaluate case strengths and weaknesses
- Serve as an expert witness
- Identify plaintiff's future medical needs and associated costs

LNCs read reports and records and determine whether the standards of care were met or breached. In general, if working for a plaintiff in a malpractice case, the LNC will look for breaches in the standards of care; if working for the defense, the LNC will look for nursing care that is given within the standards of care related to the complaint. It is essential that the attorneys be kept informed of all findings—even those that might negatively affect their case (Robson, 2009).

When providing services, the LNC may submit an *affidavit*, a written statement explaining the expert's credentials, background, and licensing or certification(s). It also provides a list of the materials read and considered in the case, and the findings of the review are summarized into a case analysis. After the submission of an affidavit, the LNC may be asked to provide a deposition. The *deposition* is a pretrial discovery process that

---

BOX 32.3   Tips for Testifying at a Deposition or in Court

Do's

- Dress professionally and conservatively.
- Tell the truth at all times.
- Listen to the complete question before responding.
- Speak slowly, clearly, and concisely when answering.
- Take a few seconds to formulate an answer before responding.
- Minimize "ums" or "uhs" by pausing at the end of sentences.
- If there is an objection, stop talking and wait for the judge to make a ruling.
- When answering questions, make eye contact with the jury members.
- Remain calm.
- Respond confidently.
- Practice difficult words.
- Avoid nervous gestures; keep your hands in your lap.

Don'ts

- Avoid saying "I think" and "I believe."
- Never interrupt.
- Do not answer a question that you do not understand; ask the attorney to repeat questions as needed.
- Do not become defensive or angry.

Data from Ruiz-Contreras A: The nurse as an expert witness, *Top Emerg Med* 27(1):27–35, 2005.

BOX 32.4   Types of Evidence

Tangible (touchable) evidence—recognized on sight:

- Weapons/tools
- Bullets, casing, wadding, gunshot residue
- Matches, lighters, or other ignition sources
- Blood, semen, saliva, tissue
- Soil, paint
- Clothing or personal effects
- Notes or messages
- Photographs

Transient evidence—temporary and may be lost, destroyed, or damaged:

- Physical findings such as bruises, swelling, bleeding, tenderness
- Odors (e.g., marijuana, alcohol, gasoline)

Trace evidence—may not be visible; identified by microscope or alternative light sources:

- Fibers
- Biological specimens: blood, semen stains
- DNA

Data from Hammer RM, Moynihan B, Pagliaro EM: *Forensic nursing: a handbook for practice*, ed 2, Burlington, MA, 2013, Jones & Bartlett Learning; Lynch VA, Duval JB: *Forensic nursing science*, ed 2, St. Louis, 2011, Elsevier/Mosby; and Safertein R: *Criminalistics: an introduction to forensic science*, ed 10, Upper Saddle River, NJ, 2010, Pearson.

---

allows the attorneys on both sides to learn more about what the courtroom testimony will be. It is given to a court reporter, and the respondent is under oath.

During the deposition, the LNC presents the facts of the case and is questioned by attorneys from both sides. This process may be quite lengthy and stressful. It is essential that the LNC be prepared, having reviewed everything thoroughly. After this process, the LNC is given a written transcript of the deposition, which needs to be carefully reviewed for accuracy. If the case goes to trial, the LNC will then testify in court (Robson, 2009; Ruiz-Contreras, 2005).

In some cases, the forensic nurse is called on to testify in court, not as an expert witness as described previously, but as a factual witness—one who has firsthand knowledge of the case in question. In these cases, the forensic nurse provides factual statements about the evidence collected and what was observed (Pagliaro and Cewe, 2013). Box 32.3 lists tips that will be helpful for nurses to review before testifying in court.

Clinical Forensic Nurse Examiner

Emergency and Critical Care

Registered nurses may be employed in EDs and critical care units as **forensic nurse examiners**. In this role they deliver care to living patients who are involved with the legal system, and their services may include several subspecialties. The term **living forensics** refers to individuals who are subject to forensic investigations, including but not limited to survivors of physical and mental trauma, toxicology emergencies, interpersonal violence, transportation crashes, and police detention (Lynch, 2011).

As illustrated in Clinical Example 32.2, the ED is frequently the initial location of the initial forensic nursing examination or medicolegal investigation (Doughtery, 2011). It is imperative

that registered nurses identify forensic patients; initiate the proper collection, preservation, and chain of custody of evidence; and then provide accurate documentation for this unique population. The recognition, collection, and documentation of evidence collected within the ED may have an important role in the investigation of crimes and can have a major impact on legal decisions. Box 32.4 lists types of evidence.

Clinical Example 32.2

A 27-year-old woman arrived at the ED with a gunshot wound of the head. Emergency medical technicians reported to the ED nurse and doctor that the client was found by her boyfriend barely breathing. The boyfriend called 911, and the client was transported to the hospital. The client arrived at the hospital in asystole and was pronounced dead within 10 minutes of arrival. The ED nurse applied her forensic knowledge and placed brown paper bags on the client's hands, securing them with tape. This procedure is performed to preserve gunpowder or primer residue. Gunpowder or primer residue aids in the identification of the shooter and distance of the gun. When a gun is fired, residue is released and lands on the items close to the gun, specifically the hands and clothing of the person firing it.

The police agency investigated the death. The nurse's intervention, placing paper bags over the client's hands, preserved the presence or absence of gunshot or primer residue. The police agency performed a scanning electron microscope examination for gunpowder residue and did not find any on the client's hands. This finding led police to further investigate the incident and discover that the boyfriend had shot the client, rather than the first presumption, that the gunshot wound was self-inflicted.

Organ and Tissue Donation and Transplantation

Forensic nurses also have a role in providing a detailed physical examination of patients who may be organ and tissue donors.

This area of care is complex and requires detailed understanding of related legal and ethical issues. When a patient is declared brain dead or donation after cardiac death (DCD), federal law states that the legal next of kin shall be approached for organ and tissue donation. A forensic nurse is able to conduct and provide a detailed physical examination and to collect any evidence that may be required. A thorough death investigation at the hospital may be required for sudden, unexpected, and nonnatural deaths. This involves reviewing medical records and documenting injuries, which is essential for the medicolegal investigation agency to identify acceptable candidates and potential organs and tissues for harvest. The nurse involved in this process must be knowledgeable about legal specifications related to organ donation and be familiar with agency policies and procedures for determining brain death and DCD. The nurse must also have excellent communication skills as well as the ability to relate empathetically to grieving families. In this capacity, the forensic nurse working harmoniously with organ and tissue procurement agencies can obtain release authorization for life-saving organs (Shafer, 2011).

Care of Vulnerable Populations

The youngest, oldest, and disabled populations are the most vulnerable to maltreatment. Nurses dedicating their practice to these vulnerable populations often are required to collaborate with other agencies to ensure adequate resources are available. Often advocacy groups are referred to for assistance.

Child Abuse and Neglect. Child abuse and neglect (child maltreatment) are major concerns for society; therefore the role of a forensic nurse examiner is especially imperative. The Federal Child Abuse Prevention and Treatment Act defines child abuse and neglect as minimum of:

> *Any recent act or failure to act on the part of a parent or caretaker which results in death, serious physical or emotional harm, sexual abuse or exploitation; or an act or failure to act which presents an imminent risk of serious harm.*
> **(42 U.S.C.A. §5106g, as amended and reauthorized by the CAPTA Reauthorization Act of 2010)**

In 2015, approximately 683,000 children were victims of child abuse and neglect, and nearly 77.7% of the perpetrators involved at least one parent. Furthermore, reported cases of child abuse or neglect resulting in death in were estimated to be 1670 children (U.S. Department of Health and Human Services [USDHHS], Administration for Children and Families [ACF], 2015).

States have varying definitions of what constitutes or determines child abuse and neglect. If a forensic nurse suspects that a child is being abused or neglected, the nurse should refer to the state's legislation surrounding the reporting of these suspicions. The following definitions are provided by USDHHS, ACF (2015):

Neglect: Failure of a parent, guardian, or caregiver to provide basic needs. Neglect may be physical (deprivation of adequate food, clothing, shelter, or supervision); medical (failure to provide necessary medical treatment); educational (failure to educate a child or attend to special education needs); or emotional (failure to attend to emotional needs or provide psychological care or allowing the usage of alcohol or other drugs).

Sexual abuse: Range of activities from noncontact indecent exposure to production of pornographic materials, to incest, rape, fondling, and genital contact to actual adult–child sexual intercourse.

Physical abuse: Intentional physical injury, including striking, kicking, burning, and biting.

Emotional abuse (or psychological abuse): A pattern of behavior that impairs the child's emotional development or sense of self-worth, including constant criticism, threats, and rejection.

For the well-being and safety of the child, a nurse ensures that abuse and neglect are swiftly identified and reported to the proper authorities, including the consultation of a forensic nurse examiner (Finn, 2011; Lewis-O'Connor and Latimore, 2017). The nurse obtains a thorough history and assessment, focusing on several facets of abuse and neglect. These include child–parent interaction, the child's appearance and behavior, child–child interaction, and the environment.

A forensic nurse may be employed in a variety of clinical settings that assess, diagnose, and treat children. These settings may include pediatric or general EDs, hospitals, physician offices, schools, home health, hospice, and child advocacy centers.

Elder Mistreatment. Forensic nurse examiners caring for the geriatric population play an important role similar to that of pediatric forensic nurses. Elder mistreatment is thought to be one of the most underdiagnosed and underreported crimes in the United States (Pickens and Dyer, 2016). Unfortunately, there is no exact accounting of elder mistreatment cases, for several reasons: an absence of standardized reporting systems, no consistency in state definition of elder mistreatment, and lack of national data collection (Hammer and Hammer, 2013). Regardless, elder maltreatment is an act of violence or the nonconsented withdrawal of necessary care to sustain life (Pickens and Dyer, 2016)

There are several forms of elder abuse: physical, psychological or emotional, financial, neglect, and sexual abuse (Pickens and Dyer, 2016). Physical abuse is the intentional harm or injury of another person resulting in injury, pain, or impairment (Pickens and Dyer, 2016). In a study by Acierno and colleagues (2009), 1.6% of subjects reported physical mistreatment, and family members accounted for 76% of the mistreatment; specifically, in 57% of cases the abuser was a partner and/or spouse.

Psychological or emotional abuse occurs when there is mental or emotional anguish (e.g., verbal or nonverbal infliction of anguish, pain, or distress) (Pickens and Dyer, 2016). Acierno and colleagues (2009) reported that 4.6% of elders experienced emotional abuse, and for 25% of them, the abuse came from the partner and/or spouse. Financial exploitation occurs when the elder person's financial assets, property, or funds are utilized for another person's benefit without the elder's consent. In the study by Acierno and colleagues (2009), more than 5% of subjects reported being a victim of financial exploitation.

Sexual abuse is the nonconsensual contact of any kind with an elderly person (Pickens and Dyer, 2016). The elder population is at risk for sexual abuse because of inability to resist pursuit or inability to recognize the abuse due to mental illness or other advanced disease processes. Less than 1% of respondents in the study by Acierno and colleagues (2009) reported sexual abuse, and for 40% of those who did report the abuse, the partner and/or spouse was responsible.

Lastly, neglect is the most common form of elder abuse, whether it is caregiver neglect or self-neglect. Caregiver neglect occurs when the obligated caregiver fails to provide appropriate clothing, food, or health services either via refusal to fulfill these requirements or abandonment of the elder client (Pickens and Dyer, 2016). Self-neglect occurs when the elder discounts personal well-being—this could be the result of medical or mental illnesses. Acierno and colleagues (2009) report that 5.1% of elders experienced caregiver neglect.

The elderly client may be hesitant to report abuse, ask for assistance, or acknowledge the maltreatment because the abuser might be a spouse and/or partner, child, or close relative, or because the disclosure would possibly result in litigation and institutionalization (Pearsall, 2011). Forensic nurses may be employed in any setting, treating or seeing elder clients. Some settings are EDs, hospitals, physician offices, nursing homes, home health agencies (Clinical Example 32.3), and geriatric day care centers.

Clinical Example 32.3

A home health care nurse has received a referral from the hospital for a 80-year-old female residing at her home with her son. The patient had been discharged from the hospital with the diagnosis of urinary tract infection and pneumonia. Her son reports she was confused and coughing for 2 months before he took her to the hospital. Her past medical history includes dementia, impaired mobility, and dysphasia from a prior stroke. Upon arrival at the residence, the nurse greets the patient, who is lying in bed. The home is cluttered and dirty, with visible roaches, and the refrigerator/freezer is filled with meat, cheese, milk, and beer. The nurse's assessment findings include the following: clothing is loose fitting and adult brief is soiled, strong body and urine odor present, body is emaciated with upper and lower extremity contractures, contusions of various coloring are located on the upper thighs and posterior torso, stage II decubitus ulcers are present on the right hip and sacral areas (both are covered with soiled dressing), and dentition is poor. The son explains that the patient obtained the contusions because at times she becomes confused and strikes out, hitting things. Furthermore, this happens during times that he attempts to bathe and turn the patient.

Upon leaving the residence, the nurse contacts her supervisor to discuss the findings and her concerns about physical and sexual abuse and neglect. The supervisor agrees, and the patient is returned to the ED for a forensic nurse examination, at which time the forensic nurse places a call to Adult Protective Services for further evaluation and investigation. The hospital is also contacted to discuss why the patient was discharged back into this environment.

Disabled Population. It is well documented that children and elderly with disabilities are more likely to be mistreated. Mandatory laws addressing the reporting of abuse or neglect of a disabled person aged 18 to 64 years varies within states. Throughout their life span, the risk for one or more forms of mistreatment of individuals with disabilities is three times higher than that for individuals without disabilities (Harrell, 2012).

Forensic Psychiatric Nurse

The forensic psychiatric nurse bridges the gap between the criminal justice, legal, and mental health systems. Forensic psychiatric nurses apply the nursing process to clients who await a criminal hearing or trial while maintaining a neutral, objective, and detached position (Mason, 2011). Forensic psychiatric nurses collect evidence by determining intent or diminished capacity in the client's thinking at the time of the incident. To do so, they often spend several hours interviewing and observing the client, carefully documenting conversations and observations.

The forensic psychiatric nurse may be called to court to testify as an expert witness in a mental health issue; therefore it is imperative that the nurse have an understanding of mental illnesses and personality disorders. Roles filled by or activities performed by psychiatric forensic nurses include the following (Mason, 2011):

- Sanity or competency evaluation (for legal purposes)
- Assessment of violence potential
- Assessment of capacity to formulate intent
- Parole and probation considerations
- Assessment of racial or cultural factors in crime
- Assistance in jury selection
- Sexual predator screening
- Provision of expert witness testimony

❓ ACTIVE LEARNING

Spend a few hours working with a forensic nurse in a clinical setting. Observe the nurse's interventions and processes related to assessment, evidence collection and preservation, documentation, and collaboration with, for example, police officers. Take note of the techniques used for interviewing and counseling.

CORRECTIONAL NURSING

Correctional nursing is a specialized subset of forensic nursing. It requires a significant amount of knowledge as well as an understanding and awareness of the unique needs and perspective of the clients served. Several issues specific to correctional nursing and related issues are described in this section.

Unlike in any other care setting, clients are inmates, and care is negotiated and provided with recognition of safety and security issues for the nurse and the constitutional right of prisoners to receive adequate and timely health care. The primary goal in correctional facilities is to maintain a safe, secure, and humane environment for inmates. Health care, including nursing care, is a necessary and essential part of that environment.

Maintenance of a Safe Environment

Correctional facilities are violent environments, and nurses practicing in correctional settings must continually negotiate personal safety and nursing care (Clinical Example 32.4). Nurses in this setting must be aware that medical supplies issued to inmates can be a safety threat to the environment. For example, a simple elastic bandage can be used to improve the grip on a homemade weapon. Virtually any prescribed medication can have value on the prison "black market." Furthermore, nurses are subject to manipulation by inmates, who may seek nursing care for reasons other than health. As the following clinical example illustrates, the nurse must maintain an escape route to use if a situation of personal violence is imminent. In addition, no nursing care in a correctional environment requires a nurse to be locked in an enclosed environment with an inmate. Although it might appear that providing humane, therapeutic nursing care in an environment of potential violence is contradictory, it is ultimately a prerequisite for nursing practice in correctional settings.

Clinical Example 32.4

Safety in Correctional Facilities

In a county jail in Michigan in 2014, a nurse was attacked by an inmate who was pretending to be sick. Deputies on duty became aware of the possible problem. The nurse was leaving the inmate's cell when he attacked. The nurse was not seriously injured; however, this incidence illustrates the risk within the environment and the need to be alert (http://www.wnem.com/story/23782972/surveillance-video-shows-nurse-being-attacked-by-inmate).

🔊 RESEARCH HIGHLIGHTS

Public Health Role in Death Investigation

Drake et al. (2015) assessed the practice differences of the public health role of two death investigation systems in Texas. The authors utilized a previously validated instrument adapted from the Public Health Essential Services and sent it to 723 justice of the peace offices and 12 medical examiner offices in the 254 counties of Texas. Ten medical examiners and 112 justices of the peace responded. The study found that medical examiners are more likely than justices of the peace to fulfill the essential medicolegal death investigation services. Specifically, the researchers indicated that medical examiners have formal processes and follow set guidelines for carrying out their role versus the justice of the peace. In terms of formally evaluating or trending quality and effectiveness of their work product, no statistical differences were found between the two systems. Drake and colleagues proposed improving the Texas medicolegal death investigation system by restructuring it into a regionalization system. This could ensure optimal standards, accreditation, training, education, and quality and economy of scale service were being provided to the public.

Drake SA, Cron S, Giardino A, Nolte KB: Comparative analysis of the public health role of two types of death investigation in Texas: application of the essential services. *J Forensic Sci* 60(4): 914–919, 2015. https://doi.org/10.1111/1556-4029.12748.

HEALTH ISSUES IN PRISON POPULATIONS

Today's prison inmate often enters prison with health care issues. Nurses employed in the correctional setting are likely to see health care problems that are similar to those in an acute care setting or a community outpatient clinic. The daily operation of a correctional clinic includes management of acute and chronic illness. Most health care clinics in correctional environments screen each inmate upon entry into the facility. The health care triage process generally includes a physical and a mental health history. Many significant health care issues are recognized during the screening process, often for the first time.

Chronic and Communicable Diseases

The most critical heath care issues among the incarcerated population are chronic and communicable diseases. Of continuous concern are HIV, hepatitis, and tuberculosis. According to the Bureau of Justice Statistics, the rate of HIV infection decreased slightly from 146 cases per 10,000 inmates in 2010 to 143 per 10,000 at year end in 2012 (Maruschak et al., 2015), but remains very high. Likewise, hepatitis is a serious health care issue in correctional facilities. According to the Bureau of Justice Statistics, 6.5% of inmates reported hepatitis as a health problem in 2012 (Maruschak et al., 2015). The rate of these and other communicable diseases among the incarcerated population is associated with high-risk behaviors, including current and previous drug use, unprotected sexual intercourse, and tattooing.

Of growing concern are the increased rates of chronic conditions such as hypertension and diabetes (Maruschak et al., 2015). Additionally, in 2012 about one quarter of inmates were of normal weight, with the majority being overweight (46%) to morbidly obese (2%).

As it is for the general population, managing inmates with multiple chronic conditions, including infectious and noninfectious, will continue to be a major threat to the health of those incarcerated.

Women in Prison

By 2014, the number of incarcerated women reached 215,332 (The Sentencing Project, 2015). In 2014, women in state prisons were incarcerated for drug offenses 24% versus 15% for males (Carson, 2015). Of the estimated 74 million children under the age of 18 in 2007, 2.3% had a parent incarcerated, of which 8% were mothers (Glaze and Maruschak, 2010). Approximately 8 in 10 women with a prior mental health diagnosis reported physical or sexual abuse before imprisonment: 57.2% were physically abused and 39% sexually abused (CSOSA, 2014).

Drug use and victimization, combined with the stress associated with being separated from their children, put incarcerated women at risk for many mental and physical health problems, including the risk of HIV infection and other sexually transmitted diseases. Unfortunately, health care providers in correctional facilities have limited experience and training to meet the health care needs of women in prison, and quality of care is adversely affected. For example, women who have been sexually assaulted are often reticent about obtaining regular gynecological examinations. The National Commission on Correctional Health Care (NCCHC, 2014) confirms that routine gynecological examinations are not consistently apart of health screening for women upon entry into a correctional facility or a routine part of ongoing health care. The NCCHC (2014) offers the following to guide the provision of health care for women:

- Correctional institutions' health care intake procedures should include comprehensive gynecological examinations.
- Comprehensive health care services should be available to incarcerated women that give special consideration to the

reproductive health needs of women, the high rate of victimization among incarcerated women, counseling related to parenting issues, and accessibility to drug or alcohol treatment.

ETHICAL INSIGHTS

Inmates' Refusal of Medications

An inmate's right to refuse treatment is a legal and ethical issue that nurses working in a correctional environment sometimes experience. The right to refuse treatment and the state's power to enforce treatment are both highly charged legal and political issues and have gained attention in state and local courts. The issue of forced medication and competence to stand trial is of particular concern. The legal and ethical principles that guide forced treatment against the will of an inmate have historically been potential safety issues toward self or others in the environment. The Supreme Court decision in *Harper v. Turner* in 1987 permits the violation of the rights of the incarcerated so long as the prison policy is reasonably related to repressing violence within the prison system (Black, 2008).

Unlike in nursing practice with the general population, prison inmates who refuse health care do not leave the facility and return home. Nurses practicing in correctional facilities continue to provide care and address the consequences of an inmate's refusal of treatment. For example, an inmate who refuses to adhere to treatment protocols for schizophrenia may affect the safety of the environment and in fact create a "ripple effect," thus undermining prisoner administration (LGIT, 2009). Nurses are obliged to treat any resultant health issues. However, individuals who are incarcerated by the state have a constitutional right to refuse and receive health care. Nurses practicing in correctional settings must recognize that involuntary medical treatment is undertaken after internal review and judicial proceedings; however, a hearing is not necessary.

Adolescents in Prison

Increasing numbers of adolescents are committing violent crimes, and many states have lowered the age limit at which adolescents may be tried and sentenced as adults. Consequently, adolescents who have been convicted of violent crimes are often incarcerated in adult facilities. Incarcerating adolescents in an adult population presents barriers to meeting the distinct developmental needs of adolescents. These developmental needs include rapid physical and emotional growth and nutritional needs, all influenced by environment, genetics, and family experiences. Adult correctional facilities are not generally equipped to deal with the challenges of adolescent development. Adolescents in an adult correctional facility are the highest at risk than any other group (Campaign for Youth Justice, 2011). Juveniles in adult correctional facilities are 36 times more likely than the adult population and more likely than juveniles in the juvenile center to commit suicide.

To ensure the safety of adolescents in an adult facility, the nurse must be aware of their individual vulnerability. A mechanism for adolescents to access medical and mental health care is essential. Services and interventions should be provided that consider the developmental stage and the experience of adolescence.

🔍 ACTIVE LEARNING

Spend a day in a jail or correctional facility working with a correctional forensic nurse. Pay particular attention to differences in care delivery related to legal and ethical issues unique to this subspecialty. Develop impressions into a paper.

MENTAL HEALTH ISSUES IN CORRECTIONAL SETTINGS

Approximately 34% of state inmates, 24% of federal inmates, and 17% of jail inmates received treatment for mental health problems (James and Glaze, 2006). Being in prison with a mental illness such as schizophrenia, bipolar affective disorder, major depressive disorder, or personality disorder makes adjustment to incarceration extremely difficult. The great number of inmates with mental illnesses in today's prisons makes it difficult to meet the needs of this population.

In the late 1950s and early 1960s, deinstitutionalization moved people with mental illness out of state hospitals into communities that were often ill prepared to care for them. As a result, many people with a mental illness reside in nursing homes, residential homes, prisons, or jails. People with mental illness are more likely to encounter law enforcement than health care providers when in the midst of acute mental distress. This results in more than 2 million people a year going to jails, with the vast majority not the result of criminal activity (National Alliance for the Mentally Ill [NAMI], 2017).

According to NAMI, most jail inmates with symptoms of mental illness are charged with minor crimes. A far smaller number of inmates with severe mental illness commit more serious crimes, again frequently a consequence of either inadequate or no treatment. NAMI (2017) takes the position that many dangerous or violent acts by people with severe mental illness are a result of inappropriate or inadequate treatment. The following strategies have been proposed to address the criminal justice and forensic issues facing mental illness:

- Train police officers to recognize severe mental illness in the community and to respond appropriately to people who are experiencing psychiatric crises.
- Divert nonviolent offenders with severe mental illnesses away from incarceration into appropriate treatment.
- Establish "mental health courts" to hear all cases involving individuals with severe mental illness charged with misdemeanors or nonviolent felonies in order to divert as many as possible away from incarceration and into treatment and services.
- Create specialized units within departments of parole and probation to coordinate services for people with severe mental illness on probation.

In 2009, over half of all state offenders and nearly half of all federal offenders had acute symptoms or chronic history of mental illness (e.g., depression, schizophrenia, or bipolar disorder) (Human Rights Watch, 2009).

Nurses employed in correctional settings must always be aware of the vulnerabilities of people with mental illness who are incarcerated. Depression, schizophrenia, bipolar disorder, and other neurobiological disorders can be readily treated with newer-generation psychiatric medications that reduce or ameliorate symptoms, but the unique vulnerabilities of incarceration often remain. Nurses should also be aware that once released from imprisonment, these individuals are at substantial risk of mental illness relapse and reinstitutionalization (Perdue et al., 2016).

ACTIVE LEARNING

Attend a session of local or state mental health court (court proceedings to determine the status of an individual's mental status and disposition—e.g., confinement to a mental institution or release in the care of a guardian or family member). Report on the experience to classmates.

EDUCATION AND FORENSIC NURSING

According to Kent-Wilkinson (2011), because of the amount and depth of knowledge and skills needed by forensic nurses, whatever their subspecialty area, simply completing a continuing

TABLE 32.1   Basic Curricula for Forensic Nursing Programs

Subject	Topic(s)
Fundamentals for forensic nursing	Evidence collection
	Documentation
	Interviewing skills
	Basic criminal, procedural, and constitutional law
	Scope of practice
	Interdisciplinary collaboration
	Testifying in court as an expert witness
Forensic law	Legal concepts (culpability, burden of proof, rationale for punishment, mitigating circumstance)
	Defense issues (justification, insanity, entrapment, duress)
Forensic science	Collection and preservation of evidence
	Interpretation of DNA and laboratory reports
	Forensic chemistry and toxicology
	Cause and manner of death
	Blood spatter interpretation
	Mechanism of injury; wound identification

Data from Burgess AW, Berger AD, Boersma RR: Forensic nursing: investigating the career potential in this emerging graduate specialty, *Am J Nurs* 104(3):58–64, 2004.

education course is not adequate for practice. As a result, several colleges and universities offer a variety of programs to educate practitioners, future educators, and researchers of forensic nursing. The core curriculum for forensic nursing was published recently (Price and Maguire, 2016) to provide guidance across settings. This is the direct result of the identified need and growing knowledge base for practice of this specialty area. Table 32.1 gives an overview of basic curricula for forensic nursing programs. In addition, during the formal programs of study, the student usually completes a minimum specified number of supervised clinical hours; a clinical internship or fellowship also may be required.

For those interested in seeking additional education in the growing specialty of forensic nursing, Box 32.5 lists nursing colleges and universities that have programs in forensic nursing. It should be noted that some of these programs offer a certificate in forensic nursing, whereas others provide a minor or concentration, and still others grant a graduate degree (typically a master of science in nursing degree) or postgraduate certificate.

The American Nurses Credentialing Center offers an Advanced Forensic Nursing certification (AFN-BC). To become eligible to obtain an AFN-BC, a nurse must (1) hold an active RN license, (2) have practiced at least 2 years as a full-time registered nurse, (3) have obtained a graduate degree in nursing, (4) have practiced a minimum of 2000 hours within a specialty area of forensic nursing within the last 3 years, (5) have completed a minimum of 30 continuing education hours within the specialty forensic nursing area, and (6) have fulfilled two of the professional development categories specific to forensic nursing (six academic credits, presentations, publication or research, preceptor, or professional service) (ANCC, 2017).

BOX 32.5   Schools Offering Programs in Forensic Nursing (Graduate and Certificate Programs)

California
University of California at Riverside, Riverside, California—*online*

Colorado
University of Colorado at Colorado Springs, Beth-El College of Nursing, Colorado Springs, Colorado

Georgia
Emery University, Atlanta, Georgia

Massachusetts
Boston College, Chestnut Hill, Massachusetts
Fitchburg State College, Fitchburg, Massachusetts—*online*

New Jersey
Fairleigh Dickinson University, Teaneck, New Jersey
Monmouth University, West Long Branch, New Jersey—*online*

New York
Binghamton University, Binghamton, New York—*online*

Ohio
Cleveland State University, Cleveland, Ohio—online
Xavier University, Cincinnati, Ohio

Pennsylvania
Duquesne University, Pittsburgh, Pennsylvania—online
Drexel University, Philadelphia, Pennsylvania-online
University of Pennsylvania, Philadelphia, Pennsylvania-online
University of Pittsburgh, Pittsburgh, Pennsylvania

Texas
The University of Texas Health Science Center at Houston School of Nursing, Houston, Texas-online
Texas A&M, College Station, Texas

Washington
University of Washington, Seattle, Washington

CASE STUDY Application of the Nursing Process

Correctional Nursing

Mr. Smith is a 65-year-old African American male serving a sentence for aggravated assault. Mr. Smith has a medical history of diabetes mellitus, hypertension, coronary artery disease, and peripheral vascular disease. Three weeks ago, his right foot was amputated because of gangrene. Mr. Smith has been admitted to the infirmary six times since the procedure, stating, "I'm not feeling well; can you double-check my sugar?"

The incision site is healing well, and his diabetes mellitus is under control with medication. Mr. Smith takes his medications as prescribed, and his doctor believes he is doing well and continues with his current medication regimen.

Mr. Smith's daughter visits him only once every 6 months because she lives out of state. His son is also in prison but at another location. Mr. Smith's wife recently died from a motor vehicle accident, and he was unable to attend the funeral.

Assessment

Mr. Smith has a flat affect and does not make eye contact. He constantly looks at the ground and does not speak clearly when asked questions. Many times the nurse must ask him to repeat himself. According to medical records, he has lost approximately 18 pounds since surgery and he says, "I'm not hungry, that's why I don't eat." When asked about his sleeping habits, Mr. Smith states he sleeps all day except when the guards make him get up. He says he has not played cards with his buddies in more than a week. He also reports that he has been buying Soma "from them" and has not taken a bath in 3 days.

Diagnosis

Individual

- Despair, gloom, hopelessness
- Inability to overcome mental and emotional difficulties
- Powerlessness

Family

- Situational crises

Community

- Lack of mental health services

Planning

Mr. Smith will set goals with the health care provider and will ask for assistance with communication with his daughter and son.

Individual

Long-Term Goal

- Client will reestablish positive relationships with fellow inmates within 2 weeks.

Short-Term Goal

- Client will verbalize and recognize his feelings.
- Client will participate in diversion activities of his choice (e.g., playing cards).

Family

Long-Term Goal

- Family will demonstrate coping skills appropriate to the situation.

Short-Term Goal

- Family will verbalize and recognize feelings.

Community

Long-Term Goal

- Program will be available for all individuals.

Short-Term Goal

- Begin mental health programs, utilizing forensic nurses.

Intervention

Individual

- Mr. Smith will be encouraged to express his feelings in an open and nonjudgmental environment, allowing for the development of a therapeutic relationship.
- The forensic nurse will schedule several visits to the clinic and encourage Mr. Smith to participate in activities, such as card playing, with his friends.

Family

- Mr. Smith's daughter will be included in the plan of care and encouraged to express her thoughts and feelings relating to her father's imprisonment.

Community

- The forensic nurse will arrange several activities for inmates suffering from mental illnesses, including group activities and group talk.

Evaluation

Individual

Mr. Smith slowly engaged the forensic nurse individually and in group therapy. He gained 5 pounds over 2 weeks and was able to make eye contact. Mr. Smith expressed his grief for the death of his wife. He gradually stopped buying Soma and spent more time with his friends.

Family

Mr. Smith's daughter continued to visit only once every 6 months, but was able to fully explain her thoughts and feelings about her father's incarceration. The time the daughter spent with her father increased and was more meaningful.

Community

A forensic nurse was on constant duty to assist inmates with mental health illnesses.

Levels of Prevention

Primary

- Encourage interaction with colleagues and family.
- Promote participation in prison activities.

Secondary

- Screen for depression.
- Provide outreach services to inmates with mental illness.

Tertiary

- Encourage therapy to reduce symptoms of mental illness.

CASE STUDY Application of the Nursing Process

Forensic Nursing

Transcript of a 911 telephone call:
- *Emergency operator:* "This is 911, what is your emergency?"
- *Caller:* "My son isn't breathing, he's not moving, I need help!"
- *Emergency operator:* "We will send an ambulance and police to assist you."
- *Caller:* "Thank you, please hurry!"

Emergency medical personnel arrived at the house to discover James Oats, a 14-year-old white male, lying face up on his bed. The young man was unresponsive and not breathing. Emergency medical personnel immediately began lifesaving interventions, but despite all efforts, they were unsuccessful. James Oats was pronounced dead at his house.

Police officers arrived at the residence during the rescue attempt and secured the scene. They then notified homicide detectives and the medical examiner's office. Teresa Fernandez, a forensic nurse death investigator (FNDI), was dispatched to the residence to work in collaboration with the homicide detective, Pete Smith, to investigate the death.

The police determined that there was no indication of foul play. The house was in order, there was no evidence of a robbery, and all the doors and windows were locked. A PlayStation was attached to the television, various clothes were strewn about the room, and schoolbooks were on the desk.

The decedent's mother, Jane Oats, informed the FNDI that James was in fine health. She explained that he had undergone a physical examination last week for athletics and that the findings were unremarkable. James had an older brother and younger sister, both in excellent health. James's father has hypertension and a history of heart disease, and diabetes and cancer were present in grandparents.

Teresa (the FNDI) tried to comfort Mrs. Oats, who was extremely upset; she was crying and hyperventilating. Teresa turned to Mr. Oats, who was also present. In answer to Teresa's questioning, Mr. Oats reported that other parents and teachers had been concerned about rumors of the increasing use of "bars" in area schools. Teresa was alarmed by this information and questioned him further about what he meant; he confirmed that the school kids were reportedly using the antianxiety medication Xanax.

Assessment

Teresa performed an assessment of the decedent. James was wearing blue jeans, a yellow shirt, and socks. Her findings: "Livor mortis is consistent with body position and blanchable; rigor mortis is breakable in the jaw, arms, and legs. Frothy white foam cone was present at mouth and within bilateral nares. There are no visible signs of trauma."

The decedent was removed from the residence by the medical examiner's office, and an autopsy was performed the next day. The pathologist reported that the physical findings from the autopsy were unremarkable. During the autopsy, toxicology samples were collected from the heart, liver, and stomach.

Toxicology results were returned and were positive for an extremely large amount of alprazolam (Xanax). The final official cause of death for James Oats was alprazolam toxicity; the manner of death was accidental.

Along with James's parents and Detective Smith, Teresa was informed of the cause and manner of death. Mr. and Mrs. Oats were devastated by the news and, upon questioning, stated that they did not understand how James had obtained the Xanax pills. They assured the detective and the FNDI that the only prescription medications in the residence were locked in the master bedroom cabinet and that James had no access to them.

Mr. Oats reported that Mrs. Oats has not been eating and had lost 25 pounds in 3 weeks. She had not been able to return to work, cried continuously, and did not care for their other children. Mr. Oats reported that the entire family was withdrawn; the younger child was misbehaving in school and received detention several times. Mr. Oats expressed exasperation with the need to provide all child care, perform routine chores, and go to work; he admitted that he did not know how much more he could handle.

Mr. Oats told the investigators that community and church members were extremely helpful and sensitive to the family. The school officials and area churches agreed to support and offer programs to encourage children to say no to drugs; these programs were to focus more attention on prescription medications. Furthermore, the school James attended was investigating drug and alcohol abuse. The school social worker told Mr. Oats that a support group was being formed to assist students with James's death.

Detective Smith interviewed several of James's classmates and discovered that Xanax was used by many of them. From the information that he was able to gather, it appeared that this was the first time James had tried the drug. Detective Smith discovered that some of the students were obtaining Xanax from their parents and selling it to their peers. Furthermore, he learned that students are trying the "bars" because "it's cool."

Diagnosis
Family
- Mental and emotional distress
- Grief
- Lack of family support
- Excessive stress

Community
- Readiness for healing

Planning
Family
- The Oats family will initiate counseling to assist with acceptance of and coping with James's death.

Long-Term Goal
- Family will identify need for outside support and seek such support.

Short-Term Goals
- Family will verbalize and recognize feelings surrounding the death.
- Family will express feelings honestly.

Community
Long-Term Goal
- Members of the community will establish a plan to deal with problems and stressors, including premature deaths.

Short-Term Goal
- Members of the community, including school personnel and students, will identify positive and negative factors affecting management of current and future problems and stressors.

Intervention
Family
Teresa Fernandez:
- Listened to the family's comments, remarks, and expression of concerns, noting nonverbal behaviors and responses
- Encouraged family members to verbalize feelings openly and clearly
- Referred family to appropriate resources for assistance as indicated (e.g., counseling, psychotherapy, spiritual guidance)

Community
With police, school personnel, and community leaders, Ms. Fernandez:
- Reviewed the community plan for dealing with substance abuse problems among schoolchildren and assessed the related stressors
- Determined the community's strengths and weaknesses

continued

Forensic Nursing

- Identified available resources
- Established a mechanism for self-monitoring of community needs and evaluation of efforts

Evaluation
Family
- The Oats family began family counseling and slowly accepted James's death.
- James's siblings began educating fellow classmates about the ill effects of abusing prescription medications.

Community
- The community implemented quarterly meetings for grieving families that included licensed counselors.
- The community members employed "just say no" rallies focusing on school-aged children.

Levels of Prevention
Primary
- Initiate drug teaching in middle and high schools, focusing on drug resistance training, social skills, and personal management.

- Support programs that encourage students to role-play and apply life skills to deal with peer pressure.
- Provide life-skills training (e.g., skills to cope with peer pressure, improve self-esteem/confidence).

Secondary
- Organize group sessions in school to discuss illegal prescription medication abuse.
- Provide information to school personnel and parents on how to identify or screen for evidence of use of drugs and alcohol among school-aged children.
- Provide information on area groups that provide support for students who want to avoid using drugs or want to stop using drugs.
- Reduce or stop harm that is done to individuals or groups while they are using drugs.

Tertiary
- Reduce risk that additional students will abuse prescription medication.
- Provide support to those who are abusing such substances.
- Refer to support systems (e.g., Narcotic Anonymous).

SUMMARY

Forensic nursing is a broadly expanding specialty that combines multiple aspects of nursing science into the care of patients and families with forensic or legal concerns. Most often, the forensic nurse is employed in a hospital, clinic, correctional facility, or medicolegal death investigation setting. Specialized knowledge, competency, and skills are essential to the practice and require advanced education and training.

As mentioned previously, assessing for evidence of violence and intervening as needed are fundamental requirements of care that all health professionals must perform. Therefore every nurse has the potential to interact with a client, patient, or population with forensic needs, regardless of the client population or setting of care. Forensic nurses are faced with the challenge of meeting nursing needs while ensuring legal aspects are objectively ensured for living or deceased, and the need for practitioners in this specialty area is expected to grow.

EVOLVE WEBSITE

http://evolve.elsevier.com/Nies/community
- NCLEX Review Questions
- Case Studies

BIBLIOGRAPHY

42 U.S.C.A. §5106g), as amended and reauthorized by the CAPTA Reauthorization Act of 2010.

Acierno R, Hernandez-Tejada M, Muzzy W, et al.: *National elder mistreatment study*, 2009. Available from: <https://www.ncjrs.gov/pdffiles1/nij/grants/226456.pdf>.

Amar AF, Sekula LK: *A practical guide to forensic nursing incorporating forensic principles into nursing practice Sigma Theta Tau International*, 2017.

American Association of Legal Nurse Consultants: *What is an LNC?*, 2017. Available from: <http://www.aalnc.org/page/what-is-an-lnc>.

American Board of Medicolegal Death Investigators (ABMDI): *Board certification (advanced)*, 2017. Available from: <http://www.abmdi.org/board_certification>.

American Legal Nurse Consultant Certification Board (ALNCC): *Eligibility criteria*, 2017. Available from: <http://www.aalnc.org/page/become-an-lnc>.

American Nurses Association: *Scope and standards of forensic nursing practice*, Washington, DC, 2009, American Nurses Publishing.

American Nurses Association: *Code of ethics with interpretive statement*, Washington, DC, 2014, American Nurses Publishing.

American Nurses Credentialing Center: *Advanced forensic nursing certification eligibility criteria*, 2017. Available from: http://www.nursecredentialing.org/AdvForensicNursing-Eligibility.aspx>.

Black L: Forced medication of prison inmates, *Virtual Mentor AMA J Ethics* 10(2):106–109, 2008.

Burgess AW, Berger AD, Boersma RR: Forensic nursing: investigating the career potential in this emerging graduate specialty, *Am J Nurs* 104(3):58–64, 2004.

Campaign For Youth Justice, 2011. Retrieved at: http://www.campaignforyouthjustice.org/documents/KeyFactsonYouthinAdultJailsandPrisons.pdf.

Carson EA: *Prisoners in 2014*, Washington, DC, 2015, Bureau of Justice Statistics.

Court Services and Offender Supervision Agency (CSOSA), 2014. Retrieved at: http://www.csosa.gov/newsmedia/factsheets/statistics-on-women-offenders-2014.pdf.

Coalition for Juvenile Justice: *Childhood on trial: the failure of trying and sentencing youth in adult criminal court*, 2005. Available from: <http://www.juvjustice.org/media/resources/public/resource_115.pdf>.

Collins SE, Halpern KJ: Forensic nursing: a collaborative practice paradigm, *J Nurs Law* 10(1):11–19, 2005.

Dole PJ: Forensic nursing in correctional care. In Lynch V, Duval JB, editors: *Forensic nursing science*, ed 2, St. Louis, 2011, Mosby.

Doughtery CM: Evidence collection in the emergency department. In Lynch V, Duval JB, editors: *Forensic nursing science*, ed 2, St. Louis, 2011, Mosby.

Ferrell J, Caruso C: Sexual assault evidence recovery. In Lynch V, Duval JB, editors: *Forensic nursing science*, ed 2, St. Louis, 2011, Mosby.

Finn O: Child maltreatment: forensic biomarkers. In Lynch V, Duval JB, editors: *Forensic nursing science*, ed 2, St. Louis, 2011, Mosby.

Geissler-Murr A, Moorhouse MF: Legal nurse consulting. In Lynch V, editor: *Forensic nursing*, St. Louis, 2011, Mosby.

Glaze LE, Maruschak LM: *Parents in prison and their minor children*(Bureau of Justice Statistics Rep No NCJ 222984), 2010. Available from: <https://www.bjs.gov/content/pub/pdf/pptmc.pdf>.

Hammer TC, Hammer RM: Crimes against the elderly. In Hammer RM, Moynihan B, Pagliaro EM, editors: *Forensic nursing: a handbook for practice*, ed 2, Burlington, MA, 2013, Jones and Bartlett.

Hanzlick R: *Death investigation systems and procedures*, Boca Raton, FL, 2007, CRC Press.

Hanzlick R, Hunsaker III JC, Davis GJ: *National association of medical examiners: a guide for manner of death classification*, 2002. Available from: <https://netforum.avectra.com/Public/DocumentGenerate.aspx?wbn_key=38c0f1d2-11ec-45c7-80ca-ff872d0b22bc&SITE=NAME>.

Harrell E: *Crime against persons with disabilities: 2009-2011 statistical tables*(Bureau of Justice Statistics Rep No NCJ240299), 2012. Available from: <http://bjs.ojp.usdoj.gov/content/pub/pdf/capd0911st.pdf>.

Human Rights Watch: *Mental Illness, human rights, and US prisons*, 2009. Retrieved at: https://www.hrw.org/news/2009/09/22/mental-illness-human-rights-and-us-prisons.

International Association of Forensic nurses: *Sexual assault nurse examiner (SANE) educational guidelines handbook*, 2015. Available from: http://c.ymcdn.com/sites/www.forensicnurses.org/resource/resmgr/2015_SANE_ED_GUIDELINES.pdf.

James DJ, Glaze LE: *Mental health problems of prison and jail inmates*(Bureau of Justice Statistics Rep No NCJ 213600), 2006. Available from: <www.ojp.gov/bjs/pub/pdf/mhppji.pdf>.

Kent-Wilkinson A: Forensic nursing educational development: an integrated review of the literature, *J Psychiatr Ment Health Nurs* 18(3):236–246, 2011.

Ledray LE: Sexual violence. In Lynch V, Duval JB, editors: *Forensic nursing science*, ed 2, St. Louis, 2011, Mosby.

Ledray LE, Arndt S: Examining the sexual assault victim: a new model for nursing care, *J Psychosoc Nurs* 32(2):7–12, 1994.

Local Government Insurance Trust (LGIT): *Right of inmates to refuse medical treatment*, 2009. Retrieved at: http://www.lgit.org/DocumentCenter/Home/View/356.

Lewis-O'Connor A, Latimore A. In Amar AF, Sekula LK, editors: *A practical guide to forensic nursing incorporating forensic principles into nursing practice Sigma Theta Tau International*, 2017.

Lynch V: Evolution of forensic nursing science. In Lynch V, Duval JB, editors: *Forensic nursing science*, ed 2, St. Louis, 2011, Mosby.

Lynch V: Forensic nursing science. In Hammer RM, Moynihan B, Pagliaro EM, editors: *Forensic nursing: a handbook for practice*, ed 2, Burlington, MA, 2013, Jones and Bartlett.

Lynch V, Koehler SA: Forensic investigation of death. In Lynch V, Duval JB, editors: *Forensic nursing science*, ed 2, St. Louis, 2011, Mosby.

Pickens S, Dyer CB: Elder abuse in America, *Open Med J* 3:188–193, 2016. https://doi.org/10.2174/1874220301603010188.

Maruschak LM: *HIV in Prisons, 2001-2010*(Bureau of Justice Statistics Rep No NCJ238877), 2012. Available from: <http://bjs.ojp.usdoj.gov/content/pub/pdf/hivp10.pdf>.

Maruschak LA, Berzofsky M, Unangst J: *Medical problems of state and federal prisoners and jail inmates, 2011-12* (Bureau of Justice Statistics Rep No NCJ 248491). February 2015. Available from: https://www.bjs.gov/content/pub/pdf/mpsfpji1112.pdf<>.

Mason T: Psychiatric forensic nursing. In Lynch V, Duval JB, editors: *Forensic nursing*, ed 2, St. Louis, 2011, Mosby.

Mitchell S, Drake SA: Death investigation. In Amar AF, Sekula LK, editors: *A practical guide to forensic nursing incorporating forensic principles into nursing practice Sigma Theta Tau International*, 2017.

National Commission on Correctional Health Care: *Women's health care in correctional settings*, 2014. Available from: <http://www.ncchc.org/filebin/Positions/Womens_Health_Care_in_Correctional_Settings.pdf>.

National Alliance for the Mentally Ill [NAMI]: *NAMI warns senate about criminalization of mental illness*, 2017. Available from: https://www.nami.org/Press-Media/Press-Releases/2016/NAMI-Warns-Senate-about-Criminalization-of-Mental. http://www.nami.org/About-NAMI/Policy-Platform/10-Criminal-Justice-and-Forensic-Issues.

Office for Victims of Crime, 2017. Available from: https://www.ovcttac.gov/saneguide/introduction/what-is-a-sane/.

Pagliaro EM, Cewe BRB: The forensic nurse witness in the American justice system. In Hammer RM, Moynihan B, Pagliaro EM, editors: *Forensic nursing: a handbook for practice*, ed 2, Burlington, MA, 2013, Jones and Bartlett.

Pearsall C: Elder maltreatment: forensic biomarkers. In Lynch V, Duval JB, editors: *Forensic nursing science*, ed 2, St. Louis, 2011, Mosby.

Perdue GL, Murray MC, Rivera WA: In Price B, Maguire K, editors: *Core curriculum for forensic nursing*, Lippincott Williams & Wilkins, 2016.

Price B, Maguire K: *Core curriculum for forensic nursing*, Lippincott Williams & Wilkins, 2016.

Potter PA, Perry AG: *Fundamentals of nursing*, ed 9, St. Louis, 2016, Mosby.

Robson B: From emergency nurse to legal nurse consultant and independent practitioner: legal nurse consulting? What is that? *NENA Outlook* 32(2):24–26, 2009.

Ruiz-Contreras A: The nurse as an expert witness, *Top Emerg Med* 27(1):27–35, 2005.

Shafer TJ: Organ donation. In Lynch V, Duval JB, editors: *Forensic nursing science*, ed 2, St. Louis, 2011, Mosby.

The Sentencing Project Research and Advocacy for Reform, 2015. Available at http://www.sentencingproject.org/wp-content/uploads/2016/02/Incarcerated-Women-and-Girls.pdf.

U.S. Department of Justice/Bureau of Justice Statistics [USDOJ/BJS]: *Criminal victimization*, 2012.

U.S. Department of Health and Human Services; Administration for Children and Families; Administration on Children; Youth and Families Children's Bureau: *Child maltreatment*. Author: Washington, DC, 2015. < https://www.acf.hhs.gov/sites/default/files/cb/cm2015.pdf.

U.S. Preventive Services Task Force: Screening for intimate partner violence and abuse of elderly and vulnerable adults: clinical summary of U.S. *Preventive Services Task Force recommendation*, 2013. Available from: <http://www.uspreventiveservicestaskforce.org/uspstf/uspsipv.htm>.

33

Faith Community Nursing

Beverly Cook Siegrist

OBJECTIVES

Upon completion of this chapter, the reader will be able to do the following:

1. Understand the potential role of faith communities in improving the health of Americans.
2. Describe the philosophy and historical basis of faith community nursing.
3. Define the roles, functions, and education of the faith community nurse.
4. Discuss faith communities as clients of the community health nurse.

5. Describe the role of the faith community nurse in the spiritual health and wellness of faith communities.
6. Discuss contemporary issues in faith community nursing, such as working with vulnerable populations and facing ethical and legal issues.
7. Apply the nursing process to a case study related to a faith community practice.

KEY TERMS

CIRCLE Model of Spiritual Care	faith factor	personal health counselor
coordinator of volunteers	Granger Westberg	referral agent
developer of support groups	health advocate	spiritual distress
facilitator	health educator	spirituality
faith community	integrator of health and healing	

The purpose of this chapter is to present an overview of faith community nursing and to explore the challenges and opportunities nurses face when providing nursing care to faith communities. On the basis of centuries-old philosophies from churches and religious groups, nurses are applying the science of nursing and caring to address the biopsychosocial health needs of individuals and groups in church congregations and faith communities across the country. Clinical Examples 33.1 and 33.2 illustrate models of faith community nursing found in the United States and suggest the unique ways that faith community nurses (FCNs) provide nursing care.

Clinical Example 33.1

Sandra Mills began her FCN practice as a volunteer when her parish priest recruited her to help establish a cancer support group and coordinate classes for caregivers. Within 6 months, her church's social concerns committee established a paid position on their ministry team and employed her as a full-time, paid staff member. After completing a faith community nursing program through a local university, she began to develop a health ministry in her church. She describes her days as full and rewarding. Each day, she visits ill or homebound parish members and provides support through prayer, education, and listening. She is challenged to locate and provide references to community resources, provide health education to church groups (e.g., mothers' day out and the over-55 group), and coordinate the efforts of other volunteers in the church. She is practicing holistic nursing for the first time in her 15 years of practice. She has found that the church, as a healing community, allows her to focus on the body–mind–spirit connection she believes is necessary to improve the health of congregation members.

Clinical Example 33.2

Marilyn Michaels is a former home care and hospice nurse who works as an FCN coordinator for St. Luke's Hospital, which is a 400-bed medical center serving a Midwestern rural population. Her position was created to assist community churches in developing and maintaining parish nurse programs. She supervises 12 registered nurses employed by the hospital, who provide nursing through a contract to area congregations until the churches' budgets can support a nurse's salary. She also works with churches that have a volunteer model of health care ministry. She coordinates educational programs, including a 34-hour preparation program for beginning FCNs, an advanced program for FCN coordinators in individual churches, and monthly educational programs offered through an FCN support group. Marilyn developed the support group and facilitates communication among the 200 nurses and 100 church communities that St. Luke's Hospital serves. She also assists the many faith community programs by connecting them with other services that the hospital and community agencies provide (e.g., screening, support groups, and speakers). The program at St. Luke's Hospital is self-supporting through grants and educational programs.

These examples illustrate how faith community nursing is evolving in the United States and worldwide, from its beginning with fewer than a dozen nurses in Chicago. The practice now involves in excess of 30,000 nurses in more than 29 countries (Westberg Institute, 2017). The growing number of registered nurses (RNs) in faith community nursing evidences this practice as a significant role for the community health nurse. FCNs are now recognized as leaders with the ability to positively impact the health and wellness faith communities.

Community health nursing has evolved from early church efforts to provide care for the sick and disenfranchised. Modern faith community nursing focuses on the global health and wellness issues of all people and has its roots in more recent efforts to encourage the reemergence and blending of health care roles into the healing ministry of faith communities (Hickman, 2007; Patterson, 2004; Solari-Twadell and McDermott, 1999).

FAITH COMMUNITIES: ROLE IN HEALTH AND WELLNESS

Former President Jimmy Carter, faculty and founding member of Strong Partners Interfaith Health Program at Emory University in Atlanta, Georgia, understands the importance of faith communities for Americans. President Carter is quoted as follows on the Interfaith Health Program website (http://www.interfaith.emory.edu):

What if churches, mosques, and temples worked together to improve the health of their communities? If faith groups adopted one small area and made sure that every single child was immunized…that every person had a basic medical exam…that every woman who became pregnant would get prenatal care? Are these possible? We believe the answer is yes.

(Interfaith Health Program, 2005)

Throughout history, church communities have provided care for the indigent and disenfranchised, meeting basic human needs for food, clothing, and basic health care. The majority of the world's populations belong to organized faith communities. Approximately one third of the people in the world (1.6 billion, or 31.5%) identify themselves as Christians, followed by Muslims (1.6 billion, 23%), Hindus (1 billion, 15%), Buddhists (500 million, 7%), and Jews (14 million, 0.2%) (Pew Research Center, 2012). All of these religions have traditions and rituals related to health and healing, including specific prayers and practices. Some of the religions give specific guidelines for ministering to the ill, homebound, or dying members. All of the major religions describe the relationship among health, healing, and wholeness. The Old Testament discusses Shalom, or God's desire for health and wholeness for the earth and its people. The New Testament documents the healing activities of Jesus, restoring health to people. The Talmud describes the importance of maintaining physical health and vigor so that Jewish people will understand God's will in their lives. Followers of Buddhism believe that health and healing are interconnected and that illness occurs when there is an imbalance between life and the environment (International Parish Nurse Resource Center [IPNRC], 2013).

Koenig et al. (2012), in the *Handbook of Religion and Faith*, cite a positive correlation between religion and health that has recently been termed the **faith factor**. These writers also note that more than 1800 research studies have been completed since 2000 studying longevity and religiosity. Williams and Sternthal (2007) completed a meta-analysis of studies related to spirituality, religion, and health. In 17 studies, individuals who reported intrinsic religion (internalized or regularly practiced) and regular attendance at a religious service reported decreased stress. In 147 studies, these researchers found that there was an inverse relationship between religiosity and depression. They found evidence in another 49 studies indicating that people who practiced religious coping had lower levels of anxiety, depression, and stress and coped more positively with many chronic diseases, such as HIV, hypertension, and cancer. One reason for this variance may be that the people who reported the highest level of religious involvement also reported practicing healthier lifestyles, including exercising more and smoking less (Myers, 2004, 2008; Tsuang et al., 2002). Eckersley (2007) suggests that "religion provides things that are good for health and well-being, including social support, existential meaning, a sense of purpose, a coherent belief system and a clear moral code" (p. S54). Myers (2008) and Koenig and George (2004) suggest that faith communities contribute to the well-being of their members through support, prayer, and providing a sense of hope. The importance of stress management in health promotion and disease management is well documented.

Organized religions are attempting to meet the needs of members in many nontraditional ways, such as exploring Internet church services, developing support groups, and including modern music and drama in traditional worship services to improve intergenerational communication. FCNs, because of their educational preparation and goals, are ideal health professionals to ensure that the health information provided in congregations is accurate and accessible. FCNs also understand the importance of **spirituality** in health and healing. The role of the FCN therefore complements the ministry of health found in faith communities.

FOUNDATIONS OF FAITH COMMUNITY NURSING

The Reverend Granger Westberg, a Lutheran minister, is considered the founder of the modern faith community nursing movement. Educated as a chaplain and minister, he worked with nurses in hospitals, medical schools, and church communities. Westberg was a visionary, with an understanding of the possibilities that church leaders, health care professionals, and congregational members could make in improving whole person health (body–mind–spirit). In one sermon he noted, "the church has not assumed its share of the responsibility for the health of the community" (Solari-Twadell and McDermott, 2006, p. 6). He later proposed to the W. K. Kellogg Foundation and the Department of Preventive Medicine of the University of Chicago College of Medicine the founding of "wholistic health centers" where family physicians provided primary health care in churches with a team of nurses and clergy (Holistic Health Centers, 1976). These projects were implemented with success in various Illinois communities over the next decade. Evaluators later identified that a major reason for the success of the centers was the nurses, who could act as bridges between the ministers and the physicians because they understood both the science of medicine and the importance of religion in health and wellness (Holistic Health Centers, 1976). Impressed with the nurses' ability in viewing the physical, emotional, and spiritual challenges of human illness, Westberg described parish nursing as the culmination of his lifelong work in relating theology and health care. In 1984, he first proposed a parish nurse program to Lutheran General Hospital (LGH) in Chicago. Westberg envisioned a partnership between the hospital and all church congregations in the hospital's community. He proposed that participating churches would make contributions to fund a nurse's salary and identified seven roles the nurse could use to provide services to faith communities, discussed later (Hickman, 2007; O'Brien, 2003; Patterson, 2004).

In 1985, six FCNs were hired in the Chicago area. Initially, LGH and the participating churches' contributions primarily funded the nurses' salaries. As the program grew and the IPNRC became a reality, oversight was provided by the Lutheran-rooted Advocate Health Care System. Located in Park Ridge, Illinois, the center offered education, development guidance, and contact with parish nurses nationally and internationally. In 2001, ownership of the IPNRC moved from Advocate Health Care System to the Deaconess Foundation of St. Louis, Missouri. The Deaconess ministries in the United States have their roots in the Deaconess service movement founded in Germany in the mid-1800s. Deaconess Foundation has been involved in faith community nursing since the late 1980s and, as the Deaconess

Parish Nurse Ministries, is a leader in the specialty in the United States. The Deaconess Parish Nurse Ministries served as the parent organization of the IPNRC until 2011 (IPNRC, 2009; Westberg, 2007).

In 2011, the IPNRC became the newest section of the community outreach division of the Church Health Center located in Memphis, Tennessee. The Church Health Center was founded in 1987 by Scott Morris, family practice physician and ordained United Methodist minister, to provide quality and affordable health care for working, uninsured people and their families. His vision is to "reclaim the Church's biblical commitment to care for our bodies and spirits" (Church Health Center, n.d.). The organization is now the largest faith-based health care organization of its type in the country. Using a volunteer interprofessional team of nurse practitioners, dentists, and others, the Church Health Center currently provides care to more than 58,000 patients without government funding. Patients pay an average of $25 per visit on a sliding-fee scale. A wellness model of care is the foundation for all programs of the Church Health Center. The philosophy of the IPNRC and the Church Health Center is a complementary one related to a belief in the importance of the role of the church in health and wellness. Fig. 33.1 illustrates the wellness model that is the basis for the vision, mission, and programs related to the Church Health Center. Part of the community outreach of the Center is to build congregational relationships and to "encourage, educate and equip" people to live healthier lives. Additionally, Morris has a personal knowledge of Westberg's vision for faith community nursing. He had previously met and discussed faith community nursing with Westberg as he was developing his plan to merge church and health. The Church Health Center has the resources to move faith community nursing to the next level.

In 1998, the American Nurses Association (ANA), in collaboration with the newly formed Health Ministries Association, Parish Nurse Division, published the first *Scope and Standards of Parish Nurse Practice*. This was a landmark publication for parish nurses, officially recognizing their practice as a nursing specialty. ANA revised the standards in 2012, providing a clearer definition of the practice, including advanced nursing practice and changing the name of the specialty from parish nurse to faith community nurse. While acknowledging the importance of the Judeo-Christian basis of the practice, the authors of *Scope and Standards* believed that the change better reflected the diversity now found in the specialty.

To celebrate the twenty-fifth anniversary of the founding of modern FCN, the IPNRC in 2016 was renamed the Westberg Institute for Faith Community Nursing (WI) (Westberg Institute for FCN [WI], 2016). The mission of the WI is to be a resource to FCNs focusing on "high quality, outcomes-based FCN practice" through research and connections with FCNs worldwide. As previously mentioned, the WI (2017) reports that faith community nursing is now practiced in more than 29 countries, including Australia, Bahamas, Canada, England, Ghana, Kenya, South Korea, Madagascar, Malawi, Malaysia, New Zealand, Nigeria, Pakistan, Palestine, Scotland, Singapore, South Africa, Swaziland, Ukraine, United States, Wales, Zambia, and Zimbabwe, serving Muslim, Jewish, and Christian faith

The Church Health Center
Model for Healthy Living

Faith Life
Friends & Family
Nutrition
Movement
Your Life
Medical
Emotional
Work

 Faith Life

Building a relationship with God, your neighbors, and yourself.

 Movement

Discovering ways to enjoy physical activity.

 Medical

Partnering with your healthcare provider to manage your medical care.

 Work

Appreciating your skills, talents, and gifts.

 Emotional

Managing stress and understanding your feelings to better care for yourself.

 Nutrition

Making smart food choices and developing healthy eating habits.

 Family & Friends

Giving and receiving support through relationships.

FIG. 33.1 The Church Health Center model for healthy living. (From Church Health Center: *Model for healthy living,* n.d. Accessed 2017. <http://www.chreader.org/contentPage.aspx?resource_id=712&listWebPage_id=1>.)

communities. Many FCNs continue to identify themselves as parish nurses in deference to Westberg and the origins of the practice. For this reason, the terms are used interchangeably in the literature and at conferences. Other FCNs may be known

as *congregational nurses* or *church nurses,* choosing to identify themselves in the manner most accepted by their individual faith communities.

Important to the continued growth of the nursing specialty was the development of the first professional nursing specialty membership organization, Faith Community Nursing International (FCNI). Chartered by a small group of FCNs from across the country in 2013, the group became incorporated in 2014 and established the mission of connecting, supporting, and promoting a global community of FCNs to positively affect the health of faith communities and the community as a whole (ANA, 2017). Working groups of members are currently building new networks to promote FCN research, education, and policy. The organization's publication is the *International Journal of Faith Community Nursing,* which is an open-access online journal (FCNI, 2017).

⚗ RESEARCH HIGHLIGHTS

Health Coaching in Faith-Based Community Diabetes Education

A significant health burden exists related to type 2 diabetes. Evidence-based solutions through research are needed to improve diabetes outcomes. Faith community diabetes education can be utilized to provide the knowledge needed to manage the disease. The purpose of the current study was to determine if a faith-based community diabetes education program including health coaching can increase self-efficacy in people with type 2 diabetes.

This pilot study used a pretest/posttest format for data collection. After providing diabetes education for all participants, half of the group received health coaching and the other half had no further intervention. A survey consisting of two evidence-based tools, the Short Diabetes Knowledge Instrument and the Diabetes Self Efficacy Scale, along with demographic data, was utilized for the pretest. Data analysis included t-tests and Pearson correlation.

Although there was no significant difference between the intervention and control groups, the results showed diabetes knowledge levels and self-efficacy were significantly improved from pretest to posttest in all participants through t-test analysis (n 16, t –2.45, p 0.027; n 16, t –2.44, p 0.028). Within the intervention group, there was also improved diabetes knowledge from pretest to posttest (n 8, t –2.38, p 0.05). A positive correlation was found between diabetes knowledge on the pretest and the posttest self-efficacy (r 0.67, t 0.004).

From Meyer JL, Holland BE: Health coaching in faith-based community diabetes education. *IJFCN* 2(1):2016:14–20. http://digitalcommons.wku.edu/ijfcn/vol2/iss1/3/

Solari-Twadell and McDermott (1999) and Westberg (1990) described the philosophical basis of parish nursing as encompassing the following five key elements:
1. The spiritual dimension is central to the practice.
2. The role balances nursing science and technology with service and spiritual care.
3. The nurse's clients are members of the faith community defined by the church and its public service philosophy.
4. Parish nursing services are built upon principles of self-care and capacity building, with a focus on understanding the connection between health and the individual's relationship with God, faith traditions, nursing, and the broader society.

5. The parish nurse understands that holistic health is a dynamic process that requires connections among the person's spiritual, psychological, physical, and social dimensions.

These beliefs direct the parish nurse in planning nursing care and defining health not only as wellness but also as wholeness of body and spirit. They also emphasize spiritual health as a motivating factor in seeking wellness care, participating in education, and enhancing self-care capabilities (Hickman, 2007; Patterson, 2004; Smith, 2003). The IPNRC (2009) identifies a vision that "every faith community in the future will have access to a FCN." The defining characteristics and roles of the FCN in any setting may arise from these philosophical foundations.

The following current mission statement for parish nurses was developed and approved in 2000 by more than 600 attendees at the Fourteenth Annual Westberg Symposium:

> *Parish nursing (aka faith community nursing) is the intentional integration of the practice of faith with the practice of nursing so that people can achieve wholeness in, with, and through communities of faith in which the parish nurse serves. Parish nurses educate, advocate, and activate people to take positive action regarding wellness, prevention, appropriate treatment of illness, and social and spiritual connections with God, members of their congregations, and their wider community.*
>
> **(Patterson, 2004, p. 32)**

The WI (2017) describes the philosophy of FCN as "embracing four major concepts: spiritual formation, professionalism, shalom as health and wholeness; and community, incorporating culture and diversity."

Evident in all of these examples is that the uniqueness of faith community nursing as a community/public health practice is the setting for practice in faith communities and the importance of spirituality as an underpinning in the practice focusing on the intentional care of the spirit to assist clients in reaching maximum health and wellness.

 HEALTHY PEOPLE 2020

Faith Community Nursing

Topic Area

Educational and community-based programs

Goal

Increase the quality, availability, and effectiveness of education and community-based programs designed to prevent disease and improve health and quality of life.

Faith community nursing practice may vary depending on the needs of the faith community served. Programs and services may contribute to many *Healthy People 2020* goals. The topic area Educational and Community-Based Programs directs public health agencies to form partnerships with many community-based organizations, including faith communities, to improve the quality and effectiveness of health education programs. A free toolkit is available for faith communities to implement some of the ideas from the top 60 faith community nursing programs and community programs in the Let's Move Initiative selected as the best in the United States at promoting activity in all ages of Americans. It can be downloaded at https://www.hhs.gov/sites/default/files/lets_move_toolkit.pdf.

ROLES OR FUNCTIONS OF THE FAITH COMMUNITY NURSE

The faith community nursing practice focuses on health promotion and wellness. It is based on a holistic nursing practice that holds the spiritual dimension central to health and healing within the context of the faith community. In the nursing process, the FCN improves the health of a faith community by implementing interrelated roles or functions, including those of health educator, personal health counselor, referral agent, health advocate, coordinator of volunteers, developer of support groups, and integrator of health and healing (Hickman, 2007; IPNRC, 2013a), as summarized in Box 33.1.

As a health educator, the FCN provides or coordinates educational offerings for people of all ages and developmental stages. The educational efforts may target lifestyles, values, and wellness and may incorporate the spiritual aspects of individual and community well-being. The educator role includes educating the church leaders and members about the roles and purposes of a parish nurse. Educational efforts are based on the church community's priorities and *Healthy People 2020* (U.S. Department of Health and Human Services [DHHS], n.d.). Because the faith community membership includes people of all ages, church-based educational programs can address all 10 major health indicators (IPNRC, 2013a; King and Tessaro, 2009). Early in the development of a parish nurse program, and periodically thereafter, the parish nurse should assess the health status and needs of the congregation members to determine educational priorities. The FCN should complete an assessment on each population group served by the congregation and should include children grouped by developmental stages. Examples of educational efforts are teaching cardiopulmonary resuscitation to new mothers; teaching signs and symptoms of hypertension and stroke to adults in the congregation; educating lay church ministers visiting homebound individuals on the signs and symptoms of acute illness; and teaching basic health and safety to school-age children. With increasing frequency, FCNs are implementing comprehensive wellness programs.

BOX 33.1   Westberg's Seven Key Roles of the Faith Community Nurse

- Integrator of faith and health: helps patients understand the interrelationship between spiritual, physical and mental health, and healing within their faith tradition.
- Health educator: increases patient understanding of the relationship between lifestyle choices, faith, and health.
- Personal health counselor: listens to patient concerns and offers counsel to help them make informed decisions about health care issues.
- Facilitator of support groups: organizes support groups according to the needs of the congregation.
- Coordinator of volunteers: trains volunteers to support health ministries according to the needs of the congregation.
- Health care advocate: Assists individuals in the understanding of medical information to help them choose a care plan within their faith.
- Referral agent: provides information and access to needed community services.

One such program is "Get My People Going," developed by the IPNRC. It provides an 8-week healthy lifestyle program based on the Exodus story that includes exercise, nutrition, and community support (IPNRC, 2009).

As a **personal health counselor**, the FCN discusses health problems with individuals and families within the church community. The nurse may focus on self-care issues such as explaining a prescribed medical regimen; assessing the need for further resources and referrals; or making visits to homes, nursing homes, or hospitals (McGinnis, 2008).

The FCN utilizes referral skills and knowledge of community resources to guide individuals as they access available resources. The nurse may function as a liaison and, with the client's approval, may provide referrals to resources or health care providers. The FCN recognizes the difficulties encountered by vulnerable populations within the faith community and helps them maneuver the health care maze to access needed resources. These vulnerable populations may include non–English-speaking individuals, those who speak English as a second language, individuals living in poverty, individuals without health care insurance, and individuals living with complicated chronic or catastrophic illness.

In the role of **health advocate**, the FCN "facilitates clients' efforts in obtaining needed health services and appropriate care management plans, promotes community awareness of significant health problems, lobbies for beneficial public policy, and stimulates supportive action for health" (Clemon-Stone et al., 2002, p. 45). Advocacy can present challenges for the nurse in any setting. The nurse must always remember that the client (individual, family, or group) has the right to self-determination. The FCN's role may be that of educating clients to make the best choices or empowering them to speak for themselves. The nurse also must understand the policies and beliefs of the congregation in relation to specific health issues. Church doctrine may guide members to adopt values and beliefs that are in conflict with current health care recommendations. Individuals may request that the parish nurse provide education and support in making decisions related to issues of infertility, stem cell technology, birth control, and sex education for teens and youth. Although assuming the role of advocate implies a commitment to change, the parish nurse must understand that the politics of working within the faith system require acceptance of individual and system values and beliefs.

The role of **coordinator of volunteers** involves recruiting, training, and directing volunteers to work with the faith community nursing program or health ministry. The nurse may work with other nurses and laypeople within the congregation. The faith community nursing program may encompass all programs related to the health of the church community. For example, the community needs assessment may identify the need for development of a transportation committee or respite program. These services affect the ability of church members to access health and related services, and these programs may be delegated to the nurse. As a coordinator of volunteers, the nurse would plan, implement, and direct these programs. Many FCNs work through existing health ministry frameworks within their churches, such as health or social welfare committees. The membership of these committees may be interdisciplinary or representative of the entire church congregation. The FCN may be delegated the responsibility for developing specific health-related programs and activities. In the **facilitator** role, the nurse would also connect the church with existing resources and programs to meet identified health and educational needs. For example, the nurse might facilitate available health screenings, flu shots, or immunizations through the local public health department.

The role of **developer of support groups** requires skills in assessment, and the FCN uses community assessment and program evaluation skills. The nurse may practice within a community rich in resources and support groups or one with few health-related resources. Support groups are people who meet for support and sharing of issues related to common problems. Examples are bereavement groups and new mother groups. Support groups are different from self-help groups, which focus on personal growth (e.g., Alcoholics Anonymous). Some individuals prefer support groups to be physically located within their faith community, where they have existing support systems and can network with individuals who have common values and beliefs. The FCN must evaluate the need for a support or self-help group within the faith community. Situations that might indicate the need for support groups include the increased incidence of a sudden and shared experience by members—for example, the death of five or more members from cancer in a short time frame, several incidences of suicide, or eating disorders within a teen group. A needs assessment of the faith community also might indicate the need for development of a support group. There are many models that the parish nurse may use as guidance in the development of groups. For example, the University of Kansas provides a Community Tool Box to help with creating and facilitating support groups (http://ctb.ku.edu/en/tablecontents/). If acceptable to the client, an individual referral may be made to an existing community group. It is also important to remember that groups usually have an anticipated "life expectancy." After the needs of a particular support group are met through education or support, there may no longer be a need for the group. The FCN should document the history of the group and move forward toward new goals.

As an **integrator of health and healing**, the nurse acknowledges and integrates spirituality as the basis of his or her nursing practice. For example, in teaching a class on healthy aging, the nurse will discuss lifestyle, compliance with prescribed medical treatment, attitudes, and values and their connections to well-being. In a home visit to a terminally ill person, the nurse will explore the meaning of healing versus cure and provide emotional support and encouragement. In certain faith communities, the nurse may lead or contribute to healing services as a member of the health ministry team. A basis for successful integration of health and healing in faith community nursing practice is an understanding of spirituality as a foundation for parish nurse practice. The importance of spirituality to faith community nursing practice and health is discussed later in the chapter.

These examples illustrate the diversity and autonomy found in faith community nursing. Depending on the needs of the church community and its members, the roles may be implemented in a variety of ways and through various organizational structures. Some organizational models use volunteer and paid nurses in the role of parish nurse. Hospitals provide parish nurses to community churches through grants, contracts, and public service. Many faith communities have incorporated positions for part-time and full-time nurses within their ministerial teams. Job descriptions and programs vary; examples can be found online at websites for individual parish nurse programs or at the IPNRC website (http://www.churchhealthcenter.org/fcnhome).

EDUCATION OF THE FAITH COMMUNITY NURSE

A baccalaureate-prepared RN with several years of experience in clinical practice is best prepared to implement the roles of the FCN; however, many schools of nursing provide faith community nursing education in baccalaureate prelicensure, RN to bachelor of science in nursing, and master of science in nursing programs. The self-direction and independent decision making required by the autonomous roles of the FCN require a nurse experienced in clinical nursing and community-based nursing practice. The educational preparation of the baccalaureate nurse in community health nursing provides the theoretical basis needed to plan and implement programs for diverse populations in a congregational setting and to function as a beginning member of a pastoral team (Westberg Institute, 2016.) All FCNs should complete a formal program of study (Church Health Center, n.d.; IPNRC, 2013b; Smith, 2003; Solari-Twadell and McDermott, 1999; Westberg and McNamara, 1990). Universities, hospitals, and faith community nursing programs now offer hundreds of courses that nurses may take for college credit, continuing education, or postgraduate certification. Courses are offered online, in seminars, and in regular classrooms. More than 136 international educational partners offer parish nurse courses. A list of these educational providers can be found on the IPNRC website.

Many universities are incorporating existing basic preparation programs into advanced nursing degree programs. Programs are generally offered at beginning and advanced levels and consist of approximately 38 to 40 contact hours of planned classroom instruction, self-study, or clinical experiences at each level. Box 33.2 provides an example of the curriculum content for a beginning faith community nursing program as suggested by the IPNRC. The curriculum is currently being revised and is expected to be more flexible. The revised curriculum incorporates other topics needed to provide comprehensive nursing care and health promotion for specific faith communities, such as disaster management, care of families, and special needs of rural congregations. As faith community nursing programs grow in number and in the services they provide to faith communities, continuing education programs will increase in availability and in diversity of content. The IPNRC conference held annually at the Westberg Symposium provides the greatest opportunity for education and networking among FCNs in the world.

Implementation of the FCN's roles requires the use of the nursing process to plan nursing interventions in wellness and

---

BOX 33.2   Suggested Core Curriculum Content for Beginning Parish Nurse Program

Spirituality
- History and philosophy of faith community nursing
- Self-care
- Healing and wholeness
- Professionalism
- Ethical issues
- Documenting practice
- Legal issues
- Beginning a faith community nursing ministry
- Communication and collaboration

Holistic Care
- Health promotion
- Transforming life issues—family violence, suffering, loss, grief

Community
- Assessment
- Resources
- Advocacy
- Care coordination

Modified from International Parish Nurse Resource Center: *Role of parish nurse, mission and resources*, Park Ridge, IL, 2009, Author.

---

physical, emotional, and spiritual health. Other chapters in this text provide useful information concerning health promotion and planning activities to promote physical and mental health. Spirituality, as a major focus of nursing care, presents different challenges for the nurse.

THE FAITH COMMUNITY NURSE AND SPIRITUALITY

Westberg (2007) described the ideal FCN as one who is spiritually mature and able to apply spiritual aspects to the health care of congregation members. Many FCNs find the need for further education to develop spiritual assessment skills, acquire theological knowledge, and learn the nurse's role in healing.

Wright (2005) defines spirituality as "the human desire for a sense of meaning, purpose, connection, and fulfillment through intimate relationships and life experiences" (p. xviii). In nursing, spiritual distress is more often the focus of care. The North American Nursing Diagnosis Association (1992) defines spiritual distress as "a disruption in the life principle that pervades a person's entire being and that integrates and transcends one's biological and psychosocial nature" (p. 46). Spirituality is the basis of nursing care in the church setting. The Joint Commission, the International Council of Nursing, and the National Council of State Boards of Nursing and related National Council Licensure Examination for Registered Nurses (NCLEX) include as important "religious and spiritual influences on health" and list spiritual care as a characteristic in indicators of "quality care" (McEwen, 2005).

Many models are available to help nurses assess the spiritual dimensions of care, including the HOPE Model and the JAREL Spiritual Well-Being Scale (McEwen, 2005). The FCN should learn to use a tested model that facilitates his or her practice, because knowledge deficiencies are identified as a major barrier to spiritual nursing care (McEwen, 2005). Schnorr (1988, 2003) suggests the CIRCLE Model of Spiritual Care. This model illustrates the following concepts of care that guide nursing practice and interventions:

Caring

Intuition

Respect for religious beliefs and practices

Caution

Listening

Emotional support

Caring includes caring practices and attitudes. Swanson (1991) provided an understanding of the caring processes through her early research, which identified five caring processes: knowing (trying to understanding what events mean to the patient); being with (both emotionally and in person); doing for (as needed); enabling (helping through transitions and life stages); and maintaining belief (helping the person sustain faith or hope). These processes were later further defined and identified as caring behaviors. The top caring behaviors in nursing as derived from the literature are attentive listening, comforting, honesty, patience, responsibility, providing information so the patient can make an informed decision, touch, sensitivity, respect, and calling the patient by name (Swanson, 1991; Watson, 1998; Wolf, 1986; Wolf et al., 2004). Nurse theorist Jean Watson described caring as "professional, ethical, scientific, esthetic, personalized giving-receiving behaviors that allow for contact between the nurse and client" (quoted in Dossey, 1999, p. 45). Intuition requires acting on instinct, hunches, or "gut feelings." Benner (1984) described intuitive abilities as responses that expert nurses have after several years of experience; these abilities enable the nurse to "read between the lines." Schnorr (1988) described respect as understanding the importance of religious beliefs and practices. The nurse allows time for prayer and sacrament and supports and encourages religious activities. Caution in spiritual care advises the parish nurse to avoid proselytizing or "preaching" religion to clients. The ANA's (2012) *Code of Ethics for Nurses* also provides the nurse with direction to avoid judgments and respect the client's right to self-determination. Listening is a skill that is highly developed in most experienced nurses. It allows an understanding of spoken and unspoken words and feelings, encourages open communication, and supports and empowers patients to communicate needs and desires. Emotional support is the link between the physical and spiritual. Among the emotional interventions, Schnorr (1988) includes working with feelings, showing love, and using appropriate touch and empathy.

Prayer is a commonly used spiritual intervention that can provide comfort and support. Many nurses are not comfortable with sharing individual or group prayer. Clients may ask FCNs to offer prayer for healing or recovery (Clinical Example 33.3). Many faith traditions, such as Catholic and Jewish, have traditional prayers that the parish nurse can read or memorize.

A guideline to follow is to keep the prayer simple and offer the request to the client's higher power. The nurse may have a poem for healing that is meaningful, which may be also be used. Silence may also be used after a simple prayer, or the nurse may request that the client offer his or her own prayer. Hickman (2007) suggests that through prayer, spiritual assessment, and hope and faith, the FCN facilitates important client outcomes for spiritual health and well-being, including self-esteem, self-actualization, hope, trust, and peace.

Clinical Example 33.3

During a meeting of the health ministry committee, the FCN nurse learned that Mrs. James, a church member, had been diagnosed with end-stage breast cancer. Mrs. James is a 45-year-old wife and mother of two school-age children. She returned home after surgery and had to decide whether to seek further treatment within the following weeks. Her husband attended church with his family although he was a member of another faith community. A home health nurse was involved with Mrs. James's postoperative care, and it was possible that a referral to hospice would occur after her decisions regarding further treatment. The nurse called Mrs. James and offered to make a home visit to assess how the FCN and church community could support and care for the family's well-being. Mrs. James welcomed the visit. Showing respect for their faith beliefs, the nurse offered prayer and waited for a request from the couple. The nurse's instincts and experience in working with patients with cancer and their families guided her in using listening as a nursing intervention during this initial visit and in using caution when Mrs. James asked for guidance in making treatment decisions. The nurse further explored the home situation, the needed educational support, and the physician's prognosis and treatment options with the patient. Emotional support was important for Mrs. James, and the FCN offered support through touch and words of concern. This model helped develop an initial nurse–client relationship of trust and open communication.

ISSUES IN FAITH COMMUNITY NURSE PRACTICE

The practice of faith community nursing is affected by many issues common to community health practice as well as issues specific to parish nursing. Selected issues discussed in this section include working with vulnerable populations and the legal and ethical issues of confidentiality and accountability. Other issues identified as important by the IPNRC are end-of-life and family violence issues; these are required content in faith community nursing courses.

Providing Care to Vulnerable Populations

The philosophical foundations of faith communities related to caring, outreach, and support of vulnerable populations place the parish nurse in a position to positively influence the health of diverse groups. Historically, churches have been among the first groups to sponsor and support refugees, develop programs for homeless individuals and families, offer assistance and resources to low-income families, and provide resources to entire communities during disasters (e.g., floods and tornadoes). FCNs are able to provide care for diverse populations using skills in assessment, planning, and interventions.

FCNs can be instrumental in helping diverse populations access services; however, nurses should not attempt to meet the population's many needs alone (Boss, 1996; Hickman, 2007). When one is using available health resources, "more is not necessarily better." The nurse in the educator role can assess the needs of vulnerable populations and teach the faith community about the people and their spiritual, emotional, and physical needs. A community of caring that can collectively meet the many needs of vulnerable populations will emerge from the congregation. Boss (1999) called this the *Nehemiah approach,* meaning that people collectively share their talents and desire to do the work. The FCN works as a member of a caring church community to meet the health and related needs of vulnerable populations. For example, as Hispanic populations grow in rural populations, the need for churches to meet the needs of this population also grows. Established churches may provide resources for Hispanic populations to form their own churches. The FCN may serve an outreach church in addition to the parent church.

End-of-Life Issues: Grief and Loss

Faith communities have long been the first-line provider of support related to loss, grief, and dying. The aging population, the increased prevalence of chronic diseases such as cardiovascular disease and cancer, and public awareness have contributed to the need for improved end-of-life care. FCNs become partners with hospice and home care nurses in providing palliative care to congregation members. The IPNRC suggests that the FCN needs a theoretical base that includes an understanding of grief and loss from a developmental and social perspective, knowledge of the manifestations of normal and complicated grief, and nursing interventions to facilitate healthy grieving.

FCN activities related to end-of-life care may include educational sessions on drawing up living wills, establishing health care surrogates, and understanding hospice and palliative care; providing home visits to dying congregational members and emotional support to family and survivors; and developing grief support groups.

Family Violence Prevention

Education and prevention of family violence directly relate to *Healthy People 2020* objectives, and all nurses must be informed in this area (IPNRC, 2009; Smith, 2003). The FCN must have an understanding of risk factors for family, child, and elder abuse; knowledge of the cycle of abuse; and assessment skills to identify individuals and families at risk for violence. Family violence affects all racial, ethnic, religious, and socioeconomic classes in the United States.

In intimate partner violence (IPV) (also known as *domestic abuse, spouse abuse, domestic violence, courtship violence, battering, marital rape,* or *date rape*), it is important to understand that the main issue is an imbalance of power. There are no standard reporting laws across the United States related to IPV; however, it is essential that the FCN recognize signs and symptoms of IPV and have an intervention plan that includes providing support, establishing a trusting relationship, discussing safety issues, making appropriate referrals for shelter and counseling, and documenting the abuse according to the organization's policy (IPNRC, 2013a).

Child abuse and neglect are reportable in all 50 states:

All 50 States, the District of Columbia, and the U.S. territories have enacted statutes specifying procedures that a mandatory reporter must follow when making a report of child abuse and neglect. Mandatory reporters are individuals who are required by law to report cases of suspected child abuse or neglect. In most States, the statutes require mandatory reporters to make a report immediately upon gaining their knowledge or suspicion of abusive or neglectful situations. In all jurisdictions, the initial report may be made orally to either the child protection services agency or to a law enforcement agency.

(U.S. Department of Health and Human Services [DHHS], n.d.)

Nursing interventions for suspected or actual child abuse include the following:
1. Report to the appropriate authority.
2. Provide resources and referrals.
3. Establish a trusting relationship with the child or adolescent.
4. Provide presence.
5. Listen.
6. Document according to policy, law, or both.

The National Center on Elder Abuse (2013) reported that 13% of the U.S. population, or 40.3 million people, were aged 65 years or older (based on the 2010 U.S. Census) and possibly as many as 10% experienced some type of abuse in 2010. Women were more likely to be exploited than men, and major financial exploitation may occur at the rate of 41 per 1000 individuals. Elder abuse includes not only physical abuse but also psychological neglect, with or without verbal threats; violation of personal choice or rights; financial theft or misuse of the elder's money; and failing to provide basic needs (food, shelter, clothing, and medical care). The parish nurse or another church volunteer may be the first individual to identify signs and symptoms of elder abuse. The nurse's role may also include educating church volunteers on identifying abuse and making reports and referrals. The nurse must have skill in recognizing symptoms of abuse and must possess assessment or screening questions to identify specific problems. Specific nursing interventions include the following:
1. Recognizing that all states have laws against elder abuse but that reporting varies from state to state so it is important to know state laws
2. Establishing a trusting relationship with the elder and being a presence (being with the elder as needed)
3. Providing appropriate referral and resources
4. Documenting the abuse according to policy, law, or both

ETHICAL INSIGHTS

Principles of Applied Ethics in a Faith Community

Applied ethics refers to the utilization of ethical principles in real-life situations. The values and beliefs of faith communities raise additional ethical considerations for the parish nurse. Actions of the parish nurse may result in a conflict between established nursing interventions and beliefs of the faith community. The IPNRC (2009) identifies these potential areas of ethical conflict:

- Infertility treatment
- Organ donations
- Blood transfusions
- Proper dress or behavior
- Withdrawal of and withholding nutrition
- DNR (do not resuscitate) orders
- Prolife versus prochoice
- Use of advance directives
- Distribution of scarce resources
- Competency for decision making
- Clergy sexual conduct

The FCN's roles include understanding the scope of practice for parish nurses related to ethical practice and the values and beliefs of the community served. The nurse must understand his or her own beliefs and values that are in conflict with the faith community's beliefs. It is necessary that the parish nurse know when to seek help, when to refer, and when to remove himself or herself from the ethical decision-making process (O'Brien, 2003).

Confidentiality

The *Code of Ethics for Nurses* (ANA, 2008) and the *Scope and Standards of Faith Community Nursing Practice* (Health Ministries Association and ANA, 2012) provide ethical guidance to parish nurses. FCNs are accountable to state boards of nursing, employing agencies (i.e., including churches), and the faith communities they serve. Many ethical and legal issues are generic to clinical practice settings; however, confidentiality issues have the potential to be problematic in a church community. Nurses who volunteer in faith communities, as in any other community organization in which they use the title nurse or employ nursing skills, must maintain active licenses as required by the state in which they reside. Many state boards of nursing provide practice guidelines related to the accountability and responsibility of the RN as a volunteer. Basically the nurse should assume he or she is accountable and responsible for knowing and following established policies and procedures.

Concerned church members may identify individuals in need and refer them to the parish nurse. In the role of health minister, the parish nurse may receive private and sensitive information. The nurse does not act in the role of minister or priest. Congregation members should not relate information in the form of confession or repentance; however, the connection with the church ministry team may put the nurse in a position to hear this type of sensitive information.

The nurse should protect clients' rights to confidentiality in relation to information concerning their health or health-related condition. Although the nurse must share information with the church minister in certain instances, the nurse should share confidential information with other church ministry leaders (or prayer groups) only when given permission by the client.

Exceptions are found in religious sects or congregations that require the public confession of members' behaviors or conditions so that members may benefit from divine intervention and forgiveness. As a care provider, the FCN should be aware of these rituals and practices before counseling members of the faith community (Fowler, 1999). General guidelines for medical record management should be followed by the FCN. Policies and procedures for managing and storing records and sharing and requesting medical information must be established. Faith community nursing programs within faith communities generally are not required to follow Health Insurance Portability and Accountability Act (HIPAA) guidelines related to medical records and confidentiality, because churches are not in the category of identified health care providers. An exception is parish nurse services provided by a licensed health care provider such as a hospital; in this instance, HIPAA regulations do apply (IPNRC, 2009).

Accountability

The FCN is a licensed RN and must comply with the professional standards and state board of nursing regulations for nursing practice. Due to the independent practice of the FCN, it is essential that the nurse maintain professional malpractice insurance. Additionally, the Westberg Institute (2017) provides the following suggestions to decrease FCN liability:

- Create and maintain a strong line of communication between the parish nurse and the church, staff, client, client's family, and any other stakeholder.
- Have a well-defined job description for the position in the faith community.
- Comply with boundaries/functions of the *Faith Community: Scope and Standards of Practice.*
- Maintain a documentation system that supports the actions of a faith community nurse (WI, Professional Liability, 2017, para 4).

Sister Mary Angela Shaughnessy (1998) provides direction for the FCN by listing the following information related to church law:

- Volunteers in a church are held to the same degree of accountability as are paid employees.
- The doctrine of separation of church and state does not exempt churches from discrimination laws.
- Ministers, both ordained and nonordained, may be required to disclose confidential information in court.

As volunteers or paid employees, nurses are accountable to the nursing standards and civil laws designed to protect individuals from abuse, neglect, and discrimination. FCNs, as nonordained ministers, do not have client–professional privileges and should be aware of appropriate standards in documenting provided services. In documenting parish nurse services, "less is better." Many churches may not have the facilities to store medical records in a secure locked area. In this instance, the nurse should have a file storage system that locks and can be kept in a secure location. Simple records of blood pressure screenings or health education programs could include only numbers of attendees or blood pressure results categorized by American Heart Association standards as hypertensive, borderline, or normal. Also included in the documentation could be numbers of individuals referred for services. Faith community governing boards or committees need not have the names of individual clients but will be interested in the types of services and numbers of clients served. Individual client services require a nurse's note or assessment and development of a nursing care plan. Before beginning a faith community nursing program, the nurse should develop and follow general policies and guidelines for record keeping and storage. Shaughnessy (1998) provides further information related to contract law. The handbooks, brochures, or programs that church-related institutions offer are contracts. The FCN should ensure that health information is current and based on accepted practices and standards. These suggestions are not intended to limit the parish nurse's creativity or scope; rather, they emphasize that the professional nurse is accountable for his or her practice in any role.

? ACTIVE LEARNING

1. Speak with a minister, priest, rabbi, or church leader in the community from a faith belief system different from your own. Explore the philosophical basis for the church's role in health and healing.
2. Visit websites devoted to faith community nursing and identify the models of faith community nursing programs or read the descriptions of their practice. Share these with the clinical group.

CASE STUDY APPLICATION OF THE NURSING PROCESS

Needs Assessment of a Faith Community

Nancy Elliot, an FCN at Living Hope Baptist Church, just completed a needs assessment of her faith community of 200 families. Nancy is new to the faith community nursing role, having recently been hired. Living Hope, considered a moderate-sized church, is located in a rural community of 40,000. Nancy decided to perform the needs assessment of the congregation and community before planning programs and services for the faith community.

Assessment

The community has one hospital and a variety of voluntary and official community agencies. Many private practitioners are available, either in the town or within a 1-hour drive in a larger city. Recently the town was awarded a grant to develop community parks and recreational facilities. Nancy is surprised by the demographic picture she finds after completing an assessment. Young families with toddlers to young school-age children comprise more than 70% of the congregation. She notes that these families are in the childbearing developmental stage of family growth and development. The remaining 30% of the members are elders, more than half of whom are 80 years or older. The survey indicates that the members are most interested in health screening and educational opportunities presented at the church. Only 3% of the members reported having no health insurance.

A discussion with the minister provides additional information. Two new industries have recently relocated to the area. The parent home of both of these industries was formerly located in distant states. Many new members have relocated to the area. Nancy understands that these young families may have decreased family and social support and little knowledge of existing community resources. The minister also informs her that the current church ministries focus on the elderly members and that new services are needed. Nancy schedules a meeting with the young parents after a church social gathering. Fifty mothers and fathers attend the session to discuss the health-related needs of the families. They identify that a "mothers' day out" program is a priority and also request information on community resources, parenting classes, and health and wellness programs for the children and parents. On the basis of the needs assessment and sessions with the parents, the FCN determines the following goals, nursing diagnoses, and population-focused nursing interventions.

Diagnosis
Individual

- Readiness for health promotion, as evidenced by requests for health information related to parenting, health, and wellness
- Potential for parent support, as evidenced by developmental stage of families, requests for education, and presence of new community members with limited knowledge of community resources

- Potential for community building, as evidenced by individual concerns related to limited social support and lack of social networks

Family

- Potential need for family support, related to recent relocation to new community and lack of social network

Community (Faith Community)

- At risk for community (congregation) disorganization, related to recent change in membership demographics, lack of developed resources, and new or developing faith community nursing role

Planning

A plan of care is developed to address the needs of the individuals, families, and the Living Hope faith community. Goals suggested by the FCN are mutually agreed upon by the ministerial team and congregational members.

Individual
Long-Term Goals

- Monthly educational programs will be offered addressing current issues in parenting and health and wellness of young families.
- Congregation will establish a social network for young parents.
- Ministerial leaders will dedicate funds to increase resources for children and young adults.

Short-Term Goals

- Establish parent steering committee for educational program ideas, identification of parent talents (assist with education programs).
- Explore development of mothers' day out program.

Family
Long-Term Goals

- Parent members will report increased social networks.
- Parent members will identify adequate resources to support growing family.

Short-Term Goal

- Identify community and congregation support for new and growing families.

Community (Faith Community)
Long-Term Goal

- Programs will be established to support growing families.

continued

CASE STUDY APPLICATION OF THE NURSING PROCESS—cont'd

Needs Assessment of a Faith Community

Short-Term Goal
- Implement one new program (educational, social) or resource for families each quarter of the church year.

Interventions

Nancy utilized diverse interventions to meet the goals established for families of Living Hope.

Individual

Nancy asked the parents to complete a talent survey to identify the resources available within the families of Living Hope. From this survey, Nancy identified two RNs willing to help provide educational programs and three previously certified early childhood teachers. The teachers were willing to develop a committee to explore the development of a mothers' day out program, a playgroup, and a new parent support group. Additional members were willing to begin a ministry to provide meals to new parents. Community resources were identified at the local health department to help teach parenting classes and provide immunizations. A plan was established to begin the mothers' day out program part-time within 2 months. The playgroup and educational programs were implemented immediately.

Family

The ministerial team and a parent advisory group were formed to identify family needs. Family social events were planned, including a church picnic. Planning was made for age-appropriate activities, such as the development of a soccer team for the youth, a softball team for the young adults, and a literary club for those interested. The advisory committee developed a budget to submit to the ministerial team, requesting financial support to develop a playground for the children attending the mothers' day out program and the hiring of a part-time employee to supervise the related activities. The families reported greater feelings of support from the faith community, increased social support and networks, and a feeling of belonging to the greater community.

Community (Faith Community)

The faith community developed a budget to support individual and family requests. Monthly health education programs became the standard, with topics noted on the monthly calendar. Members reported increased feelings of "community" not only among the young families but also across generational lines, as new members increasingly participated in leadership roles within the congregation. The minister documented an increase in weekly attendance, which had a positive impact on the long-range goals identified by the congregational members.

Evaluation
Individual and Family

Attendance at the health and wellness and parenting sessions increased with each educational session offered. Initial attendance was 5 to 7 people for each session, and after 6 months, the average attendance was 15 to 20 people for each session. The request from attendees changed from offering additional educational sessions to planning intervention programs such as a yoga class and a weight reduction program. The playground was completed in less than the planned time because of the increased budget. The mothers' day out program, which began as a part-time, 3-day-per-week program, grew to a Monday-through-Friday program within 12 months. The program became self-sufficient by the end of the year because of established fees, parent volunteers, and donations. Men and women verbalized an increased satisfaction with their spiritual growth and support from the faith community. Nancy developed a health ministry committee of volunteers from within the church and was able to increase the number and variety of related parish nurse activities.

Community (Faith Community)

The health and wellness activities attracted the attention of sister churches, and a grant was offered to increase the number of family support services and wellness programs offered within the church. Health and wellness programs were expanded to include additional methods for reaching congregational members, such as through a website. The greater attendance and participation of congregational members positively affected all members, who benefited from the leadership and positive environment. The educational offerings and intervention programs were developed on the basis of *Healthy People 2020* goals, in particular, increasing activity and exercise, healthy eating, and obesity prevention (DHHS, 2010).

Levels of Prevention

The roles of the FCN direct the interventions and programs planned for faith communities. The following are examples of all three levels of prevention applied to this case study.

Primary
- Assessment and teaching about parenting, health, and wellness
- Development of programs and social support systems to prevent social isolation and increase resources for successful parenting and healthy behaviors

Secondary
- FCN assessment and screening to identify individuals and families at risk
- Congregational resources and educational programs developed to meet individual and family needs

Tertiary
- FCN either provides or refers to resources for rehabilitation for families coping with children with disabilities or chronic health problems (parents and children).

▌ SUMMARY

This chapter provided an overview of the FCN's role in providing nursing care for faith communities, and it explored the historical and philosophical foundations of the modern faith community nursing practice. Traditional roles of the nurse are used in unique ways to allow the FCN to provide nursing care to church communities. The FCN's role in the development of spiritual health and well-being becomes significant and requires the nurse to focus on the spiritual needs of congregation members. The CIRCLE Model for planning spiritual nursing may be used to guide nursing interventions. Faith community nursing offers new opportunities for increasing the health and wellness of clients and requires the nurse to refocus skills and knowledge.

Many educational programs are available throughout the United States to provide faith community nursing education after basic nursing education. These programs are offered as continuing education and through formal university courses as part of degree programs. Church law, nursing ethics, and standards are the basis for the legal and ethical faith community nursing practice. As a relatively new area of community health nurse practice, faith community nursing offers the RN many opportunities to improve the health of faith communities through a holistic nursing practice that connects the body, mind, and spirit in the celebration of health and healing.

ⓔ EVOLVE WEBSITE

http://evolve.elsevier.com/Nies/community
- NCLEX Review Questions
- Case Studies

BIBLIOGRAPHY

American Nurses Association: *Faith community nursing: scope and standards*, ed 2, Silver Springs, MD, 2017, Author.

Benner P: *From novice to expert*, Menlo Park, CA, 1984, Addison-Wesley.

Boss J: Lesson learned over time: great teachers—St. Francis, St. Clare, and Eleanor, *Health Dev* 2:7–19, 1996.

Boss J: Parish nursing with under organized, underserved, and marginalized clients. In Solari-Twadell PA, McDermott MA, editors: *Parish nursing: promoting whole persons health within faith communities*, Thousand Oaks, CA, 1999, Sage.

Church Health Center: *About us: Our mission*, 2013. Available from: <http://www.churchhealthcenter.org/>.

Clemon-Stone S, McGuire S, Eigsti D: *Comprehensive community health nursing*, ed 6, St. Louis, 2002, Mosby.

Dossey MD: Dynamics of healing and the transpersonal self. In Dossey MD, Keegan L, editors: *Holistic nursing: a handbook for practice*, Gaithersburg, MD, 1999, Aspen.

Eckersley RM: Culture, spirituality, religion and health: looking at the big picture, *Med J Aust* 186(Suppl 10):S54–S56, 2007.

Fowler M: Ethics as a context for the practice. In Solari-Twadell PA, McDermott MA, editors: *Parish nursing: promoting whole persons health within faith communities*, Thousand Oaks, CA, 1999, Sage.

Health Ministries Association and American Nurses Association: *Faith community nursing: scope & standards*, Washington, DC, 2012, American Nurses Association.

Hickman JS: *Faith community nursing*, Philadelphia, 2007, Lippincott Williams & Wilkins.

Holistic Health Centers: *Survey research report*, Hinsdale, IL, 1976, Society for Holistic Medicine.

Interfaith Health Program: *Strong partners: interfaith health program*, Atlanta, GA, 2005, Emory University.

International Parish Nurse Resource Center: *Basic parish nurse preparation curriculum*, St. Louis, 2013, Deaconess Parish Nurse Ministries.

King MA, Tessaro I: Parish nursing: promoting health lifestyles in the church, *J Christ Nurs* 26(1):22–24, 2009.

Koenig HG, George L: Religion, spirituality, and health in hospitalized older patients, *J Am Geriatr Soc* 52A:532–541, 2004.

Koenig HG, King D, Carson VB: *The handbook of religion and health*, ed 2, New York, 2012, Oxford.

McEwen M: Spiritual nursing care, *Holistic Nursing Practice* 19:161–168, 2005.

McGinnis DL: The emerging role of faith community nurses in prevention & management of chronic disease, *Policy Polit Nurs Pract* 9(3):173–180, 2008.

Mendelson SG, McNeese-Smith D, Koniak-Griffin D, et al.: A community-based parish nurse intervention program for Mexican-American women with gestational diabetes, *JOGN* 37(4):415–425, 2008.

Myers DG: Stress and health: spirituality and faith communities. In Myers DG, editor: *Psychology*, ed 7, New York, 2004, Worth Publishers.

Myers DG: Religion and human flourishing. In Eid M, Larsen R, editors: *The science of subjective well-being*, New York, 2008, Guilford.

National Center on Elder Abuse: 2013. Available from: <www.ncea.aoa.gov/ncearoot/Main_Site/pdf/publication/FinalStatistics050331.pdf>.

North American Nursing Diagnosis Association: *NANDA nursing diagnosis: definitions and defining characteristics*, Philadelphia, 1992, Author.

O'Brien ME: *Parish nursing: healthcare ministry within the church*, Sudbury, MA, 2003, Jones and Bartlett.

Patterson D: Parish nursing: a beneficial partner for clergy, *The Clergy Journal* 53:32–33, 2004.

Pew Research Center: *Religion and public life: The global religious landscape*, 2012. Available from: http://www.pewforum.org/2012/12/18/global-religious-landscape-exec/.

Schnorr MA: *Spiritual nursing care: theory and curriculum development*, Doctoral dissertation, DeKalb, IL, 1988, Northern Illinois University. (Dissert Abstr Int 50:601-A, DA8912525).

Schnorr MA: Parish nurse pedagogy or andragogy. In: *Proceedings of the 17th Annual Westberg Parish Nurse Symposium*. St. Louis, MO, 1998, 2003, International Parish Nurse Resource Center.

Shaughnessy MA: *Ministry and the law: what you need to know*, New York, 1998, Paulist Press.

Smith SD: *Parish nursing: a handbook for the new millennium*, New York, 2003, Haworth Pastoral Press.

Solari-Twadell PA, McDermott MA: *Parish nursing: promoting whole person health within faith communities*, Thousand Oaks, CA, 1999, Sage.

Swanson KM: Empirical development of a middle range theory of caring, *Nursing Research* 40(3):161–166, 1991.

Tsuang MT, Williams WM, Lyons MJ: Pilot study of spiritual and mental health in twins, *Am J Psychiatry* 159:486–488, 2002.

U.S. Department of Health and Human Services: *Healthy people 2010*. Washington, DC, Government Printing Office. <www.healthypeople.gov>.

U.S. Department of Health and Human Services (DHHS): National Center on Elder Abuse, Administration on Aging: *Statistics and data*, n.d. Available from <www.ncea.aoa.gov/library/Data.index.aspx#problem>.

Watson MF: New dimensions in human caring theory, *Nursing Science Quarterly* 1(4):175–181, 1998.

Westberg G: *The parish nurse: providing a minister of health for your congregation*, Minneapolis, 1990, Augsburg.

Westberg G: A personal historical perspective of whole person health and the congregation. In Williams DR, Sternthal MJ, editors: *Spirituality, religion and health: evidence and research directions*, *Med J Aust*, 186(10 Suppl):S47–S50, 2007.

Westberg Institue: *International parish/faith community nursing*, 2016. Available from: https://westberginstitute.org/international-al-faith-community-nursing/.

Westberg Institute: *Philosophy of parish nursing*, 2017. Available from: https://westberginstitute.org/philosophy-of-parish-nursing/.

Williams DR, Sternthal MJ: Spirituality, religion and health: evidence and research directions, *Med J Aust* 186(10 Suppl):S47–S50, 2007.

Wolf ZR: The caring concept and nurse identified caring behaviors, *Topics in Clinical Nursing* 8(2):84–93, 1986.

Wolf ZR, Zuzelo PR, Costello R, et al.: Development and testing of the caring behaviors: inventory for elders, *International Journal of Holistic Care* 8(1):48–54, 2004.

Wright LM: *Spirituality, suffering and illness*, Philadelphia, 2005, FA Davis.

34

Home Health and Hospice

Carrie L. Buch and Mary A. Nies

OBJECTIVES

Upon completion of this chapter, the reader will be able to do the following:

1. Define home health care.
2. Discuss the purpose of home health services.
3. Differentiate between the purpose of a public health nursing visit, a home health nursing visit, and a hospice nursing visit.
4. Use the nursing process in outlining the steps involved in conducting a home visit.
5. Identify the types of home health agencies.
6. Apply the nursing process to a home health client situation.

KEY TERMS

advance directive
durable power of attorney
home health care
living will

Home visits have been an integral part of nursing for more than a century, originating with Florence Nightingale's "health nurses" in England. Following Nightingale's vision, Lillian Wald founded the Henry Street Settlement in 1893. In addition, Wald, the "mother of public health nursing," launched the Visiting Nurse Service of New York, which has become the nation's largest nonprofit home- and community-based health care organization (Ruel, 2014).

Home health care includes a wide range of health care services provided to people in their homes to help them through an illness or injury (Medicare.gov, 2016a). Home health care is typically more affordable than and just as effective as care that people receive in a hospital or skilled nursing facility. In addition, home health care is more convenient for people and their families, as the care they need is brought to them. Examples of home health care services include wound care, education, IV therapy, nutrition therapy, follow-up with a patient after discharge from the hospital, and monitoring of an unstable or chronic illness. The goal of home health care is to help people get better in their own homes to regain as much independence as possible (Medicare.gov, 2016a).

Hospice care focuses on caring for people facing a terminal illness when the goal is no longer curing the disease (National Hospice and Palliative Care Organization [NHPCO], 2016). Most hospice care occurs in the home with support given to clients and their families. The goal of hospice care is that each person will die pain free and with dignity. Ongoing support is provided to the family after the patient dies (NHPCO, 2016)

PURPOSE OF HOME HEALTH SERVICES

The primary purpose of home health services is to provide nursing care to individuals and their families in their homes. The specific objectives and services nurses offer vary according to the type of agency providing services and the population served. Nurses who work for public health departments, visiting nurse associations, home health agencies, hospice agencies, or school districts usually provide home visits. Nurses who make home visits receive referrals from a variety of sources, including the patient's physician, nurse practitioner or nurse midwife, hospital discharge planner or case manager, schoolteacher, and clinic health care provider. The patient or the patient's family can also originate requests for nursing visits to assess and assist in the client's health care.

Nurses from clinics or health departments often conduct home visits as part of patient follow-up. These public health nurses make visits to follow patients with communicable diseases and to provide health education and community referrals to patients with identified health problems. Home health nurses who work for home health agencies that are affiliated with hospitals or nursing registries often make home visits to assist patients in their transition from the hospital to home. In addition, health care providers in private practice may order these visits when patients experience exacerbation of chronic conditions.

The focus of all home visits is on the individual for whom the referral is received. In addition, the nurse assesses the individual–family interaction and provides education and interventions for the family and the client. The nurse evaluates how the individual and family interact as part of an aggregate group in the community. The nurse identifies the need for referrals to community services and performs the referrals as necessary.

Home health care has changed dramatically in the last 20 years in relation to changes in Medicare home health reimbursement. "The Balanced Budget Act of 1997 (BBA) (Public Law 105–33), which was enacted on August 5, 1997, significantly changed the way Medicare pays for home health services" (Department of Health and Human Services [DHHS], 2017, p. 3). Prior to the BBA, home health care agencies (HHAs) were reimbursed using a retrospective payment system for services rendered. HHAs are now reimbursed using the home health prospective payment system (PPS). Under the PPS, HHAs receive a fixed amount of money based on reasonable cost given the client's diagnosis and plan of care. Since the PPS was implemented in 2000, the Centers for Medicare & Medicaid Services (CMS) made revisions in 2008 and 2012. The changes included providing coverage for more diagnosis groups and certain secondary diagnoses, different resource costs depending on the timing of the home health episodes as well as certain wound and skin conditions, and changes to the therapy schedule from a single 10-visit threshold to multiple thresholds to allow for more visits if needed (DHHS, 2017).

Home health care services have changed to address the needs of the population. Home health nurses visit clients of all ages and races. They visit clients who are acutely, chronically, or terminally ill; were recently discharged from the hospital or a rehabilitation facility; need wound care or intravenous therapy; have a feeding tube or tracheostomy; or high-risk pregnant women. Home health care continues to focus on the care of sick patients and is expanding to include health promotion and disease prevention interventions, including client and family education. Currently, most reimbursement for nursing services is based on the patient's need for skilled nursing. On each patient visit, the nurse must document that the care provided is of a skilled nature that requires the knowledge and assessment skills of a nurse and must verify that the patient or a family member could not provide the same level of care.

Services coordinated in the home include not only skilled nursing care provided by registered nurses (RNs), but also the services of physical, occupational, and speech therapists; social workers; and home health aides. The broader home care industry definition of *home health care* includes supportive social services, respite care, community nursing centers, group boarding homes, homeless shelters, adult day care, intermediate-skilled extended care facilities, and assisted living facilities (American Nurses Association [ANA], 2008).

In addition, telephone support services are becoming an increasingly important aspect of home health care (Kelly and Godin, 2014). In telephone support programs, nurses contact clients through regularly scheduled telephone calls to assess how the client is doing, how well they are following the plan of care, and if they need additional support services or a home visit. Telephone support programs are beneficial in improving client outcomes and decreasing hospitalizations (Kelly and Godin, 2014).

TYPES OF HOME HEALTH AGENCIES

Home health agencies differ in financial structure, organizational structure, governing board, and population served. The most common types of home health agencies are official (i.e., public), nonprofit, proprietary, chains, and hospital-based agencies. The number of freestanding proprietary agencies has grown faster than that of any other type of Medicare-certified home health agency. Freestanding proprietary agencies now account for 62% of all home health agencies, and hospital-based agencies for 12% of all certified home health agencies (National Association for Home Care and Hospice [NAHC], 2010).

There continues to be an increase in the number of managed care agencies, which may have any type of financial structure. Managed care agencies contract with payers, such as insurance companies, to provide specified services to the enrolled clients at predetermined prices. Managed care agencies receive payment before offering services and are responsible for taking the financial risk of providing care to patients within the budgeted allotment. This arrangement works well with large numbers of enrolled clients, because the financial risk is spread across a larger number of people, many of whom are healthy and will not require skilled services.

Official Agencies

Local or state governments organize, operate, and fund official (i.e., public) home health agencies. These agencies may be part of a county public health nursing service or a home health agency that operates separately from the public health nursing service but is located within the county public health system. Taxpayers fund official home health agencies, but the agencies also receive reimbursement from third-party payers such as Medicare, Medicaid, and private insurance companies.

Nonprofit Agencies

Nonprofit home health agencies include all home health agencies that are not required to pay federal taxes because of their exempt tax status. Nonprofit groups reinvest any profits into the agencies. Nonprofit home health agencies include independent home health agencies and hospital-based home health agencies. Not all hospital-based home health agencies are nonprofit, even if the hospital is nonprofit. The home health agency can be established as a profit-generating service and serve as a source of revenue for the hospital or medical center. In this situation, the home health agency is categorized organizationally as for-profit and it pays federal taxes on the profits.

Proprietary Agencies

Proprietary home health agencies are classified as for-profit and pay federal taxes on the profits generated. Proprietary agencies can be individually owned agencies, profit partnerships, or profit corporations. Provided that the agencies make profits, investors in corporate proprietary partnerships receive financial returns on their investments in the agencies. A percentage of the profits generated are also reinvested into the agencies. Agencies within chains have a financial advantage over single agencies. The chains have lower administrative costs, because a larger single corporate structure provides many services. For example, a multiagency corporation has greater purchasing power for supplies and equipment because it purchases a larger volume. A single corporate office can provide administrative services such as payroll and employee benefits for all chain employees, thereby avoiding duplication of these services at each location. Criticism of proprietary and chain agencies includes concerns over the quality of services provided by agencies that are profit driven.

Hospital-Based Agencies

Since the implementation of the home health PPS, the number of hospital-based home health agencies has significantly increased (NAHC, 2010). This trend is not surprising in light of the fixed reimbursement under PPS and the hospitals' incentive to decrease patients' length of stay. By establishing home health agencies, hospitals are able to discharge patients who have skilled health care needs, provide the necessary services to the patients, and receive reimbursement through third-party payers such as Medicare, Medicaid, and private insurance companies. The rising number of home health agencies affiliated with hospitals indicates that these agencies are profitable endeavors that provide hospitals with an additional revenue source.

CERTIFIED AND NONCERTIFIED AGENCIES

Certified home health agencies meet federal standards; therefore they are able to receive Medicare payments for services provided to eligible individuals. Not all home health agencies are certified. The noncertified home care agencies, home care aide organizations, and hospices remain outside the Medicare system. Some operate outside the system because they provide non–Medicare-covered services. For example, they do not provide skilled nursing care and are not eligible to receive Medicare reimbursement.

 ACTIVE LEARNING

Contact a local home health agency and interview the agency director. Ask what type of agency it is, the profit status, and whether it is Medicare certified. Report findings to classmates.

SPECIAL HOME HEALTH PROGRAMS

Many home health agencies offer special, high-technology home care services. Offering high-tech services at home is both beneficial to the patient's health and financially advantageous. Through the implementation of these special programs, patients who require continuous skilled care in an acute or skilled nursing institution are able to return to receive care in their homes. From the financial perspective, skilled services provided at home are less costly than hospitalization.

Examples of special services are home intravenous therapy programs for patients who require daily infusions of total parenteral nutrition or antibiotic therapy, pediatric services for children with chronic health problems, follow-up for premature infants who are at risk for complications, ventilator therapy, and home dialysis programs. The key to the success of all these programs is the patient's, family's, or caregiver's ability to learn the care necessary for a successful home program and the motivation of these individuals to provide the care. If family or caregiver support is not available in the home, the patient cannot be a candidate for any of these programs, and other arrangements for care must be found.

Home dialysis programs are a growing trend. Through such programs, patients learn how to do dialysis at home with a helper who is often a family member or friend. Patients and their helpers receive 3 to 8 weeks of training from the dialysis clinic to learn how to use the equipment, monitor their vital signs, and keep good records of their treatment. The clinic provides the machine and all of the supplies and furnishes 24-hour telephone support. The patient follows up at the clinic monthly to ensure that treatments are working and to discuss any issues or concerns (National Kidney and Urologic Diseases Information Clearinghouse [NKUDIC], 2016).

REIMBURSEMENT FOR HOME CARE

Any individual older than 65 years who is homebound, under the care of a physician, and requires medically necessary skilled nursing care or therapy services may be eligible for home care through a Medicare-certified home health agency. These services must be intermittent or part-time and require physician authorization and periodic review of the plan of care. The only exception is hospice care. Any individual older than 65 years who is certified by a physician or a nurse practitioner (NP) to be terminally ill with a life expectancy of 6 months or less is eligible to receive the Medicare Hospice Benefit (DHHS, 2016). There is no requirement for the individual to be homebound or in need of skilled care or for the services to be intermittent or part-time. The hospice physician or hospice NP must recertify the patient after the first 90 days and then every 60 days to determine whether he or she is still eligible for hospice care (DHHS, 2016).

The rapid growth of the home health market is reflective of the following:

- Increasing proportion of people aged 65 years and older
- Lower average cost of home health care compared with institutional costs
- Active insurer support for home care
- Medicare promotion of home health care as an alternative to institutionalization

Patient or family payments comprise 46% of the private financing (12% of total spending) for home health services. Private health insurance and nonpatient revenue pay the remaining private financing. Private health insurance includes managed care plans that often involve preapproval of services and referrals from primary care providers. Private insurance companies require precertification to verify patient eligibility for services. The home care RN speaks to the RN at the insurance company, who determines the number of visits that the insurance company covers. In contrast, for Medicare patients, the home care RN determines the schedule and number of visits without calling Medicare to get preapproval. Medicare pays the home care agency a predetermined amount based on the health condition and needs of the patient. Medicare pays for home care services based on 60-day episodes. If a patient is still eligible for home care services after the first episode, a second episode can begin. There are no limits to the number of episodes for each patient. However, if the patient receives four visits or fewer per episode, the HHA is paid a standardized per-visit amount instead of an episode payment. These payment adjustments are called *low utilization payment adjustments* (CMS, 2016).

Between 1967 and 1985, the number of home health agencies certified to provide care to Medicare recipients tripled, from 1753 to 5983 (NAHC, 2010). In the mid-1980s, this number leveled off at 5900 as a result of an increase in the volume of paperwork required and unreliable payment policies. This led to a lawsuit against the Health Care Financing Administration (HCFA) charged by Representatives Harley Staggers (D-WV) and Claude Pepper (D-FL) and a coalition of members of the U.S. Congress, consumer groups, and the NAHC. The successful conclusion of the lawsuit gave NAHC the opportunity to participate in rewriting the Medicare home care payment policies. New payment policies brought an increase in the home health benefit and increased the number of Medicare-certified home health agencies to more than 10,000. The number is now declining as a direct result of the changes in Medicare home health reimbursement enacted as part of the Balanced Budget Act of 1997. However, because of this decline, the CMS enacted a new payment system whereby home care agencies are reimbursed on a prospective payment system based on the patient's diagnosis. The amount provided to home health agencies is determined on the basis of the average national cost of treating a home health client for 60 days. The goal of this system is to encourage efficient use of home health services without sacrificing quality (NAHC, 2010).

OASIS

The Outcome and Assessment Information Set (OASIS) is a data set that determines Medicare pay rate and measures outcomes for adult home care patients to monitor outcome-based quality improvement (CMS, 2008). The data set includes sociodemographic, environmental, support system, health status, and functional status attributes of adult patients as well as information about service utilization. These items are used to monitor outcomes, plan patient care, provide reports on patient characteristics for each agency, and evaluate and improve clinical performance. Nurses must use OASIS for all patients receiving skilled care that is reimbursed by Medicare and Medicaid (CMS, 2008).

NURSING STANDARDS AND EDUCATIONAL PREPARATION OF HOME HEALTH NURSES

According to the ANA (2008), the generalist home care nurse should be educated at the baccalaureate level because of the autonomy and critical thinking skills that are necessary in home care. The generalist home health nurse must have community health assessment skills to assess client and caregiver needs, provide client and caregiver education, perform nursing actions following the client's plan of care, manage resources to facilitate the best possible outcomes, provide and monitor care, collaborate with other disciplines and providers to coordinate client care, and supervise ancillary staff and caregivers. In home care, the nurse has a primary function of managing an interdisciplinary team that includes physical therapists, occupational therapists, social workers, nurse assistants, chaplains, and so on. In addition, the responsibilities of the generalist home health nurse include, but are not limited to, performing holistic, periodic assessments of client and family/caregiver resources; participating in performance improvement activities; collecting and using research findings to evaluate the plan of care; educating clients and families on health promotion and self-care activities; being a client advocate; promoting continuity of care; using the *Scope and Standards of Home Health Nursing Practice* to guide clinical practice; and identifying ethical issues and exploring options with the necessary individuals and staff members to achieve resolution (ANA, 2008).

In addition to the ANA standards, home health nurses should use the competencies developed by the QSEN (Quality and Safety Education for Nurses) Institute as a guide for best practices in home care (QSEN Institute, 2014). The QSEN competencies were developed by a national advisory board that included distinguished faculty to establish effective teaching approaches to ensure that nurses graduate with essential competencies in (1) patient-centered care, (2) teamwork and collaboration, (3) evidence-based practice, (4) quality improvement, (5) safety, and (6) informatics. These six competencies in QSEN are being used by several health care institutions to monitor and ensure that their nurses are providing safe, high-quality patient care (QSEN Institute, 2014).

The advanced practice home health nurse has a master's or doctoral degree in nursing and can perform all of the duties of the generalist home health nurse (ANA, 2008). In addition, the advanced practice nurse contributes significant clinical expertise to home health patients and their families; demonstrates proficiency in care management and consultation; and is an expert in implementing and evaluating health programs, resources, services, and research for clients with complex conditions. The duties of the advanced practice home health nurse include, but are not limited to, prescribing pharmacological and nonpharmacological treatment to manage chronic illnesses, providing consultation and serving as a resource to the generalist home health nurse, participating at all levels of quality improvement and research, educating all members of the health care team about emerging trends in home health care, performing direct care of the client and family, managing and evaluating the care the client is receiving from caregivers, monitoring trends in reimbursement for home health services, consulting with staff about any ethical issues that may arise, managing an interdisciplinary team, and disseminating practice and research findings to colleagues (ANA, 2008).

Albrecht's conceptual model (1990) for home care clearly identifies educational content areas for students in undergraduate and graduate nursing programs that have specialties in home health care. An underlying premise of the model is that professional satisfaction and effective patient outcomes depend on the education and experience of the home health nurse. Implications that are apparent in the model include the following (Albrecht, 1990, p. 125):

- Nursing programs at the undergraduate and graduate levels must prepare competent providers of home health care.
- Curricula must include concepts related to the suprasystem, health service delivery system, and home subsystem, which includes structural, process, and outcome elements.
- Students at the undergraduate level need at least one clinical observation or experience in a home care agency.
- Graduate-level students need specific courses that cover concepts present in the model, including knowledge of education; preventive, supportive, therapeutic, and high-tech nursing interventions for home health care; a multidisciplinary

approach to home health care; health law and ethics; systems theory; economics covering supply, demand, and productivity; and case management and coordination.

The home health nurse serves as a case manager for patients who receive care either from the staff of the home health agency or through contract services. The success of the case management plan is contingent upon the nurse's ability to use the nursing process to develop a plan of treatment that best fits the individual needs of the patient and the patient's family or caregiver. Patient and family assessment is the first step in developing the treatment plan and nursing care plan.

The Albrecht nursing model for home health care provides a framework for nurses, patients, and their families to interact and identify mutual goals of interventions and promote the patient's self-care capability at home (Fig. 34.1) (Albrecht, 1990). Three major elements for measuring the quality of home health care patient outcomes are structural, process, and outcome elements.

Structural elements include the client, family, provider agency, health team, and professional nurse. The process elements include the type of care, coordination of care, and intervention. Outcome elements consist of patient and family satisfaction with care, quality of care, cost-effectiveness of care, health status, and self-care capability.

In the Albrecht model for home care, the relationship between the structural elements and the process elements directs the interventions. The nurse executes the nursing process, including assessment, nursing diagnosis, planning, intervention, and evaluation, and then the nurse coordinates patient care (Albrecht, 1990).

CONDUCTING A HOME VISIT

Visit Preparation

It is important that the nurse prepare for the home visit by reviewing the referral form, which should furnish the purpose of the visit, the geographic residence of the family, and any other pertinent information. The first home visit gives the nurse the opportunity to establish a trust relationship with the client and family to establish credibility as a resource for health information and community referrals in a nonthreatening environment.

The Referral

The referral is a formal request for a home visit. Referrals come from a variety of sources, including hospitals, clinics, health care providers, individuals, and families. The type of agency that receives the referral varies, depending on the necessary client services. Home health referrals are requested to provide clients with short-term, intermittent, skilled services and rehabilitation. Visits can last from 30 to 90 minutes and are scheduled on an intermittent basis according to the specific needs of the client. For example, a client who had a stroke requires skilled nursing assessments, physical therapy visits for gait training, speech therapy for speech deficit improvement, and occupational therapy for retraining in activities of daily living (ADLs) such as bathing and cooking.

By reviewing the referral form before the first visit, the community health nurse (CHN) obtains basic information about

FIG. 34.1 Albrecht nursing model for home health care. (Based on Albrecht MN: The Albrecht model for home health care: implications for research, practice, and education. *Public Health Nurs* 7:118–126, 1990. Reprinted by permission of Blackwell Scientific Publications, Inc.)

the client, such as name, age, diagnosis or health status, address, telephone number, insurance coverage, and reason for the referral. The form also specifies the source of the referral—clinician, health care provider, communicable disease service, hospital, client, or client's family. Additional information provided in the home health referral includes current client medications, prescribed diet, physician's orders, care plan goals, and other disciplines involved in the client's care. This information is important because it helps the nurse become familiar with the client's condition.

Public health referrals are made for clients who are in need of health education (e.g., infant care education and resource allocation) or for follow-up of clients with communicable diseases.

Public health referrals usually provide information on the client's condition that necessitates public health nurse (PHN) visits. For example, for a client who is positive for tuberculosis (TB), the PHN is notified of the client's place of residence, type and location of employment, and any known contacts, including family and friends. Another example of a public health referral is one to a 16-year-old girl for antepartum visits because she is 7 months' pregnant and has just initiated prenatal care.

Initial Telephone Contact

The nurse contacts the client and informs him or her about the service referral. The first telephone contact with the client or family consists of an exchange of essential information, including an introduction by the nurse, identification of the agency that received the referral, and the purpose of the visit. After the initial exchange of information, the nurse informs the client of his or her desire to make the home visit, the client gives permission, and the group sets a mutually acceptable time for the visit. The nurse is a guest in the client's home; therefore it is important that the client agrees to the visit. The nurse then verifies the client's address and asks for specific directions to the client's home.

During a home health visit, the nurse requests proof of insurance, such as a Medicare, Medicaid, health maintenance organization membership identification, or insurance card. The nurse should forewarn the client so the client or family can locate the information before the visit. If the client is unable to provide this verification, the nurse assists with locating the information during the visit. Clients who receive a public health home visit do not require evidence of insurance coverage because these services are not billed directly. County public health budgets or state or federally funded programs generally cover these visits.

Not all clients have telephones. For a client without one, the nurse should check the referral for a telephone number where messages can be left. It is also worthwhile to contact the health care provider who made the referral to see whether the telephone number was omitted unintentionally. If the client does not have a telephone, the nurse may choose to make a drop-in visit. This type of visit consists of an unannounced visit to the client's home, during which the nurse explains the purpose of the referral, receives the client's permission for the visit, and appoints a time for a future visit with the client. The client may agree to have the first visit while the nurse is there.

If the client is not at home for the drop-in visit, the nurse should leave an official agency card and a brief message asking the client to contact the agency to schedule a nursing visit. The nurse informs the referring agency that the visit was attempted but that the client was not available for contact. A formal agency letter, identifying the agency and the reason for the referral, is often sent to clients who are difficult to contact. The nurse's primary responsibility, when he or she has been unsuccessful in locating the client, is to keep the clinic, physician, or referring agency informed of efforts to establish contact with the client.

Environment

An environmental assessment begins as the nurse leaves the agency and travels to the client's home. While driving, the nurse should observe the area surrounding the client's home. The nurse should look for the location of grocery stores, drug stores, gas stations, etc., in relation to the client's home. The nurse should observe the condition of the client's home as well as the surrounding neighborhood. In addition, the nurse should note the client's dwelling; for example, whether the client lives in a single-family home, in a single room in a home or hotel, in an apartment, or in a shared apartment or house.

Upon arrival to the client's home, the nurse should note the accessibility of the home relative to the client's condition such as stairs, railings, handicapped facilities, lighting, etc. In addition, the nurse should note potential trip hazards, including uneven pavement, cracked cement, small rocks, etc. The nurse should also observe potential safety concerns, such as the client lives alone, the neighborhood has a high crime rate, the building or home is not secure, trip hazards inside the home (such as rugs, clutter on the floor), unclean environment, etc. It is also important for the nurse to note if the client's home has hot running water, heat, sanitation facilities, and adequate ventilation. The nurse should also observe if the client has food in the home and should make note of the client's primary caregiver and support system.

Improving Communication

When the nurse meets with the client, whether in the home or at another mutually agreeable location, the initial conversation revolves around social topics. The nurse assumes a friendly manner and asks general questions about the client, the client's family, and health care services that will benefit the client. These questions help the nurse assess the client's needs and create a comfortable atmosphere for communication.

Building Trust

Many clients in need of nursing visits do not trust the health care system and are uncomfortable with the representative from an agency visiting their home. For example, a client who is pregnant and does not have legal status in the United States will be hesitant to allow a nurse to visit; the client will be afraid of being reported to immigration authorities. The nurse's role in visiting this client is to focus on the health and safety of the client and her fetus. The nurse must build a trust relationship early in the visit or the client will not allow additional visits. If a trust relationship is not established and the client believes that the nurse will report her to immigration authorities, it is highly probable that the client will move to another location to avoid future contact.

DOCUMENTATION OF HOME CARE

Many home health nurses would probably identify documentation issues as the most frustrating part of providing home health care. The nurse documents assessment data and interventions for all home visits. The patient record also contains a copy of the nursing care plan. "A patient MUST meet these Conditions of Participation to qualify for home health care: 1) confined to home, 2) under the care of a physician, 3) receiving services under a plan of care established and reviewed by a physician, and 4) need of skilled nursing care on an intermittent basis" (Acello and Brown, 2015, p. 8). It is critical that the nurse document that the patient meets all of these criteria at each visit.

Medicare holds a prominent position as a home health care payer; therefore the HCFA's regulations determine the home health industry's documentation. Correct and accurate completion of required Medicare forms is the key to reimbursement. For more information, the reader should visit http://www.cms.gov/Medicare/CMS-Forms/CMS-Forms/CMS-Forms-List.html. Payment or denial of payment for visits is based on the information presented on the forms. If the nurse does not clearly document the provided skilled care in the electronic nursing notes, the fiscal intermediaries will argue that the care was either unnecessary or not performed and will deny reimbursement. The home health nurse must have an excellent clinical foundation and the ability to identify and document actual and potential patient problems that require skilled nursing interventions (Acello and Brown, 2015).

Documenting the care provided to record the patient's quality of care is just as important as documenting for reimbursement purposes. The documentation of home visits records the nurse's observations, assessments of the patient's condition, provided interventions, and the patient's and family's ability to manage the care at home. In addition, documentation of patient visits serves as a formal communication system among other home health professionals who also interact with the patient and family.

APPLICATION OF THE NURSING PROCESS

Assessment

During the first home visit, the type of client assessment will vary depending on the purpose of the home visit. The home health nurse assesses the client's knowledge of his or her health status. The nurse identifies knowledge deficits and uses this information to develop a care plan.

Subjective information is obtained from the client and the client's family and includes the client's perception of the situation and what the client identifies as problems. The nurse assesses whether the client is isolated from others physically or socially and whether the client is a member of a close-knit, nurturing, supportive family or kinship network. The amount of support the client perceives as available may or may not be accurate; therefore the nurse asks several questions about the client's family, friends, and daily routine to assess the client's level of social support.

During the first home visit, the home health nurse assesses the client's health knowledge; his or her physical, functional, and psychosocial status; physical environment; and social support. The nurse collects information through observations and questions the patient and family or caregivers in the home environment. It is not unusual to find inconsistencies between information the patient provides during hospitalization about the amount of physical and emotional support available to the patient in the home and the amount of help actually available to the patient in the home. The nurse validates or modifies the referral information to reflect the actual home situation. Home health nurses often use contracts that the nurse, patient, and family jointly develop to delineate the responsibilities of the patient in the home.

The client's physical assessment is generally performed in the home health visit and includes a review of all systems, with an emphasis on the systems affected by the client's present condition. The nurse obtains objective data through the use of essential physical assessment skills such as observation, palpation, auscultation, and percussion. The physical assessment also includes information regarding the client's functional status. Assessment of the functional status is important for Medicare reimbursement and for the development of an individualized plan of care. This assessment includes information regarding the client's ability to ambulate, to perform ADLs independently, and to use an assistive device such as a cane or wheelchair. Specific functional limitations, such as shortness of breath and muscle weakness, are assessed at this time.

Information obtained during the assessment phase is used to identify nursing diagnoses and develop a plan of care. Data collection continues while the patient receives home health services. Changes in the patient's condition, environment, or social structure necessitate modifications in the treatment plan and the nursing care plan.

There are differences between the treatment plan and the nursing care plan. The plan of treatment includes the type of home health services received, the projected frequency of visits by each discipline, and the necessary interventions (Medicare.gov, 2016b). The nursing care plan addresses specific nursing interventions designed to treat the patient's actual or potential problems and includes identified goals with measurable outcomes.

Diagnosis and Planning

Develop a Plan for the Client and Family

After the assessment phase of the home visit, the nurse identifies the nursing diagnoses that address the patient's problems and identifies actual or potential problems. The identification of nursing diagnoses serves as the basis for the nursing care plan. This plan is developed in consultation with the client and the family. The plan identifies short-term and long-term goals and measurable outcomes for the patient. Goals are identified that the client is willing to work toward with the nurse's assistance. The plan identifies nursing interventions that are necessary and additional home health services that are appropriate to help the patient achieve the identified goals. To maximize the plan's success, it is important that the patient and family are involved in the planning process and that they access community resources. Planning is a dynamic process that continues while the patient receives nursing services. The plan is modified as needed, depending on the patient's condition, until the identified goals are met.

Outline the Client and Family Roles

The goal of home visits for both public health and home health nursing is to involve the client and family in taking an active role in health promotion. The nurse is careful not to allow the client to become dependent on the nurse's interventions, because the nurse's involvement is short term. The nurse leaves a written copy of the plan of care with the client as a reminder for the client and family of their role as well as the nurse's role in the plan of care.

Intervention

Implementation of the plan of care begins during the first home visit. The nurse begins to provide the client and family with health information concerning the client's health status and informs them about the availability of and access to community resources. In the case of the home health visit, the nurse provides skilled nursing care. At the end of the initial home visit, the nurse discusses the need for another home visit. The nurse and client discuss the goal of the next visit; specifically, they discuss what the client should do before the visit. The nurse informs the client and family about any information or skills he or she will provide during the next visit, and the nurse and client agree on a day for the next visit.

Referral for Community Services

During the first visit, the nurse provides the client and family with information regarding community resources, including the purpose of the resources, their eligibility for the services provided, any involved expense, and agency telephone numbers. Referrals depend on the availability of community resources, the client's eligibility for the services, the client's and the family's willingness to use the services, and the resources' suitability for the client and family. Examples of such services are immunization clinics for children in the family; adult day care or senior centers for elderly clients who could benefit from socialization; adult education classes or continuation of high school for pregnant teen clients who have dropped out of high school; Meals on Wheels (MOW) services for clients who are not able to prepare meals; homeless shelters for men, women, and families; soup kitchens; resources for clothing and housing; mental health clinics; resources for battered spouses; and primary care clinics for low-income clients with and without insurance.

If necessary, the client or client's family may request the nurse's assistance in contacting the community resources. The client and family are encouraged to make the contacts, but if the client and family are unable to make the calls or do not speak English, the nurse needs to intervene on behalf of the client. By providing referral information during the first home visit, the nurse can follow up on the client's or the family's success in contacting and using community services.

Terminating the Visit

The nurse terminates the first visit when the assessment is completed and a care plan has been established with the client. The average visit should not exceed 1 hour. The client receives a great deal of information during that hour, and the nurse collects a great deal of information. Most clients are tired at the end of a 1-hour visit and often cannot retain additional information. It is preferable to set a date for another home visit to reinforce the information provided and to work progressively toward achieving goals.

Evaluation

Evaluation of Progress toward Goals

The evaluation phase occurs when the nurse can determine whether the mutually established goals are realistic and achievable for the patient and the patient's family. The evaluation process is continuous and allows the nurse to determine the success or progress toward the patient's identified goals. The nurse can identify the need for revisions in the nursing care plan and treatment plan through the collection of additional data during the evaluation phase. The nurse can intervene to make necessary changes. An example is an elderly wife who, during the initial home visit, stated that she preferred to provide the physical care for her frail, nonambulatory husband. On a subsequent visit, the nurse assessed that the patient was not receiving the care required for the patient's personal care, specifically bathing. The nurse discussed the problem with the wife and presented her with available options. These included the services of a home health aide to provide personal care and bathing three times a week. A new plan was developed, and it included the home health aide. The plan was implemented and evaluated during future visits. Input from the client is critical to determine whether the goals established are realistic and achievable for the client.

Modification of the Plan as Needed

The evaluation process also allows the nurse and client or family to discuss what is working well and where modifications are necessary in the plan. Evaluation occurs through open communication between the nurse and client, and the nurse asks questions about specific parts of the care plan. If a trust relationship exists, the client feels comfortable telling the nurse about problems in the care plan.

When Goals Are Achieved

The overall purpose of home visits is to assist the client with necessary information and nursing care to enable the client to function successfully without nursing interventions. When the plan-of-care goals are achieved, the client does not need the nurse any longer. The client knows what community resources are available and how to access health care services for primary, secondary, and tertiary interventions.

Formal and Informal Caregivers

Formal caregivers include professionals and paraprofessionals who provide in-home health care and personal services. They are compensated for the services they provide. The largest number of employees consists of home care aides and RNs. Informal caregivers are family members who are caring for the client. The presence or absence of an involved family member can make the difference between the successful completion of the plan of treatment, with the patient remaining in the home, and the need to transfer the patient to an extended-care facility or board-and-care facility. When a capable family member or caregiver is available to assist the patient, the home health nurse spends much of the visit assessing the skills of the caregiver. The home health nurse instructs the caregiver in the correct procedures for providing care and in recognizing the signs and symptoms of problems that must be reported to the health care provider. The goal of the home health nurse's instruction is to provide the caregiver with the skills necessary to care for the patient successfully in the home without intervention of the nurse or other members of the home health team.

The home health nurse faces a special challenge with patients who lack a family member or caregiver capable of learning and providing necessary care. When the patient lives alone and does not have caregivers, the nurse explores other resources available to supplement the patient's self-care activities in the home. For example, if the patient has extensive physical care needs and sufficient financial resources, the nurse may suggest hiring an attendant. Medicare and private insurance companies do not pay for attendant care. If the patient's income is low enough, in-home county support services may be an option. The nurse may consider other services for the patient, such as MOW for nutritious meals delivered to the patient's home. Friendly Visitors, a volunteer service, sends a volunteer to the patient's home once a week or more to provide socialization for the patient. Other options that are available in some communities are adult day health centers and senior service centers. Both of these options require arranged patient transportation to and from the centers. A variety of transportation methods are available in different communities; volunteers may transport patients to the centers, or public transportation systems may be available, such as minivans, that provide door-to-door service. Selected services and referrals are based on the patient's individual needs and on the patient's level of functional ability.

ETHICAL INSIGHTS
Home Health and Hospice Care

- Most legal and ethical issues in home health care involve the care of terminally ill patients.
- Early education about these issues is essential to the prevention of problems.
- Early education also gives patients the opportunity to make decisions for themselves and to communicate those decisions to family members and health care providers.

Continued

Home Health and Hospice Care

- All competent adults have the right to make decisions that will direct health care providers in the type of care they administer.
- This communication can occur through the completion of advance directives, durable power of attorney for health care, and living wills.

Advance Directive

An **advance directive** is a written document in which a competent person gives instructions about future health care in the event that the individual is unable to make decisions. These directives are completed on a voluntary basis. Medicare-certified health care agencies must ask patients about advance directives and must provide the patient with the advance directive form if the patient is interested in completing it.

Durable Power of Attorney for Health Care

A **durable power of attorney** for health care is one type of advance directive. Also called a *health care proxy*, the durable power of attorney for health care gives another person the power to make medical decisions related to care of the patient. This person, as identified by the patient, acts as the patient's agent in all decisions regarding health care, personal care, and custody in the event that the patient becomes incompetent or disabled and is unable to make decisions.

Living Will

A **living will** is a written document in which a patient voluntarily informs doctors and family members about the type of medical care desired should the patient become terminally ill or permanently unconscious and unable to communicate. In the living will, the patient can describe the type of care desired, depending on the clinical situation. For example, if the patient is terminally ill and unconscious, the patient can direct the health care team to perform only those measures that will provide comfort and nothing further. The patient can specifically indicate his or her opposition to lifesaving measures; for example, the patient may request the denial of cardiopulmonary life support in the event of a cardiac arrest. Other examples are indicating the exclusion of chemotherapy, blood transfusions, and respirator use in an attempt to prolong life.

HOSPICE HOME CARE

Hospice and palliative nursing care is becoming increasingly important, as there is a tremendous need to improve end-of-life care for the terminally ill. Nurses who work with the terminally ill seek to enhance the patient's quality of life by focusing on relieving suffering throughout the illness, supporting the patient and family through the dying process, and providing grief support to the family after the patient has died (ANA, 2007). Hospice and palliative care nurses have a holistic approach to their patients and are responsible for taking a comprehensive health history and physical examination, including an evaluation of mental status; evaluating functional abilities; performing appropriate laboratory and diagnostic studies; determining effective pharmacological and nonpharmacological therapies to manage symptoms; identifying patient and/or family/caregiver goals; providing culturally competent care that is consistent with the patient's health beliefs, values, and practices; evaluating the patient's emotional state and the response to his or her illness and impending death; identifying coping strategies and support systems; evaluating financial resources; and conducting a spiritual assessment (ANA, 2007).

The advanced practice hospice and palliative nurse is an important role for nurses with a master's degree or higher in nursing (ANA, 2007). The advanced practice hospice and palliative nurse functions as an expert clinician who performs the duties of the generalist hospice nurse in addition to assuming the responsibilities of advanced-level care, which may include prescribing pharmacological treatment to manage symptoms. It is recommended that all advanced practice hospice and palliative nurses obtain certification in advanced practice hospice and palliative nursing (ANA, 2007).

Patients are admitted into hospice care when they have a life expectancy of 6 months or less, and the focus of care shifts from curative to comfort care. However, many patients with terminal illnesses want to continue curative treatments and are not ready to be admitted into a hospice program. Those patients who do not have a life expectancy of 6 months or less and/or want to continue curative treatment can receive the benefits of palliative care. Palliative care focuses on symptom management while the patient is still receiving other treatments, such as chemotherapy. It is important to note that Medicare fully covers all hospice-related expenses, including medications, related to the terminal diagnosis. However, Medicare does not cover any expenses, including medications, related to other diagnoses.

Hospice and palliative nursing care is provided in a variety of settings, including hospitals, nursing homes, residential homes, and palliative care clinics. For the patient receiving hospice services in the home, the goal is to keep the client as comfortable at home as long as possible and to provide support and instruction to caregivers. Some patients stay home until they die, and for others their caregivers decide whether they should remain at home or be admitted to an extended-care facility or a hospital. Each family unit has different needs, and each must be supported in its decisions. Home death should not be the standard that determines excellence in any case, nor should home death be the ultimate measure of "successful" home care. It is vital to realize that caring for a terminally ill person also includes caring for the family or caregivers. Not all caregivers want their loved one to die at home, and not all caregivers are capable of allowing that to happen. The goal of having a home death must be the goal of the patient and family, regardless of the nurse's personal preference.

When caring for a terminally ill person at home, the hospice nurse must be skilled in physical and psychosocial care for both the patient and the caregiver. The patient is viewed as a whole person, not as an isolated disease. Caring for a terminally ill person at home demands that the nurse view the family system as a unit. In addition, it is important to note that hospice care is a team approach. Each patient has a physician, a nurse, a social worker, a nurse assistant, and a spiritual counselor to provide a multidisciplinary, holistic approach to caring for that patient and his or her family. The team coordinates care with each other and additional resources, such as pain management, as necessary. Furthermore, many hospice agencies have weekly interdisciplinary meetings in which the various members of the hospice team meet to discuss the patients and work together to resolve issues and make sure the patients are receiving the best possible care.

Caring for the Caregiver

Although the dying patient is the focus of all skilled nursing care, the experienced home care nurse knows that a careful assessment of the caregiver's mental and physical health is important. The spouse, lover, children, friends, and neighbors who have made the commitment to stay until the end need the nurse's time and attention as much as, if not more than, the patient. Although the patient's wishes are important, all decisions regarding care are made considering the health of the caregivers. Camak (2015) found that caregivers are at increased risk for developing mental and physical health problems. Caregiver burden is a significant concern; therefore nursing interventions must be directed toward preventing a decline in the caregiver's health.

Caregivers need reassurance that their judgment is sound, and they need reminders that they cannot do anything "wrong" if it is done for the patient's comfort. The caregivers must understand that they will not mistakenly overdose the patient, and they must be reminded repeatedly that the patient will not die from something they did or did not do. Caring for the terminally ill requires that the home care nurse is willing to nurse the entire family. In addition, the nurse must involve all members of the hospice team to ensure that the caregivers receive the care they need.

Pain Control and Symptom Management

Pain control is an important goal for hospice nurses and their patients. Hospice nurses perform regular pain assessments that involve asking patients the following questions about their pain: (1) history; (2) character (such as sharp, dull, aching); (3) severity or intensity, which is most commonly rated on a pain intensity scale from 0 to 10 with 0 being no pain and 10 being the worst pain imaginable; (4) location; (5) effects on quality of life; (6) precipitating factors; and (7) relieving factors (Norlander, 2008). It is vital that the hospice nurse not only performs regular pain assessments but also remembers that pain is highly subjective and every person experiences pain differently and uniquely; therefore the patient's pain is whatever he or she says it is, regardless of the nurse's objective evaluation of the situation.

Pain medication is administered in doses sufficient to keep the patient free of pain and is administered on a regular schedule to prevent pain from recurring before the next dose. Hospice methods of pain control are particularly well suited to home care. The vast majority of patients can be pain free until their deaths. The key to successful pain control for the terminally ill is to persuade patients to take their medications on a regular basis, not just when they "can't stand it any longer." Generally, these medications are long acting and are administered every 8 to 12 hours. In addition, patients have fast-acting pain medications to take for "breakthrough pain," which happens when the patient experiences an increase in pain before it is time for the next dose of scheduled pain medication. The fast-acting medications are generally administered every 1 to 2 hours as needed.

Many patients, especially the elderly, are afraid of becoming "junkies" or "druggies" and want to delay using pain medication until they "get really bad." Many people believe that using these medications signals "the end of the line," and they are amazed to learn that patients do well while receiving such agents for months, even years, before death occurs. Almost every family must learn that addiction is not the same as tolerance and that their physicians will not "cut off the supply" if they "take too much."

In addition to pain control, hospice nurses help in managing other symptoms such as nausea and vomiting, constipation, diarrhea, fatigue, and decreased appetite. Nurses assist patients in management of these symptoms through medications and/or strategies to help cope with the symptoms. Strategies include such things as increasing fluids to prevent constipation, frequent rest periods to minimize fatigue, and eating small amounts as desired to cope with the decrease in appetite. In addition, the nurse educates the patient and family that some of these symptoms, such as fatigue and decreased appetite, are related to the dying process and are signs that the patient is declining.

Furthermore, the nurse, along with other members of the hospice team, provides emotional support to patients and families as they adjust to the patient's impending death. The nurse educates the patient and family about what physical symptoms the patient will most likely experience as he or she approaches death. In addition, the nurse, along with the social worker and spiritual counselor, provides emotional support and helps the patient and family work through any anxiety or fears they have about dying. Finally, the nurse is there to support the family immediately after the patient dies, and hospice provides bereavement support to families up to a year after the patient's death.

Cultural Differences Related to Death and Dying

When caring for patients and their families in hospice, the nurse must remember that beliefs, attitudes, and values about death, dying, grief, and loss are influenced by society and culture (Cancer.net, 2015). However, these societal and cultural influences are often difficult to recognize. Furthermore, many individual differences within a cultural group, such as spirituality, age, and gender, affect a person's interpretation about the meaning of death. Although there are these individual differences, some general characteristics regarding death and dying are common to people of a certain cultural group. It is important to understand some of these differences to provide culturally sensitive care and ensure a peaceful and dignified death.

For example, among African Americans, health status should be reported to the eldest family member, spouse, or parents, and there is often open and public displays of emotion, although this possibility varies from person to person. African Americans generally care for dying elders at home until death is imminent and then they bring their loved one to the hospital, because some believe that death in the house brings bad luck. Among Mexican Americans, the extended family takes care of the sick and dying person, and there are often several family members present at the same time. In general, Mexican Americans prefer to die at home because the hospital environment may be too restrictive in meeting the needs of the extended family and because some believe that their spirit may get "lost" if they die at the hospital. In comparison, among American Indians, some tribes prefer to remain close to the dying person, but other tribes avoid contact with the dying. Similarly, those tribes that prefer to avoid contact may prefer that their loved one dies in the hospital, whereas those tribes that prefer to remain close may prefer to have the person die at home.

These are just some examples of cultural characteristics that influence death and dying beliefs and practices. It is important to understand and respect the differing values and beliefs of patients and their families. Furthermore, it is essential to ask patients and/or families about their beliefs and practices to avoid overgeneralizations and to ensure that nursing care is patient centered and culturally sensitive.

ACTIVE LEARNING

1. Make arrangements to accompany a PHN, a home health nurse, and/or a hospice nurse on home visits.
2. Interview a PHN about the types of client referrals received, and ask what interventions are usually performed. Repeat this activity with a home health nurse and a hospice nurse. Ask the nurses what they like best about their jobs.
3. Attend a team meeting in a home health agency or a hospice program to see how the roles of the various team members blend together to provide family-centered care.
4. Interview a PHN and a home health nurse, and ask how the community affects the care they provide.

CASE STUDY Public Health Visit

Communicable Disease Follow-Up

The PHN received a referral from the county hospital to see Ray, a 57-year-old white man with newly diagnosed TB. The first purpose of the referral was for the PHN to meet with the client to ensure that he received the appropriate information about TB and received follow-up medical care on a regular basis. The second purpose of the referral was for the PHN to meet with Ray and identify the people with whom he had been in close contact. The nurse then established contact with these people, notified them that they had been exposed to TB, and encouraged them to have follow-up tests for TB.

The nurse contacted Ray and established a time for the home visit. The nurse noted that he resided in a residential hotel in a lower-middle-class neighborhood of a large urban area. During the initial visit, the nurse discovered that the client was an unemployed construction worker. He did not know where he might have contracted TB. Ray assured the nurse that he was taking his medication as directed. He gave the nurse the names of the friends he played poker with every week at a hotel and told the nurse that he advised his friends to be tested for TB. The nurse made a note of the names and later talked with them individually by telephone. During these subsequent conversations, the nurse was very careful to maintain the client's confidentiality. The nurse informed these individuals that they could have been exposed to TB and that they should seek testing through their health care providers or through their local health department.

Ray indicated that he did not have family and he had minimal contact with other people besides his friends at the hotel. The nurse recorded this information on the communicable disease form and returned the information to the public health department's communicable disease division.

Assessment

The PHN's assessment of the client with a communicable disease involved the individual, family, and community. The PHN assessed whether the client received appropriate information and regular medical care for TB and whether the client followed the prescribed treatment regimen.

Although Ray stated that he did not have family, his friends in the hotel constituted a working support network. The PHN knows that the client's support network is whomever the client identifies. Nursing assessment of Ray's support network involved determining whether the members were tested for TB. In addition, the PHN assessed the client's network for the following:

- Network composition
- Network's knowledge of TB
- Functional capacity
- Network stressors
- Network strengths and weaknesses
- Network's ability to provide support for Ray
- Health beliefs and practices
- Use of health services

The PHN was aware that the number of new cases of TB in the community had increased over the past 12 months. The PHN further noted that there was an increase in the number of area residents immigrating from various developing countries and that this population might be at increased risk for development of TB.

Diagnosis
Individual
Lack of awareness regarding the disease process and transmission of TB

Family
Lack of awareness regarding the disease process and transmission of TB, location of communicable disease clinics, and the importance of screening those exposed to TB

Community
Potential for development of TB among community residents, indicated by an increased incidence of new cases of TB over the past 12 months

Planning
A plan of care is established with mutually agreed-upon goals based on the nurse's assessment of the individual, family, and community.

Individual
Long-Term Goal
- Client will perform self-care activities related to treatment of TB and follow up as necessary with appropriate health care professionals.

Short-Term Goal
- Client will verbalize knowledge of transmission of TB; signs and symptoms of complications of TB; purpose, administration schedule, and side effects of medications.

Family
Long-Term Goal
Support network members with positive test results will receive appropriate treatment

Short-Term Goal
Support network members will demonstrate basic knowledge of cause and transmission of TB and will agree to be tested for TB.

Community
Long-Term Goal
Incidence of TB in the community will decrease over the next 3 years.

continued

CASE STUDY   Public Health Visit—cont'd

Communicable Disease Follow-Up

Short-Term Goal

Community members will demonstrate knowledge of increased incidence of TB in their community and of available community resources for treatment and prevention of TB.

Intervention

Implementation of the plan of care for the client with TB occurs at the individual, family, and community levels.

Individual

The PHN referred Ray to the communicable disease clinic at the local health department. TB is a reportable communicable disease; therefore the PHN obtained information from the client regarding people with whom he had been in close contact.

Family

The PHN contacted members of Ray's support network and referred them to the communicable disease clinic as appropriate. The nurse provided these people with information concerning TB transmission and the importance of early treatment and follow-up.

Community

The PHN met with professionals from the communicable disease clinic and the health department and with members of the community to establish a program to raise public awareness about the increased incidence of TB in the community. The public was informed about the importance of preventive measures, the availability of community screening services for TB, and the existing health care resources in the community.

Evaluation
Individual

The client's knowledge of the disease process, transmission, treatment, and signs and symptoms of TB is an indicator in evaluating the care plan. Confirmation of the client's follow-up with the communicable disease clinic can also be used for evaluation.

Family

The support network's knowledge of the disease process, transmission, treatment, and signs and symptoms of TB is an indicator in evaluating the care plan. Confirmation of the support network's follow-up with the communicable disease clinic can also be used for evaluation.

Community

The incidence rate of TB in the community and the rate at which TB clinics and related resources are used are measures that can be used to evaluate the effectiveness of interventions at the aggregate level.

Levels of Prevention

The PHN is actively involved in all three levels of prevention through education programs, early detection programs, and appropriate referrals for patients with TB. Examples of each of these levels of prevention are as follows:

Primary

Goal: Prevention of specific disease occurrence such as TB.
- Development of programs that increase public awareness of the disease process and of the transmission, diagnosis, and treatment of TB.

Secondary

Goal: Early detection of existing conditions.
- Tuberculin skin testing and subsequent follow-up of positive test results.

Tertiary

Goal: To reduce the effects and spread of TB.
- Referral for early, effective treatment and education of clients for self-care.

CASE STUDY

Public Health Home Visit: Antepartum Client

The PHN received a referral to see a 17-year-old African American woman named Ali, who was referred by the county prenatal clinic. Ali was 5 months pregnant with her third pregnancy within the past year. Ali miscarried the previous two pregnancies during the first trimester.

When the nurse made the home visit, she noted that Ali was 5 feet 9 inches tall and weighed 120 lb. She resided in a two-room apartment with her boyfriend, who was the father of the baby. The nurse began the first visit with social talk, asking Ali general questions about her employment, education, and the duration of her residence in the area. Ali appeared to be pleased that the nurse was interested in her. Once a trusting relationship was initiated, the nurse asked Ali how she felt about the pregnancy. Ali revealed that she was happy about the pregnancy but was worried that there would be problems because she had had two previous miscarriages. She had not planned any of the pregnancies, but she did not use contraceptives to prevent the pregnancies either. Ali's boyfriend worked and was able to pay the rent and buy food for her. Ali dropped out of high school during her junior year, but she wanted to complete her high school education. She had Medicaid coverage for her health care.

During the initial home visit, the nurse assessed that Ali was underweight and had several knowledge deficits in the areas of prenatal nutrition, infant care, breastfeeding, and contraception. The nurse also identified the need for a referral to the public school for the continuation of Ali's high school education. The nurse briefly discussed her assessment with Ali in a nonthreatening, nonjudgmental manner. The nurse informed Ali that, if she was interested, she could schedule future home visits to provide Ali with more information and answer her questions. Ali agreed to receive future visits to discuss the topics the nurse identified during the assessment phase. They mutually agreed upon the plan for future visits. As the visits progressed, the nurse and Ali modified the plan on the basis of progress evaluation.

The nurse terminated home visits with Ali when the mutually established goals were achieved. The nurse scheduled a postpartum visit with Ali after the baby was born to assess infant care and answer any questions Ali had concerning infant care.

Assessment

Although it was important to perform an individual assessment of Ali, the PHN assessed Ali as a member of a family and as a member of the community. *Community* in this case referred to the aggregate of publicly insured adolescent pregnant women. Assessment of Ali revealed an underweight 17-year-old pregnant woman who was unable to demonstrate knowledge of nutrition in pregnancy, infant care, breastfeeding, contraception, or educational options for pregnant teenagers.

Public Health Home Visit: Antepartum Client

An individual assessment of Ali mandated the need for an assessment of the composition and function of Ali's family. The PHN assessed the following factors with regard to Ali's family:

- Family composition and support network
- Family's and support network's attitude toward mental and physical health and use of health care services
- Family's and support network's attitude toward Ali's physical, mental, social, spiritual, and economic support

Family's and support network's beliefs and attitudes regarding infant care, breastfeeding/bottle feeding, immunizations, and nutrition

Attitude of infant's father regarding involvement with Ali and their baby, his health beliefs, and his ability to assume the role of parent

The PHN was aware of the need to see the larger, aggregate picture. Identifying the aggregate as the pregnant adolescent community, the PHN used the following techniques in an ongoing assessment (Lewenson and Truglio-Londrigan, 2010)

- Observations
- Resource analysis
- Key informant interviews
- Environmental indexes

Using these techniques, the PHN gathered information regarding the following:

- Educational and employment options for pregnant teens and teens with infants
- Availability of health services targeting low-birth-weight infants
- Availability of support groups for this aggregate
- Availability of teen parenting classes

Diagnosis

The PHN formulated nursing diagnoses based on thorough individual, family, and community assessments.

Individual

- Lack of awareness regarding nutrition in pregnancy, infant care and feeding, contraception, availability of community resources, and educational options for pregnant teenagers
- Inadequate nutritional support related to low-income status and inadequate knowledge of nutritional requirement for pregnancy

Family

- Lack of family support related to Ali's living away from home
- Altered family communication patterns related to role confusion among family members

Community

- Minimal availability of health care services, parenting classes, contraception counseling, and educational opportunities for pregnant teenagers
- Lack of coordination of existing services

Planning

Planning health services and interventions for pregnant teenagers involves formulation of mutually agreed-upon short-term and long-term goals for the individual, family, and community.

Individual
Long-Term Goal

- Ali will carry her infant to term without evidence of maternal or fetal complications.

Short-Term Goals

- Ali will gain at least 3 lb per month.
- Ali will demonstrate knowledge of community resources for pregnant adolescents by the next nursing visit.

Family
Long-Term Goal

- Ali, her partner, and other family members will be able to perform mutually determined role responsibilities.

Short-Term Goal

- Ali and her partner will attend teen parenting classes.

Community
Long-Term Goals

- Establishment of effective, comprehensive prenatal health, contraception, and education services for pregnant teenagers
- Decline in rate of teen pregnancies and birth of compromised neonates over the next 24 months

Short-Term Goals

- Increased community awareness of resources for pregnant teenagers
- Increased awareness of contraception counseling services for adolescents

Intervention
Individual

Implementation of Ali's individual care plan involved visits by the PHN with a referral to existing prenatal services for pregnant teenagers.

Family

Family intervention was composed of Ali's and the father's referral to a support group for pregnant teenagers and partners.

Community

Implementation of the care plan for the aggregate of adolescent pregnant women included the following:

- Meeting with community leaders
- Meeting with local school administrators and faculty to disseminate information for pregnant teenagers
- Formation of community organizing groups

Evaluation
Individual

Evaluation included measures of the client's nutritional status and her use of support groups and educational and nutritional services.

Family

Evaluation included measures of the family's use of support groups and educational and services.

Community

Evaluation of the effectiveness of interventions at the aggregate level focused on measurement of available options for pregnant teenagers, measures of teen awareness and use of services, and determination of changes in incidence rates of teen pregnancy and compromised neonates.

Levels of Prevention

The PHN not only works with the patient and the patient's support network, but also provides care to the entire community through education and intervention programs. The PHN is actively involved in working with individual teenagers, their friends and families, and the community in reducing the incidence of teenage pregnancy and assisting pregnant teenagers with prenatal care and available resources. Examples of providing care at the three levels of prevention are listed here.

Primary

- Activities that prevent teen pregnancy from occurring, such as individual and family counseling and school and community education programs

Secondary

- Interventions for early detection of teen pregnancy and early intervention, such as counseling for prenatal care

Tertiary

Goal: To reduce the effects of adolescent pregnancy

- Provision of prenatal education in areas such as nutrition, parenting, and infant care

CASE STUDY

Hospice Home Visit

Anne McMillan is 80 years old and is terminally ill with metastatic breast cancer. She has been a widow for 5 years and has three daughters and two sons. All of her children are married with kids of their own, except one son who is handicapped and lives with Anne. Anne is too weak to care for herself and is moving in with her youngest daughter. Her daughter's house is a colonial with all bedrooms upstairs. There is a first-floor bathroom. During her first visit, the hospice nurse talks with Anne and her daughter and explains what hospice is all about. The nurse then admits Anne into the hospice program and begins her initial assessment. Anne's primary physical complaints are back pain and constipation. She is still eating and drinking regularly. The nurse immediately recognizes that Anne will need a hospital bed. Anne already has a walker, but the nurse informed Anne and her daughter that they could have a bedside commode if needed in the future as Anne becomes weaker. Anne's biggest concern is her handicapped son, saying, "He can't be by himself for long and I don't know where he can go now that I can't take care of him." Except for the handicapped son, all of her children and many of her grandchildren are active in her care.

Assessment

On her initial visit, the hospice nurse collects the following data about Anne, her family, and her community. In this case, the community consists of Anne's social support outside of her family, such as her neighborhood and church.

- Pain assessment, including history, character, severity, location, effects on quality of life, precipitating factors, and relieving factors
- Other physical symptoms, such as fatigue, nausea, vomiting, constipation, diarrhea, decreased appetite, and decreased mobility
- Client and family fears, anxiety about dying and the dying process
- Support network and family dynamics
- Client's anxiety about situation concerning handicapped son
- Additional support network outside of family
- Effect of diagnosis and prognosis on Anne's social support, including her neighbors and her church community

Diagnosis

Individual

- Pain related to disease process
- Potential for constipation and discomfort related to decreased mobility
- Apprehension related to concerns about safety and well-being of handicapped son

Family

- Strong support system indicated by active family participation in Anne's care

Community

- Anticipatory grieving related to social isolation after leaving neighborhood and moving in with daughter

Planning

Individual

Long-Term Goals

- Pain will remain controlled until client expires.
- Client will have regular bowel movements for the next 2 months.
- Client will verbalize satisfaction about resolution of situation concerning handicapped son.

Short-Term Goals

- Pain will be well controlled within 24 to 48 hours.
- Client will have a bowel movement within 24 to 48 hours.
- Client will have decreased anxiety about handicapped son within 24 to 48 hours because the social worker will have found a place for the son to live.

Family

Long-Term Goals

- Family will remain active in Anne's care until she is buried.
- Family will provide a support network for each other and use hospice services for continued support through Anne's death and burial and for months afterward.

Short-Term Goal

- Family will actively participate in Anne's care.

Community

Long-Term Goal

- Client will continue to receive support from friends.

Short-Term Goal

- Client will verbalize feelings about moving in with daughter and leaving friends behind.

Intervention

Individual

After talking with the doctor, the hospice nurse starts Anne on methadone 20 mg daily and Roxanol 5 mg as needed for breakthrough pain. The nurse explains to Anne and her daughter that she is constipated because of her decrease in mobility. The nurse obtains an order for a stool softener and instructs Anne to take it twice daily. The nurse also explains to Anne and her daughter that, as Anne declines, her appetite will decrease and she will eat less and less and may not have bowel movements very frequently. Anne should let the nurse know if she ever feels uncomfortable because she has not had a bowel movement in a few days. The nurse talks to the social worker, who finds a group home for Anne's handicapped son.

Family

The nurse and social worker talk with the family and help them develop a system so that Anne always has someone with her and to help ensure that all of the responsibility for Anne's care does not fall on one person. They also inform the family about resources to support them.

Community

Anne has a nurse, social worker, spiritual counselor, and nurse assistant assigned to her care. Each of these hospice workers helps Anne discuss her feelings about her situation and works with her to continue to receive support from her friends and neighbors.

Evaluation

Individual

All of Anne's goals are met, because she has good pain control until she dies, she no longer experiences discomfort and problems with constipation, and she expresses less anxiety and worry about her handicapped son. Although she still has some concerns, she feels much better about the situation.

Family

The family's goals are met, because they remain active in Anne's care until she dies. In addition, they use hospice resources appropriately and as necessary, and they support one another through the entire process.

Community

The goals are met, because Anne expresses her feelings about her situation, and her closest friends remain supportive to Anne through visits and phone calls.

CASE STUDY—cont'd

Hospice Home Visit

Levels of Prevention

In this case, the three levels of prevention focus on helping the client and family through all phases of hospice care from admission until death. Some examples are as follows.

Primary

- Anticipating needs and intervening early on to prevent problems such as skin breakdown and lack of pain control
- Educating the client and family about hospice and the dying process

Secondary

- Responding quickly to needs as they arise
- Continued education about the hospice and dying experience

Tertiary

- Assisting the client and family through the active phase of dying
- Providing follow-up bereavement support to the family

SUMMARY

This chapter presents information on performing public health, home health, and hospice nursing visits to clients in their homes. A general overview of the nursing process for clients in the home setting is presented and expanded to include the individual, family, and community. Case studies involving communicable disease, teen pregnancy, and terminal cancer are described. The home visit is the foundation of community health nursing and provides a forum for important interventions with individuals, families, and communities. The CHN is responsible for bringing the concerns of individuals and families into the community.

Ⓔ EVOLVE WEBSITE

http://evolve.elsevier.com/Nies/community

- NCLEX Review Questions
- Case Studies

BIBLIOGRAPHY

Acello B, Brown LR: *Home health assessment criteria: 75 checklists for skilled nursing documentation*, 2015. Available from: https://hcmarketplace.com/aitdownloadablefiles/download/aitfile/aitfile_id/1678.pdf.

Albrecht MN: The Albrecht nursing model for home health care: implications for research, practice, and education, *Public Health Nurs* 7:118–126, 1990.

American Nurses Association: *Scope and standards of hospice and palliative nursing practice*, Washington, DC, 2007, Author.

American Nurses Association: *Scope and standards of home health nursing practice*, Washington, DC, 2008, Author.

Camak DJ: Addressing the burden of stroke caregivers: a literature review, *J Clin Nurs* 24(17/18):2376–2382, 2015. https://doi.org/10.1111/jocn.12884.

Cancer.net: *Understanding grief within a cultural context*, 2015. Available from: http://www.cancer.net/coping-with-cancer/managing-emotions/grief-and-loss/understanding-grief-within-cultural-context.

Centers for Medicare and Medicaid Services: *Home health PPS*, 2016. Available from: http://www.cms.gov/Medicare/Medicare-Fee-for-Service-Payment/HomeHealthPPS/index.html?redirect=/homehealthpps/.

Department of Health and Human Services: *Centers for Medicare and Medicaid Services: Home health prospective payment system*, 2017. Available from: https://www.cms.gov/Outreach-and-Education/Medicare-Learning-Network-MLN/MLNProducts/Downloads/Home-Health-PPS-Fact-Sheet-ICN006816.pdf.

Department of Health and Human Services: *Centers for Medicare and Medicaid services: Hospice payment system*, 2016. Available from: https://www.cms.gov/Outreach-and-Education/Medicare-Learning-Network-MLN/MLNProducts/downloads/hospice_pay_sys_fs.pdf.

Kelly R, Godin L: The effect of a "surveillance nurse" telephone support intervention in a home care program, *Geriat Nurs* 36:111–119, 2014. https://doi.org/10.1016/j.gerinurse.2014.11.004.

Lewenson SB, Truglio-Londrigan M: *Public health nursing assessment tool*, 2010. Available from: http://samples.jbpub.com/9780763766542/41764_trugliolondrigan_appendix.pdf.

Medicare.gov: *What's home health care?* 2016a. Available from: https://www.medicare.gov/what-medicare-covers/home-health-care/home-health-care-what-is-it-what-to-expect.html.

Medicare.gov: *What's a home health care plan?* 2016b. Available from: https://www.medicare.gov/what-medicare-covers/home-health-care/home-health-plan-of-care.html.

National Association for Home Care and Hospice: *Homecare online: Basic statistics about home care*, 2010. Available from: <http://www.nahc.org/assets/1/7/10HC_Stats.pdf>.

National Kidney and Urologic Diseases Information Clearinghouse: *Home hemodialysis*, 2016. Available from: <http://www.kidney.niddk.nih.gov/kudiseases/pubs/homehemodialysis/>.

National Hospice and Palliative Care Organization: *Hospice care*, 2016. Available from: http://www.nhpco.org/about/hospice-care.

Norlander L: To comfort always: *a nurse's guide to end of life care*, Indianapolis, IN, 2008, Sigma Theta Tau International.

QSEN Institute: *QSEN competencies*, 2014. Available from: <http://qsen.org/competencies/>.

Ruel SR: Lillian Wald: A pioneer of home healthcare in the United States, *Home Healthcare Nurse* 32(10):597–600, 2014. https://doi.org/10.1097/NHH.0000000000000153.

HealthyPeople.gov: *Healthy People 2020: Topics & objectives*. Available from: <http://www.healthypeople.gov/2020/topicsobjectives2020/default.aspx>.

INDEX

Note: Page numbers followed by "f" refer to illustrations; page numbers followed by "t" refer to tables; page numbers followed by "b" refer to boxes.